THE CHALLENGE OF EPIDEMIOLOGY
Issues and Selected Readings

Discussed and compiled by:

Carol Buck
Alvaro Llopis
Enrique Nájera
Milton Terris

D1616714

Scientific Publication No. 505

PAN AMERICAN HEALTH ORGANIZATION
Pan American Sanitary Bureau, Regional Office of the
WORLD HEALTH ORGANIZATION
525 Twenty-third Street, N.W.
Washington, D.C. 20037 USA

1988

Published also in Spanish (1988) as:
El desafío de la epidemiología: problemas y lecturas seleccionadas
ISBN 92 75 31505 1

ISBN 92 75 11505 2

CONTENTS

D. CASE CONTROL STUDIES

E. COHORT STUDIES

F. EXPERIMENTAL STUDIES

PART V. PERSPECTIVES AND PROSPECTS

PREFACE

Epidemiologists, health planners, and administrators from countries throughout the Americas Region, among others, met at a seminar in Buenos Aires, Argentina in November 1983, to discuss and analyze the role of epidemiology in the developing countries of the Western Hemisphere. After formulating and analyzing ideas and initiatives on the use and future prospects of epidemiology in Latin America, the participants made important recommendations for adjusting epidemiology's practice to current needs.[1]

They agreed that the most important epidemiological issue in the Region has been the change in the health profile of the population as a result of the social, economic, environmental and demographic changes. While communicable diseases persist in most countries of the Americas, they have been increasingly joined by noninfectious diseases that strike mostly adults and the elderly, by accidents, and by illnesses linked to the workplace and to environmental pollution.

For the industrialized nations, the evolution of patterns of disease spanned more than a century and fell into three fairly distinct stages. The first, marked by infectious diseases associated with poverty, malnutrition, and poor environmental and personal hygiene, gradually gave way thanks to better housing and sanitation, greater availability of safe drinking water, and vaccination services. In the second stage, degenerative diseases such as heart disease, cerebrovascular accidents, and cancer gradually began to replace infectious diseases as the leading causes of death. Finally, the third stage reflects a growing concern with health problems caused by exposure to environmental pollution and to changing social conditions in families, communities, and the workplace which foster violence, alcohol abuse, and drug addiction.

One of the distinguishing features of the health situation in developing countries is that, whereas developed nations went through all three stages in more than a century, developing countries must face all three at once. Consequently, health conditions in the Americas have become a veritable epidemiological mosaic.

---

[1] The report and the working documents of the Buenos Aires seminar were published in 1984, in PAHO publication PNSP 84-47.

As a response to this complex health situation, and as part of their effort to attain the goal of health for all by the year 2000, the countries of the Region have expanded and reorganized their health service systems, frequently combining programs and activities in order to improve their equity, efficiency, and efficacy. But much remains to be done: the health sector must compete with other sectors for extremely scarce financial resources, and limited access to health care still leaves vast segments of the population with insufficient or without any health coverage at all.

The organization of services represents a major challenge for the health sector. On the one hand, some objectives which involve providing services to the population at large—such as health promotion and primary prevention—can be achieved only through cooperation with other sectors like education, water supply and sanitation, and agriculture. On the other, the delivery of services requires the mobilization of many different resources within the health sector, including a wide range of types of personnel, health centers, and general and specialized hospitals.

The countries of the Region must also address improving the administration of health care service systems. For the effective administration of health care systems involves much more than managing facilities and support services; it includes setting priorities, allocating resources based on the health needs of targeted populations, and evaluating the impact of the services—a capability that continues to be very limited in most developing countries.

Epidemiology—its concepts and its methods—has a major role to play in this process. Besides its importance and usefulness in disease surveillance and prevention, epidemiology has an even more critical function to carry out—the gathering of knowledge for understanding the health-disease process. It can anticipate needs, identify risk conditions, and orient the definition of priorities and the use of available resources for planning and administering health systems. In short, by analyzing and evaluating health problems and health services, and their contexts, epidemiology can go beyond considering just specific health problems; it can help bring us closer to considering society as the source for explaining health problems and their solutions.

The participants at the Buenos Aires seminar recommended that the practice of epidemiology be reoriented to realize the discipline's full potential for improving knowledge, achieving more effective prevention of health problems, and evaluating health care services. Accordingly, the Pan American Health Organization has redirected its technical cooperation activities in epidemiology, emphasizing the promotion of research, the reorientation of training programs, and the dissemination of information in order to broaden the scope of the practice of epidemiology in the Region. In addition, to address one of the seminar's conclusions that public health workers' and students' "lack of access to scientific medical literature . . . adds to the difficulties experienced in training and carrying out research, and hinders the overall development of epidemiology," PAHO is organizing a bibliography on epidemiology which will be made available to the main health institutions in the Region.

This volume is an important step in making technical material more accessible to public health workers. It traces the evolution of epidemiology through writings selected because of their enduring value, because they highlight the importance of epidemiology in unconventional areas, or because they defined trends or advanced knowledge. By highlighting the historical framework of epidemiology's evolution both as a discipline and as a tool to elucidate health problems in society, this book will give a sense of what epidemiology has meant in the past, how it developed, what it means, and the challenges it faces now and will face in the future.

Carlyle Guerra de Macedo
Director

INTRODUCTION

The Challenge of Epidemiology represents the culmination of a collaborative effort. Two units of the Pan American Health Organization, Health Situation Analysis and Trend Assessment and Health Manpower Development, worked on the book. Dr. Clovis H. Tigre, an epidemiologist with the former, coordinated its production, and a working group of editors comprised of four eminent epidemiologists—Carol Buck of the University of Western Ontario, Alvaro Llopis of the Central University of Venezuela, Enrique Nájera of the University of Seville, and Milton Terris of the *Journal of Public Health Policy*—selected works for the anthology and provided the background discussions for each section. These discussions, designed to provide a framework for the anthologized works, were taped and transcribed from actual sessions held by the editors. They have been kept in their original style to preserve the editors' opinions and the spirit of their discussions.

The editors first met to discuss objectives and overall procedures. At that time it was decided that selections for the anthology of the book would be chosen from suggested entries submitted by experts in epidemiology from throughout the world. Letters were sent to approximately one hundred such individuals[1] asking them to nominate up to ten works which they considered landmarks in the development of the discipline, outstanding contributions to the field, or examples of the advancement of an innovative concept. From this vast storehouse of articles, chapters of books, and excerpts of works, the four editors would then carefully select most of the anthology, seeking a well-balanced, final version. The remaining submissions would be integrated into an extensive epidemiology bibliography.

At a subsequent meeting the editors organized the selected articles in five sections. The first two, "Historical Development" and "From the Old to the New Epidemiology," trace the historical evolution of the discipline. Section 3, "Etiologic Investigations," and section 4, "Health Services and Health Policies," address the application of epidemiology. Section 5, "Perspectives and Prospects," offers the editors' views on the future of epidemiology. The first four sections contain both discussions and a collection of reprinted

---

[1] A list of these contributors appears as an appendix in this book.

works arranged chronologically; the last section contains only discussions. A Spanish version of this book is also being prepared. The translation of the discussions and the articles was conducted by the staff of the department of Preventive and Social Medicine, Faculty of Medicine, University of Seville, Spain.

We hope that, in addition to providing valuable information, this book will also stimulate debate on the history and development, scope and limitations, and uses and perspectives of epidemiology. In this way, this book would become a useful tool for both students and professionals—as well as providing a much needed frame of reference for reorienting the practice of epidemiology in the Region.

PART I

HISTORICAL DEVELOPMENT

DISCUSSIONS

NAJERA: Perhaps we could begin by exploring why, how, when, and where the concept of epidemiology originated. As far as we know, "epidemic" and "endemic" derived from *epidemeion* and *endemeion*. Hippocrates used these words at the School of Cos 2400 years ago, as a way of incorporating a community outlook into the understanding of diseases. Their purpose at that time, and their correct etymology, was to differentiate diseases that visit the community—the verb *epidemeion* meaning "to visit"—from those that reside in it, without the added meaning of an unusual or severe occurrence. We should, therefore, keep this characteristic of "visitor" in mind, because of its usefulness in creating a methodology for studying health problems in the community.

LLOPIS: In addition to using the words "epidemic" and "endemic" in his *Airs, Waters, Places*, Hippocrates also referred to what is now the basis of epidemiological investigations: the distribution of disease in terms of time, space, and the people affected by it. In his aphorisms he studied the distribution of diseases according to season and age. In other works he also emphasized the influence of other conditions such as climate, individual body-build, and habits.

NAJERA: My students and I have been trying to find where and when the word epidemiology was first used, yet we have only been able to discover that it was already in use in Spain in the late sixteenth century. Angelerio, a physician of that time, wrote a study on plague entitled *Epidemiología*. The second edition of this work was published in Madrid in 1598.

Although we have searched in different countries for other books or studies using the word epidemiology, we have not been able to find any further use of the term until the beginning of the nineteenth century. In 1802 it was used in the title of a book written by the Spanish physician, Villalba. This book, *Epidemiología Española*, compiled all epidemics and outbreaks in Spain dating from the fifth century B.C. up to 1801. Although plague is the most frequently described epidemic, all other epidemic diseases are also carefully accounted for. Malaria, for example, is

3

one disease worth mentioning, since it is a typical epidemic disease with deep roots in people's socioeconomic development. *Epidemiología Española* includes some very interesting observations carried out during the Middle Ages concerning the presence of malaria in rice growing areas. These observations showed that when rice was grown in a previously malarious area, no malaria occurred; yet when grown in a non-malarious area, malaria usually ensued. You see, if the area was already malarious, then it meant it was a wet area. When rice growing started, it became dry for certain periods, thus interrupting the mosquito's life cycle. But when dry areas were irrigated in order to grow rice, malaria occurred because these areas became wet. Those were wonderful conclusions to arrive at in those days. You see, these observations were of extraordinary importance and could be interpreted as one of the first observations of the kind which allow us to arrive at epidemiological interpretations.

The other major Spanish contribution I can think of comes from Casal, a physician who lived and worked in northern Spain, in Asturias, during the first half of the eighteenth century. At that time a new disease, that people called *mal de la rosa* (disease of the rose) because of the dermatitis it produced, was occurring. Later on this disease would be known by its Italian name, pellagra. Casal began looking at why this disease was there and why people said it was new. He concluded that the disease must be a result of diet, since the people most affected were the poorest people in the area. When he looked at the diet, he saw that those who contracted the disease ate no meat or eggs or anything costly at all. They ate corn—the cheapest thing available at the time. Corn had been introduced recently from America as animal feed, which made it very inexpensive, and the poor ate it almost exclusively. In his book, Casal even gives the clinical description of the disease. By studying what he called the natural history of the disease, he discovered that the dementia was the last stage of the *mal de la rosa*, rather than a different disease as had been thought.

TERRIS: Some time after Casal, during the nineteenth century, the theoretical debate was whether diseases were caused by contagion or by miasma. Up to 1874 the miasmatists were dominant; theirs was the accepted theory. The question of miasma versus contagion was also a political struggle. The contagionists, with few exceptions such as the liberal Henle, were conservatives and reactionaries, representatives of the old regime, who eventually turned out to be correct. The liberals and radicals like Virchow in Germany, Villermé in

France, and Alison in Scotland, who blamed disease on poverty and other social conditions, and the miasmatists like Farr and Simon in England, turned out to be wrong in their opposition to contagionism. The fact that in 1854, at least 20 years before this theory was accepted, Snow used the germ theory of disease to explain cholera, is a remarkable feat—a fascinating demonstration that epidemiologists could be ahead of microbiologists and everyone else.

What happened after 1874 was very interesting. Now medicine had another theory, the germ theory, that was the dominant one. Everything was explained on the basis of this theory. There are marvelous examples, such as beriberi, where the data didn't fit the germ theory, yet they still tried to explain the findings on that basis, just as Farr had tried to explain cholera by the miasma theory. But the first real breakthrough for noninfectious disease didn't come until 1912, when Casimir Funk enunciated the "deficiency" theory of disease. This was the first noninfectious theory of disease, and its acceptance became the basis for development of the whole area of nutritional diseases.

Public health in the modern sense, however, had really started in the early nineteenth century in France, not in England or Germany. This was attested to by the English. Richardson, Snow's colleague, noted in 1855 that the English were far behind the French public health workers, since the latter had a highly developed public health literature based on scientific investigation. Furthermore, the French workers were concerned with all aspects of public health, not merely the epidemic diseases. Perhaps the leading spirit in this movement was Villermé, who wrote on the conditions in the textile factories and clearly demonstrated the relation of economic status to mortality. In 1826, he wrote *On Mortality in the Different Sections of Paris*, which linked poverty and disease. Farr also did work in this area, describing mortality in the different social classes. Farr follows Villermé; they are very much alike. These issues are relevant because an important trend in Latin America today is social epidemiology, the relationship of poverty and occupation with illness and health.

NAJERA: I think, to continue with Terris's line of thought, that one could say that the French Revolution brought the community's interests into the social organization of the state for the first time. Before, the king was the state; his interests and those of the nobility were the only considerations in the organization of the state. The French Revolution brought in the community's interests, so that people like Guillotin or Pinel could work for the people. You see, in a sense, public health existed before. One could claim that the quarantine measures of the fourteenth century were public health measures, and isolating the sick was done even earlier. But these public health measures were not developed to protect all of the community, just some part of it: the nobility, the king, or trade. These measures were always very limited in scope. The French Revolution broadened this scope, marking the beginning of public health for the community as a whole. This is what I think made the big difference, and what differentiated the new type of work from that of the eighteenth century which was mostly research work: Lind's was really a piece of research and Casal was also mainly a research investigator, but Guillotin and Villermé were really doing public health.

TERRIS: I think we have to discuss the impact of the Industrial Revolution. A big impetus to all the French epidemiologists, and then to the English, was industrialization—the inhuman working conditions, the miserable housing and overcrowding in the cities, the terrible situation that resulted. The French were particularly concerned with the factories because they considered them to be the main source of the deterioration in health status. Villermé stated this in his major treatise, *A Description of the Physical and Moral State of Workers Employed in Cotton, Wool, and Silk Mills.* It was the Industrial Revolution that brought about public health in a very real sense.

NAJERA: Well, Villermé was concerned with the workers' conditions because nobody cared about them. A century had elapsed since industrialization started before steps were taken to improve the health of the population. The Industrial Revolution started during the second half of the eighteenth century, but it went very slowly and its effects were not really seen for quite some time. By the beginning of the nineteenth century, industry had developed so much that they needed more people, more workers.

For example, in England, where there was a very special social environment, the New Poor Law was enacted so that poor people would receive medical relief at the working place rather than at the parishes. The classes in power abolished the Old Poor Law so the poor would be forced to come to the towns to work in the factories. This was a very important social change, and it is so interesting to read how Chadwick, who has been considered one of the big names in public health, was responsible for abolishing the Old Poor Law. The situation was completely schizophrenic: on the one hand he was trying to make things better for the people with public health, but on the other he was putting people to work under horrible conditions.

TERRIS: It was not schizophrenic, it was Benthamite. It's hard to
            believe, but if you read Chadwick's *Report on the Sanitary
            Conditions of the Laboring Population of Great Britain*, you
            discover that his rationale for sanitary reform was to miti-
            gate the trouble caused by "young. . . passionate and dan-
            gerous" workers engaged in labor demonstrations. He pro-
            posed that working-class people should be allowed to
            become old enough to mature and acquire a sense of re-
            sponsibility. That way they would not be supportive of
            trade unions, anarchism and so on—in his own words,
            "anarchical fallacies . . . trade unions . . . the violence of
            strike after strike." He also conceived and administered the
            Poor Law Amendment Act of 1834, which mandated that
            there would be no more home relief. People either had to
            go to the workhouse—the hated Bastille as the poor soon
            learned to call it—or get no medical relief at all. The poor
            were forced into the cities, and the industrialists got the
            labor they wanted. It was all of a piece. Chadwick a human-
            itarian? Not as far as I am concerned.

NAJERA: He was a man of his time. He knew exactly what he wanted
            and he served the establishment. He served those in power.
            Chadwick was the prime force behind England's public
            health movement, and since he lived to a very old age his
            influence was felt almost throughout the nineteenth cen-
            tury. He was born in 1800 and lived to the end of the
            century, 1890, in fact.

BUCK: I think he was a contemporary of Charles Dickens, who, by
            the way, although also concerned with the appalling condi-
            tions, probably did not like Chadwick very much. The story
            I have heard is that Chadwick became very much disliked
            and they really wanted to get rid of him, so they pensioned
            him off. They gave him quite a handsome pension for those
            days, and he got his revenge by living yet another 30 years.

TERRIS: He was called "the most hated man in England."

NAJERA: I think we also need to consider the shift between the
            eighteenth and the nineteenth centuries, especially in the
            latter part of the nineteenth, from people like Baker and
            Casal to people like Finlay, Chagas, and Carrión. With the
            industrial revolution, infectious diseases became the big
            problem. They resulted from poor living and working con-
            ditions, from overcrowding, and from lack of sanitation in
            the slums created for poor laborers in industrialized towns.
            From the middle to the end of the nineteenth century,
            everything became infectious diseases and microorganisms.
            These diseases were prominent, while malnutrition, low

salaries, and other social factors were forgotten. Panum, Snow, Finlay, Chagas, Carrión, Takaki, Haffkine all looked at infectious diseases. The other diseases practically disappeared from the focus of research and attention, although certainly not from reality. Villermé had shown that there was a strong relationship between poverty and disease, but only a few decades later a shift had occurred. Suddenly no one thought of this link anymore; everyone was trying to discover those new, "socially neutral," biologic agents—the microbes.

TERRIS: I am not sure I accept what you are saying. I think the time when infectious disease became all important was after Pasteur and Koch, because then they could do something about it. Then the whole field became infectious disease. It was the success that created the interest, not the existence of the problem. The reason that the Latin Americans today think only in terms of infectious diseases is that they can do something about them.

Let me put it another way. Noninfectious diseases existed long before 1940, but there was no noninfectious disease epidemiology of any great significance until after some successes were achieved—until, for example, the relation of cigarette smoking to lung cancer was discovered and the risk factors for coronary heart disease were demonstrated. Once there was some success, everyone jumped on the bandwagon.

I don't accept the thesis that it was the Industrial Revolution which caused an emphasis on infectious diseases. They were the most important diseases long before the Industrial Revolution. Look at plague. Look at all the great epidemics of the Middle Ages. They dominated the field. As a matter of fact, look at the early books like *Epidemiología Española*, they are all about *pestes*, plagues. It's all infectious disease; it never was anything else. The only time they get into occupational disease and toxicology is with the Industrial Revolution.

NAJERA: Well, we could talk a lot about this. But what you said about the focus shifting to noninfectious diseases in the 1940s is more complicated. And the reason being success? Not necessarily. Take cancer and smoking. It's been 40 years since the epidemiological discoveries, and we still are about the same. It's not that we have had actual success, but, rather, we have the *possibility* of success.

And as far as infectious diseases not becoming important until Koch and Pasteur, it's not that clear cut. Snow's work was with infectious diseases, and that was 30 years before

Koch. So, by the time of Koch and Pasteur the shift had already occurred.

TERRIS: Was it really a shift?

NAJERA: Except for the work of Panum, Budd, and Snow, we don't have examples of good epidemiology in other diseases in the mid nineteenth century, and yet there had been quite a few a century before. In any case, in the 1840s or 1850s, the attention focused on infectious diseases because they had become really predominant. Before the epidemics of cholera, typhoid, or respiratory diseases such as tuberculosis or scarlet fever, infectious diseases were not such a terrible problem. This is why I think that the social conditions of the industrial revolution made infectious diseases so predominant that attention was shifted to them. Why was Snow studying cholera? Not because of the possibility of success, but because cholera was important. And why was cholera important? Because of the overcrowding in London, as a result of the process of industrialization.

Long before Pasteur, infectious diseases were so important that they even generated international health measures at the first International Sanitary Conference held in Paris in 1851. The participants debated whether diseases like cholera were miasmatic or contagious; even political considerations entered into the positions adopted by some of the countries. It was to England's advantage for these diseases to be miasmatic, whereas Spain wanted them to be infectious so it could set trade barriers against England. All of this was between 1850 and 1890. The controversy ended when it was demonstrated that these diseases were infectious, that the germs were there. Then the approach shifted from changing the social conditions to the development of vaccines as a means of prevention.

TERRIS: I couldn't disagree with you more. If you read Hecker's *The Epidemics of the Middle Ages,* the main diseases before the Industrial Revolution were infectious diseases. They didn't know about any other diseases, all they knew about was infectious diseases. Only the fact that the Industrial Revolution intensified some of them is true.

NAJERA: I am talking of the shift in the late eighteenth and nineteenth centuries.

TERRIS: But there was little or no interest in noninfectious diseases before then. Look at the plague, the "Black Death" which wiped out a quarter of the population of Europe in the fourteenth century. Look at syphilis, an enormous problem long before the Industrial Revolution. But I do think you are right about the intensification of some infectious diseases in the big cities after the Industrial Revolution.

NAJERA: Well, if you take plague, for instance, it is very interesting to discuss why it intensified during the Middle Ages. This wasn't a new disease, and yet it became the great epidemic from the fourteenth to the seventeenth centuries. Then, long before anything could be done about it, plague disappeared. All of a sudden there were no more plague epidemics. I believe this was because the process of urbanization affected the rats, and the Norwegian rat replaced the black rat.

TERRIS: I could also argue that another big factor, long before the Industrial Revolution, was the commercial revolution. The extension of trade on a world scale brought disease from all over the world. This was a major factor.

NAJERA: There were no new diseases, or very few new diseases. Some said syphilis came from America, but that has never been proven.

TERRIS: It isn't a question of new diseases. Disease spread because of the development of international trade which we associate with the commercial revolution. And the commercial revolution preceded the Industrial Revolution by at least 200 years.

NAJERA: Not that much.

TERRIS: Well, 1492 started an era of worldwide discovery and trade.

NAJERA: But long distance trade began long before, for example trade with China. Trade grew with the incorporation of America, it was another big door opened to knowledge, but what can be considered important is the social change that was brought about by the Industrial Revolution. The people who came from the villages into the towns to become laborers. I think this is what created the extraordinary overcrowding of the big towns like London, Manchester, Paris, or Berlin.

TERRIS: I agree with that, it is true they didn't have sanitation in the big cities.

NAJERA: And they were absolutely overcrowded. Take cholera, for example, and all the discussion about whether cholera was really a new and imported disease or if it was an exacerbation of "cholera nostras."

TERRIS: The difference in our positions is that you claim there was a shift toward infectious diseases as a result of the Industrial Revolution, whereas I say that all that really happened was that infectious diseases, which were the main causes of disease, were intensified by the Industrial Revolution.

NAJERA: No, the shift that I refer to is a shift in attention, not a shift in the diseases. Both types of disease existed before. Chronic diseases were there and epidemic, or infectious, diseases were there, but attention was not focused on the infectious diseases until the Industrial Revolution. What happened then was that they were intensified.

Why did Snow study cholera? Because it was something that was obvious, it was there, people were dying like flies in London, in Soho. This was something that had not occurred before, because the living and working conditions of the people were worse than ever.

TERRIS: They were dying like flies from infectious diseases all through the Middle Ages. The difference is that they weren't able to deal with them. Science hadn't developed, technology hadn't developed. It was during the Industrial Revolution that it was possible to develop a totally new approach.

NAJERA: In any case, the fact that Snow was able to deal with cholera through sanitation because he discovered the key role of the contaminated water pump, is good. But sanitation was known to be the fundamental thing to avoid epidemics by the Greeks in the fifth century B.C. and even by the Indus Valley civilizations of Mohenjo-daro, Harappa, or Taxila some five or six centuries before that. Yet sanitation had only been applied to the very rich. But since overcrowding was not a problem, they could manage—epidemics came and went. But the overcrowding of the nineteenth century was terrible.

Why did Dickens write his stories? Because the conditions of the people were different. They were living worse than ever in these industrial-town slums. There are descriptions of families of 12 living in one room. This had not happened before. True, there had always been poor people, but most of them lived in rural areas where there was more space.

TERRIS: Well, I must tell you that the plagues of the Middle Ages were much more devastating than the plagues of the Industrial Revolution. If you look at the Great Plague, whole cities were practically wiped out in Asia and Europe. I've read the accounts and it was much worse than what happened during the Industrial Revolution.

NAJERA: This may be, but the descriptions of the Middle Ages and even of some later periods were narrative accounts without any data, and most probably were quite exaggerated.

LLOPIS: I don't think I agree that these were only stories, since these narratives gave all the historical and economic contexts of the plague epidemics of the fourteenth century. And, as Terris has said, whole cities were wiped out. The economic impact of these epidemics was major. So many people died that goods and properties, the entire community's wealth, were left for far fewer people. The standard of living rose after each one of these great outbreaks.

NAJERA: All I'm saying is that there was much better data in the nineteenth century than before. Besides, the fact that plague was an important infectious disease from the fourteenth to the seventeenth centuries isn't relevant in the context of the effects of the Industrial Revolution. The plague epidemics of the Middle Ages were a consequence of a different kind of revolution, one that happened when overcrowding started in the medieval towns. These burghs were different than the Roman towns. The houses in the Roman towns had separate living and storage sections. But the houses in the medieval towns had no sanitation and had a loft where the grain for the whole year was stored. This loft made an ideal dwelling for the black rat. The black rats lived in the house and so it was possible for plague to spread from rat to rat and, therefore, from house to house. So, these epidemics really resulted from the urban revolution. And I agree that there was also a correlation with economics. The price of wheat, for instance, went down after a very good harvest. When the price went down, people stored more grain in order to have an ample supply or to speculate while they waited for prices to go up. Since they kept more grain in the houses, the rats thrived and multiplied—and with them the intensity of plague. Plague epidemics followed good harvests, which is opposite from what one would think.

TERRIS: I would still want to emphasize that there was no shift of concern from noninfectious disease to infectious disease because of the Industrial Revolution. People were always concerned with infectious diseases; this was the major area of concern. Infectious diseases increased as a result of the

Industrial Revolution and that is why they tried to do something about them, but there was no shift. There was no change. No one was working on noninfectious diseases and then shifted to infectious diseases.

LLOPIS: These men were not talking about infectious disease or chronic disease. In some cases they did not know what they were dealing with. Some of these diseases were studied in order to establish their modes of transmission, because investigators felt they might be communicable diseases. In other cases they were just trying to find out anything they could. Actually, their work was more in the line of research. They could be classified as researchers, investigators, etiological researchers, really.

NAJERA: Perhaps it would be useful, at this point, to review some of the important, early works. Take Lind, for example. After he did his work on scurvy in the first half of the eighteenth century, nothing happened. Nobody paid attention to him, and for the next 50 years people continued to die of scurvy. It was only after the work of Gilbert Blane and the publication of his "Observation on the Diseases of Seamen" in 1789, that the English Navy would take action. Blane based his work on Lind's and Cook's experience because he believed strongly in prevention.

TERRIS: Kamahero Takaki was the James Lind of beriberi. By 1882, Takaki's observations as director of the Tokyo Naval Hospital led him to attribute beriberi to poor diet. He persuaded the skeptical Japanese admiralty to initiate massive dietary reforms. Crews were given more fresh meat and vegetables and at some meals they were given barley instead of rice. The effects were incredible. In 1882, there were over 400 cases of beriberi for each 1000 men. In five years the disease was completely eliminated.

LLOPIS: Another important investigator was Panum, who addressed the question of incubation periods in his "Observations made during the Epidemic of Measles in the Faroe Islands". He discovered that the age distribution of the disease in those islands where the virus had not circulated for a long time was different than in those where it had. In the former it was the adults who had the measles, which, under normal conditions they didn't have.

NAJERA: Think, too, how interesting it is to compare, for example, Snow and Farr, how formative. If one analyzes Farr today, it is possible to conclude that he was also right. Snow had the success, he dealt with the disease, but theoretically and methodologically it was Farr who was right. Farr was much more logical, much more of an epidemiologist. Snow, by luck or chance, found out that the pump was the key to the spread of cholera, and, therefore, had the success. But it was Farr who was really closer to the sociological roots of the disease. By looking at people according to income he came closer to the problem, without, of course, the possibility of coming up with a solution.

TERRIS: I do not agree. What Farr did was to publish a paper showing that as altitude above the Thames increased, cholera decreased. That was based on the miasma theory, and the paper was published to buttress this theory. If you read Snow's book carefully, you'll find that it is a profound sociological document. He showed that cholera was the disease of the poor because it flourished among people who were crowded together. The eating room and the sleeping room were the same. He showed that the rich did not have that problem, since they had separate rooms for eating and sleeping. He even included occupational epidemiology because he pointed out that the miners had so much cholera because they had to defecate and eat in the same space and it was impossible for them to escape this. Yes, it was a profound sociological document. Farr was too busy with altitude because he held to the miasma theory. The real pioneer of "social" epidemiology was Snow, not Farr.

BUCK: I believe that Najera was thinking of another work of Farr, one where he showed the difference in mortality between the country and the city and developed the idea of the minimum mortality which might be obtained in every segment of the country.

NAJERA: If one looks at the way that Baker studied lead poisoning in Devon in the first half of the eighteenth century, that was also very impressive. He undertook this study after the problem was considered solved. Someone else, Huxham, had attributed the disease to cider, but Baker knew that in France they had had a similar colic and there was no cider there, only wine. So he deduced that it couldn't be the cider. It was neither the cider nor the wine, but the lead that was present in both. Acute poisoning in the case of the Devon colic and chronic in the gout in France.

We could also mention the famine in Ireland in 1845, where practically half the population died and a third emigrated to the United States—the Kennedys and most of the Irish families came to the United States at this time. Ireland was a British colony that grew potatoes as a monoculture. Heavy rains promoted an extraordinary growth of a fungus—the potato blight—that practically destroyed the year's crops. As a result of this, a famine ensued, and people, millions of poor people, died of hunger. This was analyzed very well by René Dubos.

BUCK: There also was a beautiful etiological mistake in that. When it was suggested that the typhus fever which broke out among the Irish coming in ships to the New World was a communicable disease, people laughed; they were certain that the disease was caused by malnutrition.

NAJERA: Another good example was Jenner's work with smallpox vaccination. In the eighteenth century people were becoming more and more variolated through the technique of using direct inoculation. This technique was imported from China and was becoming more and more common, especially for the rich, for the nobility. When he was practicing in Devonshire, Jenner apparently saw that many variolated people had the same type of lesions as some milkmaids, and people confirmed that these milkmaids never had smallpox. So he thought that this must be a similar, but not exactly the same, thing. His line of thought was that smallpox was one thing, variolation a second, and the milkmaid's immunization a third similar thing. So it occurred to him that he could experiment, and he set up an experiment with only one subject, a boy. You see, it was still an experiment. After all, Lind's experiment on scurvy had only 12 subjects. Lind took 12 sailors and put six groups of two people in six different treatments. So it was not much of an experiment with two subjects in each group.

BUCK: Jenner avoided the problem of random allocation.

TERRIS: He didn't go beyond that one experiment?

NAJERA: Well, from the experiment with the boy he concluded that the results were good, and everybody accepted them. So he introduced a new method, vaccination, as it was later called. Immediately people were opposed to him, especially the church, because it could not accept the idea of introducing an animal substance into the human body. A big battle began. The big problem was, and this is the most interesting thing, that after the first experiment with the boy, most of the people that were vaccinated died from the inoculation. It was described in detail by several people in England, from the late 1790s up to 1820 or so. It was a big mess. Some of the vaccines were very good and nobody died, but they still did not protect people against smallpox. Some people have concluded that what probably happened was that when Jenner saw that people were dying from the vaccine, he went back to variolation without telling anyone. Two or three books have been published recently on this subject in England. They have copied comments made at the time about people who died and ones who did not; what was happening and why; whether the method was good or not, etc. It was a very, very complicated beginning for this method. Perhaps Spain backed it more than most countries, and organized the expedition of Dr. Francisco Balmis that carried the vaccine around the world. This expedition should be designated as the first international health program.

TERRIS: So there was reason for the opposition.

NAJERA: Sure there was reason for the opposition; people were being killed by the inoculation. But what is interesting is that Jenner developed the vaccine.

BUCK: If we use Jenner in this book, I think the only part we want to include would be the passage that describes the rarity of the disease in the milkmaids. That's the epidemiological part isn't it?

NAJERA: That's a good point. After that they had technical problems.

TERRIS: I think we should also include Carlos Finlay and yellow fever.

NAJERA: Yes, sure, and we should also mention Daniel Carrión, the Peruvian who described a rare disease in Peru. It is a severe disease called *verruga peruana*, Peruvian wart, transmitted by Phlebotomus, sandflies. While he was still a medical student, Carrión set out to prove that the disease was infectious and that the systemic manifestations, which had been considered to be another disease, were part of the same disease. He set up an experiment where he had himself inoculated with material from a wart. He subsequently developed the systemic manifestations, made the clinical description of the disease as he became sicker, and proved that it was infectious—then he died.

TERRIS: He died?!

NAJERA: Yes, I think it's important to emphasize in closing this section that the motivation in all the people we have mentioned was to question what was known, to question the established truth. This is what makes them real investigators. Baker, for instance, was not happy with an explanation that didn't fit his observations of colic in England, so he started to investigate. Casal did the same thing. All of them, I think, except Villermé. Villermé is something different from the others in the sense that his work was more of an observation of the social and political context.

BUCK: By the way, I suddenly realized we have overlooked Semmelweis, haven't we?

LLOPIS: His investigations of childbed fever made in a Vienna maternity clinic in 1846 constitute a solid piece of epidemiological research.

BUCK: Yes, his study of the harmfulness of interventions is the first epidemiological study of iatrogenic illness. It also has a sort of lesson indicating how difficult epidemiological investigations of health services are. He was literally driven to his death, I think, by the reception of that paper.

TERRIS: In the old days, epidemiologists were willing to take serious risks in order to answer questions. Take Lazear of the Walter Reed Commission. There is a fairly widespread opinion that he experimented on himself, that his death wasn't accidental. Self-experimentation was a real tradition. For example, when Goldberger and Anderson of the United States Public Health Service were studying typhus fever in Mexico, Anderson slept in a bed in which a person with typhus fever had died, to see if the disease could be transmitted in that way. The United States Public Health Service had a number of martyrs to various diseases, either through self-experimentation or because they caught the disease inadvertently and died. For all these early investigators there was a tradition of real heroism, a willingness to put their lives on the line.

AIRS, WATERS, PLACES

Hippocrates

I. . . . Whoever wishes to pursue properly the science of medicine must proceed thus. First he ought to consider what effects each season of the year can produce; for the seasons are not at all alike, but differ widely both in themselves and at their changes. The next point is the hot winds and the cold, especially those that are universal, but also those that are peculiar to each particular region. He must also consider the properties of the waters; for as these differ in taste and in weight, so the property of each is far different from that of any other. Therefore, on arrival at a town with which he is unfamiliar, a physician should examine its position with respect to the winds and to the risings of the sun. For a northern, a southern, an eastern, and a western aspect has each its own individual property. He must consider with the greatest care both these things and how the natives are off for water, whether they use marshy, soft waters, or such as are hard and come from rocky heights, or brackish and harsh. The soil too, whether bare and dry or wooded and watered, hollow and hot or high and cold. The mode of life also of the inhabitants that is pleasing to them, whether they are heavy drinkers, taking lunch, and inactive, or athletic, industrious, eating much and drinking little.

II. Using this evidence he must examine the several problems that arise. For if a physician know these things well, by preference all of them, but at any rate most, he will not, on arrival at a town with which he is unfamiliar, be ignorant of the local diseases, or of the nature of those that commonly prevail; so that he will not be at a loss in the treatment of diseases, or make blunders, as is likely to be the case if he have not this knowledge before he consider his several problems. As time and the year passes he will be able to tell what epidemic diseases will attack the city either in summer or in winter, as well as those peculiar to the individual which

are likely to occur through change in mode of life. For knowing the changes of the seasons, and the risings and settings of the stars, with the circumstances of each of these phenomena, he will know beforehand the nature of the year that is coming. Through these considerations and by learning the times beforehand, he will have full knowledge of each particular case, will succeed best in securing health, and will achieve the greatest triumphs in the practice of his art. If it be thought that all this belongs to meteorology, he will find out, on second thoughts, that the contribution of astronomy to medicine is not a very small one but a very great one indeed. For with the seasons men's diseases, like their digestive organs, suffer change.

III. I will now set forth clearly how each of the foregoing questions ought to be investigated, and the tests to be applied. A city that lies exposed to the hot winds—these are those between the winter rising of the sun and its winter setting—when subject to these and sheltered from the north winds, the waters here are plentiful and brackish, and must be near the surface, hot in summer and cold in winter. The heads of the inhabitants are moist and full of phlegm, and their digestive organs are frequently deranged from the phlegm that runs down into them from the head. Most of them have a rather flabby physique, and they are poor eaters and poor drinkers. For men with weak heads will be poor drinkers, as the after-effects are more distressing to them. The endemic diseases are these. In the first place, the women are unhealthy and subject to excessive fluxes. Then many are barren through disease and not by nature, while abortions are frequent. Children are liable to convulsions and asthma, and to what they think causes the disease of childhood, and to be a sacred disease. Men suffer from dysentery, diarrhoea, ague, chronic fevers in winter, many attacks of eczema, and from hemorrhoids. Cases of pleurisy, pneumonia, ardent fever, and of diseases considered acute, rarely occur. These diseases cannot prevail where the bowels are loose. Inflammations

Source: Excerpted from Hippocrates, *Airs, Waters, Places,* ed. W.H.S. Jones. Cambridge, Harvard University Press, 1948. By permission of the publisher.

of the eyes occur with running, but are not serious; they are of short duration, unless a general epidemic take place after a violent change. When they are more than fifty years old, they are paralyzed by catarrhs supervening from the brain, when the sun suddenly strikes their head or they are chilled. These are their endemic diseases, but besides, they are liable to any epidemic disease that prevails through the change of the seasons.

IV. But the following is the condition of cities with the opposite situation, facing the cold winds that blow from between the summer setting and the summer rising of the sun, being habitually exposed to these winds, but sheltered from the hot winds and from the south. First, the waters of the region are generally hard and cold. The natives must be sinewy and spare, and in most cases their digestive organs are costive and hard in their lower parts, but more relaxed in the upper. They must be bilious rather than phlegmatic. Their heads are healthy and hard, but they have in most cases a tendency to internal lacerations. Their endemic diseases are as follow. Pleurisies are common, likewise those diseases which are accounted acute. It must be so, since their digestive organs are hard, and the slightest cause inevitably produces in many patients abscesses, the result of a stiff body and hard digestive organs. For their dryness, combined with the coldness of the water, makes them liable to internal lacerations. . . .

VII. . . . I wish now to treat of waters, those that bring disease or very good health, and of the ill or good that is likely to arise from water. For the influence of water upon health is very great. Such as are marshy, standing and stagnant must in summer be hot, thick and stinking, because there is no outflow; and as fresh rainwater is always flowing in and the sun heats them, they must be of bad colour, unhealthy and bilious. In winter they must be frosty, cold and turbid through the snow and frosts, so as to be very conducive to phlegm and sore throats. Those who drink it have always large, stiff spleens, and hard, thin, hot stomachs, while their shoulders, collar-bones and faces are emaciated; the fact is that their flesh dissolves to feed the spleen, so that they are lean. With such a constitution they eat and drink heavily. Their digestive organs, upper and lower, are very dry and very hot, so that they need more powerful drugs. This malady is endemic both in summer and in winter. In addition the dropsies that occur are very numerous and very fatal. For in the summer there are epidemics of dysentery, diarrhoea and long quartan fever, which diseases when prolonged cause constitutions such as I have described to develop dropsies that result in death. These are their maladies in summer. In winter young people suffer from pneumonia and illnesses attended by delirium, the older, through the hardness of their digestive organs, from ardent fever.

AN INQUIRY INTO THE NATURE, CAUSES, AND CURE OF THE SCURVY

James Lind

PREFACE

The subject of the following sheets is of great importance to this nation; the most powerful in her fleets and the most flourishing in her commerce of any in the world. Armies have been supposed to lose more of their men by sickness than by the sword. But this observation has been much more verified in our fleets and squadrons where scurvy alone, during the last war, proved a more destructive enemy, and cut off more valuable lives, than the united efforts of the French and Spanish arms. It has not only occasionally committed surprising ravages in ships and fleets, but almost always effects the constitution of sailors; and where it does not rise to any visible calamity, yet it often makes a powerful addition to the malignity of other diseases. It is now above 150 years since that great sea-officer, Sir Peter [Richard] Hawkins, in his observations made in a voyage to the South sea, remarked it to be the pestilence of that element. He was able, in the course of twenty years in which he had been employed at sea, to give an account of 10000 mariners destroyed by it. But I flatter myself that it will appear from the following treatise that the calamity may be prevented and the danger of this destructive evil obviated; nor is there any question but every attempt to put a stop to so consuming a plague will meet with favourable reception from the public. . . .

OF THE CAUSES OF SCURVY

I had the opportunity in two Channel cruises, the one of ten weeks, the other of eleven, *ann.* 1746 and 1747 in his Majesty's ship the *Salisbury*, a fourth rate, to see the disease rage with great violence. And here it was remarkable that

Source: Excerpted from James Lind, *A Treatise of The Scurvy in Three Parts, Containing an Inquiry into the Nature, Causes and Cure of That Disease, together with a Critical and Chronological View of What has been published on the subject.* Edinburgh, Sands, Murray, and Cochran, 1753.

though I was on board several other long Channel cruises, one of twelve weeks particularly, from the 10 August to the 28 October, yet we had but one scorbutic patient, nor on the other that I remember had we the least scorbutic appearance. But in those who I have mentioned the scurvy began to rage after being a month to six weeks at sea, when the water on board, as I took particular notice, was uncommonly sweet and good, and the state of provisions such as could afford no suspicion of occasioning a general sickness, being the same in quality as in former cruises. And though the scorbutic people were by the generous liberality of that great and good commander, the Hon. Captain George Edgcumbe, daily supplied with fresh provisions, such as mutton broth and fowls and even meat from his own table, yet at the expiration of ten weeks we brought into Plymouth 80 men out of a complement of 350 more or less afflicted with this disease.

Now it was observable that both these cruises were in the months of April, May and June, when we had, especially in the beginning of them, a continuance of cold, rainy and thick Channel weather, as it is called, whereas in our other cruises we had generally very fine weather, except in winter, when, during the time I was surgeon, the cruises were but short. Nor could I assign any other reason for the frequency of this disease in these two cruises and our exception from it at other times but the influence of the weather; the circumstances of the men, ship and provisions being in all other respects alike. I have more than once remarked that after great rains or a continuance of close, foggy weather, especially after storms with rain, the scorbutic people generally grew worse; but found a mitigation of their symptoms and complaints upon the weather becoming drier and warmer for a few days. And I am certain it will be allowed by all who have had an opportunity of making observations of this disease at sea, or will attentively consider the situation of seamen there, that the principal and main predisposing cause to it is a manifest and obvious quality of the air, viz., its moisture. The effects of this are perceived to be more immediately hurtful and pernicious in certain constitutions; in those who are much weakened by preceding sickness; in those who, from a lazy inactive disposition, neglect to use proper exercise; and in those who indulge a discontented melancholy humour; all which may be reckoned the secondary disposing causes to this foul and fatal mischief.

As the atmosphere at sea may always be supposed to be moister than that of the land, hence there is always a greater disposition to the scorbutic diathesis at sea than in a pure dry land air. But supposing the like constitution of air in both places, the inconveniences which persons suffer in a ship during a damp wet season are infinitely greater than people on land are exposed to; these latter having many ways of guarding against its pernicious effects by warm dry clothes, fires, good lodging, etc., whereas sailors are obliged not only to breathe in this air all day, but sleep in it at night, and frequently in wet bed clothes, the ship's hatches being necessarily kept open. And indeed one reason for the frequence of the scurvy in the above cruises was no doubt the often carrying up of the bedding of the ship's company to quarters, where it was sometimes quite wet through and continued so for many days together when, for want of fair weather, there was no opportunity of drying it.

No persons sensible to the bad effects of sleeping in wet apartments or in damp bed clothes and almost in the open air without anything sufficiently dry or warm to put on will be surprised at the havock the scurvy made in Lord Anson's crew in passing the Cape Horn, if their situation in such uncommon and tempestuous weather be properly considered.

During such furious storms the spray of the sea raised by the violence of the wind is dispersed over the whole ship, so that the people breathe, as it were, in water for many weeks together. The tumultuous waves, incessantly breaking in upon the decks and wetting those who are upon duty as if they had been ducked in the sea, are also continually sending down great quantities of water below; which makes it the most uncomfortable wet lodging imaginable and from the labouring of the ship it generally leaks down in many places directly upon their beds. There being here no fire or sun to dry or exhale the moisture, and the hatches necessarily

kept shut, this moist, stagnating, confined air below becomes most offensive and intolerable. When such weather continues long, attended with sleet and rain as it generally is, we may easily figure to ourselves the condition of the poor men who are obliged to sleep in wet clothes and damp beds, the decks swimming with water below them; and there to remain for four hours at a time, till they are again called up to fresh fatigue and hard labour and again exposed to the washing of the sea and rains. The long continuance of this weather seldom fails to produce the scurvy at sea.

As to its breaking out so immediately in those ships upon their leaving the coast of Mexico, it was not only to their finding so few refreshments, especially fruits and vegetables fit to be carried to sea at the harbour of Chequetan, but also to the incessant rains they had in their passage to Asia and the great inconveniences that necessarily attend so long a continuance of such weather at sea. To which it may be added that by observations made on this disease it appears that those who are once infected with it, especially in so deep a degree as that squadron was, are more subject to it afterwards than others. I remember that many of them who returned to England with Lord Anson and afterwards went to sea in other ships were much more liable to scurvy than others.

* * *

It will be now proper to inquire into the diet which mariners are necessarily obliged to live upon at sea. And as it appears to be the principal occasional cause of their malady it may be worthwhile to consider sea provisions in their best state, it being found by experience that, notwithstanding the soundness and goodness of both water and provisions, the calamity often rages with great fury and can be removed only by change of diet. Now, if in this case they appear to have so great an influence in forming the distemper, what ill consequences may not reasonably be expected from a much worse state of them, as from putrid beef, rancid pork, mouldy biscuit and flour, or bad water, which are misfortunes commonly at sea? All which must infallibly have bad effects in so putrid a disease.

It must be remarked in general that the sea diet is extremely gross, viscid and hard of digestion. It consists of two articles, viz., the sweet farinaceous substances unfermented, and salted or dried flesh and fish.

But more particularly in our Royal Navy, whose provisions for goodness and plenty exceed those of any other ships or fleets in the world, every man has an allowance of a pound of biscuit a day, which in the manner it is baked will be found more solid and substantial food than two pounds of ordinary well baked bread at land. And this is a principal article of their diet. But the sea biscuit undergoes little or no fermentation in baking and is consequently of much harder and more difficult digestion than well leavened and properly fermented bread. For it must be here understood that the mealy parts of vegetable seeds dissolved only in water are by experience found to make too viscid an aliment to be constantly used by the generality of mankind, whereas by fermentation and the acid in the leaven the glutinous viscidity and tenacious oils of those mealy substances are broken and subdued; and they become easily dissolvable afterwards in water, with which before they would only make a paste or glue, and are now miscible with all the humours of the body. Well baked bread, which had undergone a sufficient degree of fermentation, is of light and easy digestion, and indeed the most proper nourishment for man, as it is adapted by its acescency to correct a flesh diet; whereas on the contrary sea biscuit, not being thus duly fermented, will in many cases afford too tenacious and viscid chyle, improper for nourishment of the body where the vital digestive faculties are weakened and impaired.

The next article in their allowance of what is called fresh provisions is one pound and a half of wheat flour in the week, which is made into pudding with water and a certain proportion of pickled suet. This last does not keep long at sea, so that they have often raisins or currants in its place. But flour and water boiled thus together form a tenacious glutinous paste requiring the utmost strength and integrity of the powers of digestion to subdue and assimilate it into nourishment. We find that weak, inactive, valetudinarian people cannot long bear such food. . . .

OF THE PREVENTION OF THE SCURVY

I shall conclude the precepts relating to the preservation of seamen with showing the best means of obviating many inconveniences which attend long voyages and of removing the several causes productive of this mischief.

The following are the experiments.

On the 20th May, 1747, I took twelve patients in the scurvy on board the *Salisbury* at sea. Their cases were as similar as I could have them. They all in general had putrid gums, the spots and lassitude, with weakness of their knees. They lay together in one place, being a proper apartment for the sick in the fore-hold; and had one diet common to all, viz., water gruel sweetened with sugar in the morning; fresh mutton broth often times for dinner; at other times puddings, boiled biscuit with sugar etc.; and for supper barley, raisins, rice and currants, sago and wine, or the like. Two of these were ordered each a quart of cyder a day. Two others took twenty five gutts of elixir vitriol three times a day upon an empty stomach, using a gargle strongly acidulated with it for their mouths. Two others took two spoonfuls of vinegar three times a day upon an empty stomach, having their gruels and their other food well acidulated with it, as also the gargle for the mouth. Two of the worst patients, with the tendons in the ham rigid (a symptom none the rest had) were put under a course of sea water. Of this they drank half a pint every day and sometimes more or less as it operated by way of gentle physic. Two others had each two oranges and one lemon given them every day. These they eat with greediness at different times upon an empty stomach. They continued but six days under this course, having consumed the quantity that could be spared. The two remaining patients took the bigness of a nutmeg three times a day of an electuary recommended by an hospital surgeon made of garlic, mustard seed, *rad. raphan.*, balsam of Peru and gum myrrh, using for common drink barley water well acidulated with tamarinds, by a decoction of which, with the addition of *cremor tartar*, they were gently purged three or four times during the course.

The consequence was that the most sudden and visible good effects were perceived from the use of the oranges and lemons; one of those who had taken them being at the end of six days fit for duty. The spots were not indeed at that time quite off his body, nor his gums sound; but without any other medicine than a gargarism of elixir of vitriol he became quite healthy before we came into Plymouth, which was on the 16th

June. The other was the best recovered of any in his condition, and being now deemed pretty well was appointed nurse to the rest of the sick. . . .

As I shall have occasion elsewhere to take notice of the effects of other medicines in this disease, I shall here only observe that the result of all my experiments was that oranges and lemons were the most effectual remedies for this distemper at sea. I am apt to think oranges preferable to lemons, though perhaps both given together will be found most serviceable. . . . I am informed it was principally oranges which so speedily and surprisingly recovered Lord Anson's people at the island of Tinian, of which that noble, brave and experienced commander was so sensible that before he left the island one man was ordered on shore from each mess to lay in a stock of them for their future security. . . . Perhaps one history more may suffice to put this out of doubt.

"In the first voyage made to the East Indies on account of the English East India Company there were employed four ships commanded by Captain James Lancaster, their General, viz. the *Dragon,* having the General and 202 men, the *Hector* 108 men, the *Susan* 82 and the *Ascension* 32. They left England about 18 April; in July the people were taken ill on their passage with the scurvy; by the first of August all the ships except the General's were so thin of men that they had scarce enough to hand the sails; and upon a contrary wind for fifteen or sixteen days the few who were well before began also to fall sick. Whence the want of hands was so great in these ships that the merchants who were sent to dispose of their cargoes in the East Indies were obliged to take their turn at the helm and do the sailors duty till they arrived at Saldanha [near Cape of Good Hope]; where the General sent his boats and went on board himself to assist the other three ships, who were in so weakly a condition that they were hardly able to let fall an anchor without his assistance. All this time the General's ship continued pretty healthy. The reason why his crew was in better health than the rest of the ships was owing to the juice of lemons of which the General having brought some bottles to sea, he gave to each, as long as it lasted, three spoonfuls every morning fasting. By this he cured many of his men and preserved the rest; so that although his ship contained double the number of any of the others yet (through the mercy of God and to the preservation of the other three ships) he neither had so many men sick, nor lost so many as they did."

Here indeed is a remarkable and authentic proof of the great efficacy of juice of lemons against this disease, as large and crowded ships are more afflicted with it and always in a higher degree than those that are small and airy. This little squadron lost 105 men by the scurvy. Upon its afterwards breaking out among them when in the East Indies in a council held at sea it was determined to put directly into some port where they could be supplied with oranges and lemons, as the most effectual and experienced remedies to remove and prevent this dreadful calamity.

ABOUT THE DISEASE COMMONLY CALLED "MAL DE LA ROSA" IN THIS PROVINCE

Gaspar Casal

After carefully observing, in many years of practice, all the symptoms associated with this disease, and seeing that it is the most terrible and refractory of all endemics in this region, I feel I should write its history.

Although the symptoms of this disease are many and cruel, as will soon be seen, only one of them is given the common name: a terrible scab that, though at first only reddens the affected spot and covers it with a somewhat rough crust, eventually degenerates into an extremely dry, rough, and blackish scab, broken by deep cracks that penetrate to the living flesh and produce acute pain, a burning sensation, and discomfort.

To merit the name of "mal de la Rosa," this malignant crust must be attached only to the metacarpus or metatarsus on the hands or feet, so that no affliction of any kind, appearance, or condition whatever in this region can be given that name if these scabs do not form on the aforesaid parts. Therefore, though they may appear on the soles of the feet, the palms of the hands, the elbows, arms, head, face, belly, thighs, or legs, and though they may be red and rough, may appear as scabs or erysipelas (also called "rosa"), and though to these be added all the other symptoms distinctive of "mal de la Rosa," in no wise may they be termed such if said scabs are not located on the metacarpus or the metatarsus. It is well to know that these scabs develop almost always near the spring equinox, and very rarely at any other time. In the summer they are usually sloughed off, perhaps by moisture and sweat, and then the places where they were are left perfectly free of any scab, but the red stigma remains, exquisitely fine and resplendent, like the scars that usually remain when burns have healed; so that, while the other surfaces of the metacarpus and metatarsus may have a thin, wrinkled, and hairy skin, as is generally the case in the old, the part that had been covered by the crust is seen to be smooth, hairless, and free of wrinkles, but it is tighter or flatter than the rest of the skin. It is probable that the name "rosa" derives from the color and brilliance of the scar.

These marks persist throughout the life of those who harbor the disease. It may well be described as anniversary, for it returns every year in the spring, like the swallows. In those in whom the disease is recent, the scabs are not as horrible nor do they leave so visible a scar when they are sloughed off. Nor does the disease always attack both hands, for some patients have it only in one, others in both, yet others in both hands and one foot, and others in both hands and both feet. The scabs never form on the palms of the hands or on the soles of the feet, but only on the backs of the feet and hands. Sometimes the crust covers all the metacarpus and metatarsus, but is then not so widespread.

In some patients, though not in all, there is another visible sign of this disease, which is a darkly ashen, crusty roughness on the lower front of the neck which extends, in the form of a collar, from one side to the other of the neckline over the clavicles of the chest and the manubrium of the sternum at the upper end; it is about two fingers wide, like a narrow band, and almost always leaves the posterior part of the cervix intact, touching at its extremes only the two sides of the trapezius muscle without extending beyond it. From the middle of this muscle a kind of appendix of the same width descends over the sternum to the middle of the chest. . . . I have never seen this sign in any man, whether healthy or ill, save those who suffered from "mal de la Rosa," and hence I believe, though not all agree, that it occurs only in those who suffer this illness.

HISTORY OF THIS DISEASE

As I have already said, I have long endeavoured to examine all the symptoms of this dis-

Source: Excerpted from *Memorias de la Historia Natural y Médica de Asturias, 1762*. Reprinted and annotated by A. Buylla y Alegre and R. Sarandeses y Alvarez. Oviedo, Escuela Tipográfica del Hospicio, 1900.

ease with utmost diligence, but thinking to myself that from none could I get more exact word on them than from the patients themselves, in 1735 I began examining them and writing down whatever answers they gave to my questions, whether proper or improper. . . .

ON THE SYMPTOMS OF THIS DISEASE

From the facts presented and many others I have been able to acquire after careful examination, it is possible to infer the phenomena of this disease; however, since some of them are proper and exclusive to it while others are common to it and other diseases, I will treat first of the former.

The proper and exclusive symptoms of this disease are:

1. Constant shaking of the head which, while common to all, is in some so incessant that for not an instant are they free from irregular motion of the whole body. In this city's Hospital of Santiago I cured a poor woman (and, if necessary I would so affirm under oath) whose body, particularly the upper half, waved like a swallow contending against a fitful wind, so that, to remain upright, she had to move her feet with extreme rapidity in order to avoid falling to the ground at any moment.

2. A painful, burning sensation in the mouth, blisters on the lips, and foulness on the tongue.

3. A disagreeable weakness of the stomach and weakness throughout the body, particularly in the legs, and a strange lassitude and indifference.

4. The crusts on the metacarpi and metatarsi and the collar of a sort in the upper part of the neck.

5. The burning heat that torments them, while in bed.

6. That smoothness or delicate fineness of the skin that can withstand neither heat nor cold, and

7. The depression that, with no known cause, assails them and makes them break out in piteous weeping, a phenomenon which of itself is pathognomonic to this disease. . . .

OTHER STAGES AND FINAL OUTCOME OF THE DISEASE

There is another metastasis or stage of this disease, fairly frequent and no less terrible, but which does not happen in any season, but more particularly during summer, when the heat of the sun is most intense. Then, many of those in whom the "mal de la Rosa" is already rooted, fall into melancholy, and these poor victims, impelled not so much by fury as by anguish, fall into fits of taunts and insults and, deserting their homes, wander through woods and solitary places, even sinking into despair. It is therefore likely that the cause or ferment of this disease is intense heat which, as I have already said, patients of this kind can barely withstand.

Some will be struck with what I have several times observed, which is that most of those whose melancholy derived from this disease died sooner than maniacs and melancholics whose conditions arose from a different source; however, if we examine with careful judgment the causes that speed the death of these sufferers, we shall find nothing to wonder at, for there is undoubtedly a great difference between primitive diseases and those that spring from sympathy, epigenesis or metastasis, even though very few outward differences may be visible. . . .

CAUSE OF THIS DISEASE

It may be in the temperature or in the constitution of the atmosphere, or in the food. Since in *Historia Físico Médica* (Physical-Medical History) of this region, which I wrote with my own hand and still have in my home, I have dealt sufficiently with temperature, I will treat here only foods.

The principle food of almost all sufferers of this affliction is maize and millet, since from their flour they make their bread; they also prepare *papas* which, mixed with milk or butter, constitute their ordinary fare. They also eat eggs, chestnuts, lima beans, turnips, cabbages, milk, lard, cheese, apples, pears, nuts, hazelnuts, and other fruit of trees. They almost never eat fresh meat and only seldom eat salt meat, for almost all those who suffer this disease are poor peasants, who not only have no salt pork, but also no salt meat from any other animal for every day, not even for every ten days. The millet bread is generally unleavened, without yeast, and cooked in a small oven. They drink water, and their dresses, their shirts, their beds, and their dwellings are the same as their food. . . .

TREATMENT FOR THESE ENDEMICS

. . . Regarding the cure of "mal de la rosa," I can only speak of the dietary, pharmaceutical, and surgical remedies that I have learned from experience. I have constantly observed that changing the ordinary foods for more substantial and nutritious ones was most useful to diminish this disease and, on careful examination of the matter, it is indeed so. The ferment, or whatever one may call what constitutes the immediate cause of this disease, among other small qualities that appear to distinguish it, results in a pronounced emaciation, which is confirmed *first* by all the phenomena described before: *second,* the transition of this disease to other diseases; *third,* the lack of nutritive substances in the ordinary diet. The bread is not baked in large ovens but in very small ones, or in the embers of the hearth, and, according to Hippocrates, "bread baked in those ovens or in embers is exceedingly dry, in the latter because of the ashes and in the former because it loses its juice owing to the smallness of the oven." Milk, which owing to the fat it contains undoubtedly could undo the emaciation caused by the ordinary foods, is generally taken after that fat is extracted, for the poor extract and sell it in order to purchase other needed foods, so that they only have the whey and some cheesy part for their own table.

As I have been told by a reliable person, a woman is still alive who, having suffered the transition of "mal de la rosa" to dementia, fell into the mania (either impelled by the disease or by an impulse of the same nature) of craving and eagerly seeking butter, and buying as much as she could find and eating it to satiety as her only daily sustenance; and by this diet alone, which she kept for some time, she recovered fully not only from "mal de la rosa," but also from her dementia. It is inferred, therefore, from the foregoing what kind of diet is suitable for these patients.

In order for the surgical-pharmaceutical treatment to provide more effective relief for the patient, it must be adjusted to the manifestations of the disease and to the particular disposition of the patient. Many have been relieved by gentle purgatives, bleedings and also, at times, vomitives and, lastly, certain antiscurvy infusions of fumaria, agrimony, chickory, sorrel, etc., and others by bark infusions; yet others by purgatives made of certain leaves and flowers, such as those of aniseed, fennel, black hellebore; oak bark, violet, borage and bugloss and, lastly, others by pills and syrups of cress, fumaria, sorrel and chickory.

AN ESSAY CONCERNING THE CAUSE OF THE ENDEMIAL COLIC OF DEVONSHIRE

George Baker

It seems. . . . not to have been without suffi-cient foundation, that I have for some time sus-pected, that the cause of this Colic is not to be sought for in the pure Cyder; but in some, either fraudulent, or accidental, adulteration.

Upon inquiry, I find that the disease is very common all over the county of Devon; but that it particularly infests those parts of the county, where the greatest quantities of Cyder are made. I likewise find that it is not only common among the lower class of inhabitants; but that it is much more frequent among people of all ranks, than in other parts of England; and that it is not intirely confined to the autumnal sea-son. . . .

According to my information, eighty Pa-tients, under the effects of the Devonshire colic, were admitted into the Bath-hospital in the course of the last year; forty of whom are said to have been cured, and thirty-six sent away greatly relieved. I likewise am informed from the Bath-hospital, that the proportion of such Patients from Devonshire, to that from the counties of Hereford, Gloucester, and Worcester, is gener-ally as eight to one.

In some letters, which I have lately received from Dr. Wall, of Worcester, the following facts are mentioned. "The counties of Hereford, Gloucester, and Worcester, are not, so far as I know, subject to the colic of Poitou, or any other endemic illness, unless it may be the rheu-matism; which, I think, the inhabitants of Here-fordshire are more liable to, than those of some other counties. There is no Lead, which can give occasion to that colic, used in any part of the *apparatus* for grinding or pressing the ap-ples, or fermenting the liquor. Once indeed, in a plentiful year of apples, I knew a Farmer, who, wanting casks, filled a large leaden cistern with new cyder, and kept it there, till he could procure hogsheads sufficient to contain the li-quor. The consequence was, that all who drank of it were affected by it as the Lead-workers usually are. We had eleven of them, at one time, in our Infirmary.

"I have lately had two or three Patients in that distemper, occasioned by their having drunk cyder made in a press covered over with Lead. But this fact of a cyder-press covered with Lead, is a singular, and perhaps the only instance of the kind in this part of England. It happened in a part of the county of Worcester, adjoining to Warwickshire, where very few apples grow; and the bed of the press being therefore cracked by disuse, the sagacity of the Farmer contrived this covering, to prevent a loss of his liquor. In gen-eral, the cyder-drinkers with us are healthy and robust; but for the most part lean. The liquor is clear, and passes off readily by urine and per-spiration; which enables the common people to drink immense quantities of it when at labour, to the amount of several gallons in a day. I have heard it observed by a Physician, late of this place, who was much concerned in the cure of Lunatics, that more of those unhappy Persons came to him from Herefordshire, than any other place. The fact, if true, may possibly arise from the quantity drunk, rather than the qual-ity."

Were the *apparatus* for making cyder the same in all the cyder-counties, it would appear very remarkable, that the inhabitants of one county should experience such terrible effects from the use of this liquor, while those of the other coun-ties drink it with impunity. But, if we inquire into the method of making cyder in the county of Devon, we shall be able to conjecture with some degree of probability, what it is that occa-sions such a difference. The large circular trough, in which the apples are ground, is gen-erally composed of several pieces of moor-stones, cramped together with iron, some melted Lead being poured into the interstices. It frequently happens, that these stones, which are thus to be joined, are unequal, and do not correspond with each other; so that consider-

Source: Excerpted from George Baker, *An Essay concerning the Cause of the Endemial Colic of Devonshire.* London, J. Hughs, near Lincoln's-Inn-Fields, 1777.

able chasms are left between them; and these chasms are filled up with Lead. In this case the apples, ground by the pressure of the roller, immediately come in contact with no small quantity of this poisonous mineral.

It is likewise common, in several parts of the county, either to line the cyder-presses entirely with Lead, in order to prevent their leaking; or to make a border of Lead quite round the press, in order to receive the juice of the apples, and to convey it into a vessel, made of wood or stone, placed underneath. And in many other places, where these methods are not used, it is common to nail sheet-lead over any cracks or joints in the presses; and likewise to convey the juice of the apples from the presses in leaden pipes. Moreover I am informed, that it is the practice of some Farmers, in managing their weak cyder, made early in the year, before the apples are ripe, to put a leaden weight into the casks, in order to prevent the liquor from growing sour; and that this cyder is the common drink of their servants and labourers. But I am willing to believe, that this pernicious method of adulteration (against which severe laws have been enacted, as well in France as in Germany, and which crime, in both countries, is deservedly punished by death) is not often practised by our countrymen.

Dii meliora piis, erroremque hostibus illum!

Dr. Wall informs me, that in some parts of the counties of Hereford, Gloucester, and Worcester, the mills, in which the apples are ground, being 16, 18, or 20 feet in diameter, consist of several pieces of stone or timber, joined together with cramps of iron, fastened with Lead: but that these cramps are fixed in the *bed* of the mill, or on the outside of the curb, and not in the groove where the apples are ground. The same Gentleman observes, that, if many apples, full of juice, lie long on the *bed* of the mill (where the apples are placed in an heap, that they may be ready to be thrown into the groove), some of which may perhaps be rotten, others bruised in the gathering, and a moisture spread over the whole, from the fermentation and sweating of the fruit, it may perhaps be doubted, whether some part of the Lead, used in the cramps, may not be dissolved; tho' it must be, at most, in a quantity extremely small; there being but very little Lead used in the junctures; and the surface exposed to the apples being almost imperceptible. But I am informed by

another person, that in many parts of Herefordshire, and the neighbouring counties, the stones of the mills, are joined together with putty; (which is whiting, mixed with oil into a tough paste) and that neither iron nor Lead are originally used in the construction of them; but that, if any of the joints, in wearing, happen to start (which is sometimes the case) they are repaired with iron cramps fastened with lead.

These facts having been well ascertained, I determined to make use of the first opportunity, which might occur, of informing myself by experiment, whether or no there are really marks of solution of Lead in the cyder of Devonshire. Being therefore, in the month of October 1766, at Exeter, I procured some of the expressed juice of apples, as it flowed from a cyder-press, lined with Lead, in the parish of Alfington. On this I made and repeated several experiments by means of the *atramentum sympatheticum*, or *liquor vini probatorius* described by *Neuumann*; and of the volatile tincture of sulphur. These experiments intirely satisfied me, that the Must contained a solution of lead. The same experiments were made on some cyder of the preceding year. This likewise shewed evident signs of lead contained in it; but in less proportion than in the Must.

But, being unwilling to make any positive assertion, solely on the authority of my own trials, more especially as I had been under the influence of a preconceived opinion; I brought with me to London some of the same Must, which I had examined at Exeter. This Must, together with some Devonshire cyder of the preceding year which I purchased of the maker (who assured me that he used no Lead in any part of the *apparatus* for making cyder, except only what is necessary for composing the trough, as was mentioned above), were the subject of some experiments, in making which, Dr. Saunders, an ingenious Gentleman, who teaches Chemistry, kindly gave me his assistance. . . .

Experiment I.

A small quantity of Devonshire cyder being exposed upon clean paper to the fumes of the volatile tincture of sulphur, became immediately of a darkish colour, approaching to black. And we could only imitate this colour by exposing a dilute solution of *Saccharum Saturni* to the same fumes. A small quantity of cyder, made in the county of Hereford, exposed in like manner to the same fumes, exhibited no such appearance, until a few drops of a solution of *Saccharum Saturni* were added to it.

Observation I.

From this experiment we are to understand that the acid, before united with the Lead in the cyder, and the volatile alkali in the tincture of sulphur, mutually attracted each other; and that it was the precipitate of the Lead united with the sulphur, which produced the dark colour above-mentioned.

Experiment II.

A small quantity of *Hepar Sulphuris* (prepared by digesting together in a sand-heat one ounce of orpiment, and two ounces of quick-lime, with twelve ounces of water, in a close vessel) being added to some Devonshire cyder, in a few minutes occasioned a darkish colour in the body of the liquor, approaching to black; and the whole became very opake. No such change was produced in the cyder of the county to Hereford, until a few drops of a solution of *Saccharum Saturni* were added; when the same appearance, which was produced in the Devonshire cyder, was perceived.

Observation II.

The reasoning, made use of in the former observation, is applicable here. The decomposition of the *Saccharum Saturni* and of the *Hepar Sulphuris* was effected by the same laws of elective attraction.

Experiment III.

To a small quantity of Devonshire cyder a few drops of *Hepar Sulphuris* (prepared by boiling equal parts of fixed vegetable alkali and sulphur together in water) were added; and a precipitation of a very dark colour was produced.

When some Herefordshire cyder was treated in the same manner, the precipitate produced was as white as milk; and it was only upon the addition of a few drops of a dilute solution of *Saccharum Saturni*, that a precipitate of the same colour with the former could be obtained.

Observation III.

There is some nicety required in making this experiment. The *Hepar Sulphuris* is not to be added in any large quantity; for as all the lead is precipitated upon the first addition, it is easy to perceive the several successive shades of colour in the precipitate, until all the lead is separated; and then the precipitate, upon a farther addition of *Hepar Sulphuris,* assumes the whiteness of the precipitate obtained from the Herefordshire cyder, which intitles it to the appellation of *Lac Sulphuris.* If a large quantity of *Hepar Sulphuris* be at once added, the whiteness of the too copious precipitate is such, as to render the dark colour of what is first precipitated imperceptible.

Experiment IV.

Some Devonshire cyder was examined by means of the volatile tincture of sulphur, as in Experiment III. A very dark coloured precipitate was obtained. A similar precipitate could only be obtained from Herefordshire cyder, after that a weak solution of *Saccharum Saturni* was added to it.

Some of the Must (taken from the press in the parish of Alfington, as was mentioned above) treated in the same manner with the cyder, produced precipitates of a deeper black colour. This sufficiently shews, that the solution of Lead in the Must was stronger than that in the cyder.

It is a matter of no consequence, whether the Lead, the existence of which is proved, was applied to the cyder in its state of Must, or in that of a vinous liquor. However, as the must afforded more considerable signs of impregnation than the cyder, it would seem probable that the lead was added to the Must; and that, as the acid, during the fermentation, is in a great measure converted into alcohol, a proportional quantity of lead will consequently be precipitated.

The same experiments were afterwards tried on several other specimens of Devonshire and the Herefordshire cyder. The result of them was constantly and uniformly the same as has been described.

It has been proposed by several Authors, to detect such adulterations of wines by means of the vitriolic or of the muriatic acid; which, by uniting with the lead, will make it precipitate.

But it is ascertained by the experiments, made by Professor Gaubius, that trials, made with the acids, are less conclusive than those which have been described.

Experiment V.

In order to leave the matter entirely without doubt, an extract from 18 common quart bottles of Devonshire cyder (first strained through a cloth) which had been in my cellar more than three months, was prepared. This extract, being assayed with the black flux, a quantity of Lead, weighing four grains and an half, was found at the bottom of the crucible. These experiments were made in October 1766. . . .

* * *

May not I presume to hope, that the present discovery of a poison, which has for many years exerted its virulent effects on the inhabitants of Devonshire, incorporated with their daily liquor, unobserved, and unsuspected, may be esteemed by those, who have power, and who have opportunities to remove the source of so much mischief, to be an object worthy of their most serious attention? I have long lamented, that a County, which is distinguished by some peculiar blessings, should likewise be distinguished by a peculiar calamity, as it were in consequence of its fertility. The subject therefore having appeared to me important, I have spared no pains in this investigation; and I am insured of my reward in the consciousness of having endeavoured to preserve my countrymen and fellow-creatures from one of the most dreadful diseases, incident to the human body.

This essay will probably be hereafter published in a medicinal collection. Some copies of it are now printed, with a particular view of giving to the inhabitants of the county of Devon the earliest intimation of their danger; in order that they may take the proper steps to preserve their health, and to secure the value of their property.

AN INQUIRY INTO THE CAUSES AND EFFECTS OF THE VARIOLAE VACCINAE

Edward Jenner

In this Dairy Country a great number of Cows are kept, and the office of milking is performed indiscriminately by Men and Maid Servants. One of the former having been appointed to apply dressings to the heels of a Horse affected with *the Grease,* and not paying due attention to cleanliness, incautiously bears his part in milking the Cows, with some particles of the infectious matter adhering to his fingers. When this is the case, it commonly happens that a disease is communicated to the Cows, and from the Cows to the Dairy-maids, which spreads through the farm until most of the cattle and domestics feel its unpleasant consequences. This disease has obtained the name of the Cow Pox. It appears on the nipples of the Cows in the form of irregular pustules. At their first appearance they are commonly of a palish blue, or rather of a colour somewhat approaching to livid, and are surrounded by an erysipelatous inflammation. These pustules, unless a timely remedy be applied, frequently degenerate into phagedenic ulcers, which prove extremely troublesome.[1] The animals become indisposed, and the secretion of milk is much lessened. Inflamed spots now begin to appear on different parts of the hands of the domestics employed in milking, and sometimes on the wrists, which quickly run on to suppuration, first assuming the appearance of the small vesications produced by a burn. Most commonly they appear about the joints of the fingers, and at their extremities; but whatever parts are affected, if the situation will admit, these superficial suppurations put on a circular form, with their edges more elevated than their centre, and of a colour distantly approaching to blue. Absorption takes place, and tumours appear in each axilla. The system becomes affected—the pulse is quickened; and shiverings, with general lassitude and pains about the loins and limbs, with vomiting, come on. The head is painful, and the patient is now and then even affected with delirium. These symptoms, varying in their degrees of violence, generally continue from one day to three or four, leaving ulcerated sores about the hands, which, from the sensibility of the parts, are very troublesome, and commonly heal slowly, frequently becoming phagedenic, like those from whence they sprung. The lips, nostrils, eyelids, and other parts of the body, are sometimes affected with sores; but these evidently arise from their being needlessly rubbed or scratched with the patient's infected fingers. No eruptions on the skin have followed the decline of the feverish symptoms in any instance that has come under my inspection, one only excepted, and in this case a very few appeared on the arms: they were very minute, of a vivid red colour, and soon died away without advancing to maturation; so that I cannot determine whether they had any connection with the preceding symptoms.

Thus the disease makes its progress from the Horse to the nipple of the Cow, and from the Cow to the Human Subject.

Morbid matter of various kinds, when absorbed into the system, may produce effects in some degree similar; but what renders the Cow-pox virus so extremely singular, is, that the person who has been thus affected is for ever after secure from the infection of the Small Pox; neither exposure to the variolous effluvia, nor the insertion of the matter into the skin, producing this distemper. . . .

Case VIII.

Elizabeth Wynne, aged fifty-seven, lived as a servant with a neighbouring Farmer thirty-eight years ago. She was then a dairymaid, and the Cow Pox broke out among the cows. She

Source: Excerpted from Edward Jenner, *An Inquiry into the Causes and Effects of the Variolae Vaccinae.* London, Sampson Low, 1798.

[1] They who attend sick cattle in this country find a speedy remedy for stopping the progress of this complaint in those applications which act chemically upon the morbid matter, such as the solutions of the Vitriolum Zinci, the Vitriolum Cupri, &c.

caught the disease with the rest of the family, but, compared with them, had it in a very slight degree, one very small sore only breaking out on the little finger of her left hand, and scarcely any perceptible indisposition following it.

As the malady had shewn itself in so slight a manner, and as it had taken place at so distant a period of her life, I was happy with the opportunity of trying the effects of variolous matter upon her constitution, and on the 28th of March, 1797, I inoculated her by making two superficial incisions on the left arm, on which the matter was cautiously rubbed. A little efflorescence soon appeared, and a tingling sensation was felt about the parts where the matter was inserted until the third day, when both began to subside, and so early as the fifth day it was evident that no indisposition would follow.

Case IX.

Although the Cow Pox shields the constitution from the Small Pox, and the Small Pox proves a protection against its own future poison, yet it appears that the human body is again and again susceptible of the infectious matter of the Cow Pox, as the following history will demonstrate:

William Smith, of Pyrton in this parish, contracted this disease when he lived with a neighbouring Farmer in the year 1780. One of the horses belonging to the farm had sore heels, and it fell to his lot to attend him. By these means the infection was carried to the cows, and from the cows it was communicated to Smith. On one of his hands were several ulcerated sores, and he was affected with such symptoms as have been before described.

In the year 1791 the Cow Pox broke out at another farm where he then lived as a servant, and he became affected with it a second time: and in the year 1794 he was so unfortunate as to catch it again. The disease was equally as severe the second and third time as it was on the first.[2]

In the spring of the year 1795 he was twice inoculated, but no affection of the system could be produced from the variolous matter; and he has since associated with those who had the Small Pox in its most contagious state without feeling any effect from it.

---

[2] This is not the case in general—a second attack is commonly very slight, and so, I am informed, it is among the cows.

A DESCRIPTION OF THE PHYSICAL AND MORAL STATE OF WORKERS EMPLOYED IN COTTON, WOOL, AND SILK MILLS

Louis R. Villerme

A BRIEF SUMMARY OF THE THREE SECTIONS[1]

In view of the amount and scope of the information presented in this volume, I feel compelled to summarize it here in a few pages. This summary will present a kind of comparative description of the main characteristics of workers in wool, cotton, and silk industries as well as the similarities and differences in workers of the same trade but who work in different locations and those in workers of the same industry but who work on different trades. This chapter, then, will attempt to summarize the information presented in the preceding chapters. . . .

Weavers, who represent a large class, normally work at home in the cellar or in damp, poorly ventilated ground floors. Most of them live in the country. They are frequently involved in agriculture, and, generally speaking, they are orderly, thrifty, and of good moral character. However, except for a small number of weavers who produce "fashion" fabrics and dry goods, their earnings are very modest and their eating habits, health, and housing leave much to be desired. . . .

Workers at mechanized spinning and cloth mills work in common areas, where the mixture of sexes and ages frequently has a negative impact on their inclinations and habits, particularly when they live in a large city or when they do not return home to their families in the evening. This work, in addition to being unhealthy for an excessive number of small children, is oftentimes remunerated with very low wages, which are all the more insufficient considering that these workers have no other source of income and almost never have standing or savings.

The condition of cotton workers is worst in Lille and in the Department of the Haut-Rhin. Horrible indigence, destitution, depravity, and marked degradation have been documented in Lille, as well as many workers who are poorly sheltered, poorly dressed, ill-nourished, pale, thin, and exhausted from fatigue in the Haute-Alsace. However, most of these workers, who have been given the odd and expressive epithet of "white negroes" in Thann and Mulhouse, deserve the compassion of respectable persons in view of their good qualities and the cause of their misery.

LENGTH OF THE WORKING DAY[2]

The working day is very long, except in times of crisis. Workers employed in cotton and wool mills work between 15 and 15½ hours each day, of which an average of 13 work hours are required.

To support this statement I could state the starting and closing times of the various mills that I visited, but I prefer to let the manufacturers speak for themselves. During the 1834 commercial and industrial survey, whose results were published by order of the Ministry of Trade, many spinning-mill workers made statements.

One of them reported that in Roubaix the working day was 14½ hours, including 2 hours for meals and rest; children worked as long as adult men and, among the former, there were *six-year-olds and many eight-year-olds*.

Two others stated that at their factories in Rouen the working hours, not the length of the working day, were 13½ hours year round.

Another stated that in the Departments of the Haut-Rhin and the Bas-Rhin, the working day is 13 hours.

Others stated that in the city of Saint-Quentin

Source: Excerpted and translated from Louis R. Villerme, *Tableau de L'Etat Physique et Moral des Ouvriers Employés dans les Manufactures de Coton, de Laine et de Soie.* Paris, Jules Renouard et Cie, Libraires, 1840.

[1] From Volume I.

[2] From Volume II.

all workers, regardless of age or sex, work 13 hours per day.

Furthermore, the length of the working day, which is more or less the same throughout France, does not seem to be any shorter in spinning mills in Belgium, at least in Ghent. I did find it to be shorter, however, in the Swiss districts of Zurich and Argovie, particularly in Zurich.

The 1834 survey also showed that the work day in cloth mills lasted 13 hours out of a 15-hour day in Elbeuf, 13 hours in Abbeville, 13 in Louviers, and 15 in Sedan, but it lasted 12 hours in Carcassonne and only 8 to 10 hours in Lodève.

A report done for the Société industrielle de Mulhouse, dated 29 February 1827, established the length of a work day in spinning mills at ordinarily 13 to 14 hours, for children as well as for adults; another report done for the same company and dated 31 May 1837 contains the following surprising statement: "Some mills in France keep their workers 17 hours a day; the only time they have for rest during those 17 hours is one-half hour for lunch and one hour for supper, which leaves 15½ hours of actual work". . . .

When there are large or rush orders, work at the mills sometimes goes through Saturday night. This is an exception, however, and rather than have the workers spend the night at the factory, they are normally made to come back Sunday morning and work until noon. Lastly, there are some mills, although their number is very limited, that operate seven days a week, 24 hours a day; in these cases, they operate with two shifts which normally alternate one week of day work with one week of night work.

These periods seem quite long, I might even say excessively so, especially considering that they are the same for all workers regardless of their age. As a result, they are one of the causes, if not the major one, of the state of suffering of the children and of some of the poorest adults.

Regardless of how sad the condition of the adults is, the children who are employed in great numbers in our mills should move us in particular, for they are all too often victims of the irresponsibility and improvidence of their parents, and, in any case, do not deserve their sad situation.

In Alsace, many of these unfortunate children come from Swiss or German families who have been entirely ruined, and who, drawn by hopes for a better future, come to compete with the local residents. Their first concern after procuring a job is to find lodging; however, the high rents in the cities and nearby villages where the mills are located, often force them to live a league and sometimes even a league-and-a-half away.

As a result, the children, many of whom are barely seven years old, and some even younger, lose sleep and rest because they have to cover this long and tiring route twice a day: in the morning to go to the factory and in the evening to return home.

More than anywhere else this cause of suffering can be observed in Mulhouse, a city which despite its rapid growth is not able to provide housing for all of the workers who come in response to the unending call of the mills. It is indeed a very sad sight to see the workers arriving from all directions each morning. It is hard to imagine the multitude of gaunt children, clothed in rags, who trudge barefoot through the rain and mud, carrying in their hand or, if it is raining, under their coat that has become waterproof from all of the oil that has fallen from the looms, the morsel of bread that is all they have to eat until they return home that evening.

It is true that the children employed in the other cotton and spinning mills in the Haut-Rhin and in similar establishments in other parts of France are not so badly off; they are, however, pale, enervated, slow in their movements, withdrawn when they play, and have an outward appearance of misery, suffering, and exhaustion. This contrasts with the rosy complexion, stoutness, liveliness, and all other signs of good health that can be seen in children of the same age when one leaves manufacturing areas and enters a farming district.

These evils are even more deplorable considering that the marvelous machines of present-day mills make it possible to substitute many adults with children, thereby necessarily increasing the number of children in factories at the same time as it produces a drop in the availability of farm hands. However, as mentioned above, industry, when concentrated in the cities, creates a new class whose fortune is more unstable than that of farm workers, since it is subject to all kinds of variations, all kinds of crises related to trade; this class would, however, be better off than farm workers during ordinary times if it had better habits and methods, and a spirit of foresightedness.

So as to give a better idea that the working day for children is, in fact, too long in the mills, I would like to mention here that usage and legislation have established for all kinds of work, including forced labor, a working day of 12 hours, reduced to 10 hours of actual work with 2 hours of meals. For the workers under consideration here, the length of the working day is between 15 and 15½ hours, of which 13 to 13½ are actually spent working. What a difference! . . .

CHILDREN EMPLOYED IN FACTORIES

The manufacture of cotton and wool thread and fabric used to be spread throughout the countryside, in private homes, as is still the case today throughout France and in almost all of Europe for flax or hemp thread and fabric. However, the Arkwright loom and other more advanced, modern machinery used for spinning and weaving have resulted in a concentration of cotton and wool mills in large factories that run on fire-run pumps or water-power. Horses are only rarely, if at all, used. This change has brought about others: many adults have been replaced with children and this system has resulted in the serious abuses described in the preceding chapter and has given rise to very vocal complaints in Great Britain since the end of the nineteenth century. These complaints, whether or not exaggerated, threw light on the lamentable status of children in cotton mills. It was natural that it should be in England, the largest manufacturing country in the world and the country that has surpassed all others in the art of spinning, that the consequences of this new system should first be felt.

I do not wish to repeat known facts here, but in order not to omit any facts on children, I would now like to examine the report mentioned above from the Bureau of Mills of our Trade Ministry. I have deleted those passages that do not modify already known facts.

Wages for children vary between 25 and 75 centimes, according to age, strength, and skills. It is normally increased by 1 sou per day for each year until the age of 17 or 18.

Generally, night work for children is a cause of great demoralization. I believe it has been shown that children who are not under the supervision of their parents in the factories are more prone than others to accept wayward ideas and disorderly habits, particularly if they earn good wages.

Children who work with their parents in the factories represent between one-tenth and one-half of the young working force, or an average of one-third. Even they, however, do not entirely support or help their parents. Furthermore, many parents place their children in other factories than where they themselves work so that if the parents' factory stops working, the entire family will not be out of work at the same time.

All available information indicates that children who begin working at factories at the age of 6 have no education whatsoever; and normally those children who begin working before 10 or 11 years of age are not able to read or write. Although some evening and Sunday schools have been opened, children who work 12 to 14 hours a day, or who have worked the night before, are too exhausted to attend classes. Moreover, the indifference of parents in this respect is normally very high. Religious instruction, we have been assured, is generally accorded the necessary time. . . .

GENERAL CONSIDERATIONS

It has been said that whenever a great number of persons are kept together in a closed area, their health suffers. If we were to extend this statement to factories, the facts stated above would still not confirm this. No disease is exclusively characteristic of a given kind of factory, although some are more frequent when the conditions in which the workers live promote their development.

In cotton-spinning mills, for example, coughing, pulmonary inflammations, and the dreaded phthisis attack and debilitate many workers employed in the threshing or in the initial carding stage; according to my information, these same diseases also have a strong impact on the workers who fasten, sweep, or unplug wadding, those who inhale cotton dust and fluff, and among the hand weavers.

Even though there are many victims of pulmonary inflammations and phthisis, their premature deaths do not seem to me any more deplorable than the development of scrofula among the working masses at our factories. We know the broad extent of this scourge which marks children and young persons with swellings, scars, disabilities, and hideous deformities, particularly in certain areas such as the large cities where poor people gather in the street or in dark, dirty, poorly ventilated lodgings where sunlight does not enter. It particularly attacks weavers and their families. Besides these grievous effects, one must add the small and lank stature, the weakness, and pitiful debilitated condition of the populations ravaged by scrofula. Compare these people, bent over their looms each day, arising in shadows, wilting, one might say, like plants; compare them to other residents of the same places or to farmers who work and live in the open air with bright sunlight and you will be amazed by the difference.

This difference is enormous and is well known to the officials in charge of army recruitment; unfortunately no one has yet compiled and described observations of this which would remove all doubts. This is what led me to undertake research in this respect. However, the time available only enabled me to carry out this work for the city of Amiens. My results show that the men aged 20 to 21 who were most often found unfit to serve in the army by reason of their size, constitution, or health, often came from the poorer classes, one could even say from the *factory working class.* In order to find 100 men fit for military service, 193 men have to be drafted in the more comfortable classes and up to 343 have to be drafted in the poorer classes. . . .

With respect to workers in spinning and weaving mills, who show the highest mortality rates for all age brackets (depending on the age, this is one third, one half, or even higher than that for the class including cotton print workers, mill operators, manufacturers), it has not been forgotten how badly off they are: pale, thin, and weakened from hardship and poverty. I say *poverty* because they are far from able to obtain sufficient good food in exchange for their work. It is, therefore, not surprising that for all age groups, their mortality rates are higher than in the other classes. This class includes many families who used to work in the fields and who prefer a low-level job to the shame of begging for bread. This abrupt and total change from life in the fields to life in the city, from open air jobs to jobs in closed factories, often produces a devastating effect on their constitution, besides

all the troubles that preceded and that will follow said change.

The excessive mortality among families of workers employed in the cotton spinning and weaving mills in Mulhouse mainly affects the younger age groups. In fact, one-half of the children born to the class of manufacturers, businessmen, and factory managers reach the age of 29, whereas one-half of the children of weavers and factory workers in the spinning mills will die, as hard as it may seem to believe, before the age of 2. . . .

No one will deny that there are some professions that are essential and that are just as unhealthy as cotton threshing: the skinner of rabbit and hare pelts, the miner who extracts mercury from the earth, the night watchman, the sewerman, the preparer of white lead and other chemical reagents, etc. These professions, everyone would agree, are neither less dirty, nor less toilsome, nor do they always give those who perform them a happier outlook, a broader horizon, more space, cleaner air, or better wages than many of the jobs in the manufacturing sector.

Professions most often affect the health of persons and their families in an indirect, mediate way through the conditions involving food, clothing, lodging, fatigue, duration of work, customs, etc. in which the workers exist. This rule should be regarded as a general one. The danger presented by dust to some workers that inhale it in cotton-spinning mills would be an exception, as would be the rather frequent accidents that occur during the work day. These are normally injuries to hands and fingers that are caught in machines or gears. Sometimes bones are broken, limbs are severed, or even death can occur. These accidents are always the fault of either the manufacturer who has neglected to isolate or surround the dangerous parts of machines with a casing or screen, or of the workers themselves, especially children, who neglect to take safety measures. I do not know how frequent they are, but I believe that the very serious ones are not very numerous and generally result from oversight on the part of the victims. Most of these could be prevented by use of the screens that I mentioned above. Some manufacturers have already made this expense, however, others, and these are the majority, have not taken this safety measure. Legislation should be passed to make this compulsory.

OBSERVATIONS MADE DURING THE EPIDEMIC OF MEASLES ON THE FAROE ISLANDS IN THE YEAR 1846

Peter Ludwig Panum

Measles had not prevailed on the Faroes since 1781; then it broke out early in April, 1846. As I intend to offer in another section some observations about this disease, I shall limit myself here to mentioning the effect of this epidemic on the mortality. Of the 7782 inhabitants, about 6000 were taken with measles in the course of about half a year, in that the first case appeared, in Thorshavn, on the 4th or 5th of April, and after the 17th of September only a few cases were still occurring on Sandø. From the beginning of the year to the middle of September, a total of 255 persons died, of whom at least 102 died of measles or its sequelae. But as I have no very accurate statistical data for Suderø, which Mr. Manicus has taken care of, I shall here give account only of the other islands, comprising six parishes, with 6626 inhabitants, of whom about 5000 had measles last year. From the beginning of the year 1846 until the epidemic had ended, 215 persons died in these parishes, of whom 164 died during the epidemic, the duration of the latter having been calculated separately for each village, and, of these, seventy-eight were victims of measles or its results. It must, however, be observed withal that the number of those who died of measles seems to be set too low as far as Sydströmø is concerned. The fact is that for this parish I was able to refer only to the records which I found in the church registers, where measles is given as the cause of death in but twelve instances. But since the church registers also show that of sixty-eight individuals who died on Syndströmø from the first of the year to July 30th, sixty-four died between April 21st and July 21st, just in the space of time during which measles prevailed there, whereas, according to the average count for the years 1835–1845, only 23⁹/₁₁ persons usually die yearly in Sydströmø, it is unlikely that only twelve should have been carried off by measles. This is the more extraordinary, because, of the sixty-four dead, forty-five had lived in Thorshavn (with about 800 inhabitants), where both physicians of the country live, and, in accordance with instructions, report the causes of death to the priests, who record them in the church registers. In all the other parishes where I had been able by personal presence to obtain more reliable information, it was found that between a third and a half of those who died in the course of the year were carried off by measles or its sequelae, except in Sandø, however, where measles demanded no sacrifices. Therefore, even if we ascribe to an influenza epidemic beginning with the arrival of the ship some effect upon the mortality, it appears to me as probable that the actual number of deaths from measles was between 78 and 164; in the first case, there would have been one death among 64 measles patients, and in the other one among 30½. Whereas the ratio of deaths to the total number of people, which in Denmark, according to the average calculation for 1801 to 1834, is 1:41.22, and on the Faroes, according to the average computation for 1835 to 1845, is usually 1:64.66, it is here found to be 1:31.07 in only the first two-thirds of the year 1846.

It is a remarkable fact, indicative of the serious character of measles among grown people, that the yearly average age of death, namely, 44⅛ years (usually 44⅔ years), was practically unaltered. Table 1 serves to show the mortality in the respective ages during the measles epidemic of 1846, and a comparison of these rates with those usual on the Faroes.

This review shows that measles, perhaps associated with the epidemic of influenza which prevailed with it in the spring, was destructive to the young children under one year of age, but, on the other hand, did not remarkably increase the mortality between the first and twentieth years of life, because the disease was less dangerous in this period; and that the mor-

Source: Excerpted from Peter Ludwig Panum, *Observations made during the Epidemic of Measles on the Faroe Islands in the Year 1846*, trans. Ada Sommerville Hatcher. N.p., Delta Omega Society, 1948.

Table 1. Mortality in the respective ages during the measles epidemic of 1846, and a comparison of these rates with those usual on the Faroes.

Ages	From 1835-1845 inclusive, died yearly, by average computation at the respective ages	In the first two-thirds of the year 1846 died	Percent of persons of the resp. ages taken by death yearly, for 1835-1845, reckoned from the census of 1845	Percent of persons of the resp. ages died in first two-thirds of 1846, counted from census of 1845 and my own notes	Number of times mortality in first two-thirds of 1846 was greater than that usual in an ordinary whole year.
Under 1	18 1/11	50	10 9/11	30	About 2 9/11
1–10	7 3/11	6	6/11	6/11	0
10–20	5 5/11	5	5/11	4/11	÷
20–30	6 6/11	8	11/22	15/22	About 1 4/11
30–40	6 2/11	13	17/22	2 1/11	About 2 1/2
40–50	7 4/11	18	1 1/11	2 8/11	About 2 1/2
50–60	5 5/11	28	10/11	4 4/9	About 5
60–70	8 2/11	31	2	7 8/11	About 3 3/4
70–80	14 10/11	30	6 5/10	13 1/11	About 2
80–100	16 9/11	26	16 9/11	26	About 1 1/2
Total	96 3/11	215			

tality rose from the thirtieth year, until it became greatest for the ages between the fiftieth and sixtieth years, that is, five times as great as usual; it then descended again after the sixtieth year, not because the disease was less dangerous for those still older, which was by no means the case, but because it was precisely sixty-five years ago that measles had last prevailed on the Faroes, and those who had recovered from the disease at that time were now spared.

Table 2 shows how the measles epidemic on the Faroes—irrespective of the difference which might arise from the fact that no age was ex-

empt, whereas in Denmark measles ordinarily attacks only children—contributed to make the mortality in 1846 more like that of Denmark than usual. Accordingly, it might appear as if the singular way in which measles affected the mortality rate on the Faroe Islands had something in common with the way in which a number of simultaneously occurring epidemics affects the mortality of Denmark and other countries.

The influence which the epidemic of measles of 1846 exerted on the mortality rates of the Faroes may serve as an example to illustrate the

Table 2. Comparison of mortality rates from measle epidemics in the Faroes and in Denmark.

Ages	Mortality on the Faroes (except Suderø) in the first two-thirds of the year 1846, reckoned on 1000 individuals, instead of on the actual mortality of 215	Mortality in Denmark in the years 1829-1833 incl. reckoned for 1000 males.	Mortality on the Faroes (except Suderø) in the years 1835-1845 incl., reckoned for 1059 individuals of whom 60 were stillborn or died within 24 hours
Under 1	233 ⎱ 261		199 ⎱ 279
1–10	28 ⎰	366	80 ⎰
10–20	23	43	60
20–30	37	56	72
30–40	60	60	68
40–50	84	77	81
50–60	130	105	60
60–70	144	123	90
70–80	140	113	164
80–100	121	57	185

tendency of epidemics as a whole to decimate the population of a country. Of course, measles is not wont under ordinary conditions to menace any but children, but on the Faroes it evidently attacked almost the entire population without respect to age; and the epidemics in the aggregate, which prevail in other countries but partially spare the Faroes, also threaten the entire population, without respect to age. I believe that I have established that the most essential cause of the favorable rates of mortality on the Faroes may be looked for in the freedom of these islands, because of their situation as well as their isolated condition as regards commerce, from many diseases which in other places, in Denmark, for instance, very considerably increase the mortality. . . .

As to the *length of the incubation period,* accurate and satisfactory observations have hitherto been lacking, as far as I know, since some authors regard it as eight days, others as from ten to fourteen days, and others again assume no definite stadium contagii latentis. This is not strange, however, inasmuch as observations in regard to the subject could not well be made where a very lively intercourse goes on among the people, and where each individual comes into contact with a large number of other individuals, each of whom may be carrying the material of infection with him. Here in Copenhagen, for instance, it can very rarely be said of a measles patient that he was exposed to infection only once, on this or that day; for it can hardly ever be proved that he was not in anywise exposed earlier or later, without knowing it, to the influence of the contagion of measles. To be able to arrive at some definite result in reference to this question would call for special circumstances which might render it possible to make accurate observations, and these circumstances were offered on the Faroe Islands. The isolated situation of the villages, and their limited intercourse with each other, made it possible in many, in fact in most, cases to ascertain where and when the person who first fell ill had been exposed to the infection, and to prove that the contagion could not have affected him either before or after the day stated. . . .

. . . On the 4th of June a boat with ten men from Tjörnevig had taken part in a catch of grind at Vestmannhavn; and on the 18th of June, precisely the fourteenth day following, the measles exanthem had broken out on all ten

men, after they had been feeling ill from two to four days, and had been suffering with cough and smarting of the eyes. The ten men mentioned had not been together at all except at the grind catch referred to, and none of them had been at any place where they could have happened to be exposed in the remotest way to the infection, which they dreaded and shunned. In Vestmannhavn, on the other hand, they had not only been in contact with many men who had recently got up after measles (perhaps some of them still florid with the exanthem), but had also been staying for some time in houses where persons had to go to bed on the next day with an eruption of the measles exanthem. From twelve to sixteen days after these ten men had taken measles (counting from the appearance of the rash), the exanthem broke out on nearly all the other inhabitants, except some few individuals, who were not attacked until twelve to sixteen days after the first general outbreak.

These facts might suggest that the contagion of measles produces no visible effect for quite a long time, usually ten to twelve days, after its reception into the organism, since the catarrhal prodromal stage began just after this lapse of time, and the exanthem first appeared on the fourteenth day after the reception of the infective matter. If this supposition were confirmed, then the observation that the second and third general outbreaks ensued each after about fourteen days' interim would make it probable that measles is most infectious during the stage of eruption and efflorescence, and not, as generally supposed, during that of desquamation.

In order to investigate as to whether or not these suppositions were well-founded, I decided to undertake in each village to which I came, a brief inquiry, as exact as possible, in regard to the origin, mode of introduction and of spread of the disease. In this manner I obtained, for fifty-two villages, the names of the persons who first took measles, the circumstances and dates of their exposure to infection, the dates on which the exanthem appeared on them, and the time that elapsed thereafter before other residents broke out with the exanthem. It would become too tedious to review this for every single village, especially since I found the suppositions set forth above confirmed everywhere, and I did not encounter any instances to prove that there were exceptions to the rule. I shall, therefore, present here only some cases by which these conclusions were substantiated in most remarkable fashion.

In Velberstad, on Sydströmø, I obtained statements which contradicted my assumption of a stage of incubation of a definite length, inasmuch as there appeared to have been, in the case of a certain patient, only ten days between the time on which the patient was exposed to the infection and the day on which the exanthem appeared. Since it was a very reliable man who stated this to me, and the patient concerned was his own wife, I thought I had found here an exception to the rule. But on Olai (July 29th), the same man sent me a message by his nephew, Pastor Djurhuus, to the effect that his statement had not been correct, but that it was exactly fourteen days, instead of ten, that had intervened between the time that his wife had been exposed to the infection and the day on which she broke out with the exanthem. Shortly before my arrival the man had lost at the same time his beloved wife and a sister, and his grief had distracted him.

The other case in which I thought I had found an exception to the rule was in Hattervig, on Fuglø. A young man, the first person who had developed measles there, declared to me that he had not been outside Hattervig except on Whitmonday (June 1st) when, together with another man, he was in Arnefjord, on Bordø, where at that time measles had not broken out, but where, as he had learned later, a man had developed the exanthem on the 3rd of June, and two others on the 8th.[1] The first young man asserted that in his case the exanthem had appeared on the 11th of June, but in his companion's not until the 14th. Although I explained to him that it was of great importance to other people that he should tell me the truth, and that there was no question of any responsibility for him, he would not admit that he had been exposed any earlier to the infection. But in the evening, when I was sitting in the smoke-room, attired in Faroese clothes, he came to me and begged my pardon because he had not recollected correctly; the fact was that he had

been also in Klaksvig, on the 30th of May, and being in an intoxicated condition, had been in several houses where there was measles. The procedure that I had followed, somewhat resembling an examination, had made the young man from that isolated Fuglø uneasy, and had induced him to conceal the truth.

In Selletraed, on Østerø, I was told that a young man had been infected on June 4th at the grind haul in Vestmannhavn, and that on June 9th he had broken out with the exanthem, and that his younger brother and other folk in the village had been infected by him, and had broken out with the exanthem on June 17th. I asked for the almanac, and inquired where the older brother had been on the 26th of May (fourteen days before the exanthem broke out on him). They told me that on that very day he had been in Nord-Øre, where measles was prevailing, and that on the way home he had spent the night of the same day in Sydre-Göthe, and had slept in the bed with the servant-man of P. Johnson's widow; but that in Nord-Øre he had not been in any house, and there was no measles in Sydre-Göthe at that time. By looking at my notes afterwards, I found that the servant-man mentioned was the first person who took measles in Sydre-Göthe, and that the exanthem had spread over his whole body a few days later. Then I learned that only those folk in the village who had broken out with the measles exanthem at the same time as the younger brother had been along with the brothers at the grind catch at Vestmannhavn. It was now clear to me that the elder brother had been infected in Göthe (or possibly in Nord-Øre), and the younger, together with the others, in Vestmannhavn.

In Fuglefjord, on Østerø, on account of my observations, I acquired the reputation of being able to prophesy. On my first arrival there, the daughter of Farmer J. Hansen, churchwarden, had recently had measles, but had then got up, and, except for a slight cough, was almost entirely well. All the other nine persons in the house were feeling well in every respect and expressed the hope that they would escape the disease. I inquired as to what day the exanthem had appeared on the daughter, asked for the almanac, and pointed to the fourteenth day after that on which the exanthem had been noticed on the daughter, with the remark that they should make a black line under that date,

---

[1] This was related correctly. On the 20th of May, one man had been at the trading-place, Klaksvig, where the measles was prevailing, and he broke out with the exanthem on June 3rd; on the 25th of May the two others had been at the same place and the exanthem appeared on them on June 8th.

for I feared that on it measles would show itself on others in the house; if this did not happen on that day, they might perhaps have some hope of being exempt. As it turned out I was summoned to Fuglefjord again ten days later and was met with the outcry: "What he said was correct! On the day he pointed out the measles broke out, with its red spots, on all nine." . . .

. . . Similarly, towards the end of the epidemic, the disease attacked very slowly in Kunø, Midtvaag, and Sandevaag. At the height of the epidemic, in Tjörnevig, for example, about fourteen days after one or several persons had caught measles, the majority of the residents of the village were attacked, and only a relatively small number were spared until fourteen days after the great onset; but the people in the last-named villages fell ill gradually, so that only a few were attacked fourteen days after those who took the disease first; fourteen days later, others; about fourteen days after these, still others, and so on; thus the disease lingered longer in the villages last attacked than in those that were infected earlier. Nevertheless, measles preserved withal, at least as far as my experience went, its definite period of development (from the reception of the infection to the appearance of the exanthem); and in fact, I know of no case where, after a pause of more than fourteen days, measles had appeared afresh in a village without reinfection from some other place. Nevertheless, we cannot deny the possibility that the infective material may be retained for quite a while after the cessation of measles, in wool or clothing, for instance, or in other things that are capable of harboring it.

The rule *that the contagion of measles does not produce any symptoms of illness at all, for a considerable time after it has been received into the organism, and then, according to my observations, after an indefinite prodromal period, brings forth the well-known exanthem* always on the thirteenth or fourteenth day, has thus proved constant for me in a significant series of accurate observations. . . .

It is known to be generally supposed that measles sometimes attacks one and the same individual twice. In this connection it is quite remarkable, however, that of the many aged people still living on the Faroes who had had measles in 1781, not one, as far as I could find out by careful inquiry, was attacked the second time. I myself saw ninety-eight such old people, who were exempt because they had had the disease in their youth. This was the more noteworthy in that a high age by no means lessened the susceptibility to measles, since, as far as I know, all the old people who had not gone through with measles in earlier life were attacked when they were exposed to infection; whereas certain young persons, although constantly exposed, were exempt. If recovery from measles sixty-five years before could insure people against taking the disease a second time, it might be supposed that still greater protection would be afforded by having recovered from it a shorter time before; and I am, therefore, inclined to assume that the cases in which measles was observed to occur the second time in the same person are attributable to erroneous diagnosis, or at least are extremely rare.

ON THE MODE OF COMMUNICATION OF CHOLERA

John Snow

It would occupy a long time to give an account of the progress of cholera over different parts of the world, with the devastation it has caused in some places, whilst it has passed lightly over others, or left them untouched; and unless this account could be accompanied with a description of the physical condition of the places, and the habits of the people, which I am unable to give, it would be of little use.

There are certain circumstances, however, connected with the progress of cholera, which may be stated in a general way. It travels along the great tracks of human intercourse, never going faster than people travel, and generally much more slowly. In extending to a fresh island or continent, it always appears first at a sea-port. It never attacks the crews of ships going from a country free from cholera to one where the disease is prevailing, till they have entered a port, or had intercourse with the shore. Its exact progress from town to town cannot always be traced; but it has never appeared except where there has been ample opportunity for it to be conveyed by human intercourse.

There are also innumerable instances which prove the communication of cholera, by individual cases of the disease, in the most convincing manner. Instances such as the following seem free from every source of fallacy.

I called lately to inquire respecting the death of Mrs. Gore, the wife of a labourer, from cholera, at New Leigham Road, Streatham. I found that a son of deceased had been living and working at Chelsea. He came home ill with a bowel complaint, of which he died in a day or two. His death took place on August 18th. His mother, who attended on him, was taken ill on the next day, and died the day following (August 20th). There were no other deaths from cholera registered in any of the metropolitan districts, down to the 26th August, within two or three miles of the above place; the nearest being

Source: Excerpted from *Snow on Cholera*. Cambridge: Harvard University Press, 1949. By permission of the publisher.

at Brixton, Norwood, or Lower Tooting. . . .

The following instances are quoted from an interesting work by Dr. Simpson of York, entitled "Observations on Asiatic Cholera":—"The first cases in the series occurred at Moor Monkton, a healthy agricultural village, situated to the north-west of York, and distant six miles from that place. At the time when the first case occurred, the malady was not known to be prevailing anywhere in the neighbourhood, nor, indeed, at any place within a distance of thirty miles.

"John Barnes, aged 39, an agricultural labourer, became severely indisposed on the 28th of December 1832; he had been suffering from diarrhœa and cramps for two days previously. He was visited by Mr. George Hopps, a respectable surgeon at Redhouse, who, finding him sinking into collapse, requested an interview with his brother, Mr. J. Hopps, of York. This experienced practitioner at once recognized the case as one of Asiatic cholera; and, having bestowed considerable attention on the investigation of that disease, immediately enquired for some probable source of contagion, but in vain: no such source could be discovered. When he repeated his visit on the day following, the patient was dead; but Mrs. Barnes (the wife), Matthew Metcalfe, and Benjamin Muscroft, two persons who had visited Barnes on the preceding day, were all labouring under the disease, but recovered. John Foster, Ann Dunn, and widow Creyke, all of whom had communicated with the patients above named, were attacked by premonitory indisposition, which was however arrested. Whilst the surgeons were vainly endeavouring to discover whence the disease could possibly have arisen, the mystery was all at once, and most unexpectedly, unravelled by the arrival in the village of the son of the deceased John Barnes. This young man was apprentice to his uncle, a shoemaker, living at Leeds. He informed the surgeons that his uncle's wife (his father's sister) had died of cholera a fortnight before that time, and that, as she had no children, her wearing apparel had been sent to

Monkton by a common carrier. The clothes had not been washed; Barnes had opened the box in the evening; on the next day he had fallen sick of the disease.

"During the illness of Mrs. Barnes, her mother, who was living at Tockwith, a healthy village five miles distant from Moor Monkton, was requested to attend her. She went to Monkton accordingly, remained with her daughter for two days, washed her daughter's linen, and set out on her return home, apparently in good health. Whilst in the act of walking home she was seized with the malady, and fell down in collapse on the road. She was conveyed home to her cottage, and placed by the side of her bedridden husband. He, and also the daughter who resided with them, took the malady. All the three died within two days. Only one other case occurred in the village of Tockwith, and it was not a fatal case." . . .

"A man came from Hull (where cholera was prevailing), by trade a painter; his name and age are unknown. He lodged at the house of Samuel Wride, at Pocklington; was attacked on his arrival on the 8th of September, and died on the 9th. Samuel Wride himself was attacked on the 11th of September, and died shortly afterwards. . . ."

It would be easy, by going through the medical journals and works which have been published on cholera, to quote as many cases similar to the above as would fill a large volume. But the above instances are quite sufficient to show that cholera can be communicated from the sick to the healthy; for it is quite impossible that even a tenth part of these cases of consecutive illness could have followed each other by mere coincidence, without being connected as cause and effect.

Besides the facts above mentioned, which prove that cholera is communicated from person to person, there are others which show, first, that being present in the same room with a patient, and attending on him, do not necessarily expose a person to the morbid poison; and, secondly, that it is not always requisite that a person should be very near a cholera patient in order to take the disease, as the morbid matter producing it may be transmitted to a distance. It used to be generally assumed, that if cholera were a catching or communicable disease, it must spread by effluvia given off from the patient into the surrounding air, and in-

haled by others into the lungs. This assumption led to very conflicting opinions respecting the disease. A little reflection shews, however, that we have no right thus to limit the way in which a disease may be propagated, for the communicable diseases of which we have a correct knowledge spread in very different manners. The itch, and certain other diseases of the skin, are propagated in one way; syphilis, in another way; and intestinal worms in a third way, quite distinct from either of the others.

A consideration of the pathology of cholera is capable of indicating to us the manner in which the disease is communicated. If it were ushered in by fever, or any other general constitutional disorder, then we should be furnished with no clue to the way in which the morbid poison enters the system; whether, for instance, by the alimentary canal, by the lungs, or in some other manner, but should be left to determine this point by circumstances unconnected with the pathology of the disease. But from all that I have been able to learn of cholera, both from my own observations and the descriptions of others, I conclude that cholera invariably commences with the affection of the alimentary canal. The disease often proceeds with so little feeling of general illness, that the patient does not consider himself in danger, or even apply for advice, till the malady is far advanced. In a few cases, indeed, there are dizziness, faintness, and a feeling of sinking, before discharges from the stomach or bowels actually take place; but there can be no doubt that these symptoms depend on the exudation from the mucous membrane, which is soon afterwards copiously evacuated. This is only what occurs in certain cases of hæmorrhage into the alimentary canal, where all the symptoms of loss of blood are present before that fluid shows itself in the evacuations. In those rare cases, called "cholera sicca," in which no purging takes place, the intestines have been found distended with the excretion peculiar to the disease, whenever an examination of the body has taken place after death. In all the cases of cholera that I have attended, the loss of fluid from the stomach and bowels has been sufficient to account for the collapse, when the previous condition of the patient was taken into account, together with the suddenness of the loss, and the circumstance that the process of absorption appears to be suspended. . . .

Diseases which are communicated from person to person are caused by some material which passes from the sick to the healthy, and which has the property of increasing and multiplying in the systems of the persons it attacks. In syphilis, small-pox, and vaccinia, we have physical proof of the increase of the morbid material, and in other communicable diseases the evidence of this increase, derived from the fact of their extension, is equally conclusive. As cholera commences with an affection of the alimentary canal, and as we have seen that the blood is not under the influence of any poison in the early stages of this disease,[1] it follows that the morbid material producing cholera must be introduced into the alimentary canal—must, in fact, be swallowed accidentally, for persons would not take it intentionally; and the increase of the morbid material, or cholera poison, must take place in the interior of the stomach and bowels. It would seem that the cholera poison, when reproduced in sufficient quantity, acts as an irritant on the surface of the stomach and intestines, or, what is still more probable, it withdraws fluid from the blood circulating in the capillaries, by a power analogous to that by which the epithelial cells of the various organs abstract the different secretions in the healthy body. For the morbid matter of cholera having the property of reproducing its own kind, must necessarily have some sort of structure, most likely that of a cell. It is no objection to this view that the structure of the cholera poison cannot be recognised by the microscope, for the matter of smallpox and of chancre can only be recognised by their effects, and not by their physical properties.

The period which intervenes between the time when a morbid poison enters the system, and the commencement of the illness which follows, is called the period of incubation. It is, in reality, a period of reproduction, as regards the morbid matter; and the disease is due to the crop or progeny resulting from the small quantity of poison first introduced. In cholera, this period of incubation or reproduction is much shorter than in most other epidemic or communicable diseases. From the cases previously detailed, it is shown to be in general only from twenty-four to forty-eight hours. It is owing to this shortness of the period of incubation, and to the quantity of the morbid poison thrown off in the evacuations, that cholera sometimes spreads with a rapidity unknown in other diseases. . . .

The instances in which minute quantities of the ejections and dejections of cholera patients must be swallowed are sufficiently numerous to account for the spread of the disease; and on examination it is found to spread most where the facilities for this mode of communication are greatest. Nothing has been found to favour the extension of cholera more than want of personal cleanliness, whether arising from habit or scarcity of water, although the circumstance till lately remained unexplained. The bed linen nearly always becomes wetted by the cholera evacuations, and as these are devoid of the usual colour and odour, the hands of persons waiting on the patient become soiled without their knowing it; and unless these persons are scrupulously cleanly in their habits, and wash their hands before taking food, they must accidentally swallow some of the excretion, and leave some on the food they handle or prepare, which has to be eaten by the rest of the family, who, amongst the working classes, often have to take their meals in the sick room: hence the thousands of instances in which, amongst this class of the population, a case of cholera in one member of the family is followed by other cases; whilst medical men and others, who merely visit the patients, generally escape. The *post mortem* inspection of the bodies of cholera patients has hardly ever been followed by the disease that I am aware, this being a duty that is necessarily followed by careful washing of the hands; and it is not the habit of medical men to be taking food on such an occasion. On the other hand, the duties performed about the body, such as laying it out, when done by women of the working class, who make the occasion one of eating and drinking, are often followed by an attack of cholera; and persons who merely attend the funeral, and have no connexion with the body, frequently contract the disease, in consequence, apparently, of partaking of food which has been prepared or handled by those having duties about the cholera patient, or his linen and bedding. . . .

The involuntary passage of the evacuations in

---

[1] In the so-called secondary fever there is toxicohemia, arising from suppressed excretion by the kidneys.

most bad cases of cholera, must also aid in spreading the disease. Mr. Baker, of Staines, who attended two hundred and sixty cases of cholera and diarrhœa in 1849, chiefly among the poor, informed me, in a letter with which he favoured me in December of that year, that "when the patients passed their stools involuntarily the disease evidently spread." It is amongst the poor, where a whole family live, sleep, cook, eat, and wash in a single room, that cholera has been found to spread when once introduced, and still more in those places termed common lodging-houses, in which several families were crowded into a single room. It was amongst the vagrant class, who lived in this crowded state, that cholera was most fatal in 1832; but the Act of Parliament for the regulation of common lodging-houses, has caused the disease to be much less fatal amongst these people in the late epidemics. When, on the other hand, cholera is introduced into the better kind of houses, as it often is, by means that will be afterwards pointed out, it hardly ever spreads from one member of the family to another. The constant use of the hand-basin and towel, and the fact of the apartments for cooking and eating being distinct from the sick room, are the cause of this. . . .

The mining population of Great Britain have suffered more from cholera than persons in any other occupation,—a circumstance which I believe can only be explained by the mode of communication of the malady above pointed out. Pitmen are differently situated from every other class of workmen in many important particulars. There are no privies in the coal-pits, or, as I believe, in other mines. The workmen stay so long in the mines that they are obliged to take a supply of food with them, which they eat invariably with unwashed hands, and without knife and fork. The following is a reply which I received from a relative of mine connected with a colliery near Leeds, in answer to an inquiry I made:

"Our colliers descend at five o'clock in the morning, to be ready for work at six, and leave the pit from one to half-past three. The average time spent in the pit is eight to nine hours. The pitmen all take down with them a supply of food, which consists of cake, with the addition, in some cases, of meat; and all have a bottle, containing about a quart of 'drink'. I fear that our colliers are no better than others as regards cleanliness. The pit is one huge privy, and of course the men always take their victuals with unwashed hands."

It is very evident that, when a pitman is attacked with cholera whilst at work, the disease has facilities for spreading among his fellow-labourers such as occur in no other occupation. That the men are occasionally attacked whilst at work I know, from having seen them brought up from some of the coal-pits in Northumberland, in the winter of 1831–2, after having had profuse discharges from the stomach and bowels, and when fast approaching to a state of collapse. . . .

If the cholera had no other means of communication than those which we have been considering, it would be constrained to confine itself chiefly to the crowded dwellings of the poor, and would be continually liable to die out accidentally in a place, for want of the opportunity to reach fresh victims; but there is often a way open for it to extend itself more widely, and to reach the well-to-do classes of the community; I allude to the mixture of the cholera evacuations with the water used for drinking and culinary purposes, either by permeating the ground, and getting into wells, or by running along channels and sewers into the rivers from which entire towns are sometimes supplied with water.

THE ETIOLOGY, CONCEPT, AND PROPHYLAXIS
OF CHILDBED FEVER

Ignaz Semmelweis

AUTOBIOGRAPHICAL INTRODUCTION

Medicine's highest duty is saving threatened human life, and obstetrics is the branch of medicine in which this duty is most obviously fulfilled. Frequently it is necessary to deliver a child in transverse lie. Mother and child will probably die if the birth is left to nature, while the obstetrician's timely helping hand, almost painlessly and taking only a few minutes, can save both.

I was already familiar with this prerogative of obstetrics from the theoretical lectures on the specialty. I found it perfectly confirmed as I had the opportunity to learn the practical aspects of obstetrics in the large Viennese maternity hospital. But unfortunately the number of cases in which the obstetrician achieves such blessings vanishes in comparison with the number of victims to whom his help is of no avail. This dark side of obstetrics is childbed fever. Each year I saw ten or fifteen crises in which the salvation of mother and child could be achieved. I also saw many hundreds of maternity patients treated unsuccessfully for childbed fever. Not only was therapy unsuccessful, the etiology seemed deficient. The accepted etiology of childbed fever, on the basis of which I saw so many hundreds of maternity patients treated unsuccessfully, cannot contain the actual causal factor of the disease.

The large gratis Viennese maternity hospital is divided into two clinics; one is called the first, the other the second. By Imperial Decree of 10 October 1840, Court Commission for Education Decree of 17 October 1840, and Administrative Ordinance of 27 October 1840, all male students were assigned to the first clinic and all female students to the second. Before this time student obstetricians and midwives received training in equal numbers in both clinics.

The admission of maternity patients was regulated as follows: Monday afternoon at four o'clock admissions began in the first clinic and continued until Tuesday afternoon at four. Admissions then began in the second clinic and continued until Wednesday afternoon at four o'clock. At that time admissions were resumed in the first clinic until Thursday afternoon, etc. On Friday afternoon at four o'clock admissions began in the first clinic and continued through forty-eight hours until Sunday afternoon, at which time admissions began again in the second clinic. Admissions alternated between the two clinics through twenty-four hour periods, and only once a week did admissions continue in the first clinic for forty-eight hours. Thus the first clinic admitted patients four days a week, whereas the second clinic admitted for only three days. The first clinic, thereby, had fifty-two more days of admissions [each year] than the second.

From the time the first clinic began training only obstetricians until June 1847, the mortality rate in the first clinic was consistently greater than in the second clinic, where only midwives were trained. Indeed, in the year 1846, the mortality rate in the first clinic was five times as great as in the second, and through a six-year period it was, on the average, three times as great. This is shown in Table 1.

The difference in mortality between the clinics was actually larger than the table suggests, because occasionally, for reasons to be examined later,[1] during times of high mortality all ill maternity patients in the first clinic were transferred to the general hospital. When these patients died, they were included in the mortality figures for the general hospital rather than for the maternity hospital. When the transfers were undertaken, the reports show reduced mortality, since only those who could not

Source: Excerpted from Ignaz Semmelweis, *The Etiology, Concept, and Prophylaxis of Childbed Fever,* trans. K. Codell Carter. Madison, The University of Wisconsin Press, 1983.

We have omitted the bracketed page references to the original German version which appeared in the above-cited source. Ed.

[1]See below, pages 50ff.

Table 1. Annual births, deaths, and mortality rates for all patients at the two clinics of the Vienna maternity hospital from 1841 to 1846.

	First Clinic			Second Clinic		
	Births	Deaths	Rate	Births	Deaths	Rate
1841	3036	237	7.7	2442	86	3.5
1842	3287	518	15.8	2659	202	7.5
1843	3060	274	8.9	2739	164	5.9
1844	3157	260	8.2	2956	68	2.3
1845	3492	241	6.8	3241	66	2.03
1846	4010	459	11.4	3754	105	2.7
Total	20 042	1989		17 791	691	
Avg.			9.92			3.38

be transferred because of the rapid course of their illness were included. In reality, many additional victims should be included. In the second clinic such transfers were never undertaken. Only isolated patients were transferred whose condition might endanger the other patients. . . .

. . . What is the origin, then, of the difference in mortality between the clinics? Hyperinosis [excessive fibrin in the blood], hydremia [excessive water in the blood], plethora [an excessive quantity of blood], disturbances caused by the pregnant uterus, stagnation of the circulation, inopexia [spontaneous coagulation of the blood], delivery itself, decreased weight caused by the emptying of the uterus, protracted labor, wounding of the inner surface of the uterus in delivery, imperfect contractions, faulty involutions of the uterus during maternity, scanty and discontinued secretion and excretion of lochia [a vaginal discharge during the first few weeks after delivery], the weight of secreted milk, death of the fetus, and the individuality of patients are causes to which may be ascribed much or little influence in the generation of childbed fever. But in both clinics these must be equally harmful or harmless and they cannot, therefore, explain the appalling difference in mortality between the clinics.

While I was still unable to find a cause for the increased mortality rate in the first clinic, I became aware of other inexplicable circumstances. Those whose period of dilation was extended over twenty-four hours or more almost invariably became ill either immediately during birth or within the first twenty-four or thirty-six hours after delivery. They died quickly of rapidly developing childbed fever. An equally extended period of dilation in the second clinic did not prove dangerous. Because dilation was usually extended during first deliveries, those delivering for the first time usually died. I often pointed out to my students that because these blossoming, vigorously healthy young women had extended periods of dilation, they would die quickly from puerperal fever either during delivery or immediately thereafter. My prognoses were fulfilled. I did not know why, but I often saw it happen. This circumstance was inexplicable, since it was not repeated in the second clinic. I speak here of the period of dilation, not of delivery; thus the trauma of delivery is not under consideration.

Not only these mothers but also their newborn infants, both male and female, died of childbed fever. I am not alone in speaking of puerperal fever of the newborn.[2] With the exception of the genital areas, the anatomical lesions in the corpses of such newborn infants are the same as the lesions in the corpses of women who die of puerperal fever. To recognize these findings as the consequence of puerperal fever in maternity patients but to deny that identical findings in the corpses of the newborn are the consequence of the same disease is to reject pathological anatomy.

But if the maternity patients and the newborn die from the same disease, then the etiology that accounts for the deaths of the

---

[2] Semmelweis was not alone, but he was in the minority. There was a discussion of infant puerperal fever in French medical literature in 1855. The discussion was reviewed in the *Monatsschrift für Geburtshülfe* 7(1856): 152f., and in the *Wiener medizinische Wochenschrift, Journal Revue*, no. 3 (1856):22f. Carl Braun also mentioned that "the unmistakable influence of puerperal fever epidemics on the mortality of fetuses has been recognized in the Viennese maternity hospital for years"; he then notes that the French refer to such cases as puerperal fever of fetuses. Carl Braun, *Lehrbuch der Geburtshülfe* (Vienna: Braumüller, 1857), pp. 589f.

Table 2. Annual births, deaths, and mortality rates for newborns at the two clinics of the Vienna maternity hospital from 1841 to 1846.

	First Clinic			Second Clinic		
	Births	Deaths	Rate	Births	Deaths	Rate
1841	2813	177	6.2	2252	91	4.04
1842	3037	279	9.1	2414	113	4.06
1843	2828	195	6.8	2570	130	5.05
1844	2917	251	8.6	2739	100	3.06
1845	3201	260	8.1	3017	97	3.02
1846	3533	235	6.5	3398	86	2.05

mothers must also account for the deaths of the newborn. Since the difference in mortality between the maternity patients in the two clinics was reflected in the mortality rates for the newborn, the accepted etiology for childbed fever no more accounts for the deaths of the newborn than for the deaths of the maternity patients. Table 2 gives the mortality rates of the newborn at the two clinics.

Because their mothers died or were otherwise unable to nurse, many of the newborn were sent directly to the foundling home. Later we will consider their fate.[3]

The occurrence of childbed fever among the newborn can be explained in two ways. Childbed fever may be caused by factors operating on the mother during the intrauterine life of the fetus, and the mother can then impart the disease to the infant. Alternatively, the causes may affect the infant itself after birth, in which case the mother may or may not be affected. Thus the infant dies, not because the disease has been imparted, as in the first case, but rather because childbed fever originates in the infant itself. If the mother imparts childbed fever to the infant during intrauterine life, then the difference in infant mortality between the two clinics cannot be explained by the accepted etiology, because this etiology inadequately explains the origin of the disease in mothers. If the cause of childbed fever operates directly on the infant independently of the mother, then it is still impossible for the accepted etiology to explain the difference in infant mortality rates. [Given the accepted theories], one would expect the mortality in the second clinic to have been either equal to or greater than that of the first. Of course, many of the causal factors that purportedly explain childbed fever among maternity patients are simply impossible with regard to infants—infants would not, in all probability, fear the evil reputation of the first clinic, their modesty would not be offended by having been delivered in the presence of men, etc.

Childbed fever is defined as a disease characteristic of and limited to maternity patients, for whose origin the puerperal state and a specific causal moment are necessary.[4] Thus when this cause operates on a person who is predisposed by the puerperal state, childbed fever results. However, if this same cause operates on persons who are not puerperae, some disease other than puerperal fever is generated. For example, some believe that maternity patients in the first clinic, knowing of the countless deaths occurring there each year, are so frightened that they contract the disease. Thus the disposing factor is the puerperal state, and the precipitating factor is fear of death. We can assume that many soldiers engaged in murderous battle must also fear death. However, these soldiers do not contract childbed fever, because they are not puerperae and so they lack the disposing factor.

If an individual is openly examined for the instruction of males, her modesty is offended and, because she is predisposed by the puerperal state, she contracts childbed fever. But female modesty can be offended in many ways, and if the offended young woman is not in the puerperal state, she does not contract childbed fever because she is not predisposed. Something else occurs; for example, she may swoon. Chilling brings childbed fever in puerperae, but in

---

[3] See below, pages 57ff.

[4] Among Semmelweis's contemporaries the causal explanation of a specific instance of some disease was usually divided into predisposing and exciting factors. Different diseases were believed to result from the operation of a constant, exciting cause if the persons on whom that cause operated had been differently predisposed. In this and the following two paragraphs Semmelweis is subjecting this doctrine to ironic criticism.

other persons it causes rheumatic fever. In puerperae, mistakes in diet induce childbed fever. In others, similar mistakes cause only gastric fever.

Becoming convinced that childbed fever is not restricted to puerperae and that it can begin during birth or even in pregnancy, one may ignore the puerperal state and focus on the unique composition of the blood during pregnancy. But even if we adopt such an approach, what predisposes the newborn to puerperal disease? Surely not the puerperal condition of their genitals. Do both male and female have the blood composition uniquely characteristic of pregnancy? The occurrence of childbed fever among the newborn shows that the very conception of puerperal fever is erroneous.

Because Vienna is so large, women in labor often deliver on the street, on the glacis,[5] or in front of the gates of houses before they can reach the hospital. It is then necessary for the woman, carrying her infant in her skirts, and often in very bad weather, to walk to the maternity hospital. Such births are referred to as street births. Admission to the maternity clinic and to the foundling home is gratis, on the condition that those admitted be available for open instructional purposes, and that those fit to do so serve as wet nurses for the foundling home. Infants not born in the maternity clinic are not admitted gratis to the foundling home because their mothers have not been available for instruction. However, in order that those who had the intention of delivering in the maternity hospital but who delivered on the way would not innocently lose their privilege, street births were counted as hospital deliveries. This, however, led to the following abuse: women in somewhat better circumstances, seeking to avoid the unpleasantness of open examination without losing the benefit of having their infants accepted gratis to the foundling home, would be delivered by midwives in the city and then be taken quickly by coach to the clinic where they claimed that the birth had occurred unexpectedly while they were on their way to the clinic. If the child had not been christened

and if the umbilical cord was still fresh, these cases were treated as street births, and the mother received charity exactly like those who delivered at the hospital. The number of these cases was high; frequently in a single month between the two clinics there were as many as one hundred cases.

As I have noted, women who delivered on the street contracted childbed fever at a significantly lower rate than those who delivered in the hospital. This was in spite of the less favorable conditions in which such births took place. Of course, in most of these cases delivery occurred in a bed with the assistance of a midwife. Moreover, after three hours our patients were obliged to walk to their beds by way of the glass-enclosed passageway. However, such inconvenience is certainly less dangerous than being delivered by a midwife, then immediately having to arise, walk down many flights of stairs to the waiting carriage, travel in all weather conditions and over horribly rough pavement to the maternity hospital, and there having to climb up another flight of stairs. For those who really gave birth on the street, the conditions would have been even more difficult.

To me, it appeared logical that patients who experienced street births would become ill at least as frequently as those who delivered in the clinic. I have already expressed my firm conviction that the deaths in the first clinic were not caused by epidemic influences but by endemic and as yet unknown factors, that is, factors whose harmful influences were limited to the first clinic. What protected those who delivered outside the clinic from these destructive unknown endemic influences? In the second clinic, the health of the patients who underwent street births was as good as in the first clinic, but there the difference was not so striking, since the health of the patients was generally much better.

This would be the place to exhibit a table showing that the mortality rate among those who delivered on the street was lower than among those who delivered in the first clinic. While I had access to the records of the first clinic I felt that such a table was unnecessary because no one denied these facts. Thus I neglected to complete a table. Later when I was no longer assistant, these facts were denied, as was the existence of a significant difference in mortality between the clinics. Because of Table 1,

---

[5] While Semmelweis was in the first clinic, Vienna was still surrounded by medieval fortifications. The glacis was a broad earthwork that sloped away from the city and that constituted part of the fortifications. Between 1857 and 1865 the city walls were demolished and were replaced by gardens, boulevards, and public buildings.

however, this difference is undeniable. In 1848 Professor [Josef] Skoda[6] proposed that the faculty of the Viennese medical school nominate a commission that, among other things, would construct such a table. The proposal was adopted by a great majority, and the commission was immediately named. However, as a result of protests by the Professor of Obstetrics, higher authorities intervened and the commission was unable to begin its activity.[7]

In addition to those who delivered on the street, those who delivered prematurely also became ill much less frequently than ordinary patients. Those who delivered prematurely were not only exposed to all the same endemic influences as patients who went full-term, they also suffered the additional harm of whatever caused the premature delivery. Under these circumstances, how could their superior health be explained? One explanation was that the earlier the birth, the less developed the puerperal condition and therefore the smaller the predisposition for the disease. Yet puerperal fever can begin during birth or even during pregnancy; indeed, even at these times it can be fatal. The better health of patients who delivered prematurely in the second clinic conformed to the general superior health of full-term patients in the clinic.

Patients often became ill sporadically. One diseased patient would be surrounded by healthy patients. But very often whole rows would become ill without a single patient in the row remaining healthy. The beds in the maternity wards were arranged along the length of the rooms and were separated by equal spaces.

---

[6] Josef Skoda (1805–81) was head of the department for thoracic diseases, and from 1846 until 1871 he was Professor of Medicine at the University of Vienna. Skoda pioneered auscultation and repercussion as diagnostic techniques, and popularized the use of the stethoscope. He supported Semmelweis at the beginning, but seems never to have accepted Semmelweis's strategy of characterizing diseases etiologically. After Semmelweis left Vienna for Budapest in 1850, Skoda apparently never again mentioned Semmelweis or his works—not even in lectures on puerperal diseases.

[7] The Professor of Obstetrics was Johann Klein. The proposal was, in fact, adopted unanimously, which means that even Klein approved of having a commission investigate Semmelweis's findings. But when the commission was named, Klein was not included. Thus, he would not have been a member of the commission that was to investigate work done in his own clinic. This may have led him to protest to the ministry. Erna Lesky, *Ignaz Philipp Semmelweis und die Wiener medizinische Schule* (Vienna: Hermann Böhlaus, 1964), pp. 11–35.

Depending on their location, rooms in the clinic extended either north-south or east-west. If patients in beds along the north walls became ill we were often inclined to regard chilling as a significant factor. However, on the next occasion those along the south wall would become ill. Many times those on the east and west walls would become diseased. Often the disease spread from one side to the other, so that no one location seemed better or worse. How could these events be explained, given that the same patterns did not appear in the second clinic where one encountered the disease only sporadically?

It was my firm conviction that childbed fever was not contagious and did not spread from bed to bed. Later we will consider the proof for this conviction. For now, it is sufficient to note that the disease appeared only sporadically in the second clinic. If childbed fever were contagious, from the sporadic cases whole rows would become ill as the disease spread from bed to bed.

The authorities did not remain indifferent to the disturbing difference in mortality rates between the two clinics. Commissions repeatedly investigated and conducted hearings to determine the cause of the difference, and to decide whether it was possible to save a larger number of those patients who became ill. To achieve this last goal, from time to time all the diseased patients were transferred to the general hospital. But in spite of the change in physicians, rooms, and medical procedures, etc., the patients died almost without exception. The commissions would conclude that the cause of the great mortality rate was one or another or several of the endemic factors previously discussed. Various suitable measures were adopted, but none succeeded in bringing the death rate within the limits set by the second clinic. The failure of these measures proved that the factors identified were not, in fact, the relevant causes.

Toward the end of 1846 an opinion prevailed in one commission that the disease originated from damage to the birth canal inflicted during the examinations that were part of the instructional process. However, since similar examinations were part of the instruction of midwives, the increased incidence of disease in the clinic for physicians was made intelligible by assuming that male students, particularly foreigners, were too rough in their examinations. As a result of this opinion the number of students was reduced from forty-two to twenty. Foreigners were almost entirely excluded, and examinations were reduced to a minimum. The mortality rate did decline significantly in December 1846, and in January, February, and March of 1847. But in spite of these measures, fifty-seven patients died in April and thirty-six more in May. This demonstrated to everyone that the view was groundless. To further the reader's understanding, Table 3 shows the mortality figures for 1846 and for the first five months of 1847. We will come back later to the fact that from December 1846 through March 1847 the mortality rate declined, and that it climbed back up again in April and May 1847.[8]

Recommendations based on studies of the cause of the great mortality in the first clinic all involved one inexplicable contradiction: given the concept of an epidemic, and given that the commissions did not have the power to change the atmospheric-cosmic-terrestrial conditions of Vienna, they should have concluded that no remedies were possible. But they did not draw this conclusion, even though they considered the deaths an epidemic. What does one do to shorten the duration or to prevent the recurrence of a cholera epidemic? They attributed the disease to one or more of the previously identified endemic causes. They did not, however, identify it as an endemic disease, which would have been appropriate, but rather as an epidemic. In general, the unfortunate confusion in the concepts of epidemic and endemic disease delayed discovery of the true cause of childbed fever.

In classifying puerperal disease as epidemic or endemic, one must disregard entirely the number of patients who become ill or die. The cause of the illness or death determines whether the disease is epidemic or endemic. Epidemic puerperal fever is induced by atmospheric-cosmic-terrestrial influences; the concept of an epidemic does not stipulate whether one or one hundred persons become ill. If puerperal fever is caused by endemic factors— that is, by factors whose operation is limited to a specific location—then puerperal fever is endemic, and it is immaterial whether one or one hundred individuals become ill. This follows

Table 3. Monthly births, deaths, and mortality rates for all patients at the first clinic of the Vienna maternity hospital from January 1846 to May 1847.

	Births	Deaths	Rate
1846			
Jan.	336	45	13.39
Feb.	293	53	18.08
Mar.	311	48	15.43
Apr.	253	48	18.97
May	305	41	13.44
Jun.	266	27	10.15
Jul.	252	33	13.10
Aug.	216	39	18.05
Sept.	271	39	14.39
Oct.	254	38	14.98
Nov.	297	32	10.77
Dec.	298	16	5.37
1847			
Jan.	311	10	3.21
Feb.	912	6	1.92
Mar.	305	11	3.60
Apr.	312	57	18.27
May	294	36	12.24

from the concepts of epidemic and endemic disease. In classifying the disease one way or the other, however, the commissions did not consider the purported cause but only the number of cases. Because many patients became ill and died, it was identified as an epidemic.

I was convinced that the greater mortality rate at the first clinic was due to an endemic but as yet unknown cause. That the newborn, whether female or male, also contracted childbed fever convinced me that the disease was misconceived. I was aware of many facts for which I had no explanation. Delivery with prolonged dilation almost inevitably led to death. Patients who delivered prematurely or on the street almost never became ill, and this contradicted my conviction that the deaths were due to endemic causes. The disease appeared sequentially among patients in the first clinic. Patients in the second clinic were healthier, although individuals working there were no more skillful or conscientious in their duties. The disrespect displayed by the employees toward the personnel of the first clinic made me so miserable that life seemed worthless. Everything was in question; everything seemed inexplicable; everything was doubtful. Only the large number of deaths was an unquestionable reality.

[8] See below, pages 58 and 59.

The reader can appreciate my perplexity during my first period of service when I, like a drowning person grasping at a straw, discontinued supine deliveries, which had been customary in the first clinic, in favor of deliveries from a lateral position. I did this for no other reason than that the latter were customary in the second clinic. I did not believe that the supine position was so detrimental that additional deaths could be attributed to its use. But in the second clinic deliveries were performed from a lateral position and the patients were healthier. Consequently, we also delivered from the lateral position, so that everything would be exactly as in the second clinic.

I spent the winter of 1846–47 studying English. I did this because my predecessor, Dr. Breit, resumed the position of assistant, and I wanted to spend time in the large Dublin maternity hospital. Then, at the end of February 1847, Dr. Breit was named Professor of Obstetrics at the medical school in Tübingen. I changed my travel plans and, in the company of two friends, departed for Venice on 2 March 1847. I hoped that Venetian art treasures would revive my mind and spirits, which had been so seriously affected by my experiences in the maternity hospital.

On 20 March of the same year, a few hours after returning to Vienna, I resumed, with rejuvenated vigor, the position of assistant in the first clinic. I was immediately overwhelmed by the sad news that Professor [Jakob] Kolletschka, whom I greatly admired, had died in the interim.

The case history went as follows: Kolletschka, Professor of Forensic Medicine, often conducted autopsies for legal purposes in the company of students. During one such exercise, his finger was pricked by a student with the same knife that was being used in the autopsy. I do not recall which finger was cut. Professor Kolletschka contracted lymphangitis and phlebitis [inflammation of the lymphatic vessels and of the veins respectively] in the upper extremity. Then, while I was still in Venice, he died of bilateral pleurisy, pericarditis, peritonitis, and meningitis [inflammation of the membranes of the lungs and thoracic cavity, of the fibroserous sac surrounding the heart, of the membranes of the abdomen and pelvic cavity, and of the membranes surrounding the brain, respectively]. A few days before he died, a metastasis also formed in one eye. I was still animated by the art treasures of Venice, but the news of Kolletschka's death agitated me still more. In this excited condition I could see clearly that the disease from which Kolletschka died was identical to that from which so many hundred maternity patients had also died. The maternity patients also had lymphangitis, peritonitis, pericarditis, pleurisy, and meningitis, and metastases also formed in many of them. Day and night I was haunted by the image of Kolletschka's disease and was forced to recognize, ever more decisively, that the disease from which Kolletschka died was identical to that from which so many maternity patients died.

Earlier, I pointed out that autopsies of the newborn disclosed results identical to those obtained in autopsies of patients dying from childbed fever. I concluded that the newborn died of childbed fever, or in other words, that they died from the same disease as the maternity patients. Since the identical results were found in Kolletschka's autopsy, the inference that Kolletschka died from the same disease was confirmed. The exciting cause of Professor Kolletschka's death was known; it was the wound by the autopsy knife that had been contaminated by cadaverous particles. Not the wound, but contamination of the wound by the cadaverous particles caused his death. Kolletschka was not the first to have died in this way. I was forced to admit that if his disease was identical with the disease that killed so many maternity patients, then it must have originated from the same cause that brought it on in Kolletschka. In Kolletschka, the specific causal factor was the cadaverous particles that were introduced into his vascular system. I was compelled to ask whether cadaverous particles had been introduced into the vascular systems of those patients whom I had seen die of this identical disease. I was forced to answer affirmatively.

Because of the anatomical orientation of the Viennese medical school, professors, assistants, and students have frequent opportunity to contact cadavers. Ordinary washing with soap is not sufficient to remove all adhering cadaverous particles. This is proven by the cadaverous smell that the hands retain for a longer or shorter time. In the examination of pregnant or delivering maternity patients, the hands, contaminated with cadaverous particles, are brought into contact with the genitals of these individuals, creating the possibility of resorption. With resorption, the cadaverous particles are introduced into the vascular system of the patient. In this way, maternity patients contract the same disease that was found in Kolletschka.

Suppose cadaverous particles adhering to hands cause the same disease among maternity patients that cadaverous particles adhering to the knife caused in Kolletschka. Then if those particles are destroyed chemically, so that in examinations patients are touched by fingers but not by cadaverous particles, the disease must be reduced. This seemed all the more likely, since I knew that when decomposing organic material is brought into contact with living organisms it may bring on decomposition.

To destroy cadaverous matter adhering to hands I used *chlorina liquida*. This practice began in the middle of May 1847; I no longer remember the specific day. Both the students and I were required to wash before examinations. After a time I ceased to use *chlorina liquida* because of its high price, and I adopted the less expensive chlorinated lime. In May 1847, during the second half of which chlorine washings were first introduced, 36 patients died—this was 12.24 percent of 294 deliveries. In the remaining seven months of 1847, the mortality rate was below that of the patients in the second clinic (see Table 4).

In these seven months, of the 1841 maternity patients cared for, 56 died (3.04 percent). In 1846, before washing with chlorine was introduced, of 4010 patients cared for in the first clinic, 459 died (11.4 percent). In the second clinic in 1846, of 3754 patients, 105 died (2.7 percent). In 1847, when in approximately the middle of May I instituted washing with chlorine, in the first clinic of 3490 patients, 176 died (5 percent). In the second clinic of 3306 patients, 32 died (0.9 percent). In 1848, chlorine washings were employed throughout the year and of 3556 patients, 45 died (1.27 percent). In the second clinic in the year 1848, of 3219 patients 43 died (1.33 percent). The mortality rates for the individual months of 1848 are shown in Table 5.

In March and August 1848 not a single patient died. In January 1849, of 403 births 9 died (2.23 percent). In February, of 389 births 12 died (3.08 percent). March had 406 births, and there were 20 deaths (4.9 percent). On 20 March Dr. Carl Braun[9] succeeded me as assistant.

As mentioned, the commissions identified various endemic factors as causes of the greater mortality rate in the first clinic. Accordingly, various measures were instituted, but none brought the mortality rate within that of the second clinic. Thus one could infer that the

Table 4. Monthly births, deaths, and mortality rates for all patients at the first clinic of the Vienna maternity hospital from June to December 1847.

	Births	Deaths	Rate
1847			
Jun.	268	6	2.38
Jul.	250	3	1.20
Aug.	264	5	1.89
Sept.	262	12	5.23
Oct.	278	11	3.95
Nov.	246	11	4.47
Dec.	273	8	2.93
Total	1841	56	3.04

Table 5. Monthly births, deaths, and mortality rates for all patients at the second clinic of the Vienna maternity hospital from January to December 1848.

	Births	Deaths	Rate
1848			
Jan.	283	10	3.53
Feb.	291	2	0.68
Mar.	276	0	0.00
Apr.	305	2	0.65
May	313	3	0.99
Jun.	264	3	1.13
Jul.	269	1	0.37
Aug.	261	0	0.00
Sept.	312	3	0.96
Oct.	299	7	2.34
Nov.	310	9	2.90
Dec.	373	5	1.34
Total	3556	45	
Avg.			1.27

[9] Carl Braun (1822–91) was Klein's assistant from 1849 until 1853. He succeeded Klein as Professor of Obstetrics at the University of Vienna and became Rector of the University. Braun was consistently hostile to Semmelweis; he was not conscientious in using the prophylactic measures necessary to prevent childbed fever, and he did not accept Semmelweis's etiological characterization of the disease.

factors identified by the commissions were not causally responsible for the greater mortality in the first clinic. I assumed that the cause of the greater mortality rate was cadaverous particles adhering to the hands of examining obstetricians. I removed this cause by chlorine washings. Consequently, mortality in the first clinic fell below that of the second. I therefore concluded that cadaverous matter adhering to the hands of the physicians was, in reality, the cause of the increased mortality rate in the first clinic. Since the chlorine washings were instituted with such dramatic success, not even the smallest additional changes in the procedures of the first clinic were adopted to which the decline in mortality could be even partially attributed. The instruction system for midwives is so instituted that pupils and instructors have less frequent occasion to contaminate their hands with cadaverous matter than is the case in the first clinic. Thus, the unknown endemic cause of the horrible devastations in the first clinic was the cadaverous particles adhering to the hands of the examiners.

In order to destroy the cadaverous material, it was necessary that every examiner wash in chlorinated lime upon entry into the labor room. Because students in the labor room had no opportunity to contaminate their hands anew, I believed one washing was sufficient. Because of the large number who gave birth each year in the first clinic, patients were seldom alone in the labor room; as a rule several were there simultaneously. For purposes of instruction, those in labor were arranged and examined sequentially. I regarded it as sufficient that after each examination the hands were washed with soap and water only. Within the labor room, it seemed unnecessary for the hands to be washed with chlorine water between examinations. Once the hands had been cleaned of cadaverous particles, they could not become contaminated again.

In October 1847, a patient was admitted with discharging medullary carcinoma [cancer of the innermost part] of the uterus. She was assigned the bed at which the rounds were always initiated. After examining this patient, those conducting the examination washed their hands with soap only. The consequence was that of twelve patients then delivering, eleven died. The ichor from the discharging medullary carcinoma was not destroyed by soap and water. In

the examinations, ichor was transferred to the remaining patients, and so childbed fever multiplied. Thus, childbed fever is caused not only by cadaverous particles adhering to hands but also by ichor from living organisms. It is necessary to clean the hands with chlorine water, not only when one has been handling cadavers but also after examinations in which the hands could become contaminated with ichor. This rule, originating from this tragic experience, was followed thereafter. Childbed fever was no longer spread by ichor carried on the hands of examiners from one patient to another.

A new tragic experience persuaded me that air could also carry decaying organic matter. In November of the same year, an individual was admitted with a discharging carious left knee. In the genital region this person was completely healthy. Thus the examiners' hands presented no danger to the other patients. But the ichorous exhalations of the carious knee completely saturated the air of her ward. In this way the other patients were exposed and nearly all the patients in that room died. The reports of the first clinic indicate that eleven patients died in November and eight more in December. These deaths were largely due to ichorous exhalations from this individual. The ichorous particles that saturated the air of the maternity ward penetrated the uteruses already lacerated in the birth process. The particles were resorbed, and childbed fever resulted. Thereafter, such individuals were isolated to prevent similar tragedies.

The maternity hospital in Vienna was opened on 16 August 1784. In the eighteenth century and in the early decades of the nineteenth century, medicine was concerned with theoretical speculation, and the anatomical foundations were neglected. Thus in 1822, of 3066 patients only 26 died (.84 percent). In 1841, after the Viennese medical school adopted an anatomical orientation, of 3036 patients 237 died (7.7 percent). In 1843 of 3060 patients 274 died (8.9 percent). In 1827, of 3294 patients 55 died (1.66 percent). In 1842 of 3287 patients 518 died (15.8 percent).[10] From 1784 until 1823, over a period of twenty-five years, less than 1 percent of the patients cared for in the maternity hospital died. This is shown in Table 6.

---

[10] The figures for 1841, 1842, and 1843 are for the first clinic only, see Table 1.

Table 6. Annual births, deaths, and mortality rate for all patients at the Vienna maternity hospital from 1784 to 1848.

Year	Births	Deaths	Rate	Year	Births	Deaths	Rate
1784	284	6	2.11	1817	2735	25	0.91
1785	899	13	1.44	1818	2568	56	2.18
1786	1151	5	0.43	1819	3089	154	4.98
1787	1407	5	0.35	1820	2998	75	2.50
1788	1425	5	0.35	1821	3294	55	1.66
1789	1246	7	0.56	1822	3066	26	0.84
1790	1326	10	0.75	1823	2872	214	7.45
1791	1395	8	0.57	1824	2911	144	4.94
1792	1574	14	0.89	1825	2594	229	4.82
1793	1684	44	2.61	1826	2359	192	8.12
1794	1768	7	0.39	1827	2367	51	2.15
1795	1798	38	2.11	1828	2833	101	3.56
1796	1904	22	1.16	1829	3012	140	4.64
1797	2012	5	0.24	1830	2797	111	3.97
1798	2046	5	0.24	1831	3353	222	6.62
1799	2067	20	0.96	1832	3331	105	3.15
1800	2070	41	1.98	1833	3907	205	5.25
1801	2106	17	0.80	1834	4218	355	8.41
1802	2346	9	0.38	1835	4040	227	5.61
1803	2215	16	0.72	1836	4144	331	7.98
1804	2022	8	0.39	1837	4363	375	8.59
1805	2112	9	0.40	1838	4560	179	3.92
1806	1875	13	0.73	1839	4992	248	4.96
1807	925	6	0.64	1840	5166	328	6.44
1808	855	7	0.81	1841	5454	330	6.05
1809	912	13	1.42	1842	6024	730	12.11
1810	744	6	0.80	1843	5914	457	7.72
1812	1419	9	0.63	1844	6244	336	5.38
1811	1050	20	1.90	1845	6756	313	4.63
1813	1945	21	1.08	1846	7027	567	8.06
1814	2062	66	3.20	1847	7039	210	2.98
1815	2591	19	0.73	1848	7095	91	1.28
1816	2410	12	0.49				

This table provides unchallengeable proof for my opinion that childbed fever originates with the spread of animal-organic matter. At the time when the educational system limited opportunities for spreading decaying animal-organic matter, the patients cared for in the maternity hospital were much healthier.

As the Viennese medical school adopted an anatomical orientation, the health of the maternity patients worsened. When the number of births and of students became so great that one professor could not supervise the births and give instruction, the maternity hospital was divided into two clinics. At that time the same number of male and female students were assigned to each clinic. On 10 October 1840, by imperial decree, all males were assigned to the first clinic and all female students to the second. I am not able to say in which year the maternity hospital was divided. Colleagues who taught obstetrics in the second clinic when male students were still admitted report that there was, at that time, no significant difference in mortality between the clinics. The consistently unfavorable health of patients in the first clinic dates from 1840, when all male students were assigned to the first clinic and all female students to the second. After what has been reported, it would be superfluous to explain these facts further.

Table 1 indicates the difference in mortality rates between the patients of the two clinics after the first was devoted exclusively to training obstetricians and the second to training midwives. This would be the place to provide a similar table for the years during which female and male students were divided equally between both clinics. It would show that during this time the mortality rate was not consistently larger in the first clinic. However, I do not have

Table 7. **Annual births, deaths, and mortality rates for all patients at the two clinics of the Vienna maternity hospital for 1839 and 1840.**

	First Clinic			Second Clinic		
	Births	Deaths	Rate	Births	Deaths	Rate
1839	2781	151	5.4	2010	91	4.5
1840	2889	267	9.5	2073	55	2.6

access to the necessary data. The reports were prepared in triplicate in both clinics. One copy remained in the institution; one copy was sent to the governmental administration. Those who now have these reports would do a service to science if they would release them to the public.[11] I possess the reports of both clinics only for 1840, when the male and female students were separated, and for the preceding year (see Table 7). The variation in mortality for both clinics can be traced to the activities of those in the process of becoming physicians. I was obstructed in disclosing this information because at the time it was construed as a basis for personal denunciation.

Professor Skoda assigned various responsibilities to the above mentioned commission of the Viennese medical college. Among these were the construction of a table showing, as far as the data was available, the number of deliveries and of deaths month by month, and a list of the assistants and students in the sequential order in which they served and practiced in the maternity hospital. Professor [Karl] Rokitansky[12] has directed the pathological-anatomical division since 1828. From his recollections, and from autopsy reports, and with the help of other physicians and of the assistants and students who participated in the examination of corpses, it would be possible to determine whether the number of diseased patients corresponded to

the activities of assistants and students in the autopsy room. As mentioned above, higher authorities prevented the commission from carrying out this assignment.

In consequence of my conviction I must affirm that only God knows the number of patients who went prematurely to their graves because of me. I have examined corpses to an extent equaled by few other obstetricians. If I say this also of another physician, my intention is only to bring to consciousness a truth that, to humanity's great misfortune, has remained unknown through so many centuries. No matter how painful and oppressive such a recognition may be, the remedy does not lie in suppression. If the misfortune is not to persist forever, then this truth must be made known to everyone concerned.

After it was realized that the additional deaths in the first clinic were explained by cadaverous and ichorous particles on the examiners' contaminated hands, various unexplained phenomena could be accounted for quite naturally. In the morning hours the professor and the students made general rounds; in the afternoons the assistant and the students made rounds. As part of their instruction, the students examined all patients who were pregnant or in labor. The assistant was also obliged, before the morning visit of the professor, to examine those in labor and to report on them to the professor. Between these visits the assistant and the students would assume responsibility for necessary examinations. When, therefore, dilation extended over a long period and the patient spent one or more days in the labor room, she was certain to be examined repeatedly by persons whose hands were contaminated with cadaverous and ichorous particles. In this way childbed fever was induced, and as I have mentioned, these individuals died almost without exception. Once the chlorine washings were adopted and the patients were examined only by persons with clean hands, patients with

---

[11] On page 139, German edition, . . . Semmelweis reports that he has just obtained this information and proceeds to give the table that he here omits. He refers back to this page and apologizes for not including the information where it was first needed. The figures for 1839 and 1840 were made public in Carl Haller's report on the operation of the Vienna General Hospital published in the *Zeitschrift der k. k. Gesellschaft der Ärzte zu Wien*, 5, no. 2 (1849): 535–46.

[12] Karl Rokitansky (1804–1878) was Professor of Pathological Anatomy at the University of Vienna from 1844 until 1875 and was Rector of the University in 1853. He was one of the outstanding anatomists of the century—he is said to have performed more than 30 000 autopsies. Rokitansky also supported Semmelweis against the older members of the faculty until Semmelweis left Vienna in 1850.

extended periods of dilation stopped dying, and extended labor was no more dangerous than in the second clinic.

In order to make my next point intelligible, I must partially explain how I conceive of childbed fever. For now it is sufficient to observe that foul animal-organic particles are resorbed, and that in consequence of this resorption, disintegration of the blood [*Blutentmischung*] sets in. We have already noted that those with extended periods of dilation contracted rapidly developing childbed fever either during birth or directly thereafter. In other words, the resorption of foul animal-organic particles and the resulting disintegration of the mother's blood occurred at a time when the fetal blood was in organic exchange through the placenta with the blood of the mother. In this way, blood disintegration, from which the mother was suffering, was transmitted to the child. In consequence the newborn, whether female or male, died from a disease identical to that of the mother and in numbers equal to the mothers. Childbed fever originates in the mother because foul animal-organic matter is resorbed and leads to blood disintegration. In the infant the situation is somewhat different. The fetus, as yet unborn and in the birth canal, does not resorb foul animal-organic matter when it is touched by the examiner's contaminated fingers, but only when its blood is organically mixed with the mother's blood that has already become contaminated. This explains why an infant never dies of childbed fever while the mother remains healthy; childbed fever does not arise in the newborn through direct resorption. Both become ill while the child and mother are in organic interchange through the placenta and when the blood of the mother has disintegrated through the resorption of foul animal-organic matter. The mother can become ill while the child remains healthy if the organic interchange between them is ended by the birth process before disintegration of the mother's blood has begun.

As I have said, cadaverous particles adhering to the hands were destroyed by chlorine washings. In this way, the incidence of disease among maternity patients was brought within the limits set in the second clinic. Chlorine washings had the same effect on the incidence of disease among the newborn. Healthy mothers could no longer impart childbed fever to their infants.

In 1846, without chlorine washing, of 3533 infants in the first clinic, 235 died (6 percent). In the second clinic, of 3398 infants 86 died (2.5 percent). In 1847, during the last seven months of which we washed with chlorine, of 3322 infants 167 died (5.02 percent). In the second clinic, of 3139 infants 90 died (2.8 percent). In 1848, when chlorine washings were practiced during the entire year, of 3496 infants 147 died in the first clinic (4.2 percent). In the second clinic 100 infants died, out of 3089 (3.2 percent). These infant deaths were not from childbed fever.

If a mother died before her child, or if a mother, for whatever reason, could not nurse her child, the child was taken to the foundling home. In the foundling home, many nursing infants died of childbed fever. After the introduction of chlorine washings, nursing infants in the foundling home ceased to die of childbed fever. Dr. [Alois] Bednar, then head physician of the Imperial Foundling Home in Vienna, wrote: "Sepsis of the blood of newborns has become a great rarity. For this we must thank the consequential and most noteworthy discovery of Dr. Semmelweis, emeritus assistant of the Viennese first maternity clinic. His work fortunately explained the cause and the prevention of the formerly murderous ravages of puerperal fever."[13] Where I speak of childbed fever of the newborn, Dr. Bednar correctly speaks of sepsis of the blood; he thus remains consistent with ordinary usage.

Once the cause of the increased mortality in the first clinic was identified as cadaverous particles adhering to the hands of the examiners, it was easy to explain why women who delivered in the street had a strikingly lower mortality rate than those who delivered in the clinic. This was so because once the infant was born and the placenta separated, there was generally no longer opportunity for instruction; thus there were no examinations. A bed was assigned to such patients, and they generally left it in good health. There was no reason for their genitals to be touched by contaminated hands; therefore they did not contract childbed fever. Also, women who delivered prematurely became ill less often because they were not examined ei-

---

[13] [Alois] Bednar, *Die Krankheiten der Neugeborenen und Säuglinge vom klinischen und pathologisch-anatomischen Standpunkte bearbeitet* (Vienna: Gerold, 1850), p. 198 [author's note].

ther. The first requirement in premature births is to delay birth if possible. Consequently, these persons were not used for open instruction, and decaying organic matter was not conveyed to their genitals.

The sequential appearance of disease was also easy to explain. Because of the large number of births in the first clinic, several individuals were often in the labor room simultaneously. These persons were examined at least twice a day—during the morning rounds of the professor, and during the afternoon rounds of the assistant. Everyone in labor was examined for instruction sequentially in the order of their beds. When, therefore, the examiners' hands were contaminated with cadaverous particles, the genitals of several individuals were simultaneously brought into contact with cadaverous particles. This meant that the germ [*Keim*] for childbed fever was planted through resorption in several individuals at once. The patients were placed back in the maternity ward in the order in which they had delivered. Thus it often happened that those who were together in the labor room delivered at about the same time and thereafter remained in the same sequential order in the maternity clinic. In the labor room they were examined in rows by persons whose hands were contaminated with cadaverous particles, the germ of the future puerperal fever, and the disease occurred among them sequentially. After chlorine washing was instituted, sequential cases of the disease ceased.

I mentioned that toward the end of 1846, because of the prevalence of childbed fever in the first clinic, yet another commission was instituted—I have no idea how many times this had already been done—in order to identify the cause of these deaths. This commission identified the cause as injury to genitals inflicted during instructional examinations. But because the same examinations were conducted for the instruction of midwives, the commission explained that male students, particularly foreigners, examined too roughly. Consequently, the number of students was reduced to a minimum. Table 3 shows how great the mortality was before this measure was adopted, how it then declined, and how, in the months of April and May, it increased again in spite of the preventive measures. I will now explain these phenomena. Before I do, however, one item must be discussed.

As an aspirant for the position of assistant in the first clinic, later as provisional assistant and then, finally, as actual assistant, it was not possible for me to study gynecology at the gynecological division of the Imperial Hospital. However, such study was highly desirable for an obstetrician. As a substitute, as soon as I had decided to devote my life to obstetrics I examined all the female corpses in the morgue of the Imperial General Hospital. From 1844 until I moved to Pest in 1850, I devoted nearly every morning before the professor's rounds in the obstetrical clinic to these studies. I very much appreciate having enjoyed the friendship of Professor Rokitansky. Through his kindness I secured permission to dissect all female corpses, including those not already set aside for autopsy, in order to correlate the results of my examinations with autopsies.

For reasons that do not concern us here, the assistant of the first clinic seldom visited the morgue in the months of December 1846 and January, February, and March 1847. The Austrian students, whose number was reduced to eighteen, followed his example. The opportunity for them to contaminate their hands with cadaverous particles was thereby greatly reduced. Restricting examinations to the minimum also reduced the opportunity for the genitals of patients to be touched by contaminated hands. For these reasons, mortality in the first clinic was reduced during these months.

On 20 March 1847, I reassumed the position of assistant in the first clinic. Early that morning I conducted my gynecological studies in the morgue. I then went to the labor room and began to examine all the patients, as my predecessors and I were obliged to do, so that I could report on each patient during the professor's morning rounds. My hands, contaminated by cadaverous particles, were thereby brought into contact with the genitals of so many women in labor that in April, from 312 deliveries, there were 57 deaths (18.26 percent). In May, from 294 deliveries there were 36 deaths (12.24 percent). In the middle of May, without noting the exact day, I instituted chlorine washings. Thus, the great mortality in the first clinic was not caused by injuries in rough examinations—a completely false assumption—but by contaminated fingers that contacted the genitals of the patients. During April and May, when again so many died, the clinic remained the same as in earlier months, yet the mortality rate increased significantly because I intervened, my fingers contaminated with cadaverous particles.

After chlorine washings were conducted for a longer period with such beneficial results, the number of students was again increased to forty-two. One no longer took account of whether they were Austrian or foreign. The examinations were resumed as was expedient for instruction. Nevertheless, the first clinic lost the dismal distinction of having the greater mortality rate. In December 1846 and in January, February, and March of 1847, I functioned as provisional assistant and simultaneously conducted gynecological studies in the morgue, yet in these months the mortality rate remained low. The reason is that as provisional assistant I had the right, but not the duty, to examine all patients in labor. After three years in so large a maternity hospital, it was no longer instructive for me to examine all the patients. I examined only exceptional cases—that is, I examined very seldom. When I became the actual assistant, it was my duty to conduct all examinations before the professor's morning rounds. Thereafter, it was necessary for me to examine nearly all the women in labor for the purpose of instructing the students. This occasioned the great mortality rates in April and May of 1847.

Native students are those who completed their education at an Austrian university [*Hochschule*]. Foreign students are those who were educated elsewhere and who then did further work at the great University of Vienna. In Vienna one can meet physicians from all the countries of the civilized world. The course in practical obstetrics lasted two months. The influx of students into this, the largest maternity hospital in the world, was so great that to accept simultaneously all who sought admission would have excessively disrupted the patients. Applicants were assigned numbers, and were accepted sequentially to replace departing students, regardless of whether they were native or foreign. Each student was free to repeat the course as often as he felt it necessary for his own obstetrical training. However, in order that those who wished to repeat the course would not remain constantly enrolled, precluding others from taking it at all, it was necessary that one wait three months after completing the course before enrolling again. The commission charged the foreigners with being more dangerous than the natives because they were rough in examinations and, consequently, at any one time only two foreigners were allowed to attend the course in practical obstetrics. Everyone, even those who do not share my opinion, will agree that the commission acted groundlessly in imputing guilt to the foreigners. In fact, I alone held that foreigners *were* more dangerous than natives, but not because they examined more roughly. The reasons that foreigners were more dangerous than natives lies in the following considerations.

Foreigners come to Vienna to perfect medical training already begun in their own universities. They visit pathological and forensic autopsies in the general hospital. They take courses in pathological anatomy, in surgery, obstetrics, microscopic surgery of cadavers, they visit the medical and surgical wards of the hospital, etc. In a word, they utilize their time as efficiently and educationally as possible. They have, therefore, many opportunities for their hands to become contaminated with foul animal-organic matter. Thus, it is no wonder that foreigners, busy in the maternity hospital at the same time, are more dangerous for patients. Natives take the course in practical obstetrics after completing two difficult examinations in order to attain the degree of Doctor of Medicine. The law stipulates that the minimum preparation time for these examinations is six months. Thus the natives have already toiled excessively before they are admitted into the maternity hospital, and they regard the time there as a rest. While enrolled in practical obstetrics, natives do not concern themselves with other activities that would contaminate their hands. Indeed, while working at the maternity hospital, they concern themselves even less with other aspects of medicine because, after completing the course, they can perfect their knowledge of medicine to the highest possible degree. Since the foreigners are generally able to remain in Vienna only a few months, they are compelled to work simultaneously in more than one aspect of medicine. Even so, one cannot impute guilt to the foreigners any more than to me or to all the others who undertook examinations with contaminated hands. None of us knew that we were causing the numerous deaths.

THE MOSQUITO HYPOTHETICALLY CONSIDERED AS THE AGENT OF TRANSMISSION OF YELLOW FEVER[1]

Carlos J. Finlay

Some years ago I had the honor to submit to your consideration the results of my alkalimetric experiments, by which I think I have definitely demonstrated the excessive alkalinity which prevails in the atmosphere of Havana. Some of the Members now present, may perhaps remember the relations which I then attempted to establish between that peculiarity and the development of yellow fever in Cuba. Much however has been done since that time, more accurate data have been obtained, and the etiology of yellow fever has been more methodically studied. In consequence thereof I feel convinced that any theory which attributes the origin and the propagation of yellow fever to atmospheric influences, to miasmatic or meteorological conditions, to filth or to the neglect of general hygienic precautions, must be considered as utterly indefensible. I have, therefore, been obliged to abandon my former ideas, and shall now endeavor to justify this change in my opinions, submitting to your appreciation a new series of experiments which I have undertaken for the purpose of discovering the manner in which yellow fever is propagated.

In this paper I shall not concern myself with the nature or form of the morbific cause of yellow fever, beyond postulating the existence of a material, transportable substance, which may be an amorphous virus, a vegetable or animal germ, a bacterium, etc., but, at any rate, constitutes something tangible which requires to be conveyed from the sick to the healthy before the disease can be propagated. What I propose to consider is the means by which the morbific cause of yellow fever is enabled to part from the body of the patient and to be implanted into that of a healthy person. The need of an external intervention, apart from the disease itself, in order that the latter may be transmitted is made apparent by numerous considerations; some of them already pointed out by Humboldt and Benjamin Rush since the beginning of this century, and now corroborated by recent observations. Yellow fever, at times, will travel across the Ocean to be propagated in distant ports presenting climatic and topographic conditions very different from those of the focus from which the infection has proceeded, while, at other times, the disease seems unable to transmit itself outside of a very limited zone, although the meteorology and topography beyond that zone do not appear to differ very materially. Once the need of an agent of transmission is admitted as the only means of accounting for such anomalies, it is evident that all the conditions which have hitherto been recognized essential for the propagation of the disease must be understood to act through their influence upon the said agent. It seemed unlikely, therefore, that this agent should be found among Micro or Zoophytes, for those lowest orders of animal life are but little affected by such meteorologic variations as are known to influence the development of yellow fever. To satisfy that requisite it was necessary to search for it among insects. On the other hand, the fact of yellow fever being characterized both clinically and (according to recent findings) histologically, by lesions of the blood-vessels and by alterations of the physical and chemical conditions of the blood, suggested that the insect which should convey the infectious particles from the patient to the healthy should be looked for among those which drive their sting into blood-vessels in order to suck human blood. Finally, by reason of other considerations which need not be stated here, I came to think that the mosquito might be the transmitter of yellow fever.

Source: Excerpted from *Carlos J. Finlay—Obras Completas,* compiled by César Rodríguez Expósito. Havana, Academia de Ciencias de Cuba, 1965.

[1] Read before the Royal Academy of Medical, Physical and Natural Sciences, session of August 14th, 1881. Translated by Dr. Finlay from the *Anales de la Academia de Ciencias Médicas, Físicas y Naturales de la Habana,* Vol. XVIII, p. 147. Vide also *Revista de la Asociación Médico-Farmacéutica de la Isla de Cuba,* January 1902, p. 273.

Such was the hypothesis which led me to undertake the experimental investigation which I shall here relate. . . .

Although mosquitoes are found in all latitudes, their abundance varies in different localities. Humboldt and Bonpland, in their *Travels in Equinoctial America* wrote: "The annoyance suffered from mosquitoes and *zancudos* in the torrid zone is not so general as most people think. On the high plateaux more than 400 toises (2500 feet) above the sea-level, and in very dry plains, far from large rivers, such as Cumana and Calabozo, gnats are not much more abundant than in the most populous parts of Europe." The influence of dryness and of a long distance from water-courses, pointed out by those travels, is easily understood, inasmuch as the larvae and pupae of the mosquitoes are aquatic, and the winged insect requires water for the laying and hatching of its eggs. The impediment to their propagation at high levels may consist in the exaggeration of the difficulty which those insects must always experience in flying upwards after they have filled themselves with blood; a difficulty which will be much more marked in a species having such small wings as those of the *C. mosquito*. The rarefaction of the atmosphere at those great heights necessarily increases that difficulty, and, under those circumstances, the mosquito will instinctively shun those localities. The above mentioned travelers also relate that a missionary priest, Bernardo Zea, had built himself a room over a scaffolding of palm boards, and they used to go there at night to dry their plants and to write their Diary, adding: "The missionary had rightly observed that those insects are more numerous in the lower strata of the atmosphere, within 12 to 15 feet from the ground." Further on they write: "As one proceeds towards the plateau of the Andes, those insects disappear and the air one breathes becomes pure . . . at a height of 200 toises (1500 feet) mosquitoes and zancudos are no longer feared."

Historically the mosquito is one of the insects most anciently observed. Aristotle and Pliny refer to its proboscis which serves both for piercing the skin and for sucking the blood. The Greek historian Pausanias, according to Taschenberg, mentions the city of Myus, in Asia Minor, situated on a bay which had formerly communicated with the sea but was afterwards cut off from it: when the water in the lake which

was thus formed ceased to be salt, such a plague of mosquitoes was developed that the inhabitants had to abandon the city and betook themselves to Miletus. So also in the Decades of Herrera, we read that Juan Grijalva when he first discovered the coast of New Spain (Mexico), in 1518, landed with his men on an islet which he named San Juan de Ulua, and they had to build their huts "at the top of the highest sand-mounds which they could find in order to avoid the importunity of mosquitoes." Seven days later, Diez del Castillo had to seek protection in some Indian places of worship, "unable to stand the mosquitoes." Finally, in 1519, on the same spot where Veracruz now stands, according to Herrera "the long-legged mosquitoes and the small one which are still worse used to worry the people who went with Cortes." . . .

It is well known that only the female mosquitoes bite and suck blood, while the males feed on vegetable juices, principally the sweet ones; but I have not found it mentioned in any author that even the females never bite before having been fertilized. This, at least, I infer from the following experiments:

A female *C. mosquito*, caught soon after breaking loose from its pupa-case, and kept alive during three days, cannot be got to bite during that space of time. I have several times repeated the experiment and always with a negative result.

Female mosquitoes which are caught pairing, bite and suck blood readily very soon after they are parted.

Finally, those which are caught in the act of biting and sucking blood will, as a rule, lay eggs after a few days, while the fertilized females which have not been allowed to suck blood die without ever laying any ova.

We are thus led to infer that the craving of the female mosquito for live blood is not meant to supply an indispensable article of food. Indeed it seems improbable that for the nourishment of so small a body, such a disproportionate quantity of rich blood should be needed. I have come to the conclusion that the sucking of blood is intended for another object connected with the propagation of the species. The likeliest hypothesis seems to be that the feed of blood acts through the degree of heat which it procures. If, for instance, the maturation of the ovules contained in the ovaries of the mosquito demands a temperature of 37° C., the latter could

scarcely be obtained by any other means so
readily as by the insect filling itself with a fair
amount of blood of that temperature; and
sometimes it may be more convenient for the
mosquito to bite a patient attacked with fever,
whose blood at 39° or 40° may prove more
efficacious in hastening the process of ovulation. It will thus be understood why large insects like the *zancudo* are able to absorb with a
single bite the amount of blood required for the
maturation of all the 200 to 350 ova which they
lay at one sitting, while the smaller species, like
the *C. mosquito,* have to bite and fill themselves
several times with blood before beginning to lay,
and generally require several sittings before all
their ova are laid.

After the female mosquito has filled itself
with blood it requires two, three or four days,
according to the species (*and the season of the
year*) to complete the digestion of its feed; and,
during that time, remains out of sight spending
hours in a curious performance the object of
which Réaumur did not understand, having
only observed it in the open. When the insect is
confined in a glass tube, it is easy to see that the
performance consists in besmearing every part
of its body with a secretion which is picked up
from the anal extremity with its hind legs and
smeared successively upon the legs, the abdomen, the wings, the thorax, the head and
even the proboscis. As suggested by Felipe Poey,
facile princeps among our Cuban Naturalists, the
object of this operation is probably to make the
mosquito waterproof before it goes to the water
to lay its eggs. During the digestion, the mosquito also drops some bloody particle or excrement which present the peculiarity of being
extremely soluble in water, even after being
kept in a dry condition during several months.
This is probably due to the admixture of the
blood with the saliva poured out during the
process of biting, and which is generally believed to render the blood more fluid while it is
being sucked by the insect. As a rule, after a
complete, uninterrupted feed of blood, the
mosquito does not bite again, and even shuns
the contact of the bare skin (perhaps because
the heat of it becomes at that time disagreeable),
until the digestion of the blood has been completed. With the *zancudo* (night-mosquito) it is at
that time that its ova are laid. . . .

Evidently, from the point of view which I am
considering, the *Culex mosquito* is admirably

adapted to convey from one person to another a
disease which happens to be transmissible
through the blood; since it has repeated opportunities of sucking blood from different
sources, and also of infecting different persons;
so that the probabilities that its bite may unite all
the conditions required for the transmission will
thereby be greatly increased. On the other
hand, inasmuch as the *C. cubensis* absorbs a
larger quantity of the infectious blood at each
feed, its mouth-parts may retain a larger
amount of virus, and perhaps produce a graver
inoculation when it happens to attack a non-
immune a few moments after having bitten the
patient, its first bite having been interrupted. In
that case, a graver infection might result but the
chances of its occurring would be much
less. . . .

It is a well-known fact that, while mosquitos
are never wholly absent from Havana, they are
much more abundant at some seasons of the
year. It appears to me that they increase in numbers from April or May till August, and thereafter gradually decrease till February or March.
Another point, however, requires to be borne in
mind, inasmuch as it affords an explanation of
the recurrence, hitherto unaccounted for, of
yellow-fever epidemics without new importation
in localities previously considered as immune. I
allude to the hibernation of mosquitoes, a phenomenon which is not observed in our climate,
at least in all its phases; but which constitutes,
according to the best authorities, the regular
mode by which the species is propagated in cold
climates during winter. Taschenberg informs us
that: "the fertilized females of the last generation hibernate during winter in out-of-the way
places such as the cellars of dwellings, and set
about propagating their species the following
spring."

Among the conditions which favor the development of mosquitoes may be mentioned: heat,
moisture, the vicinity of stagnant waters, low,
dark localities sheltered from the wind, and the
summer season. It is necessary, however, to bear
in mind Humboldt's observation that the abundance of mosquitoes is not always in accordance
with recognizable meteorological or topograph-
ical conditions.

I have already referred to the difficulty which
our mosquito, by reason of its comparatively
small wings, must experience in its upward
flight after it has filled itself with blood. It will

also be hindered by the same cause, from going far from the place where it has accomplished its last bite, and, in general, from traveling any considerable distance through the air without resting. This circumstance will not prevent, however, its being conveyed, hidden among clothes, caught under a hat, inside of a traveling bag, etc., to considerable distance, after a recent bite, perhaps carrying upon its mouth-parts the inoculable germ of the disease. . . .

After this long, but necessary account of the habits of our Cuban mosquitoes, and of the *Culex mosquito* in particular, let us consider by what means that insect might transmit the yellow fever, if that disease happens to be really transmissible through the inoculation of blood. The first and most natural idea would be that the transmission might be effected through the virulent blood which the mosquito has sucked, amounting to 5 and even to 7 or 9 cubic milli- meters, and which, if the insect happens to die before completing its digestion, would be in ex- cellent conditions to retain during a long time its infecting properties. It might also be sup- posed that the same blood which the mosquito discharges, as excrement, after having bitten a yellow-fever patient, might be dissolved in the drinking-water, whereby the infection might be conveyed if the latter were susceptible of pen- etrating by the mouth. But the experiments of Firth and other considerations arising from my personal ideas regarding the pathogenesis of yellow fever, forbid my taking into account ei- ther of those modes of propagation, as I shall now explain. When the U. S. Yellow-fever Com- mission took their leave, two years ago, they presented us with a valuable collection of micro- photographs from preparations made by our corresponding Member, Dr. Sternberg, showing what, to me, appeared to be a most striking feature, namely, that the red blood-globules are discharged unbroken in the hemorrhages of yellow fever. This fact taken in connection with the circumstance that those hemorrhages are often unattended with any perceptible break in the blood-vessels, while, on the other hand, they constitute a most essential clinical symptom of the disease, led me to infer that the principal lesion of yellow fever should be sought for in the vascular endothelium. The disease is trans- missible, it attacks but once the same person, and always presents in its phenomena a regular order comparable with that observed in the

eruptive fevers, all of which circumstances sug- gested to my mind the hypothesis that yellow- fever should be considered as a sort of eruptive fever in which the seat of the eruption is the vascular endothelium. The first period would correspond to the initial fever, the remission to the eruptive period, and the third period would be that of desquamation. If the latter phase is accomplished under favorable conditions, the patient will only show evidence of an exagge- rated transudation of some of the liquid ele- ments of the blood through the new endo- thelium; if the conditions are unfavorable, a defective endothelium will have been produced, incapable of checking the figured elements of the blood: passive hemorrhages will occur and the patient may find himself in imminent dan- ger. Finally, assimilating the disease to small- pox and to vaccination, it occurred to me that in order to inoculate yellow fever it would be nec- essary to pick out the inoculable material from within the blood vessels of a yellow-fever patient and to carry it likewise into the interior of a blood vessel of the person who was to be inocu- lated. All of which conditions the mosquito sat- isfies most admirably through its bite, in a man- ner which it would be almost impossible for us to imitate with the comparatively coarse instru- ments which the most skillful makers could pro- duce.

Three conditions will, therefore, be necessary in order that yellow fever may be propagated: 1. The existence of a yellow-fever patient into whose capillaries the mosquito is able to drive its sting and to impregnate it with the virulent particles at an appropriate stage of the disease. 2. That the life of the mosquito be spared after its bite upon the patient until it has a chance of biting the person in whom the disease is to be reproduced. 3. The coincidence that some of the persons whom the same mosquito happens to bite thereafter shall be susceptible of con- tracting the disease.

The first of these conditions, since Dr. Am- brosio G. del Valle has been publishing his valu- able mortuary tables, we may be sure has never failed to be satisfied in Havana. With regard to the 2d and 3d, it is evident that the probabilities of their being satisfied will depend on the abun- dance of mosquitoes and on the number of susceptible persons present in the locality. I firmly believe that the three above mentioned conditions have, indeed, always coincided in years when yellow fever has made its greatest ravages.

Such is, Gentlemen, my theory: and I consider that it has been singularly strengthened by the numerous historical, geographical, ethnological and meteorological coincidences which occur between the data which I have collected regarding the mosquito and those which are recorded about the yellow fever; while, at the same time, we are enabled by it to account for circumstances which have until now been considered inexplicable under the prevailing theories. Yellow fever was unknown to the white race before the discovery of America, and according to Humboldt, it is a traditional opinion in Veracruz that the disease has been prevailing there ever since the first Spanish explorers landed on its shores. There also, as we have seen, the Spaniards since their first landing have recorded the presence of mosquitoes; and with greater insistence than in any other place in America, in the identical sand-mounds of San Juan de Ulúa (the present site of Veracruz). The races which are most susceptible to yellow fever are also the ones who suffer most from the bites of mosquitoes. The meteorological conditions which are most favorable to the development of yellow fever are those which contribute to increase the number of mosquitoes; in proof of which I can cite several local epidemics regarding which competent authorities assert that the number of mosquitoes during the prevalence of the yellow fever was much greater than on other occasions; indeed, it is stated in one instance that the mosquitoes were of a different kind from those which were usually observed in the locality, having gray rings around their bodies. Regarding the topography of the yellow fever, Humboldt points out the altitudes beyond which mosquitoes cease to appear, and in another passage gives the limits above the sea-level within which the yellow fever may be propagated. Finally, in the notorius case of the U. S. Steamship Plymouth, in which two cases of yellow fever occurred at sea, after the vessel had been disinfected and frozen during the winter, four months after the last previous case had occurred on that vessel (the preceding November), the facts can be readily accounted for by the hibernation of mosquitoes which had bitten the former yellow fever patients, and, which, upon finding themselves again within tropical temperatures, recovered from their lethargic condition and bit two of the new men of the crew.

Supported by the above reasons, I decided to submit my theory to an experimental test, and, after obtaining the necessary authorization, I proceeded in the following manner.

On the 30th of last June, I took to the Quinta de Garcini a mosquito which had been caught before being allowed to sting, and there made it bite and fill itself with blood from the arm of a patient, Camilo Anca, who was in the fifth day of a well characterized attack of yellow fever of which he died two days later. I then picked out F. B., one of twenty healthy nonimmunes who have continued until now under my observation, and made the same mosquito bite him. Bearing in mind that the incubation of yellow fever, in cases which allow its limits to be reckoned, varies between one and fifteen days, I ordered the man to be kept under observation. On the 9th of July, F. B. began to feel out of sorts, and on the 14th he was admitted in the Military Hospital with a mild attack of yellow fever perfectly characterized by the usual yellowness, and albumin in the urine which persisted from the third till the ninth day.

On the 16th of July, I applied a mosquito at the same Quinta de Garcini, to a patient, Domingo Rodríguez, in the third or fourth day of yellow fever; on the 20th, I allowed the same mosquito to bite me and, finally, on the 22d I made it bite A. L. C., another of the 20 men who are under observation. Five days later, this man was admitted at the Hospital with fever, severe headache, pain in the loins and infected eyes; these symptoms lasted three days, after which the patient became convalescent without having presented any yellowness nor albuminuria. His case was, however, diagnosed as "abortive yellow fever" by the physician in charge.

The 29th of July, I made a mosquito bite D. L. R. who was going through a severe attack of yellow fever at Quinta de Garcini, being then in its third day. On the 31st, I made the same mosquito bite D. L. F., another of my 20 men under observation. On the 5th of August, at 2 a.m., he was attacked with symptoms of mild yellow fever; he subsequently showed some yellowness but I do not think that he developed any albuminuria; his case was, nevertheless, diagnosed "abortive yellow fever."

Finally, on the 31st of July, I applied another

mosquito to the same patient, D. L. R. at Quinta Garcini, his attack having then reached its fifth day and proving fatal on the following one. On the 2d of August I applied this mosquito to D. G. B., another of my twenty nonimmunes. Till the present date (12th), this last inoculation has not given any result; but, as only 12 days have elapsed, the case is still within the limits of incubation.[2]

I have to state that the persons mentioned above are the only ones who were inoculated with mosquitoes in the manner described; and that since June 12th, till now (in the course of seven weeks), barring my first three inoculated men, no other case of confirmed or abortive yellow fever has occurred among the twenty nonimmunes whom I have had under observation.[3]

These experiments are certainly favorable to my theory, but I do not wish to exaggerate their value in considering them final, although the accumulation of probabilities in my favor is now very remarkable. I understand but too well that nothing less than an absolutely incontrovertible demonstration will be required before the generality of my colleagues accept a theory so entirely at variance with the ideas which have until now prevailed about yellow fever. In the meantime, I beg leave to resume in the following conclusions the most essential points which I have endeavored to demonstrate.

CONCLUSIONS

1. It has been proved that the *C. mosquito*, as a rule, bites several times in the course of its existence, not only when its bite has been accidentally interrupted, but even when it has been allowed to completely satisfy its appetite; in which case two or more days intervene between its successive bites.

2. Inasmuch as the mouth-parts of the mosquito are very well adapted to retain particles that may be in suspension in the liquids absorbed by that insect, it cannot be denied that there is a possibility that said mosquito should retain upon the setae of its sting some of the virulent particles contained in a diseased blood, and may inoculate them to the persons whom it afterwards chances to bite.

3. The direct experiments undertaken to decide whether the mosquito is able to transmit yellow fever in the above stated manner, have been limited to five attempted inoculations, with a single bite, and they have given the following results: One case of mild yellow fever, perfectly characterized, with albuminuria and icterus; two cases diagnosed as "abortive yellow fever" by the physicians in charge; and two ephemeral fevers without any definite characters. From which results it must be inferred that the inoculation with a single bite is insufficient to produce the severe forms of yellow fever, and that a final decision as to the efficacy of such inoculations must be deferred until opportunity is found for experimenting under absolutely decisive conditions, outside of the epidemic zone.

4. Should it be finally proven that the mosquito-inoculation not only reproduces the yellow fever, but that it constitutes the regular process through which the disease is propagated, the conditions of existence and of devel-

---

[2] This inoculated man D. G. B., came to my office on the 17th of August to be inspected, stating that during the previous six days he had been suffering from headache, loss of appetite and general malaise. On the 24th I found that he had fever (Pulse 100, Temperature 30,1) and he stated that it had been higher on the previous day and also that same morning. The fever however was never severe, and the patient did not report himself sick nor took any medicine. The fever ceased, but the pain in the head continued a few days longer.

Another of my 20 nonimmunes was bitten on the 15th of August by a mosquito which, 2 days before, had bitten a patient at the Military Hospital, in the 5th day of yellow fever. This inoculated man does not appear to have been sick so far (September 1st). I have not been able to see him since his inoculation, and it is only from hearsay that I have been informed that he had felt poorly on the 24th and 25th of August; but did not report himself sick.

[3] There was a fourth case which was also diagnosed as "abortive yellow fever" at the Military Hospital, but regarding whose diagnosis Dr. Delgado and I were doubtful. He was one of the 20 nonimmunes of our group, and a different kind of inoculation was tried upon him, the particulars of which will be considered of some interest at the present day.—On the 28th of June 1881, 7 a.m., a night-mosquito (*C. pungens*) was found inside the mosquito-net of a fatal case of yellow fever in the 5th day of attack. Placed in a glass cage, the *pungens* discharged some black blood upon the sides of the tube the following day. On the 26th of July, a couple of drops of sterilized, distilled water were used to dissolve the dry bloody excrement, and the same was soaked up with a small bit of sugar which looked thereafter as if it had been soaked in black coffee. A freshly caught *C. mosquito* was now introduced in the phial, and went greedily for the sugar. A little more water was now added, turning the sugar into a reddish brown syrup, from which the same *C. mosquito*, in the course of ½ hour had taken a good feed.—On the 29th of July, 2 p.m., L. G. P. one of my 20 nonimmunes, was bitten by this *C. mosquito*.—On the 31st of July this man was admitted to the Military Hospital, with fever, flushed face, cephalalgia, pain in the back, epigastralgia, infected eyes.—On the 3d of August he had neither fever nor albumin.

opment for that dipterous insect would account for the anomalies hitherto observed in the propagation of yellow fever, and while we might, on the one hand, have the means of preventing the disease from spreading, nonimmunes might at the same time be protected through a mild inoculation.

My only desire is that my observations be recorded, and that the correctness of my ideas be tested through direct experiments. I do not mean by this that I would shun the discussion of my opinions; far from it, I shall be very glad to hear any remarks or objections which my distinguished colleagues may be inclined to express.[4]

---

[4]N.B. The notes do not belong to the original paper.—C.F.

MORTALITY OF MINERS: A SELECTION FROM THE REPORTS AND WRITINGS OF WILLIAM FARR[1]

MORTALITY OF MINERS, 1848-1853, CORNWALL

From the evidence given before us by Dr. Farr, F.R.S., Chief of the Statistical Department of the General Register Office, and from a Return prepared for us by the Registrar General and printed in the Appendix, we are enabled to show the rates of mortality prevailing among the miners of Cornwall at different periods of life, as compared with those prevailing among the non-mining population of the same districts, for the five years 1849–53 inclusive, and also for the more recent triennial period 1860–62 inclusive.

The districts selected for the purposes of this comparison were those of Liskeard, St. Austell, Truro, Helston, Redruth, and Penzance. The death-rates were computed from the aggregate numbers of males, and of deaths of males of the two classes respectively in the whole six districts taken together. Table 1 shows the rates of mortality from all causes during the earlier period 1849–53, among the two sections of the population, for the several successive decennial periods of life, from the age of 15 up to that of 75 years.

From the figures in Table 1 it appears that the rates of mortality among the miners are not materially different from those prevailing among the non-mining males of the same districts until after the age of 35 years, after which there is a large and progressive excess of mortality among the mining section of the male population. If we assume the rate of mortality among the non-mining males at each decennial

Table 1. Average annual number of deaths per 1000 miners, and per 1000 males exclusive of miners, in Cornwall, from all causes, during the five years 1849–53 inclusive.

Ages	Metal miners	Males, exclusive of miners
15–25	8.90	7.12
25–35	8.96	8.84
35–45	14.30	9.99
45–55	33.51	14.76
55–65	63.17	24.12
65–75	111.23	58.61

period of life to be represented by 100, then that among the miners would be represented by 125 between the ages of 15 and 25 years, by 101 between 25 and 35, by 143 between 35 and 45, by 227 between 45 and 55, by 263 between 55 and 65, and by 189 between 65 and 75 years. That the large and progressive excess of mortality among the miners between the ages of 35 and 65 years must be due to unwholesome conditions incident to their occupation may be inferred from the fact that it does not commence until they have had full time to operate. The somewhat higher rate of mortality among miners between the ages of 15 and 25 years probably arises from the circumstance that many of the boys are put to work in the mines at too early an age.

That the excessive mortality among the miners in Cornwall is not caused by the mere working underground in dark galleries, a necessary condition of the miner's occupation, and must therefore be mainly due to other causes, is clearly proved by some statistics relative to the coal miners of Durham and Northumberland, also given in evidence by Dr. Farr. Table 2 shows the rates of mortality among the coal miners of Durham and Northumberland during the five years 1849–53 inclusive, for each decennial period of life, from the age of 15 up to that of 75 years, compared with the rates among the Cornish miners already quoted.

Source: Excerpted from *Vital Statistics: A Memorial Volume of Selections from the Reports and Writings of William Farr,* introduction by Mervyn Susser and Abraham Adelstein. Metuchen: Scarecrow Press, 1975. Courtesy of The New York Academy of Medicine Library.

[1] This extract is a summary of Dr. Farr's evidence given before the Royal Commission on the Condition of Mines in 1864, of which Lord Kinnaird was Chairman, and is reprinted from the Commissioners' Report, together with some of the Tables furnished by Dr. Farr, the remainder of which will be found in the Appendix to that Report.

Table 2. Average annual number of deaths per 1000 Cornish metal miners, and per 1000 Northern coal miners, from all causes, during the five years 1849–53 inclusive.

Ages	Cornish metal miners	Northern coal miners
15–25	8.90	8.50
25–35	8.96	8.49
35–45	14.30	10.13
45–55	33.51	16.81
55–65	63.17	24.43
65–75	111.23	65.16

Assuming, on the authority of the previous table, the rate of mortality among the coal miners at each period of life to be represented by 100, then that among the Cornish miners would be represented by 105 between the ages 15 and 25 years, by 106 between 25 and 35, by 141 between 35 and 45, by 199 between 45 and 55, by 258 between 55 and 65, and by 171 between 65 and 75 years. The rates of mortality among the Cornish miners from the age of 35 years upwards are thus shown to have been almost as much in excess of the rates which prevail among the coal miners in the selected districts of Durham and Northumberland, as they were above the rates prevailing among the non-mining male population of Cornwall.

The evidence regarding the more recent period 1860–62 shows that the great excess of mortality among the Cornish miners still continues, although the proportions are slightly different. Table 3 shows the rates of mortality among the two sections of the male population respectively, from all causes, during the three years 1860–62, for the same periods of life as the former Table.

Again, assuming the rate of mortality at each period of life among the non-mining males to be represented by 100, then the rate among the miners would be represented by 126 between the ages of 15 and 25, by 115 between 25 and 35, by 150 between 35 and 45, by 238 between 45 and 55, by 317 between 55 and 65, and by 207 between 65 and 75 years.

From Dr. Farr's evidence, supplemented by the Registrar General's Return, it further appears that the excessive rate of mortality among the Cornish miners is mainly caused by the large number of deaths from pulmonary consumption and other diseases of the lungs. As, however, deaths which are registered in some districts as due to consumption are registered in other districts under different names, such as asthma and bronchitis, it is best for statistical purposes to throw all the diseases of the lungs into one class under the general name of Pulmonary Diseases, an arrangement which enables the rates of mortality from diseases of the lungs in different districts to be more accurately compared with each other than if the several diseases of these organs were nominally kept separate. The class of pulmonary diseases thus formed comprises, phthisis, laryngitis, bronchitis, pleurisy, pneumonia, asthma, and all cases returned as "diseases of the lungs."

Table 4 shows the average annual rate of mortality per 1000 persons from pulmonary diseases among miners, and also among males exclusive of miners, during the three years 1860–62 inclusive, for each decennial period of life between the ages of 15 and 75 years.

Assuming as before that the rate of mortality among the males exclusive of miners is represented at each period of life by 100, then that among the miners would be represented by

Table 3. Average annual number of deaths per 1000 miners, and per 1000 males exclusive of miners, in Cornwall, from all causes, during the three years 1860–62 inclusive.

Ages	Metal miners	Males, exclusive of miners
15–25	9.44	7.50
25–35	9.57	8.32
35–45	15.12	10.08
45–55	29.74	12.50
55–65	63.21	19.96
65–75	110.51	53.31

Table 4. Average annual number of deaths per 1000 miners, and per 1000 males exclusive of miners in Cornwall, from pulmonary diseases, during the three years 1860–62 inclusive.

Ages	Metal miners	Males, exclusive of miners
15–25	3.77	3.30
25–35	4.15	3.83
35–45	7.89	4.24
45–55	19.75	4.34
55–65	43.29	5.19
65–75	45.04	10.48

Table 5. Average annual number of deaths per 1000 miners in Cornwall from all causes and from pulmonary diseases in 1849–53 and 1860–62.

Ages	All causes		Pulmonary diseases	
	During the five years 1849–53	During the three years 1860–62	During the five years 1849–53	During the three years 1860–62
15–25	8.90	9.44	3.05	3.77
25–35	8.96	9.57	4.42	4.15
35–45	14.30	15.12	8.47	7.89
45–55	33.51	29.74	24.31	19.75
55–65	63.17	63.21	44.46	43.29
65–75	111.23	110.51	55.87	45.04

114 between the ages of 15 and 25 years, by 108 between 25 and 35, by 186 between 35 and 45, by 455 between 45 and 55, by 834 between 55 and 65, and by 430 between 65 and 75 years. It is therefore evident that pulmonary diseases are the chief cause of the excess of mortality among the Cornish miners; and that these diseases are due to the conditions incident to the miners' labour may also be confidently inferred, as in the case of the death-rates from all causes, from the fact that the excess of mortality arising from them does not reach its acme until after the middle of life, when these conditions have had full time to produce their effect on the health of the miners. A much greater discrepancy will be observed between the rates of mortality from pulmonary diseases among the miners and non-miners than has been shown to exist between the rates of mortality from all causes among the two sections of the population respectively. This is undoubtedly due to the fact that exposure to the peculiar evils incident to the occupation causes many miners to die of pulmonary diseases who in different circumstances would have died of other complaints.

Table 5 contrasts the rates of mortality among miners at the two periods 1849–53 and 1860–62, both from all causes and from pulmonary diseases.

It will be seen in the above table that the only material difference in favour of the more recent period is that existing between the 45 and 55 years. A comparison of the rates of mortality from all causes among the non-mining section of the male population also shows a similar improvement in favour of the more recent period.

Yorkshire and Northern Counties

From a return prepared at our request by the Registrar General, and printed in the Appendix, it appears that, as has been shown to be the case in Cornwall, so also in these northern districts the rates of mortality are much higher among the mining than among the non-mining section of the male population.

The districts comprised in the return are the lead-mining districts of Northumberland, Durham, Cumberland, Westmoreland, Yorkshire, and Lancashire. But inasmuch as the numbers of miners, and of course the numbers of deaths of miners, in some of these counties were too small, taken separately, to justify any deductions with regard to the comparative health of the mining and non-mining sections of the population, we shall only quote from the return of the death-rates as computed from the aggregate numbers of males, and of deaths of males of the two classes respectively, in all the lead-mining districts of the six counties taken together. In order to show the comparative health of the two sections of the population at the present time, the rates of mortality comprised in the return have been calculated for the three years 1860–62 inclusive; these years have been selected because the last Census was taken in 1861, the middle year of the term which renders the calculations as nearly accurate as possible. Table 6 shows the average annual rates of mortality per 1000 miners, and per 1000 males exclusive of miners, from all causes, for the several successive decennial periods of life from the age of 15 up to that of 75 years.

The figures in Table 6 show that at all ages from 15 years upwards the miners die in larger proportions than the men of the same districts

Table 6. Average annual number of deaths per 1000 lead miners, and per 1000 males exclusive of miners, from all causes, during the three years 1860–62 inclusive.

Ages	Metal miners	Males, exclusive of miners
15–25	9.53	7.57
25–35	12.38	9.19
35–45	17.64	10.13
45–55	33.11	16.18
55–65	78.34	29.38
65–75	127.52	66.10

not employed in mining, and also that this excess of mortality among the miners increases largely and progressively with increasing age, up to that period of life after which few miners continue to work underground. Thus if it be assumed that the rate of mortality among the non-mining section of the male population at each successive period of life quoted in the table is equal to 100, then the rate among miners between the ages of 15 and 25 years would be 126; between 25 and 35 years, 135; between 35 and 45 years, 174; between 45 and 55 years, 205; and between 65 and 75 years, 193.

From the return prepared by the Registrar General it also appears that this excess of mortality among miners is mainly due to the greater prevalence and fatality of pulmonary diseases among them, as compared with that among the non-mining section of the male population. Table 7 shows the average annual rates of mortality per 1000 miners, and per 1000 males exclusive of miners, from pulmonary diseases, for the several successive periods of life from the age of 15 up to that of 75 years.

With regard to Table 7, if it be again assumed that the rate of mortality from pulmonary diseases among the non-mining section of the male population at each successive decennial period of life is equal to 100, then the rate among miners between the ages of 15 and 25 years would be 88; between 25 and 35 years, 124; between 35 and 45 years, 334; between 45 and 55 years, 445; between 55 and 65 years, 574; and between 65 and 75 years, 308.

Thus it appears not only that the rate of mortality from pulmonary diseases among the lead miners in these counties is higher than that among the male inhabitants of the same districts who do not work in the mines, but also

that this excess of mortality does not begin until after the age of 25 years, when the unwholesome conditions contingent on working in the mines have had sufficient time to exercise a sensible influence on the health of the miners. The smaller rate of mortality from pulmonary diseases which will be observed to exist among miners between the ages of 15 and 25 years, as compared with that among the non-mining section of the male population at the same ages, may be presumed to arise from the very probable fact that youths with known tendency to diseases of the lungs are not usually put to labour in the mines. On the other hand, the much larger discrepancy between the rates of mortality among miners and among other males from pulmonary diseases, as compared with that between the respective rates of mortality from all causes, is undoubtedly due to the fact that exposure to the peculiar conditions attendant on their occupation causes many miners to die of pulmonary diseases who in different circumstances would have died of other complaints, and therefore the great excess of deaths from pulmonary diseases does not in the same proportion raise the general rate of mortality, although, as has been seen, it does so to a very large extent.

North Wales

The returns of mortality relating to North Wales, prepared for us by the Registrar General, have reference only to the district of Holywell. Table 8 shows a very considerable excess in the rates of mortality from all causes among the lead miners, as compared with the

Table 7. Average annual number of deaths per 1000 lead miners, and per 1000 males exclusive of miners, from pulmonary diseases, during the three years 1860–62 inclusive.

Ages	Metal miners	Males, exclusive of miners
15–25	3.40	3.97
25–35	6.40	5.15
35–45	11.76	3.52
45–55	23.18	5.21
55–65	41.47	7.22
65–75	53.69	17.44

Table 8. Average annual number of deaths per 1000 lead miners, and per 1000 males exclusive of lead miners, from all causes, in the District of Holywell during the three years 1860–62 inclusive.

Ages	Lead miners	Males, exclusive of lead miners
15–25	6.04	7.46
25–35	15.72	10.52
35–45	18.05	12.57
45–55	25.74	15.19
55–65	55.19	28.11
65–75	86.96	75.78

other section of the male population, during the three years 1860–62 inclusive.

Assuming, as in the previous sections, that the rates of mortality among the males, exclusive of lead-miners, are represented at each period of life by 100, that among the lead miners will be represented by 81 between the ages of 15 and 25, by 149 between 25 and 35, by 144 between 35 and 45, by 169 between 45 and 55, by 196 between 55 and 65, and by 115 between 65 and 75 years.

As in the other metal-mining districts referred to in this report, so also in this district, the excess of mortality among the metal miners, over that which prevails among the other section of the male population, is mainly due to the excess of deaths from pulmonary diseases. Table 9 shows the mortality from these diseases, among the two sections of the population respectively, for each decennial period of life from the age of 15 up to 75 years.

Again, assuming the rates of mortality among the male population not engaged in lead mining to be represented at each age by 100, then that among the lead miners would be represented by 89 between the ages of 15 and 25, by 72 between 25 and 35, by 196 between 35 and 45, by 208 between 45 and 55, by 289 between 55 and 65, and by 285 between 65 and 75 years.

The excess of mortality among the lead miners of the Holywell district over that which

Table 9. Average annual number of deaths per 1000 lead miners, and per 1000 males exclusive of lead miners, from pulmonary diseases, in the District of Holywell during the three years 1860–62 inclusive.

Ages	Lead miners	Males, of lead miners
15–25	3.02	3.39
25–35	4.19	5.79
35–45	10.62	5.41
45–55	14.71	7.06
55–65	35.32	12.21
65–75	48.31	16.96

prevails among the other section of the male population is thus evidently much less striking than has been shown to be the case in the Cornish and Northern metal-mining districts, both as regards the deaths from pulmonary diseases and those from all causes. Nevertheless, the above statistics clearly indicate that the Holywell lead miners suffer from some causes of disease and premature death from which the rest of the male population are exempt. Reasoning from analogy, it is therefore but fair to presume that in this as in the other metal mining districts, the excess of mortality among the miners arises in some way from conditions incident to their occupation. (Report of Royal Commission on Condition of Miners, 1865; pp. x–xxxvi.)

NOTES ON VERRUGA PERUANA[1]

Daniel Carrión

Synonyms

Verruga de sangre.—Verruga blanda.—Verruga andícola (Dr. Salazar).—Verruga de Castilla, de zapo ó de quinua.—Verruga mular.

Definition

Verruga is an irregular, noncontagious, endemic and anemia-causing fever, chiefly characterized by pains and muscular contractions (cramps), arthralgias with infarct and more or less severe ostealgias. It produces a polymorphous eruption; it has a generally lengthy but variable cyclic course, which is not affected by treatment; and it also can give rise to numerous complications.

Etiology

The action of the verruga-generating agent is limited to the site where it emerges.

Emergence of verruga is not influenced in the slightest by age, sex, race, etc.; however, I will make the point that, just as there are resistant individuals, there are also predispositions in individuals that favor the development of verruga, and to these can be added fatigue, the weakness in some persons due to their own constitution or previous illness, and, finally, an individual's lack of acclimatization to those localities where the disease prevails.

Not even animals are immune from this disease, which appears in cattle, pigs and, most of all, horses; hence the name of verruga *mular* given to manifestations of the disease in these animals.

Symptoms

The course of this disease may be divided into four distinct stages: 1) incubation; 2) invasion, subdivided into the prodrome and the invasion proper; 3) eruption; and 4) dessication, regression or atrophy, or mortification, depending on the course taken by the verrucous tumor.

First Period: Incubation.

In our present state of knowledge it is difficult to determine accurately the boundaries of this first period; while this is true, it is no less true that this unfortunate uncertainty will be dispelled when the practice of inoculation is extended to the disease that concerns us. In spite of everything, it can be said on the basis of some observations that the period runs from 8 to 30 or 40 days.

Second Period: Invasion.

As we have already stated, this second stage comprises two subperiods, as follows:

1. Prodrome. Consisting of discomfort, dejection, curvature, lassitude, yawning and aversion to any movement, to which are sometimes added the symptoms of dyspepsia; and

2. Invasion proper. This is, as a rule, gradual, marked by an accentuation of the phenomena assigned to the prodrome, plus those described in what follows.

Pain. Bone and joint pains, rachialgia and contusive pains almost everywhere in the body are the hallmark of verruga, and also the most characteristic and constant sign of the disease from its onset.

These pains are generally rheumatoid and worsen at night. They invade the joints one by one, usually starting in a knee or one of the small joints of foot or hand. They spread and intensify in proportion to the severity of the disease, its duration, and the climate in which the victim finds himself, and it has been noted that the pains are excruciating in cold places.

The rachialgia and myalgias, which rank second among the *algias,* are at times so intense as to make some muscles rigid, which then results in torticollis, opisthotonos, and more or less permanent contracture of upper and/or lower

Source: Excerpted from Casimiro Medina, *La Verruga Peruana y Daniel A. Carrión.* Lima, Imprenta del Estado, 1886.

[1]It must be borne in mind that Carrión had not yet completed nor reviewed these notes.

limbs which, together with the arthralgias which immobilize the joints, lock victims in unnatural positions.

In the more severe cases, many patients cannot endure the pain without crying out or moaning; every worsening of the pain provokes new and vivid suffering. . . .

Now we will concern ourselves with other, no less important, symptoms which complete the characteristic picture of the period of the invasion proper.

The verrucous agent undoubtedly attacks the blood, for nutrition in those suffering from this disease is profoundly changed to the extent of producing cachexia. This is manifested by the anemia that develops at more or less galloping speed and with greater or lesser energy, depending on the individual. Unfortunately, I know of no study that has determined the total number of red cells destroyed by the etiologic agent.

The skin becomes pale and muddy; the mucosae, particularly the palpebral and gingivolabial, lose their color and become waxy.

The heart beats weakly, and in most cases a murmur of greater or lesser intensity can be heard.

Movements become languid, without energy or definition, and walking is unsteady.

There is ringing in the ears, confusion, bewilderment, and insomnia.

More or less rapid serous suffusions usually occur on many occasions.

In most cases the spleen is considerably enlarged, at times descending into the left iliac fossa (as with the patient in history No. 10); in addition, the spleen is hard and so it is easy to locate by palpation if there is no ascites. In many cases the liver is found to be infarcted.

The anemia becomes more pronounced as the disease takes its course.

Finally, during this period women experience menstrual disorders.

Third period: Eruption.

The eruption begins to appear after a period that varies between twenty days following the poisoning or invasion and six or even eight months thereafter.

The eruption begins on the limbs, face, etc., spreading immediately to the rest of the body, and invading some mucosae as well.

During this period the general symptoms improve considerably, particularly if the eruption is somewhat rapid and complete. Only the anemia may persist and increase, particularly when the hemorrhage that ensues with rupture of the verrucous tumors is repeated frequently, which is very common.

Is the eruption constant? Yes, as constant as that of other eruptive fevers, this being the most characteristic phenomenon, the most fully pathognomic symptom of the disease. It is also remarkable for its constancy, its duration, its termination and, finally, for many other particularities that I will mention hereafter.

Passing now to an examination of verrucous tumors in all their phases, I will say that, of course, their form and development and the sites at which they appear are most varied. They emerge now on the surface of the skin, now beneath it in the subcutaneous form, both varieties constituting what we could call the *external eruption* of the disease, which also includes eruptions on the surface of the mucosae, such as those of the mouth, nose and eyelid. . . .

Fourth period:

The end of the disease varies with the course taken by the tumor.

I will, therefore, say a few words about how the verrucous neoplasm terminates in its various forms.

When the eruption takes place on the surface of the skin, the tumor, as indicated above, is no larger than a pea. Having grown to this size, it remains stationary for some time and then shrinks very, very slowly, sometimes taking several months to disappear altogether. Meanwhile, its color changes from deep red to a very markedly blackish red. As the tumor regresses or reabsorbs, the skin flattens and all that can be seen are small blackish spots similar to moles, which first turn yellowish and then lose more and more color until all that is left are small whitish spots clearly distinguishable from the rest of the skin and covered with scales that soon fall away leaving no trace whatever.

As to the large tumors that break, mortify and ulcerate the skin, I will say that they are generally excised by a surgeon, an operation that is sometimes easy because the neoplasm is supported only by a thin pedicle.

The end of the disease, therefore, depends

on the disorders produced by the tumor and the general condition of the individual.

Diagnosis

The diagnosis of the disease is as difficult to establish at the onset of the disease as it is easy to confirm during the eruptive period. Indeed, we frequently see experienced practitioners mistake for an attack of malaria in its various forms, or for articular, muscular or osseous rheumatism, what is but the first or second stage of Verruga Peruana.

Of course, I will note that one of the principal difficulties in distinguishing this disease from malaria is that in most of the areas where it exists, malaria is also dominant, and the two diseases can attack together or separately.

In the present state of our knowledge, there is, in my humble view, only one fact on which we may safely rely to suspect Verruga Peruana before its eruptive phase. I refer to knowledge of the place or places where the patient has been or passed through. If we observe fever, whether continuous, remittent or intermittent, and articular and muscular pains accompanied by cramps in an individual who arrives from Matucana, for example, we can assert almost without fear of error that we are in the presence of Verruga Peruana.

However, I am forced to say that the symptomatology of the incubation stage of this fever, indigenous to our land, is still too sketchy for the practitioner who desires to establish his diagnosis from the beginning in order to apply a suitable therapy. These obscurities, these uncertainties, will be dispelled, I am sure, on the day that the practice of inoculation becomes established among us; and this inoculation would, moreover, make clear to us many other most important particularities about the innermost nature of the pathogeny of the verrucous agent.

Pathogeny

As I see it, Verruga Peruana is a miasmatic, and probably a parasitic disease. Its essential nature is still in question owing to the shortage of serious studies on the matter.

THE PRESERVATION OF HEALTH AMONGST THE PERSONNEL OF THE JAPANESE NAVY AND ARMY[1]

Baron Takaki[2]

LECTURE I.*

Mr. Treasurer and Gentlemen, I am here today owing to an invitation from the staff of St. Thomas's Hospital and Medical College. I feel that it is a great honour to me personally and also a great compliment paid to the medical profession of the Japanese empire, and I thank you all on their behalf for your cordial and friendly feeling towards us. . . .

Here I have Table 1 showing various details from 1878–1888 and I am now going to explain all the details. From 1888 to the present day there have been no important changes. In looking over this table we find the average number of general diseases during 1878, 1879, and 1880 to be just over 4327 per 1000—that is, one sailor suffered 4.32 times every year. The death-rate averaged 16.34 per 1000 and the invaliding-rate 8.75. The number of beri-beri (kak'ke) patients was 349.33 per 1000. Those who died from it averaged 7.96 and those invalided 2.45. Therefore, the number of sailors lost through death and made invalid owing to general diseases was 24.09 per 1000 and those lost through death and invaliding from beri-beri 10.43 per 1000. If we now subtract 10.43 from 24.09 only 13.66 remain. Therefore it was clear that if beri-beri could be wholly exterminated the number of losses from illness would decrease to 13.66.

From 1881 to 1883 the number of cases of illness slightly decreased. In 1884 the general aspect of the health of the navy suddenly changed for the better and the number of general diseases as well as cases of beri-beri markedly decreased. The number of general diseases was 1865.02 per 1000—that is, one person became ill 1.8 times a year. Deaths per 1000 decreased to 7.98 and invalids to 7.80.

The number of beri-beri cases averaged 127.35 per 1000. Deaths from it decreased to 1.42. Therefore, the average of deaths and invalids from general diseases decreased to 15.78 and that of beri-beri to 1.60 per 1000. Similarly in 1885 the number of general diseases decreased to 992.48 per 1000 and deaths to 7.08 per 1000. Beri-beri decreased to 5.93 per 1000 without death. So the number of deaths and invalids decreased to 12.14. In 1886 general diseases per 1000 averaged 577.46, deaths 7.43, and beri-beri 0.35, without death or invaliding. In 1887 general diseases per 1000 were 434.22, deaths 6.04, and invalids 6.15. In 1888 general diseases per 1000 averaged 400.59, deaths 7.08, and invalids 9.15. In short, the number of losses through deaths and invalids per 1000 in 1884 was 15.78, in 1885 12.14, in 1886 12.57, in 1887 12.19, and 1888 16.33. If we now compare these five years with three years from 1878 to 1880 we find a marked decrease of general diseases and disappearance of beri-beri with corresponding decrease in the loss of sailors year by year. . . .

The first time I heard of the fearful nature of beri-beri was 44 years ago. At that time guards were despatched by several Daimios to Kyoto to act as protectors of the Imperial Palace and my father being one of them stayed there for over a year. On his return he told me of the disease called beri-beri which killed many of these men. They attributed the cause to food and called a provision box the "beri-beri box." Later, in 1868, that is, in the year of the Meiji Revolution, I served for eight months in the army of Prince Shimadzu but did not see any beri-beri. As I said before, I entered the navy in 1872 and began to treat beri-beri patients for the first time. Up to May, 1875, I had seen several hundreds of beri-beri cases at the Naval Hospital. In the summer several acute cases appeared daily. Often five or six cases had to be treated at the same time and attending officers had to work very hard both day and night. At that time the beri-beri patients constituted three fourths

* **Source:** Excerpted from *Lancet*, 1369–1371, May 19, 1906.
[1] Three lectures delivered at St. Thomas's Hospital, London, on May 7th, 9th, and 11th, 1906.
[2] Director-General of the Medical Department of the Imperial Japanese Navy.

75

Table 1. Showing the general health of the navy.

Year	Strength	Cases of disease or injury	Ratio of cases per 1000 of strength	Average ratio of cases per person per annum	Died	Ratio of deaths per 1000 of strength	Invalided	Ratio of invalided per 1000 of strength	Cases of kak'ke	Ratio of cases of kak'ke per 1000 of strength	Died	Ratio of deaths per 1000 of strength	Invalided	Ratio of invalided per 1000 of strength
			All diseases and injuries						Cases of kak'ke or beri-beri					
1878	4528	17 788	3928.45	3.93	56	12.37	44	9.72	1485	327.96	32	7.07	19	4.20
1879	5031	22 426	4413.70	4.41	119	23.42	39	7.68	1978	389.29	57	11.20	8	1.57
1880	4956	22 819	4604.32	4.60	63	12.71	43	8.68	1725	348.06	27	5.45	9	1.82
1881	4641	15 766	3397.12	3.40	81	17.45	29	6.25	1163	250.59	30	6.46	16	3.45
1882	4769	12 074	2531.77	2.53	103	21.60	30	6.29	1929	404.29	51	10.69	17	3.56
1883	5346	16 380	3063.97	2.90	85	15.90	28	5.24	1236	251.20	49	9.17	4	0.75
1884	5638	10 515	1865.02	1.81	45	7.98	44	7.80	718	127.35	8	1.42	1	0.18
1885	6918	6866	992.48	0.91	49	7.08	33	4.77	41	5.93	—	—	1	0.14
1886	8475	4874	577.46	0.52	63	7.43	52	6.14	3	0.35	—	—	—	—
1887	9016	3954	434.22	0.40	55	6.04	56	6.15	—	—	—	—	—	—
1888	9184	3679	400.59	0.40	65	7.08	48	9.15	—	—	—	—	—	—

of the whole number of patients. Various forms of treatment were adopted: purgatives and digitalis for œdema, palpitation, &c.; strychnine, iron, &c., for numbness and paralysis; tincture of aconite for hyper-sensibility of muscles; and purgatives and venesection for acute cases. These forms of treatment were general and there was no definite opinion as regards the food.

Conditions being such, it became my fixed desire to discover the cause and treatment of beri-beri. But I thought that with my insufficient knowledge of medical science I could not possibly discover them, and from then on the desire to go abroad in order to fit me for attaining my object never left my thoughts even for a moment. At last, in June, 1875, the desire was fulfilled and I started for England. I reached London in July and entered St. Thomas's Hospital Medical School in October. After staying there for over five years I returned to Japan in November, 1880, and was made the director of the Tokyo Naval Hospital in December. Thus, I got an opportunity to treat beri-beri patients again. The general conditions on my return were exactly the same as before I went to England and with subsequent increase of sailors more beri-beri cases appeared. At times, when the disease was in full force, we found the hospital too small and often had to use neighbouring temples. Moreover, acute cases were many and medical officers had a very busy and hard time. Such conditions used to strike my heart cold

whenever I came to think of the future of our Empire, because, if such a state of health went on without discovering the cause and treatment of beri-beri our navy would be of no use in time of need.

As a first step towards the cause and cure of this disease I began to note the localities and seasons and to examine sailors in ships, barracks, &c., and I obtained the following facts:—
1. Beri-beri occurred mostly from the end of spring to summer, but it was not limited to the warm season, sometimes occurring during the severe cold of winter. 2. The occurrence of the disease varied in different ships, barracks, &c. 3. Even in the same ship it appeared in some stations, not in others, and was never certain. 4. It occurred from time to time without regard to the state of quarters or clothing. 5. I found out that although clothing, food, living, &c, were not quite the same in all stations, yet they were almost similar.

With these facts I could not easily discover the cause and I went on with further investigations with the following results:—1. As regards the class of patients in general, I found that sailors, soldiers, policemen, students, shop-boys, and so on, were those who suffered most. The upper class rarely became affected. 2. The people living in the same place suffered unequally—that is, some suffered and others did not. 3. Although it occurred mostly in large cities, like Tokyo, Osaka, and Kyoto, yet it sometimes appeared in smaller towns as well. Thus with such results and without discovering the cause of beri-beri the time quickly passed to the year 1882. In February of the year 1882 I was appointed the Vice-Director of the naval Medical Bureau.

About that time it was found to be necessary to provide an extra medical officer besides the usual number on board the training ships going for long cruises on account of the abundance of beri-beri cases among the men during the voyage. In 1882 there was a critical state of affairs with Korea and three warships were sent to Ninsen (Chemulpo) and Saibutsu Bay. They stayed there only 40 days but owing to shortness of hands caused by the prevalence of beri-beri among sailors the officers felt quite unfit for battle and it was a very anxious time for those in positions of responsibility because those three ships would have been of no fighting value in the critical moment. For example, in one of the ships 195 out of 330 were down with beri-beri. As a consequence I handed to the chief of the Naval Medical Bureau on June 24, 1882, a memorandum describing the facts. Following this, in August, 1882, H.I.M.S. *Fuso,* in spite of anchoring off Shinagawa Bay, had to send half of its crew ashore in turns for the treatment of beri-beri. Continuing still further, I examined the reports of the Tokyo and Yokohama naval hospitals for 1881 and found out that three-fourths of the patients had suffered from beri-beri.

In 1883 I received permission from the Minister of the Navy to examine the hygienic conditions of ships, barracks, schools, &c., belonging to the navy. I found that although working hours, clothing, dwelling-houses, &c., were similar everywhere, yet in food there was a great deal of difference. So I now asked the head of each sectional department to send me in the reports describing the details of food taken three times daily for a week. From this I discovered the following facts: 1. Nitrogenous substances contained in the food were not sufficient to make up for the amount of nitrogenous substances discharged from the body. 2. On the contrary, the food contained too much carbohydrates. If we now look into the table recognised by scientists showing the comparative amounts of nitrogen and carbon discharged daily by a fair-sized adult we shall see that carbon equals 310 grammes and nitrogen equals 20 grammes—i.e., nitrogen is to carbon as 1 is to 15.5. 3.

The food taken by our sailor showed nitrogen 1 to carbon 17–32. 4. The greater the difference in these proportions the more beri-beri occurred, and the lesser the difference the less.

After obtaining these important facts I came to think that:—1. Beri-beri is caused by the disproportion of nitrogenous and non-nitrogenous elements (nitrogen and carbon) in food—that is, the amount of the nitrogenous was insufficient and that of the non-nitrogenous excessive. 2. The symptoms of beri-beri patients are really due to these causes and the good results obtained by purgatives are due to their powers in getting rid of the abundant carbohydrates. 3. The pathological changes occurring in nerves, muscle, &c., are the result of inability of the tissues to repair the waste owing to the insufficiency of nitrogenous substances in the food and the above changes are further aggravated by the presence of the large quantity of carbohydrates in the food.

In October, 1882, I submitted a proposal to the Minister of the Navy, the late Count Kawamura, the chief object of which was to change the old dietary system. When this proposal was put forward before a meeting there was a good deal of opposition. They said that the change was too radical and instanced the great disturbances caused by the change of diet in the Italian navy some years before. They also called attention to the new system of fixing the amount of food by quality and quantity instead of by monetary value as in the old. . . .

LECTURE II.*

The Methods for Investigating the Cause of Beri-Beri.

1. As we could not discover the true origin of beri-beri in spite of examination of symptoms, pathology, &c., we must use some other means. 2. In order to examine the food necessary for nourishing the human body it is important to know the comparative scale of nutritive elements—that is, proteids, fat, carbohydrates and salts, and of carbon and nitrogen. 3. On examining the food taken by those suffering from beri-beri it is found that the proportion of these

* **Source:** Excerpted from *The Lancet*, 1451–1454, May 26, 1906.

elements is not correct. 4. The causes of this disease are due to the loss of equilibrium in the proportion of nutritive elements and also to the deficiency of a certain element—that is, the composition of food is not correct. 5. The occurrence of beri-beri due to the deficiency of a certain element—that is, proteids—is shown in the examples of the long voyages of the *Asama, Tsukuba, Ryujo,* &c. The disease does not occur if the food is well supplied; for example, it does not occur among men having a sufficient supply of food or among officers, and in voyages with long stoppages at ports and short sailings. From 1882 to 1883 when the *Ryujo* went for long voyages, the disease disappeared completely as soon as she arrived at Hawaii and was supplied with fresh articles of food. 6. High temperature, moisture, marshy air, over-crowding, hard labours, nervous exhaustion, coarse food, &c., cannot be considered the chief causes of beri-beri, because if they are the causes both Europeans and Americans ought to suffer, but on the contrary they do not. 7. On considering the question both from theoretical and practical points it seems quite reasonable therefore to suppose that the true cause of beri-beri lies in a wrong method of diet. In December, 1883, instead of the very simple rules of the previous year, I compiled a new book of instructions consisting of 77 articles and 22 blank forms, and had it used throughout the navy, with the approval of the Minister of the Navy. . . .

In 1883, after my proposal to reform the diet system on Nov. 26th, I made a great effort in order that the *Tsukuba* should go over the same route as the *Ryujo.* There was opposition to this from various points and the permission could not be obtained easily but in the end after much discussion all difficulties were overcome, except that of expense. So with the knowledge of the Minister of the Navy I consulted Hakubun Ito, Councillor of the Imperial Household, and Seigi Matsugata, the Minister of Finance, and finally obtained my object by the special allowance of 60,000 yen (about £6000) from the Treasury. Before the sailing of the *Tsukuba* a special committee for investigation was put on board and consisted of the following gentlemen: Captain S. Arichi, Lieutenant Y. Matsumara, Surgeon T. Aoki, and Paymaster N. Kataoka. The food-supply was ordered according to the new system. The vessel sailed on Feb. 2nd, 1884, and returned to Shinagawa on Nov.

16th. The result obtained was good. . . .

When the good report ("no beri-beri") of the experimental voyage of the *Tsukuba* became known the principal men in the navy for the first time began to support me in my fixed purpose. They said that they had always opposed me in their hearts and only obeyed the new regulations because they were ordered by the Minister, but they would give in now after such powerful practical proofs. In January 1885, on looking through the reports of 1884, I was greatly satisfied with the results as shown in Table 1. The number of general diseases was nearly halved and that of beri-beri was considerably decreased without a death.

On Feb. 13th, 1885, I made a new proposal for using barley and rice in equal proportion instead of rice alone and of having this adopted from March 1st, as the season of beri-beri was approaching, under the following rules—that is, from March 1st to 15th, only once at breakfast; from March 16th to 31st, twice a day, morning and evening; after April 1st, at every meal. I did this for the following reason. Although the number of cases of beri-beri in the navy decreased considerably (almost half the number in the year before) and the deaths had become almost unprecedentedly few since the formation of our navy owing to the new food regulations of February, 1884, yet the disease had not yet disappeared completely and we were obliged to make further efforts to exterminate it. Then I thought of the plan of using barley instead of bread alone, as the men could eat the former better than the bread. From this I expected better results. The Minister of the Navy ordered the addition of the word "barley" amongst the articles of food and its practical application on Dec. 21st throughout the whole navy. . . .

On March 19th, 1885, I obtained the honour of an interview with His Majesty the Emperor and presented the reports of the following items: 1. The results of beri-beri investigation on board the *Ryujo.* 2. The decrease of beri-beri from the gradual improvement of diet since Jan. 15th, 1884. 3. A great probability of exterminating the disease from the navy in a few years.

On March 28th, 1885, I for the second time spoke on the preventive measures of beri-beri before the meeting of the Hygienic Society of Japan, the chief items of which were: 1. The report of the investigation committee placed on board the training-ship *Ryujo* during its voyage in 1883. 2. The report of the experimental voyage of the *Tsukuba* in 1884. 3. The results obtained through the examination of food supplied in 1883—that is, the very small quantity of nitrogenous food as against the large amount of carbohydrates, the proportion being 1 of nitrogen to 28 of carbon. In addition, the occurrence of numerous beri-beri and general diseases during that year. 4. The good results obtained by improved diet since 1884 and the difference brought about in the proportion of nitrogen and carbon by various changes in the proportion of diet.

On August 24th, 1885, I made a proposal to change bread and biscuit for equally proportioned barley and rice which had been supplied since March of that year, because I recognised its necessity owing to the great difficulties in cooking during rough weather, even in time of peace. In November of that year my proposal was taken up and its application was at once ordered. . . .

By the beginning of 1890 the reformed diet was crowned with a complete success, and not only was the beri-beri wholly exterminated but also the general diseases became greatly decreased. In the same year the Imperial Ordinance for the reformed diet was issued and thus my original object was fulfilled.

All through these years of hardships I tried to explain my views to others by comparing the food to gunpowder. I said that the former is the primary force of the human body as is the powder in the case of the gun, so it is just as important to select the food suitable for sailors as the powder for guns and rifles.

A NEW DISEASE ENTITY IN MAN: A REPORT ON ETIOLOGIC AND CLINICAL OBSERVATIONS

Carlos Chagas

First, a quick review of the background: while working in a malaria-control campaign in the northern section of the state of Minas Gerais, we came across a large bug locally called "barbeiro," which, like the bedbug, infests homes and attacks man at night, when the lights are out.

Since this was a blood-sucking insect and such insects are of importance in human and animal pathology as vectors of disease, we examined "barbeiro" specimens and found in their hindguts a flagellate of crithidial morphology. The next step was to ascertain whether this flagellate was just a parasite of the insect or a stage in the life cycle of a parasite of vertebrates.

In almost all marmoset (*Callithrix penicillata*) specimens from the same region, we had found a parasitic trypanosome. We suspected that the "barbeiro" was the intermediate host, and the flagellate forms in its gut were stages in the life cycle of this parasite, *Trypanosoma minasense* Chagas. Because of this, we sent specimens of the bug to our director and teacher Dr. Oswaldo Cruz, who had them feed on a marmoset. Dr. Cruz succeeded in infecting this marmoset with a hemoflagellate which, being quite different in morphology from *Trypanosoma minasense*, we named *Trypanosoma cruzi*.

I studied the new parasite and found, through repeated experiments, that the insect was indeed the intermediate host, and that it took at least eight days after a bite for transmission to take place. I then made another trip to Minas Gerais for the purpose of establishing the definitive habitual host of the flagellate. The habits of the "barbeiro" suggested a situation of intradomiciliary infection; we were most impressed by the poor state of health of those who lived in infested houses. After conducting physical examinations, we found that the affected persons, especially the children, showed symptoms of a chronic disease unlike those already known and described.

These symptoms included some that occur in trypanosomiasis in man and household animals, such as generalized lymph node enlargement, edema, swollen face, etc. We then recalled many patients in that area who had sought me out earlier, sometimes with and sometimes without fever, and these patients always presented the same intense morbid condition and symptoms for which I was then unable to diagnose the cause. Their fever did not yield to quinine, and no malaria parasites could be found in their blood.

Our first breakthrough was finding a cat with parasitic hemoflagellates in a house where "barbeiros" were abundant. The first examinations of fresh blood from chronic sufferers were without result. When we were later called to treat a child in grave condition, febrile, with very pronounced swelling in the face, many enlarged nodes in different regions, and thyroid hypotrophy, we found numerous flagellates in freshly drawn blood. By staining them I was able to identify them as the same parasite transmitted by the "barbeiro" to laboratory animals.

Examination of guinea pigs inoculated with blood from this first patient revealed a development of the same process previously observed, and in the lungs we found a schizogony of eight units identical to those observed in our studies of the life cycle of *Schizotrypanum cruzi*. We obtained more positive results by inoculating guinea pigs with blood from chronic patients. This procedure established the new human-disease entity produced by *Schizotrypanum cruzi*. We communicated the results of our work to Dr. Oswaldo Cruz, the director of the Manguinhos Institute, who sent a preliminary report to the National Academy of Medicine. Due to other commitments, we could not begin the detailed clinical study of the disease until ten months after these findings.

The transmitting insect is a heteropterous hemipteran, species *megistus*, genus *Conorhinus*,

Source: *Carlos Chagas: Coletânea de Trabalhos Científicos.* Brasilia, Editora Universidade de Brasília, 1981.

family Reduvidae (sic). Dr. Arthur Neiva has recently published a detailed study of its biology in the *Memorias do Instituto Oswaldo Cruz*. *Conorhinids* invade homes, where they actively multiply, becoming exceedingly numerous and troublesome to the occupants.

The many cracks in the mud walls of primitive, grass-thatched huts are the preferred habitat of the bug, where it greatly multiplies. Even better-built houses, if they offer suitable hiding places, are infested with the bug. The bug can find shelter in the cellars of houses, and enters occupied rooms at night through cracks in the floor. On small farms in the region, we found *Conorhinids* in different outbuildings such as carriage-houses, storerooms, stables, etc. The bug frequently is found in chicken coops, where it feeds on chicken blood.

In the contaminated areas where we worked, we never found a bug-free hut among the rural population. New houses, built in remote spots far from other dwellings, are very quickly invaded by *Conorhinus*, despite the difficulty of infestation from another home.

In areas where the "barbeiro" is present, recently settled small towns are quickly infested. A case in point is Lassance, a village that came into being with the arrival of the railroad. In the first two years after it was established, infested houses were few and far between. Today, four years later, *Conorhinus* is found in almost every house of Lassance, and schizotrypanosis is rampant.

The bug bites only at night. In the dark, when the lights have been turned off, it leaves its hiding place and crawls down the walls in search of man. Adults can reach beds and mosquito nets in short flights. During the day, *Conorhinids* do not leave their hiding places. However, if a person leans for some time against a wall, he is sometimes bitten, as happened in our presence to a companion on an excursion to an infested house. We report this as a warning against prolonged contact with the walls of suspect houses.

The bug's bite is almost painless and leaves no betraying mark at the site, nor is it followed by any inflammation whatever. I watched children sleeping undisturbed while about 20 nymphs and adults of *Conorhinus* sucked blood from their bodies.

Conorhinus megistus transmits the disease as a larva, as a nymph, and as a winged insect. A young larva is no larger than a bed bug and can be carried along in laundry, luggage, etc. This fact is very important for prophylaxis, and may account for the appearance of sporadic cases in homes where "barbeiros" are not present. We should also state the possibility of the disease being transported by larvae to other parts of the country when frequent communication has been established with infested regions.

PART II

FROM THE OLD TO THE NEW EPIDEMIOLOGY

DISCUSSIONS

BUCK: The title of this section implies a transition from the "old" to the "new" epidemiology, and I am not exactly sure what we mean by transition. In the first section we discussed early works that represented the old epidemiology. By new do we mean, then, the application of epidemiology to new problems? Perhaps a good beginning for this section would be for us to try and define this transition.

NAJERA: In this second section, I see us starting in the early twentieth century, when there already was a fairly well established, scientifically sound, infectious disease epidemiology, and then moving on to a broader application of epidemiology to all health problems. This would be what I would call the difference between the "old" and the "new" epidemiology: the shift of interest and concern that occurred in the 1940s and 1950s.

LLOPIS: In my opinion, this transition may have peaked in the 1940s, but it had already started in the previous decades. A case in point is that, as early as 1914, Goldberger's work was more rigorously scientific, more methodologically sound, than the work of any of the people we mentioned in the historical discussion.

TERRIS: I agree with you. The truth is, if you really look at it closely, that a lot of things were already happening before the 1940s. As you mentioned, Goldberger's work on pellagra began in 1914. Even earlier, beginning in 1910, the Public Health Service in the United States did a good deal of work on occupational disease epidemiology. In the late 1920s, the Massachusetts State Legislature, responding to the concerns of the public, actually ordered the State Health Department to begin studies in chronic disease epidemiology. And the National Cancer Institute was organized in the United States in the thirties, before the war. I am sure that if you looked at England, you would find that they, too, were doing a fair amount of cancer epidemiology in the twenties and thirties, which is why Major Greenwood could include the subject in his text in 1935. We don't have any occupational health specialists here, but if we did, they would undoubtedly point out some key occupational studies. I know that Winslow and Greenburg were doing studies of occupational disease in the twenties. So there was a lot of work leading up to this transition, and what happened is that it came to fruition in the forties. It was like Pasteur and Koch. If you read carefully, you find out that all during the 1850s and 1860s there was a tremendous development of animal microbiology, and that this was the basis on which Pasteur and Koch arrived at their epoch-making discoveries.

I think we need to discuss all the factors that came together to influence the transition. For instance, I would like to comment on the ideological aspect because I think it is rather interesting. In both England and the United States there was a rediscovery of the sociological school of epidemiology. It was a rebirth of the views of Villermé, Virchow, and the others who thought there was much more to health problems than sanitation, that poverty was important. The reason they had failed to demonstrate their point was that in this century they didn't have the methodology; the movement ended up with rhetoric. It was only in the twentieth century, when sociological epidemiology developed further, that the necessary methodological tools were available to carry through the needed research.

I would like to suggest that what is happening in Latin America today—this ideological ferment of social epidemiology which is somewhat political in orientation— is, in a sense, a preparation for work. Another example is the South African school of social medicine, a group of liberal and radical young people who were very much influenced by Henry Sigerist. Unfortunately, South Africa did not have an epidemiological tradition, so they turned to sociology and anthropology. When a number of them emigrated to the United States, they had to learn their epidemiology here.

My view is that the period of transition starts as a real movement in 1943 with John Ryle. His story is a dramatic one. Here was a distinguished British professor of medicine who resigned his position as the Regius Professor at Cambridge to become the first Professor of Social Medicine at Oxford. He stated his concept of social medicine very clearly: a transition to noninfectious disease epidemiology. As I said earlier, Ryle represented a throwback to the sociological school of the nineteenth century. Like Alison in Scotland and Virchow in Germany, he believed that disease is caused by poverty and other social conditions. The British school in the forties thought that there must be something in society that causes infectious diseases. It was this simple logic that led to the shift in epidemiology from the study of infectious diseases to the study of noninfectious diseases.

Now we are concerned with the epidemiology of injuries, with occupational diseases, with environmental hazards, and we are beginning to use epidemiology to evaluate the validity of clinical procedures and the effectiveness of health services. There has been a tremendous growth in epidemiology, and I think that this book has to give a sense of all this change, development, and expansion.

BUCK: I would like to go back one generation before Ryle, to a work whose content would be very appropriate. I am thinking of Major Greenwood, who preceded Bradford Hill at the London School of Hygiene. In 1935, he published a book called *Epidemics and Crowd Diseases*, and that book not only contains chapters on tuberculosis and other contagious diseases of great concern, but also chapters on cancer and psychological causes of illness. Greenwood made it clear that epidemiological concepts were transferable from one kind of disease to another.

TERRIS: You are right about Major Greenwood; the movement had already started in the thirties.

I mentioned Ryle because it was such a dramatic thing, one of the outstanding clinicians of Great Britain deciding to leave clinical medicine to work in epidemiology. It was unheard of. I might add, as a postscript, the curious irony that many years later, Richard Doll, one of the world's outstanding epidemiologists, was appointed Regius Professor of Medicine at Oxford. Isn't that a marvelous turnabout?

NAJERA: Defining a transition period is very complicated. It started long before the forties and developed quite slowly. We should also try to address the reasons behind Ryle's change of mind. I think the transition came as a consequence of looking at health problems comprehensively. People like Ryle, who had a comprehensive knowledge of medicine, and people who knew statistics started to realize that the social aspects of most diseases were more important than either the specific agent that caused them, or whether they were classified as infectious or noninfectious. I think that is what Ryle said in the preface of his book, that infectious diseases also have sociological roots. Therefore, to be a doctor he had to do social medicine; he had to consider the social factors because they were more important.

I think that the development of health services was also a major factor in the transition. This was also the major difference between the rest of Europe and England. France, Italy, Denmark, the Scandinavian countries, and everyone copied the German insurance system, but the British developed their own. For centuries, England has had a tradition of providing services for everyone that, in my opinion, no other country has had. This tradition probably stemmed from the fact that Henry VIII took for the state the social responsibilities that the church used to have. Also, statistics developed in England around the seventeenth century. They were called "political arithmetic," and they were a way to use mathematics to make information available to the state, to the ruling power. And so, the use of statistics as a way to evaluate health conditions (which started with Petty and Graunt who were the first to look at mortality) prompted people to think that the state should provide health care for everybody. From there, people went on to suggest that the state, the government, be organized in ministries, including a ministry of health. Of course, these ideas weren't fully developed until later, but this is where one sees the earliest signs of the concept that the state has to care for the health of everybody.

The socialist movement in England was also different from the socialist movement in the rest of Europe. You see, I believe that Bismarck introduced the health insurance system in Germany not as a means of developing social services, but as a way of curtailing the development of social ideology. John Peter Frank had done the same a century before. But in England, the development of health services was profoundly rooted in a social ideology. In this sense, British politics played an important role in the development of health services by establishing participation by the people much earlier than in other countries of Europe. One could say that this political development started in Spain, but that the Catholic Church prevented it from continuing. That is why neither Spain nor France continued to develop along these lines, whereas England did. The English health service development began a long time ago and continued unabated. This is probably why, although health services in other European countries may have been comprehensive by the beginning of this century, the way in which they developed in England was different.

Another influencing factor which should be considered in the early twentieth century is the Russian Revolution. The Russians also developed, for the first time in their history, a comprehensive health service. What Semashko, the Soviet Union and the world's first minister of health, did in 1918 was closely watched and commented on by radicals in Europe. In 1919, as a result of what was happening in the Soviet Union, England improved its health services by reorganizing its Ministry of Health. So, my contention is that the development of public health services greatly influenced the transition in epidemiology and that this, too, is probably what sets England and the United States apart from the rest of Europe. A country's political development serves as background.

Spain is somewhere in between, because at the beginning of the twentieth century it was influenced by the Rockefeller Foundation and the development of public health services along American or English lines. In 1924, Spain established its National School of Public Health, one of the first in Europe (the second, I believe, after the London School of Hygiene), and introduced a public health component into its already comprehensive rural medical care network. A real school of thought in epidemiology started there between the late 1920s and the Spanish Civil War in the late 1930s. That was quite a development. This could help explain why there is more epidemiology in Spain than in many other countries in Europe.

BUCK: Going back to the comments on Ryle, I feel I should point out that John Cassel's work is another influential example of the important principle that a variety of diseases can have a common cause. I think that several of his papers were landmarks in the sense that they made that point and illustrated it with fairly convincing evidence.

TERRIS: I have often puzzled over why it was England that pioneered in the noninfectious diseases. Why not Sweden, where the problems of noninfectious disease were felt earlier because of an aging population. Yet Sweden never developed this field. The big development was in Britain and the United States. The question is why, and I am not sure I have all the answers to that. I once discussed this with Abe Lilienfeld, who thought that it occurred because of the development of vital statistics in England. My own interpretation is that political factors are important. The reason the movement began in Britain, and it is difficult to say why it did not happen elsewhere, was that much of the leadership of the British movement for social medicine was influenced by labor and socialist ideology. Major Greenwood was a founding member of the Socialist Medical Association (SMA) in 1930; Richard Doll was an active member; and Ryle himself had close ties to the SMA. Jerry Morris was certainly pro-labor. J.A.H. Lee once told me at an International Epidemiological Association meeting in Yugoslavia that those who went into social medicine in Great Britain fulfilled at least two of three criteria: one, they were pro-labor; two, they were Scots; and three, they had done something else before going into medicine. I do not know if this is true, but he was making the point that the sociological orientation really came out of a political consciousness. This was also true to some extent in the United States, but more so in Britain. Why it did not happen in the rest of Europe would be the subject of a long discussion.

Now, these were not new ideas. Alison, a Scottish epidemiologist at the time of Farr and Chadwick who was very critical of Chadwick's work, agreed with Virchow, Villermé, and others of the sociological school of the 1840s and 1850s in Europe. They all believed that disease was not just caused by emanations, bad sanitation, miasma; it was also caused by poverty, the miserable social conditions. The difference, as I have said before, is that in the nineteenth century they didn't have the methodological tools to get at the specific agents. It is not enough to come up with the general statement that society is the cause of disease. I keep hearing that all diseases are social, and that if the social order could be changed then disease would disappear. We already know that this is not true, and this rhetoric has to be replaced by specific research and action. In the 1840s Virchow said it was the old reactionary system and the attendant misery of the peasants that caused the epidemics of typhoid fever in Silesia. This was true, but it wasn't enough to say that it was the social system; he could not get at the specific agents. After all, in the 1840s, they did not have the background of a hundred years of science, statistics, and methods in epidemiology. In the twentieth century they were able to find specific factors such as cigarettes, toxins, and saturated fats.

BUCK: Just to add a comment to the idea of the specifics, I think it is important to stress that the theory was very general and evidence was hard to come by. The specifics are just now beginning to flower, especially in the area of psychoimmunology. Cassel, for example, looked at the effects of abrupt cultural dislocation on such physiological specifics as blood pressure and blood lipids. He recognized that there could be even more subtle influences than the purely dietary. That was one of the beginnings, which happened to be contemporaneous with Seeley work on stress. People then began to go back to the physiological work of Walter Cannon and to see it in an epidemiological context for the first time.

As you say, the notion that societal forces cause disease does not necessarily mean that a simple reordering of something as vague as society would provide the solution. In other words, the term "societal causes of disease" has to be refined so that it includes specific mechanisms and specific individual responses, perhaps even analogous to the immune reactions to infectious disease.

NAJERA: Isn't it also possible that an important factor in the transition rested with the development of trade unions in England, since they developed alongside the socialism of labor? What I think played an important part in the shift toward chronic or noninfectious diseases, was that when the union members started to demand their rights, their health problems were not chickenpox nor any of the infectious diseases with the exception of, perhaps, cholera. Consequently, people started concentrating on those diseases that affected adults, or almost only adults, since infectious diseases were mostly restricted to children. This is what I think caused noninfectious diseases to gain importance. And this, in turn, allowed Ryle and others to consider the importance of sociological factors even for infectious diseases.

BUCK: How much was the transition to chronic disease epidemiology, apart from the obvious rising importance of chronic disease, due to the fact that a lot of these physician-epidemiologists of the period had been internists?

NAJERA: It is possible that this was a factor, but I think that the key was this radical or socialist ideological thrust, and that its impact was the extent of health services coverage that began with the insurance system.

Health service coverage, along with the sanitation movement of the nineteenth century, seemed to be enough. The nineteenth century sanitation theory postulated that providing safe water was enough sanitation for disease control. At the same time, the workers' conditions forced the expansion of health coverage to include all diseases. At first, only accidents were covered, but by the forties, most diseases were covered by the insurance system. By the twenties or thirties, those countries that had better services, like England, looked beyond infectious diseases.

TERRIS: I don't agree. Most countries with highly developed insurance systems didn't do anything in this area. Sweden didn't experience this change, neither did France or Germany. Yet the United States, which had no government health insurance, played a leading role in the development of noninfectious disease epidemiology.

NAJERA: Yes, but England did the most. They started the whole thing.

TERRIS: They may have started the movement, but I don't think it was because of insurance. If this were true, it should have happened all over Europe, but it did not. In Germany, national health insurance for all diseases started in 1884. It began in England in 1911, and included only wage earners, not their families. It was a limited program. The German system was more comprehensive.

No, it wasn't insurance that led to the new epidemiology. The European countries which had insurance did not develop chronic disease epidemiology. It happened in England and the United States for reasons which had nothing to do with insurance but had a great deal to do with an independent public health movement as exemplified both by the School of Hygiene in London and the Public Health Service in the United States. It had nothing to do with medical care insurance. If it had, why didn't it develop in the Soviet Union? They had a comprehensive national health service which covered all diseases, and yet they did not develop chronic disease epidemiology. And that was true of the other socialist countries.

NAJERA: Perhaps in the Soviet Union the system evolved too early— it was at the beginning of the century. And the other socialist countries followed the Soviet Union's model.

TERRIS: No, I think the reason is very different. What the socialist countries have done is to develop a very powerful medical care system which has come to dominate the health services. Why did the movement for noninfectious disease epidemiology occur essentially in England and the United States? I believe the reason it did not happen elsewhere in Europe was that the health services were all clinically dominated. There was no strong independent tradition of epidemiology and public health. This was true of Sweden, France, Germany, the Soviet Union—all of Europe, both East and West. Medicine overshadowed public health. But then why did it happen in England, which also was dominated by clinical medicine except for the London School of Hygiene? Remember the field was called social medicine; the movement for noninfectious disease epidemiology developed within the medical schools.

There are two other issues, two revolutions in thinking, which I think may also have influenced this transition. The first was the discovery that infection is not the same as disease, that there are inapparent infections. Early in this century, Chapin got rid of fumigation in the United States because he pointed out that epidemiology teaches us that there is no use in fumigating. Disease is spread mainly by healthy carriers, not by cases. That was a tremendous leap forward, based on the understanding that infection is not synonymous with disease. The second big revolution was the discovery—which resulted from mass X-ray surveys and other screening procedures—that disease and illness are not synonymous. Through X rays we found out that people could have a chest full of disease and yet look perfectly healthy, without illness or symptoms. Another example is the Pap smear: a woman seems perfectly healthy but is found to have carcinoma in situ.

BUCK: You could say the same for hypertension.

TERRIS: Well, you can argue whether hypertension is a disease. But I think that those two discoveries were terribly important in the way we think about the natural history of disease. Our concept of disease was changed by microbiology and epidemiology, by mass surveys and screening. The whole idea of finding disease before it resulted in illness was a discovery of the twentieth century.

BUCK: I work a lot with academic people who practice family medicine, and, of course, they have opened my eyes to the fact that a substantial part of what the primary care physician treats is not even a diagnosable condition. I do not mean it is imaginary; it is genuine enough ill health. It just does not fit our mode of disease classification at all, but is much more compatible with the psychosocial taxonomy. This, of course, takes us back to Ryle, Cassel, and the others.

TERRIS: Going back to the transition, in the United States the schools of public health succeeded in making the change. When I studied at the Johns Hopkins School of Hygiene in 1943, not a single noninfectious disease was mentioned in the course in epidemiology. This was the country where Goldberger had done his classic studies on pellagra, but his work was never discussed at Hopkins then. It was only infectious disease that was studied. But now epidemiology at Hopkins is concerned primarily with noninfectious diseases, perhaps too much so. The same was true of medical care. In 1943 we had all of three sessions on medical care by a visiting lecturer, while now this area dominates the field of health administration at Hopkins. The same transition took place in all of the United States schools of public health.

BUCK: We were wondering why England seems to have been ahead. When I was taking my D.P.H. at the London School of Hygiene in 1950–1951, we had chronic disease epidemiology, we had public health administration, and we had what I guess you would call medical care topics, but we had no laboratories in bacteriology. They had already made the switch by 1950. There was almost nothing that came up later in North America that they had not forecast for me in the London School of Hygiene.

It is also necessary to recognize that statistics certainly helped to influence this transition. But, as you say, once the political momentum got rolling, the London School of Hygiene was to medicine what the London School of Economics was to some other fields. They are only about four blocks apart. There was an *avant garde* spirit there which went beyond the political side of medicine and into the epidemiological side. You see, Bradford Hill, Doll, and Donald Reid already were working in the Department of Epidemiology and Medical Statistics in 1950; they weren't in any medical school. Most of the medical schools in London were small and none of them at that time had a department of preventive medicine. They did not want to, I am quite sure. They were strictly clinical, hospital schools, and they made little attempt to teach anything in the line of public health. Nobody was worried about that because the big positions in public health could be taken by the bright young people who were being attracted into the London School of Hygiene.

TERRIS: In their epidemiologic studies, as I recall, the British worked very closely with the health departments. They did not have money, like we had in the United States, to set up their own studies, so they had to go to the health department of the hospital for their study populations.

This section should emphasize that in this transition, epidemiology moved from concentrating exclusively on infectious diseases to looking at all disease and injury, even "positive" health. In other words, that this transition resulted in the expansion of epidemiology. Methodological problems were being solved on the way, and they are not all solved as yet, by any means. Confounding variables still confound us. The important point was the shift in interest and concern to a whole new area. Epidemiology stopped being limited to infectious disease and became concerned with all the factors that influence the health of populations. And other than the deficiency theory of disease which, as mentioned earlier, was first developed by Casimir Funk, in general it was Great Britain and the United States that developed noninfectious disease epidemiology.

Take cigarette smoking and lung cancer. The first papers appeared in the United States early in 1950, when Wynder and Graham, and Levin, Goldstein, and Gerhardt published their work in the *Journal of the American Medical Association*. Then, in England, in September of the same year, Doll and Hill's paper appeared in the *Lancet*. That was the starter gun for noninfectious disease epidemiology. It developed almost simultaneously in the United States and Great Britain. These two countries became the center, and from there noninfectious disease epidemiology began to spread everywhere.

My theory about why it happened first in England and the United States and not in the rest of Europe is that in other countries they had no public health as an independent discipline. They never worked with statisticians, they never developed groups of interdisciplinary teams. In England, the London School of Hygiene was the focal point of the epidemiologic revolution: Major Greenwood had been both an epidemiologist and a statistician; they had epidemiologists like Richard Doll, Jerry Morris, and Donald Reid, and statisticians like Bradford Hill and Peter Armitage. Theirs was an interdisciplinary group made up of more than just physicians. And the United States, too, had such a powerful group of epidemiologists coming out of the Public Health Service: Rosenau, Goldberger, McCoy, Anderson, Frost, and many others. There was a fantastic growth of epidemiology in the United States; that is why the United States became a leader in this field.

NAJERA: This is a good point. In other countries there was no true *public* health in the sense of a discipline with profound community objectives.

TERRIS: I must say that I am biased on this question, because I am convinced of the need for both an independent public health movement and for schools of public health. I want to get the field out from under the medical milieu; it gets stifled in the medical profession. It has to be multidisciplinary, even though physicians play a tremendous role.

BUCK: I could propose another theory to you: that it is almost chance that determined in which country epidemiology flourished. Maybe it wasn't the things you were mentioning about politics and so on. It may be that it was a kind of rare phenomenon that arose in a few places, akin to a genetic mutation. Seriously, though, I am not sure we have the answer.

TERRIS: Well, think of it. There was a tremendous need for noninfectious disease epidemiology because of the aging population, and because infectious diseases were being conquered. It became very clear that noninfectious diseases were the major problems.

BUCK: If we take that tack, I see no problem with it. If we limit ourselves to defining the transition as the application of epidemiology to noninfectious diseases, with the methodological implications of that switch, then I think we are on solid ground. But if we try to account for it rather than just to describe it, we may be over our heads.

TERRIS: But it is very important to discuss this whole question. I think the future depends on this. We now see a retrogressive movement in the world. The medical profession is trying to recoup its fortunes. That is why we have clinical epidemiology; they are trying to stop this development of prevention and public health. Europe was held back because it was under the domination of physicians; they had no independent epidemiology and no public health. I'm willing to take the position that this is what really happened.

NAJERA: If you begin with the last century, there is a logical flow when you trace where and why public health started, how it developed, and why some countries were left behind.

TERRIS: Why are the Latin American countries now becoming interested in noninfectious disease? It's very simple. Heart disease is the leading cause of death in 28 countries of the Americas, cerebrovascular disease in 3, and cancer in 1, compared with diarrhea and enteritis in only 5, and influenza and pneumonia in only 2. Injuries are second in Costa Rica and fourth in Mexico. Latin American countries now have the same problems as the industrial nations. That is why they are becoming more interested in the noninfectious diseases.

BUCK: Leaving that aside for the moment, couldn't you still argue that the new epidemiology developed in countries in which noninfectious diseases first began to rise in prominence?

TERRIS: Not really. If that were the case, France and Sweden should have been the first because they had the most old people.

BUCK: I think it's a multicausal thing. I don't think there is a single explanation. I think, first, that the rise in noninfectious diseases had to occur. Second, as you are saying, there had to be some structure for encouraging this new interest. I am wondering, in many of these countries that went ahead, if that structure that had served them very well during the infectious disease era—the Public Health Service being an example in the United States—was for some reason flexible enough to take on and lead in the new issues. Now, I am not sure what the British counterpart was. It may have been the School of Hygiene and Tropical Medicine. So I am putting it to you that the countries which had both the early rise of chronic diseases and the structure would perhaps be the leaders.

TERRIS: I agree. That is true. It's both. They had the problem and they had the structure, the capability to deal with it.

You know what is crucial in the whole thing? I am now convinced that it was the collaboration of epidemiologists and statisticians. At the London School of Hygiene and Tropical Medicine they had Doll and Hill, and Major Greenwood himself was both epidemiologist and statistician. In the United States Harold Dorn set up a statistical unit at the National Cancer Institute which included half-a-dozen of the most brilliant young statisticians in the country— including Jerry Cornfield and Nathan Mantel—who were put to work to develop the methodology.

BUCK: If we attribute what happened in England to their School of Hygiene and Tropical Medicine can we find any counterpart institutions in Germany and France?

TERRIS: No, all they had were medical schools. They didn't do epidemiology. It was mainly legal medicine.

LLOPIS: I agree. For example, in France they tended to look at demographic problems, and statistical work was, therefore, mostly related to demography. They were always concerned with maintaining a demographic balance with neighboring countries. So, when epidemiology began its development in the 1950s, they used statistics and demography as a starting point. They had no counterpart institutions.

NAJERA: That's right; they didn't exist. If you look at some of the German textbooks of epidemiology, they deal exclusively with infectious diseases: they explore all modes of transmission, including 20 or more ways to spread respiratory disease. As an aside, I would like to suggest that we do not use the term "chronic," but instead use the term noninfectious, because tuberculosis is a chronic disease and so are syphilis and leprosy.

BUCK: In 1979, Elizabeth Barrett-Connor wrote a paper on the epidemiology of infectious and noninfectious disease, where she made the point that the difference between the epidemiology of infectious and noninfectious diseases is not that big, since we have one epidemiology that allows us to study both kinds of disease. I think that this idea, that the difference is more quantitative than qualitative, is an important one, because it shows how the epidemiological transition was possible. Part of her argument also was that noninfectious disease epidemiologists tend to look down on infectious disease epidemiologists. Everyone notices, for example, that the infectious disease papers rarely come first in the *American Journal of Epidemiology*.

TERRIS: It didn't use to be that way.

BUCK: Well, it's been that way for about 10 years. I notice it every month. Barrett-Connor pleaded for a stop to this two-class system, pointing out that infectious disease epidemiology takes some know-how too.

TERRIS: We should include her paper in this section, perhaps as the last paper, to say, "look, you have made the transition, but don't go too far." Because what has happened is that most of the current American textbooks of epidemiology do not even discuss infectious disease.

BUCK: The real truth of the matter is that the complexity of the epidemiology of some infectious diseases such as leishmaniasis, schistosomiasis, and leprosy makes the epidemiology of cancer and heart disease look simple. Actually, couldn't tuberculosis represent the transitional disease, the one infection that had so much in common with noninfectious chronic disease that it required chronic disease methods?

CONSIDERATIONS ON PELLAGRA

Joseph Goldberger

THE ETIOLOGY OF PELLAGRA*

The writer desires to invite attention to certain observations recorded in the literature of pellagra, the significance of which appears entirely to have escaped attention.

At the National Conference on Pellagra held in Columbia, S. C., November 3, 1909, Siler and Nichols in their paper on the "Aspects of the pellagra problem in Illinois" state that certain facts "would seem to indicate that the exciting cause of the disease is present within the institution" (Peoria State Hospital), and add that "at the same time no nurses, attendants, or employees have shown the disease."

Manning, medical superintendent of the asylum at Bridgetown, Barbados, on the same occasion, in arguing against the identity of a disease that he called psilosis pigmentosa with pellagra, but which undoubtedly is this disease, states that he had never seen it develop in an attendant.

At the same conference, Mobley, from the Georgia State Sanitarium, in the course of his discussion of the relation of pellagra to insanity, presents data showing that at the Georgia State Sanitarium a considerable proportion of the cases of pellagra develop in inmates who have been residents therein for considerable periods, mentioning one case in an inmate after 10 years residence. In this connection he remarks, what must have struck him, as it no doubt must have appealed to Siler and Nichols at the Illinois institution, as a curious fact, that "so far as can be ascertained there has never been a case of pellagra to develop among the nurses, white or colored, while employed as such in the Georgia State Sanitarium."

Sambon (1910) in his "Progress report" states that in Italy "no precautions are ever taken to avoid propagation of the malady in any of the pellagrosari, locande sanitarie, hospitals, insane asylums, and other institutions in which very numerous pellagrins are collected every year.

* **Source:** *Public Health Reports* 29:1683–1686, 1914.

Long experience has taught that there is no danger whatever of transmission from the sick to the healthy in any collective dwelling within urban precincts."

Sambon's statement is confirmed by Lavinder, who in a personal communication states that on careful inquiry while visiting a large pellagrosario near Venice, one in which some 300 to 500 pellagrins are constantly present and cared for by a large number of Sisters of Charity and other employees, he was assured that no employee had ever developed the disease at the institution.

The results of personal inquiry at some of our State asylums in which pellagra occurs confirm the reported observations above cited. Thus at the South Carolina State Hospital for the Insane, where Babcock (1910 Ann. Rept.) states that cases of pellagra develop in patients who have been there for years, no case so far as the writer was able to ascertain has occurred in the nurses or attendants. It may be of interest to recall in this connection that in his annual report for 1913 Babcock states that a total of about 900 pellagrins had been admitted to his institution during the preceding six years.

At the State hospital for the insane at Jackson, Miss., there have been recorded 98 deaths from pellagra for the period between October 1, 1909, and July 1, 1913. At this institution cases of institutional origin have occurred in inmates. Dr. J. C. Herrington, assistant physician and pathologist, told me at the time of my visit of a case in an inmate after 15 and in another after 20 years' residence at the institution. No case, so far as I was able to learn, has developed in a nurse or attendant, although since January 1, 1909, there have been employed a total of 126 who have served for periods of from 1 to 5 years.

In considering the significance of the foregoing observations it is to be recalled that at all of these institutions the ward personnel, nurses, and attendants spend a considerable proportion of the 24 hours, on day or night duty, in close association with the inmates; indeed, at many of these institutions, for lack of a separate building or special residence for the nurses, these live right in the ward with and of necessity under exactly the same conditions as the inmates.

It is striking therefore that although many inmates develop pellagra after varying periods of institutional residence, some even after 10 to 20 years of institutional life, and therefore it seems permissible to infer, as the result of the operation within the institution of the exciting cause or causes, yet nurses and attendants living under identical conditions appear uniformly to be immune. If pellagra be a communicable disease, why should there be this exemption of the nurses and attendants?

To the writer this peculiar exemption or immunity is inexplicable on the assumption that pellagra is communicable. Neither "contact" in any sense nor insect transmission is capable of explaining such a phenomenon, except on the assumption of an incubation or latent period extending over 10 to 20 years. In support of such an assumption there exists, so far as the writer is aware, no satisfactory evidence.

The explanation of the peculiar exemption under discussion will be found, in the opinion of the writer, in a difference in the diet of the two groups of residents. At some of the institutions there is a manifest difference in this regard; in others none is apparent.

The latter would seem to be a fatal objection to this explanation, but a moment's consideration will show that such is not necessarily the case. The writer, from personal observation has found that although the nurses and attendants may apparently receive the same food, there is nevertheless a difference in that the nurses have the privilege—which they exercise—of selecting the best and the greatest variety for themselves. Moreover, it must not be overlooked that nurses and attendants have opportunities for supplementing their institutional dietary that the inmates as a rule have not.

In this connection brief reference must be made to two other epidemiological features of pellagra. It is universally agreed (1) that this disease is essentially rural, and (2) associated with poverty. Now there is plenty of poverty and all its concomitants in all cities, and the question naturally arises why its greater predilection for rural poverty? What important difference is there between the elements of poverty in our slums and those of poverty in rural dwellers? It is not the writer's intention to enter at this time into a detailed discussion of these questions; he wishes to point out one difference only. This difference relates to the dietary. Studies of urban and rural dietaries (Wait—Office of Experiment Stations, Bull. 221, 1909) have shown that on the whole the very poor of cities have a more varied diet than the poor in rural sections. "Except in extreme cases, the city poor . . . appear to be better nourished than the mountaineers" of Tennessee.

With regard to the question of just what in the dietary is responsible, the writer has no opinion to express. From a study of certain institutional dietaries, however, he has gained the impression that vegetables and cereals form a much greater proportion in them than they do in the dietaries of well-to-do people; that is, people who are not, as a class, subject to pellagra.

The writer is satisfied that the consumption of corn or corn products is not essential to the production of pellagra, but this does not mean that corn, the best of corn, or corn, products, however nutritious and however high in caloric value they may be, are not objectionable when forming of themselves or in combination with other cereals and with vegetables, a large part of the diet of the individual.

In view of the great uncertainty that exists as to the true cause of pellagra, it may not be amiss to suggest that pending the final solution of this problem it may be well to attempt to prevent the disease by improving the dietary of those among whom it seems most prevalent. In this direction I would urge the reduction in cereals, vegetables, and canned foods that enter to so large an extent into the dietary of many of the people in the South and an increase in the fresh animal food component, such as fresh meats, eggs, and milk.

It may be of interest to add that intensive studies along the lines so strongly suggested by the observations above considered are being prosecuted by several groups of workers of the United States Public Health Service.

THE CAUSE AND PREVENTION OF PELLAGRA*

Because of the prevalence of pellagra throughout a considerable part of the United

---

* **Source:** *Public Health Reports*, 29:2354–2357, 1914.

States, and the fact that this disease has so far baffled all attempts to ascertain its cause and means of prevention, the following letter from Surg. Joseph Goldberger, in charge of the Government's pellagra investigations, is of interest.

Evidence seems to be accumulating to show that pellagra is due to the use of a dietary in which some essential element is reduced in amount or from which it is altogether absent, or to the use of a dietary in which some element is present in injurious amount.

UNITED STATES PUBLIC HEALTH SERVICE,
Washington, September 4, 1914.

The SURGEON GENERAL,
Public Health Service.

SIR: As indicated in my progress report of June 5, 1914, the primary object of the pellagra studies that are being conducted under my general direction is the determination of the essential cause of the disease.

Although pellagra has been known and studied abroad for nearly two centuries, not only is its essential cause not known, but the broad question of whether it is to be classed either as a dietary or as a communicable (contagious or infectious) disease has never been satisfactorily determined.

Abroad, the spoiled-maize theory of Lombroso has for many years been the dominating one. Its adequacy, however, has on various grounds been repeatedly questioned.

In the United States, with the progressive and alarming increase in the prevalence of the disease, there has developed both in the lay and in the medical mind the opinion that pellagra is an infectious disease. This opinion has received important support, first, from the Illinois Pellagra Commission and, second, from the Thompson-McFadden Commission (Siler, Garrison, and MacNeal). In planning our investigations, therefore, due consideration was given to these two distinct possibilities, and the problem was attacked from both points of view.

From the point of view that we might be dealing with an infection, a comprehensive series of inoculations in the monkey was begun last fall by Drs. C. H. Lavinder and Edward Francis. Although every kind of tissue, secretion, and excretion from a considerable number of grave and fatal cases was obtained and inoculated in every conceivable way into over a hundred rhesus monkeys, the results have so far been negative.

At my suggestion Dr. Francis is making a culture study of the blood, secretions, and excretions of pellagrins by the newer anaerobic methods. This has been in progress about six weeks, but has so far given only negative results.

Epidemiologic studies were begun and have been in progress at the Georgia State Sanitarium in immediate charge of Dr. David G. Willets, and at an orphanage in Jackson, Miss., in immediate charge of Dr. C. H. Waring. These studies have brought out facts of the very greatest significance.

In a paper published in the Public Health Reports of June 26, 1914, I called attention to certain observations which appear inexplicable on any theory of communicability. These observations show that although in many asylums new cases of pellagra develop in inmates even after 10, 15, and 20 years' residence, clearly indicating thereby that the cause of the disease exists and is operative in such asylums, yet at none has any one of the employees contracted the disease, though living under identical environmental conditions as the inmates, and many in most intimate association with them.

In order to obtain precise data bearing on these observations, Dr. Willets is making a careful study of the records of the Georgia State Sanitarium. These show that of 996 patients admitted during 1910—excluding those that died, were discharged during their first year, or had pellagra on admission or within a year of admission—there remained at the institution after one year 418, and of this number 32, or 7.65 percent, have developed pellagra since that time. Of the present employees of this asylum, 293 have been in more or less intimate association with pellagrins and have lived in substantially the same or in identical environment as the asylum inmates for at least one year. If pellagra had developed among these employees at the same rate as it has among the inmates, then 22 of them should have the disease. As a matter of fact not a single one has it.

The studies at the orphanage at Jackson show that on July 1, 1914, of 211 orphans 68, or 32 percent, had pellagra.

The distribution of these cases with respect to age developed the remarkable fact that practically all of the cases were in children between the ages of 6 and 12 years, of whom in consequence over 52 percent were afflicted. In the group of 25 children under 6 years of age there were two cases and in the group of 66 children over 12 years of age there was but one case. Inasmuch as all live under identical environmental conditions, the remarkable exemption of the group of younger and that of the older children is no more comprehensible on the basis of an infection than is the absolute immunity of the asylum employees.

A minute investigation has been made at both institutions of all conceivable factors that might possibly explain the striking exemption of the groups indicated. The only constant difference discoverable relates exclusively to the dietary. At both institutions those of the exempt group or groups were found to subsist on a better diet than those of the affected groups. In the diet of those developing pellagra there was noted a disproportionately small amount of meat or other animal protein food, and consequently the vegetable food component, in which corn and sirup were prominent and legumes relatively inconspicuous elements, forms a disproportionately large part of the ration. Although other than this gross defect no fault in the diet is appreciable, the evidence clearly incriminates it as the cause of the pellagra at these institutions. The inference may therefore be safely drawn that pellagra is not an infection, but that it is a disease essentially of dietary origin; that is, that it is caused in some way such as, for example, by the absence from the diet of essential vitamins, or possibly, as is suggested by Meyer and Voegtlin's work, by the presence in the vegetable-food component of excessive amounts of poison such as soluble aluminum salts.

One-sided eccentric diets such as were consumed by the affected groups above referred to are in the main brought about by economic conditions. Poverty and the progressive rise in the cost of food oblige the individual, the family, and the institution to curtail the expensive elements—meat, milk, eggs, legumes—of the diet and to subsist more and more largely, especially in winter, on the cheaper cereal (corn), carbo-hydrate (sirup, molasses), and readily procurable vegetables and fats ("sow belly"). In the well-to-do, more or less well-recognizable eccentricities of taste may cause the individual,

without himself realizing it, to subsist on a one-sided or eccentric diet. Somewhat similar eccentricities of taste are more or less common in the insane, some of whom, indeed (as the demented), because of apathy and indifference, will not eat at all. These, for the most part included in the "untidy" class, require special care in feeding. The poorer the institution, the fewer and of lower grade is likely to be its attendant personnel and therefore the greater the danger that these very trying and troublesome types of inmates will receive inadequate attention, and so be improperly (one-sidedly) fed. It has repeatedly been noted by observers that at insane asylums the "untidy" (the group in which my observations show scurvy and beriberi most likely to develop) were the most afflicted with pellagra. By some this supposed excessive susceptibility is explained as dependent on the untidiness which favors filth infection. The true explanation, however, is that both the untidiness and the supposed excessive susceptibility of these inmates are primarily dependent on the apathy and indifference typical of most of this group. The deteriorated mental condition causing apathy and indifference results not only in untidiness of person, but passively or actively in an eccentricity in the diet. I believe that in this, in conjunction with a diet admittedly low in the animal protein component we have the explanation of the excessive prevalence of the disease at the Peoria State Hospital, a hospital almost all of whose inmates in 1909 were of the "hopeless, untidy, incurable" class, drawn from the other Illinois institutions.

While confident of the accuracy of our observations and of the justice of our inferences, there is nevertheless grave doubt in my mind as to their general acceptance without some practical test or demonstration of the correctness of the corollary, namely, that no pellagra develops in those who consume a mixed, well-balanced, and varied diet, such, for example, as the Navy ration, the Army garrison ration, or the ration prescribed for the Philippine Scouts.

Respectfully,
Jos. GOLDBERGER,
Surgeon in Charge of Pellagra Investigations.

CANCER AND OTHER CHRONIC DISEASES IN MASSACHUSETTS

George H. Bigelow[1] and Herbert L. Lombard[2]

THE PROBLEM AND OUR CONCLUSIONS

The problem of chronic disease will not be downed. Health officers, legislators and physicians may prefer to turn their backs on it, vaguely hoping that it will solve itself as sewage-burdened streams were expected to purify themselves. ("Let Nature take its course!") But the burden of pollution became too great, people died in conspicuous numbers, and sanitation became general. So this thing called "civilization" is working poor old Nature overtime. Increasingly great numbers of people are ill, crippled and dying from chronic disease, and so the problem thus created will not be downed.

Since it will not be downed, we must consider whether it may down us if we do not do something about it. To formulate any plan of action there must be an objective around which the plan may be organized. In the whole field of health and disease what is our objective? Would we wipe out completely all sickness and death and have people, after an indefinite term of years, spontaneously disintegrate like Oliver Wendell Holmes' one-horse shay, or else go on forever? The prospect of inevitable immortality in this imperfect world might, of all things, be the most intolerable. Again, radical curtailment of deaths without a corresponding curtailment of disease would multiply suffering shockingly and would place on society a growing burden of sickness which would eventually reach a volume that could not be supported. If, then, our theoretical objective is not the elimination of all deaths, nor even a reduction of deaths without a corresponding or even greater reduction of sickness, what is it that we are after?

We take it that any serious social program aims at increasing the total volume of serenity among the peoples of the world. This serenity is a composite of moral, psychological and physical factors. On the physical side we desire that every child shall be born with as few handicaps due to heredity, prenatal environment and the exigencies of parturition as is practical. We desire that during infancy, growth and nutrition shall be as untrammeled as possible, with as little damage from the environment as is at all reasonable. During late adolescence, and early and middle adult life, when the work of the world is done, we strive for a people whose effectiveness shall be as little impeded by the shackles of disease as possible. And at the end, what? Is it not that we would have, after a span of years passed in reasonable serenity, a reduction to a minimum of the span of crippling and painful terminal illness, and then a humane departure, which can certainly be faced with more assurance than could an irrevocable guarantee of immortality here. If anything like the above can be accepted generally, we see that the complete elimination of sickness and death may not be even theoretically desirable, but rather some conscious and rational control of sickness and death. Such an attitude makes the approach to chronic diseases even more complex since they occur largely in an age group where we might not, if we could, entirely eliminate disease and death, but would rather delay them and make them more humane.

Again, for any considered program against crime, cyclones or chronic disease we must have knowledge and, as we found to our belated sorrow when developing a cancer program under a legislative mandate, knowledge is the least of our burdens in chronic disease. Such studies as there are have been made on selected and limited groups. For the population as a whole we know nothing of the relative or absolute prevalence of the varied chronic diseases, their duration, degree and proportion of crippling, their age and economic distribution, the ade-

Source: Excerpted from George H. Bigelow and Herbert L. Lombard, *Cancer and Other Chronic Diseases in Massachusetts.* Cambridge, The Riverside Press, 1933.
[1] Commissioner, Massachusetts Department of Public Health; Lecturer, Public Health Administration, Harvard School of Public Health.
[2] Director, Division of Adult Hygiene, Massachusetts Department of Public Health; Assistant Professor of Hygiene and Public Health, Tufts College Dental School.

quacy and extent of resources and their utilization, to say nothing of the medical babel as to whether or not we know for each of the diseases anything that can be used effectively for prevention, early diagnosis, cure or even alleviation. As a result of some years of labor in this field we have produced perhaps a mouse. But compared with nothing a mouse is relatively a gigantic beast. So in this book we offer our findings, such as they are, in the hope that they may in some slight way help others striving to find a solution, and not a hollow panacea, for the present chronic disease dilemma.

The Inevitableness of the Chronic Disease Problem

We are theoretically touched by what sickens and kills people thousands of miles away or on the other side of the globe, and give grudging pennies to the Red Cross or our missionaries with the platitude that "we are all brothers" and then forget it all as promptly as possible. But the things that really motivate are those that sicken and kill our own families and those of our neighbors, and that is just what chronic disease is doing. There is hardly a family in Massachusetts without immediate experience with cancer, heart disease, or rheumatism (we prefer this term as more inclusive than "arthritis"), and therefore immediate realization of the inadequacies of our resources and their utilization. It is out of the emotional impetus roused by such a widespread experience with futility that action in a democracy and revolution in an autocracy spring, and, unguided, such emotional action may result tragically in even more costly futility than before.

Social Aspects

In the aggregate our population is growing older, and approximating more and more that of the Old World. The frontier community is largely one of young adults. As the frontier recedes, sociological maturity, if not senescence, follows. Hence the chronic disease problem is more pressing in the older parts of this country.

Also, immigration restrictions have speeded up this aging process since immigrants, largely spurred on by youth and adventure, are for the most part young adults. Further, both our birth and death rates are falling, which means a population of relatively fewer youths and more aged

people. In fifty years our death rate has dropped 25 percent while our birth rate has correspondingly fallen 30 percent. Another evidence of this phenomenon of the aging of our population is shown by the fact that over the last two generations the average age of our population has increased one year each decade and, if anything, this rate of aging may speed up in the near future. This results in the population over fifty years of age increasing about one percent each decade.

A very sobering way of expressing the sociological effect of all this is that sixty years ago (1870) there were seven persons in the productive ages of twenty to sixty years for every one who was over sixty. Seven to share the burden of the dependent aged through kinship, philanthropy or taxes, while now that figure has shrunken to 5.4—a 23 percent shrinkage in the burden carriers in sixty years.

The curtailment of immigration has other influences on this problem than merely the aging of the population. In Massachusetts all the chronic diseases appear to have a somewhat higher death rate among the foreign born and their first generation than among those of native born parents. For certain specific diseases their rate here seems to be higher than the corresponding rate in their native country, though such comparisons are hazardous because of lack of uniformity of figures. Contrast with this, however, the results of our sickness survey that the incidence of chronic disease is higher among the native than among the foreign born. Fewer cases but more deaths should mean a shorter duration and higher case fatality among the foreign born. And this we have found to be true. But we have no answer as to why the average duration of these diseases should be greatest among the native born, next among the foreign born, and least among the first generation of the foreign born. Again, the high mortality may not be due to nativity but to poverty as was reported in England in relation to cancer. We also found a higher chronic disease incidence among the lower economic groups. This is all confusing, if you will, but suggests that the influence of retarded immigration on this whole matter may be considerable and varied.

Again, in cancer and to a lesser extent in the other diseases, there has been and is vast discussion as to whether the increase in rates is apparent rather than real. The doubters must, of course, admit an actual increase since the number of aged people subject to these diseases has enormously increased, but they do question an increase in rates. The apparent increase they attribute to more people in the susceptible ages and improvement in diagnostic accuracy. The results of our studies lead us to feel that over and above these factors there has been an actual increase in the rates of many of the chronic diseases studied, though in cancer, with the flattening of the curve in some of the younger age groups, and perhaps in some of the other diseases, the peak of the increase may not be too far distant. Schereschewsky, in an exhaustive study of this question in relation to cancer, comes to the conclusion that about two-thirds of the increase must be considered real. It would seem the height of folly to refuse to face the problem under the sophistry that the increase is apparent but not real.

There is reason to suppose that with so large a proportion of the population living in restricted quarters in the cities, with the decrease in the size of families, and the general entrance of women into gainful employment, the average family is less able to adjust itself to the care of chronic sickness than formerly. The aunt or cousin who was never happier than when taking command during sickness now is likely to have a job. The trained nurse is usually too expensive for protracted illness, only 3.2 percent of the families studied having had one during the year preceding the survey, and those for an average of only three months. The trained nurse does not seem to be largely considered in such cases, as only one percent more said they would have liked one. Then, too, there is the problem of putting her up in cramped quarters unless she comes by the day. The visiting nurse may more and more fill a need here though as yet she has not figured prominently.

The pressure, then, is for more and more institutionalization of these cases, which will be considered at length later. Here we might consider briefly the sociological effect of freeing the home from direct responsibilities in the care of illness and particularly illness in older members of the family. More and more of the functions of the home are being taken over elsewhere; recreation, education, religious and moral instruction, raising foodstuffs, even such homely activities as cooking, washing, freezing

ice cream and the like. It is said that if the home ceases to be a haven for the sick members, another fundamental tie will be severed. With the peak of income for the worker falling below the age of forty (the optimum being usually eighteen to thirty-five) the father is in a psychological dilemma in maintaining his position as head of the family if one or more of his children earns more than he. If we add to this a general feeling that the home has little or no responsibility for caring for the old people when sick, a profound reversal in our social attitude will have taken place.

On the other hand, many physicians and others have seen daughters' lives and health wrecked through devoted attendance on a parent during a lingering and painful illness. Through devotion, families may take on financial obligations that will be burdensome for years. The toll of jangled nerves and broken spirits may menace the integrity of a home long after the invalid has passed on. The answer is discriminating social study of each problem. There are many cases of chronic sickness happier and better off in the home, and some that surely need other resources. Our study indicated that 11 percent of all chronic disease cases were in homes totally inadequate to care for them and that 11 percent represents 55 000 cases in Massachusetts.

Economic Aspects

In chronic disease we are dealing with a problem, on the surface at least, predominantly of late middle and old age. When you have diseases that are forty times as common over eighty as under twenty years of age, with frequency increasing with the age of the group studied, you are obviously faced with a problem where the investment of large sums of money is of questionable value except in terms of the humanities. Overwhelmingly, most of the work of the world is done by people in the age groups twenty to forty ("unemployed at forty") or shall we say fifty or sixty. But chronic disease bears heaviest after fifty-five or sixty. Perhaps the most economically sound place for a high death rate is in the cradle since there the community has made but slight investment, unless we can talk of hopes and aspirations and love in terms of investment. But very properly the community is shocked at a high infant mortality with its loss of potential good to the state, and demands vigorous steps to control such a death rate.

The least economical time for a high death rate is the late teens and early twenties where tuberculosis is still so prominent. Here the public investment in sustenance and education has been very large and there has been little or no opportunity for a return to be made on this investment except through their value as consumers, a value of which we are now becoming acutely conscious. But when we come to high incidence over fifty-five or sixty, what is to be said? We all know of astonishingly competent people who after sixty have much to give in the way of wisdom, and art, and administrative and manual skill. But these are exceptions even with the present multiplication of the aged. The work of the world is done by younger adults.

On the other hand, it can be said that long before crippling and death, the effectiveness of those who will be recognized as the chronic sick is impaired. The onset is insidious and extends back into the younger years with concomitant lost time and ineffectiveness. A group of diseases which afflicts 18.5 per 1000 of the population under twenty is not negligible even at that age. While the etiology of chronic disease is far from known, it is recognized that general hygienic measures are promising prophylactics, and this would warrant the support of infant, child, school, college and industrial hygiene programs. Also, we must give care to these younger groups with chronic disease. It is true that the old will seek this care too, but so they do for tuberculosis, mental disease, orthopedic conditions, and the like, even though in these fields we recognize that it is the young who should command the first of our attention.

Perhaps, but these arguments do not convince us. From the economics alone it would seem that tuberculosis, pneumonia, and other communicable diseases, the acute causes of sickness and death in pregnancy, childhood and young adult life, the accidents and homicides, these squanderously young terminations of considerable investment, should first arrest our attention. But we have said that the emotional demands of chronic disease will not down. There are half a million cases, and that is the reason, in this State, why this is so. Also, since all great movements are emotional and not rational, we may stop baying the moon, recognize that any large program is uneconomical but

perhaps inevitable, and devote our energies to determining just what that program should be.

Perhaps the most popular solution of any pressing problem of sickness is more hospital beds. They are specific but hideously expensive. We do not know how many beds we need, and what proportion should be expensive, as in general hospitals, or economical, as in nursing homes. We do not know what the average stay should be. If it is three months, it is one thing; if it is three years, it is quite another. At our cancer hospital at Pondville we roughly estimated in advance that the average stay would be three months, but, as the alleviatory part of the work has bulked vastly larger and the terminal part less than we expected, the average stay has been but one month. That gives us three times as many beds, and yet at this moment we need fifty more.

In this connection it is important to note that not only do chronic diseases make up two-thirds of all deaths in Massachusetts, whereas fifty years ago they were but one-third, but also from the duration as noted on the death returns there is a marked increase in the length of the chronic disease that kills. In twenty years the duration of such diseases in persons over fifty years of age has increased 2.6 times. This is a vague figure. The onset of a chronic disease is usually difficult to state precisely, as is even the onset of symptoms. Yet we know of no reason why the error should not be essentially constant. If it cannot be brushed aside, this increased duration has great significance in the institutionalization problem.

This consideration of the economic aspects of care of terminal illness suggests that a person dying of an acute illness has been less of a community burden, so far as his care is concerned, than one dying of a chronic illness. From this point of view, since preventive medicine has contributed so much more to the control of acute than chronic disease, its contributions have been uneconomical. But, of course, the problem is not as simple as this. Many of the acute illnesses are communicable and the financial burden as well as the disease may be spread to others. Again, the fatalities from acute disease bulk larger in the younger age groups where deaths are more uneconomical. Therefore, we can hardly indict preventive medicine because its major contributions have been in fields where the diseases are of short duration.

The losses from chronic disease can never be accurately estimated and yet have a vast bearing on the economics of the question. The time lost by wage-earners with chronic disease in Massachusetts in one year represents the time of one man for 34 000 years. At an average wage of four dollars per day this amounts annually to $40 million or nearly the cost of our State government for the same period. If we add to this the money spent for care, the service given through philanthropy or taxes, the loss to other wage-earners in caring for the sick person, and the vast ramifications of the indirect by-products of sickness, we would certainly get a figure of twice that or enough to run the government of the Commonwealth of Massachusetts for two years. A serious consideration of economics in this field would seem imperative.

Such colossal cost accounting of sickness has become popular in this country of late, usually to rationalize hardly less colossal expenditures. Their critical consideration is often prevented by the very weight of their cumulated digits. Their value is often impaired by the inaccuracy or uncertainty of their initial premise. Also, a pertinent question is often evaded. Granted, the cost of illness is very great, but what would the cost of prevention or mitigation be? For the chronic diseases at present, the vagaries of personal hygiene are all that we have to offer in the way of prevention, so that the cost of mitigation is what we need to consider directly. A hospital bed costs from three to six thousand dollars (perhaps just now a little less) to construct. Convalescent and nursing home beds cost somewhat less. Let us take, then, three thousand dollars as a conservative average figure. Let us again be conservative and say each bed can serve three cases a year. (Since the service we are now considering is largely terminal and since the duration of untreated cases of chronic disease runs from two years (cancer) to some fourteen years (rheumatism), an average terminal hospitalization of four months is almost foolishly conservative.) Let us also take the figure from our surveys of 55 000 persons in Massachusetts in homes totally unable to care for them. We find we need 18 000 beds at a minimum cost of construction of $3000 each. For maintenance, a thousand per bed per year is certainly not excessive. This leaves us with an initial investment of $55 million and a maintenance cost of $18 million. Of this latter, experi-

ence would suggest that we might expect to collect from not more than one-half of the patients not more than one-half the cost, giving a net maintenance cost of $13 million. All this would be greatly increased if the cost of more adequate extramural care of those not imperatively needing hospitalization were considered.

Such nebulous calculations as these have led us to the conclusion that early recognition in offices and clinics with short-term careful study of selected cases in adequately equipped and staffed institutions with the fullest possible employment of curative and alleviatory knowledge, to reduce the volume and duration of terminal hospitalization, should be employed. While adequate approximations of such costs are even more tenuous, it is suggested from our limited experience with cancer that an initial investment of some $5 million with annual maintenance of $500 000 to $750 000, might well be needed in this field.

And so it goes like an inverted pyramid tottering to a fall. To continue as at present costs tens of millions. To give what the humanities will demand would increase this to many tens of millions, and that only for Massachusetts. To give what would seem to be the most intelligent service in the field of recognition, cure and alleviation costs hundreds of thousands to millions. But curiously enough, the people will complacently tolerate indefinitely that nothing be done. Then, when aroused they will demand that complete service to the dying be given. What will appeal to them least is a middle course which is less expensive and more promising in the ultimate control of suffering and death.

Medical Aspects

Any medical approach to control a disease problem has five aspects in the following order of importance as far as the public is concerned: (1) prevention; (2) early diagnosis; (3) cure; (4) alleviation; and (5) terminal care. But with chronic disease the medical conservative will say that in the field of prevention we know little or nothing with assurance, that early diagnosis is uncertain and difficult, cure infrequent, alleviation doubtful and terminal care costly. And after all that, where are you? That is precisely what we said to the Legislature considering a cancer program, and one sincere and impatient member said, "Stop complaining! The medical profession and the Department of Public Health have had ten years, during which this subject has been under discussion, to give us a program. Yet all you have said is 'Wait!' Now we, the Legislature, have decided on a program. We have piped and all you have to do is dance!" The medical conservative will never call the tune, and yet if a dance is to be well danced one wants some assurance as to the music. Then, too, every program of medical social significance in tuberculosis, mental disease or what-you-will has been decried by these same medical conservatives.

Our surveys suggest a number of predisposing factors, all of which have been suggested before at one time or another. They are prior acute infections, failure to eat protective foods such as milk, fruit and green vegetables, nervous temperament, confirmed lack of exercise, and continued indigestion and use of laxatives. When parents or grandparents were reported as dying of any of the chronic diseases under consideration the incidence in families was about 50 percent higher than when such was not the case. Again, when brothers or sisters or other members of the household were said to have chronic disease the rate doubled over those households where such sickness in relatives or households was denied. This is of course crude and might perhaps implicate environment as much as heredity. But certainly the suggestion of familial vulnerability of blood vessels and other organs to wear and tear has been often suggested and these findings might substantiate it. Unexpectedly enough, abnormalities of weight seemed to be less significant as influencing rates of chronic diseases than some of the other factors. This certainly differs from popular medical and lay opinion but lack of exercise and improper food may be conducive both to overweight and illness.

The above is enough to justify a program of adult hygiene as at least decreasing certain predisposing factors to chronic disease. Even more important is probably the personal hygiene in childhood and adolescence and the whole health education program in the schools; first, because the seeds of later disease are probably sown there, and also that is the age when health habits may really become a part of life. The confirmed dietary and other hygienic abominations in adults can no more be altered than can the number of hairs encasing the same adult head.

Early diagnosis is difficult in any field. The easy thing in any field is late diagnosis. To recognize diseased conditions soundly before they have given much of any symptoms is the modern challenge to the medical profession, and is the most difficult challenge ever thrown down to any profession. On the one hand, the sincere physician must not be a chronic alarmist, nor on the other must he be a fatuous optimist. We are told that by the time there are signs in the chest, tuberculosis is no longer early. Yet some would seem to expect the unaided, single-handed physician to so recognize tuberculosis. Of course he must have lavish access to X-ray resources to succeed. So with other diseases. We must have organization of special resources and special medical skills through private hospitals, in urban and rural centers, health centers, industries, schools, colleges, governmental hospitals and clinics—by all known means until the most effective formula has been devised. It may be that the best formula will differ in different types of communities in different parts of the country. But at the heart of any of them there must be sound medical direction, and always the principal filter through which these resources will be reached will be the private practitioner. And the role of an intelligent filter in any complex matter is difficult, to hold back the non-essential and with discrimination to let the essential through!

But all this is of no account unless the people present themselves early. To be willing to pay for the absence of pain is the height of popular medical wisdom. If the onset of all chronic disease were as flamboyant as a boil, success would be easy. But its very insidiousness militates against success. The principal reason given for delay in seeking medical advice for cancer was that the symptoms were thought to be trivial. This reason was more frequently given by men than by women. Popular education as to early signs and symptoms must be accepted as essential.

Cure or relief of these diseases raises endless medical discussion. Some purists prefer the term "arrested" to "cured," as is used in tuberculosis. But for the person with cancer, adequately treated, who lives fifteen years without return of symptoms and then dies of something else, cure is the appropriate term. He can leave it to the academicians to haggle over lexicographic niceties. Then relief is enormously important and is sometimes difficult to distinguish from cure. If through short-term and intermittent hospital admissions, as we find at our hospital for cancer at Pondville, a person can be improved and kept at work for months or years, and perhaps admitted for a short stay terminally, how much more economical and humane than long-term admission for merely custodial care. Medically discriminating short-term expensive service may in the aggregate cost less than indiscriminate long-term cheaper service.

Certainly, when we find that of the 138 000 cases of rheumatism in Massachusetts 70 percent or over 90 000 are getting no care, on the one hand, while adequate medical centers assure us that 70 percent could be cured or definitely benefited, it does not take a course in higher mathematics to realize that the public is not getting what in our present knowledge it is entitled to. When it realizes this, it will get it and, depending on the adequacy of medical direction, what it gets will be good, bad, or indifferent.

What shall be said as to terminal hospital care? In the first place, do not segregate the dying. Few institutions can keep their good names with a death rate over 30 percent. Then, too, medical interest cannot be held by exclusively advanced terminal cases. They shnould be cared for in small groups in other institutions preferably near their own homes. Most people, like certain wounded animals, have instincts that bring them home to die. Until through prevention and cure we can reduce their volume, let us in this way handle our terminals as economically and humanely as possible.

Of course, critically in these fields we need more knowledge. But even beyond that we need ability to put such knowledge as we have and will have to work for the benefit of the people.

The Relative Importance of the Different Chronic Diseases

As in the field of communicable disease the problem of the control of diphtheria is approached in one way and that of typhoid fever in quite another, so we may expect in the field of chronic disease that the problems of rheu-

matism, heart disease and cancer, for example, will require different approaches. It is well, then, to consider the relative importance of these different diseases before making a selection.

Mortality

Heart disease furnishes about 20 percent of all deaths, cancer about 10 percent, and so on, in receding importance. In all, chronic diseases cause 66 percent of all deaths while fifty years ago it was 33 percent. In general the death rates are somewhat higher among the foreign born and their first generation, and except for tuberculosis which is highest in the smallest communities, the rates increase with density of population. This latter phenomenon is not true of rheumatism.

In the past, death rates, because of their ready availability and dramatic appeal, have perhaps influenced too much our thinking as to the relative importance of various diseases. There are other factors of disease of even more moment, as we shall see.

Morbidity and Disability

A conservative estimate reached in more than one way is that there are about 500 000 persons with chronic disease in Massachusetts, varying all the way from no disability to complete crippling. This represents about 12 percent of the population. About 45 percent of these are partially disabled (225 000 persons), while nearly 5 percent are totally disabled (22 500 persons). The incidence is 50 percent higher among the poor than among those that are better off. This means a high chronic disease rate in families cared for by public welfare departments. Families with such sickness require about twice the money benefits of those without, so that chronic disease is costly to departments of public welfare.

Among the individual diseases, rheumatism leads with 138 000 cases at any one time, of which 5600 are totally disabled; heart disease comes next with 84 000 cases and 2600 completely disabled; then arteriosclerosis with 64 000 cases and 1800 completely disabled; digestive diseases, 29 000 cases and 500 completely disabled; diseases of the eye and ear with 24 000 cases and 350 completely disabled; apoplexy and tuberculosis with about 16 000 cases each and 3800 of the former completely disabled; diabetes, 15 000 cases with 800 completely disabled; cancer, 11 500 cases, and so on.

Here we see that rheumatism displaces heart disease which leads as a cause of death, and rheumatism exceeds all others in total numbers completely disabled. Thus, while rheumatism does not kill, it does attack large numbers, with heavy disability rates.

Duration

The average untreated case of cancer lives some twenty-one months, let us say, for round numbers, two years. The heart case lives some seven to nine years, while the rheumatic lives fourteen years or more. The rheumatics in the survey who had complete disability had had this same disability for an average of two years. As these cases were all alive the average complete disability for rheumatics before death is presumably at least twice this, or four years. If we add a preceding period of partial disability we see that the problem of the crippled rheumatic becomes staggering. Neurasthenia was the only disease considered which gave longer complete disability, but these cases number less than 10 percent of the rheumatics. Heart disease crippled for only half as long and in only half as many cases.

Rheumatism, then, cripples in the largest number of cases, and kills in the smallest. This very ability to cripple without killing would seem to put it in the lead of all other chronic diseases as of pre-eminent social, economic and medical importance.

What Might Be Done

Before discussing what might be done, let us see what the survey revealed as to the treatment actually being received by the cases found. Nearly half of all the cases had received no treatment or merely self-medication during the year. This medically neglected group ran from about one-eighth of the diabetics to about two-thirds of the rheumatics. The principal reasons given for failure to obtain treatment were that approximately 60 percent felt doctors could not help or they had no faith in them, 33 percent felt that the condition was not serious, and 13 percent gave economic reasons. Certainly, here the restraint is far more profound than merely

economics. Those in the country had doctors as frequently as those in the cities but fewer had attended clinics. Interestingly, the native born of native born parents went less to clinics, used less self-medication, but did patronize more Christian Science healers. Only 3.2 percent had used trained nurses during the year while 4.3 percent had been to a hospital. Ninety-eight percent were cared for in their homes and in 11 percent of the cases the homes were grossly inadequate for such care. Among the poor, 43 percent of the homes were unsuitable.

This is enough to indicate the enormous inadequacy of care for these cases. But what is to be done? The general points have already been reviewed. First, we must have general education as to personal hygiene and the importance of early detection. Second, every effort must be made through the private office, the clinic and the hospital to extend the adequacy of early diagnosis and discriminating therapy to benefit the patient and to overcome the blighting hopelessness as to what modern medicine can accomplish in chronic disease (think of 13 percent of the diabetics without medical care for a year!). The medical profession should lead first in widespread postgraduate education, since the pall of hopelessness among the profession in regard to effective therapy of many of these diseases is even more atrophying that that of the public; and second, through directing the organization of resources. But the profession alone cannot handle this enormous problem, nor will it. All resources, private, philanthropic and governmental must be enlisted. Complacency is wicked and dangerous.

What Can We Learn From the Massachusetts Cancer Program?

Our five years' experience with a governmental cancer program is reviewed elsewhere in this book. While specific accomplishments are still largely quantitative rather than qualitative we can draw certain conclusion. It has been developed with the co-operation of the medical profession, and under the direction of outstanding physicians and lay people. It shows that:

(a) When aroused, the legislature will demand service for a chronic disease;
(b) The services of our best medical and lay citizens can be commandeered to develop and guide a program;

(c) Physicians will respond to educational opportunities and will send their patients to clinics and hospitals if such institutions can get their confidence;

(d) Patients will come in large numbers to private offices, clinics and hospitals when told of the need of utilizing such services;

(e) There is some evidence that they will utilize these services earlier if repeatedly importuned;

(f) All methods of public information must be employed interminably;

(g) Under governmental direction, clinic and hospital service can be developed of a quality not heretofore available;

(h) There are preventive, diagnostic, curative, alleviatory and terminal aspects to the cancer problem as to all others;

(i) There would seem to be no reason until some better plan is enunciated, why similar services under such auspices should not be developed for other of the important chronic diseases;

(j) There is reason to suppose that if someone else does not take the initiative, the people through their legislature will again do so, to the great shame of the medical and public health professions.

The Relation Of Health Departments To All This

A recent letter to all the state and provincial health officers of the United States and Canada on this subject brought the reply, with three inspired exceptions, that they were doing nothing about adult hygiene and chronic disease and that many hoped they never would. One of the frequent reasons given was fear of antagonizing the medical profession. But they seemed to have no fear of antagonizing the public on whose good will their livelihood depends.

It may well be argued that it is not a function of public health; that it is inevitably too much involved in diagnosis and treatment and too little in prevention; that hospital administration is no proper function of a health officer, etc., etc. But what department of government should handle it if and when the people determine that something shall be done? There are no departments of public disease. The departments of public welfare are perhaps the nearest but in general they are not sufficiently sophisticated medically to assure adequacy. An institutional department is too concerned with the hotel aspects of institutions to readily appreciate the professional niceties that must differentiate one type of hospital from another if it is to be more than an expensive nursing home.

It will be said that it is no proper function of government. Very well, we wish it were not. But we feel that any activity which the people insist shall be a function of government will be a function of government. Until some other agency comes forward more actively to fill this gap between our knowledge and its general application for the people, we feel that health officers must actively prepare themselves to enter more and more this field. It may sink them, but so may failure to prepare. When that other agency does present itself (and we doubt if it ever will) let the health officer be the first to welcome it and to hand over to it the key of the citadel of chronic disease control. But until such time the health officer would do well to feel that that key is definitely committed to him and let the people not find him wanting in his stewardship.

ON THE EPIDEMIOLOGY OF CANCER

Major Greenwood[1]

Our consideration of the epidemiology of tuberculosis carried us some way from the conventional field of old textbook epidemiology, but there was at least a thread of connection inasmuch as tuberculosis is known to be an infectious disease. When we approach the study of cancer that thread snaps, because, using the word "infectious" in any ordinary sense, there is no reason whatever to think that cancer is infectious.

From the statistical point of view there is no doubt that cancer is one of the most important crowd-sicknesses, and, if we were able to take statistical records at their face value we should have to conclude that it is a sickness which increases with the spread of material civilization.

In civilized States the mortality ascribed to cancer is far greater than among primitive races, and in any one civilized State the mortality now ascribed to cancer is far heavier than a generation ago. The Table 1 of English experience is typical.

Statisticians are, however, a cautious race, and very few of them have been prepared to accept these figures at their face value. Forty years ago King and Newsholme in a very valuable paper initiated a discussion which still goes on. The most striking part of their work was an analysis of the experience of Frankfürt-am-Main, where deaths from cancer had been classified by site of occurrence for many years. It was found that between 1860 and 1889 mortality from cancer of those parts of the body in which the disease was readily detected had not increased. They urged that the general increase of mortality from cancer was consistent with the causal factor being not a greater number of deaths from cancer but a more accurate specification of the

Source: Major Greenwood, *Epidemics and Crowd Diseases, An Introduction to the Study of Epidemiology.* New York: The MacMillan Company, 1935.
[1] President of the Royal Statistical Society; Professor of Epidemiology and Vital Statistics in the University of London (London School of Hygiene and Tropical Medicine); formerly Medical Officer in the Ministry of Health.

Table 1. Annual mortality from cancer (all forms) per 100 000 living in successive decennia, England and Wales.

	All ages standardized	Ages							
		0-	15-	25-	35-	45-	55-	65-	75 and upwards
Males:									
1851-1860	20.5	1	2	6	18	42	93	150	174
1861-1870	25.6	1	2	6	21	54	121	187	227
1871-1880	33.3	1	2	7	24	71	159	261	299
1881-1890	46.7	2	3	8	30	100	230	376	393
1891-1900	63.5	2	4	10	38	130	316	533	582
1901-1910	78.2	2	4	11	41	155	390	668	787
1911-1920	89.6	2	4	11	42	168	444	800	973
1921-1930	100.4	2	5	12	42	163	472	955	1276
Females:									
1851-1860	43.8	1	2	14	60	128	186	236	233
1861-1870	52.1	1	2	16	67	154	230	281	280
1871-1880	61.9	1	2	17	79	176	277	352	352
1881-1890	73.9	1	3	17	86	205	338	453	460
1891-1900	88.2	2	3	18	89	232	410	583	638
1901-1910	94.0	2	2	17	85	232	441	666	790
1911-1920	96.0	2	3	16	79	227	438	711	919
1921-1930	98.8	2	4	16	76	214	424	774	1131

causes of death. Twenty-three years later another eminent statistician, Dr. Willcox, of Cornell University, continued the analysis of the Frankfürt data down to 1915, and surveyed the whole field. In his judgment this wider survey confirmed the opinion of King and Newsholme. In his words: "The cumulative evidence that improvements in diagnosis and changes in age composition explain away more than half, and perhaps all, of the apparent increase in cancer mortality rebuts the presumption raised by the figures, and makes it probable, although far from certain, that cancer mortality is not increasing."

A year or two later, however, Dr. T. H. C. Stevenson recorded in the annual report of the Registrar-General for 1917 the results of some analyses which are not easily reconciled with Dr.

Willcox's general conclusion. Dr. Stevenson took for his basis the 685 142 deaths from cancer recorded during 1897-1917 in England and Wales, and inquired whether the increase of mortality were really concentrated upon "inaccessible" or difficult diagnosible sites (see Table 2). As a basis of classification he availed himself of an inquiry made by the Bureau of the Census of the United States of America in 1914. In the United States the practitioners reporting 52 420 deaths from cancer registered in that year were invited to state whether the diagnosis was or was not certain. For the sites classified by Dr. Stevenson as "accessible" the highest proportion of uncertain diagnoses was 0.6 percent (rectum). In the "inaccessible" group the proportion of uncertainty ranged from 15.3 percent (ovary and Fallopian tubes) to 72.0 percent

Table 2. Accessible and inaccessible sites of fatal cancer: mortality per 1 million living 1901-1917, England and Wales.[a]

| | | All Ages | | | | | | | | | 85 and |
		Crude	Standardized	0-	25-	35-	45-	55-	65-	75-	upwards
Males:											
Accessible	1901-1902	200	211	—	25	—	429	996	1819	2380	2485
	1916-1917	367	285	—	35	—	508	1320	2509	3517	4589
Inaccessible	1901-1902	440	461	—	60	—	921	2373	4052	4178	2512
	1916-1917	776	598	—	78	—	1056	2868	5521	6749	3810
Indefinite	1901-1902	54	55	—	13	—	108	260	369	550	682
	1916-1917	68	56	—	19	—	115	227	324	429	325
All Sites	1901-1902	694	727	—	98	—	1458	3629	6240	7108	5679
	1916-1917	1211	939	—	132	—	1679	4415	8354	10 695	8724
Females:											
Accessible	1901-1902	484	463	4	102	550	1376	2064	2600	3235	3962
	1916-1917	563	486	4	75	500	1388	2180	2951	4214	5038
Inaccessible	1901-1902	457	433	11	65	293	937	2141	3615	3857	2364
	1916-1917	576	493	11	59	283	950	2400	4295	5493	4228
Indefinite	1901-1902	45	44	8	13	36	91	155	264	400	687
	1916-1917	31	28	8	11	23	53	107	160	215	309
All Sites	1901-1902	986	940	23	180	879	2404	4360	6479	7492	7013
	1916-1917	1170	1007	23	145	806	2391	4687	7406	9922	9575
Persons:											
Accessible	1901-1902	347	345	—	68	—	921	1565	2253	2877	3416
	1916-1917	480	391	—	78	—	964	1761	2754	3935	4879
Inaccessible	1901-1902	449	446	—	63	—	929	2249	3809	3991	2419
	1916-1917	661	541	—	73	—	1001	2628	4841	5996	4080
Indefinite	1901-1902	48	48	—	13	—	99	204	310	463	686
	1916-1917	47	41	—	14	—	83	165	234	301	314
All Sites	1901-1902	844	839	—	144	—	1949	4018	6372	7331	6521
	1916-1917	1188	973	—	165	—	2048	4554	7829	10 232	9273

[a] Taken from Annual Report of the R.G., 1917, Table LIII.

(stomach). Dr. Stevenson found that in the male sex, mortality from cancer of "accessible" sites had actually increased faster than mortality from cancer of "inaccessible" sites. The former showed an increase of 56 percent, the latter of 41 percent. Among women the position was reversed, but the general increase of mortality from cancer in women was much less than that of cancer in men. "This remarkable and quite unexpected result," wrote Dr. Stevenson, "makes it very difficult to attribute so important a share in the recorded increase in the cancer of males to improved diagnosis as has hitherto seemed probable."

These were the conclusions reached by competent authorities on the evidence available fifteen years ago. Before canvassing them it will be interesting to consider the experience of the last ten years. After the war the male rate of mortality from cancer continued to increase; it was 921 (standardized) per 1 million in 1920, 947 in

1921, and passed the 1000 in 1925, when it had reached 1023; then there was a slight decline to 1018 in 1927, a further rise to 1032 in 1928, and then practically the same rates 1031 in each of the following years. The decennial average of 1901-1910 was 784, so that the rate of 1929 or 1930 had an increase of 31.5 percent over the average of twenty-five years earlier.

Table 3 . . . gives various details. We cannot without further calculation repeat the analysis of 1917, but, taking the decennium 1911-1920 as a datum line and ranking (as in 1917) lip, tongue, mouth and tonsil, jaw, rectum, breast, rodent ulcer, penis, scrotum, other skin, larynx, and testis as "accessible," the remainder, except cancer of bones (which I omit) as "inaccessible" sites, we reach by addition the following results. In 1911-1920 the rate for "accessible" sites (males) was 269.3; in 1929 it was 281.5, an increase of 4.5 percent. In 1911-1920 the rate for "inaccessible" sites was 556.1; in 1929 it was

Table 3. Cancer mortality—rates per 1 million population (standardized) for the more important sites for each sex, 1901-1910, 1911-1920, 1921-1930, 1926, 1927, 1928, 1929, and 1930.[a]

	Males	Females	Males	Females	Males	Females	Males	Females	Males	Females
	All Sites		Lip		Tongue		Mouth and Tonsil		Jaw	
1901-1910	784	942	12.8	0.8	43.1	4.4	?	?	22.6	6.9
1911-1920	897	959	12.6	0.7	50.8	4.3	23.5	3.0	25.1	7.2
1921-1930	1004	986	11.5	0.7	46.1	3.8	28.3	3.6	20.8	6.4
1926	1011	995	10.6	0.6	43.7	3.7	29.6	4.1	21.0	6.9
1927	1018	984	11.9	1.0	46.6	4.3	29.5	3.4	21.1	6.0
1928	1032	1000	12.3	0.7	45.5	4.2	30.5	3.5	19.6	5.5
1929	1031	999	10.4	0.6	41.8	4.1	27.6	3.5	19.2	6.5
1930	1031	987	11.3	0.7	40.6	3.5	29.3	3.8	16.7	5.3
	Pharynx		Esophagus		Stomach		Liver		Gall-bladder	
1901-1910	?	?	51.2	14.6	167.2	133.0	?	?	?	?
1911-1920	10.8	3.0	60.6	16.5	186.4	139.0	87.1	98.0	6.0	11.6
1921-1930	12.6	3.0	64.2	18.1	221.1	155.5	61.0	60.9	8.8	16.6
1926	13.1	3.1	65.4	17.8	222.2	163.2	61.2	59.8	9.1	17.7
1927	13.2	2.8	60.7	18.0	229.0	157.0	55.8	52.1	8.3	17.6
1928	12.6	2.9	64.3	18.7	227.4	161.5	51.8	52.6	9.5	16.9
1929	13.8	2.8	62.3	18.3	237.2	164.6	52.3	50.6	9.4	17.6
1930	11.8	3.2	61.8	18.6	233.7	162.8	47.7	45.4	9.5	17.1
	Mesentery and Peritoneum		Intestine		Rectum		Ovary and Fallopian Tube		Uterus	
1901-1910	8.2	15.8	65.3	72.3	79.8	55.9	—	19.2	—	?
1911-1920	6.0	12.0	96.8	109.2	93.6	59.3	—	24.3	—	174.4
1921-1930	5.4	8.1	125.4	129.9	105.5	59.8	—	36.0	—	157.9
1926	5.6	9.3	131.5	135.4	107.2	59.7	—	35.7	—	156.4
1927	4.8	7.3	132.0	131.8	105.7	60.3	—	38.9	—	155.1
1928	5.8	7.3	132.5	138.5	105.7	58.0	—	39.2	—	154.9
1929	4.4	7.2	134.3	138.6	108.0	58.3	—	40.8	—	150.3
1930	4.9	6.6	136.9	138.4	110.6	59.9	—	42.3	—	143.9

Table 3. (Continued.)

	Males	Females	Males	Females	Males	Females	Males	Females	Males	Females
	Breast		Rodent Ulcer		Penis		Scrotum		Other Skin	
1901-1910	1.5	158.4	?	?	?	—	?	—	?	?
1911-1920	1.6	170.8	6.7	4.3	6.6	—	2.4	—	17.6	10.9
1921-1930	1.8	189.1	8.4	4.9	6.4	—	2.7	—	17.6	10.2
1926	1.7	184.3	7.5	4.8	6.9	—	2.7	—	18.1	9.3
1927	1.6	193.5	6.5	5.2	6.4	—	3.0	—	18.8	10.3
1928	1.9	196.2	9.0	5.7	6.1	—	3.1	—	18.2	9.9
1929	1.8	195.7	9.5	5.0	5.7	—	2.7	—	18.2	10.7
1930	2.3	194.5	9.1	4.6	6.3	—	2.3	—	16.1	9.0
	Larynx		Lung		Pancreas		Kidney and Suprarenals		Bladder	
1901-1910	?	?	10.2	7.0	14.5	11.8	8.4	7.6	?	?
1911-1920	23.9	6.0	12.7	7.0	16.7	13.1	9.1	7.2	28.2	9.7
1921-1930	31.3	7.1	25.2	9.6	26.3	19.5	11.7	8.9	30.5	11.4
1926	33.5	7.3	23.3	9.2	26.0	21.2	11.4	8.8	30.0	11.1
1927	31.7	6.9	26.8	9.7	30.3	20.4	12.2	9.6	30.5	11.6
1928	31.8	7.6	32.0	10.4	28.8	21.0	12.5	9.0	32.0	11.9
1929	31.4	7.6	33.4	11.9	30.3	20.0	13.2	9.6	32.3	12.3
1930	31.6	8.5	40.2	13.9	29.4	23.8	13.0	8.7	31.8	11.5
	Prostate		Testis		Bones		Mediastinum			
1901-1910	11.8	—	?	—	?	?	8.1	4.5		
1911-1920	26.5	—	4.9	—	15.7	12.0	9.2	4.6		
1921-1930	47.7	—	5.8	—	17.6	13.5	12.6	5.8		
1926	47.9	—	5.2	—	17.3	13.1	13.3	6.0		
1927	47.8	—	7.1	—	18.1	11.7	12.9	6.0		
1928	53.8	—	6.3	—	18.6	14.6	13.3	5.4		
1929	56.4	—	5.2	—	17.6	14.6	12.1	5.6		
1930	54.9	—	6.7	—	17.3	12.0	13.1	5.3		

[a] Taken from Statistical Review of England and Wales for 1930, Text, Table LII.

691.4, an increase of 24.3 percent. The selected causes account for 92 percent of the total mortality ascribed to cancer in 1911-1920, and for 94.3 percent of the total mortality in 1929. In the last thirteen years the mortality from "inaccessible" cancer has increased much faster than that from "accessible" cancer. This is a very different result from that found by Dr. Stevenson nearly twenty years ago. The figures quoted above are not comparable, because, in order to meet a not very important objection to the usual method, a different method of standardization was used by him. Even the table in the 1917 annual report is not strictly comparable because the sum of the "accessible" and "inaccessible" site rates in 1916-1917 has a larger proportion of the total than in our series. Still, the difference is not important enough to invalidate a comparison. These earlier figures showed an increase between 1901-1902 and 1916-1917 of 35 percent in mortality from cancer of "accessi-

ble" and of a little less than 30 percent of mortality from "inaccessible" sites. Comparing the complete decennia of 1911-1920 and 1921-1930, the "accessible" rates are 269.3 and 283.5, an increase of 5.3 percent. The "inaccessible" rates are 556.1 and 652.5, an increase of 17.3 percent. It will be noticed that the average rate for the decennium 1921-1930 is in the "accessible" group slightly higher, and in the "inaccessible" group decidedly lower, than for the year 1929 used in the last comparison. For 1930 the "accessible" rate was 282.9, the "inaccessible" rate 688.7. It will be felt that these statistical results are a little confusing. While between 1897 and 1917 "accessible" cancer was increasing faster than "inaccessible" cancer, during the last decade the relation has been reversed. Is any reconciliation possible?

In connection with the decennial analysis of occupational mortality effected on the material of the census of 1921 and the three years' death

Table 4. Standardized mortality (C.M.F.) at ages 20-65 years of all occupied and retired civilian males and of the five social classes from cancer of various sites, 1921-1923.[a]

	Occupied and retired	Standardized mortality (C.M.F.)				
		I	II	III	IV	V
All sites	128.4	102.5	118.1	127.1	123.8	157.8
1. Lip	1.0	0.3	0.5	0.7	1.4	1.7
Tongue	7.5	3.6	5.5	7.1	7.5	12.4
Mouth	2.2	1.3	1.6	2.2	2.2	3.6
Jaw	3.2	0.9	2.3	3.1	3.5	5.2
Tonsil	1.6	0.4	1.4	1.5	1.7	2.6
Pharynx	1.8	1.6	1.4	1.8	1.8	2.9
Esophagus	9.7	7.4	8.8	10.1	8.5	12.6
Stomach	29.5	17.6	24.2	29.4	31.2	38.2
2. Small intestine	0.6	0.7	0.6	0.7	0.6	0.8
Cecum	0.9	1.1	1.1	1.0	0.7	0.8
Hepatic and splenic flexures	0.4	0.1	0.5	0.3	0.5	0.3
Sigmoid flexure	2.2	3.4	2.5	2.2	1.8	2.1
Colon, part not stated	5.7	7.5	6.2	5.6	5.0	5.7
Intestine, part not stated	3.4	2.8	3.6	3.4	3.4	3.6
Large intestine	9.1	12.0	10.2	0.1	7.9	8.8
Total intestine (excluding rectum)	13.3	15.4	14.2	13.2	12.0	13.2
Rectum and anus	12.5	11.6	12.8	12.7	12.0	12.2
3. Larynx	4.6	3.3	4.4	4.3	4.4	6.2
Skin	3.0	1.9	2.2	3.0	3.6	4.5
Breast	0.2	—	0.3	0.2	0.2	0.4
4. Peritoneum, omentum, mesentery	0.9	1.3	0.8	1.0	0.9	0.9
Pancreas	3.4	3.5	3.5	3.3	3.0	3.8
Kidney and suprarenal	1.6	1.1	1.7	1.6	1.5	1.4
Bladder	3.1	3.3	3.0	3.2	2.4	3.9
Prostate	2.9	3.2	3.2	3.0	2.3	2.5
Testes	0.9	0.8	1.5	0.8	0.8	0.7
Brain	0.5	0.8	0.8	0.6	0.4	0.3
Bones	2.2	1.6	2.5	2.3	2.1	1.9
Gall-bladder	0.9	0.9	0.8	1.0	0.8	0.9
5. Lung	3.3	3.3	3.6	3.2	2.6	4.1
Liver	8.8	6.2	8.9	8.7	8.8	9.5
Abdomen	0.6	0.7	0.5	0.6	0.6	0.6
Neck	0.3	0.6	0.1	0.3	0.4	0.6
Lymphatic glands	4.1	3.6	3.4	4.2	3.6	5.6
Mediastinum	1.9	3.6	2.1	1.7	1.9	1.8
Other specified sites	2.0	2.6	2.1	2.0	1.7	2.5
Multiple	0.2	0.3	0.2	0.2	0.1	0.2
Site not stated	0.1	—	0.1	0.1	0.1	0.1
1. Upper alimentary canal	56.8	33.0	45.6	56.0	57.8	79.3
2. Intestine and rectum	25.8	27.1	27.1	25.9	24.0	25.4
3. Larynx, skin, breast	8.1	5.1	6.7	7.9	8.3	11.4
4. Deep-seated sites	16.4	16.5	17.8	16.7	14.2	16.3
5. Miscellaneous and ill-defined sites	21.2	20.8	20.9	20.8	19.8	24.9
1,3. Exposed sites	65.0	37.9	52.3	63.9	66.1	90.9
2,4,5. Other sites	63.3	64.3	65.8	63.4	57.9	66.5

[a] Annual Report of the R.G. Decennial Supplement, 1921. Occupational Mortality, p. xxiii, Table 4.

certificates of 1921-1923, Dr. Stevenson pointed out a very interesting relation between mortality from cancer and social class. The principal facts are shown in Table 4. . . .

These social classes purport to represent the following categories: Upper and Middle Classes form Class I, Intermediates form Class II, Skilled Workers form Class III, Intermediates form Class IV, and Unskilled Workers form Class V. As illustrations of the method of assignment I take first the profession to which some of my readers belong. Physicians, surgeons, registered medical practitioners, and dentists are assigned to Class I; veterinary surgeons to Class II; sick nurses, mental attendants, subordinate medical service (including masseurs, bone setters, and herbalists) to Class III. The reader will recollect that the analysis relates to *men* only. Take now a larger group, that of agricultural occupations. None are assigned to Class I. To Class II are assigned land and estate agents and managers (not auctioneers and estate agents), farmers, farmers' sons or other relatives assisting in the work of the farm, agricultural and forestry pupils (not at colleges), agricultural machine, tractor proprietors, managers, and foremen. To Class III are assigned gardeners, nurserymen, seedsmen, florists, foresters and woodmen, drainage superintendents, foremen, etc. To Class IV are assigned shepherds, agricultural machine tractor drivers and attendants, agricultural laborers, farm servants, land drainers, drainage laborers, laborers in woods and forests, other agricultural occupations. Class V receives gardeners' laborers, estate laborers, pea and fruit pickers. It would be very easy to recall individual exceptions to this classification. Bone setters have been known to bear titles and to reside in Park Lane, and estate agents to possess Rolls-Royce cars. Yet it would be perverse to deny that, as a statistical grouping, these classes from I to V do correspond to a social-economic trend from the most to the least eligible way of life in terms of the ordinary Englishman's standards of eligibility.

Refer now to the Table. It will be seen that mortality from cancer in the worst-placed social class is very much higher than in any other class. The difference between Class V and Class IV is greater than between Class IV and Class I. This contrast is much greater for particular sites than for cancer as a whole. Thus the mortality from cancer of the lip in Social Class V is more than five times as great as in Class I, and that due to cancer of the tongue is more than three times as great. On the other hand, cancer of the rectum and anus is little more fatal in Class V than in Class I, and cancer of the colon less fatal.

At the bottom of the Table those sites of cancer which may be called exposed sites, particularly the upper part of the alimentary canal, are grouped together, and it is seen how great is the contrast between Class V and Class I, while for other sites there is no difference. The striking result led Dr. Stevenson and his colleagues to write: "It thus appears that a large proportion, at least, of cancer mortality is of a highly preventable nature, for we must suppose that if the conditions of life of all sections of society could be assimilated to those of its upper ranks, mortality from cancer of the exposed sites would fall for all classes to the Class I level. Indeed, it is very possible that knowledge of the preventable causes accounting for the difference might provide the means of reducing if not eliminating these forms of cancer for all causes,[2] for these causes might well be found to apply in varying degree to all sections of society.". . .

I shall not discuss this view now, except with respect to the particular statistical issue which is perplexing us. If we believe, as I think we must, that during the last thirty to fifty years the general conditions of life of the population have improved greatly, so that the contrast between the extent of *commoda vitae*—whether quality and quantity of food, clothing, fresh air, or what one pleases—enjoyed by Classes I and V is much less than a century ago; this, then, might account for the recent stagnation or even decrease in mortality from cancer of exposed sites. Let us think for a moment of the beginning of the alimentary canal, fatal cancers of which are less frequent than before the war. I was taught that non-specific predisposing causes of, for instance, cancer of the tongue were a chronically septic mouth, the irritation due to a jagged tooth, a clay pipe, etc. One was also taught that syphilis with an associated glossitis was an important precursor. That splendid teacher, the late H. L. Barnard, used to tell us in outpatients

---

[2] The quotation is exact but perhaps for "causes" we should read "classes."

that it might be all very well to smoke and all very well to get syphilis, but that a prudent man contented himself with one or other enjoyment, for their combination might lead to cancer of the tongue. I suppose it is not too optimistic to believe that in the last generation mouths have become cleaner, prophylactic dentistry commoner, the smoking of foul pipes and the suffering from ill-treated syphilis decidedly rarer than in the past. We must add, although—for reasons to be given later on—it is not, perhaps, a factor of numerical importance yet, that the surgical and radiological treatment of malignant disease of these sites has steadily improved. But, at any rate within the terms of the passage I have just quoted from the report on Occupational Mortality, the facts that mortality from cancer of the stomach is increasing and that cancer of the stomach is one of the forms of cancer of an exposed site for which the contrast in mortality between Class I and Class V is very great are unfavorable to the optimistic explanation of the previous paragraph. It will be seen that with the help of statistical analysis and starting from plausible etiological hypotheses, one reaches results interesting but incomplete. At this point it will be convenient to recur to the purely statistical aspects of the matter.

Waiving for the moment the question whether rates of mortality from year to year are materially comparable, can we from examination of the secular graphs of mortality make any reasonable guess as to the future trend? The graph of age-standardized mortality among males certainly does suggest a slackening rate of increase, but he would be a bold man who would prophesy the value of the rate of mortality which will be ultimately attained. Across the chart (Figure 1) has been drawn the locus of a function, the simple logistic function, which has often proved a good means of describing the evolution of biological processes, such as the growth of population. It will be seen that, although not so bad a representation of the general trend, it certainly does not describe the "law" of change. The equation of this particular curve is:

$$y = \frac{1027.6}{1 + e^{-\frac{(5.376 + t)}{8.074}}}$$

where y is the annual rate of mortality in year t (origin 1901). It postulates a rate of mortality

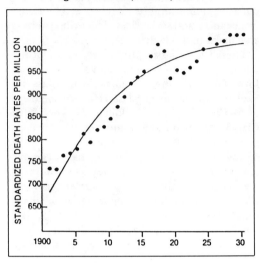

Figure 1. Cancer, all sites, males.

never in finite time attaining 1027.6 per million. In each of the years 1928-1930 (inclusive) the attained rate was higher than this. I think we may have a good deal of faith that the standardized mortality-rate in our generation will not exceed 1050, and that it will certainly not increase fast. But we cannot be more precise than that.

The course of mortality in females is still more refractory to any mathematical polishing process. It is, indeed, a strange picture, suggesting some queer speeding up of the rate of increase just before the war, leading to a falling away which has been replaced by a fairly steady or at worst slightly increasing trend. Mainly owing to the facts that the mortality from cancer in women is not increasing, or at least is only very slowly increasing, while the mortality in males is now definitely greater than in females, most people seem to be more interested in doing sums with the data for males. But from the educational point of view the mortality from cancer in women is more interesting. At the present time more than a third of the whole mortality from cancer in women is accounted for by recorded primary cancers of the breast or uterus, and these rates for sites which lend themselves to relatively easy diagnosis have changed greatly in the present generation. In 1901, when the all-sites rate was 943 per 1 million (these are age-standardized rates), the rate for the breast was 148.9 and for the uterus

223.8. In 1930, when the general rate was 987, the breast rate had risen to 194.5 and the uterus rate had fallen to 143.9. Yet, as one knows, the operative treatment of cancer of the breast is one of the triumphs of modern surgery, a much less dangerous and more successful treatment than that of the uterus—in spite of great improvements in the latter field.

Up to a certain point the explanation of this change is adequate. It was shown first by the late Dr. T. H. C. Stevenson that the death-rate of single women from cancer of the breast was much higher and from cancer of the uterus much lower than that of married women.

Since his original demonstration of the broad facts it has been shown that the higher incidence of fatal cancer of the breast is correlated with incomplete functioning of this sexual organ, i.e. that those who do not become pregnant have a greater liability. It has been shown that the higher liability of married women to uterine cancer is confined to cancer of the neck of the uterus, and that this liability does not increase with the number of children born, although associated with the bearing of children, i.e. that the contrast is between parturients and women who have borne no children. Some writers have even gone so far as to say that multiparae are more favorably situated than women who have only borne one or two children.

Further, it has been shown that, even now, the number of women suffering from malignant disease of either organ who present themselves at so early a stage of the morbid process that really radical surgery can be used is a disappointingly small proportion. Hence, although

we should expect treatment already to influence rates of mortality we should not be surprised to find that the effect is still but small.

All this is satisfactory enough to anybody who likes explanations, but there is a good deal left wholly unexplained. For instance, if we make comparison between countries on the same cultural level, and compiling statistics with equal accuracy, we find very great differences between the rates of mortality from cancer of the breast and uterus.

Tables 5 and 6, comparing the experiences of England and Wales and the Netherlands (with some other countries), bring this out. Here we have two countries suffering not widely dissimilar tolls of total mortality from malignant disease, yet contrasting greatly in respect of cancer of the female breast and sexual organs. An expert committee of the Health Organization of the League of Nations spent much time and labor in seeking to explain this discrepancy. The investigation verified the facts; it made it clear that no simple explanation (such as better facilities, or better use of facilities, for radical treatment) was adequate, and it got no further. If we could explain this discrepancy we should, I imagine, be near the center of the cancer maze. That we cannot is a warning to those who would solve the problems of malignant disease from an armchair. I suppose to most readers this is an unsatisfactory account. We seem to know a little about a great many things of importance and a great deal about a few things of no special importance, but the epidemiological-statistical method has, so far, reached no clear-cut conclusion which is of general etiological

Table 5. Cancer mortality in females of the genital organs and breast. Rates per 10 000.

Year	Genital organs			Breast		
	England and Wales	Italy	Holland	England and Wales	Italy	Holland
1905	—	1.50	1.29	—	0.57	0.80
1906	—	1.63	1.24	—	0.59	0.89
1907	—	1.59	1.24	—	0.56	1.03
1908	—	1.57	1.43	—	0.57	0.89
1909	—	1.56	1.28	—	0.59	0.97
1910	—	1.60	1.40	—	0.58	1.00
1911	2.43	1.48	1.17	1.84	0.55	0.98
1912	2.46	1.40	1.27	1.97	0.59	1.19
1913	2.55	1.50	1.40	2.02	0.59	1.08
1914	2.50	1.51	1.31	1.99	0.59	1.10
1916	2.47	1.49	—	2.11	0.56	—

Table 6. Cancer mortality at ages expressed as rates per 10 000.

		50-60					60-70					70 and upwards			
		England and Wales	Sweden	Holland	Italy	Prussia	England and Wales	Sweden	Holland	Italy	Prussia	England and Wales	Sweden	Holland	Italy	Prussia
1911	Male	27.85	23.88	37.48	15.36	25.58	59.52	52.63	97.26	30.67	52.34	87.87	70.27	109.47	42.91	62.74
	Female	31.85	22.27	34.73	19.64	25.98	55.64	43.10	77.44	33.57	46.68	83.50	59.43	96.45	48.23	58.06
1912	Male	28.35	22.41	37.77	14.06	24.36	60.63	54.24	95.20	31.08	53.57	91.93	65.89	97.61	43.20	67.61
	Female	33.37	23.98	37.98	19.33	25.44	56.63	42.35	77.80	31.82	46.60	87.39	60.04	92.59	45.15	60.13
1913	Male	28.62	23.27	36.89	14.88	24.42	63.31	50.61	97.98	31.65	54.77	92.86	67.84	112.59	45.26	65.68
	Female	33.65	23.05	35.19	20.18	26.66	60.04	45.85	81.72	32.46	47.32	86.84	61.69	94.41	46.02	60.77
1914	Male	28.68	24.54	35.87	15.47	23.67	63.98	52.04	98.51	31.08	54.33	97.06	71.39	103.43	48.15	65.85
	Female	33.36	24.57	35.05	19.58	25.69	58.84	44.32	78.34	33.30	47.27	88.03	68.95	101.52	46.85	85.58
1915	Male	28.99	25.04	36.68	—	23.70	62.20	53.12	97.52	—	53.38	95.00	76.25	113.36	—	62.05
	Female	33.34	23.04	33.70	—	24.08	58.85	45.50	83.23	—	45.41	86.60	68.34	95.74	—	54.98
1916	Male	28.66	24.03	32.86	15.77	23.55	63.71	54.49	104.62	30.64	50.95	95.85	75.72	112.85	47.07	65.95
	Female	33.43	23.39	35.96	20.23	25.51	58.79	45.94	81.41	31.89	45.00	86.97	67.35	113.76	47.27	41.75
1917	Male	29.11	24.00	34.75	15.38	22.89	63.58	58.39	102.22	29.70	47.01	100.12	73.61	118.18	45.38	61.59
	Female	34.05	25.05	36.01	19.29	24.39	59.97	46.26	83.12	31.53	43.41	89.79	61.31	100.90	46.21	57.13
1918	Male	29.25	—	34.70	—	23.63	62.44	—	101.10	—	50.78	93.86	—	108.17	—	60.51
	Female	33.19	—	35.02	—	24.86	59.81	—	85.34	—	44.74	88.17	—	111.94	—	56.06

importance. That is, I think, a just criticism, yet I am not pessimistic.

The answer to the young lady's question to Babbage, of calculating machine fame: "Please, Mr. Babbage, if you ask the wrong question, will it give you the right answer?" is still "No." Even in this country approximately accurate statistical data of mortality from cancer are a product of less than a generation. The accuracy is still only approximate.

* * *

Here my sketch of crowd-diseases must end. A great many important objects have been brought into the picture, but many have been omitted.

Among crowd-diseases in the grand manner, malaria does not yield in importance to plague; among crowd evils always with us, whooping-cough is not less deadly than measles, while traffic accidents (which surely come within my definition of a crowd-disease) are a good deal more deadly. The trouble is that when one enlarges the definition of epidemiology one is theoretically committed to a treatise on *all* the bad

habits of mankind, and so must practice an illogical moderation.

Perhaps, however, enough has been said to enable an interested reader to go further by himself. I hope to have taught him that this is a field of study not only as important but as interesting as others universally agreed to be within the circle of general culture. The subject is one which the non-professional reader has no excuse for neglecting on the ground that it is dry and technical. If and when all educated persons are as familiar with this kind of medical history as they are with political history, the level of discussion of social legislation will be raised and less attention will be paid to the dicta of "experts," "well-known Harley Street specialists" or even "professors," to the benefit of all concerned.

RECOMMENDATIONS FOR FURTHER STUDY

My "Review of Recent Statistical Studies of Cancer Problems" (*Cancer Review*, March 1928) gives a slightly fuller account and numerous references. I advise the student to read, *first*, the discussions of cancer statistics printed in the annual reports of the Registrar-General, beginning with that contained in the report for 1911.

"SOCIAL MEDICINE" AND "PUBLIC HEALTH"

John A. Ryle

I have scarcely as yet had time to familiarize myself with the organization of research and teaching in the field of preventive medicine in American universities, and I may appear to have overemphasized the distinctions between what we have long called 'public health' and what we now call 'social medicine'. The main differences, however, would seem to be these:

1. Public health, although in its modern practice attaching an ever-increasing importance to the personal services, for a long time and at first for very sufficient reasons, placed the emphasis on the *environment*. Social medicine, deriving its inspiration more from the field of clinical experience and seeking always to assist the discovery of a common purpose for the remedial and preventive services, places the emphasis on *man*, and endeavours to study him in and in relation to his environment. Furthermore, the immediate material environment, in the shape of housing, drainage, and water supplies, is today extended to include the whole of the economic, nutritional, occupational, educational, and psychological opportunity or experience of the individual or the community.

2. Public health, in the first instance, and again for obvious reasons, has been largely preoccupied with the communicable diseases, their causes, distribution, and prevention. Social medicine is concerned with all diseases of prevalence, including rheumatic heart disease, peptic ulcer, the chronic rheumatic diseases, cardiovascular disease, cancer, the psychoneuroses, and accidental injuries—which also have their epidemiologies and their correlations with social and occupational conditions and must eventually be considered to be in greater or less degree preventable.

3. Where hospital practice (as distinct from preventive theory and practice) is concerned, social medicine properly takes within its ambit the whole of the work of a modern almoners' department; this includes social diagnosis and social therapeutics—the investigation of conditions, the organization of after-care, and the

readjustment of the lives of individuals and families disturbed or broken by illness. The almoner or medical social worker also has an important part to play in teaching and in the follow-up activities of a clinical research unit. . . .

THE FUTURE

I come lastly to the most important and yet the most difficult question which I have set myself to try to answer. Speculation is not my habit, but this great centenary gathering, this hour in history which we all hope to look back upon as a moment of pause between two eras— a bad one and a better—tempt me to invite my native optimism and emergent ideas to go into partnership for the occasion. "What", I have asked, "may be the larger influence of these new directives for medical and social thought and action? How, possibly, will they assist the general evolution of Medicine in the new age that lies ahead of us?"

Our great contemporary biologist and humanist, Julian Huxley . . . , has discussed the transition now in progress from the age of 'economic man' to the age of 'social man'. Our profession, which is so particularly concerned with man and his welfare, must assist this transition with all the scientific and humanist wisdom at its command. Hitherto, our science, like our practice, has evolved along individualist lines. Whatever the several countries may do with regard to the modification of their systems of practice and of service, it seems to me that the scientific study of health and disease in man— the most complex of all social animals—must henceforward concern itself to an ever-increasing degree with the interactions and correlations of disease and health with changing social circumstance. Socially, industrially, politically, we are creating a new age. With it, inevitably, we alter the whole character and distribution of diseases and set ourselves new problems for solution in the fields of medical science, practice, and administration.

Source: John A. Ryle, *Changing Disciplines.* London, Oxford University Press, 1948. By permission of Oxford University Press.

Some of my friends have rebuked me for leaving the clinical fold. I reply in effect that I have merely taken the necessary steps to enlarge my field of vision and to increase my opportunities of etiological study. My allegiance to human medicine is in no whit broken. I wish I could convey to them and to others some of the sense of stimulation and rejuvenation that my close association with statisticians and medical social workers and with men and women in the public health and industrial health services has brought to me. Thirty years of my life have been spent as a student and teacher of clinical medicine. In these thirty years I have watched disease in the ward being studied more and more thoroughly—if not always more thoughtfully—through the high power of the microscope; disease in man being investigated by more and more elaborate techniques and, on the whole, more and more mechanically. Man, as a person and a member of a family and of much larger social groups, with his health and sickness intimately bound up with the conditions of his life and work—in the home, the mine, the factory, the shop, at sea, or on the land—and with his economic opportunity, has been inadequately considered in this period by the clinical teacher and hospital research worker. The medicine of the teaching schools has, as I have suggested, undergone a gradual conversion to a highly technical exercise in bedside pathology and therapeutic method. The morbid "material" of the hospital ward consists very largely—if we exclude the emergencies—of end-result conditions for which, as a rule, only a limited amount of relief repays the long stay, the patient investigation, and the anxious expectancy of the sick man or woman. With etiology—the first essential for prevention—and with prevention itself, the majority of physicians and surgeons have curiously little concern. Nor have they at present the opportunity, nor yet the appropriate types of training or assistance, requisite for the study of etiology or prevention. Their material is mainly selected by four factors: the gravity, the difficulty or the rarity of their cases, or their suitability otherwise for admission to a hospital. Some of the most common diseases, the less lethal diseases, and the beginnings of disease are even considered as providing "poor teaching material". Health and sickness in the population and their possible correlations with significant and mea-surable social or occupational influences are outside their province. . . .

PREVENTION OR CURE?

For a very long time we have accepted the old adage "Prevention is better than cure". In our new era the belief in it—for of its truth there can be no doubt—must be made ever more manifest in our research and its directives and in our teaching. The most conspicuous interest of the student ten or twenty years hence will, I hope, no longer be in the rare or difficult and too often incurable case, but in the common and more understandable and preventable disease. May the daily questions on his lips become not "What is the treatment?" but "What are the causes?" and "If preventable, then why not prevented?"

The study of the ultimate causes of disease—the procatarctic causes, without which the specific factors can never find their opportunity—goes hand in hand with the study of the causes of health, and how much we have still to learn of the meaning and measurement of health. When social pathology and hygiology come into their own we may witness a return—but this time with fuller scientific authority for the guidance of the people and their teachers and rulers—of that ancient pride in health as a cultural objective which has been largely in abeyance since the days of the old Greek civilization.

The training of the doctor, which began with observations on and the care of the sick individual, is due now for a great forward stride. Observations on whole communities, whether great or small (or on appropriate samples), and improved health provisions for them, must henceforward become the prior objective. The individual is not likely to suffer neglect in the process, for all communities are composed of individuals. For generations yet we shall doubtless continue to build our costly hospitals and clinics, and require our armies of practitioners and ancillaries, but meanwhile we must at least embark upon the crusade which will end in the steady reduction of waiting-lists and the closure of hospital wards, and which will eventually put the physical, mental, and moral health of peoples before their material wealth. In that crusade—whether by our researches, by realistic reforms in teaching, by the better education of the people or direct representations to government—it is our first duty as physicians to explore and prepare the way.

I submit that we can only do this effectively by electing to pursue the study of social man in sickness and in health as assiduously as we have hitherto pursued the study of individual man in the isolation of the consulting room or the hospital bed, when health has finally passed him by. The quality of our actions and our practice and of our leadership in social reformation will depend, as in the past, on many disciplines, but not least, perhaps, upon the science whose history I have briefly sketched and whose province I have endeavoured to define.

SICKNESS AND STRESS IN OPERATIONAL FLYING

D. D. Reid

To the medical branch of an air force, the social or environmental conditions of pressing importance are the psychological stresses inevitable in air warfare. Only in war is it possible to observe the effects of such factors as acute hazard and intensive operational effort, with their resultant anxiety and fatigue, on the performance and well-being of such a highly selected population as the air crews of the Royal Air Force. Both the immediate effects of these stresses on efficiency and the long-term results in health were, therefore, the urgent concern of those whose duty it was to minimize these effects by every means open to the medical branch of a combatant force. The central issue was one of limitation of spells of duty—either short-term, where the effects of hours of prolonged attention were to be forestalled, or long-term, where the limits of an operational tour had to be set at a level high enough to ensure an adequate operational return for the training investment made yet not so long as to endanger health and morale. The problems of peacetime practice in social and industrial medicine are hardly as dramatic, yet the essential mechanism of the adjustment of men to the less hazardous but frequently harassing conditions of post-war life are identical. This account of some typical studies of sickness in relation to measurable environmental and personal factors is given in the hope of displaying the potentialities of the methods used in the study of problems of sickness and morale in an industrial population.

Research on duty limitation in the R.A.F. during the war had a tripartite approach by clinical, laboratory, and field surveys. The clinical studies have been described by Symonds (1), the laboratory work by Russell Davis (2); in the present paper is set out an application of statistical methods to data collected in the course of active operations in the field.

Source: *British Journal of Social Medicine.* 2:123–131, 1948.

BACKGROUND OF PRESENT STUDY

The background to the present studies may be briefly sketched. In the world war 1914–18, work was mainly along clinical lines, the opinions expressed (3) being intuitive judgments based on extensive experience with cases of neurosis occurring in the operational squadrons. The importance of the hazardous, fatiguing, and often physically exhausting nature of flying duties was recognized, but the issue was clouded by a preoccupation with the cumulative effects on health and performance of the physical stresses specific to flight, such as oxygen lack, and others less specific, such as cold, noise, discomfort, and glare. A tendency to overstress the importance of the presumed cumulative effects of the stresses of air fighting as a cause of breakdown in flying men persisted until the world war 1939–45, and with it the implication that a simple relation existed between the number of hours' flying done and the resultant degree of deterioration in health and efficiency. Thus in the short-term context, efficiency would fall off towards the end of an operational sortie, while in the long run, signs and symptoms of impending breakdown were to be looked for after a prolonged tour of many sorties.

Contrary indications, however, came from laboratory experiments recently described by Russell Davis (2) where, in a complex and distracting experimental situation analogous to flying, no progressive deterioration in efficiency was observed. On the other hand, it became clear that anxiety and tension had much more serious effects on the level of performance. This was strikingly confirmed by an analysis of the errors made by navigators of bomber aircraft during sorties against German targets (4, 5). The effect of anticipatory anxiety was seen in a steady deterioration in efficiency on the outward journey, particularly over the enemy coast, and on approaching the target. This effect reached a maximum in the acute anxiety engendered by heavy enemy fighter opposition and persisted as long as the aircraft was over enemy territory. Compared with this, any effect of "fatigue," in its conventional sense of deterioration at the end of prolonged activity, was minimal. Similarly, Bradford Hill and G. O. Williams (6) showed that landing accidents were no more common after long sorties than after much shorter ones.

Clinical studies by Symonds and D. J. Williams (7) on the histories of cases of neurosis arising in the operational Commands demonstrated that the bulk of them were men of neurotic predisposition who broke down early in their operational career. There did remain, however, many instances of breakdown after prolonged stress among men of the toughest fibre. Tour limitation, therefore, was essential, and in the formulation of policy in this matter the precision of statistical methods complemented the insight of the clinical approach. A search for objective measures of the process of adaptation to stress during the course of an operation tour showed that the critical nature of the early part of the tour was revealed by a simultaneous increase in the incidence of psychological disorder and the frequency of reporting sick and a fall in the average weight of a large group of flying men (4, 5). As adjustment to the strain took place, these three indicators tended to stabilize at a new level and showed no sign of deterioration towards the end of a tour limited to thirty bomber sorties. The possibility of using such measures in the determination of optimum tour limits was thus evident, but there remained the task of discerning the relative importance of such measurable environmental factors as hazard, experience, and effort in the maintenance of health in men exposed to their effects. These relationships could then be taken into account in laying down the broad principles of tour limitation.

OUTLINE OF METHOD

In such a study, the effects of these measurable external factors in health and morale were assessed by the varying incidence of neurosis and venereal disease among the flying crews. Men react differently to strain; some find refuge in neurotic illness, while in others the weakening is one of morals rather than of morale. With the monthly incidence of these two types of illness as criterion, then, the relative impor-

tance of any environmental factor can be gauged by the closeness of the association between its varying intensity and the fluctuations in the incidence of nervous and venereal disease.

As Bomber Command formed the largest body of men in the R.A.F. engaged in operational flying of a particularly hazardous and strenuous character, the vital and operational statistics of the five major Groups of this Command were studied for a period of twenty months from June, 1943, to January, 1945, inclusive. Product-moment coefficients of correlation were calculated between the criteria and various items believed to indicate the magnitude of the several environmental factors of importance. The conventions adopted may be briefly set out.

CRITERIA OF EFFECTS OF STRESS

Neurosis. The incidence of psychological disorder is taken as the percentage of the average aircrew strength for any month who were referred during that month for psychiatric opinion because of psychological disorder. It might have been preferable to assign these cases to the month in which they became non-effective. As the delay between the latter date and the date of the first psychiatric interview is normally fairly short, however, this should affect the extent rather than the nature of the relationships between the incidence of neurosis and the items investigated. Similarly, it was impossible to account for cases of psychological disorder dealt with on the stations without being referred to the psychiatrist. This, too, may lessen the closeness of the correlation, but it should not hide any striking relationship which does exist.

Venereal Disease. Similarly, the incidence of venereal disease is taken as the percentage of the average air crew strength reported as fresh cases of venereal disease during the month in question.

MEASURES OF ENVIRONMENTAL FACTORS

Hazard. The hazard or degree of personal danger to which crews are subject in any month is best measured by the casualty rate through operational causes, i.e. in battle or in flying accidents, in that month. This hazard rate is the percentage of the average monthly crew strength who become casualties during the month. The cumulative effect of hazard is taken into account by calculating the correlation coefficient between the neurosis incidence in one month and the casualty rate both in the same month and in the month before.

An alternative method of measuring the degree of hazard is to calculate the average number of aircraft lost through enemy action in the course of every hundred sorties carried out by the Bomber Group in the month. This percentage has been termed the "missing per sortie" rate. It depends in part, of course, both on the effectiveness of the enemy opposition and on the skill of the crews' defensive tactics. To some extent it is thus a measure of their operational efficiency. It is also a measure of the *rate* at which casualties are occurring rather than the *total* casualties suffered during the month.

Inexperience. The level of operational experience of the Group is quite easily measured by calculating the percentage of the average crew strength for the month who have been posted into the Group, on completion of training, during the month. In other words, this percentage expresses the proportion of the squadrons' strength who are novices to operational flying.

Effort. The cumulative effect of long hours of highly skilled activity should be reflected in an association between the incidence of neurosis and features of squadron employment to which fatigue is often attributed. Among these are the average number of flying hours per individual in each month and/or the frequency and average duration of the sorties occurring during that month. The total number of hours, operational and non-operational, flown each month by all the aircraft in the Group, and the average number of men on board being known, it is easy to calculate the mean number of flying hours done by each man in each month. The frequency with which each man operated, i.e. the average number of sorties per man per month, is calculated in the same way from the total number of aircraft sorties carried out by the Group in the month in question. Similarly, the number of operational hours and the number of sorties carried out by the Group in any one month being known, simple division of the former by the latter gives the average duration of sortie during that month. As when dealing with the effect of hazard, the cumulative effect of the operational effort from one month to the next

can be gauged by the correlation between the flying time and sortie duration and frequency averages for one month and the incidence of neurosis in the next.

SUMMARY OF RESULTS

For security reasons it is unfortunately impossible to give in detail the figures upon which these measures are based, but they derive from the experience of the whole of Bomber Command at a period of its maximum strength. The correlation coefficients indicating the relationship between these measures and the criteria are given in Table 1 where they are arranged in order of their magnitude under the headings as previously defined.

For venereal disease, similar results were obtained; the only significant correlations were between the venereal disease incidence and the casualty and inexperience groups of items (Table 2).

It would appear from these correlation coefficients that only hazard and inexperience are significantly related to the selected criteria of the effects of operation strain. There is no evidence of such a clear relationship between the criteria in the "effort" group of items; yet these items may be fairly termed "fatiguing" in that they might be expected to have a cumulative effect on the mental health of the crews. It is clear that the monthly variation in "effort" in this study has not had an appreciable effect on the monthly incidence of neurosis.

Some allowance must be made for the association between the influx of new crews in any one month and the heavy casualty rate sustained by these operationally inexperienced men in the succeeding month. At the same time, in the latter month, these men reach the critical stage in their tour when breakdown is most likely. The association between the neurosis rate and the casualty rate in any month may therefore be merely an expression of their common relationship to the novice rate in the previous month. Fortunately this possibility can be taken into account by calculating the partial or net correlation between the casualty rate and the neurosis rate in any month when the novice rate in the previous month is kept constant. The value obtained ($r = 0.3734$) shows that the casualty rate in any month is significantly more closely associated with the neurosis rate than might be ex-

Table 1. Correlation between items and neurosis rate.

	r =
A. *"Hazard" group of items*	
1. Casualty rate (in same month)	0.4194[a]
2. Casualty rate (in previous month)	0.3312[a]
3. Missing per sortie rate (in previous month)	0.2455[b]
4. Missing per sortie rate (in same month)	0.2404[b]
B. *"Inexperience" group of items*	
1. Novice rate (in same month)	0.2906[a]
2. Novice rate (in previous month)	0.2869[a]
C. *"Effort" group of items*	
1. Total flying hours per man (in previous month)	0.1163
2. Total flying hours per man (in same month)	0.1157
3. Average sortie duration (in previous month)	0.0933
4. Average sortie duration (in same month)	0.0351
5. Operational flying hours per man (in previous month)	0.0323
6. Average frequency of sorties per man (in previous month)	0.0267
7. Average frequency of sorties per man (in same month)	0.0029
8. Operational flying hours per man (in same month)	0.0019

[a] denotes highly significant relationship, $P < .01$.
[b] denotes a significant relationship, $P < .05$.

plained by their common relationship to the proportion of inexperienced crews. Similarly, there exists a significant net correlation between the novice rate in any month and the neurosis rate in the next, even after eliminating the effect of simultaneous variations in the casualty rate ($r = 0.2044$). The experience in venereal disease is analogous; the net correlation between the casualty rate in one month and the venereal disease rate in the next is, when the novice rate is kept constant, significantly high ($r = 0.3546$). On the other hand, the net relationship between the novice rate and the venereal disease rate becomes insignificant ($r = 0.1292$) when simultaneous fluctuations in the casualty rate are taken into account.

The position may be summarized by suggesting that although correlation, particularly in a time series such as this, does not necessarily mean causation, the hazard of operational flying has both an immediate and delayed effect on the incidence of both neurotic and venereal disease. The immediate effect is most marked on neurotic illness; the delayed effect, probably as the result of the delay in obtaining opportunities for infection and the incubation period of gonorrhoea (the most frequent type), was more definite in venereal disease. Further, the immediate response to the realization of the dangerous nature of their duty was reflected in an increase in neurosis, particularly among the inexperienced men, but the rise in venereal dis-

Table 2. Correlation Between Operational Factors and V.D. Rate.

	r=
A. *"Hazard" group of items*	
1. Casualty rate (in previous month)	0.4109[a]
2. Casualty rate (in same month)	0.2972[a]
B. *"Inexperience" group of items*	
1. Novice rate (in same month)	0.2399[b]
2. Novice rate (in previous month)	0.0350

[a] denotes highly significant relationship, $P < .01$.
[b] denotes a significant relationship, $P < .05$.

ease was not particularly frequent among operational novices.

PRACTICAL CONSEQUENCES OF RESULTS

Of the measurable environmental factors affecting health and morale, operational hazard is thus clearly of decisive importance. Conversely, factors such as the number of flying hours done by each man and the frequency of operating do not produce the cumulative effect on mental health which conventional ideas about "fatigue" might have led one to expect. In laying down a policy of tour limitation, therefore, the duration of the operational tour to be expected from those who survive long enough to become due for relief must take these facts into account. No arbitrary number of flying hours can be taken as the optimum limit in all types of flying. Since the number of hours flown does not in itself determine the incidence of neurosis, it would be unrealistic to translate a tour limit of x hours from, say, long-range flying boat sea patrols to the conditions of intensive fighter operations. Tour limits may be *expressed* in flying hours, but they had to be framed to take into account the hazard involved in the particular type of flying in question. The basic principle adopted was the setting of the limit at a level giving the individual a chance of surviving the particular hazards entailed which could be faced without breakdown in health and morale by the resolute type of man who elected to serve in the air. Exactly what that limit should have been was difficult to assess. Within the range of casualty rates experienced by Bomber Command during the period reviewed, there appeared to be no point beyond which a sudden serious deterioration took place. The physical measures of health already mentioned gave no indication of a decline in health among those who survived the initial period of adaptation. On the other hand, the hazard of bomber operations was such that the incidence of neurosis in Bomber Command was higher than in any other Command of the Royal Air Force (7). The "expectation of life" prevailing in that Command could, therefore, be taken as a minimum rather than an optimum for general application and the duration of the operational tour in other forms of combat flying set to ensure that the individual pilot had at least the same chance of survival as was general in the bomber offensive against German targets.

SICKNESS ON SORTIES: A SPECIFIC ENQUIRY

Useful as these general indications were, the size of the multiple correlation coefficient between neurosis, and hazard and inexperience ($R = 0.4585$) suggests that these factors accounted for only about 21 percent of the total amount of variance in the incidence of neurosis. They take no heed of intangibles such as squadron leadership and personal morale. Tour limits can be laid down very broadly, but in their application to an individual case the complex of relevant personal and environmental features must be resolved by the squadron commander, aided by his medical officer, in determining the best time of relief from further operational duties.

Typical of the problems met with by the squadron doctor was the case of sickness causing the abandonment or cancellation of an operation sortie. This was an unusual event (it happened about once in every 5575 person-sorties), so that no single medical officer could acquire the body of clinical experience needed to frame a sound prognostic judgment. Yet, if no obvious physical reason for the sickness was present, two questions rose urgently in the mind of the squadron doctor:

(*a*) Is this sickness likely to be a portent of impending breakdown?

(*b*) Does the return to full duty of this man, whose morale and efficiency may be suspect, entail an increased hazard for the aircraft in which he is flying?

To assess the prognostic significance of the basic patterns of reaction observed, statistical studies were made of a series of such cases occurring in Bomber Command.

OUTLINE OF METHOD

The nature of the two critical questions implies that some follow-up of the subsequent operational careers of the sick men is required. Not only must their own medical and operational histories be obtained and analyzed, but a suitable standard of comparison must be afforded. This was effected in practice by making a series of paired comparisons between the "sick" case and a corresponding "control" man selected from among the others in the squadron. From the Squadron Weekly Aircrew List for the week in which the sickness occurred was selected a "pair" for the man whose illness during or just before a sortie had caused its abandonment or cancellation. This "control" man was selected as far as possible so that each pair was comparable in respect of these items in the following order of priority: (1) crew duty; (2) number of sorties performed before the date of the sickness; (3) squadron; (4) officer or non-commissioned officer status. Thus it was hoped to control the influence on morale and efficiency of such factors as the stresses specific to the task in the air, operational experience, squadron leadership, and living conditions. In other words, during their subsequent careers in the squadron, both the "sick" man and his "control" were subject to the same environmental influences and differed only in the one respect of this particular type of sickness. In a group of such pairs, the differences between their subsequent performance should therefore be due mainly to differences in the psychological qualities of the individuals themselves, since both men in each pair are equally likely to be affected by the chances and hazards of flying in war.

The subsequent operational career of each of the men thus paired was followed up through the records of the Personnel Staff sections in each Group Headquarters. Two features were examined in particular:

(1) the cessation of flying duties through illness, whether physical or psychological;
(2) the survival time subsequent to the date of sickness, measured for each man of the pair by the number of sorties completed.

These features were recorded, together with all the relevant medical data about the sick case, on cards which could then be sorted into groups. The manner of this division depended on the factor being studied, for example, nature of symptom pattern, previous operational experience, etc. Inter-group as well as inter-pair differences could thus be investigated and the relative prognostic importance of both sickness in general and of some additional factor, such as experience, assessed. The statistical methods involved are detailed in the appropriate tables in each section.

In the clinical assessment of the likelihood of a psychological basis for the complaints which necessitated the return of the aircraft, full weight would be given to definite physical signs of disease; but in so many of these cases no such definite aid is forthcoming and the medical of-

ficer must rely upon a subjective account of the symptoms. In order to assay the relative prognostic importance of various types of symptom pattern, the pairs of sick cases and their controls were divided up on the basis of an arbitrary grouping of the presenting symptoms.

1. *Syncope.* All cases where the patient lost consciousness were taken separately. These cases were divided into:

(a) those where the fainting was clearly due to a failure of the oxygen supply;
(b) those where no defect of the oxygen apparatus could be found. Fainting was here usually preceded by dizziness, defective vision, and vomiting, and often followed by stupor.

2. *Nervous.* Cases in which fainting did not occur but where symptoms referable to the nervous system were complained of, were next classified together. These symptoms fall broadly into two groups, the first dealing with intellectual and emotional disturbance and the second with more specific physical complaints. These grades may be described in more detail:

(a) inability to concentrate, lack of confidence in his ability to carry out his duty, frank admissions of panic or fear, feelings of anxiety or acute depression perhaps accompanied by weeping;
(b) dizziness, blurring of vision, complaints of confusion, fatigue or "muzziness," faintness without loss of consciousness, neuritic pains, muscular weakness, backache, "pins and needles," sweating and rapid breathing.

3. *Alimentary.* Nausea, epigastric pain, heartburn, waterbrash, vomiting, colic.

4. *Airsickness.* Cases were classified as airsickness only when there was a clear previous history of airsickness.

5. *Respiratory* (and ear, nose, and throat). Painful ears, sinus pains, cough, breathlessness, asthma.

6. *Injuries.* Usually minor injuries, received just before take off.

In following up the operational careers after the date of sickness, particular note was taken of the reasons for cessation of full flying duties. Medical reasons for becoming non-effective might be physical or psychological. "Psychological reasons" have here been extended to include not only frank neurotic disorder but also executive disposal, for example, on grounds of "lack of moral fiber." The prognostic importance of

Table 3. Physical and psychological wastages in symptom groups.

	No. of pairs	Physical wastage				Psychological wastage			
		Sick		Control		Sick		Control	
		No.	%	No.	%	No.	%	No.	%
"Syncope"	19	0	0.0	0	0.0	15	78.9	0	0.0
"Nervous"	31	2	6.5	2	6.5	9	29.0	0	0·0
"Alimentary"	47	1	2·1	1	2.1	6	12.8	0	0.0
"Airsickness"	7	0	0.0	1	14.3	1	14.3	0	0.0
"Oxygen lack"	9	0	0.0	0	0.0	2	22.2	1	11.1
"Respiratory"	34	7	20.6	1	2.9	3	8.8	0	0.0
"Injuries"	8	0	0.0	0	0.0	0	0.0	0	0.0
Totals	155	10	6.5	5	3.2	36	23.2	1	0.6

any feature of the group being studied will therefore be indicated by the disparity between the proportion of subsequent psychological failures in the "sick" and "control" series of paired cases.

SUMMARY OF RESULTS

Table 3 shows the wastage rates for physical and psychological reasons in each of the symptom pattern groups already described.

Inspection of the final percentages in Table 3 shows that although the wastage for physical reasons in the "sick" group (6.5 percent) is larger than in the "controls" (3.2 percent), this disparity is not nearly so striking as the difference between the corresponding psychological wastage rates of 23.2 percent. and 0.6 percent. Prognostic importance being measured by the extent of this disparity, the syndrome sets can be classified by the size and significance of the difference in psychological wastage rates between the "sick" and "control" group in each syndrome set. Table 4 shows how the syndromes may be thus divided into those which are significantly related to the chance of subsequent psychological failure and those where the differences might well be due to chance. Further, the former group may be placed in order of importance by the extent of this disparity.

Table 4 shows that although there is a consistent tendency for those who have been sick on a sortie to incur a later psychological disability, this tendency is only significant in three syndrome groups—"syncope," "nervous," and "alimentary"—in that order. It should also be noted that only the first of these is anything like a certain indicator of psychological breakdown.

Other features of each individual case, operational experience and time of onset, must therefore be considered as in Tables 5 and 6.

This division of the cases into groups according to the number of sorties completed prior to

Table 4. Symptom pattern and disparity in psychological wastage rates.

Syndrome type	No. of pairs	Difference %	S.E. of difference %
Significant			
"Syncope"	19	78.9	±9.4
"Nervous"	31	29.0	±8.2
"Alimentary"	47	12.8	±4.9
Not significant			
"Airsickness"	7	14.3	a
"Oxygen lack"	9	11.1	a
"Respiratory, etc."	34	8.8	±4.9
"Injuries, etc."	8	0.0	±0.0

[a] Exact treatment of these small samples shows the difference to be insignificant.

Table 5. Interrelation of operational experience and subsequent history.

Operational experience in sorties	No. of pairs	Psychological wastage			
		Sick		Control	
		No.	%	No.	%
0–3	39	10	25.6	0	0.0
4–9	41	15	36.6	0	0.0
10–19	46	9	19.6	1	2.2
20+	29	2	6.9	0	0.0
Total	155	36	23.2	1	0.7

Table 6. Time of onset and subsequent history.

Stage in sortie (flying time in minutes)	No. of cases	% of total cases	Psychological wastage	
			No.	%
0–9	45	29.0	7	15.6
10–29	20	12.9	3	15.0
30–39	23	14.9	6	26.1
40–59	27	17.4	6	22.2
60–90	27	17.4	9	33.3
90 +	13	8.4	5	38.5
Total	155	100.0	36	23.2

the date of sickness shows that the psychological wastage rates rise to a maximum early in the tour, that is, that sickness occurring during the first ten sorties is much more likely to be psychogenic than if it arises later in the tour (a table comparing the numbers of wastages among sick men who had done less than ten sorties and the remainder gives $\chi^2 = 5.0763$, n = 1, .05>P>0.02). This, of course, is in keeping with the previous work which demonstrated the increased effects of stress on the operationally inexperienced.

Similarly, the importance of the stage in the particular sortie at which symptoms arose is evident in Table 6. The original reports of these sicknesses showed not only the time of take-off but also the time of onset of symptoms. The difference between those times thus indicates the stage in the sortie or distance out from base when the symptoms were first observed.

Table 6 shows that although most of the sickness occurs early in the sortie, the chance of subsequent psychological failure rises consistently in each successive stage of the sortie. This suggests (although the χ^2 value of 5.3679, n = 2, ·10>P>.05 is barely technically significant) that illness arising later in the sortie is more likely to have a psychological basis than sickness occurring either at take-off or in the first half-hour. In the previous study on navigator performance it was observed that efficiency fell off as the enemy coast was approached, presumably due to the increasing effects of anticipatory anxiety. It seems likely that this effect is becoming apparent in the increased likelihood of psychogenic upset occurring as the sortie progresses.

All three factors, then, symptom pattern, operational experience, and stage in sortie, are probably related to the likelihood of psychological failure in the subsequent flying career. Despite this association, however, it does not necessarily follow that each of these factors can be taken as independent items of clinical evidence in formulating a prognostic judgment. If one factor overlaps much with another, for example if *all* cases of syncope occurred in the later stages of the sorties, then taking stage of sortie into account would not enhance the accuracy of a prognosis based on our experience of syncope cases alone. On the other hand if the two are not related, then one can legitimately consider the stage of sortie as additional information of prognostic value. The contingency tables giving the relationships between each of the three factors are not reproduced, but they suggest that there is no significantly close relationship between them; this is confirmed in each instance by the χ^2 test. It follows, then, that in any individual case the information relevant to each of these three aspects can be combined in framing an estimate of the likely outcome of the patient's subsequent operational career.

The risk entailed in allowing a man who has suffered from a sickness which might well be psychogenic to go back to operational duty can be measured by the difference, if any, in the number of sorties subsequently completed by the "sick" compared with the "control" member of the pair in the same squadron at the same time. Any gross disparity in favour of the controls would imply that the return of the "sick" men to their operational duties entailed an increased hazard for the aircraft in which they flew. The differences actually observed are given in Table 7.

As Table 7 indicates, there is a slight adverse difference in the total number of sorties subsequently performed in the group who went on

Table 7. Comparison of subsequent operational survival time in sorties.

	No. of cases	Sorties subsequently completed ("Sick" v. "Control")	
		Mean difference	S. error of difference
S.N.A.[a]	63	− 1.35	±1.48
Others	42	+ 2.14	±1.68

[a] S.N.A.—"Syncope," "Nervous," and "Alimentary" disorders.

operating even after a sickness of a type normally associated with a liability to psychological failure. The "t" test for the significance of this mean difference between pairs indicates, however, that the difference might easily have occurred by chance. Further subdivision of the cases was hardly justified by the numbers involved, so that it must be concluded from these results that if a man carried on without breakdown after an illness in the air which might well have been psychogenic in origin, his presence in the crew did not seem to affect appreciably the aircraft's chance of safe return in subsequent sorties.

DISCUSSION

These studies are typical of the field research which formed a useful complement to clinical and laboratory work in war medicine. They are important for the confirmation which they gave in this instance to the suggestion that anxiety was more important than prolonged effort as a cause of deterioration in health and operational efficiency. Essentially statistical in methodology, they show how the numerical approach can be a useful adjunct to the clinical or impressionistic methods which rely upon the intuitive judgments of the skilled observer and to laboratory work where realism must so often be sacrificed to technical convenience.

The recognition and measurement of the effects of the mental stresses inherent in the operational environment is important in war; the physical conditions of battle may change, but the principles of action in human behavior remain. But these methods and results, though useful in war, may be none the less useful in peace. Admittedly we have dealt with the effects of particularly severe strain on a highly selected group, but the principles probably hold for the results in the less resilient population of a factory of the far from negligible emotional stresses of industrial life. The many-sided aspect of the reaction to stress—the failing efficiency, the objective signs of physical deterioration, and the characteristic symptom patterns—calls for an equally varied taste in the methods used in such studies.

If Service experience such as here described be taken as a guide, it would appear that the convergent attack on a single problem by workers skilled in clinical, laboratory, and statistical field research is a useful approach to the difficulties of investigation in social medicine.

SUMMARY

This paper describes typical field studies, carried out in Bomber Command of the Royal Air Force during the war 1939–45, on the effects of operational stresses both on the incidence of certain diseases and in individual cases of sickness occurring in the course of bomber operational sorties.

A study of the relationship between the incidence of neurosis and venereal disease and various indices of operational hazard and effort suggests that the acute anxiety caused by a high casualty rate had a much more decisive effect on health and morale than had prolonged or intensive operational effort.

Operational inexperience, which also plays a part in determining the incidence of neurosis, is shown to be relevant in the prognosis of cases of sickness occurring in conditions of acute stress on operational sorties. The chance of subsequent psychological failure in such cases is also seen to have been related to the type of presenting syndrome and the stage in the sortie at which the sickness appeared. Fainting and symptoms referable to the nervous and alimentary systems, particularly if they arose some time after take-off, were indicative of impending breakdown. In those instances where this did not occur, however, no extra risks to the aircraft in which he flew were incurred by allowing the man to continue on operational duty.

These suggestions of the predominant effects of anxiety over "fatigue" (in the sense of the end results of prolonged effort) can be related to the findings of laboratory and clinical research done in the Royal Air Force. The value of simple statistical methods in field research as a complement to laboratory and clinical studies is discussed.

I am indebted to Air Marshal Sir Harold Whittingham, Director General of Medical Services of the Royal Air Force during the war, for his encouragement, to the Consultants in Neuropsychiatry and Medical Statistics, Sir Charles Symonds and Prof. A. Bradford Hill for their direction and advice, and to the present Director General of Medical Services, Royal Air Force, Air Marshal P. C. Livingston, for permission to publish this work. My thanks are also due to Miss O. M. Penfold, formerly Corporal W.A.A.F., for secretarial and computing assistance.

References

(*1*) Symonds, C.P. *Br Med J* 2:703 and 740, 1943.
(*2*) Davis, D. Russell. Pilot error. Air Ministry A.P. 3139a. H.M.S.O., 1948.
(*3*) Birley, J.L. *Lancet* 1:1147, 1920.

(*4*) Reid, D.D. Some measures of the effect of operational stress on bomber crews. Air Ministry A.P. 3139: 245–258. H.M.S.O., 1947.
(*5*) Reid, D.D. Fluctuations in navigator performance during operational sorties. Air Ministry A.P. 3139: 321–329. H.M.S.O., 1947.
(*6*) Hill, A. Bradford, and G.O. Williams. Investigation of landing accidents in relation to fatigue. *Flying Personnel Research Committee Report* No. 423 (m), 1943.
(*7*) Symonds, C.P., and D.J. Williams. Clinical and statistical study of neurosis precipitated by flying duties. Air Ministry A.P. 3139: 140–172. H.M.S.O., 1947.

EPIDEMIOLOGY—OLD AND NEW[1]

John E. Gordon[2]

The changes in the social and economic structure of the world that have taken place during the past one hundred years have had a fundamental effect on existing attitudes in epidemiology. The position is such as to require re-examination of the scope of interests to be included within that field and a fresh assessment of the place of epidemiology in the practice of preventive medicine and public health. Of the many factors that have led to this situation, two are outstanding. The first is that of this shrinking world (1)—that measured in terms of travel time, the world becomes progressively smaller, and that it tends to become more and more a single epidemiologic universe. The second influence is that of an aging population, a state of affairs that now characterizes most modern civilizations.

This Shrinking World

Since earliest historical times, trade and travel have been recognized as factors contributing to the frequency and seriousness of disease processes. In ancient times, the contacts of peoples were necessarily peripheral and indirect, except as they resulted from invasion or conquest or the forced migration of populations. The numbers that moved about were small, and progress was slow.

A progressive change has been under way since the fifteenth century, a change that experienced a marked impetus in the nineteenth century and in the past twenty-five years has brought alterations that are no less than astounding (2). Those associated with the airplane are obvious. No place in the world is now more than three to five days removed from Detroit or Grand Rapids, considering only com-

mercially available and wholly ordinary means of transport. The change in sea travel has been less evident and of slower evolution, but compared with the days of sailing vessels is no less striking. The effects brought about by the modern technology of transport and travel are not limited to international considerations. Those within countries are just as marked. They have brought about a mingling of peoples that is of even greater moment epidemiologically than those which concern nations.

More is involved than the matter of speed. As distances shrink, the amount of travel tends to increase and with it a greater interdependence of peoples one on the other. A direct result of the introduction of rapid transport is the growth and multiplication of great cities and the industrialization of whole areas, of such moment as to approach the practical reality of huge groups of people with one water supply, one milk supply, and one food supply. The transportation of the world has not only changed the world itself but also the course of civilization.

Although the ultimate has not been reached, the world tends to fuse into a single epidemiologic universe. The trend is so definite that today it is difficult to recognize the separate epidemiologic units that existed not so long ago, units that were marked by continental if not by national boundaries. The tropics are no longer the remote areas of a generation ago. People go there in the course of their ordinary activities; they acquire the diseases there prevalent, and often they bring them home with them.

An Aging Population

Since 1850 the population of the United States has shown an increasing proportion of people in the older age groups, and correspondingly fewer children and young adults. Persons aged more than fifty years included 13.3 percent of the population in 1900; the proportion is now almost twice as great, and the

Source: *Journal of the Michigan State Medical Society.* 49:194–199, February, 1950.
[1] Presented at the Eighty-fourth Annual Session of the Michigan State Medical Society at Grand Rapids, September 22, 1949.
[2] Department of Epidemiology, Harvard University School of Public Health, Boston 15, Massachusetts.

estimate for the year 2000 is 33.0 percent (*3*). Children aged less than fifteen years made up 41.6 percent of the population of 1850, but by 1950 the proportion had dropped to 25.7 percent. These changes characterize the people of modern civilizations generally and throughout the world. They are less marked in primitive regions but will become more evident just as surely as an improved public health leads to a lesser cost from communicable disease and fewer deaths from infection in childhood.

The diseases of an older population are not those of a younger people, especially when that older population is subjected to the continuous salting with infection which is characteristic of modern metropolitan populations.

THE CHANGING CHARACTER OF MASS DISEASE PROBLEMS

The mass disease problems that affect modern communities have been notably altered within a century. The causes are many, a great many more than the two just presented. They relate both to man as an organism and to the environment in which he lives. Some diseases now have far less significance; others have come from an inconsequential position to rank among the leading causes of death or as major factors in lost efficiency or disabling illness. What has happened, however, is more than a matter of differences in relative importance of the numbers of persons involved. In many instances, the nature and character of a mass disease has changed. Less often, new problems have been introduced by reason of the shifting ecological state. The communicable diseases provide the best illustration of these several considerations, principally because custom has long marked this group as the type of mass disease problem.

Communicable Disease

Comparing present conditions with those that existed a hundred years ago, the changes that have occurred among the communicable diseases are so great as to constitute almost another world. Intestinal infections are far less frequent. Diseases transmitted through discharges of the upper respiratory tract find a much more important place among infections in general. The situation is less definite for diseases spread by direct contact, although the trend in incidence is that of the respiratory diseases, with the result that these conditions likewise become of greater moment as the agglomeration of peoples becomes more pronounced. The venereal diseases, as representative of the class, still remain the problem they always were. An improved control of arthropod-borne disease has been an outstanding accomplishment of recent years, so successful as to have restricted measurably the frequency of those conditions. Among diseases of man originating from animals, more has been done about infections associated with domestic animals than those where wild animals are the reservoir. No reason exists for believing that the actual frequency of diseases of animal origin has increased, but relatively they become more important among classes of communicable disease because of the lesser numbers arising from other sources.

One or other of two general means is useful in judging quantitatively the changes that have taken place in the frequency of communicable diseases. The first is through comparing computed rates of incidence in terms of units of population. The second is through examining the relative standing among mass diseases as causes of death.

In 1900 the ten leading causes of death in the United States included five infectious diseases. The current list has only two. First place in 1900 was occupied by an infectious disease, tuberculosis. By 1946 the highest rank held by a communicable process was sixth, for pneumonia of all forms. An examination of the two lists of diseases responsible in 1900 and in 1946 for the greatest numbers of deaths will demonstrate that the advances made have had to do with the communicable diseases where prevention rests largely on community measures. The current problems are provided by those other diseases where prevention depends so much on individual initiative and on the activities of the private practitioner of medicine. As for the communicable diseases themselves, an increasing tendency is seen toward an established equilibrium in clinical behavior and in community frequency, of the type which has been so satisfactory and so long continued with mumps.

With some caution it may be suggested that the days of the great epidemics are over. This appears likely if environmental conditions remain as they are or continue to follow the trend they now do. If the environment is altered materially or new factors are introduced, such as another French Revolution, almost anything could happen, including reversion to epidemic situations that characterized the world of a century ago. The composite experience of the past hundred years and especially that of the recent global war supports the opinion of a favorable future in respect to major world outbreaks. The history of a typical American city, Philadelphia, is examined with profit. The greatest epidemic of modern times, the pandemic of influenza of 1918, was a small affair in terms of deaths compared with the earlier epidemic visitations on that city. The experience is not unique. A similar course of events has characterized other representative American cities, Boston, New Orleans, Chicago and New York.

The greatest attention and the principal interest in epidemiology continues to be directed toward the communicable diseases, not because these diseases are dominantly important, for actually they are of lesser relative moment than some others. It is largely because they are better and longer understood. It is therefore reasonable for the communicable diseases to continue to be the fundamental concern of epidemiologists. The gains that have been made must be held. Perhaps the more important consideration is that these diseases offer the most favorable opportunity to gain familiarity with the epidemiologic method. The reasonable approach to the broader and less well explored fields of mass disease is through expansion and transfer of that method.

Noncommunicable Organic Disease

The important community health problems of the present are concerned with those organic diseases which are not communicable from man to man and not caused by a specific infectious agent. This is just as true if judgment is based on another of the major criteria, not on deaths but on defect or disability.

Heart disease now ranks as the first cause of death in the United States; and deaths from cancer, from circulatory disturbances, from metabolic diseases, nutritional disturbances, and the degenerative diseases are well up on the list. A direct relation is seen with the altered social and economic conditions of the present

century. Many of the changes have been brought about by the newer age characteristics of the population. With fewer deaths from communicable disease, people now live longer, and long enough to acquire conditions which are so largely limited to older people. This is a natural evolution. Disease, and particularly communicable disease, is an unnatural means through which to govern population numbers. The natural means of elimination is through old age and accident.

The practical result of this shifting situation is an established and increasing trend among public health workers to accord greater emphasis to diseases characteristic of old age and less to the health problems associated with communicable disease. This is a reasonable attitude, as the evidence already introduced has demonstrated. However, a satisfactory perspective and a balanced judgment are necessary in the newly developed enthusiasm about geriatrics. The health of children is still the important consideration among public health problems, admittedly not because of communicable disease but because of nutrition, growth, development and the varied psychiatric disturbances. The child has a life expectancy of many years; that of the older group is brief. The greater profit in years of healthful living is alone sufficient reason for greater stress on the mass diseases of childhood. The kind of years that are gained is of equal significance: for the child these are years of productive and creative effort; for the older person they are likely to be not only few but relatively unproductive.

Functional Disease

Of all mass health problems of communities, more interest has been given to organic disease than to functional disturbances (4). A number of reasons account for this difference. There is greater ease of recognition, a more ready establishment of cause, and a greater availability of methods for measuring both cause and effect. It is just being appreciated that mental disorders, the problems of addiction to alcohol and tobacco, and the social diseases concerned with occupation, recreation, and the intellectual pursuits of man, also constitute group as well as individual problems. As a field in epidemiology, these mass diseases of functional origin have scarcely been touched. There is every indication of a developing activity within the immediate future (5).

Injuries

With the advent of a modern practice of medicine some fifty years ago, the duties of a physician came to be understood as something more than the care of the sick and the injured. The obligations of the doctor were defined as "first to prevent disease; if that is not possible, to cure; and if that is impossible, to alleviate." The newer concept of prevention, as it developed, was applied almost wholly to disease, to the sick. The injured were largely forgotten until the recently aroused interest in the civilian problem of accidents and such military conditions as trench foot, battle casualties, and the ordinary injuries of military life. Collectively, these are the problems in an epidemiology of trauma.

Accidents of all forms, as judged by data of 1947, ranked fourth among causes of death in the United States. The traumatic injuries after accidents can be demonstrated to conform to the same biologic laws as do disease (6). They are amenable to the same epidemiologic approach, and, what is least well appreciated, they are preventable and controllable. Instead of something set apart from disease and scarcely to be considered within the scope of preventive medicine, injuries are as much a public health problem as measles.

CURRENT DIRECTION OF EPIDEMIOLOGIC INTERESTS

Evidence has been presented of the wide range of pathologic conditions included within modern ideas of mass or community disease. The approach to solution of problems concerned with mass disease, as typified by the communicable diseases, has been through epidemiology, a biologic discipline concerned with disease as it affects groups of people. Medicine and public health would thus appear called upon to alter existing interpretations of the field of usefulness of the epidemiologic method. A limitation to the communicable diseases is no longer warranted by present-day conditions. The larger problems of public health lie with other diseases, both organic and functional, and with injuries. The validity of

that concept depends upon the assumption that all mass diseases and injuries conform to the same biologic laws of ecology as do communicable processes. It is believed they do.

If an etiologic interpretation of disease and injury is the basis of modern practice, and it surely is, then the agents that give rise to the many pathological conditions must be variously viable and nonviable, sometimes transmissible and sometimes not. If morbid conditions of man are the result of a reaction between the human host and his environment, then all disease conditions can be interpreted in terms of three principal factors. The first is the agent, either an inanimate object or substance, or a living thing that directly gives rise to the condition. The second is the host, the living organism affected or injured; and man, of all living things, is the most important host. The third factor is the environment in which host and agent exist, an environment which has much to do with determining the qualities and activities of both, and additionally has a strong influence on the nature and effectiveness of the interaction that takes place between the two. Thus looked upon, disease and injury, and also the physiologic state, are recognized as ecologic phenomena and amenable in their group manifestations to the methods of epidemiologic analysis. Epidemiology is seen as a biologic discipline applicable to all diseases where groups of persons or things are involved, to include both plant and animal.

The development of new knowledge or the introduction of new conditions commonly calls for a change in methods or a shift in emphasis. Evidence has been presented that the world tends to become one epidemiologic universe, that it is experiencing a changing character of population, that the social and economic environment has been markedly altered. This has resulted in altered values among mass disease problems. To meet its obligations to preventive medicine and public health, epidemiology needs to broaden its interests. As expressed by Dr. Joseph Mountin (7), it is high time that epidemiologists escaped their Broad Street pump fixation. The reference, of course, is to the classical studies of Snow (8) on cholera, where the foundation was laid for the field method in epidemiology and from which developed the established association of epidemiology and communicable disease. The implication in this trite remark is that restriction to a concern of communicable disease, to the neglect of more pressing problems, is no longer justifiable. That epidemiology should give more attention to the mass problems of organic and functional disease generally, and less to communicable disease, may be accepted as principle, applying with little reservation to the countries of North America and Western Europe. It is in line with the altered conditions of the modern world. For many countries the communicable diseases still remain the first consideration. Little doubt exists, however, that this is the epidemiology of the future, to become increasingly applicable in most countries of the world.

EPIDEMIOLOGY IN RELATION TO MEDICINE AND PUBLIC HEALTH

Epidemiology is understood to be an independent general biologic discipline, the basic science of public health. The function of public health services is accepted as "the application of the sciences of preventive medicine through government for social ends, the purpose not to salvage the individual but to understand and reduce sickness of any kind of a community or group." Here is a clear separation of interests. The prevention of disease in the individual, which is the function of preventive medicine and of the medical practitioner, is distinguished from the prevention of disease in the group or community, which is the concern of public health and of public health workers. If public health is a branch of knowledge distinct from medicine, and the separation is believed well made, then public health must rest on some fundamental discipline which is characteristic of its activities and individual to it. Public health deals with groups of people, and epidemiology is the study of disease behavior as manifested by groups. For this reason epidemiology is stated to be the basic science of public health. It occupies no exclusive position, for all of the sciences of preventive medicine come into play, and other disciplines are of greater importance in the control and management of community disease. It is basic in the sense that it is the point of departure, the means by which mass disease is recognized and appraised. It is perhaps best understood as the counterpart of diagnosis in clinical medicine.

The study of disease as a mass phenomenon differs from the study of disease in the individual primarily in respect to the unit of investigation. It is early appreciated that the herd, the crowd or the community is not a simple aggregate of the persons comprising that grouped population, but that each universe of people is an entity, a composite that possesses as much individuality as does a person. The methods and techniques used in the study of the herd likewise differ from those applied to the individual, to such an extent that Greenwood (9) has well remarked that a man highly skilled in individual diagnosis and treatment may be wholly unskilled in generalization. The differences and the similarities in the approach to problems of health and disease as they concern the group and the individual may be examined with profit.

Fundamental to all activities in clinical medicine is a knowledge and a familiarity with rather an imposing array of sciences. Medicine these days has use for scientific disciplines of a wide order. The list starts with what are commonly termed the medical sciences. Included are the disciplines which have been a part of medicine from its earliest history: anatomy and physiology, histology and embryology, with pathology occupying the central position, and then the newer disciplines of biochemistry and bacteriology. All are supported by the natural sciences, principally physics and chemistry. To exclude the mathematical sciences would be to leave doubt that medicine is the science it surely is. The broadening interests of medical practice within recent years require addition to this list of a number of social sciences—economics, sociology, and psychology—and, with little debate, the less directly applicable biological sciences such as anthropology and genetics. The list is by no means exhausted, for medicine, in furtherance of its broader obligations of prevention as well as therapy, progressively finds need for most of the physical and biological sciences and increasingly those of the social group. With the principal objective of the physician the prevention and cure of disease and injury, it is reasonable that the primary interest in these disciplines is more utilitarian and indirect, rather than fundamental and as a matter of specific concern. They occupy the place they do in clinical thought for a single reason, and that is the degree to which they contribute to a central discipline called diagnosis. This is the means by which disease of the individual is recognized, evaluated and judged as to final outcome. Clinical medicine revolves about diagnosis, for this is the branch of knowledge that directs and determines the ultimate objective, the proper management and treatment of the patient.

The approach to the problems of the group is much the same. The fundamental need for the basic sciences is no less. Some few, such as biostatistics and toxicology, receive greater emphasis; others, such as anatomy, somewhat less. Again, the concern with the fundamental sciences stems from the same need, that is to say, the aid they contribute to a central discipline that is also concerned with the recognition, evaluation and prognosis of disease, but this time as it affects communities rather than individuals. This discipline, epidemiology, is the counterpart of diagnosis and bears precisely the same relationship to public health practice as does diagnosis to clinical management. Epidemiology and public health practice act for the group as do diagnosis and treatment in disease of the individual.

This concept of itself suggests that epidemiology is a discipline with implications more far reaching than the study of epidemics. In the first place its usefulness is not limited to the professional worker in public health. Although dealing with smaller units, the clinician makes use of the methods of epidemiology in applying preventive medicine to family groups. Almost no individual illness fails of an impact on the persons who surround the patient. Such practice of small group epidemiology differs not at all in principle from the activities of the public health worker in the broader problems where the population group is that of a city, a state or a nation. Other applications of the epidemiologic method to purely clinical problems are less well appreciated. One of the most practical is a substitution of epidemiological analysis and mathematical interpretation for the clinical impression derived from case reports. It serves thus in the evaluation of new drugs and methods of treatment, in determining the usefulness of suggested diagnostic procedures and in precise definition of the clinical course and behavior of a disease or injury. The epidemiological method would appear the reasonable approach in search for a better definition of the precan-

cerous and the prediabetic states upon which more than anything else rational and successful prevention depends. It provides the ultimate means for testing the value of results from experimental microbiologic research in such matters as the causes of communicable disease or in modes of transmission. A passing familiarity with the medical literature of the day suffices to show the increasing extent to which the epidemiologic or group approach is being incorporated into modern clinical practice and investigation.

The uses to which epidemiology is put by the professional public health worker are better known. The traditional application is in the study of epidemics, but even for the communicable diseases such limitation has long since passed. Far more effort is directed towards the study of infections as they occur under ordinary circumstances, with the result that endemiology, or study of the long continued behavior of a disease through field survey in a community, far outweighs the effort expended on the accidental and bizarre epidemic. Epidemiology thus progressively becomes more a study of the whole natural history of disease than of its unusual manifestations.

The field method of epidemiological study has other uses in applied public health than the direct investigation of disease. The administrator turns the method to his purposes in determining the necessary provisions for hospital care of community populations (*10*). It is the accepted procedure in appraisal of the accomplishment attained in programs for prevention and control of a disease (*11*).

Research in the field, through study of disease as it manifests itself in nature, is an important and independent approach to solution of medical problems. Modern medical progress has been so thoroughly associated with research in the biological laboratory, and it has been so largely a development of the experimental method, that this other and older method has come in recent years to be overshadowed. Progress through experiment is oftentimes slow, and dead ends are met, with the result that an increasing tendency becomes evident, to try the new and yet old approach through field epidemiologic methods. This is by no means limited to the communicable diseases, for the value of contributions from the field is so definite that similar methods are being turned toward other areas of mass disease, such as cancer (*12*), and specifically cancer in industry (*13,14*). There is much activity in the field of nutritional disturbances (*15*), with dental metabolic diseases (*16*), and currently in diabetes (*17*), and thyrotoxicosis (*18*). Even such unusual fields as the congenital anomalies (*19*) now engage the attention of the experimental epidemiologist.

With full appreciation of the contributions made to modern medical progress through skilled observations by the individual practitioner, there is nevertheless an increasing appreciation of the extent to which knowledge of a total problem can be enlarged through analysis and study of the facts accumulated by many observers; that benefit is to be derived through investigation of disease processes as they affect groups of people, as a means of supplementing clinical study of the individual patient and the knowledge to be derived from experiment. It likewise becomes increasingly evident that to understand fully all the variations which disease may show, it is necessary to draw on the experience of the world and not to reason too broadly from results obtained in a small section of a single country. Disease shows many peculiarities under the multiple influences of varying environment and that applies not alone to the communicable diseases. Diphtheria and cancer are almost universally described in terms of the clinical and epidemiological behavior they evidence in north temperate climates. What occurs in the tropics is often widely different. An international viewpoint becomes increasingly necessary for a full and clearer comprehension of disease.

References

(*1*) Staley, E. *This Shrinking World*. Chicago, World Citizen's Association, 1939.

(*2*) Davis, D.J. *IMJ* 88:186–194, 1945.

(*3*) United States Department of Commerce, Bureau of the Census. *Forecasts of the Population of the United States, 1945–1975*.

(*4*) Wearn, J. F. *JAMA* 134:1517–1520, 1947.

(*5*) Halliday, J.F. *Psychosocial Medicine*. New York, W.W. Norton & Co., 1948.

(*6*) Gordon, J.E. *Am J Public Health* 39:504–515, 1949.

(*7*) Mountin, J. Personal communication, 1947.

(*8*) Snow, J. *On the Mode of Communication of Cholera*. Ed. 2. London, John Churchill, 1855.

(*9*) Greenwood, M. *Epidemics and Crowd Diseases*. New York, Macmillan Co., 1935.

(*10*) Bourke, J.J., and M. Bullowe. *Am J Public Health* 31:926, 1941.

(*11*) Bell, J.A. *JAMA* 137:1276–1281, 1948.

(*12*) Levin, M.L. *Cancer* 1:489–497, 1948.

(*13*) Hueper, W.C. *Occupational Med.* 5:157, 1948.

(*14*) Hueper, W.C. *JAMA* 139:335, 1949.

(*15*) Milam, D.F. *NC Med J* 2:6–11, 1941.

(*16*) Dean, H.T. *J Am Coll Dent* 12:50–53, 1945.

(*17*) Wilkerson, H.L.C., and L.P. Krall. *JAMA* 135:209, 1947.

(*18*) Iverson, K. *Am J Med Sci* 217:121–130, 1949.

(*19*) Ingalls, T.H., and J.E. Gordon. *Am J Med Sci* 214:322–328, 1947.

INFECTIOUS AND CHRONIC DISEASE EPIDEMIOLOGY: SEPARATE AND UNEQUAL?

Elizabeth Barrett-Connor[1]

For some time I have been confused and irritated by the division of epidemiology and epidemiologists into the subspecialties of infectious disease and chronic disease. Those who doubt this division need only to look at the curricula of schools of public health, chapter headings in standard textbooks of epidemiology, and job descriptions as they are advertised in various media. Although the division has historical rationale and is perpetuated by current federal funding, as outlined below, I believe the distinction is arbitrary and detrimental to epidemiologists and to the epidemiologic study of disease.

How did this division come about? Over half a century ago epidemiologic observations had already been made about chronic diseases of non-infectious cause, such as pellagra in the poor and scrotal cancer in chimney sweeps. However, most earlier epidemiologic investigations were concerned with the study of infectious diseases. Then, in the 1940s, many prominent epidemiologists stressed the importance of applying the tools of epidemiology to the study of chronic diseases and decried the limitation of epidemiology to the field of infectious disease. As Murphy (1) has noted, a major act of faith in the epidemiologic work of the past thirty years has been that methods which worked well in infectious disease could be successfully applied to chronic diseases. The successes of chronic disease epidemiology support the assumption but have been paradoxically divisive.

DEFINITIONS

As applied to disease or illness, the word "chronic" means slow progression and long du-

ration. It is the opposite of "acute," a term which implies a swift onset and short course. Despite the simplicity of definition, no one has satisfactorily classified all diseases on the basis of duration. Indeed, most diseases on any list are sometimes acute and sometimes chronic. A cerebrovascular accident may be immediately fatal or produce sequelae which persist for months or years. Heart disease, usually classified as chronic, is acute for those myocardial infarct victims who die before reaching the hospital. The tendency to consider infection as synonymous with acute is equally misleading. Many infections or their sequelae are chronic: sinusitis, cystitis, syphilis, tuberculosis, paralytic poliomyelitis, congenital rubella and rheumatic heart disease, to name a few.

Acuteness or chronicity are often not permanent attributes of a disease. An acute disease may be redefined when scientific advances permit identification of the pre-clinical phase. A chronic condition may be transformed into an acute illness when early treatment aborts sequelae. In the Baltimore study of chronic disease (2), one in ten "substantial conditions" would have had complete recovery with appropriate care.

Latency

A long interval between exposure to the putative risk factor(s) and disease onset is believed to characterize most chronic illnesses. But many infections appear after latent periods as long as those proposed for chronic diseases. Thus, infection with a tubercle bacillus acquired in childhood is often first manifest in late adult life. Herpes zoster represents reactivation of childhood chickenpox in many, if not all, cases. A large proportion of infections in the compromised host undoubtedly reflects activation of dormant infection. Indeed, the incubation period for the majority of infections afflicting adults today is either delayed or poorly defined.

Source: *American Journal of Epidemiology* 109:245–249, 1979.
[1] Departments of Medicine and Community Medicine, University of California, San Diego, La Jolla, CA 92093.

Transmissibility

Many infectious diseases are propagated from person to person. However, this is by no means true of all infectious agents: food poisoning caused by preformed toxins, Legionnaires' disease and coccidioidomycosis are not transmitted from person to person. Some chronic diseases of as yet unknown etiology may turn out to be transmissible. Clusters of leukemia and lymphoma suggest a transmissible agent as do the recent studies of residents of households in which victims of multiple sclerosis reside (3). It would be premature to divide epidemiologists into those who deal with transmissible or non-transmissible conditions. If leukemia, cervical cancer, multiple sclerosis, arthritis and diabetes prove to be caused by a transmissible agent, as many now suspect, persons now classified as chronic disease experts may find themselves to be infectious disease epidemiologists.

Etiology

At the turn of the century, infectious disease was the major area of research in medicine. The discoveries of specific agents which produced specific diseases were straightforward and satisfying, and led to one of the basic tenets of medicine: a single disease process has a single causation. Clinical observation, bacteriologic investigation and the development of the antimicrobials in the early 1940s led to the preeminence of infectious disease as a medical problem whose etiology and management were established. In contrast, chronic disease epidemiology has attended the study of diseases of unknown cause, conditions which are increasingly recognized as multifactorial in origin. Thus, the dichotomy became cause-known/unifactorial vs. cause-unknown/multifactorial.

Although it is true that the necessary cause of most acute diseases is a known agent, and the necessary cause of most chronic diseases remains unknown, this is surely more a function of the state of the art than the nature of disease. All diseases have multiple causes. The necessary microbial agent is not the sole determinant of outcome. As Stewart (4) has written, "If two susceptible subjects are exposed to equal doses of the same germ, and one develops infection while the other does not, the factor governing the development of the infection clearly lies outside the germ."

For most diseases, the frequency of exposure exceeds the frequency of illness. Only the availability of the necessary agent has provided the reagents required to demonstrate that most of those infected with the tubercle bacillus or the polio virus are not sick. We are just at the threshold of understanding why most of those who smoke cigarettes do not develop lung cancer (5). Heritable and environmental determinants of chronic disease may well precede comparable discoveries in the arena of infection.

Behavioral considerations

Evidence accumulated during the last twenty years indicates that the most important chronic diseases are caused by a variety of personal and social habits, such as improper diet, excessive drinking and smoking, lack of exercise, and unsafe driving and working practices. Behavioral considerations also determine the distribution of many infectious diseases. For example, venereal disease, the most important epidemic infection in the United States today, does not occur among the chaste, and active tuberculosis is disproportionately frequent among those who abuse alcohol.

In neither acute, infectious, nor chronic disease is a complete understanding of cause required for prevention. Smallpox was prevented before isolation of the bacterium; lung cancer can be prevented before identification of the specific carcinogen in cigarette smoke. When an infectious disease is transmitted or maintained because of attitudes, behavior or surroundings, a purely germ-oriented approach is unlikely to provide effective control.

Study design

No study design is unique to any branch of epidemiology. The epidemiologic study of both acute and chronic conditions usually requires a denominator and/or a comparison group, can be done retrospectively or prospectively, and can examine prevalence or incidence. The search for causality in a food poisoning outbreak, examining the attack rates of those with and without exposure to the suspect food, applies the same principles as those used in a comparison of the incidence of uterine cancer among those with and without the suspect hormone. Cross-sectional or case-control comparisons are used to validate or refute clinical tenets of acute and chronic disease. Such studies led to the delayed recognition that most of the symptoms attributed to pinworm are equally frequent in uninfected children (6), that splinter hemorrhages traditionally attributed to bacterial endocarditis are equally common in hospitalized patients without endocarditis (7), and that the symptoms attributed to gallbladder disease are equally prevalent in women without gallbladder disease (8). The same principles of study design that apply to clinical trials of vaccines or prophylactic antimicrobials apply to the study of lipid lowering drugs or antihypertensive agents.

A major tool of the chronic disease epidemiologist has been the population survey, a prototype of which has been the Framingham Study (9). In community-based studies, entire populations of persons, including a majority who are presumably well, are examined for a variety of characteristics and diseases. Cross-sectional studies define the usual, if not normal, and prospective studies define putative risk factors. Observations such as those made in Framingham led to the recognition that blood pressure and plasma cholesterol were important predictors of coronary artery disease.

In the past, infectious disease epidemiologists worked from the vantage of sick persons. Epidemics were described in terms of the ill, and the well population was used primarily for age- and sex-specific denominator data. But community-based studies of the distribution of disease and its precursors are by no means the purview of chronic disease epidemiologists alone. The Seattle Virus Watch Study (10), which has added important information to our knowledge of the transmission and frequency of respiratory infections, is a case in point.

Analytic methodology

One phenomenon which perhaps best distinguishes the chronic from the infectious disease epidemiologist is the use of more sophisticated mathematical methods feasible with computer-assisted analysis. Because neither the etiology of chronic disease nor its management was as simple or obvious as the situation which appeared to exist in infectious disease, progressively sophisticated mathematics were developed by epidemiologists and bio-statisticians, at a time when most research in the field of infectious disease involved clinical observations or experiments conducted in the laboratory. The danger is that goodness of fit sometimes substitutes for common sense or biologic plausibility (11). Chronic disease epidemiologists are often in the awkward position of analysis without hypothesis. In the absence of either an agent or a unique outcome, they must perform hypothesis-seeking exercises. The pitfalls of data dredging greatly exceed those of hypothesis testing. The multiple possible analyses render almost a certainty that some variables will be significantly associated with some diseases.

In the days before linear regression and multiple logistic function, many infectious disease epidemiologists personally gathered and manually tabulated their data. This experience clarified the sometimes remarkable limitations of data—which by virtue of categorization and computerization may gain unwarranted credibility. Experiences gained in the shorter time-frame of some infectious processes also provided valuable insights about the hazards of early assumption. Farr (12) demonstrated a remarkable correlation of cholera mortality and altitude in nineteenth-century London but failed to consider water as the variable of interest. A recent report (13) of an excess of hepatitis among young women using oral contraceptives would have profited by a consideration of the probable differences in lifestyle among women who chose oral contraceptives as compared to those without such contraceptive practices.

Many infectious disease epidemiologists come from the ranks of clinicians and laboratorians, and lack the skills traditionally considered in the purview of the chronic disease epidemiologist. These skills are now essential to the discovery of those variables which, in the presence of the necessary agent, determine infection, disease and outcome. Whereas the infectious agent can usually be isolated and enumerated with precision, the extraneous factors which determine morbidity and mortality are more difficult to quantify. It is the task of epidemiology to find other methods to assess with precision the contribution of these factors to infectious disease. The arbitrary separation of infectious disease from chronic disease epidemiology in teaching and research does disservice to this need.

Money, research and training

The increase in life expectancy in the U.S. since 1900 can be traced to the decline of infectious diseases. Improvements have been small since 1950. Chronic conditions are the major causes of morbidity and mortality in the developed world.

The pre-eminence of chronic diseases has led to targeted research as a major source of federal funds for scientific inquiry. Money is specified for the training of heart disease, cancer, diabetes and arthritis epidemiologists, to name a few. In contrast, infectious disease epidemiology has not been a major area of targeted training or research, although there are a few exceptions such as nosocomial infection and venereal disease. The limited resources presently allocated to infectious disease epidemiology, as compared with chronic disease epidemiology, have determined the career choices of epidemiologists, because they find it to their advantage to designate themselves as chronic disease specialists. Funding allocations not only determine the direction of research, they also determine the titles of the workers!

CONCLUSION

Some scientific disciplines are best able to answer certain questions in medicine. Much of modern epidemiologic effort has been directed toward investigating problems regarding which the rest of science has few useful leads. Any disease, acute or chronic, which lacks either a logical structure or a plausible hypothesis is difficult to study. But the identification of a necessary agent, microbial or otherwise, does not answer all relevant and important questions any more than demonstration of an associated variable confirms causality or predicts prevention.

Epidemiologically, acute diseases differ from chronic diseases in two major aspects: immediacy of response and uniqueness of observation. The lessons learned in infectious disease, where the agent and outcome were more readily available to test predictions, must be shared with those epidemiologists who—in their haste to assign causality—sometimes abandon biologic wisdom in favor of quantitative ideology.

Many of the unanswered questions in acute/infectious disease epidemiology need to be addressed by those techniques currently attributed to and taught with chronic disease epidemiology. Acute and chronic disease epidemiologists have important lessons to offer each other. A sharing of experience and methodologies could avert the unfortunate plethora of truly terrible data analyzed ad nauseum, or good data poorly interpreted. Once these lessons have been learned, we should discard the qualifiers and call an epidemiologist an epidemiologist. Acute and chronic disease epidemiologists are not separate and unrelated species, any more than acute and chronic diseases can be neatly categorized.

References

(1) Murphy, E.A. Epidemiological strategies and genetic factors. *Intl J Epidemiol* 7:7–14, 1978.
(2) Commission on Chronic Illness. Chronic illness in a large city—The Baltimore Study. In *Chronic Illness in the United States*. Vol. IV. Cambridge, Mass., Harvard University Press, 1957.
(3) Schocket, A.L., and H.L. Weiner. Lymphocytotoxic antibodies in family members of patients with multiple sclerosis. *Lancet* 1:571–573, 1978.
(4) Stewart, G.T. Limitations of the germ theory. *Lancet* 1:1977–2081, 1968.
(5) Emery, A.E.H., R. Anand, N. Danford, et al. Arylhydrocarbonhydroxylase inducibility in patients with cancer. *Lancet* 1:470–471, 1978.
(6) Weller, T.H., and C.W. Sorenson. Enterobiasis: Its incidence and symptomatology in a group of 505 children. *N Engl J Med* 224:143–146, 1941.
(7) Kilpatrick, Z.M., P.A. Greenberg, and J.P. Sanford. Splinter hemorrhages—their clinical significance. *Arch Intern Med* 115:730–735, 1965.
(8) Price, W.H. Gallbladder dyspepsia. *Br Med J* 2:138–141, 1963.
(9) Dawber, T.R., W.B. Kannel, and L.P. Lyell. An approach to longitudinal studies in a community: The Framingham Study. *Ann NY Acad Sci* 107:539–556, 1963.
(10) Fox, J.P., C.E. Hall, and M.R. Cooney. The Seattle Virus Watch.II. Objectives, study population and its observation, data processing and summary of illnesses. *Am J Epidemiol* 96:270–285, 1972.
(11) Feinstein, A.R. *Clinical Biostatistics*. St. Louis, Mo., CV Mosby, 1977.
(12) Langmuir, A.D. Epidemiology of airborne infection. *Bacteriol Rev* 25:173–181, 1961.
(13) Morrison, A.S., H.O. Jick, and H.W. Ory. Oral contraceptives and hepatitis. A Report from the Boston Collaborative Drug Surveillance Program, Boston University Medical Center. *Lancet* 1:1142–1143, 1977.

PART III

ETIOLOGIC INVESTIGATIONS

DISCUSSIONS

NAJERA: Perhaps we should start by emphasizing the interrelated-
ness of the factors that cause disease. Today, everybody
talks of multicausation, but if you read the studies, most
researchers still search for "a cause," they still think in terms
of a single or a few simple causes of disease. They haven't
really begun to understand disease as a result of the interaction of factors working within a real web. It was Mac-
Mahon who first talked of a "web of causation," but too
often this is still interpreted as a complicated but linear
chain of causation rather than a complicated interre-
lationship of many factors. A web really means interrelation. I think we have to emphasize this.

BUCK: But, you see, it is so hard to keep the web in mind when you
are actually looking for a cause. When we were debating the
causes of the epidemiologic transition we fell into exactly
the same trap. It is still so easy to fall into this trap.

NAJERA: True, it is easier to talk about a web than to work with it. I
remember a very good paper by Capra that traced the great
evolution in physics from Newton to the theory of relativity
and compared it with the relative lack of such development
in the applied sciences. In medicine, for example, we are
still stuck with a Newtonian approach. This is why we still
think of the causes of disease in terms of one or two, at
most a few, factors. We really can't understand the web of
causation because this would be comparable to understanding the concept of relativity. We should know at least a little
more of modern physics. When we were children we were
taught Newtonian physics; we know very little, if anything,
of relativity, Einstein, and quantum physics. We have to
force ourselves to think differently. Even if it is very difficult for us to understand the meaning of interrelations, of a
real web, we have to change our way of thinking and working. Perhaps it will be easier for the new generations to do
so.

TERRIS: The concept of web of causation should be discussed in
contrast to single-cause and multifactorial-cause concepts.
In my basic course in epidemiology, I give a lecture called
"The Web of Causation." To illustrate the concept I give the

149

example of the long-standing prevalence of diarrhea and enteritis in India. I point out that the British occupation of India was a major factor in why India has had so much diarrhea and enteritis for so long. Not all students appreciate this kind of analysis. In fact, I recall one student who responded by launching into an emotional defense of the British Empire.

But perhaps one of the most fascinating illustrations of the web of causation is the British epidemic of gout in the eighteenth and nineteenth centuries. Before that, Portugal's flourishing textile industry had competed with the British textile industry. England, involved in the War of the Spanish Succession, signed the commercial pact known as the Treaty of Methuen. The treaty allowed British textiles to enter Portugal duty-free; in exchange, the British allowed Portuguese wine to enter Britain with a lower duty than French wine. The treaty resulted in the destruction of the Portuguese textile industry. This is one of the reasons that Portugal failed to develop as an industrial country.

The British, at war with France at the time, could then substitute Portuguese wine for French wine. But in order to preserve the wines for the long voyage from Portugal to Britain, they were fortified with alcohol that presumably had been distilled or stored in lead vessels. The Portuguese wines apparently contained large amounts of lead that caused the gout. This possible scenario was described by two clinicians from the University of Alabama in an article published in the *Bulletin of the History of Medicine*. The article reported an outbreak of 37 cases of gout in moonshiners who distilled their illegal whisky in old automobile radiators which had been repaired with lead. They drank leaded alcohol and developed gout as a result. The authors of the article described this sequence of events and hypothesized that a similar process had occurred in England.

BUCK: Did they have other symptoms of lead poisoning in eighteenth-century England?

TERRIS: The lead content was not enough to produce massive poisoning, just enough to damage the kidneys and raise the uric acid in the blood.

To test their hypothesis, the Alabama clinicians went to England and analyzed four bottles of port dating from the late eighteenth and early nineteenth centuries. They found large amounts of lead in the old wine, but only traces in new wine. Who would have thought that the Treaty of Methuen would have had a hand in the eighteenth-century gout epidemic? Yet it all fits epidemiologically: only the rich were affected; they ate a lot of meat, drank a lot of port wine, and they suffered from gout.

NAJERA: Using a play as a metaphor is another good way to understand how the concept of the web of causation differs from other approaches of disease causation. For example, in some plays one actor, one main character, practically carries the whole play. This would be analogous to thinking of disease causation in terms of one agent that is more prevalent, more necessary, more important. In other plays, however, there are many actors with equally important roles; you need all of them to reach the play's outcome. This is comparable to approaching disease causation in terms of how people and other factors interrelate in a complicated web of causation. Some factors would be more important than others, of course, just as in most plays you can have many actors but fewer lead roles. Investigations should aim at understanding all the factors involved. This should facilitate separating confounding factors in the analysis.

TERRIS: There's another way to look at this: "The agent is necessary, but not sufficient."

NAJERA: When we say "necessary but not sufficient," however, I think it is important that we analyze necessary for what. In many of the acute diseases, the infectious diseases, we say that the specific agent is "necessary but not sufficient" because we need the specific agent to name the disease. But in the noninfectious diseases, which agents are necessary? In many cases, we don't really know.

TERRIS: Yes we do. Cigarette smoking is necessary.

NAJERA: Not for lung cancer. There is lung cancer without cigarette smoking.

TERRIS: Very little. Cigarette smoking is almost always involved.

NAJERA: But the fact is that there is some lung cancer without cigarette smoking. If you have lung cancer without cigarette smoking, then it is not necessary.

TERRIS: Air pollution, chromates, uranium: there are a number of agents that cause lung cancer.

NAJERA: Sure, there are a number of agents, but no single one is necessary in the same way we were talking about in infectious diseases.

TERRIS: But that is also true of infectious diseases. You can have a respiratory infection caused by 30 different viruses; there is no single agent.

NAJERA: This is what I wanted to come to: the condition of "necessary" is not so clear, even for the infectious diseases. For instance, tuberculosis mycobacteria are necessary for a diagnosis of tuberculosis only because we don't call the disease tuberculosis if there are no mycobacteria. But, after all, what is the real difference between a chronic pulmonary disease with mycobacteria and a chronic pulmonary disease without? Not much, except perhaps in the way we study and describe it, or in how we treat it—if there is a specific treatment for a specific agent, that is. Aside from this, most infectious diseases could be considered in a completely different manner. We could reclassify acute respiratory diseases epidemiologically, rather than accepting pathological or therapeutical classifications.

BUCK: Not entirely. I don't think the complexity of causation comes into infectious diseases in terms of whether there is a "necessary" cause. Just as you pointed out, disease nomenclature says there is a necessary cause. We name the disease by what we regard as the necessary agent. I think that what Terris is talking about is a *sufficient* cause. It is never enough just to have the agent, because a substantial proportion of people do not develop the illness. So the web comes more into the problem of sufficiency of causation.

NAJERA: Yes, yes. I wanted to emphasize that there are very few necessary lead roles in the "plays." Unless you have a very, very severe toxin such as strychnine. Strychnine is enough; it is the only cause. You take it and you die. But there are very few things like this.

TERRIS: But in certain noninfectious diseases, I could say that a vitamin deficiency is a necessary cause.

NAJERA: Sure, but even deficiency diseases can warrant further analysis. Say there is a vitamin deficiency; isn't it just as important to establish *why* there isn't a satisfactory supply?

TERRIS: Well, that is a situation where the agent is not sufficient. Given the basic epidemiologic triad of agent-host-environment as a conceptual framework, if you don't think in terms of the web of causation, you are forgetting about the host and you are forgetting about the environment. The agent must reach the host in sufficient quantities to cause trouble, and the host must be susceptible. That is the key to the whole process.

NAJERA: Yes. What's important is how and why—under which environmental conditions including social ones—these factors can reach the host to cause disease. It is not enough to accept the concept of agent-host-environment, one should also consider what factors influence these agents to go through the environment and reach the host. This becomes much clearer with chronic diseases. Here you find factors—you could call them "through factors"—that give origin to the agents and also influence the host. In my opinion, these are mostly social factors. Given this, one can discuss the non-validity of the so-called lifestyles. After all, lifestyle is a product of the environment, the social environment.

TERRIS: To return to our discussion on the web of causation, my guess is that there are very few lectures about it in today's epidemiology courses.

NAJERA: I teach it.

BUCK: Me, too.

TERRIS: You teach it? Very few teachers give that lecture. My students don't like it. It is too theoretical for them.

NAJERA: I am often called *maraña*. In Spanish, the word for web is *trama*, but I prefer *maraña*, which means tangled web. I am always talking about the importance of thinking in the *maraña epidemiológica*, the tangled web of causation.

TERRIS: I might say that much of the epidemiology taught in the United States is single-cause oriented, both for noninfectious and for infectious diseases. Take cigarette smoking. According to this approach, the tobacco companies have nothing to do with it, just the cigarette is to blame.

NAJERA: Also, nowadays people rely too much on statistics as the only method, forgetting that statistics should be only a helpful tool to ascertain whether events occurred by chance. Yet everyone maintains that things have been scientifically proven if they have been statistically proven. The truth is that you can never prove anything statistically. All you can do is try to eliminate chance, although it can never be completely eliminated—even if it is only one chance in a million.

TERRIS: Besides, if the results are not statistically significant, it may only mean that you don't have a big enough sample. That's all it means. People don't understand that.

NAJERA: Exactly. This is very important, because in epidemiology you have to search for relationships, even if they are not very apparent. This is the way to learn more. We have to be careful not to eliminate good theories simply because they are not statistically significant, or replace them with something else just because that is statistically significant. This margin of 95 percent or 5 percent that seems to be the basis for everything, does not really mean anything. On what basis can we say that 6 percent or 10 percent is bad and 5 percent is good?

TERRIS: As we all know, traditionally mortality has been the most highly developed measure of health status, because it is easy to measure the fact of death. However, there are a number of issues to discuss regarding the measurement of mortality. For instance, I think the recent development of the "years of life lost" concept as an alternative to the old approach of mortality rates is important, as is the question of age adjustment. By the way, did you know that it was a Hungarian statistician who first brought age adjustment to the United States? He gave a paper in Chicago at a national meeting of statisticians. Soon after, everyone began to do age adjustment. It caught on.

BUCK: As far as years of life lost goes, I suspect this may have been established as a methodological approach by Farr when he used Halley's life table concept.

NAJERA: Did you know that this Halley was the famous astronomer for whom the comet that has just "visited" us again was named? You are right, Carol, his mortality tables for the city of Breslau, published in 1693, were one of the first to relate mortality and age.

TERRIS: Another problem in measuring health status is accuracy in diagnosis. For example, the British found that coronary heart disease was more prevalent in the professional classes than in the working classes, that there was a socioeconomic gradient. One of John Ryle's mistakes was to look at this finding and say it was because the upper classes had more anxieties and responsibilities than the lower classes. Abe Lilienfeld wrote a beautiful paper in which he analyzed the English data for coronary heart disease and showed that indeed it was higher in the upper classes. Then he turned around and did the analysis for degenerative heart disease and it went the other way; it was higher in the lower classes. He then combined the two diagnoses and found that the death rate was the same for all social classes. Of course, the difference was not in the diseases but in the doctors. The upper classes had young, bright internists and cardiologists who knew all about coronary heart disease, whereas the working class had the old general practitioners who all their lives had called the disease degenerative heart disease and were not about to change. That is where the difference was. Lilienfeld's paper is important because it points to the problem of inaccuracy of the death certificate and the basic data.

Ruth Puffer also did a very important study for PAHO on the accuracy of diagnosis in San Francisco, Bristol, and some Latin American cities. To test the accuracy of death certificates in these cities, they very carefully evaluated all death certificates for a given time period. It was a fascinating study that really dealt with the question of accuracy of the basic data. And the interesting part of this study, for me, was that in the Latin American cities examined, diagnoses were as accurate as those in San Francisco and Bristol. The problem in Latin America was accuracy in diagnosis in the rural areas. Of course, the problem of accuracy in morbidity data is much worse than in mortality data, and it is even more difficult when we try to look at the epidemiology of health rather than of disease.

BUCK: It would be worthwhile to mention, at this point, that Sydenstricker's early surveys in the United States probably constitute the landmarks in measurement of morbidity.

In terms of measuring health, some years ago a study done in the United States compared two groups of children with different degrees of positive health. It wasn't sick versus controls in the usual sense, instead the study looked for determinants of the more positive health of one group. The idea is good because we seldom ever investigate health, great or good health versus all other levels. We are still so disease oriented. There is a problem, of course, in studying the determinants of good health—the problem of the direction of causality. Hours of sleep, for example, could be either the result or the cause of your state of health.

TERRIS: There was a study of Guatemalan children that linked maternal and child nutrition to performance. It would seem to me that this, too, is positive health, because it measures performance rather than illness. And another study, done by the Institute of Nutrition of Central America and Panama (INCAP), measured the ability to function. They took two groups of adult Guatemalan peasants doing hard physical labor and supplemented the diet of one group. It was found that those in the group without the dietary supplement lived in negative balance: they did not get enough calories and so they lost weight. They also didn't have much energy. Both groups would work in the fields, but after the work was done, those with the supplemented diet went out and played soccer or socialized, while the ones without the supplemented diet slept or rested at home. They were simply so fatigued because of malnutrition that they couldn't really live beyond the working day. I have calculated from their data that if this is really true, most of humanity in Asia, Africa, and a good part of Latin America loses one-quarter of active life because of malnutrition. This shows that the issue of the epidemiology of health is not merely a luxury or fringe benefit for industrialized nations; it is a crucial question for the developing world.

BUCK: There also was a study comparing the intelligence of Guatemalan children with that of American children. This study showed that the difference between Guatemalan and American infants increased steadily after birth. This suggested that the difference in intelligence did not have a prenatal origin; rather, it was the post-natal nutrition which was the important factor. Speaking of intelligence reminds me that mental health is one of the most difficult areas to measure. To quote Susser: "psychiatric researchers, aware of the problem, tried at least to specify caseness, a condition a psychiatrist would judge in need of treatment." He was trying to bring together survey-detected, self-reported, and psychiatric measures of mental illness. That is interesting, because I don't believe that problem has been solved yet.

TERRIS: Going back to your comment on the early use of "years of life lost," I believe that the landmark paper is not in those early writings. This concept is a wholly new approach which had never been used in the past 50 to 100 years. It was either the United States or Canada that first used it and it has now caught on.

Do you know how "years of life lost" came to be used? When heart disease, cancer, and stroke legislation was proposed as a major priority in the United States, the people in Maternal and Child Health (MCH) were furious because the legislation did not take into account years of life lost. In light of this protest, people began to think of redoing mortality to take account of the years-of-life-lost concept. When they applied the concept in Toronto, it showed that suicide in that city was much more important than everyone had thought it was.

NAJERA: That was in the seventies.

BUCK: Well, I think it goes back further than that, though. People have been working for a long time on what they call "health status indicators." The idea of the years of quality life rather than just life was put forward by Daniel Sullivan earlier than the seventies.

TERRIS: But he did not develop the method.

BUCK: Well, Sullivan did have a method consisting of a double life table: there was a column for mortality and there was a column for disability; by using the two columns simultaneously he was able to calculate the expectancy of years of nondisabled life.

John Last's "The Clinical Iceberg," was also a key paper in health status measurement. Much of the earlier morbidity data had come from treatment services: mental illness information from hospitals and other illness data from general practitioners. Last's paper showed that only a tiny fraction of people's illness turned up in the doctor's office. This is common knowledge now, but Last's paper showed that measuring morbidity on the basis of treatment wouldn't work. We had to do surveys of some sort.

I would like, for a moment, to go back to the web of causation discussion and have us consider the factors that may be involved in heart disease. Ancel Keys found something very, very provocative in his international study. He used regression equations containing suspected causal variables. There were two equations, one for the northern countries and one for the southern countries. When the northern equation was used to predict coronary disease in the southern countries, it predicted too many cases. When the southern equation was applied to the northern countries it predicted too few. For me, this showed that, in addition to the variables in the regression equation, there were other important factors, for example, occupation.

TERRIS: Why should you call it occupation?

NAJERA: Well, perhaps occupation and environment.

BUCK: I didn't say we have shown it.

TERRIS: But what in the environment?

NAJERA: What else could it be?

BUCK: Well, it could be genetic variables because different ethnic groups were involved in the international study of heart disease.

      I think that we also need to look at old problems in new and imaginative ways. Take, for example, Rosenman and Friedman's work. They were the first who had the nerve to spend a lot of money looking at the psychological factors in heart disease, while everybody else was happy looking at fat consumption, cholesterol, smoking, and blood pressure. I know that recently some doubt has been cast on the whole thing by the Multiple Risk Factor Intervention Trial (MRFIT) Research Group study, but I wouldn't rush to discredit the idea. Experimental evidence, some of which already came in, will settle the issue.

TERRIS: I think the whole thing is still up in the air, the relation of stress and heart disease.

BUCK: Well, I see it as a new kind of variable being introduced here.

TERRIS: Stress is the oldest variable there is in heart disease.

BUCK: Yes, but the new variable brought to light by the study is not so vague. The concept of Type A behavior is different from the global kind of variable called stress, isn't it? However, I agree that we're not yet sure about Type A, and that this poses an interesting question about whether something can be significant if it is still up in the air. I don't know. You could argue both ways.

TERRIS: Irrespective of that, I feel that you are giving that issue a credence I am not willing to give it. Besides, having a lot of stress management courses to prevent heart disease is ridiculous. What we have to do is work on the important things, like saturated fats and high blood pressure and smoking. Stress management is a gimmick now, and a good deal of money is being spent on it. First of all, how are you going to control stress with this stress management business? There's no proof that stress management does a damn thing. It's a fad, as far as I'm concerned. The relation of heart disease to psychological factors has always been a fad.

BUCK: You may be right, but I doubt it.

TERRIS: Yet I must admit they *may* be right. But at this point, it's a little bit like fiber and cancer of the colon; I don't accept that. I don't accept salt and hypertension, either. If you really look at the data, it's very unclear what the facts are.

BUCK: But one thing you have to think of (and I'm not saying that this book is the place to put the position forward) is that a lot of these other factors—diet, fiber, salt, calcium, and all that sort of thing—may protect target organs from developing a disease that is really a response to stressors. We may not get the best results if we try to prevent disease by manipulating these factors one by one. It's conceivable that if the basic stressors or the stress response can be modified, the target organs would remain healthy.

TERRIS: That's a global hypothesis which I don't accept. I must tell you that many people will not accept a global hypothesis.

BUCK: It's another way of looking at disease. I have an idea that disease is like a fire: you stamp it out here and it breaks out somewhere else.

TERRIS: That is a basic issue. I've heard this said too many times now. For instance, I've heard people at meetings say, "Well, if you cut out one disease, something else takes its place." It's not true. If you look at the data, nothing takes its place. There is a decline in the death rate. It was true of infectious diseases and it's true of noninfectious diseases. People die much later. Fries is right, there is a compression of morbidity.

BUCK: No, not necessarily a compression of morbidity, although there is a postponement of mortality. Fries may be indulging in wishful thinking when he talks about a compression of morbidity.

TERRIS: But that's not true, either. This is a basic question. When you have primary prevention you're not only postponing mortality, you're preventing morbidity.

BUCK: You're right, but only if you really have achieved primary prevention.

TERRIS: But that's what we're doing with heart disease, cerebrovascular disease, accidents. It's all primary prevention. It's not secondary prevention.

BUCK: What's the primary prevention of cerebrovascular disease?

TERRIS: Hypertension control.

BUCK: By what method?

TERRIS: By drugs.

BUCK: I see.

NAJERA: That's not primary prevention.

TERRIS: It is primary prevention of stroke.

BUCK: Maybe "secondary primary."

TERRIS: What would you do with risk factors? As far as I am concerned, hypertension is not a disease but a risk factor, just like high serum cholesterol. If you control serum cholesterol, we know this will lower mortality *and* the incidence of coronary heart disease will also decrease. The same is true of stroke: if you decrease the prevalence of hypertension, the mortality and the incidence of stroke will be lower. This is compression of morbidity. I have criticized the United States Social Security Administration because they publish statements that if mortality goes down, people who get older will have more morbidity. It is not true. You can also reduce morbidity because you're preventing stroke, you're preventing heart disease, you're preventing accidents.

BUCK: A lot of this is still theoretical.

NAJERA: You will not have later death in a pure sense, though. The average age at death will remain unchanged. What you will have is more people reaching that age, but later death, real later death, you will not have.

TERRIS: Sure you will.

NAJERA: Up to when?

TERRIS: Up to the average lifespan, which Fries has estimated to be about 85 years, with individual variations falling almost entirely within the range of 70 to 100 years.

NAJERA: O.K. We will have an age curve that shows that all people will die at the same time, at the end of the lifespan.

TERRIS: Right.

NAJERA: O.K. Then you have prevented all this morbidity, and all this mortality. People will live healthy lives. . . .

TERRIS: . . . until they've reached the end of the lifespan; then they'll die.

BUCK: They'll go out like light bulbs, I suppose.

TERRIS: We may completely disagree, but I think we all recognize that these issues are terribly important.

NAJERA: They are very important.

TERRIS: I don't buy the idea that if we lower the mortality and the incidence of a disease, something else will take its place. Nothing else takes its place.

NAJERA: You're right, it should not. It has not happened with the diseases affecting the young. Nothing has taken their place.

TERRIS: Manning Feinlieb showed this very well at one of the International Epidemiological Association meetings. He said that if you look at the rates, they are going down. That's all there is to it. But let's go back to the topic at hand; we were talking about etiologic investigations and I would like to go back to Goldberger. I think he was important because his studies show the similarity between infectious and noninfectious disease methodologies. Goldberger was a master of observation and experiment.

While he was working in entomology in the United States Public Service, there was an outbreak of a skin disease called Schamberg's disease. Goldberger was sent to solve the problem, which he did in a few days. He discovered that the disease only struck people who slept on straw mattresses. He then experimented on himself and other volunteers by sleeping on contaminated straw mattresses—they all contracted the disease. Then he sifted particles from the straw into two clean Petri dishes. The contents from one of the dishes was applied to the left axilla of a volunteer, and the skin eruption appeared. The other dish was exposed to chloroform vapor, and its contents then applied to the right axilla; there was no eruption. They examined siftings and found five very small mites which they applied to the axilla of another volunteer; the characteristic eruption appeared. They identified the mite and solved the problem.

Goldberger also was part of one of the three groups that raced to demonstrate that typhus fever is louse-borne:

there was a French group, Rickett's group in Mexico, and Anderson and Goldberger's group, also in Mexico. The French group won, by the way, not Ricketts, and not Anderson and Goldberger. But the wonderful thing was Anderson and Goldberger's analysis—based on the epidemiology of the disease and the characteristics of the possible insect vectors—of why the disease had to be louse-borne. It is that same reasoning, based on epidemiological facts, that Goldberger later used to conclude that pellagra had to be a nutritional disease.

Goldberger was an experimenter. He applied the experimental approach to a mite-borne disease, a louse-borne disease, and a noninfectious nutritional disease. You have to realize that epidemiology, before it became so observational under the influence of Wade Hampton Frost, was experimental. Epidemiologists came out of a microbiological background, and they experimented on themselves. With pellagra, Goldberger did a whole series of experiments. First of all, he did animal experiments, many of them. Then he did human experiments trying to infect U.S. Public Health Service volunteers, including himself, with the blood, nasopharyngeal secretions, skin lesions, urine, and feces of pellagra patients.

BUCK: It proved that pellagra wasn't infectious.

TERRIS: Nobody got pellagra. Then he did the studies in the orphanages and the insane asylums. He fed the inmates a good diet and pellagra disappeared.

BUCK: Did he have a control group?

TERRIS: He never had a perfect control. Now this really raises the question of whether you always need a perfect control. My answer is no. Although Goldberger did have some lucky breaks: in one orphanage, for example, they went back to the old diet and pellagra reappeared. They reintroduced the experimental diet and the disease disappeared again.

BUCK: In modern parlance, that would be called a very high-level quasi-experiment. Quasi-experiments can come pretty close to experiments.

TERRIS: But that's the danger in all this insistence on refusing to accept evidence except from randomized trials. When the Soviet Union carried out its polio immunization program, millions of people were immunized and polio practically disappeared. That was all the proof needed, as far as I'm concerned. I don't care that there was no control.

BUCK: I know what you mean, so I'm not going to argue.

TERRIS: Going back to Goldberger, his studies on pellagra also dealt with a very difficult methodological problem—the confounding variable. He discovered the connection between pellagra and a lack of meat and milk in the diet of the affected households. The problem was figuring out whether meat or milk was responsible. After all, the two were connected. Which was primary? Which secondary?

Goldberger did a very simple thing. He categorized households that consumed very little meat according to their milk consumption, showing that with a minimum of meat the incidence of pellagra declined as the milk consumption increased. Then he turned around and categorized households with very little milk consumption according to their meat consumption. It turned out that meat, too, was an independent variable. Both variables contributed to the disease. It was a very simple approach to unraveling the confounding variable.

The other approach which I think is very good was used by Doll in his work on cervical cancer. Since age at first marriage and number of pregnancies are both associated with the disease, he adjusted on age at first marriage and the association with number of pregnancies disappeared. Then he adjusted on number of pregnancies and the association with age at first marriage persisted. It was a beautiful demonstration.

There are a number of papers that deal with the issue of confounding variables, illustrating different ways of approaching one of the key problems in noninfectious disease epidemiology. For example, there is the method of multiple regression, and also the method of matching. I did a study on cancer of the mouth, pharynx, larynx, and esophagus. We matched on tobacco and showed a relation to alcohol. Then, when we got through with the study, we thought it could be the other way around, because tobacco and alcohol consumption are very closely related. So we matched on alcohol, and the tobacco relationship held up. They both held up. There are at least four different ways of dealing with confounding variables.

BUCK: To close on this theme, I think we should try to discuss experimental studies, highlighting behavioral change as a means to remove risk factors. Experience has convinced me that in the study of behavioral change the experimental approach is very difficult because of non-compliance and control-group contamination. Bradford Hill once said that you could not do an experiment on the value of breast-feeding.

LLOPIS: The principal characteristic of experimental epidemiology is that it introduces a new variable—intervention. And the only two possible intervention experiments are prophylactic measures and new treatment. These are the only possible experiments in epidemiology.

BUCK: And the fact is, you know, that experimental studies of that sort can run into serious problems with sample size because the randomization is of groups of people rather than individuals. In this type of experiment you have to make allowances for clustering, and that leads to much larger sample sizes.

TERRIS: One of the major experimental studies was the recent Lipid Research Clinic's study where they used a drug, cholestyramine resin, that lowers serum cholesterol by increasing the removal of low-density lipoproteins from the blood, but is not absorbed from the gastrointestinal tract. The study was organized by the U.S. Public Health Service, and showed very clearly that if you lower the serum cholesterol level, you lower the incidence of coronary heart disease. It really clinched it for serum cholesterol.

BUCK: I must say that I'm not convinced that lowering serum cholesterol provides an overall benefit. Coronary disease is just one part of morbidity.

TERRIS: No, I really think that study clinched it. At that point, people stopped arguing about the role of serum cholesterol.

BUCK: We're digressing now, but I think the real problem, now that you put your finger on it, is that since most people are convinced that cholesterol has a role, they feel that these experimental studies are trying to evaluate a preventive program, rather than trying to establish a cause.

TERRIS: No, it turned the tide. People stopped arguing at that point.

BUCK: I would agree with you, if we were talking about the etiological implications.

NAJERA: There was a very well-planned project in northern Nigeria to establish the role, the importance, of every factor involved in causing malaria: social factors, climatic factors, variables in the host, variables in the vector, and so on. I think it was a very well designed experimental study, etiological only in that it tried to find the role that each factor played.

TERRIS: The treatment of syphilis by the U.S. Public Health Service Hospital in Staten Island is, in my opinion, the most interesting one of all. Three cases were treated with penicillin and the disease vanished. It was published in *The American Journal of Public Health*. Now, if you had had one of these picky epidemiologists, they would have said not to publish it because there was no control.

BUCK: Well, Bradford Hill said that you didn't need a randomized clinical trial to show that streptomycin could keep people from dying of tuberculous meningitis. No one had ever recovered, and when certainty is the outcome you sure don't need a randomized trial.

TERRIS: I think this discussion is very important because today there is such a tendency toward cookbook randomization. Clinical epidemiologists are the worst in this respect.

BUCK: Purity to the point of sterility?

NAJERA: It's probably much easier to find and to do experiments in health services than to do etiological experiments, mainly because of the ethical factor.

BUCK: Not from a statistical point of view, because the problem of group randomization so often comes up in health care experiments.

NAJERA: It is the ethical part of the experiments that constitutes the main objection to most experimental epidemiology. Epidemiological experiments like the one on malaria that I mentioned may be the only model for future experimental epidemiology. In other words, one that assesses the importance of factors in a wide variety of conditions, by changing the pattern of those factors. I remember saying in one of our first discussions that we should pay more attention to the past and try to learn from it, especially from those experiments that failed. I think we would learn more from failures than we learn from successes, but the failures are never published. We should try to understand why some studies were not successful and why some were.

BUCK: I think you've raised an interesting point. There is quite a bit that we can learn from the MRFIT experiment, for example. First, it was done too late, in the sense that people in the control group had also modified their risk factors. If we are going to avoid contamination of control groups, we have to do our experiments before the public comes to believe that a causal relationship has been proven. Timing is important. The other lesson we could learn from the MRFIT study is that it might be better to experiment with one risk factor at a time. If the study had obtained a positive result, it would be difficult to know which pieces of the risk-reduction package had contributed the most.

STATISTICS OF MORBIDITY[1]

Edgar Sydenstricker

"Morbidity" is one of the terms in the definition of which the dictionary resorts to vague synonyms. We are told that morbidity is a "diseased" or "abnormal," "not sound," "not healthy," "sickly" state, and are referred to our livers in order to illustrate its meaning. Further reflection might lead us to ask how much morbidity is "normal" reaction to environment, or what proportion of illnesses is merely an unavoidable concomitant of the wearing out of human clocks, to use Pearl's metaphor, some of which are set by heredity to run a shorter time than others. When is death "normal"? At three-score years and ten, or at the century mark, or even at Methuselah's reputed age? How much of Methuselah's life was occupied in dying?

I am afraid that purely philosophical attempts to define the term will lead to a state of obfuscation—which might well be regarded as a form of morbidity in itself. Let us concede at the outset that morbidity is not as precise a concept as the statistician would desire; that it is a relative term, since one person may feel ill, stay away from work longer, be a greater nuisance than another who has the same objective symptoms; and that morbidity is essentially a subjective phenomenon. But let us take cognizance of the fact that illness, to use the commoner and more expressive term, is an undeniable and frequent experience of every person except, of course, the favored nonagenarian who, after a career devoted to tobacco, hard liquor, and perhaps other gayer irresponsibilities, is alleged in newspaper interviews never to have been sick a day in his life. Unlike birth or death, which can come but once to an individual, illness may occur often, its frequency depending not only upon its nature, its causes, and upon the susceptibility of the person concerned, but also upon its duration in relation to the length of time

considered. Obviously the calculus of probability cannot be used in morbidity statistics in the same ways as in birth or death statistics. Yet, in spite of difficulties of reducing it to precise statistical unity, illness is a *datum* measurable in fairly exact terms of duration, degree of disability, symptoms, cause, and sequelae. From the point of view of diagnosis it has an obvious advantage over death since the ill person is still subject to observation whereas the dead are unable to give further data except through autopsies. Statistics of illness can afford an indication of vitality that is not less biologically significant and is more illuminating than mortality. They portray the condition of a people's health far more delicately than death rates. They reveal the prevalence and incidence of disease in a population in a manner that is as useful to the student of society as clinical observation of the individual patient is to the physician.

* * *

The development of morbidity statistics has been very slow, and they are yet in their infancy. Their tardy progress may be ascribed to three principal reasons. One is expressed by the truism that statistics of a given kind are not continuously collected on a large scale unless there is a sufficient demand for their use in some practical way. A second reason is that the demand has come for morbidity statistics of special kinds and for specific population groups; little, if any, standardization in morbidity statistics has been attained. A third reason follows in some sense from the second—a confusion as to the concept of morbidity arising from differences in the uses to which the statistics are put. In addition to this confusion, differences in methods of collecting data, variety in definitions of a "case" of illness, the existence of peculiar factors that affect the accuracy of the record, the time element involved, and similar difficulties, have been deterrents to the accumulation of a large body of homogeneous morbidity data. It will not be possible upon this

---

Source: Excerpted from Edgar Sydenstricker, *The Challenge of Facts*, Richard V. Kasius, ed. New York, The Milbank Memorial Fund, 1974.

[1] De Lamar Lecture in Hygiene at the School of Hygiene and Public Health, the Johns Hopkins University, December 15, 1931.

occasion to review the history or to forecast the future of morbidity statistics, but the opinion may be ventured that it is doubtful that we shall ever need, and therefore shall ever have, continuous registration of illness in accordance with standardized procedure such as has been established in the field of natality and mortality. On the other hand, the future development of morbidity data promises great usefulness in two main directions:

1) As an epidemiological method whereby population groups can be accurately observed continuously in order to ascertain how actual conditions of human society influence the incidence and spread of disease.

2) As a means of portraying from time to time and for various population groups and areas, the problems of disease in far better perspective than can be given by statistics of mortality or by any other data practicable in the near future.

Our discussion purposely will be centered on the beginnings of morbidity statistics in the second direction, although the greater opportunity for development seems to me to be in the first.

* * *

Although many kinds of morbidity statistics exist, their varieties may be classified in five general groups. I shall refer to each very briefly in order to present in somewhat greater detail some results of one study of illness.

1) *Reports of Communicable Diseases.* In a strict sense, these are not morbidity data since illness is not necessarily involved. They exist, or *should* exist, for a specific purpose, namely the notification of those diseases for which reasonably effective methods of administrative control actually have been devised. Only to a limited extent are communicable disease reports useful for epidemiological studies. As Hedrich and I have shown (*1*), not only are the reports of most diseases extremely incomplete but their incompleteness varies according to age.

2) *Hospital and Clinic Records.* These are of little use in determining the prevalence or incidence of illness in a population, either in terms of a gross rate or from any specific disease. Properly made, as they rarely are, they are valuable for clinical studies and may become more so as the tendency to hospitalization increases and as clinicians become trained in analytical methods.

3) *Insurance and Industrial Establishment and School Illness Records.* The outstanding examples are the sickness experience of European insurance systems and of absences on account of illness of workers in industrial establishments in the United States. It is essential to bear in mind that important conditions affect the content, meaning, and validity of the data, although the concept of illness is more than usually specific because of technical and arbitrary definitions imposed for administrative reasons. One condition is the inclusion of only persons well enough to be employed. Another is the exclusion of all cases except disabling illnesses. Another is the exclusion of illnesses of short durations by reason of regulations as to the "waiting period," or the period of disabling illness that must elapse before the patient begins to draw sick benefits and therefore before the record of illness begins. Thus the annual disabling illness rate among male industrial workers with a waiting period of one week was 104 per 1000, whereas the rate for males in a large public service company without any waiting period was 1044 per 1000 (*2*). Again, "if wages are lost entirely when the worker is absent on account of sickness," as Brundage has shown, "the record usually shows a much lower rate of absences of relatively short duration than when full wages are paid during sickness" (Figure 1), although malingering was not found to be an important factor in two establishments studied (*3*). Malingering undoubtedly must be regarded as a condition affecting the accuracy of statistics based upon records of disability or absence. The lad who is too sick from a headache to remain in school but finds the fresh air of the baseball field beneficial, may or may not be malingering; at any rate he is often abetted by sympathetic parents. Yet the interesting suggestion has been made by Collins (*4*), and illustrated by Downes (*5*), that records of illness involving absence from school, if kept with some degree of specificity as to the nature of the illness, profitably could be used to complement the findings of the relatively infrequent and usually unsatisfactory physical examinations as a method of referring certain children for diagnosis and treatment.

4) *Illness Surveys.* These have been made, notably by the Metropolitan Life Insurance Company, to ascertain what the *prevalence* of illness is at a given date in sample populations. The method of these surveys is a simple house-to-

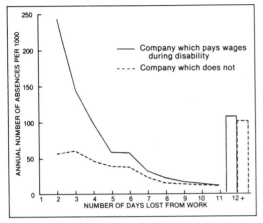

Figure 1. Frequency of absence due to disability among male employees of a company which pays wages during disability as compared with male employees of a company not paying during disability.

house canvass. The results indicate that about 2 percent of the population, including persons of all ages and at home or at work, are ill. The *incidence* of illness within a given period is not revealed by this method and, when the results are analyzed by cause, obviously the proportion of cases of long duration and of chronic type is much higher than is shown by records of incidence.

5) *Records of the Incidence of Illness in a Population Continuously or Frequently Observed.* Although this method was first employed on a considerable scale in the field of study of a single disease, pellagra, by Goldberger and myself and our associates (6), the first attempt so far as I am aware to record all illnesses continuously in a typical population on any considerable scale was made by the United States Public Health Service in Hagerstown, Maryland, in 1921-1924. The same methods, with some elaborations, have been used in several subsequent morbidity and epidemiological studies. The two main purposes of the Hagerstown study were 1) to ascertain the annual illness rate in a representative population and 2) to develop an epidemiological method whereby human populations could be observed for as complete an incidence as possible of various diseases, so far as they are manifested in illness, under actual conditions of community life.

*   *   *

Before referring to some of the results of this study from the viewpoint of general morbidity, it is important to consider the nature of the data obtained by the method of frequent and continuous observation employed in this and later similar studies.

Experience has shown that the completeness of a record of illness depends upon at least three important conditions. One is its severity and nature; the second is the length of the period for which the informant is asked to report; the third is the subjectivity of the record itself. Nearly every adult will remember an illness due to typhoid fever incident upon himself or in his family if it took place within the preceding ten or twenty years; few will recall a brief illness due to a common cold unless it occurred within a very short period immediately preceding the date of inquiry. Illnesses of a minor kind are observed and remembered when incident upon the informant himself with a greater degree of completeness than when incident upon others, even in the same family.

A few illustrations may be given. The annual incidence of illness of respiratory nature in families reported upon every half month was two attacks per person (7), whereas in families reported upon at intervals of six to eight weeks it was only about 0.7 attacks per person (8). The annual illness rate for women reporting upon themselves was 70 percent higher for respiratory conditions, 130 percent higher for nervous conditions, and 8 percent higher for digestive disorders than the rates for women reported upon by others in the same household (9). On the other hand, respiratory attack rates in families where adult males were the informants were higher for themselves than among adult females in the same families whereas all objective observations point to a higher rate among women than among men (10). Such experiences as these point to the necessity for taking influencing conditions into account that only participation in the collection of the data can possibly reveal.

*   *   *

I would have liked very much upon this occasion to have been able to bring you fresh reports upon several field studies of morbidity using or involving the recording of illness by the method of continuous observation of population groups. Unfortunately these studies either are still under way or are as yet in the process of tabulation. One is the observation of a population group of 5000 in a city of nearly 200 000 people and another is of a group of similar size in a rural area. The purposes of these studies are not merely to secure a record of the illnesses in order to depict the condition of a typical population's health in so far as it is revealed by illness, but to ascertain the extent to which illness is receiving medical service and the population itself is being served in various ways by the public health agencies, both official and unofficial. In these and other field inquires under way, the reasons why health services of different kinds are not used by the families and individuals are being ascertained in order to learn the attitude of the public and to appraise the efficiency of educational efforts. Thus the underlying method of continuous observation of a population is being applied in these two studies as a mode of measuring the effectiveness, from an important point of view, of public and private medicine—using the term "medicine" in its broad sense. A third study, in which this method is being employed, was conducted on a large scale in the United States in order to find out, with far greater accuracy than ever before, the extent to which families of different economic status actually availed themselves of medical, hospital, and other services and the actual costs of these services in detail for every illness during the period of a year. This inquiry extended into communities of different types and sizes and in many geographic areas of the country.

This particular method of the morbidity study—the continuous or frequent observation of a population—is thus being adopted for other purposes in the fields of public health and medical economics. It is essentially the method of the field zoologist, botanist, and the laboratory worker applied to the study of human populations living under conditions as they are found, but with far greater possibilities of precision in and completeness of observation than routine records made for other purposes can ever achieve. It will doubtless become a most valuable epidemiological tool as the technique of observation for specific diseases is divided and improved through experience. I need not refer here to the studies of respiratory affections conducted at the Johns Hopkins University which are notable examples of this use of the method. Epidemiological method, however, does not lie within our subject; I merely mention it in order to illustrate the fact that the study of morbidity is developing into an epidemiological mode that is both scientific and practicable.

* * *

For an illustration of morbidity studies used to depict the health of a population we may turn to the one made in Hagerstown.

The Hagerstown morbidity study (*11*) included 16 517 "years of observation," or an equivalent of a population of 7079 persons observed continuously for twenty-eight months beginning December, 1921. Illnesses were recorded as reported to experienced field investigators visiting each family every six to eight weeks, the reports being made by the household informant (usually the wife) either as experienced by herself or as she observed them in her family.

The results of the study indicated that a fairly accurate record of real illnesses was secured. Less than 5 percent of the illnesses of exactly stated durations recorded were one day or less in duration. Approximately 40 percent were not only disabling but caused confinement to bed. It is evident, therefore, that in the main the illnesses recorded were more than trivial in their character, in spite of the fact that in some instances mere symptoms were given as diagnoses. The incidence of acute attacks of specific and generally recognizable diseases was, we believe, recorded with a satisfactory degree of completeness. On the other hand, the incidence of mild attacks, as for example, of coryza, was quite incompletely recorded as judged by data on minor respiratory attacks obtained later by more intensive methods for other population groups.

For this population 17 847 illnesses were recorded in the twenty-eight month period, an annual rate of 1081 per 1000 years of life observed, or about one illness per person per year. This illness rate was over 100 times the annual death rate in the same population.

Perhaps the most interesting results of this first morbidity study of a typical population related to the variations in the incidence of illness according to age. Up to the time the

Hagerstown study was made the only data on adults came from "sickness" records of European insurance systems, English voluntary sick benefit societies, and a few American industrial employee funds. Nearly all of these records include only absences from work due to illness lasting a week or longer, and naturally indicate a rapid rise in the rate according to age because they reflected the serious illnesses only. The Hagerstown study showed that for a group composed of persons at work and at home the illness rate was high even in the younger adult ages and did not rise so quickly with age. The study also furnished data for the first time on children and adolescents with the surprising result that the peak of illness incidence was to be found in childhood and the lowest in the age period 15-24 years, a finding that has been confirmed by later studies employing similar methods (Figure 2).

This extraordinary age variation in the illness rate may be interpreted from various points of view, but before you venture any interpretations of it, certain other general considerations should be taken into account.

One is the fact that the proportion of persons suffering frequent attacks, four or more illnesses per year, was highest (45 percent) in childhood (2-9 years), lowest at 20-24 years (11 percent), rising gradually to a level of about 21 percent beginning with the age of 35. Thus the age variation in illness was partly due to the age distribution of frequently sick individuals. The proportion of persons sick once a year was about the same in every age period. On the other hand, the proportion of persons free from illness during the period was lowest in childhood (5 percent at 3-4 years), sharply rising through adolescence to a maximum of 30 percent at 20-24 years, and thereafter declining until the end of the life span (Figure 3).

A second consideration is the age variation in the severity of cases of sickness. Severity may be measured in various ways—by duration, degree of incapacitation, cause or nature of the attack, or by fatality. In order to suggest in a general way the ill person's resistance to death at different ages, a convenient mode of expression is the ratio for different age periods. The anticipated variations are clearly indicated, namely that his greatest resistance to death is in childhood, the age period 5-14; his lowest resistance is in infancy and early childhood (0-4 years) and toward the end of the natural life span. Ability to *survive* illness thus varies markedly from resistance to attacks of illness at different ages, particularly in childhood (5-14) when the average individual suffers from illness frequently but has a relatively small chance of dying, and in the older years when not only does his susceptibility to illness increase but also his chances of death. This is due partly, of course, to differences in the nature of illness occurring at these ages and partly to the diminished ability to resist the diseases which manifest themselves in morbidity (Figure 4).

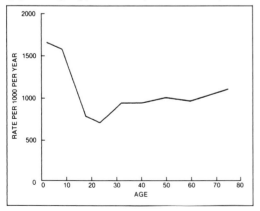

Figure 2. Age incidence of illness from all causes in Hagerstown, Maryland, as observed in a general population group, December 1, 1921–March 31, 1924.

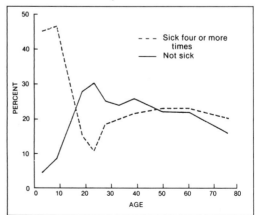

Figure 3. Proportion of persons at different ages who suffered a specified number of illnesses during twenty-six months.

Figure 4. Illnesses per death at different ages in the white population of Hagerstown, Maryland, December 1, 1921–March 31, 1924.

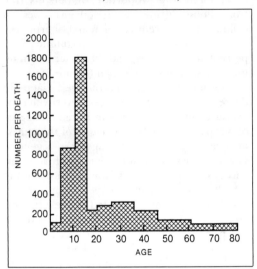

A third consideration is of basic importance—the cause or nature of illness at different ages. I can only summarize very briefly the data collected in the Hagerstown and subsequent studies. The generally known fact that each period of life is characterized by its own distribution of the causes of illness was more clearly and completely defined. In childhood, illness other than respiratory is caused chiefly by communicable diseases, diseases and conditions of the skin, ears, eyes, and teeth, and nervous and digestive disorders; in old age, illness other than respiratory is caused by the organic group of diseases and conditions, those of the circulatory system, nervous system, and kidneys. Illnesses resulting from all these causes are at their lowest level in adolescence and young adult ages. The only major cause which results in a higher rate of disability in young adult life than at any other age is the puerperal condition, and this, of course, relates to females only. Certain specific causes of illness do have their highest incidence in the young adult period of life, such as venereal diseases, typhoid fever, and pulmonary tuberculosis, except under conditions of special strain or hazard. But, by and large, this is the age most free from illness (Figures 5, 6).

The predominating importance of respiratory diseases and conditions as causes of illness at all ages is a striking fact, but their great height in childhood, their lowest level in adolescent and young adult period (15-24 years), and their gradual rise with the advance of age had not been depicted statistically. Respiratory illnesses were more frequent at both extremes of life than any other general disease group; although, with the exception of infectious diseases, circulatory diseases, and diseases of the bones and of "organs of locomotion," which so clumsily describe diseases that affect certain muscles, nearly all of the major groups of causes of illness tend to appear among the very young and among the old. In contrast to the organic troubles which so definitely begin to be manifested in middle life and which characterize old age, are the infections and the diseases and conditions affecting the skin, teeth, eyes, and ears that occur with greatest frequency in childhood.

A fourth consideration is the differential illness rates according to family economic status. After taking into account the differences in the age distribution of persons in different economic classes, the annual illness rates for Hagerstown were 991 per 1000 for the highest economic class, 1068 for the middle or "moderate circumstances" class, and 1113 for the "poor." These differences are not of the same magnitude as those found previously for infant mortality, tuberculosis, or pellagra, for example. Doubtless one reason was that the classes were not so sharply defined since the classification was based on the general impression of the investigator over two years of observation rather than upon an exact appraisal of income. A somewhat detailed analysis of the data, however, revealed the facts that the association of illness with poor economic status 1) appeared for certain causes only, and 2) was indicated in adult life and not in childhood or adolescence. An association with poor economic status was indicated for respiratory diseases, rheumatism, nervous conditions and disorders, and accidents. The commoner infectious diseases—measles, whooping cough, and chickenpox, for example—were not respectors of economic class. The lack of an association with favorable economic status with respect to diseases and conditions of the eyes and ears and of the circulatory, digestive, and eliminatory organs, may reflect the fact that such cases were more frequently attended by physicians and therefore more accurately described for the higher economic class than for the lower.

* * *

From the many interesting and suggestive data yielded by morbidity studies of this nature we may select one more fact. It is this: The general picture given by records of illness according to cause—or, more precisely, according to the *kind* of morbidity—is in sharp contrast to that given by mortality statistics. Respiratory diseases and disorders account for 60 percent of illness as against about 20 percent of deaths; the general group of "epidemic, endemic, and infectious" diseases accounts for 8 percent of illnesses, whereas only about 2 percent of the deaths were ascribable to this group; digestive diseases and disorders caused or characterized 10 percent of the illnesses as against 6 percent

of the total mortality. On the other hand, the group of "general" diseases (which includes cancer), the diseases of the nervous and circulatory systems, and the diseases of the kidneys and annexa were relatively much more important causes of mortality than of morbidity. The diseases of the heart and circulatory system show the sharpest contrast, 24 percent of deaths being ascribed to these conditions as against only 2 percent of illnesses. In other words, these diseases manifest themselves in relatively few instances of illness, although undoubtedly they shorten life and make life less efficient and enjoyable while it lasts.

* * *

I hesitate to draw the most obvious conclusion from the facts so far yielded by all studies of morbidity because I do not like to close on a

Figure 5. Causes of illnesses at different ages in a white population group in Hagerstown, Maryland, December 1, 1921–March 31, 1924. Under infectious diseases are included the "epidemic, endemic, and infectious diseases" and under "organic" the following: diseases of the eyes, ears, circulatory system, teeth and gums, kidney, and genito-urinary system.

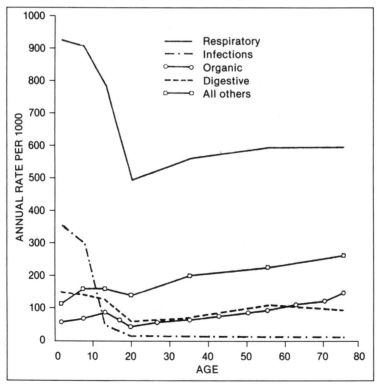

Figure 6. Variations, according to age, of certain groups of diseases which were primary causes of illness in a white population group in Hagerstown, Maryland, December 1, 1921–March 31, 1924.

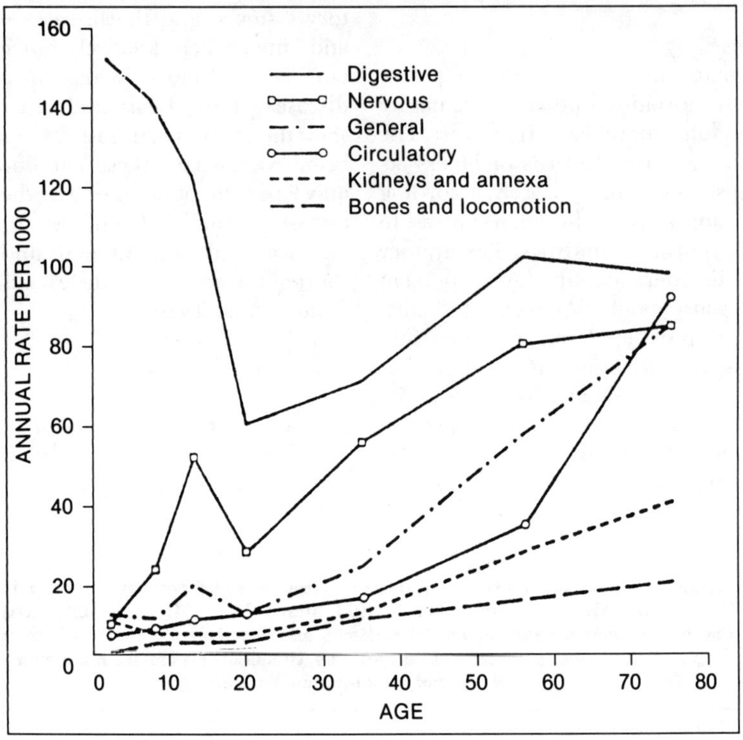

note that might be thought discouraging. I have confidence, however, in the stimulating challenge of facts. You may remember the soliloquy of *Faustus* upon the choice of a profession, written nearly 350 years ago by Christopher Marlowe, in which he weighed the success of medicine in these words:

> "Summum bonus medicinae sanitas
> The end of physic is our body's health.
> Why, Faustus, hast thou not attained that end?
> Are not thy bills hung up as monuments, whereby
> While cities have escap'd the plague, and
> Thousand desperate maladies been cured?"

So, today, we may apply to preventive medicine the test afforded by statistics of illness. It is true that some of the plagues and pestilences of Marlowe's day have been banished from a part

of the world; that many more maladies have yielded to modern treatment; that millions of people have escaped certain diseases and have lived lengthened lives. These achievements are monuments indeed to scientific discoveries and to the unselfish art of medicine. Yet undeniable morbidity experience in the twentieth century is overwhelming evidence that the goal of preventive medicine, which is a healthy people, is far from being reached. It is impossible to escape the conclusion to which these statistics drive us, that public health and the practice of medicine have as yet barely touched the task of *preventing* the conditions which manifest themselves in actual illness and all that illness implies.

References

(*1*) Sydenstricker, E., and A. W. Hedrich. Completeness of reporting of measles, whooping cough, and chickenpox at different ages. *Public Health Rep* 64(26):1537-1543, 1929.

(*2*) Brundage, D. K. The incidence of illness

among wage-earning adults. *Journal of Industrial Hygiene* 12:342, 347, 1930.

(*3*) Ibid, 340.

(*4*) Collins, S. D. The place of sickness records in the school health program. *Transactions of the Fifth Annual Meeting of the American Child Hygiene Association*, October, 1928.

(*5*) Downes, J. Sickness records in school hygiene. *Am J Public Health* 20:1199-1206, 1930.

(*6*) Goldberger, J., G. A. Wheeler, and E. Sydenstricker. A study of the relation of diet to pellagra incidence in several textile communities of South Carolina in 1916. *Public Health Rep* 35:648-713, 1920, and later publications.

(*7*) Townsend, J. G., and E. Sydenstricker. Epidemiological study of minor respiratory diseases. *Public Health Rep* 62(2):112, 1927.

(*8*) Sydenstricker, E. A study of illness in a general population group. *Public Health Rep* 61(39):12, 1926.

(*9*) Sydenstricker, E. The illness rate among males and females. *Public Health Rep* 62(30):1952, 1927.

(*10*) Sydenstricker, E. Sex difference in the incidence of certain diseases at different ages. *Public Health Rep* 63(21):1269-1270, 1928.

(*11*) Sydenstricker E. Hagerstown Morbidity Studies. A Study of Illness in a Typical Population Group. *Public Health Rep*, reprints 1113, 1116, 1134, 1163, 1167, 1172, 1225, 1227, 1229, 1294, 1303, and 1312.

THE AGE SELECTION OF MORTALITY FROM TUBERCULOSIS IN SUCCESSIVE DECADES[1]

Wade Hampton Frost[2,3]

As we pass along the age scale from infancy through childhood, to early adult life, and on to old age, the curve of mortality from tuberculosis shows a continuous movement either upward or downward. This is such a familiar fact that we are apt to take it for granted; to dismiss it as characteristic of the disease, and to pass on. But there is perhaps no single statistical record which is potentially of more significance. For every change in the rate of mortality as we pass from one age to another represents a shift in the balance established between the destructive forces of the invading tubercle bacillus, and the sum total of host-resistance. If we could accurately interpret this record, analyzing in detail each movement upward or downward and assigning to each factor its due share in the change, then we would be well on the way to knowing the epidemiology of tuberculosis.

But the record is peculiarly difficult to read with understanding, because it is immediately apparent that the most striking changes in mortality rates do not correspond to reasonably probable changes of like extent in rate of *exposure* to infection. For instance, nothing that we know of the habits of mankind and the distribution of the tubercle bacillus would lead us to suppose that between the first and the second five years of life there is, in general, a *diminution* in exposure to infection which corresponds to

Source: *American Journal of Hygiene* 30:91-96, 1939.

[1] From the Department of Epidemiology, School of Hygiene and Public Health, The Johns Hopkins University, Baltimore, Md.

[2] This material was assembled by Dr. Frost in 1936 and presented before the Southern Branch of the American Public Health Association. At the time of his death in 1938, it remained unpublished. Because of fundamental implications in regard to the interpretation of age-specific mortality rates and particularly in regard to the reaction of the human host to tuberculous infection, his notes are herewith made available, together with the table showing the basic data used in the report.

[3] The following quotation from a letter dated July 29, 1935, to the late Dr. Edgar Sydenstricker from Dr. Frost, is self-explanatory and is reproduced here as a document of scientific as well as historical interest.

" . . . Using the Massachusetts data which you so kindly sent me, extended by the calculation of corresponding rates for 1920 and 1930, I have made up the two enclosed tables which have interested me and may be of interest to you.

"In Table 1 the striking fact other than the consistent decline in mortality at every age is the progressive advancement to higher and higher ages of the peak of mortality; in 1880 the peak (or more properly the first peak) in adult life is at age 20–29, whereas, in 1930 it is in the age group 50-59. The same kind of change is, as you know, quite generally shown in other areas.

"For some years I have thought of the high mortality in later life as being related to *escape* from excessive mortality in earlier adult life. I have been thinking of the tuberculosis of today as a disease which has not the killing power to cause much mortality in the vigor of young adult life but becomes fatal in middle age or later when vital resistance has declined. It has seemed to me that it was approaching the age-selection of pneumonia—fatal chiefly at the extremes of life, non-fatal in the more vigorous ages.

"In Table 2 I have set up the mortality rates in a different way, in order to show, through successive ages, the mortality of the 'cohorts' of persons who were aged 0-9 years in 1880, 1890, 1900, etc. Thus, persons aged 0-9 in 1880 would be aged 10-19 in 1890, 20-29 in 1900 and so on until in 1930 they would be in the age group 50-59. With this rearrangement Table 2 shows what should have been but was not obvious to me from Table 1, namely, that in each *cohort*, followed through in this way, the highest mortality has been at the age 20-29. This is perhaps more readily seen from the rough pencil graph which is enclosed.

"Viewed in this light the relatively high mortality rates now exhibited in the higher age groups seem to me to have a significance quite different from what I had attributed to them. They may be interpreted as the residuum of the much higher rates which the now aged cohorts have experienced in earlier life. In general, the rule seems to be that the higher the mortality of any cohort in early life, the higher will it be in later years. Or, to have passed through a period of high mortality risk confers not protection, but added hazard in late life.

"The only other data which I have been able to study so far are for England and Wales, 1850-1930, and for the U.S. Registration Area of 1900, for the years 1900-1930. They show substantially the same relations as the Massachusetts data; also, the records for females show much the same thing, but with a more pronounced peak at the earlier age. I want to get together material for a somewhat more orderly study later.

"All of this seems to me to have a bearing on the question which is raised in the MS I sent you a few days ago—namely, how much if any we may expect adult mortality to be increased as the result of diminished infection in the favorable years of childhood—from age 3 to 12. It also seems to me to have a bearing on the moot question whether the tuberculosis of adult life is almost wholly exogenous—due to recently acquired infection—or to a considerable extent endogenous—the outcropping to clinical severity of infection which has remained latent or smoldering through the childhood years when vital resistance seems to be at its height. . . ."

the decline in mortality rate. And there is little, if any, better reason to suppose that the extraordinary rise in mortality from age 10 to age 20, 25, or 30 is paralleled by a corresponding increase in rate of exposure to specific infection.

We are forced, then, to recognize, as at least highly probable, that the predominant factor in the up-and-down movement of mortality along the age scale is change in human resistance. And this is a complex of which we have very little exact knowledge except the plain fact that age and prior exposure bring no such immunity against tuberculosis as they establish against many of the acute infections.

However, my purpose is not to attempt an interpretation of the age selection of tuberculosis; it is merely to call attention to the apparent change in age selection which has taken place gradually during the last 30 to 60 years, and to note that when looked at from a different point of view this change in age selection is found to be more apparent than real. The age-specific curve of mortality from tuberculosis for males in the United States Registration Area of 1900 is shown for the years 1900 and 1930 in Figure 1 and for Massachusetts males for the years 1880, 1910 and 1930 in Figure 2.

The tuberculosis mortality rates for Massachusetts used throughout this paper are shown in Table 1. You will note that:

1. At every age mortality is lower in the later period.

2. In each period, age selection is generally similar: mortality is high in infancy; declining

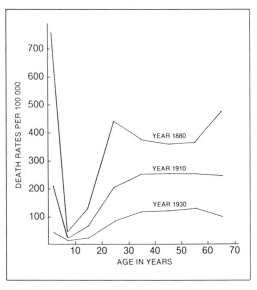

Figure 2. Massachusetts death rates from tuberculosis, all forms, males by age, 1880, 1910, 1930.

in childhood; rising in adolescence to a higher level in adult life.

3. In the later period (1930) the highest rate of mortality comes at the age of 50 to 60, whereas formerly it was at age 20 to 40.

These characteristic changes from decade to decade can be demonstrated in the records for many different areas, both for males and females.

Looking at the 1930 curve, the impression given is that nowadays an individual encounters his greatest risk of death from tuberculosis between the ages of 50 and 60. But this is not really so; the people making up the 1930 age group 50 to 60 have, in earlier life, passed through *greater* mortality risks.

This is demonstrated in Figures 3 and 4, which show for males and females in Massachusetts the death rates at specific ages in the years 1880 and 1930, and also those for each age of the cohort of 1880 or that group of people who were born in the years 1871 to 1880. These graphs indicate that the group of people who were children 0 to 9 years of age in 1880 and who are now aged 50 to 60 years (if alive) have, in two earlier periods, passed through *greater* risks. They also indicate that the age selection in the cohort of 1880 is quite different from that *apparently* indicated by the age specific mortality rates for any single year.

Figure 1. United States Registration Area of 1900, death rates from tuberculosis, all forms, males by age, 1900 and 1930.

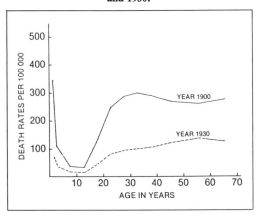

Table 1. Death rates[a] per 100 000 from tuberculosis, all forms, for Massachusetts, 1880 to 1930, by age and sex, with rates for cohort of 1880 indicated.

Age	1880	1890	1900	1910	1920	1930
Males						
0-4	760	578	309	209	108	41
5-9	43	49	31	21	24	11
10-19	126	115	90	63	49	21
20-29	444	361	288	207	149	81
30-39	378	368	296	253	164	115
40-49	364	336	253	253	175	118
50-59	366	325	267	252	171	127
60-69	475	346	304	246	172	95
70+	672	396	343	163	127	95
Females						
0-4	658	595	354	162	101	27
5-9	71	82	49	45	24	13
10-19	265	213	145	92	78	37
20-29	537	393	290	207	167	92
30-39	422	372	260	189	135	73
40-49	307	307	211	153	108	53
50-59	334	234	173	130	83	47
60-69	434	295	172	118	83	56
70+	584	375	296	126	68	40

[a] They were obtained as follows: For the years 1910, 1920 and 1930—based on U.S. Mortality Statistics—deaths from tuberculosis all forms. For the years 1880, 1890, and 1900 the rates used are calculated from data compiled by the late Dr. Edgar Sydenstricker from the state records. Because of differences of classification in deaths, it has been necessary to base the rates on the deaths recorded as "tuberculosis of the lungs" to get comparable data for these years. The rate calculated from the state records for "tuberculosis of the lungs" has been multiplied by a factor based on the proportion such deaths bore to those from tuberculosis, all forms. This factor varied with the year and age considered.

Figure 3. Massachusetts death rates from tuberculosis, all forms, males by age, in the years 1880 and 1930, and for the cohort of 1880.

Figure 4. Massachusetts death rates from tuberculosis, all forms, females by age, in the years 1880 and 1930, and for the cohort of 1880.

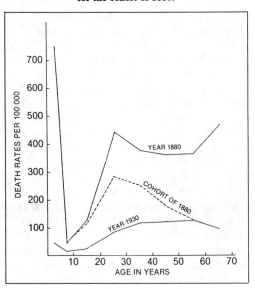

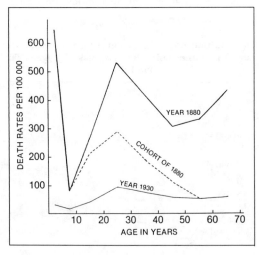

Figure 5 shows similarly for males the mortality at successive ages in cohorts of (1870), 1880, 1890, 1900, 1910. Note that "terminal" rates for these cohorts make the 1930 curve, and also that in successive cohorts the age selection has been uniform; with the mortality highest in the first five years and again from 20 to 30 years; thereafter it declines.

This fact was previously noted by K. F. Andvord (*1*). His interpretation was, in part, that this regularity of the age curve formed a basis for extending estimates of future mortality in the same cohort at higher ages. Such an interpretation is both tempting and encouraging but perhaps dangerous.

Without attempting to interpret the facts in detail, certain implications are noted.

1. Constancy of age selection (*relative* mortality at successive ages) in successive cohorts suggests rather constant physiological changes in resistance (with age) as the controlling factor.

2. If, as we may suppose, the frequency and extent of exposure to infection in early life has decreased progressively decade by decade, there is no indication that this has had the effect of exaggerating the risk of death in adult life due to lack of opportunity to acquire specific immunity in childhood.

3. Present day "peak" of mortality in *late* life does not represent postponement of maximum

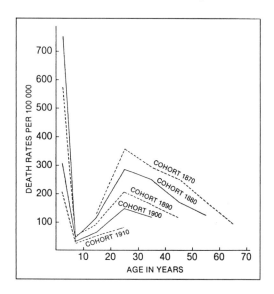

Figure 5. Massachusetts death rates from tuberculosis, all forms, males by age, in successive 10-year cohorts.

risk to a later period, but rather would seem to indicate that the present high rates in old age are the residuals of higher rates in earlier life.

Reference

(*1*) Andvord, K. F. *Norsk Mag f Laegevidenskhaben,* June, U.S. Mortality Statistics, 1930.

RECORD LINKAGE[1]

Halbert L. Dunn[2]

Each person in the world creates a Book of Life. This Book starts with birth and ends with death. Its pages are made up of the records of the principal events in life. Record linkage is the name given to the process of assembling the pages of this Book into a volume.

The Book has many pages for some and is but a few pages in length for others. In the case of a stillbirth, the entire volume is but a single page.

The person retains the same identity throughout the Book. Except for advancing age, he is the same person. Thinking backward he can remember the important pages of his Book even though he may have forgotten some of the words. To other persons, however, his identity must be proven. "Is the John Doe who enlists today in fact the same John Doe who was born eighteen years ago?"

Events of importance worth recording in the Book of Life are frequently put on record in different places since the person moves about the world throughout his lifetime. This makes it difficult to assemble this Book into a single compact volume. Yet, sometimes it is necessary to examine all of an individual's important records simultaneously. No one would read a novel, the pages of which were not assembled. Just so, it is necessary at times to link the various important records of a person's life.

The two most important pages in the Book of Life are the first one and the last one. Consequently, in the process of record linkage the uniting of the fact-of-death with the fact-of-birth has been given a special name, "death clearance."

Source: *American Journal of Public Health* 36:1412-1416, 1946.
[1] Modified form of paper given before the joint conference of the Vital Statistics Council for Canada and the Dominion Council of Health, held in Ottawa, Ontario, Canada, on May 10, 1946.
[2] Chief, National Office of Vital Statistics, U.S. Public Health Service, Federal Security Agency, Washington, D.C.

IMPORTANCE OF ASSEMBLING THE BOOK OF LIFE

There are many uses for the important records of each person, brought together as a whole. At times, even now, such a collection is of sufficient value that it is made at considerable cost in time and money. Usually, it is the individual who is made to do the work since he alone knows where his records are on file. It is much more difficult for any other person or organization to assemble the records of his life since no personal cross-index exists to lead one to all of a person's records. It is important to many people and organizations to be able to assemble this type of information easily and efficiently.

IMPORTANCE TO THE INDIVIDUAL

Sooner or later most of us need to prove facts about ourselves. The most frequent facts are concerned with birth. Sometimes other facts are needed. Many of these are recorded in the vital records of marriage, divorce, adoption, legitimation, change of name, death and presumption of death. However, it is not infrequent that facts are required from records of other types than vital records. Such types of records are those made for social security, military purposes, insurance, payment of pensions, professional licenses, hospital care, and a host of others.

At times it is necessary to prove that one is in truth the person to whom the documents refer.

After death, it becomes especially difficult for relatives to assemble even the most important pages of the Book of Life of their dead. Individuals must furnish proof before title to property is transferred or the payment of legitimate claims is made. Missing persons may be alive or dead.

IMPORTANCE TO REGISTRARS OF VITAL RECORDS

No one has a greater stake in the Book of Life than the registrar.

At the present time, he has the first page of each volume. But, although he may also have other important pages under his custody, they are scattered on different shelves of his vault. Some may be in the offices of his fellow registrars.

The registrar's primary responsibility has always been:

1. To obtain completeness and accuracy of registration.
2. To preserve records.
3. To certify from records.
4. To produce statistics from them.

The possibility of satisfying his basic responsibilities could be greatly reinforced if the registrar would take on the additional responsibility of binding the Books of Life into volumes. It is not necessary for him actually and physically to assemble the records of a particular individual and bind them into a volume. For all practical purposes, the end result will be achieved if he creates a Life Records Index indicating *where* all the most important records of an individual are filed.

The accuracy of vital records would be enhanced because of inconsistencies that would show up. The completeness of vital records would be improved because subsequent documents would show that previous records which should have been filed had not been placed on file. Certification would become more secure from fraud. For instance, birth records of dead people could not be certified for fraudulent purposes. Massive certification jobs for government, which of necessity are so often done without charge, could be handled more efficiently and less expensively through a check-off system. Statistical information would become more meaningful because it would be linked to other types of data.

It is not too rash to predict that if the registrars of the country would undertake to prepare and keep up-to-date the Life Records Index on all the people of the country and do the job systematically and efficiently, they would find themselves and their offices to be the focal point of all records concerning people through-out the country. This would probably be accomplished in a surprisingly few years because the need for such a record linkage service is very great. It should be achieved at a relatively small total cost because the mechanism of the task is a very simple one, and, in performing this service, registrars would find that they were doing a particularly fine job in carrying out their primary responsibilities of registration and statistics.

IMPORTANCE TO HEALTH, WELFARE AND OTHER TYPES OF ORGANIZATIONS

Numerous national, state, and local official organizations rely heavily on knowing certain chapters in the Life Records Index of many persons. In order to carry out their assigned tasks, organizations must ask individuals to produce proof of who they are, where and when they were born, to whom they are married, whether they served in the military forces, and a hundred other questions. Throughout all of this, the organization official must keep in mind the possibility of fraud. "Is this person really John Doe?" "Is his record as recorded true or false?"

After an individual has died, it is particularly difficult for the organization official to tap the facts concerning the records of the deceased. Frequently he does not know whether or not the individual is dead. For example, certain insurance companies systematically send to all fifty-three registration areas in the United States the names of persons with whom they have lost contact and who are presumed to be dead. The companies want to pay insurance benefits if they are due. In addition, they want to clear their books.

To know the fact-of-death whenever or wherever it occurs is of importance to every organization, official or private, that maintains an "active" file on large numbers of individuals. For example, it is costing the United States Government millions of dollars per year to maintain the millions of records of dead people in their active files. Every search for a particular record is complicated and made more costly because the files contain "dead" records. Space costs are reflected in higher rentals and upkeep.

Another reason organizations have an interest in record linkage is that it will help them obtain more meaningful quantitative knowledge about their own programs. Most organizations dealing with individuals produce some type of administrative statistics of the individuals served by them. It would greatly enhance the significance of such statistics if they could be linked to other facts about the same individuals, such as, "What sort of jobs do they hold?" "How many children do they have?" "What sort of illness do they suffer from?" "What kind of social environment do they live in?" In particular health and welfare organizations would find that this type of linked statistical analysis would open new vistas of knowledge to them.

BINDING THE BOOKS OF LIFE INTO A SINGLE VOLUME

There are many ways of binding the Books of Life into volumes. Most of the registration systems in Europe accomplish this end by a central national file. Such systems are reinforced by constant referral to this file through the exercise of police powers. In general, all such systems will find disfavor in the United States.

Several years ago Canada was forced, by the passage of legislation on family allowances, to find an economical and efficient way to link all the vital records of an individual. Annual payments of 250 million dollars required up-to-the-minute and certain proof of the ages and birth order of all children under 16 years of age. It was decided that all customary certification methods were too costly, too slow, and too open to fraud. The system as worked out in Canada has proved to be simple and relatively inexpensive. *It has worked from the start.* It has kept vital records in their proper place, i.e., under the control of public health and statistical agencies. In the near future, it will probably be expanded to include older ages.

The elements of the system are:

1. The Dominion Bureau of Statistics obtains microfilm copies of all vital records: births, deaths, marriages, divorces, adoptions, immigrations and emigrations.

2. It then produces a uniform name index punch card for all such records. The index cards so produced are decentralized by duplicating the cards or by sending printed index lists to the province of birth, regardless of what province a particular record is filed in. In this manner a printed, ledger-type Life Records Index is created for each province from the birth certificate. Each punch card is presented in this Index as a single printed line of type.

3. Massive certification jobs for governmental purposes are done by check-off against this index in the province of birth.

4. A statistical card is punched by the Dominion Bureau of Statistics at the same time as the name index card is punched.

5. The Dominion Bureau of Statistics codes and tabulates all vital statistics, and publishes the national data. Detailed provincial statistics are turned over to the province for their publication and exploitation.

6. The control of this joint federal-provincial vital records-vital statistics system is under a Council of Vital Statistics made up of the provincial registrars, the Dominion Statistician, and the Directors of Vital Statistics and Census, Divisions of the Dominion Bureau of Statistics.

7. The use of a birth card is being actively promoted throughout all Canada so that the person's identity number (birth card number) can be absorbed in all official records and thus simplify the posting of facts to the Life Records Index.

Canada has gone a long way toward producing a solution of this problem for persons under twenty years of age because of the legislation on family allowances. In addition to the great advance which Canada has made in linking the records of families having children under this age, it is now faced by problems involved in creating a nationwide prompt clearance of the fact of death.

DEATH CLEARANCE

While this is but a single step in the whole process of obtaining record linkage, it is a most important step. There is so much demand for death clearance that, whatever it cost, the earnings should pay the costs of undertaking the task on a nationwide, uniform basis.

The principal market for this national death clearance system comes from those insurance companies and social organizations and institutions, both governmental and private, which either pay out money upon the death of the individual or which have obligations that are cancelled at the death of the individual. In the aggregate, the market for this type of service is enormous. It is a multiple market, for the fact of death on one individual is needed by various organizations. Ultimately, an average of five to ten purchase orders for such information might be posted against the Life Records Index of each individual for a report of the fact of death whenever the death occurs. Since the deaths of older persons would involve a high percentage of unregistered births, it would probably be economical to handle such records on the basis of a systematic search against state death indexes.

The generalization of a record linkage system to all persons in the country depends primarily on three things:

1. *An efficient Life Records Index to the important records of an individual.* The Life Records Index should be located in the state of birth and must lead to the individual's vital records wherever they might have been placed on file. This cross-index should be arranged in birth certificate number order rather than in an alphabetical name order.

2. *An efficient and prompt inter-state exchange of essential facts* which need to be posted to the Life Records Index. This involves as a minimum the exchange of facts identifying and locating the certificates of marriage, divorce, annulment, adoption, change of name, legitimation and death, whenever they are placed on file in a state other than the state of birth.

3. *The promotion of the widespread use of the Birth Card.* This is the key to efficient record linkage. If the governmental organizations, both federal and state, absorb the birth certificate number into their own records and require that the individual produce it before they obtain services— *Services Which They Need*—people are going to carry their birth cards with them wherever they may go. If the birth certificate number becomes a part of every type of record it will greatly simplify posting to the Life Records Index. The establishment of a nation-wide system of record linkage for all persons in the country will become an invaluable adjunct to the administration of health and welfare organizations and at the same time produce coördinated statistical knowledge of great value. With the birth certificate number as the binding of the Book of Life and the Birth Card as a device to facilitate the posting to the Life Records Index, all the records on an individual will eventually become linked together. Ultimately, the birth certificate number should be requested as an item in the national decennial census. In this way the wealth of information produced by the census will be linked to the vital records listed in the Life Records Index.

A DISCUSSION OF THE CONCEPTS OF INCIDENCE AND PREVALENCE AS RELATED TO EPIDEMIOLOGIC STUDIES OF MENTAL DISORDERS[1]

Morton Kramer[2]

We need to know much more about the epidemiology of mental disorders. The research needed will prove expensive and difficult since it will depend on long observation and will involve several disciplines, but it is the way we must take to advance our knowledge of the incidence, duration and prevalence of mental diseases.

This paper gives an opportunity to acquaint epidemiologists with some of the characteristics of morbidity data on the mentally ill and some of the challenging research problems that this field presents. Because of the complex nature of the problem, epidemiologic research on the mental disorders is bringing into the public health field professional personnel from such disciplines as psychiatry, psychology, sociology, anthropology, and psychiatric social work. For the most part, persons trained in these professions have not been exposed to the philosophy underlying the epidemiologic approach to the study of disease and to the statistical methods used in such studies. This paper, therefore, will also give an opportunity to provide these professionals with some background material on two basic morbidity indexes used in studying the occurrence of disease in population groups.

DEFINITIONS

Incidence is defined as the number of new cases of a disease occurring within a specified period of time. "New case" must be carefully defined as, for example, the first or initial attack of a disease during an individual's lifetime. The incidence rate is computed by taking the ratio of the number of new cases (as defined) in the specified interval to the appropriate popu-

lation exposed to risk. This rate may be made specific for a variety of factors, such as age, sex, marital status, geographic area, and socioeconomic status.

Prevalence is defined as the number of cases of a disease present in a population group as of a specified interval of time, i.e., it is the number of cases existing at the start of an interval plus the new cases developing during the interval. As Dorn (1) points out, "the length of the interval of observation must always be specified if a prevalence rate is to be correctly interpreted, for we may speak of the number of persons who are sick at any time during a given day, week, month or other arbitrary interval." The characteristics of individuals who are to be counted as a case must be carefully defined, as for example all persons who have "active" disease within the interval of study. The prevalence rate is computed by taking the ratio of the number of cases in the specified interval to the number of people in the appropriate population group for which the rate is being determined. The rates may be made specific for age, sex, geographic area, socioeconomic status, etc.

Usually the prevalence rate can be determined more easily than the incidence rate since it can be estimated by a single case-finding survey of a population group. This is particularly true for the chronic diseases, but this should not obscure the fact that the incidence rate is the fundamental epidemiologic ratio. The fundamental nature of this rate has been emphasized by Dorn (1), Doull (2), Sartwell and Merrell (3), and others. In discussing infectious diseases Doull states, "In general terms and assuming no restrictions on exposure, incidence is dependent upon the balance which exists between

Source: *American Journal of Public Health* 47:826–840, 1957.

[1] This paper was presented before a Joint Session of the National Conference for Health Council Work and the Epidemiology and Mental Health Sections of the American Public Health Association at the Eighty-Fourth Annual meeting in Atlantic City, N. J., November 15, 1956.

[2] Chief, Biometrics Branch, National Institute of Mental Health, National Institutes of Health, Bethesda, Maryland.

resistance of the population and pathogenicity of the microorganism. This balance may be called the force of morbidity." The analogy between this concept and concepts that have been proposed with respect to the incidence of mental disorder in the population is apparent. Incidence of mental disorder would seem to be dependent upon the balance which exists between resistance of the population and those forces and stresses—biologic, cultural, psychologic—that produce mental disorder. Doull further states, " . . . prevalence is more complex. It is the resultant of the force of morbidity and those factors which determine whether the interval between onset and termination shall be long or short, whether a disease shall be acute or chronic."

In more formal terms, incidence measures the rate at which new cases are added to the population of sick persons and—in conjunction with the decrement rate, i.e., the rate at which the disease is "arrested," "cured," or at which affected individuals are removed from the population by death—determines the size and composition of the sick population. Thus, the prevalence rate of a disease is a function of the incidence rate and the duration of the disease.

HYPOTHETICAL EXAMPLES

These concepts may be illustrated by three hypothetical examples dealing with the variables incidence, duration, and prevalence. These examples show the effect of different assumptions regarding duration of disease on the resulting prevalence rate in a stationary population with a constant annual incidence rate of a specified disease.

Let us assume that there are three communities each with a stationary population of 100 000 people that have always been free of mental disorder. Suddenly, in 1940, 1000 individuals become psychotic for the first time in communities A and B and 2000 in community C. Further, to simplify the problem, let us also assume that these people all become psychotic on January 1, that they are immediately hospitalized on that day and that there is only a single type of mental disorder involved. Thereafter, on January 1 of every year, 1000 new cases of the same disorder always appear in A and B and 2000 in C. Let us also assume that the sick individuals are released from the hospital at

some specified rate and that release from the hospital is equivalent to cure of the disease, i.e., the interval between date of admission and date of release is equivalent to duration of the disease. Table 1 shows the prevalence in each community on January 1 of each year under the following assumptions with respect to the duration of illness in each cohort[3] of new cases:

Assumption 1, operating in community A: In each cohort of 1000 new cases, 100 people annually are cured.
Assumption 2, operating in community B: In each cohort of 1000 new cases, 10 percent of those still ill at the beginning of each year are cured during the following year.
Assumption 3, operating in community C: In each cohort of 2000 new cases, 40 percent of those still ill at the beginning of each year are cured during the following year.

Although the annual incidence, that is, the number of people developing a mental disorder for the first time in each year is the same in community A and B, the prevalence rates on January 1 of each year differ considerably after the first two years. For example, on January 1, 1950, in community A, the prevalence becomes stationary at 5500 patients, a prevalence rate of 5500 per 100 000 or 5.5 percent. On the other hand, in the community B, the prevalence increased steadily to 6859 or 6.9 percent on the same date. It can be shown that this rate will stabilize at 10 000 per 100 000 or 10 percent at about the year 2007. In community C, where the annual incidence rate is 2000 per 100 000 or 2 percent, twice the rate in the previous examples, the prevalence reaches 4981 cases per 100 000 population on January 1, 1950. In this population prevalence will eventually become less than in the other two examples, stabilizing at 5000 per 100 000 or 5 percent at about the year 1956.

These examples illustrate that although the prevalence of a disease differs among communities, the inference cannot be drawn that the community with the highest prevalence also has the highest incidence. Indeed, the community with the highest incidence had the lowest prevalence. Since the prevalence rate is a function of

---

[3] A cohort is a group of persons, each of whom has some common characteristic.

Table 1. Illustration of ways three hypothetical prevalence situations develop in three different communities under various assumptions of incidence and duration of disease.

Community A. Assumptions: 1000 new cases annually, each of which occurs on January 1 of specified year; 100 patients annually are cured in each cohort of such new cases. The prevalence count will stabilize at 5500 cases on January 1, 1949.

Cohort of year	Patients in hospital on January 1 of specified year										
	1940	1941	1942	1943	1944	1945	1946	1947	1948	1949	1950
1940	1000	900	800	700	600	500	400	300	200	100	0
1941		1000	900	800	700	600	500	400	300	200	100
1942			1000	900	800	700	600	500	400	300	200
1943				1000	900	800	700	600	500	400	300
1944					1000	900	800	700	600	500	400
1945						1000	900	800	700	600	500
1946							1000	900	800	700	600
1947								1000	900	800	700
1948									1000	900	800
1949										1000	900
1950											1000
Total	1000	1900	2700	3400	4000	4500	4900	5200	5400	5500	5500

Community B. Assumptions: 1000 new cases annually, each of which occurs on January 1 of specified year; 10 percent of those ill at the beginning of each year are cured during that year. The prevalence count will stabilize at 10 000 cases on January 1, 2007.

Cohort of year	Patients in hospital on January 1 of specified year										
	1940	1941	1942	1943	1944	1945	1946	1947	1948	1949	1950
1940	1000	900	810	729	656	590	531	478	430	387	348
1941		1000	900	810	729	656	590	531	478	430	387
1942			1000	900	810	729	656	590	531	478	430
1943				1000	900	810	729	656	590	531	478
1944					1000	900	810	729	656	590	531
1945						1000	900	810	729	656	590
1946							1000	900	810	729	656
1947								1000	900	810	729
1948									1000	900	810
1949										1000	900
1950											1000
Total	1000	1900	2710	3439	4095	4685	5216	5694	6124	6511	6859

Community C. Assumptions: 2000 new cases annually, each of which occurs on January 1 of specified year; 40 percent of those ill at the beginning of each year are cured during that year. The prevalence count will stabilize at 5000 cases on January 1, 1956.

Cohort of year	Patients in hospital on January 1 of specified year.										
	1940	1941	1942	1943	1944	1945	1946	1947	1948	1949	1950
1940	2000	1200	720	432	259	155	93	56	34	20	12
1941		2000	1200	720	432	259	155	93	56	34	20
1942			2000	1200	720	432	259	155	93	56	34
1943				2000	1200	720	432	259	155	93	56
1944					2000	1200	720	432	259	155	93
1945						2000	1200	720	432	259	155
1946							2000	1200	720	432	259
1947								2000	1200	720	432
1948									2000	1200	720
1949										2000	1200
1950											2000
Total	2000	3200	3920	4352	4611	4766	4859	4915	4949	4969	4981

the annual incidence and the duration of the illness, it should be clear that interpretation of differences in prevalence between communities is dependent on knowledge of these two factors.

Not only do the above considerations explain how differences in prevalence rates for a single disease develop between communities, they also explain how differences develop among prevalence rates for several diseases within the same community. Thus, if disease A has a higher prevalence rate than disease B, the difference can be accounted for as follows: (1) higher incidence for disease A associated with longer, equal, or even shorter duration for disease A than disease B; or (2) equal incidence for disease A and B associated with longer duration of disease A than disease B; or (3) lower incidence in disease A with disproportionately longer duration for disease A than for disease B.

ILLUSTRATIONS

The above principles may be illustrated by a consideration of indexes that have been used to measure the incidence and prevalence of mental disorders requiring admission to hospitals for the prolonged care and treatment of mental disorder. An index of the incidence of these mental disorders is the first admission rate, defined as the number of persons admitted for the first time to prolonged care mental hospitals per 100 000 population. An index of prevalence of these disorders is the number of persons actually resident in the hospitals for prolonged care at the end of the year per 100 000 population. These indexes may be made specific for age, sex, etc.

Both indexes have limitations discussed fully elsewhere (4–6). To illustrate, the date of first admission to a mental hospital is not necessarily coincident with the date of initial attack of mental disorder. Indeed, as more community treatment facilities develop, as the number of psychiatrists engaged in private practice increases, and as treatment methods become available that can be used by general practitioners for maintaining persons with mental disorders in the community (such as the tranquilizing drugs), considerable time may elapse between date of onset of disease and the date it may finally be found necessary to commit an individual to a mental hospital. Also, the number of patients resident in these hospitals on any one day is not

a complete count of the number of people in a community who have a psychiatric disability. Nevertheless, there are certain types of data available on hospitalized psychotics which are not available on the nonhospitalized population. For example, the time interval elapsing between date the patient is admitted to the hospital and date the patient is returned to the community or dies in the hospital gives one measure of duration of disability associated with certain hospitalized psychiatric disorders and makes it possible to illustrate how differential duration of hospitalization produces differences between resident patient and first admission rates.

Let us now consider differences between first admission and resident patient rates for all mental disorders combined, schizophrenia, and mental diseases of the senium (cerebral arteriosclerotic and senile psychoses combined) (Figure 1).

The resident patient curve for all disorders increases continuously with age from 14.1 per 100 000 in the age group under 15 years of age to 1272 in the age group 85 years and over. The first admission curve is at a considerably lower level and has a different form. Thus, the curve rises from a low of 10 per 100 000 under 15 years of age to about 84 per 100 000 in the age group 25–34 years, stays at about a level of 90 per 100 000 in the age groups 35–44, 45–54, and 55–64 years and then makes a rapid ascent to a maximum of 467 in the age group 85 years and over. Because of the large number of disorders involved and of the variations in the age at time of admission for patients with these disorders (see, for example, reference 5, page 4), the total resident patient rate is difficult to interpret. It is instructive to examine the differences between resident patient and first admission rates for two important groups of patients, the schizophrenics and patients with mental diseases of the senium.

The first admission rate for schizophrenics rises from a low of 2 per 100 000 in the age group under 15 years to a maximum of 41 in the age group 25–34 years and declines steadily with advancing age. The resident patient rate rises steadily to a peak of 318 per 100 000 in the age group 45–54 years, decreases slowly to about 285 in the age group 65–74 years, and then to 140 in the age group 85 years and over. The high resident patient rate in the older age

Figure 1. Age-specific first admission and resident patient rates per 100 000 civilian population, state hospitals for mental disease, all mental disorders and selected mental disorders, both sexes, United States, 1952.[a]

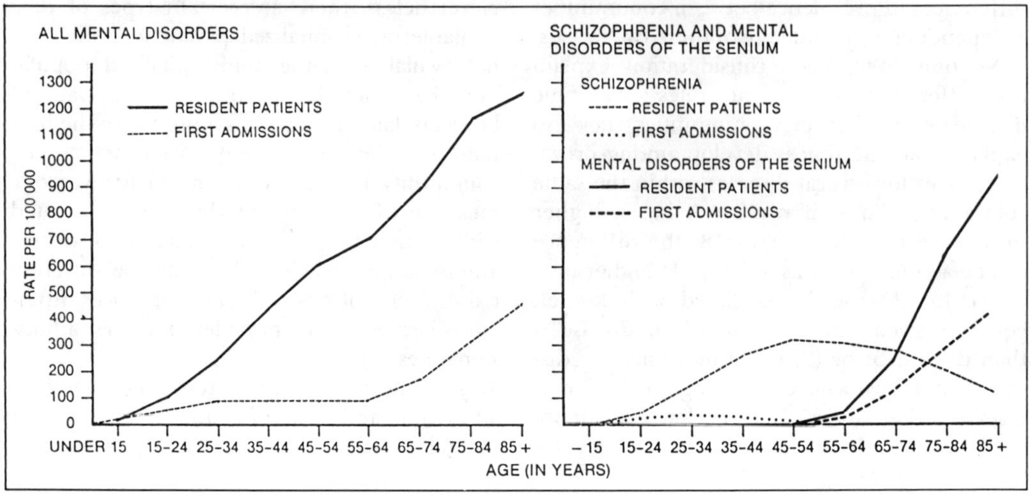

[a] Source: Patients in Mental Institutions, 1952, Part V (In preparation), National Institute of Mental Health, Public Health Service.

groups is a resultant of the accumulation of cases in the hospital. That is, the resident schizophrenics in the age groups 45 and over consist primarily of cases who have aged in the hospital rather than of new admissions in these age groups. Evidence of this fact can be obtained from Figure 2 which presents the distribution of resident schizophrenics in the New York State civil hospitals on March 31, 1955, by age and duration of hospitalization as measured by the interval between date of current admission and March 31, 1955.[4] The proportion of cases hospitalized for long periods of time increases markedly with advancing age of patient. Thus, 44 percent of the patients 15–24 were hospitalized for less than one year. This decreases to 0.4 percent for the patients 75 years of age and over. In the latter group 85 percent were hospitalized for 20 years or more.

First admission and resident rates for patients with mental disorders of the senium show a different phenomenon. Both rates rise rapidly with age. However, the high resident patient rates are accounted for primarily by the high

admission rate rather than a long duration of stay. This is apparent from Figure 2 which also presents the duration of hospitalization of resident patients with mental diseases of the senium. As will be seen later, a very high death rate following admission is responsible for short duration of stay of patients in this disease category.

It should be noted that the resident patient population is a residue population. It is a heterogeneous mixture of the residues of various cohorts of patients admitted over long periods of time—indeed from the date the hospital opened to the present day—and depleted through release and death at differential rates specific for age, sex, diagnosis, and a variety of other factors that have influenced the movement of patients during the history of the hospital.

More direct evidence on differences in duration of hospitalization and the way such differentials account for differences between distribution of diagnostic categories in first admissions and resident patients can be obtained only from studies which follow groups of first admission to determine what proportion are still in the hospital, out of the hospital, or dead within specified periods of time following admission. An example of such a study is that done on first admissions to Warren State Hospital during the period 1916–1950(5). Cohorts of patients spe-

---

[4] This interval actually represents length of time patient has been on the books of the hospital for the current admission. Although data similar to that reported by New York State are available for the patients hospitalized in 16 of the 17 Model Reporting Area States, the machine tabulations have as yet not been completed for the combined experience.

Figure 2. **Percent distribution by time on books and median time on books of patients resident in New York State Civil Hospitals for mental disease, both sexes by age and selected diagnosis, March 31, 1955.**[a]

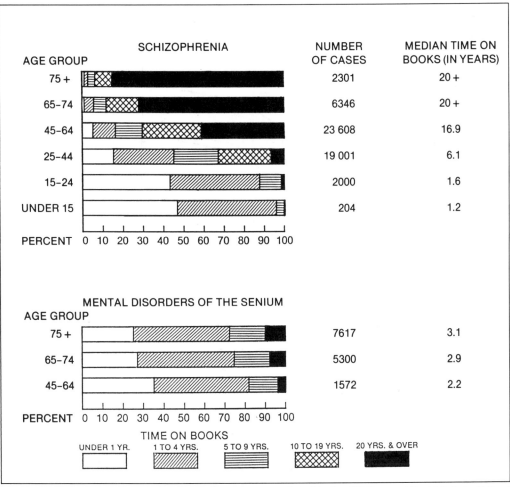

[a] Source: Unpublished data requested of model reporting area states, collected for the 1955 Census of Mental Patients, National Institute of Mental Health, Public Health Service.

cific for age, sex, and diagnosis were followed from date of admission to date of first significant release from the hospital, defined as date of first release to the community on direct discharge or convalescent care, or death in the hospital, whichever came first. An example of the retention, release, and death curves for patients admitted in the period 1936–1945 in five diagnostic categories (schizophrenia, manic depressive, involutional and syphilitic psychoses, and mental diseases of the senium) are shown in Figure 3.

The schizophrenics have the highest retention probabilities. For example, within one year following admission, 49 percent have been retained continuously in the hospital and this de-

creases to 29 percent within five years following admission. The percent of patients with mental diseases of the senium retained for one year following admission is 31 percent, decreasing to 8 percent within five years after admission. The differences in retention probabilities are a reflection of the differential rates of separation. The separation probabilities are highest for patients with manic depressive psychosis and mental diseases of the senium and lowest among the schizophrenics. However, in the manic depressive category a very high proportion of the separations are released alive and a very small proportion die in the hospital, whereas for patients with diseases of the senium the situation is reversed. Although the schizophrenics have a

Figure 3. Percent of first admissions retained in hospital, released alive and dead within specified periods following admission to Warren State Hospital, Warren, Pennsylvania, 1936–1945. Selected diagnoses, all ages, both sexes.

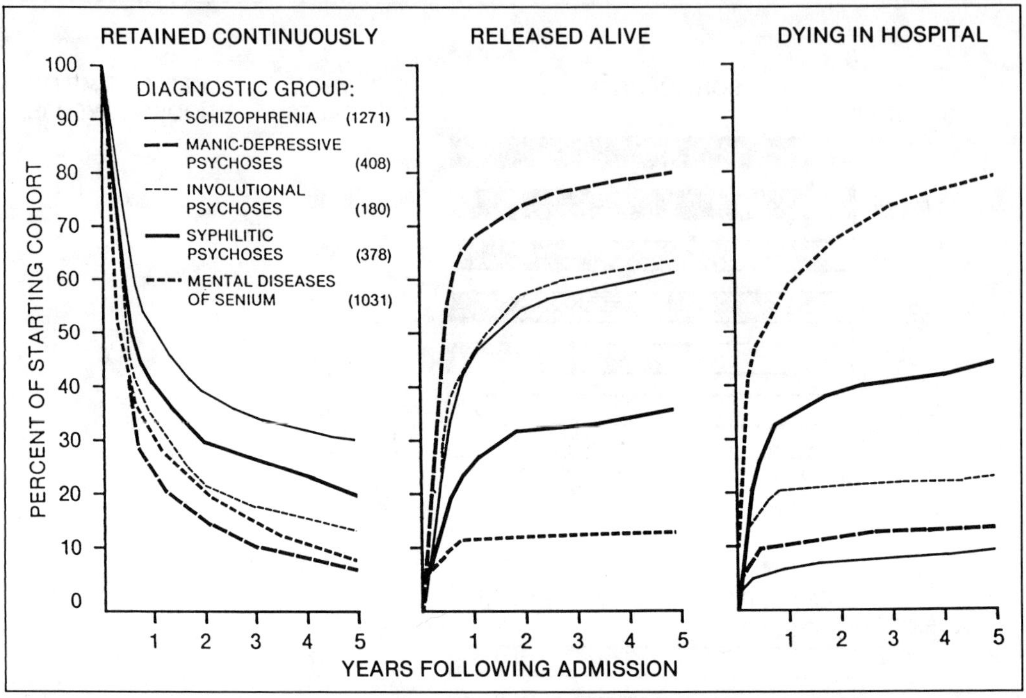

relatively high release rate, with 45 percent released within one year following admission and 61 percent released within five years, their total separation rate is lowest because of the relatively low death rate.

If we compare the percentage distribution of diagnoses at time of admission among the first admissions in the five diagnostic categories shown in Figure 3 with the corresponding distribution for those retained continuously for five years we find some striking differences. The schizophrenics constitute 39 percent of this group at time of admission and 65 percent of those hospitalized continuously for the five years, while for the mental diseases of the senium the corresponding percentages are 31 and 14 percent, respectively.

Similar differences can be shown by considering the fate of patients in relation to age at first admission. The youngest patients have the highest release rates and lowest death rates and the oldest the lowest release rates and the highest death rates (Figure 4). Variations in release and death rates by age and diagnosis are rather interesting but will not be dwelled upon here (6).

The preceding is only a partial explanation of the ways these differences occur in the composition of first admission and resident patient populations, since, following release to the community, some patients will be readmitted. Indeed, the composition of a mental hospital population is a resultant of medical, social, environmental, economic, and administrative factors which have produced current and past rates of first admission, current and past rates at which patients are released to the community or die in the hospital, and current and past rates at which patients are readmitted to the hospital. Knowledge of these rates over the years is necessary for a complete understanding of the population dynamics of these hospitals.

Time trends in the incidence and prevalence of a disease may also be affected by prevention and control programs. A major objective of the public health movement is to prevent the occurrence of disease, if possible, and to develop treatment procedures to shorten the course of a disease, or to lengthen the course by prolonging life. The effect of such programs is illustrated by considering changes in the first admission and resident patient rates for syphilitic

Figure 4. Percent of first admissions retained in hospital, released alive and dead within specified periods following admission to Warren State Hospital, Warren, Pennsylvania, 1936-1945. All mental disorders, selected admission ages, both sexes.

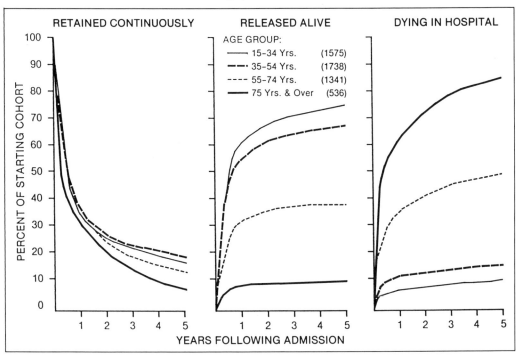

psychotics in the state hospitals of the nation in the period from 1939 to 1952 (Table 2). There has been a slight increase in the total resident patient rate during a period when the total first admission rate has decreased by 73 percent. The decrease in first admission rates has resulted in a decreased resident patient rate only in the age groups under 45 years. This has been counterbalanced by an increased accumulation of patients at the older ages, particularly 65 and over, a result of specific treatment programs which have reduced the high fatality rates once associated with this disorder.

Further evidence is obtained from the Warren State study which shows a striking change in the chances of release and death of syphilitic psychotics first admitted during the period 1916–1950 (Figure 5). There has been a consistent increase over the years in the proportion of patients retained in the hospital. This has resulted from a marked decrease in the proportion of patients dying without corresponding increases in the proportion of patients released. If the 1916–1925 cohort is compared with the

1946–1950 cohort within one year after admission, the percentage of patients released has increased from 14 percent to 39 percent and the percentage of patients dying has dropped from 56 percent to 18 percent. This has resulted in increasing the percentage of patients retained from 30 percent to 43 percent.

DISCUSSION

The preceding examples were presented to emphasize the differences between two commonly used morbidity indexes and to demonstrate that the principles that describe the dynamics of other illnesses in population groups also apply to the mental disorders. Since prevalence is a function of incidence and duration of disease, comparison of prevalence rates between various population groups, social classes, age, race, and sex groups cannot be interpreted until we know the role of the basic variables—incidence and duration—in producing a given prevalence situation.

Table 2. Age-specific first admission rates and resident patient rates for syphilitic psychoses, United States, 1939 and 1952.

	First Admission			Resident Patient		
Age	1939	1952	Percent change	1939	1952	Percent change
Total (15 years and over)			Rates per 100 000 population[a]			
Crude	8.0	2.1	− 73.8	25.9	26.0	+ 0.4
Age Adjusted[b]	8.6	2.3	− 73.3	28.0	28.7	+ 2.5
15–24	1.0	0.4	− 60.0	2.2	1.8	− 18.2
25–34	6.7	0.8	− 88.1	14.2	5.4	− 62.0
35–44	14.1	2.7	− 80.9	41.2	25.4	− 38.3
45–54	13.1	4.4	− 66.4	51.2	64.1	+ 25.2
55–64	11.0	4.1	− 62.7	45.3	57.6	+ 27.2
65 and over	4.7	2.5	− 46.8	18.7	37.1	+ 98.4
			Number of patients			
Total (15 years and over)	7781	2532	− 67.5	25 276	31 484	+ 24.6
15–24	231	71	− 69.3	533	346	− 35.1
25–34	1409	183	− 87.0	3013	1259	− 58.2
35–44	2567	594	− 76.9	7485	5573	− 25.5
45–54	2010	786	− 60.9	7857	11 492	+ 46.3
55–64	1150	568	− 50.6	4753	7997	+ 68.3
65 and over	414	330	− 20.3	1635	4817	+ 194.6

[a] Rates per 100 000 population as of July 1939 from series P45, No. 5 and 1952 from series P25, No. 121, Current Population Reports, Population Estimates, Bureau of the Census, U. S. Department of Commerce, Washington, D. C.
[b] Adjusted to age distribution of population of the United States as of July 1, 1952. Series P25 No. 121.

Figure 5. **Percent of first admissions retained in hospital, released alive and dead within specified periods following admission to Warren State Hospital, Warren, Pennsylvania, 1916-1950. Syphilitic psychoses, all ages, both sexes.**

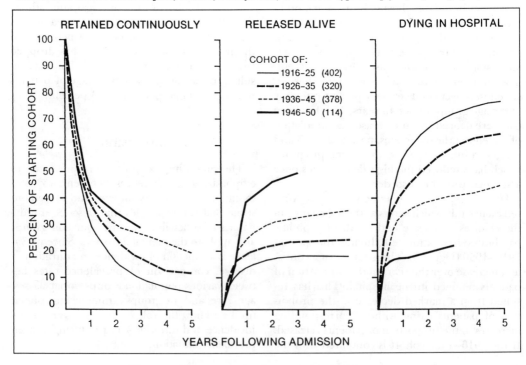

I do not wish to leave the impression that the prevalence rate is not a useful index. As Sartwell and Merrell (*3*) have said: "The kind of morbidity index which is chosen in studying a disease will depend upon the kind of information desired; thus, the medical care administrator will at times simply be interested in the prevalence of severe cases of a disease in order to estimate the number of beds needed, or the health officer may wish to know what population group will yield the most cases if a screening test is applied. The epidemiologist, however, is constantly seeking as complete a picture as possible of the distribution and course of the disease in specific segments of the population in order to arrive at an understanding of its etiology, pathogenesis, and control."

The purpose of epidemiologic investigations of the mental disorders is to discover associations that may lead to the determination of factors—biologic, psychologic, familial, socioenvironmental—that cause these disorders, and which are responsible for the disability they produce. These associations are determined by studies of the rate at which disease develops in various population groups and in various segments of these populations, and the differential duration of disease and mortality in affected individuals. The proof of etiologic relationships must then be sought through more extensive clinical or experimental investigations.

If we are to learn more about the role played by socioenvironmental variables in the production of mental disorder then we must extend our knowledge of the incidence of these disorders in various population groups. Similarly, if we are to understand the influence of these variables on the course of specific mental disorders, then we must also study variations in remission, relapse, and mortality rates. Studies of prevalence alone leave these basic questions unanswered.

These points may be illustrated by a consideration of two studies of mental disorders carried out in recent years which have investigated the relationship between social stratification, culture, and mental disorders in which the morbidity indexes have been determined from prevalence type data. The first of these projects is a study of social structure and psychiatric disorders carried out in New Haven, Connecticut, by Hollingshead, Redlich, and associates (*7, 8*), and the second, a study of mental disorders in the Hutterite population of the United States and Canada by Eaton and Weil (*9*).

The New Haven project was designed "to discover whether a relationship does or does not exist between the class system of our society and mental illnesses." Five hypotheses were being tested of which the first two are pertinent for this discussion: (1) "the prevalence of treated psychiatric disorders is related significantly to an individual's position in the class structure of his society"; (2) "the types of psychiatric disorders are connected significantly to an individual's position in the status structure."

The basic data used to test these hypotheses were derived from a psychiatric census in the New Haven area. There were 1963 persons found to be under treatment on December 1, 1950: 66.8 percent were in a state hospital; 4.2 percent in a VA [Veteran's Administration] hospital; 1.9 percent in a private hospital; 8.1 percent under treatment in a clinic; and 19.0 percent under care of private psychiatrists. The persons in the census were further subclassified into five social classes on the basis of residence, occupation, and education. Class I consists of individuals in the highest socioeconomic position and Class V in the lowest. Comparison of the distribution of persons under psychiatric treatment by social class with a similar distribution for a sample of the "normal" population demonstrated a strong inverse relationship between social class and the prevalence of treated mental disorders. There were striking differences between the proportion under various types of treatment. To use the extremes, in Classes I and II combined, 63 percent were under care of private psychiatrists and 14 percent in a state hospital, whereas in Class V the corresponding percentages were 3 and 85, respectively. The differences were statistically significant.

A point to be kept in mind in interpreting indexes of the type used in this study is that the proportion of the population with a particular type of mental disorder who are under a specified type of treatment on any one day is a function of the rate at which affected individuals come under the type of treatment and the length of time the affected individuals stay under such treatment. Our previous data on differences between diagnostic composition of first admissions to mental hospitals and resident patients may be used to illustrate this point. Although the first admission rate (i.e., the rate of coming under hospital treatment) for one disorder is high, if the separation rate is also high (i.e., average duration stay in the hospital is short), patients with this disorder may constitute a relatively small proportion of the population under treatment on any one day. On the other hand, a disorder with a relatively low admission rate may constitute a high proportion of patients under treatment because of a relatively long duration of stay. Thus, the fact that an inverse relationship exists between social class and prevalence of treated mental disorder does not mean necessarily that a similar relationship exists between the rate at which people enter into treatment and social class. Nor does it mean necessarily that a similar relationship exists between social class and the rate at which the mental disorder develops (incidence). The number of people with a particular mental disorder who are under a specific type of treatment on a given day is a resultant not only of the incidence of that disorder but also of the availability of various types of psychiatric treatment facilities and a series of medical, social, economic, environmental, personal, familial, educational, legal, and administrative factors which determine who receive treatment in the various facilities and how long they stay under such treatment. Thus, much additional research is needed to determine how much of the observed difference in prevalence of treated mental disorder between various classes of the population is due to differences in (a) incidence (the rate at which the disorder occurs), (b) the rate at which individuals come under treatment, and (c) how long they stay under the care of these treatment facilities.

The Hutterite study investigated the occurrence of mental disorders in a religious sect residing largely in North Dakota, Montana, and Manitoba. This group was reputed to be one in which mental illness was practically nonexistent. A team consisting of social scientists and a psychiatrist surveyed a large number of Hutterite villages to secure data on all known cases of mental disorder and to examine persons reported as possible cases of mental disorder. This study failed to substantiate the impression that Hutterites were almost free of severe mental illness. The morbidity index used in the analysis of the data was one termed the lifetime prevalence rate, defined as the ratio of all active

and recovered cases of mental disorders alive at the end of the enumeration period to the total population. Thus, in a population of 8542 Hutterites, enumerated as of August 31, 1951, 199 persons (23.3 per 1000 population) were found to have been affected by a mental disorder at some time during their lifetime, and were still living on the stated date. Of the cases found, 53 were cases of psychosis, yielding a lifetime prevalence rate of 6.2 per 1000 for these disorders. These rates are also presented specific for age, sex, and type of mental disorder.

In effect, this index is a determination of the proportion of a population alive on a given date who have a history of an attack of mental disorder. It should be apparent that this index is an inappropriate one to use if the focus of the research is to determine the influence of culture on the rate at which mental disorder occurs. The proportion of a population surviving to a given date with a history of a disease is a function of the incidence rate, the mortality of persons who have ever had the disease and the mortality of the nonaffected population. The fact that lifetime prevalence would differ between two or more cultural groups does not mean that incidence differs. Indeed, incidence may be equal while the duration of life following attack by the illness differs. For example, there may be two primitive cultures A and B with an equal rate of incidence of mental disorder. Culture A's attitude toward the mentally ill is a protective one and everything possible is done to prolong their lives, whereas culture B's attitude is just the opposite. Thus, in A the interval between onset of illness and death would be considerably longer than in B and as a result lifetime prevalence in A would be higher than in B.

Mortality is a factor that can not be overlooked in epidemiologic studies of mental disorder. Although little is known about mortality in psychiatric patients who have never been hospitalized, or in those who have been released from a hospital, it is known that mortality rates experienced by mental hospital patients exceed greatly mortality rates of persons of comparable age and sex in the general population (*10*). There have also been striking time trends in mortality among patients who were under 65 years of age at time of admission. To illustrate, consider the changes in mortality experienced by patients admitted to Warren State Hospital in the period 1916–1950 (Figure 6). Among patients in this age group first admitted in 1916–1925, 17 percent died in the hospital within one year following admissions and 23 percent within three years. Among patients admitted in the period 1946–1950, the corresponding percentages dropped to 6 percent and 8 percent, respectively. The above data apply to the experience of these patients during first admission status.

To obtain their complete mortality experience, i.e., to determine what proportion of the first admissions were dead within, say, three years following first admission including patients who died in the hospital and those who died in the community following release, the deaths among the patients released would also have to be determined and added to those who died in the hospital. Making a conservative estimate of the number of such deaths and adding these to the number who died in the hospital, we can state that of 100 first admissions under 65 years of age in the period 1916–1925 approximately 63 percent would still be living three years after hospitalization and 27 percent

would be dead. Among 100 first admissions in the period 1946–1950, 90 percent would still be living three years after first admission and 10 percent dead.

As can be seen from Figure 7, the mortality following admission for the patients 65 years and over is much more severe, with about 50 percent dead within one year following admission and at least 60 percent dead within three years. There has been little change in this picture over the years.

Thus, it should be clear that data on trends of survivorship as well as of incidence rates are needed in order to explain variations in lifetime prevalence rates of mental disorders between population groups.

CONCLUSION

Our knowledge of the epidemiology of mental disorders must be extended beyond that gathered through studies of mental hospital populations and the studies of either treated or true prevalence (i.e., treated plus untreated cases) of mental disorders. To accomplish this,

Figure 6. Percent of first admissions retained in hospital, released alive and dead within specified periods following admission to Warren State Hospital, Warren, Pennsylvania, 1916-1950. All mental disorders, under 65 years, both sexes.

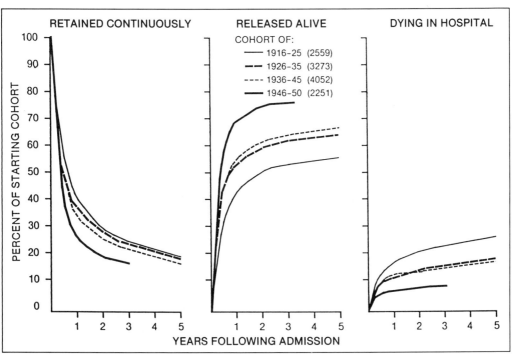

Figure 7. Percent of first admissions retained in hospital, released alive and dead within specified periods following admission to Warren State Hospital, Warren, Pennsylvania, 1916-1950. All mental disorders, 65 years and over, both sexes.

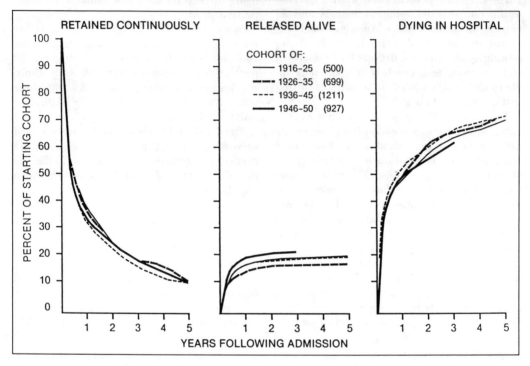

it is essential that several basic issues be resolved so that comparable data can be gathered in different population groups. The first is to obtain agreement on what constitutes a case of a specified type of mental disorder. The second is the development of standardized case-finding methods for detecting cases in the general population, and standardized methods for their classification. The third is to devise methods for measuring duration of illness, that is, the interval between onset of disease and periods of remission, and for characterizing the psychologic status, the degree of psychiatric disability, social and familial adjustment, and physical condition at various intervals following onset of disease. The fourth is to evaluate the effect of treatment on such indexes. It is to solve these major research problems that the epidemiologist and statistician need the help of the psychiatrist, psychologist, and social scientist.

Armed with the tools derived from such research it will be possible then to determine the differential rates at which the members of various population groups develop specific mental

disorders, pass through various stages of disability, achieve various stages of recovery or die. It is only through such studies that we will advance our knowledge of the incidence, duration, and prevalence of mental disorders.

References

(1) Dorn, H. Methods of measuring incidence and prevalence of disease. *Am J Public Health* 41:271–278, 1951.

(2) Doull, J.A., R.S. Guinto, et al. The incidence of leprosy in Cordova and Talisay, Cebu, P.I. *Int J Lepr* Vol. 10, 1942.

(3) Sartwell, P.E., and M. Merrell. Influence of the dynamic character of chronic disease on the interpretation of morbidity rates. *Am J Public Health* 45:579–584, 1952.

(4) Proceedings of the Conferences of Mental Hospital Administrators and Statisticians: (1) First Conference, February, 1951, PHS Pub. No. 295, 1952; (2) Second Conference, February, 1952, PHS Pub. No. 266, 1953; (3) Third Conference, April, 1953, PHS Pub. No. 348, 1954. Washington, D.C., Government Printing Office.

(5) Kramer, M., H. Goldstein, R.H. Israel, and N.A. Johnston. *Disposition of First Admissions to a State*

Mental Hospital: Experience of the Warren State Hospital During the Period 1916–1950. Pub. Health Monograph No. 32., Washington, D.C., Government Printing Office, 1955.

(6) Kramer, M., H. Goldstein, R.H. Israel, and N.A. Johnston. *Application of Life Table Methodology to the Study of Mental Hospital Populations.* Psychiatric Research Rep. No. 5, American Psychiatric Association, 1956, pp. 49–76.

(7) Hollingshead, A.B., and F.C. Redlich. Social stratification and psychiatric disorders. *Am Sociol Rev.* 18:163–169, 1953.

(8) Redlich, F.C., A.B. Hollingshead, et al. Social structure and psychiatric disorders. *Am J Psychiatry* 109:729–733, 1953.

(9) Eaton, J.W., and R.J. Weil. *Culture and Mental Disorders,* Glencoe, Illinois, Free Press, 1955.

(10) Malzberg, B. *Mortality Among Patients With Mental Disease,* Utica, N.Y., State Hospitals Press, 1934.

NUTRITION, GROWTH, AND NEUROINTEGRATIVE DEVELOPMENT: AN EXPERIMENTAL AND ECOLOGIC STUDY[1]

Joaquin Cravioto,[2] Elsa R. DeLicardie,[2] and Herbert G. Birch[3]

INTRODUCTION

This monograph is dedicated to the memory of R. A. F. Dean whose indomitable spirit did not permit severe ill health to interfere with his study of malnutrition and its importance for the production of handicap in children.

In this monograph we report the results of an experimental and ecologic study concerned with estimating some of the effects which malnutrition in early childhood may have upon neurointegrative functioning. In particular, we have been concerned with the association between malnutrition early in childhood and intersensory organization in children during the school years. A study of these relationships has derived from a concern with the possibility that inadequate food intake, particularly as represented by protein-calorie malnutrition, affects not only stature and weight, but also the capacity to learn. If this is indeed the case, then the significance of the observable and dramatic consequences of malnutrition for physical stature may be but one visible sign of functionally, perhaps, far more important non-visible handicapping. . . .

THE PRESENT STUDY

General Features

An exploration of the effects of early malnutrition on the development of neurointegrative functioning in school children can of course be carried out definitively only by means of a prospective longitudinal study of children at risk and of appropriately selected control subjects. We are currently engaged in conducting such an investigation. However, since the findings of a prospective longitudinal study become available only after a long period of delay, it was decided that a certain amount of pertinent information could be obtained through a carefully conducted cross-sectional retrospective study of neurointegrative organization in children of school age. The present monograph is the result of such an investigation.

To explore the effects of malnutrition on neurointegrative development it was decided to carry out a cross-sectional study of intersensory functioning in the total population of primary school children in a village in which detailed prior information indicated the presence of a significant prevalence level of serious acute or prolonged malnutrition during infancy and the preschool years. For purposes of the investigation malnutrition was defined retrospectively on the basis of height for age in all children ranging in age from 6 to 11 years. When the child showed a significant diminution of stature with respect to his age mates in the total village population of children, he was assumed to have an increased likelihood of having been at earlier risk of malnutrition. On this basis, at each age level, a group of children representing the lowest 25 percent of the height distribution was identified and designated as the group having the greatest likelihood of having been at earlier nutritional risk. The functioning of this group was compared with that of the children in the village who were in the tallest quartile for age and so, assuming all other factors to be equal, representing those with the least likelihood of

Source: *Pediatrics* 38(2):319, 334-359, 368-372, 1966.
[1] This work was supported in part by grants from the Association for the Aid of Crippled Children, New York, New York, the Nutrition Foundation, Inc., the Milbank Memorial Fund, and the William Waterman Fund for the Combat of Dietary Diseases. The collection of the material on intersensory functioning was done during the time Joaquin Cravioto, M.D., was officially commissioned by the Pan American Health Organization, Regional Office of the World Health Organization (WHO) as Associate Director of the Institute of Nutrition of Central America and Panama (INCAP).
[2] Group for Research on the Relationship Between Nutrition and Mental Development, Department of Nutrition II, Hospital Infantil de México, México City.
[3] Department of Pediatrics, Center for Study of Normal and Aberrant Behavioral Development NICHD (HD-00719), Albert Einstein College of Medicine, Yeshiva University, New York, New York.

having experienced a significant degree of malnutrition earlier in life. In this way groups of children with common ethnic background were identified and represented the upper and lower quartiles by height of individuals in the age groups studied.

Clearly, at least three important variables must be controlled for when height for age is being used as an index of prior nutritional risk. The first relates to parental stature and thus to familial factors affecting height. Since height at school age may reflect not only the individual's nutritional background but also his parental endowment it was necessary in designing the study to obtain anthropometric information on parents as well as on children in order to control for this variable.

A second consideration is that low stature during the years studied may represent a general maturational lag in the course of which both height and intersensory functioning may both be subnormal. To control for this possibility it was necessary to study a second sample of children of the same ages who exhibited equivalent differences in height but who had little or no likelihood of ever having been at nutritional risk.

Finally, since no integrative capacity is unaffected by environmental influences, comparative information on the social, economic, and educational status of the families from which the children derived had to be obtained. Details of the procedures used for obtaining background data on the children studied will be presented at a later point.

The indicator of neurointegrative development selected for study was intersensory organization. This was done for two reasons. In the first place a considerable body of evidence both in comparative psychology (1, 2) and evolutionary physiology (3) has accumulated which suggests that the emergence of complex adaptive capacities is underlain by the growth of increasing liaison and interdependence among the separate sense systems. Sherrington (4) in considering this process has gone so far as to argue, "The naive would have expected evolution in its course to have supplied us with more various sense organs for ampler perception of the world. . . . The policy has rather been to bring by the nervous system the so-called 'five' into closer touch with one another. . . . A central clearing house of sense has grown up. . . . Not

new senses, but better liaison between old senses is what the developing nervous system has in this respect stood for." In addition, a variety of studies (5, 6) indicate that the basic mechanism involved in primary learning (i.e., the formation of conditioned reflexes) is probably the effective establishment and patterning of intersensory organization.

The second reason for using intersensory competence as an indicator of neurointegrative development stems from the fact that Birch and Lefford (7) have shown that adequacy of intersensory interrelations improves as a clearly defined growth function in normal children between the ages of 6 to 12 years. In school children, comparable in age with the ones we were planning to study, they found that the interrelations among three sense systems— touch, vision, and kinesthesis—improved in an age-specific manner, and resulted in developmental curves that were as regular as those for skeletal growth.

Design of the Study

The design of the study was based upon the view that it was feasible to conduct a comparative study of neurointegrative functioning in school age children in whom extremes of difference in height at school ages were to be used as an index of preschool nutritional adequacy. Since height as such may with equal readiness be an indicator of maturation or constitution as of antecedent malnutrition, height as such had to be controlled for by studying a comparison sample of children who differed in stature but among whom it was most improbable that the shortest children had been subjected to nutritional stress. It was therefore decided to replicate the rural study on an upper-class urban sample of school children[4] who were most unlikely to have been at nutritional risk and whose variations in height would be unrelated to either primary or secondary malnutrition. The rural community study was ecologic in its organization and sought to relate growth achievements as well as intersensory development to the social, economic, educational, and physical characteristics of the families from which the children derived. In this connection the find-

---

[4] Thanks are expressed to the administration of the American School in Guatemala for their cooperation in permitting us to study their pupils.

ings obtained through studying the urban group could be treated not only with respect to the problem of stature but also as a device for teasing out the relations between growth and function in a socially differentiated rural group by comparing it with a socially and economically homogeneous urban group in which height differences existed but could not be related to conditions of nutrition, health, or social standing.

METHOD AND PROCEDURE

Description of the Rural Village

General Aspects of the Community

All the rural, school age children lived in the village of Magdalena, M. A. This community, inhabited by people who belong to the Cakchiquel linguistic group, is located in the Department of Sacatepéquez in the central zone of the Republic of Guatemala, C. A. It lies at an altitude of 6780 feet above sea level and is 22 miles from the capital city. The climate is characterized by two well-defined seasons, one dry and one with heavy rains, which are popularly referred to as "summer" and "winter."

The population was composed of 333 families making up a total of 1620 persons, 323 of whom were below 5 years of age. Eighty-one and six tenths percent of the population were self-identified as Indian.

The crude mortality rate was 43 per thousand during the period 1901 to 1905 and has diminished progressively reaching the figure of 15.3 in 1958-1962. The infant mortality rate (deaths in infants less than 1 year old per 1000 live births) has remained generally unchanged, although with marked annual variations, for more than 50 years. The corresponding figures for the period 1906 to 1910, and 1961-1962 were, respectively, 121 and 138. During the years 1948 to 1962 the number of deaths in the age group 6 to 12 accounted for 2.8 percent of the total deaths. Diarrhea was the main registered cause of death, followed by measles, "worms," and "dropsy" (*8*). The birth rate has been stationary around 44 births per thousand during the past 15 years.

Production and Commerce

The villagers are small farmers whose main crops are corn and beans, some greens such as

lettuce and cabbages, and vegetables including carrots and green peppers grown in small family gardens. Flowers are cultivated for commercial purposes in separate plots. There is commercial interchange between the village and the capital city, as well as with the City of Antigua, the main town in the Department.

Pattern of Food Consumption

The analysis of three dietary surveys conducted during May, June, and November of 1963 and a comparison with the data obtained for the same village in 1950 by Flores and Reh (*9*) revealed a small increase in the consumption of milk derivatives, greens, bananas, grains, roots and fats, and a reduction in the intake of corn and fruits. Nevertheless, the present diet continues to be protein poor and is not significantly more adequate than that consumed 13 years ago. Table 1 is illustrative both of the poor nutritional quality of the current diet and of this lack of improvement (*10*).

Table 1. Calorie contribution of the protein, fats, and carbohydrates consumed in Magdalena, M.A., 1950 and 1963.

Source	Percentages contributed to the total calorie value of the diet period studied			
	May 1950	May 1963	June 1963	Nov. 1963
Protein	12	12	12	12
Fats	8	11	10	10
Carbohydrates	80	77	78	78

Migration

Approximately 10 percent of the families make an annual transient emigration to the coastal region at the time of the coffee harvest. During a period of one to four weeks the whole family leaves the village. Actual emigration, that is leaving the village permanently, is so rare that it can be confidently stated that for practical purposes there is no emigration. The same is substantially the case for immigration.

Transportation

Buses to and from the capital city are available daily, and twice a week a bus runs to and from Antigua, the administrative and political head of the Department of Sacatepéquez.

Height Measurements

The standing height of all the children aged 6 to 11 was measured by two pediatricians previously trained in standardized procedures and compared one against the other through a series of exercises until they achieved replicate measurements varying by no more than 0.4 cm (*11*). All measurements were made by means of a firm wall board with a simple counterweight attached to the head block. The child was helped to stand erect with heels, buttocks, and shoulders tangentially against the wall board. The position of the child with the heels together, and feet at an angle of 45° to each other was assured by drawing the shape of them on the base of the apparatus and positioning each child to these drawings. Parents' heights were measured in the same way.

All the measurements were then arranged in decreasing order of magnitude. Quartiles were calculated for each age and sex. All the children who fell in the upper and lower height quartiles were selected to be tested for intersensory development. The number, age, and sex of children included in the rural sample are shown in Table 2.

Table 2. Age and sex distribution of the rural children studied.

Age	Boys	Girls	Total
6	6	13	19
7	21	10	31
8	11	9	20
9	16	11	27
10	16	9	25
11	9	12	21
Total	79	64	143

Child's Social and Economic Environment

A picture of the child's social, cultural, familial, and economic background was obtained by means of individual interviews of parents, observation of practices, detailed evaluations of housing and sanitary conditions, conducting a census, and through parallel anthropologic studies. . . . The general areas evaluated included the following:

(a) The family—a list of the persons making up the home and the family, civil status, age, the degree of relation with the child, their self-identification as to ethnic group, the languages spoken in and outside the home with adults and children.

(b) Factors that may influence health—such as house sanitation, personal hygiene, presence of poisonous animals and vectors of disease, crowding of adults and children, and presence of domestic animals in the home without separation from the persons.

(c) Educational background—literacy and schooling of the parents and use of such communications media as books, radio, and newspapers.

(d) Occupations and leisure time practices—sources of income for each member of the household, contribution to the home budget; the family budget for food and other purposes; the use of free time; the organizations to which they belonged; and the attachment to religious organizations and practices were determined.

(e) Availability of food in the family—the actual food produced by the family, the technique of production, the disposition of food produced, percent of produce sold, used for animal feed, left for seed, wasted because of inadequate storage; the types and amounts of food purchased were assessed.

To provide background data three dietary surveys were conducted in a sample of 57 family households, with the main objective of assessing the food consumption pattern and the adequacy of the diets in comparison to figures available for practices 13 years before.

The Urban Children

The comparison group of school age children were all students at a private school whose pupils were drawn from upper middle class and upper class families. Family income was uniformly high and educational background of the parents in all cases was beyond the secondary school level. Numbers, age, and sex of the urban children are presented in Table 3.

Procedure for Testing Intersensory Organization

The method used for studying intersensory integration was that developed and described by Birch and Lefford (*7*). Equivalence relationships among the visual, haptic, and kinesthetic sense modalities were explored for geometric form recognition. The term "haptic" is used

Table 3. Age and sex distribution of the upper social class urban children studied.

Age	Boys	Girls	Total
6	10	10	20
7	15	5	20
8	9	11	20
9	10	10	20
10	9	11	20
11	10	10	20
Total	63	57	120

here for the complex sensory input obtained by active manual exploration of a test object. Such exploration involves tactile, kinesthetic, and surface movement sensations from the subjects' fingers and hand, such as are obtained in manipulating an object. The kinesthetic sense, in this study, refers to the sensory inputs obtained through passive arm movement. In the current investigation such a motion entailed sensory input from the wrist, elbow, and shoulder joints and from the arm and shoulder musculature as its principal components.

To study intersensory equivalence in the perception of geometric forms, a paired comparison technique was utilized. A form presented to one sensory system (standard) was compared with forms presented in another sensory system (variable). Thus, a visually presented standard was compared with a series of forms presented haptically or kinesthetically. Similarly, a haptically presented standard was compared with a kinesthetically presented series. On the basis of such examination the existence of cross-modality equivalences and nonequivalences between the visual and haptic sensory systems, between the visual and the kinesthetic sensory systems, and between the haptic and kinesthetic sensory systems could be determined.

Eight blocks, selected from the Seguin Form Board, were used as the test stimuli. The forms used were the triangle, hexagon, square, hemicircle, cross, diamond, star, and circle. These forms are presented in Figure 1. The same blocks were used as the visual and haptic stimuli. As a visual stimulus the block was placed on the table directly in front of the subject. For haptic stimulation, the subject's hand, positioned behind an opaque screen, was placed on a block by the experimenter. The subject then

actively explored the form with his hand outside his field of vision. Kinesthetic information was provided by placing the subject's preferred arm behind a screen and, with the arm out of sight, passively moving it through a path describing the geometric form. This was accomplished by placing a stylus held in normal writing position in the subject's hand. The examiner gripped the stylus above the point at which it was held by the subject and then moved the stylus and hand through the path of a track describing the geometric form inscribed in a linoleum block. The track forms were made from 4 in. by 5 in. linoleum blocks in which the patterns were inscribed to a depth of ⅛ in., forming a track through which the stylus could be moved. The outline dimensions of the track were of the same size and shape as those of the various blocks used for visual and haptic stimulation.

For all sensory modalities the forms were always presented so that the long axes were paral-

Figure 1. Geometric forms used for testing intersensory integration.

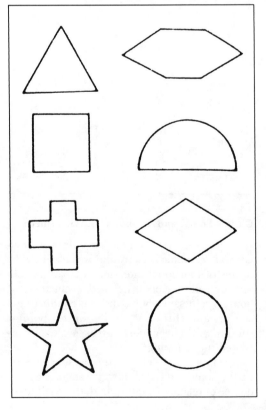

lel to the frontal plane of the subject. In a kinesthetic trial the movement was always started at the topmost point of the figure and continued in a clockwise direction for the right hand and in a counter-clockwise direction for the left hand. In putting the subject's hand through the motion, a short pause (approximately a second) was made at each point of the course where there was a change of direction. For each kinesthetic trial the subject's hand was put through only one complete circuit from topmost point to topmost point.

Three cross-modality interactions were explored for intersensory equivalences: visual and haptic interaction, visual and kinesthetic interaction, and haptic and kinesthetic interaction. Paired stimuli were presented for comparison, the first member of the pair to one sense modality and the second member of the pair to the other sense modality. In a given series of presentations the first member of the pair was held constant as a standard against which varying second members were compared successively. At the end of a complete series of trials a new standard stimulus was introduced against which the various forms presented to the other modality were compared. This procedure was repeated until the subject was examined with each of the eight forms serving as standard.

The order of presentation is given in Table 4. In this table the column headings represent either visual or haptic presentations of the standard stimuli. The stimuli listed in the columns represent successive forms which the subjects were asked to match with the standard. When the modality represented in the column heading was vision, the modality used in the comparisons was either haptic or kinesthetic. When the modality represented in the column heading was haptic, the modality used in the comparisons was kinesthetic. Thus for column 1, a visually presented triangle would be successively matched with a haptically presented square, circle, diamond, etc. When the paired comparisons represented by the first column were completed, the pairs represented by the second column were given, and so on. The second members (variable stimuli) of the pairs are in prearranged random order from column to column. The form representing the standard stimulus was represented twice among the variable stimuli. The described order of presentation was followed for visual-haptic comparisons, visual-kinesthetic comparisons, and haptic-kinesthetic comparisons.

The combination of these various factors resulted in three sets of comparative judging tasks. They were presented to the child in the following order: visual-kinesthetic series, visual-haptic series, and haptic-kinesthetic series. All subjects were tested individually in a quiet room alone with the examiner. In order to familiarize the subject with the forms, before beginning the judgments, he was given the Seguin Form Board Test. The form board was presented with the cross in the upper left-hand corner as seen from the subject's position. With the subject watching, the 10 pieces were stacked in three piles at the head of the board in a standard manner. The subject was instructed to put the blocks back into the right place. This task in effect represented a visual-visual comparison series; the form of the block and the form of the depression on the Seguin Board were visually matched by the subject. Number and kind of errors made were noted by the examiner. No time score was obtained.

Following this preliminary test, a screen was placed on the table, and the following explanation was given: "In this next game, I am going to show you a form like this circle. Then I am going to move your hand around like this." The procedure was demonstrated by moving the arm through a triangle, square, and circle. "You are to tell me if the shape your hand moves around is the same as the shape that you see in front of you. To make the game more interest-

Table 4. Order of presentation of standard and variable stimuli for testing intersensory functioning.

		Standard stimuli[a]						
		TRI	HEX	SQU	H-C	CRO	DIA	STA	CIR
		sq	st	st	cr	hx	di	tr	cr
		ci	hx	tr	hc	di	cr	di	ci
		di	cr	sq	tr	cr	hc	hc	hc
		st	hx	di	ci	tr	ci	sq	hx
Variable	stimuli	tr	ci	hx	hc	sq	hx	st	st
		hc	sq	hc	st	ci	di	hx	ci
		hx	di	sq	di	cr	tr	cr	sq
		tr	hc	ci	sq	st	sq	st	tr
		cr	tr	cr	hx	hc	st	ci	di

[a] TRI = tr = triangle; HEX = hx = Hexagon; SQU = sq = square; H-C = hc = hemicircle; CRO = cr = cross; DIA = di = diamond; STA = st = star; CIR = cr = circle.

ing, I am not going to let you see which shape your hand is going to go around. I will hold your hand behind this screen. You are not to look. We will do it like this."

The task was then demonstrated with hand behind the screen using a circle as the visual standard test object and the square, triangle and circle as kinesthetic test objects.

When the examiner was sure that the subject had understood the nature of the task, the visual-kinesthetic testing series was begun. The subject was asked for a judgment of "same" or "different" for each paired comparison presented. If the subject was doubtful, he was asked to guess. No repetitions of trials were given. No affirmations or corrections were made during the test period.

The instructions for the visual-haptic series were essentially the same as for the visual-kinesthetic except for minor changes to make the wording appropriate to the haptic stimuli. In this series the blocks were placed in the subject's hand out of his field of vision behind the screen. They were compared to the standard visual stimuli which was a block placed in the subject's field of vision on the table before him. A judgment of "same" or "different" was elicited.

For the haptic-kinesthetic series, the instructions were again the same with minor changes appropriate to the situation. In this series, however, vision was excluded by having the subjects wear a pair of darkened goggles. The standards in this series were the haptic stimuli. They were presented to the hand to which no kinesthetic stimulus was being applied. After comparison, as above, a judgment of "same" or "different" was elicited after each trial.

Judgments were scored as right or wrong. Two kinds of error were distinguished: an error made when nonidentical forms presented across modalities were judged as being the same, and an error made when identical forms were judged as being different.

RESULTS

Intersensory Integrative Development in Rural Children

The development of intersensory integrative competence with age in the whole sample of rural children is summarized in Tables 5 and 6,

Table 5. Mean and range of errors made in the recognition of identity between cross-modally presented, identical forms by the sample of rural children studied.

| | Sensory modalities tested | | | | | |
| | Visual-kinesthetic | | Visual-haptic | | Haptic-kinesthetic | |
Age	Mean	Range	Mean	Range	Mean	Range
6	5	0-15	1.06	0-8	3.67	0-13
7	3	0-10	0.28	0-2	2.0	0-8
8	1.51	0-7	0.25	0-4	1.5	0-6
9	1.28	0-7	0	0	1.0	0-4
10	1.64	0-4	0	0	1.44	0-6
11	0.66	0-4	0	0	0.76	0-3

and in Figures 2 and 3. The scores presented reflect diminution with age in the two types of errors which could be made in the course of judging whether the pairs of geometric forms, each member of which was presented to a different sensory system, were the same or different. The data presented in Table 5 and Figure 2 represent changes with age in the ability to judge cross-modally presented identical forms as being the same. Since objectively equivalent forms were judged as being nonequivalent, such errors are referred to as errors of nonequivalence.

The data presented in Table 6 and Figure 3 reflect errors that were made when objectively different forms were judged to be the same when presented across sensory modalities. Since objectively nonequivalent forms were in these instances judged to be equivalent, errors of this type are referred to as errors of equivalence.

As may be seen from these tables and figures, each of the pairs of intersensory relations im-

Table 6. Mean and range of errors made in the recognition of nonidentity between cross-modally presented, nonidentical forms by the sample of rural children studied.

| | Sensory modalities tested | | | | | |
| | Visual-kinesthetic | | Visual-haptic | | Haptic-kinesthetic | |
Age	Mean	Range	Mean	Range	Mean	Range
6	20	1-53	13.1	1-56	15.6	0-56
7	6	0-30	2.5	0-6	4.5	0-31
8	7.3	0-54	2.0	0-6	3.7	0-31
9	1.9	0-6	1.2	0-5	0.76	0-4
10	1.36	0-9	0.96	0-5	1.24	0-4
11	1.36	0-4	1.14	0-4	0.85	0-4

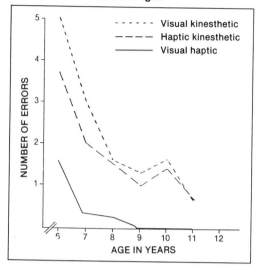

Figure 2. Mean errors for the intersensory judgment of identical geometric forms by rural children at different ages.

proved with age and had the form of a logarithmic curve of growth. As was the case for the New York suburban school children studied by Birch and Lefford (7), the different pairings of sensory interrelations did not develop to the same degree or at the same rate. In the Guatemalan rural children, as in the New York children, visual-haptic integration was significantly more effectively organized at every age than were either visual-kinesthetic or haptic-kinesthetic integrative interrelationships. The error curve for visual-haptic integration reached an asymptote between the seventh and eighth year, and performance on this task was errorless after that age. In contrast, neither visual-kinesthetic nor haptic-kinesthetic integrative performance reached an errorless level of competence within the range of ages studied.

As may be seen from Figures 2 and 3, both groups exhibited patterns of improvement with age which approximated the form of a growth function whose theoretical value may be expressed in the formula $Y = Ke^{cx}$ (where Y equals errors made, x the age of subjects in years, and e the base of the natural system of logarithms, K and c are empirical constants determined by the data.) In two cases these were not the curves of best fit and the data were assimilated to a straight line. In Table 7 the empirical equations for the development of intersensory integration with age in the two growth groups of rural chil-

dren are presented. As may be seen from Figures 4 to 9, and from Table 7 the curves of both groups are markedly similar and differ from one another primarily in the value of the constants. Further, as may be seen from the illustrations, the calculated theoretical growth curves and the empirical findings fit one another very closely.

The Relation of Intersensory Integrative Development to Height in the Rural Children

The physical growth achievements at each age level of the most stunted and the most fully grown 25 percent of the rural children are summarized in Table 8. It may be noted from this table that in the rural community at each year of age the children in the lower quartile and the upper quartile represented extremes of growth achievement. The mean difference in height across ages was 11 cm with the most striking differences manifested in the oldest age groups.

When the intersensory performances of the children in the upper quartile of growth

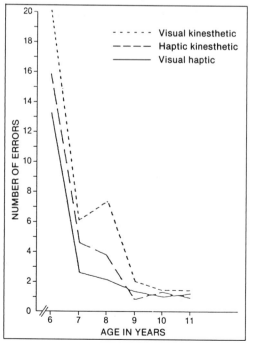

Figure 3. Mean errors for the intersensory judgment of nonidentical geometric forms by rural children at different ages.

Table 7. Empirical equations of error decrement with age, calculated from the performance of two groups of rural children with extreme differences in height.

Sense modalities tested	Quartile for height	Judgment of identical forms	Judgment of nonidentical forms
Visual-kinesthetic	Lower	$\bar{Y} = 53.9e^{-0.381x}$	$\bar{Y} - 30.34 + 2.55x^{a}$
	Upper	$\bar{Y} = 26.84e^{-0.384x}$	$\bar{Y} = 124.3e^{-0.430x}$
Visual-haptic	Lower	$\bar{Y} = 38.99e^{-0.630x}$	$\bar{Y} = 20.68 + 1.79x^{a}$
	Upper	$\bar{Y} = 960.2e^{-1.151x}$	$\bar{Y} = 12.51e^{-0.230x}$
Haptic-kinesthetic	Lower	$\bar{Y} = 29.63e^{-0.325x}$	$\bar{Y} = 241.1e^{-0.526x}$
	Upper	$\bar{Y} = 10.53c^{-0.270x}$	$\bar{Y} = 14.3e^{-0.514x}$

[a] Since the better fit for these curves of improvement with age was a straight line, they were assimilated to the equation $Y = a + bx$.

achievement are contrasted with those made by the children in the lower height quartile, differences in intersensory integrative skills are manifested for all three combinations of intersensory integration studied. These differences are particularly clear over the whole age span for the errors of nonequivalence that were made when children misjudged identical forms presented across two modalities (Figures 4, 6, and 8 and Table 9).

Differences in the number of errors of equivalence made by the two height groups in judging nonidentical forms also tended to favor the taller group of children (Figures 5, 7, and 9 and Table 10). This difference was most notable in the performances of the youngest groups of children, the 6-year-olds. Figures 10, 11, and 12 present the data on the cumulative percentage of 6-year-old children in the two height groups who made errors of equivalence and clearly indicate the lag in development of intersensory competence that was present in the shorter children during the first school year.

Figure 4. Empirical and theoretical developmental curves for visual-kinesthetic integration in two groups of rural children at extremes of height, judgment of identical forms.

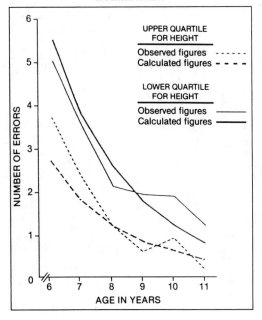

Figure 5. Empirical and theoretical developmental curves for visual-kinesthetic integration in two groups of rural children at extremes of height, judgment of nonidentical forms.

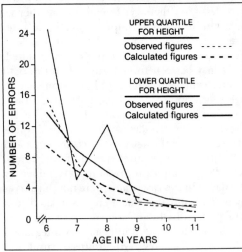

Table 8. Mean and range of height in centimeters of rural school age children at extremes of difference in stature.

Age	6	7	8	9	10	11
Lower quartile for height range	98 96-99.5	106 101-108	108 99-110	113 107-116.5	114 109-116.5	119 113-123
Upper quartile for height range	107 105-113	113 111.5-118	119 116-122	124 122-126	127 124-133	134 131-138

Figure 6. Empirical and theoretical developmental curves for haptic-kinesthetic integration in two groups of rural children at extremes of height, judgment of identical forms.

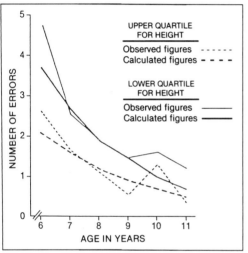

Figure 8. Empirical and theoretical developmental curves for visual-haptic integration in two groups of rural children at extremes of height, judgment of identical forms.

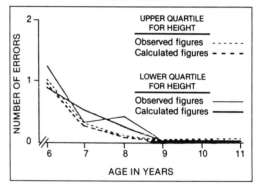

Figure 7. Empirical and theoretical developmental curves for haptic-kinesthetic integration in two groups of rural children at extremes of height, judgment of nonidentical forms.

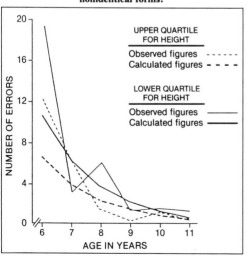

Figure 9. Empirical and theoretical developmental curves for visual-haptic integration in two groups of rural children at extremes of height, judgment of nonidentical forms.

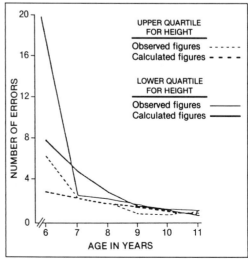

Table 9. Errors made in the recognition of identical forms by tall and short rural children.

Age	Visual-kinesthetic quartile for height				Visual-haptic quartile for height				Haptic-kinesthetic quartile for height			
	Lower		Upper		Lower		Upper		Lower		Upper	
	N	Mean	N	Mean	N	Mean	N	Mean	N	Mean	N	Mean
6	9	5 (0-15)[a]	10	3.7 (0-9)	9	1.12 (0-6)	10	1.0 (0-8)	9	4.75 (0-13)	10	2.6 (0-8)
7	17	3.53 (0-10)	14	2.35 (0-5)	17	0.29 (0-2)	14	0.28 (0-2)	17	2.53 (0-8)	14	1.64 (0-3)
8	10	2.1 (0-7)	10	1.2 (0-3)	10	0.40	10	0.10	10	1.90 (0-4)	10	1.10 (0-3)
9	16	1.93 (0-7)	11	0.63 (0-3)	16	0	11	0	16	1.46 (0-4)	11	0.54 (0-3)
10	11	1.90 (0-4)	14	0.92 (0-4)	11	0	14	0	11	1.63 (0-5)	14	1.28 (0-6)
11	10	1.20 (0-4)	11	0.18 (0-1)	10	0	11	0	10	1.20 (0-3)	11	0.36 (0-2)

[a] Figures in parenthesis show range of errors. Age is given in completed years.
N = Number of children.

In considering errors it is clear that the examination of group differences can best be explored before performance reaches a common maximum level. Since visual-haptic integration tends to reach its asymptote very early, only the youngest children showed differences in this integrative performance that are associated with differences in height. At 6 years of age the shortest of the children made a mean error of nonequivalence of 1.12 and a mean error of

Table 10. Errors made in the recognition of identical forms by tall and short rural children.

Age	Visual-kinesthetic quartile for height				Visual-haptic quartile for height				Haptic-kinesthetic quartile for height			
	Lower		Upper		Lower		Upper		Lower		Upper	
	N	Mean	N	Mean	N	Mean	N	Mean	N	Mean	N	Mean
6	9	24.50 (3-52)[a]	10	15.60 (1-53)	9	19.8 (3-56)	10	6.4 (1-21)	9	19.25 (0-56)	10	12.10 (2-26)
7	17	4.88 (0-14)	14	7.00 (0-30)	17	2.58 (0-6)	14	2.35 (0-4)	17	3.0 (0-11)	14	6.07 (1-31)
8	10	12.20 (0-54)	10	2.40 (0-7)	10	2.3 (0-6)	10	1.9 (0-5)	10	6.0 (0-37)	10	1.40 (0-4)
9	16	2.00 (0-4)	11	1.72 (0-6)	16	1.66 (0-5)	11	0.81 (0-3)	16	1.26 (0-4)	11	0.27 (0-1)
10	11	2.81 (0-4)	14	1.50 (0-4)	11	1.27 (0-5)	14	0.71 (0-5)	11	1.45 (0-2)	14	1.07 (0-4)
11	10	1.30 (0-3)	11	1.36 (0-4)	10	1.20 (0-4)	11	1.09 (0-3)	10	1.30 (0-4)	11	0.45 (0-2)

[a] Figures in parenthesis show the range of errors. Age is given in completed years.
N = Number of children.

Figure 10. Proportions of tall and short six-year-old rural children making errors of equivalence in visual-haptic judgment.

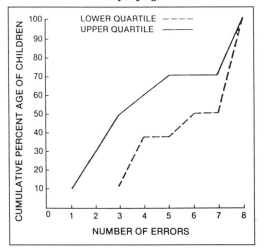

Figure 12. Proportions of tall and short six- and eight-year-old rural children making errors of equivalence in visual-kinesthetic judgment.

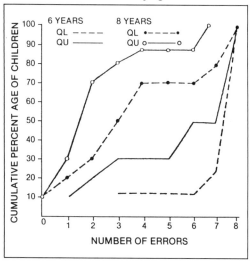

equivalence of 19.8. In contrast the tallest group made mean errors of 1.0 and 6.4 respectively. By the next year of age the asymptote for the function is approached and error differences between the two groups approached zero.

The picture for the later developing visual-kinesthetic and haptic-kinesthetic integrations is quite different. For both of these intersensory integrations significant differences in accuracy

Figure 11. Proportions of tall and short eight-year-old rural children making errors of equivalence in haptic-kinesthetic judgment.

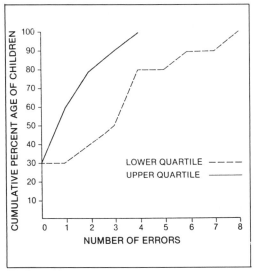

of judgment continued to exist at all but the older age levels for errors of nonequivalence. Not only were mean differences sustained but interindividual variability in performance also tended to be greater in the shorter children.

Intersensory Development in Upper Class Urban School Children

As may be seen from Table 11 the upper and lower height quartiles of the upper social class also represented extremes of growth achievement. The mean difference in height across ages for the tallest and shortest urban children was 15.5 cm, a value which was absolutely larger than that obtained between upper and lower quartiles in the rural population studied. Moreover, as may be noted by comparing the data in Table 11 with those in Table 8, the shortest urban children were comparable in height to the tallest group in the rural sample.

The errors made by the urban school children at different ages on the intersensory tasks are presented in Tables 12 and 13. As may be noted from these data and from Figures 13 and 14, the general form of the curves for age-specific performances resembles that obtained for the rural children and differs largely in that the upper social class urban children are significantly more advanced in their intersensory integrative abilities. This relationship is clearly

Table 11. Mean and range of height in centimeters of the groups of school age children of an urban upper social class tested for intersensory organization.

Age	6	7	8	9	10	11
Lower quartile for height range	111 106-115.5	115 110-118	121 119-123	130 125.5-133	130 127-132	135 32.5-137.5
Upper quartile for height range	126 124.5-129	130 128.5-135	137 132.5-141	141 137-147	147 145-150	156 155-157

manifest in Figures 3 and 4 in which the performance of the total rural and total urban groups for visual-kinesthetic and haptic-kinesthetic integration are presented. The developmental course is identical for the two groups and a simple modification of constants would clearly result in the superimposition of the age-specific error curves.

The differences between the two extreme height groups in the upper social class urban sample in intersensory integrative ability are presented in Tables 14 and 15. For neither errors of equivalence or nonequivalence, nor for

any pair of sense modalities did difference in height in this upper social stratum find a reflection in differences in the adequacy of intersensory integration. It appeared, therefore, that

Figure 13. Comparison of the age-specific error curves for visual-kinesthetic intersensory organization of rural children and upper social class urban children, judgment of identical forms.

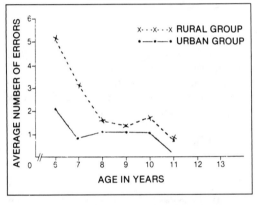

Table 12. Mean and range of errors made in the recognition of identical forms by a sample of upper social class, urban school age children.

	Sensory modalities tested					
	Visual-kinesthetic		Visual-haptic		Haptic-kinesthetic	
Age	Mean	Range	Mean	Range	Mean	Range
6	2	0-6	0.7	0-3	1.6	0-5
7	0.8	0-4	0	0	1.1	0-3
8	1.1	0-3	0.1	0-1	0.5	0-2
9	1.3	0-3	0.2	0-1	0.7	0-3
10	1.1	0-3	0.1	0-1	1.5	0-4
11	0.4	0-2	0	0	0	0-3

Table 13. Mean and range of errors made in the recognition of nonidentical forms by a sample of upper social class, urban, school age children.

	Sensory modalities tested					
	Visual-kinesthetic		Visual-haptic		Haptic-kinesthetic	
Age	Mean	Range	Mean	Range	Mean	Range
6	1.7	0-5	0.7	0-3	1.1	0-2
7	0.9	0-3	1.2	0-4	0.7	0-2
8	3.0	0-7	1.2	0-5	0.5	0-3
9	1.9	0-5	0.5	0-2	0.8	0-3
10	1.3	0-3	0.9	0-4	1.0	0-3
11	0.7	0-4	0.4	0-4	0.3	0-2

Figure 14. Comparison of age-specific error curves for haptic-kinesthetic intersensory organization of rural children and upper social class urban children, judgment of identical forms.

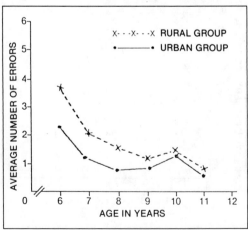

Table 14. Errors made in the recognition of identical forms by two height groups of upper social class, urban children.

Age		Visual-kinesthetic quartile for height				Visual-haptic quartile for height				Haptic-kinesthetic quartile for height		
		Lower		Upper		Lower		Upper		Lower		Upper
	N	Mean	N	Mean	N	Mean	N	Mean	N	Mean	N	Mean
6	5	2 (0-6)[a]	5	2 (1-4)	5	1.0 (0-3)	5	0.4 (0-2)	5	1.8 (0-5)	5	1.4 (0-3)
7	5	1.6 (0-4)	5	0 (0)	5	0 (0)	5	0 (0)	5	1.4 (0-3)	5	0.8 (0-2)
8	5	1.8 (0-3)	5	0.4 (0-2)	5	0.2 (0-1)	5	0 (0)	5	1 (0-2)	5	0 (0)
9	5	1.8 (1-3)	5	0.8 (0-2)	5	0.4 (0-1)	5	0 (0)	5	1 (0-3)	5	0.4 (0-2)
10	5	1.6 (0-6)	5	0.6 (0-1)	5	0 (0)	5	0.2 (0-1)	5	2 (0-4)	5	1 (0-4)
11	5	0.4 (0-2)	5	0.4 (0-1)	5	0 (0)	5	0 (0)	5	1 (0-3)	5	0.6 (0-2)

[a] Figures in parenthesis show the range of errors. Age is given in completed years.
N = Number of children.

differences in height as such, when they occurred in children who were not at risk of nutritional deprivation, did not result in differences in the rate of intersensory development or in the level of intersensory competence that was achieved at a given age. This lack of difference is illustrated by Figure 15 in which the visual-kinesthetic error performance by age of the two

Table 15. Errors made in the recognition of nonidentical forms by two height groups of upper social class, urban children.

Age		Visual-kinesthetic quartile for height				Visual-haptic quartile for height				Haptic-kinesthetic quartile for height		
		Lower		Upper		Lower		Upper		Lower		Upper
	N	Mean	N	Mean	N	Mean	N	Mean	N	Mean	N	Mean
6	5	1.4 (0-4)[a]	5	2 (0-5)	5	0.6 (0-2)	5	0.8 (0-3)	5	0.8 (0-2)	5	1.4 (0-2)
7	5	1 (0-2)	5	0.8 (0-3)	5	0.8 (0-3)	5	1.6 (0-4)	5	0.8 (0-2)	5	0.6 (0-1)
8	5	4.4 (2-7)	5	1.6 (0-5)	5	2 (0-5)	5	0.4 (0-1)	5	0.8 (0-3)	5	0.2 (0-1)
9	5	1.2 (0-2)	5	2.6 (2-5)	5	0 (0)	5	1 (1-2)	5	0.4 (0-2)	5	1.2 (0-3)
10	5	1.6 (1-3)	5	1 (0-3)	5	1 (0-4)	5	0.8 (0-3)	5	1 (0-2)	5	1 (0-3)
11	5	1.2 (0-4)	5	0.2 (0-1)	5	0.8 (0-4)	5	0 (0)	5	0.4 (0-2)	5	0.2 (0-1)

[a] Figures in parenthesis show range of errors. Age is given in completed years.
N = Number of children.

Figure 15. Visual-kinesthetic performance, by age, of tall and short children of an upper social class urban group, judgment of nonidentical forms. Quartile 1 represents the shortest children and Quartile 3 the tallest children.

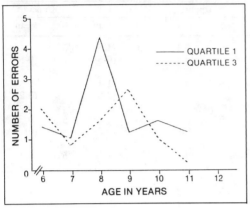

height extremes of the upper social class urban group are plotted. Similar overlapping between the two height groups occurred for the other intersensory integrations studied.

Background Factors Affecting Growth and the Development of Intersensory Integration

Two types of analysis were made of the available familial and environmental background information. The first of these was concerned with identifying factors which contributed to growth achievement. On the basis of the information collected, it was possible to analyze the relation of height at a given age to height of the parents, to the family's economic status, to housing conditions, and to parental educational level. Each of these will be considered in turn.

The mean heights of the fathers and mothers and children of the sample of rural children are presented in Table 16. As may be seen from the table, there is a tendency for the fathers of the taller children to be taller than the fathers of the children in the lowest quartile, with the mean difference in paternal height across ages 4.3 cm. However, this difference failed to meet an acceptable criterion of statistical significance. The mean heights of the mothers of the rural children in the upper and lower height quartiles were also insignificantly different from one another. Thus, parental height in the group did not appear to be significantly related to the height of the children. The height of the fathers of the upper social class urban children appeared to be more significantly related to the height of the child. The mean difference in paternal height across ages was 8.8 cm and is statistically significant (p less than 0.05, one tail). Maternal height, however, showed no systematic relation to height of offspring (Table 17).

The relation of the height of the rural children to family income, and to the percentage of the total annual expenditures spent on food, are presented in Tables 18 and 19. As may be seen from these tables, within this rural community, neither per capita nor the proportion of total expenditure devoted to food bore any systematic relation to the height of the children.

The relation of height to housing conditions is summarized in Table 20. As may be seen from the table there is a tendency for the *shorter* children to derive from families having somewhat superior housing. However, the difference is not significant at the 0.05 level of confidence.

The relation of the height of the rural child to the personal hygiene and cleanliness of himself and of his parents is considered in Tables 21, 22, and 23. The findings did not support the hypothesis that in this village conditions of personal hygiene and cleanliness, either of the

Table 16. The mean height in centimeters of two groups of rural school age children and of their parents.

Age (years completed)		6		7		8		9		10		11
Mean height	QL[a]	QU[b]	QL	QU	QL	QU	QL	QU	QL	QU	QL	QU
Children	98	107	106	113	108	119	113	124	114	127	119	134
Fathers	151	155	154	155	153	157	151	160	154	156	151	157
Mothers	143	145	143	144	141	143	143	143	144	145	144	147

[a] QL = Lower quartile for height.
[b] QU = Upper quartile for height.

Table 17. The mean height in centimeters of two groups of upper social class, urban children and of their parents.

Age (years completed)	6		7		8		9		10		11	
Mean height	QL[a]	QU[b]	QL	QU	QL	QU	QL	QU	QL	QU	QL	QU
Children	111	126	115	130	121	137	130	141	130	147	135	156
Fathers	163	176	163	163	162	175	168	174	161	178	171	175
Mothers	158	158	150	159	152	157	154	156	156	153	153	160

[a] QL = Lower quartile for height.
[b] QU = Upper quartile for height.

Table 18. Average annual per capita income in two groups of rural families with school age children showing extreme differences in height.

Age of children	6	7	8	9	10	11
Lower quartile for height	79.2[a]	85.2	101.7	132.6	107.5	116.9
Upper quartile for height	121.0	100.8	98.7	101.5	92.5	92.3

[a] Income in United States dollars.

Table 19. Mean percentage of total expenditure spent on food by two groups of rural families with school age children showing extreme differences in height.

Age of children	6	7	8	9	10	11
Families with children in lower quartile for height	66.0[a]	61.7	60.2	60.9	64.0	56.9
Families with children in upper quartile for height	56.9	60.8	61.2	61.8	65.3	62.0

[a] Percentage spent on food.

Table 20. The relation of height to housing in the rural children.

Housing conditions	Children in the lower quartile for height	Children in the upper quartile for height
Greater than the median value for the total group	40	29
Less than the median value for the total group	32	37

Difference not significant at .05 level of confidence (Chi square test).

Table 21. The relation of height to personal hygiene in the rural children.

Child's personal hygiene	Children in the lower quartile for height	Children in the upper quartile for height
Above the median for the total group	34	34
Below the median for the total group	38	31

Difference not significant at the .05 level of confidence (Chi square test).

parents or of the child, bore any systematic relation to the child's height during the school years.

The only strong positive association found between background circumstances and the child's height was between height of child and educational level of the mother (Table 24). When the mother's educational level was below the median for the sample of mothers studied, the likelihood was greater that her child would be short. Conversely, if her educational level was above the population median there was a

Table 22. The relation of height in rural children to the personal hygiene of the mothers.

Personal hygiene of mothers	Children in the lower quartile for height	Children in the upper quartile for height
Above the median for the total group	36	32
Below the median for the total group	34	34

Difference not significant at the .05 level of confidence (Chi square test).

Table 23. The relation of height in rural children to the personal hygiene of the fathers.

personal hygiene of fathers	Children in the lower quartile for height	Children in the upper quartile for height
Above the median for the total group	34	31
Below the median for the total group	34	31

Table 24. The relation of height in rural children to the educational background of the mothers.

Educational background of mothers	Children in the lower quartile for height	Children in the upper quartile for height
Above the median for the total group	28	41
Below the median for the total group	41	26

Chi 2 = 5.78.
p<0.02.

Table 25. The relation of height in rural children to the educational background of the fathers.

Educational background of fathers	Children in the lower quartile for height	Children in the upper quartile for height
Above the median for the total group	38	28
Below the median for the total group	31	35

Difference not significant at 0.05 level of probability (Chi square test).

Figure 16. Visual-kinesthetic intersensory organization, by age, of urban children, arranged according to whether the father's height was above or below the median value for the total group of fathers, judgment of identical forms.

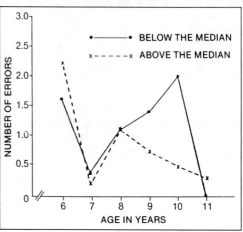

Figure 17. Visual-kinesthetic intersensory organization by age of urban children arranged according to whether the father's height was above or below the median value for the total group of fathers, judgment of nonidentical forms.

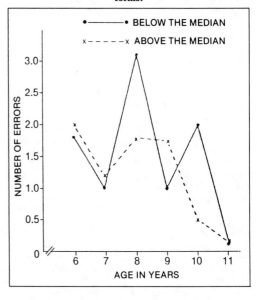

strong likelihood that her child would be in the taller segment of the population. It is of interest that no significant association was obtained between the father's educational status and the child's height (Table 25).

Since the height of the father in the urban group had been found to be related to the height of the child, it was decided to examine whether the father's height made any significant contribution to the child's intersensory performance. To carry out this analysis fathers were grouped in accordance with whether their heights were above or below the median for the sample, and the relation of the fathers' group position to the intersensory performance of the children was plotted (Figures 16 and 17). No significant association was found between the height of the fathers and the level of intersensory competence achieved by the child.

Comment

Two facts clearly emerge from the results presented. For these rural children a difference in height is accompanied by a difference in intersensory integrative ability. For the upper social class urban sample, differences in height are not associated with differences in intersensory integrative competence. Therefore, height as such cannot be considered as a determinant of intersensory integrative organization unless such difference in height occurred under circumstances in which the height differential developed from causes which affect intersensory integrative organization.

Differences in growth in the rural children are most likely to have derived from a failure to have received appropriate amounts and kinds of food (primary malnutrition), or to have been the product of infectious disease or parasitic infestations which have secondarily interfered with the individual's nutritional state either directly by increasing tissue catabolism without a compensatory increase in food intake (*12*), or indirectly through anorexia or social custom, in accordance with which, greatly reduced food consumption is deemed therapeutic in preschool children during illness and convalescence (*13*). When group differences in height do not derive from such a background set of risks, short stature is most likely to reflect familial differences in stature, and therefore, to be unassociated with disturbances in growth deriving from malnutrition. Such a view is supported by the strong relation of paternal height to height of the offspring in the upper social class urban group and the presence of a weak association in the rural population.

Whether the inadequacy in intersensory integrative performance in the rural children rep-

resents a reflection of malnutrition, or whether both poor integration and growth differences are associated with more general subcultural differences which, in an underlying way, may have contributed independently to differences in growth and to differences in intersensory functioning, is a question requiring detailed consideration. These two alternatives can most readily be analyzed if they are considered diagramatically as two consequential schemata (Figure 18). In Scheme I, malnutrition and intersensory inadequacy are hypothesized to have independent origins in a background of social impoverishment. They bear no direct relation one to the other, but are indirectly associated by virtue of a common antecedent. In Scheme II, the hypothetical causal sequence is different, and advances the view that social conditions result in malnutrition which, in its turn, has the consequences of low stature and poor intersensory integrative development. In one case, therefore, the immediately underlying process to deficiencies both in stature and neurointegrative capacity is viewed as malnutrition (Scheme II); in the other, social conditions representing an impoverished environment lead per se to poor intersensory functioning (Scheme I.)

Available evidence does not permit the rejection of either of these hypotheses. It is, however, possible to examine certain of the interferences stemming from each position and to explore them with respect to the available data. The primary inference of Scheme I is that social impoverishment, presumably including inadequate opportunities for learning, independently contributes to poor intersensory development. If this were indeed the case it would have been expected that a significant association would have been found between low stature and a variety of social factors that have been implicated as contributing to poor psychological growth. It would therefore be anticipated, if Scheme I were correct, that low stature and poor intersensory performance would have had a significant association to depressed family income, poor housing conditions, the proportion of income spent on food, personal sanitary conditions, and so on. It was, therefore, most striking to find in the data of the present study: (1) no significant association of neurointegrative function with financial status, with housing facilities, with proportion of total income, or with

Figure 18. Hypothetical relationships between social conditions, primary and secondary malnutrition, low stature, and poor intersensory development.

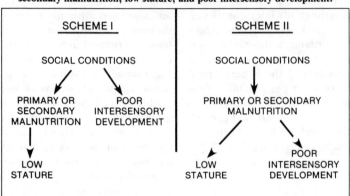

the total expenditure spent on food; (2) a weak inverse correlation with father's education; and, (3) no correlation with conditions of personal cleanliness. The only significant association with a social background factor was the correlation with the mother's educational level.

The positive relation of mother's education to intersensory adequacy must be considered in association with the distribution of responsibility within the household, and in particular with the relation of the mother to child care and child health. It is important to remember, in this respect, that in this, as in many other rural societies in Latin America, the closeness of the child to his mother during the first years of life is not confined to physical contact, but that rules and practices of health and care in the household belong to the women's world. There is, therefore, a strong possibility that the better educated female will rely less on traditional methods of feeding and child care, which are a direct cause of reduced intake of nutrients in health and disease particularly in early life.

Although these findings cannot lead to an absolute rejection of the possibility depicted in Scheme I, they certainly provide suggestive evidence that it is not a difference in general social background as such that is interfering with the child's physical growth and intersensory development. When these findings are taken together with the large body of evidence that implicates malnutrition in growth failure and with the reports of more global behavioral disturbances following malnutrition, it appears likely that malnutrition is one of the intervening variables between growth and intersensory

inadequacy. Obviously, a definite answer can be provided by anterospectively oriented longitudinal studies, wherein it would become possible to control independently for environmental circumstances and for inadequate nutritional conditions. Such studies would provide direct evidence and would not need to depend upon any inferential index of early malnutrition such as stature. . . .

If on the basis of the suggestive evidence available one accepts as a working hypothesis the possibility that malnutrition interferes with intersensory adequacy, the next issue to be considered is the set of possible mechanisms underlying the interference: Three main possibilities are apparent: (1) lack of comprehension of task; (2) sensory loss; (3) failure to develop integration among the separate sensory modalities. Each will be considered separately.

Lack of Comprehension of Task

Children can make errors simply because they may be unable to understand the verbal instructions given by the examiner. The confusion between language factors and other cognitive functions is a frequent cause of error particularly when the child is asked to make a judgment. In order to avoid this source of error a pretest was employed during which errors made because of lack of comprehension of the task were corrected. Since the items used in the pretest were identical with some of those employed during the actual testing, and since the instructions also were identical, it can safely be concluded that the errors made in judging intermodally presented forms did not stem from incomprehension of the task.

Under certain conditions individuals who are unable to discriminate on the basis of knowledge tended to make judgments by guessing. In order to eliminate this possibility a comparative analysis was made when identical and nonidentical forms were being judged. Since judgments of nonidentical pairs were more frequently demanded, if judgments were based either on random or systematic guessing, on the basis of the frequency of presented tasks, the subjects would have been expected to make three and a half times as many errors in making judgments of nonidentical forms as they made in judging identities. The findings, however, did not conform to such a pattern of chance expectation. In Table 26 the two sets of judgments are compared in terms of percentages of the maximum possible number of errors. In the great majority of instances, the percentage figures tend to be greater for judgments on identical forms and make it most unlikely that the patterns of response reflected simple random guessing.

Intrasensory Source of Error

Clearly, errors in intersensory judgment can derive from inadquacies in intrasensory functioning. Thus, an error made in the course of a visual-haptic judgment could arise as readily from the ineffectiveness of either sensory pathway as a source of information as it could from a failure to integrate the information simultaneously deriving from each of the separate sense modalities. An analysis of the data in terms of patterns of judgment makes it possible to reject such an intrasensory explanation of failure.

Since all subjects had received preliminary testing on a Seguin Form Board using the same figures as were later judged across sensory modalities and had all functioned on the former task at a level of 100 percent accuracy, and had reached with no hesitation and placed all pieces without fumbling, it could be concluded that intrasensory functioning within the visual system was adequately enough developed to permit effective discrimination of the forms by the children at all age levels studied. Analysis of the effectiveness of functioning in the haptic and kinesthetic systems can then be determined by means of an indirect analysis of judgmental patterns.

It will be recalled that for any given paired comparison of two geometric forms, the child was asked to make judgments under three intersensory conditions: visual-haptic, visual-kinesthetic, and haptic-kinesthetic. Clearly, a judgment under any one or all of these conditions could be correct or incorrect. Therefore, eight patterns of response were able to occur for any pairing under the three intersensory conditions. If the responses are ordered in the sequence visual-kinesthetic (V-K), visual-haptic (V-H), and haptic-kinesthetic (H-K), and + means correct and − incorrect, the eight possible patterns are as follows:

Pattern	V-K	V-H	H-K
I	+	+	+
II	+	−	+
III	+	+	−
IV	−	+	+
V	+	−	−
VI	−	+	−
VII	−	−	+
VIII	−	−	−

Table 26. Ratio of observed errors to maximum possible number of errors expressed as a percent (rural children).

	Intersensory modalities											
	Errors of nonequivalence quartiles for height						Errors of equivalence quartiles for height					
	Visual-kinesthetic		Visual-haptic		Haptic-kinesthetic		Visual-kinesthetic		Visual haptic		Haptic kinesthetic	
Age	Lower	Upper	Lower	Upper	Lower	Upper	Lower	Upper	Lower	Upper	Lower	Upper
6	31.2	23.1	7.0	6.2	29.7	19.2	41.9	27.8	35.4	11.4	34.4	21.6
7	22.1	14.7	1.8	1.8	15.8	10.2	8.7	12.5	4.6	4.2	5.3	10.8
8	13.1	7.5	2.5	0.6	11.9	6.9	21.7	4.3	4.1	3.4	10.7	2.5
9	12.1	3.9	0	0	9.1	3.4	3.6	3.1	3.0	1.4	2.2	0.5
10	11.9	5.8	0	0	10.2	8.0	3.2	2.7	2.3	1.3	2.6	1.9
11	7.5	1.1	0	0	7.5	2.2	2.3	2.4	2.1	1.9	2.3	0.8

The three plus signs in Pattern I indicate that the children made correct judgments under all intersensory conditions. When this pattern of response occurred it could be concluded that both intrasensory and intersensory processes were functioning completely effectively. Pattern II, + − +, occurred when the visual-kinesthetic responses were correct, but the visual-haptic response was incorrect. The presence of this pattern indicated that the child had adequate haptic and kinesthetic intrasensory functioning. Since visual intrasensory adequacy had already been independently demonstrated, the incorrect visual-haptic response need be interpreted as due to some inadequacy in visual-haptic intersensory interaction. Similarly, for Pattern III, + + −, it can be inferred that haptic and kinesthetic intrasensory functioning were adequate since each of these modalities was capable of being effectively related to vision. The incorrect haptic-kinesthetic judgment in this pattern would, therefore, indicate inadequacy in liaison between the haptic and kinesthetic sense modalities. In Pattern IV, − + +, the visual-kinesthetic response was incorrect. From this pattern of response it could be inferred that the child had adequate visual, haptic, and kinesthetic function at an intrasensory level, since, if this were not the case, the visual-haptic, and haptic-kinesthetic judgments could not have been correct. It therefore followed that the incorrect visual-kinesthetic response was due to some inadequacy in integration of information between the visual and kinesthetic sense modalities. If responses were to have occurred with high frequency in Patterns I-IV, therefore, it would be clear that intrasensory factors were not at the origin of the incorrect responses.

The average frequency with which the various patterns of response occurred in the tall and short rural children is given in Tables 27 and 28. Their evolution with age is summarized in Figures 19 and 20. As may be seen in the tables, in both tall and short subjects, the great majority of the responses fit Patterns I to IV. Thus, one can accept intrasensory adequacy in each of the sensory modalities as established, and focus attention on the analysis of the possible mechanisms through which malnutrition might influence the development of intersensory organization.

Clearly, malnutrition could act in two ways— one deriving from a direct interference with the development of the central nervous system and the other from a series of indirect effects. Let us look at the latter possibility first.

Three possible indirect effects are readily apparent:

(1) *Loss of learning time.* Since the child was less responsive to his environment when malnourished, at the very least he had less time in which to learn and had lost a certain number of months of experience. On the simplest basis, therefore, he would be expected to show some developmental lags.

(2) *Interference with learning during critical periods of development.* Learning is by no means simply a cumulative process. A considerable body of evidence exists which indicates that interference with the learning process at specific times during its course may result in disturbances in function that are both profound and

Table 27. Average frequency of occurrence of various patterns of response in two groups of rural children at extremes of height (judgment of identical forms).

Pattern V-K V-H H-K	Age in years											
	6		7		8		9		10		11	
	QL[a]	QU[b]	QL	QU	QL	QU	QL	QU	QL	QU	QL	QU
I + + +	4.22	5.5	6.29	6.14	6.3	7.1	6.31	7.63	6.81	7.21	7.3	7.81
II + − +	0.0	0.3	0.05	0.07	0.0	0.0	0.0	0.0	0.0	0.0	0.0	0.0
III + + −	0.55	0.6	0.58	0.28	0.5	0.3	0.43	0.27	0.36	0.42	0.4	0.18
IV − + +	1.00	0.9	0.82	0.57	0.9	0.3	0.50	0.09	0.54	0.21	0.0	0.0
V + − −	0.0	0.0	0.05	0.0	0.1	0.0	0.0	0.0	0.0	0.0	0.0	0.0
VI − + −	0.77	0.70	0.64	0.35	0.3	0.3	0.25	0.0	0.27	0.14	0.0	0.0
VII − − +	0.0	0.0	0.0	0.0	0.0	0.0	0.0	0.0	0.0	0.0	0.3	0.0
VIII − − −	0.44	0.0	0.0	0.0	0.0	0.0	0.0	0.0	0.0	0.0	0.0	0.0

[a] QL = Lower quartile for height.
[b] QU = Upper quartile for height.

Table 28. Average frequency of occurrence of various patterns of response in two groups of rural children at extremes of height (judgment of nonidentical forms).

Pattern V-K V-H H-K	Age in years											
	6		7		8		9		10		11	
	QL[a]	QU[b]	QL	QU	QL	QU	QL	QU	QL	QU	QL	QU
I + + +	22.33	34.6	51.35	43.64	44.1	51.8	49.62	53.18	52.27	53.07	55.4	52.90
II + − +	1.33	2.0	0.82	0.64	1.0	0.9	0.62	0.54	0.81	0.35	0.6	0.63
III + + −	1.11	2.4	1.17	1.64	0.7	0.5	0.43	0.0	0.81	0.78	0.7	0.36
IV − + +	7.22	5.6	2.82	2.14	4.6	1.3	0.75	1.63	0.72	1.07	1.0	0.81
V + − −	2.22	6.0	0.58	0.42	0.3	0.3	0.12	0.09	0.27	0.14	0.2	0.09
VI − + −	1.88	6.3	1.76	2.42	4.4	0.8	0.31	0.09	0.63	0.35	0.1	0.09
VII − − +	2.55	6.0	0.23	0.35	0.2	0.2	0.37	0.18	0.18	0.14	0.1	0.18
VIII − − −	10.77	3.1	1.00	0.71	0.5	0.3	0.43	0.0	0.09	0.07	0.2	0.27

[a] QL = Lower quartile for height.
[b] QU = Upper quartile for height.

Figure 19. Patterns of judgment for all intersensory pairings made when judging identical forms at different ages.

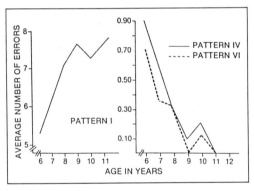

Figure 20. Patterns of judgment for all intersensory pairings made when judging nonidentical forms at different ages.

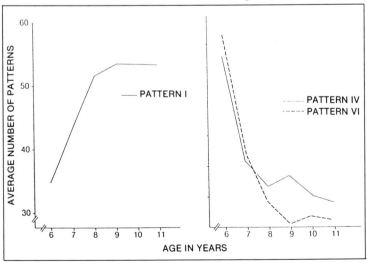

of long-term significance. Such disturbance is not merely a function of the length of time the organism is deprived of the opportunities for learning. Rather, what appears to be important is the correlation of the experiential opportunity with a given stage of development—the so-called critical periods of learning (14-16). Critical periods in human learning have not been definitively established, but in looking at the consequences associated with malnutrition at different ages one can derive some potentially useful hypotheses. Relevant to the relation between time of life at which malnutrition develops and learning may be the . . . report of Cravioto and Robles (17) who have shown that as contrasted with older patients, infants under six months recovering from kwashiorkor did not recoup their mental age deficit during the recovery period. In older children, ranging from 15 to 41 months of age, too, the rate of recovery from the initial mental deficit varied in direct relation to chronological age at time of admission. Similarly, the findings of Barrera-Moncada (18) in children, and those of Keys, et al. (19) in adults, indicate a strong association between persistence of later effects on mental performance and periods of onset and duration of malnutrition.

(3) *Motivation and personality changes.* It should be recognized that the mother's response to the infant is to a considerable degree a function of the child's own characteristics of reactivity (20, 21). One of the first effects of malnutrition is a reduction in the child's responsiveness to stimulation and the emergence of various degrees of apathy. Apathetic behavior in its turn can function to reduce the value of the child as a stimulus and to diminish the adult's responsiveness to him. Thus, apathy can provoke apathy and so contribute to a cumulative pattern of reduced adult-child interaction. If this occurs it can have consequences for stimulation, for learning, for maturation, and for interpersonal relations, the end result being significant backwardness in performance on later, more complex learning tasks.

Let us now consider the possibility that malnutrition may affect the development of intersensory organization directly by modifying the growth and biochemical maturation of the brain. It should be remembered that increase of cell cytoplasm with extension of axons and dendrites, one of the processes associated with the growth of the human brain at birth, is largely a process of protein synthesis. From the microspectrographic investigation of the regenerating nerve fibers it has been estimated that protein substance increases more than 2000 times as the apolar neuroblast matures into the young anterior horn cell. Perhaps an easier way to grasp the magnitude of this process may be simply to recall that at the time of birth the human brain is gaining weight at the rate of 1 to 2 mg per minute.

Changes in structure of the central nervous system due to feeding grossly inadequate diets to animals have been documented by Lowry (22) and Platt (23). McCance, et al. (24-28) have shown gross alterations in the content of water and several electrolytes (28) in the brain substance, and Flexner (29) and associates have advanced evidence that interference with protein synthesis in the brain produces loss of disorders in mice (29). Ambrosius, et al. (30) have reported that severely malnourished children show a distortion of the normal relation between brain weight and total body weight. They have interpreted their findings as an indication of arrested growth of the central nervous system. It may well be that so-called critical periodicity in behavior represents the responsiveness of the nervous system when it is at a given stage of biochemical organization. If this is the case nutritional inadequacy may interfere with both staging and timing of development of brain and behavior.

However, independently of the mechanism through which intersensory organization is interfered with, there can be little doubt as to the fact that there is evidence of delayed neurointegrative development in those children at nutritional risk who have grown poorly. It is, therefore, important to consider the potential significance of this type of developmental lag in so primary a process as intersensory organization for more complex psychological functioning. In this connection it is of interest to consider two significant features of learning—conditioned reflex formation and the acquisition of academic skills.

In most conditioning situations what is being demanded is the integration between two stimuli, each of which belongs to a different sensory modality. Thus, in classical salivary conditioning or in the conditioning of a leg withdrawal, a gustatory or a tactile stimulus is in effect being linked to an auditory or visual one. The process of conditioning, when effective, therefore involves the establishment of intimate equivalences between initially nonequivalent stimuli in different sensory modalities. If interrelations among sensory modalities are inadequately established the possibility exists that conditioning will either be delayed in its occurrence, or that the pairing of stimuli will be ineffective in producing conditioned reflexes. Therefore, failure for intersensory integration to occur at normal age-specific points can contribute to inadequate primary learning at the given age level.

Evidence already exists that the lag in the development of certain varieties of intersensory integrations has a high correlation with backwardness in learning to read. Thus, Birch and Belmont (*31, 32*) in their studies of reading disability in British children, and Kahn (*33*) in her study of American school children, have shown that backwardness in reading is strongly associated with inadequacy in auditory-visual integration. Evidence is also available that indicates the dependence of visual-motor control in design-copying on visual-kinesthetic integrative adequacy. In a series of investigations of preschool and school children, Birch and Lefford (*34*) have found skill in visual-kinesthetic integration to be highly and significantly correlated with design-copying in normal children. If it is recognized, with Baldwin (*35*), that such visual-motor control is essential for learning to write, the inadequacy in intersensory organization can interfere with a second primary educational skill—learning to write.

Thus, inadequacies of intersensory development can place the child at risk of failing to establish an ordinary normal background of conditionings in his preschool years and at the risk of failing to profit from educational experience in the school years.

References

(*1*) Maier, N. R. F. and T. C. Schneirla. *Principles of Animal Behavior*. New York, McGraw Hill, 1935.

(*2*) Birch, H. G. Comparative psychology. In *Areas of Psychology*, F. Marcuse, ed. New York, Harper, 1954.

(*3*) Voronin, L. G. and V. I. Guselnikov. On the phylogenesis of internal mechanisms of the analytic and synthetic activity of the brain. *Pavlov J Higher Nerv Activity* 13:193, 1963.

(*4*) Sherrington, C. S. *Man on His Nature*. London, Cambridge University Press, 1951, pp. 287-289.

(*5*) Birch, H. G. and M. E. Bitterman. Reinforcement and learning: The process of sensory integration. *Psychol Rev* 56:292 1949.

(*6*) ——————————————— . Sensory

integration and cognitive theory. *Psychol Rev* 58:355, 1951.

(*7*) ———————— and A. Lefford. Two strategies for studying perception in "brain-damaged" children. In *Brain Damage in Children: Biological and Social Aspects* (H. G. Birch, ed.). Baltimore, Maryland, Williams and Wilkins, 1964, p. 46.

(*8*) Luna-Jaspe, H., L. Vega, and J. Cravioto. Evolution of death and disease in a rural village during the past 87 years. Unpubl. manuscript.

(*9*) Flores, M. and E. Reh. *Estudios de hábitos dietéticos en poblaciones de Guatemala. I. Magdalena Milpas Altas*. Suplementos No. 2 del Boletín de la Oficina Sanitaria Panamericana, Publicaciones Científicas del Instituto de Nutrición de Centro America y Panamá, 1955, p. 90.

(*10*) García, B. Y., Girón de Meneses, and J. Cravioto. "Operación Nimiquipalg." II. Variación del consumo de alimentos en un area rural de Guatemala durante los ultimos trece años. *Guatemala Pediátrica* 4:50, 1964.

(*11*) Vega, L., J.J. Urrutia, y J. Cravioto. Estandarización de las mediciones de peso y talla en niños escolares. *Guatemala Pediátrica* 4:84, 1964.

(*12*) Wilson, D., R. Bressani, and N. S. Scrimshaw. Infection and nutritional status. I. The effect of chicken pox on nitrogen metabolism in children. *Am J Clin Nutr* 9:154, 1961.

(*13*) Cravioto, J. Consideraciones epidemiológicas y bases para la formulación de un programa de prevención de la desnutrición. *Bol Med Hosp Infant Mex* 15:925, 1958.

(*14*) Bowlby, J. Critical phases in the development of social responses in man and other animals. In *Prospects in Psychiatric Research*, J. M. Tanner (ed.). Oxford, England, Blackwell, 1952.

(*15*) Scott, J. P. Critical periods in behavioral development. *Science* 138:949, 1962.

(*16*) ———————— Critical periods. *Monogr Soc Res Child Dev* Vol. 28, 1963.

(*17*) Cravioto, J. and B. Robles. Evolution of adaptive and motor behavior during rehabilitation from kwashiorkor. *Am J Orthopsychiatry* 35:449, 1965.

(*18*) Barrera-Moncada, G. *Estudios sobre alteraciones del crecimiento y del desarrollo psicológico del síndrome pluricarencial (kwashiorkor)*. Caracas, Venezuela, Editorial Grafos, 1963.

(*19*) Keys, A., J. Brozek, A. Henschel, O. Mickelson, and H. L. Taylor. *The Biology of Human Starvation*. Vol II. Minnesota, University of Minnesota Press, 1950.

(*20*) Diller, L. and H. G. Birch. Psychological evaluation of children with cerebral damage. In *Brain Damage in Children: Biological and Social Aspects* (H. G. Birch, ed.). Baltimore, Williams and Wilkins, 1964.

(*21*) Eisenberg, L. Behavioral manifestations of cerebral damage. In *Brain Damage in Children: Biological and Social Aspects*, H. G. Birch (ed.). Baltimore, Williams and Wilkins, 1964.

(*22*) Lowry, R. S., W. G. Pond, R. H. Barnes, L. Krook, and J. K. Loosli. Influence of caloric and protein quality on the manifestations of protein deficiency in the young pig. *J Nutr* 78:245, 1962.

(*23*) Platt, B. S., C. R. C. Heard, and R. J. C. Steward. Experimental protein-caloric deficiency, Chapter 21. In *Mammalian Protein Metabolism.* New York, Academic Press, Inc., 1964.

(*24*) McCance, R. A. Food, growth, and time. *Lancet* 2:621, 1962.

(*25*) Widdowson, E. M. and R. A. McCance. The effect of finite periods of undernutrition at different ages on the composition and subsequent development of the rat. *Proc R Soc S B* 158:329, 1963.

(*26*) Pratt, C. W. M. and R. A. McCance. Severe undernutrition in growing and adult animals. 6. Changes in the long bones during rehabilitation in the cockerels. *Br J Nutr* 15:121, 1961.

(*27*) McCance, R. A. Some effects of undernutrition. *J Pediatr* 65:1008, 1964.

(*28*) Widdowson, E. M., J. W. T. Dickerson, and R. A. McCance. Severe undernutrition in growing and adult animals. 4: The impact of severe undernutrition on the chemical composition of the soft tissue of the pig. *Br J Nutr* 14:457, 1960.

(*29*) Flexner, L. B. Protein synthesis and memory in mice. *Proc Natl Acad Sci,* U.S.A. In press.

(*30*) Ambrosius, K. D. El comportamiento del peso de algunos órganos en niños con desnutrición de tercer grado. *Bol Med Hosp Infant Mex* 28:47, 1961.

(*31*) Birch, H. G. and L. Belmont. Auditory visual integration in normal and retarded readers. *Am J Orthopsychiatry* 34:852-861, 1964.

(*32*) _____ Auditory and visual integration, intelligence, and reading ability in school children. *Percept Mot Skills* 20:295-305, 2965.

(*33*) Kahn, D. A developmental study of the relationship between auditory-visual integration and reading achievement in boys. Ph.D. dissertation. Teachers College, Columbia University, 1965.

(*34*) Birch, H. G. and A. Lefford. Intersensory organization and voluntary motor control. Unpubl. manuscript.

(*35*) Baldwin, J. M. *Mental Development in the Child and the Race.* New York, The McMillan Co., 1897.

PATTERNS OF URBAN MORTALITY

Ruth Rice Puffer and G. Wynne Griffith

METHODOLOGY OF THE INTER-AMERICAN INVESTIGATION OF MORTALITY

The principal collaborator in charge of the field work in each city directed a small team consisting of one or more physicians, public health nurses, or social workers, and a secretary. Their tasks were to select the deaths to be included in the Investigation, to complete the standard form of questionnaire (Appendix 2)[1] for each death, and to transmit the forms to the central office for review and for assignment of the underlying cause of death. In addition, each principal collaborator was encouraged to utilize the data collected by his team in appropriate ways, e.g., by presenting results to professional groups in his city and by publishing those results in national journals. The methods and procedures followed consistently throughout the Investigation are described in this chapter.

Selection of Deaths

In the 12 cities the registration of deaths, at least of adults, is virtually complete. The international form of medical certificate of cause of death is always used, except in Guatemala City, where a proportion of deaths are certified by police officers, who use a special form for the purpose. In addition to the medical certificate, the forms used in all cities give the name, age, sex, place and date of death, and place of residence; and in all cities but one the civil status of the deceased is shown. The forms used in several cities include other items as well, such as occupation, date and place of birth, whether an autopsy had been performed, duration of residence at last address, and nationality or race.

The cooperation of the registration authorities in each city having been obtained, at regular intervals throughout the study period the complete set of certificates of all deaths oc-

curring in the city during the preceding period was assembled for scrutiny. The length of this interval varied from one week to one month, according to local circumstances. In 10 cities the selection of deaths to be studied could be conducted expeditiously at one central point, through which all certificates passed as a matter of routine. In Guatemala City and Lima, however, more than one registration office had to be visited on each occasion. To ensure that all certificates filed during the sampling interval were available for scrutiny, checks were made on each occasion, by noting, for example, that the sequence of serial registration numbers was unbroken.

A death was accepted as eligible for inclusion in the Investigation if, according to the information on the death certificate, two conditions were satisfied: first, the age at death was not less than 15 years or more than 74 years and, second, that the city was the normal place of residence. If the usual place of residence was not stated on the certificate, the death was regarded, provisionally, as eligible for inclusion but liable to be eliminated at a later stage if it was found that the deceased had normally resided elsewhere. The deaths of persons of no fixed residence were also retained subject to the same proviso, and this latter group eventually accounted for 5 percent of the deaths finally accepted for inclusion in the Investigation.

The aim was to investigate 2000 deaths during each of two consecutive years in each city. In four cities—Cali, Guatemala City, La Plata, and Ribeirão Prêto—all eligible deaths were investigated, for their number was not expected to exceed that target. Since in the other eight cities the number of deaths in the age group 15–74 years was expected to exceed 2000 per year, the certificates relating to deaths eligible for inclusion were systematically sampled on each occasion through the use of a constant sampling factor decided upon in advance and based on the available mortality statistics for each city. In Bogotá, 2 out of every 5 eligible deaths were selected systematically; in Bristol, 3 out of 4; in Caracas and Lima, 1 out of 2; in San Francisco,

Source: Ruth Rice Puffer and G. Wynne Griffith, *Patterns of Urban Mortality—Report of the Inter-American Investigation of Mortality*. Washington, D.C., Pan American Health Organization, Scientific Publication No. 151, 1967. Chapters II and XV.

[1] Not included in this publication.

1 out of 3; in Santiago, 1 out of 5; and in São Paulo, 1 out of 6. In Mexico City the sampling factor, originally 1 in 7, had to be changed to 1 in 5 when it was found at an early stage that the proportion of nonresidents was higher than anticipated. The sampling factor averaged 1 in 5.42 for the whole period.

Every eligible death selected was allotted a serial number, and a visit was paid to the home of the deceased person. Whenever possible, the age of the deceased was verified and a residence history obtained. If those inquiries revealed that the deceased was not eligible, either because of age or because of normal place of residence, the death was excluded. The determination of residence status did not usually present any difficulty. Duration was, of course, one criterion; of the deaths included and for which the length of residence was recorded, 96 percent had lived in the city concerned for at least 2 years immediately prior to death, and 85 percent for at least 10 years. If the duration of residence had been brief or the precise period could not be ascertained, the apparent intention of the deceased person was considered. The main source of bias to be avoided was the individual who had gone to the city to seek medical treatment and had died while residing temporarily with relatives or friends. Great care was taken to exclude any such deaths. A patient admitted from an address outside the city to a long-term institution within the city was regarded as being a resident only if he had been an inpatient continuously for at least one year.

Deaths of city residents occurring outside the city limits were traced as a matter of routine only in Bristol and San Francisco, where the existing registration practices made their investigation feasible. In the other cities mortality of residents may be underestimated, owing to the number of residents dying outside the city, but the error is thought to be small because all such cities are major hospital centers. (In the case of specialized institutions, such as hospitals for mental disorders and for tuberculosis, which accepted patients from within the city but were located outside the city, arrangements were made to trace the deaths of city residents occurring in those institutions, so that those deaths might be included on the same basis as the deaths occurring within the city limits.)

In the cities where sampling was necessary, several checks were made to ensure that the samples were representative. The distribution of deaths in the sample for a given month was compared with the distribution of all deaths for that month, with respect to three characteristics: age, sex, and the district of the city given as the usual residence of the deceased. The results were consistently satisfactory in seven of the eight cities; in Bogotá the first check showed that the method of sampling was defective, resulting in inflated numbers. The "universe" from which the defective samples had been drawn was reconstructed, and the requisite number of deaths necessary to reduce the sample to its correct size was selected by the use of random numbers. After this adjustment, the entire group was shown to be representative as regards age, sex, and district of the city.

In Caracas, where the deaths were selected weekly, a smaller sample was taken during the first six weeks of the study period (January to mid-February 1962) than in subsequent weeks, in order to allow the field investigators a short period of adjustment to the work. The study period was therefore extended into the first six weeks of 1964 to complete the number required for the overall sampling ratio.

In São Paulo, because of temporary staffing difficulties, no samples were selected for study during the months of April, May, and June 1962. To compensate for this, samples twice the normal size were drawn during the corresponding months of 1963.

In addition to the routine checks, three of which were made during the study period in all eight cities, comparisons of the complete material of both years were undertaken either by the principal collaborators or in the central office for Bogotá, Caracas, San Francisco, and Santiago, and these gave equally satisfactory results.

The central review of questionnaires afforded other, less direct and sometimes quite incidental, checks on the correctness of the sampling procedure. For instance, a batch of questionnaires from San Francisco relating to deaths occurring in May 1964 included six deaths resulting from a fire in a public building. Inquiries revealed that 16 persons had died from that fire, 15 between 15–74 years of age being residents of the city. This was consistent with the sampling factor of 1 in 3 being used in San Francisco. Other checks were provided by the fact that in any one city the numbers of deaths having a given characteristic should be approximately the same in the material of the first 12 months as in that of the second 12 months of the study period. For example, when the numbers of widowed males in the samples of the two separate years were compared, in no city did the number in the first year differ from the number in the second year to a greater extent than would have occurred as the result of random fluctuation.

Field Inquiries

During the house visit, the public health nurse or social worker not only confirmed the age and residence status of the deceased but also obtained information concerning the place of birth, the residence history, the occupations engaged in by the deceased, and the dates and places where medical attention had been given, both recently and in the past. The last items of information served as points of departure for the investigating physicians, who assembled the available clinical information relevant to establishing the cause of death. Hospital records were traced and surgical and autopsy findings were recorded, together with the results of ancillary studies such as laboratory investigations, radiology, and electrocardiography. Physicians having knowledge of the patient were interviewed. When the home visit proved unproductive for the nurse or social worker, the interviewing physician had an alternative point of departure, namely, the physician who had signed the death certificate. If death had occurred in a hospital, the record department was often the best place to start making inquiries.

Not surprisingly, the degree of success attending these efforts varied from city to city according to the nature and variety of the obstacles that had to be overcome. The home visitor had many problems. Repeated visits were often needed before a relative could be found at home. The general rule was that, if necessary, three attempts would be made to interview a likely informant. In Caracas, although deaths to be investigated were selected within one week of registration, the first home visit was frequently unsuccessful because the family had already moved to another address in accordance with an old custom. Sometimes a neighbor knew the new address, but often no trace of a relative could be found despite persistent inquiries. In the poorer quarters of some cities houses are numbered somewhat haphazardly, and it was therefore not uncommon to find houses with more than one number on the door, some of the numbers having been added by census enumerators or mosquito-spraying squads. The pertinacity of the home visitors deserves high praise.

The problems which the interviewing physician encountered depended on whether the deceased had been a patient in a hospital. If not, every effort had to be made to locate and interview a physician having knowledge of the patient. The only exceptions made were in cases in which an autopsy had established the cause of death with certainty. Finding the physician and arranging an interview sometimes proved difficult and occasionally, as when he had departed for a trip abroad, impossible. Usually the physician could produce written laboratory, radiology, and pathology reports whenever such investigations had been performed; but the doctor in private practice who kept very good clinical notes was the exception, and there were some who did not keep any. Sometimes the interviewing physician gained the impression at the interview that the clinical information was unreliable, and he indicated this when completing the questionnaire. The records of patients known to have been in a hospital, or even to have died there, were sometimes misplaced. Although records in many hospitals in several cities were of a high standard, inadequate hospital records were encountered also. In one city an immediate overhaul of the record system in a large hospital was ordered when the principal collaborator complained that no records could be traced for some of the first deaths selected for study.

When the medical and other data had been assembled, the principal collaborator summarized the findings and expressed his opinion as to the cause of death. Two copies of the completed questionnaire, together with a photocopy of the original death certificate, were then sent to the central office of the Pan American Health Organization, in Washington. Originally, a period of three months after the end of the study period was allowed for completion of the questionnaires. This time lapse proved adequate on the whole, but in all cities delays of one kind or another occurred, the most frequent having to do with reports on histological sections. The last questionnaires were received in the central office early in September 1965, 11 months after the study period had terminated in all cities. No questionnaires were lost.

Central Review Procedure

The ultimate object of the central review was the assignment of causes of death in a uniform manner for all cities, and to this end the first step consisted in dividing the questionnaires into two classes according to whether they were to be referred to the medical referees. In either case, however, all questionnaires were scrutinized by a physician, and inquiries were sent to the principal collaborator whenever an item of information required clarification or amplification. Most of this work was done by two members of the staff,[2] who in the initial stages standardized their interpretation of the criteria for referral.

Every questionnaire falling into one of the three groups listed below, eventually numbering 21 021, or 48.5 percent of the total, were studied by both medical referees, Dr. Darío Curiel and Dr. Percy Stocks, who had long experience as directors of international centers for the classification of diseases, Dr. Curiel at the Latin American Center in Caracas and Dr. Stocks at the WHO Center in London. In selecting the underlying cause of death, the medical referees took into account all information supplementing the death certificate and adhered as far as possible to the principles followed in the rules for coding death certificates as given in the *International Classification of Diseases*. For example, "mention" of a morbid condition was taken to include a well-supported statement of its presence in a hospital or autopsy record. Certain supplementary rules were developed by the referees during the pilot study, after reviewing 275 questionnaires separately and making a joint examination of the discrepancies that were found. In order to familiarize themselves further with the material, the medical referees reviewed all of the early questionnaires from several cities without preliminary sorting, and this afforded them a second opportunity to consult on their decisions. From this point on, however, they worked completely independently, so as to obviate the possibility of influencing each other's judgment.

The three groups of questionnaires on which the medical referees worked throughout were:

1. Those in which the cause of death appeared to be a condition involving the heart and circulatory system (Categories 022, 023, 330–334, 400–468, 754, of the *International Classification of Diseases*).
2. Those in which more than one cause of death appeared to be involved in the fatal sequence of events.
3. Those in which the cause of death seemed to be an ill-defined condition (Categories 780–795).

There was no difficulty in deciding which questionnaires should be seen by the medical referees, because in case of doubt the invariable rule was to refer them.

Questionnaires relating to deaths the cause of which was not in doubt were not reviewed by the medical referees (unless death was due to a cardiovascular condition). These questionnaires related to deaths from violent causes, from malignant neoplasms, from maternal causes, and from specific infections such as tuberculosis, as well as deaths from other conditions presenting a well-defined clinical picture. The assignment of the underlying cause of death was made in the central office by the reviewing physicians, and the category numbers were added by expert coders in accordance with the rules of the *International Classification of Diseases*. To ensure uniformity, these coders also assigned the category numbers of the causes of death as stated on the original death certificates accompanying all questionnaires.

For deaths from each city there were therefore at least two assignments of cause of death coded in terms of the full four-digit categories of the *International Classification of Diseases*. One was the cause of death according to the death certificate, coded by the expert coders. The other was the cause of death "on final assignment," selected by the medical referees or by the reviewing physician without reference to them. In addition, for all cities except two there was available the original coding of the death certificate made in the city concerned. On questionnaires from Cali and Guatemala City this latter coding was missing, since the inclusion of the local coding would have caused unacceptable delay. For all cities the coding of the death certificates in the central office could be compared with the coding of causes given on final assignment in the light of the information assembled by the field workers, while for 10 cities another useful comparison was possible, i.e.,

[2] Dr. Gertrud Weiss Szilard and Dr. G. Wynne Griffith, assisted for a period by Dr. Carlos Ferrero.

the local codings and those made in the central office from the same death certificates.[3]

Use of Weights in the Assignment of Causes of Death

The design of the study has an unusual feature in that a weighting system, devised by Dr. Percy Stocks, was used in the final assignment of causes of death. In the original planning undertaken by the Working Group in April 1961, the method of assignment of the underlying cause of death by medical referees received considerable attention. Although it would have been simpler to have only one person assign the underlying causes of death, this was undesirable because of the possibility that he might be unable to finish the whole series, in which event the work already done would have to be repeated by another referee replacing him. With two referees, should one fail to finish the series, it would be possible to fall back on the findings of the other. Having more than two referees, though theoretically desirable, was not practical in terms of time and cost. Fortunately, both Dr. Darío Curiel and Dr. Stocks, who in 1961 agreed to undertake the assignment, were able to complete the enormous task of reviewing some 20 000 questionnaires during the years 1962–1965.

Some arrangement was needed to combine the separate decisions of the two referees. A method commonly used is to accept agreed opinions and to have the referees discuss any disagreements, with or without a third expert. This method, which has been applied to several problems such as the interpretation of X rays, has frequently proved unsatisfactory, the end result often depending on the relative powers of

persuasion and endurance of the individuals concerned.

For the present project, involving perhaps thousands of deaths on which the referees might not agree precisely, resolution of these differing judgments by discussion was ruled out because of the cost. A method of arriving at an answer by statistical weighting of the two opinions was considered more practicable and economical, as well as better suited to the problem of choosing the underlying cause. It was recognized that the selection of a single cause of death might not always be possible, or even appropriate, where several potentially fatal pathological processes were found to coexist, particularly where the available evidence was ambiguous with respect to the terminal events. The referee's opinions would, therefore, be of two kinds. On some deaths he would have no doubt as to his choice; on others, however, he would be hesitant to make a definite choice among several alternatives, preferring to decide upon one cause as the most likely and a second as the less likely. The weighting system would take into account both the most likely and the less likely causes and yet distinguish between them. To that end, the referee would give a weight of 3 to the cause whenever he had no doubt; if he was not prepared to select a single cause, he would give a weight of 2 to the cause he considered most likely and a weight of 1 to the less likely cause.

On any given questionnaire, the two referees might agree on a single cause, in which case each referee would allot a weight of 3 to the same cause, giving it a total weight of 6; at the other extreme, if the referees differed in their selection of both the most likely and the less likely causes, as many as four separate causes might be assigned to a given death. There are a number of intermediate possibilities: for example, both referees might allot a weight of 2 to the same most likely cause, giving it a total weight of 4, but they might assign two different less likely causes, each of which would therefore have a weight of 1.

Whenever the referees did not see the questionnaires only one cause of death was involved, and this cause was always given a weight of 6. For deaths in a given city, in a given age group, or in any other group under consideration, the total weights assigned to each cause, aggregated and divided by 6, gave the "weighted" number of deaths from that cause in that group.

---

[3] One other use of the dual codings of death certificates should be mentioned. Death certificates from Bristol had been coded both in the General Register Office in London and by coders from the National Center for Health Statistics in Washington. These dual codings were compared to see whether the rules for selecting the underlying cause of death were being similarly interpreted in the two countries. A high degree of concordance was found, the codes being identical to the fourth digit in 94.5 percent of 3213 dual codings. For several important causes of death, including diabetes, lung cancer, arteriosclerotic heart disease, and bronchitis, the few disagreements that occurred would have had a negligible effect on death rates based on the certificates. Relatively more frequent were disagreements as to the interpretation of ambiguous statements on certificates where external causes were involved. Conventions to deal with these apparently differed, and death rates from accidents (other than motor vehicle accidents) and suicide would have varied by 10 percent or more, depending on which office coded the certificates.

The operation of this weighting system is in itself of considerable interest and is evaluated at length in Chapter XVI.[4] At this point, however, it might be well to stress two consequences of the system. First, in relation to any given cause (for example, the deaths assigned to tuberculosis of males in a certain city), the weighted deaths will not necessarily be an integral number, though the sum of all the weighted deaths from all the causes mentioned on final assignment in the questionnaires involved will of course be integral and equal to the number of deaths in the group. Weighted deaths by causes (to one decimal place) have always been used in calculating death rates. In the text, however, for the sake of simplicity in presentation, the weighted deaths by cause are generally shown to the nearest integer. Rounding to the nearest integer produces slight inconsistencies in some of the totals.

A second consequence of the weighting system is that the number of weighted deaths from a given cause is not always the same as the number of questionnaires in which that cause was mentioned on final assignment. Therefore, when it was necessary to relate deaths by cause to some unitary attribute, for example, civil status or occupation, depending on the cause under consideration, one of two courses was followed. The first procedure was to regard all deaths with specified weights to a given cause, as if that were the only cause involved. This was appropriate for those causes which in practice had usually been assigned alone (with a weight of 6) or assigned as the most likely cause in the joint opinion of the medical referees (with weights of 4 or 5). However, considering those causes which were often assigned as less likely ones (with weights of 3, 2, or 1), the attributes need to be weighted the same as the causes, to avoid distortion. The procedure is explained in Appendix 5.[5] In decisions on which course to use in analyses involving unitary attributes, the need to present the data clearly and simply had to be balanced against the risk of apparent inconsistencies, but the choice was governed also by the way in which the weighting system operated so far as the cause in question was concerned.

Estimates of the Populations at Risk

In each of the 12 cities a recent census was held, the dates varying between 1 April 1960 (San Francisco) to 15 July 1964 (Bogotá and Cali). Complete enumerations, by age and sex, from the latest census were obtained for all cities except Guatemala City, where the data presently available comprise a 5 percent sample of the population of the city as taken from the national census of April 1964. Through the use of the most recent enumeration and those of the preceding census, an estimate assuming a logarithmic rate of change was made of the population, by age and sex, at the midpoint of the study period in each city. These estimates are given in Appendix 6.[6] In the United States census of 1960, the population was enumerated by place of usual residence. All of the other censuses were *de facto* enumerations, and rates based on these denominators may therefore tend to underestimate the mortality of the city's residents to the extent that persons not normally resident in the area were included in the census. For some cities the effect of the resulting error on the death rate is known to be negligible, and in all instances it is certainly smaller than the effect of errors from other sources to which all census enumerations are liable.

Since the study period extended over two years, the effective population at risk for computing annual rates was twice the estimated population at the midpoint of the study period in those cities (Cali, Guatemala City, La Plata, and Ribeirão Prêto) where all deaths of residents were included. In the other eight cities allowance was made also for the fact that a sample of deaths was selected for study. The effective populations of each city by age and sex (Appendix 7),[7] used as denominators with the deaths occurring in the two-year period as numerators, give the annual death rates used in the analyses.

Standard Population

Where the structure of populations by age and sex differs widely, as in these 12 cities, comparisons of mortality are best made in separate age-sex groups. This procedure was followed whenever the numbers of deaths were

---

[4] Not included in this publication.
[5] Not included in this publication.

[6] Not included in this publication.
[7] Not included in this publication.

large enough to give reasonably stable rates. For many of the more detailed comparisons, however, inferences can be drawn more easily from the consolidated experience of the 60-year age span expressed as age-adjusted rates. Age-adjusted death rates have been calculated by the direct method, i.e., by applying the age-specific rates in each city to a standard population (Appendix 8)[8] obtained from the aggregated population of the cities in six 10-year age groups from the recent censuses. The results of the 1964 census for Guatemala City were not available until later and therefore could not be included.

The limitations of an age-adjusted rate are recognized. While such a rate has the advantage of being easier to comprehend than a set of age-specific rates, it is a fictional figure, as pointed out by Hill (1), devoid of any inherent meaning but useful because "it enables summary comparisons to be made between places . . . free from the distortion which arises from age and sex differences. . . . "

The basic data are provided in the Appendix tables,[9] so that comparisons using other methods of standardization, such as those summarized by Kitagawa (2), may be made if desired.

Statistical Interpretation

Although efforts have been made in every phase of the Investigation to ensure that the data are as accurate as possible, many of the observed differences in mortality must be interpreted with caution. The population estimates used as denominators for the age-specific rates are, so far as can be determined, the best available. But these may be subject to error. Review of the census returns for one city, for example, revealed that the exact year of age was not always known. The numbers of deaths by cause have been derived through a complicated process from which all known errors have likewise been eliminated, but it would be presumptuous to claim that the numerators of the death rates, any more than the denominators, are free from all error. Variations due to chance may assume serious proportions when rates are based on small numbers of deaths. In applying tests of statistical significance to assess the observed differences in death rates, the procedure suggested by Haenszel (3) has been found useful. The terms "significant" and "highly significant" imply that the 0.05 and 0.01 levels of probability, respectively, have been attained. With many hundreds of comparisons, a certain number must be expected to emerge as statistically significant at the given level of probability. For this reason, also, interpretation should be guarded. As will become apparent, however, the differences in mortality revealed by the Investigation were often so large that neither variations due to chance nor errors inherent in the material could reasonably account for them.

CHANGES IN ASSIGNMENT OF CAUSES: SUMMARY[10]

The deaths excluded from a broad group of causes as a result of the acquisition of detailed histories of fatal illnesses often tend to be counterbalanced by the deaths added. Thus, the effect on death rates resulting from the use of available clinical and laboratory information, in addition to the information on the death certificate, is in most instances small. For the 12 cities combined, the group of infective and parasitic diseases was increased by 5 percent, and tuberculosis, the main cause within this group, by 6 percent. The upward change in deaths from malignant neoplasms was likewise 5 percent. Diseases of the cardiovascular system decreased by 1 percent, of the respiratory system by 13 percent, and of the digestive system by 6 percent. A relatively larger number of deaths was added to maternal causes (35 percent), but deaths from accidents and violence were only 2 percent greater as a result of the Investigation.

For most cities, official death rates from broad groups of causes are probably acceptable indicators of health problems. However, for epidemiological purposes their value is more limited since even when the differences between the numbers of original and final assignments were small, changes between the two assignments involved relatively many deaths. The number of exclusions of deaths originally classified to a group, combined with the number of additions, often tends to be large in relation to the number of final assignments. Table 1 shows the percentage excess or deficit in the number

---

[8] Not included in this publication.
[9] Not included in this publication.

[10] Chapter XV of this work was prepared by Mary H. Burke.

Table 1. Number of deaths with a change in classification between original and final assignments per 100 final assignments for eight groups of diseases at ages 15–74 years, in each city, 1962–1964.

City	Infective and parasitic diseases		Malignant neoplasms		Cardiovascular diseases		Respiratory diseases		Diseases of digestive system		Maternal causes		Accidents and violence		Other causes	
	Excess or deficit	Total changes[a]	Excess or deficit	Total changes[a]	Excess or deficit	Total changes[a]	Excess or deficit	Total changes[a]	Excess or deficit	Total changes[a]	Excess or deficit	Total changes[a]	Excess or deficit	Total changes[a]	Excess or deficit	Total changes[a]
12 cities	-4.8	37.1	-4.3	11.9	0.7	27.0	15.1	68.0	6.3	42.9	-25.7	33.8	-2.3	11.7	0.7	96.1
Bogotá	-1.6	36.3	-3.3	9.8	3.6	30.5	8.5	67.5	-2.5	39.1	-37.3	39.5	-7.7	14.5	7.7	98.1
Bristol	-30.8	70.7	-6.7	9.4	5.6	15.0	3.4	40.4	-7.4	32.1	-50.0	50.0	-0.1	5.3	-9.2	78.9
Cali	2.6	42.1	-4.9	14.8	-0.6	39.5	0.5	88.9	3.4	57.7	-20.4	37.1	-0.6	12.0	10.3	123.5
Caracas	-1.9	42.4	-2.5	9.5	4.8	23.8	10.9	63.8	-0.9	49.8	-26.9	29.9	-2.6	7.3	-3.4	72.2
Guatemala City	-12.2	54.3	-14.4	31.4	-11.7	53.5	86.5	163.7	103.4	159.9	-32.6	40.1	1.0	7.4	-28.0	97.4
La Plata	-19.9	47.0	-3.2	5.9	-0.8	24.4	-3.7	57.5	-7.4	26.2	-33.0	33.0	-0.6	9.9	23.3	107.7
Lima	-2.0	18.0	-2.1	10.7	-7.4	26.9	37.0	65.9	2.6	29.1	-28.2	32.3	-0.6	7.8	10.7	87.1
Mexico City	-8.0	46.7	-6.4	15.6	-8.3	39.7	18.0	75.3	-1.7	32.5	-31.6	38.7	-17.0	44.3	21.5	96.0
Ribeirão Prêto	4.1	26.6	-8.0	13.7	-3.6	33.8	28.1	67.9	-0.4	53.8	-9.1	20.0	-3.6	11.9	7.0	97.9
San Francisco	-17.8	55.2	-5.1	7.9	6.2	17.9	33.6	72.0	-10.4	26.0	—	—	1.3	12.4	-18.9	89.8
Santiago	0.4	37.9	0.1	15.9	-1.7	29.2	13.8	64.0	0.0	23.0	-6.5	19.9	-2.2	17.0	-3.3	101.3
São Paulo	-14.5	35.8	-0.5	9.5	4.7	32.9	2.1	73.9	-3.9	42.0	-33.9	48.8	-7.6	12.9	1.6	94.8

[a] Exclusions and additions.

230

of deaths originally classified to each broad group in relation to the final assignments. For each of the same broad groups a second column in the table shows the number of changes involved per 100 final assignments, that is, the number of deaths which were in the group on either the original or the final assignment but not on both. For broad groups of causes these changes are numerous despite relatively small net increases or decreases.

Of the seven main groups shown, the largest understatement on the original classification was for maternal causes (26 percent). Respiratory diseases were not only overstated by the highest percentage (15) but they also involved the largest number of individual changes. For every 100 deaths finally assigned to the group there were 68 deaths which were in the group on only one classification, either the original or the final one. The number of changes in the group, other causes, is not comparable with those for the other groups, since a change in the former implies transfers into or out of single divisions of the group and not just between broad groups.

For the individual divisions of the broad groups far more changes occur with the use of the additional information, with less tendency toward counterbalancing. For example, the large increases in the specific forms of cardiovascular diseases (such as hypertensive and rheumatic heart diseases) and in malignant neoplasms (such as those of the cervix uteri) have previously been discussed. Clearly, death rates from defined causes were appreciably affected in many cities, and the total numbers of deaths involving changes were large.

The data presented in this chapter will be analyzed in a later report in relation to age, sex, autopsy, medical attention which the deceased received, and diagnostic procedures employed. The relationship of sudden death to causes also needs to be studied with respect to these factors. For example, for arteriosclerotic heart disease changes between original and final classifications are more numerous with increasing age and for females. Study of the material in greater depth is essential.

Only a limited number of studies have attempted to assess the reliability of medical certification of cause of death. In general, they have been studies of deaths with autopsy or of persons hospitalized during the final illness. The information assembled in this present Investigation should provide a broader view of the reliability of medical certification under differing circumstances. Comparisons with data from other studies is difficult because of variations in their design, in selection of populations, and in the criteria and methodology employed.

Moriyama et al. (4) studied a sample of deaths in Pennsylvania in 1956, querying the physicians who had signed the death certificates as to the diagnostic methods on which medical classification was based, their estimate of the certainty of diagnoses entered, and the need for revision of the medical certification. On the basis of the diagnostic evidence, the deaths in the sample were divided into four groups: (1) the death certificate provided the most probable diagnosis; (2) there was another equally probable diagnosis; (3) another diagnosis was preferred; and (4) there was no diagnostic information.

In Table 2 the agreement with the death certificate information (using categories 1 and 2, above, to signify agreement) is shown for selected causes. Also presented is the agreement between original and final assignments for San Francisco, Bristol, and the combined experience of the 10 Latin American cities. The criteria for agreement certainly differ, but the similarities by cause are apparent.

A report on the accuracy of certification has been made for England and Wales (5). In 75 hospitals a clinician who had been in close contact with the case completed a special death certificate for each death. The clinician also indicated whether the recorded cause of death was "fairly certain," "probable," or "uncertain." Following autopsy the pathologist also completed a death certificate, taking into account clinical and pathological findings. Both forms were coded in the General Register Office. The two were considered to agree if the same four-digit category of the *International Classification of Diseases* was coded for both certificates. By this stringent standard, only for 45 percent of the 9501 deaths studied was there agreement. However, for broad groups the agreement was much better and corresponded to other studies. The accuracy of medical certification was found to decrease with increasing age but not the accuracy of death rates by causes, since errors often canceled each other out. The net effect of changes produced by autopsy on mortality statistics for broad groups of diseases is compared with the present Investigation in Table 3.

A recent study (6) of deaths in Baltimore, Maryland, attempts to measure the quality of medical certification of arteriosclerotic heart disease. A stratified sample (1857 deaths) of all deaths from nontraumatic causes among residents 20-64 years of age was selected and detailed information was obtained for deaths occurring in Baltimore City. Of 478 death certificates which gave arteriosclerotic heart disease as the underlying cause of death, 26 were

Table 2. Percentage agreement of reviewers with assignment of cause from information on death certificates in a study of a sample of deaths from Pennsylvania, 1956, and in the Inter-American Investigation of Mortality, 1962–1964.

| | Pennsylvania sample[a] | | Inter-American Investigation of Mortality | | | | | |
| | | | San Francisco | | Bristol | | 10 Latin American cities | |
Cause of death	Total death certificates	Most probable diagnosis (percentage)	Death certificates	Percentage agreement	Death certificates	Percentage agreement	Death certificates	Percentage agreement
Total	2122	78.7	3865	71.4	4262	78.4	34 521	64.0
Tuberculosis (001–019)	27	85.2	39	92.3	21	81.9	1961	89.3
Malignant neoplasms (140–205)	443	85.8	809	89.1	1043	88.4	6572	77.4
Stomach and large intestine (151, 153)	120	83.3	125	95.8	174	88.4	1556	84.9
Rectum (154)	26	88.5	33	91.5	62	87.1	132	88.2
Biliary passages and liver (155)	13	92.3	11	100.0	2	50.0	86	64.3
Pancreas (157)	16	68.8	46	90.7	36	91.7	214	79.9
Larynx (161)	4	100.0	7	97.1	8	75.0	99	87.9
Trachea, bronchus, and lung (162, 163)	54	87.0	157	97.2	267	97.3	649	89.0
Breast (170)	32	93.8	72	95.8	123	98.4	429	99.0
Uterus (171–174)	28	96.4	37	98.6	34	91.2	810	95.5
Male genital organs (177–179)	21	90.5	26	88.5	32	84.4	125	82.6
Urinary organs (180, 181)	16	100.0	37	93.8	46	91.1	211	89.5
Leukemia and aleukemia (204)	13	100.0	28	96.4	25	88.0	229	88.7
Lymphomas (200–203, 205)	15	100.0	46	89.1	33	90.0	237	89.9
Diabetes mellitus (260)	61	86.9	52	62.7	36	71.7	999	74.5
Major cardiovascular-renal diseases	1406	78.2	1748[b]	71.3	2072[b]	76.9	10 155[b]	64.0
Vascular lesions affecting central nervous system (330–334)	254	85.0	279	77.1	507	90.0	2774	86.0
Rheumatic fever and rheumatic heart disease (400–416)	41	82.9	46	87.4	88	85.5	664	80.0
Arteriosclerotic heart disease (420)	692	78.6	1138	82.7	957	89.6	2740	81.3
Other heart diseases except hypertension (421, 422, 430–434)	167	66.5	72	32.4	193	33.4	1829	43.2
Hypertensive diseases (440–447)	150	76.0	213[c]	63.5	327[c]	51.3	2146[c]	50.5
Influenza and pneumonia (480–493)	31	64.5	97	41.0	165	35.7	1139	49.3

[a] Moriyama et al. (4).
[b] Cardiovascular diseases only.
[c] Hypertensive diseases and other circulatory disorders.

Table 3. Increase in deaths assigned to selected causes as result of autopsy findings in England and Wales[a] and on review of additional information in Bristol and San Francisco, 1962–1964.

	England and Wales			Bristol			San Francisco		
	Deaths assigned			Deaths assigned			Deaths assigned		
Cause of death	Before autopsy	After autopsy	Percentage change	From death certificate	Final review	Percentage change	From death certificate	Final review	Percentage change
Tuberculosis (001-019)	58	95	63.8	21	32	52.4	39	50	28.2
Syphilis (020-027)	31	31	—	8	10	25.0	9	13	44.4
Malignant neoplasms (140-205)	2283	2378	4.2	1043	1118	7.2	809	853	5.4
Stomach (151)	253	234	−7.5	115	129	12.2	52	60	15.4
Large intestine and rectum (153, 154)	288	264	−8.3	121	127	5.0	106	113	6.6
Biliary passages and liver (155)	28	69	146.4	2	4	100.0	11	14	27.3
Trachea, bronchus, and lung (162, 163)	450	534	18.7	267	294	10.1	157	171	8.9
Lymphoma and lympho-sarcoma (200-203, 205)	136	166	22.1	33	42	27.3	46	46	—
Leukemia (204)	153	147	−3.9	25	23	−8.0	28	30	7.1
Diabetes mellitus (260)	94	69	−26.6	36	46	27.8	52	62	19.2
Vascular lesions affecting central nervous system (330-334)	1096	886	−19.2	507	526	3.7	279	312	11.8
Rheumatic fever and rheumatic heart disease (400-416)	179	236	31.8	88	97	10.2	46	59	28.3
Arteriosclerotic heart disease (420)	995	1065	7.0	957	986	3.0	1138	1001	−12.0
Hypertensive heart disease (440-443)	103	160	55.3	140	125	−10.7	87	76	−12.6
Hypertension and other circulatory diseases (444-468)	455	504	10.8	187	120	−35.8	126	144	14.3
Influenza and pneumonia (480-493)	504	399	−20.8	165	71	−57.0	97	54	−44.3
Bronchitis (500-502)	217	324	49.3	294	369	25.5	15	30	100.0
Ulcer of stomach and duodenum (540, 541)	210	257	22.4	40	41	2.5	35	40	14.3

[a] Heasman and Lipworth (5).

excluded on review. Of these, 19 were reassigned to cerebrovascular disease and 7 to other causes. Supporting evidence consisted of autopsy, history of arteriosclerotic heart disease, or sudden death. Of the 488 deaths finally attributed to arteriosclerotic heart disease, autopsies had been performed for 126, electrocardiograms had been abnormal for 63, there was a history of arteriosclerotic heart disease for 213, sudden deaths without such a history accounted for 55, and there were 31 other deaths without such evidence. Of those 488 deaths, 452, or 93 percent, had been originally classified from the death certificate to the same category. Twenty-two deaths had been originally assigned to diabetes and a few to other diseases. The type of supporting evidence accepted in this study may account for the higher degree of agreement than in the present Investigation.

The effects of obtaining additional clinical and laboratory information on the fatal illness varied in magnitude in the cities of the study. In every city it is clear that medical certification can be improved, and the desirability of devising a record-linkage system to ensure the use of available hospital and autopsy information is likewise evident.

References

(1) Hill, A.B. *Principles of Medical Statistics.* 2nd Ed. London, The Lancet Limited, 1939.

(2) Kitagawa, E.M. Standardized comparisons in

population research. *Demography* 1:296-315, 1964.

(*3*) Haenszel, W., D.B. Loveland, and M.G. Sirken. Lung-cancer mortality as related to residence and smoking histories. I. White males. *J Nat Cancer Inst* 28:947-1001, 1962.

(*4*) Moriyama, I.M., W.S. Baum, W.M. Haenszel, and B.F. Mattison. Inquiry into diagnostic evidence supporting medical certifications of death. *Amer J Public Health* 48:1376-1387, 1958.

(*5*) Heasman, M.A. and L. Lipworth. *Accuracy of Certification of Cause of Death*. General Register Office, Studies on Medical Population Subjects, No. 20. London, H.M.S.O., 1966.

(*6*) Kuller, L., A. Lilienfeld, and R. Fisher. Quality of death certificate diagnosis of arteriosclerotic heart disease. *Public Health Rep* 82:339-346, 1967.

A SINGLE INDEX OF MORTALITY AND MORBIDITY

Daniel F. Sullivan[1]

A continuing interest of the National Center for Health Statistics is the development and evaluation of new health indices suited to diverse specific purposes. No one index can reflect all aspects of health, but there is considerable agreement that an index which measures some aspects of nonfatal illness as well as mortality would be desirable. A rationale for using both mortality and disability rates as the components of such an index has already been published (1).

One technique for combining mortality and morbidity rates into a single index was devised and reported by Chiang in conjunction with his development of mathematical models of illness frequency, illness duration, and mortality (2). Moriyama has discussed criteria desired in an index of health and, in view of these, reviewed some approaches proposed in the literature (3). A description and evaluation of disability concepts and measures being considered as the basis of the morbidity component of a mortality-morbidity index appeared in a recent report (4).

Another technique for merging death rates with illness rates and some illustrative results are described in this paper. A primary objective of these studies is the development of a summary measure which reflects changes over time in the health status of the nation's population. Too little is known as yet about these techniques, and in some cases about the data they employ, to permit thorough evaluation of alternative approaches to the construction of such indices. Results of studies of such measures are presented as they become available by the Center to stimulate consideration of the issues and, possibly, to stimulate further studies by those in a position to conduct related research.

Some preliminary index values based upon the techniques presented in this paper have already been published for fiscal years 1958-66

(5). The estimates in this article are also preliminary. Although they relate to only a single year, they provide previously unpublished information on whites and other persons and on sex differences. These estimates are considered more accurate than earlier computations of such values.

Results

The two related indices described in this paper are based upon a life table model. They are (a) the expectation of life free of disability and (b) the expectation of disability. Either of these measures can be calculated using various definitions of disability, and values of each index based on two alternative definitions of disability will be presented and compared.

The techniques employ a relatively simple modification of the conventional life table model to compute the expected duration of certain defined conditions of interest among the living population. Somewhat similar methods have been employed to compute expected values for conditions such as labor force participation and school enrollment (6, 7). In those applications, current mortality rates, summarized in the life table values, were combined with survey-based rates for events among the living population to produce potentially valuable measures not otherwise obtainable. Calculation of a summary measure of health status in a somewhat similar fashion was once suggested in a paper by Sanders, but the more elaborate health measures which his proposal required have not yet been developed (8).

The expectations of life and of disability presented in this paper are hypothetical values derived from a period life table. They are the values which would occur if a birth cohort of fixed size experienced, age for age throughout life, the recent age-specific mortality and disability rates used in these life table calculations. Since the age-specific rates may change considerably over the lifespan of any real birth cohort, expectations based on a period life table may

Source: *Public Health Reports* 86(4):347-354, 1971.
[1] Statistician, Office of Health Statistics Analysis, National Center for Health Statistics, Health Services and Mental Health Administration. Rockville, MD.

not reflect accurately the life experience of infants born in any specific period. Hence, these measures are intended primarily as an index for comparing the mortality-morbidity experience of different population groups and should not be construed as projections or forecasts. Methods of computing these measures are described in a subsequent section.

The modified life tables provide values of the expectation of life which omit time lost to disability. In one version of these tables, disability was defined broadly as institutional confinement for health care, prolonged incapacitation that does not include institutional care, and short-term episodes of restriction on a person's usual activities (Table 1). An alternative version eliminates only the lifetime duration of periods of bed disability (Table 2). Bed disability in this paper includes any periods spent in hospitals or other institutions for health care and also days of noninstitutional illness involving confinement to bed for more than half the daylight hours. Whichever definition is used, elimina-

Table 1. Expectations of life and approximate expectations of life free of disability and of disability, for whites and other persons by sex, at birth and at age 65, civilian resident population, United States, mid-1960s.

Color and sex	Expectation		
	Life (1965 U.S. abridged life tables)	Life free of disability	Disability
	Years at birth		
All persons	70.2	64.9	5.3
Male	66.8	61.6	5.2
Female	73.7	68.4	5.3
White	71.0	65.8	5.2
Male	67.6	62.5	5.1
Female	74.7	69.4	5.3
All other persons	64.1	58.2	5.9
Male	61.1	55.1	6.0
Female	67.4	61.4	6.0
	Years at age 65		
All persons	14.6	11.3	3.3
Male	12.9	9.4	3.5
Female	16.2	13.1	3.1
White	14.6	11.5	3.1
Male	12.9	9.5	3.4
Female	16.3	13.3	3.0
All other persons	14.0	9.3	4.7
Male	12.6	7.5	5.1
Female	15.5	11.2	4.3

Table 2. Expectations of life and approximate expectations of life free of bed disability and of bed disability, for whites and other persons by sex, at birth and at age 65, civilian resident population, United States, mid-1960s.

Color and sex	Expectation		
	Life (1965 U.S. abridged life tables)	Life free of bed disability	Disability
	Years at birth		
All persons	70.2	68.2	2.0
Male	66.8	65.2	1.6
Female	73.7	71.4	2.3
White	71.0	69.1	1.9
Male	67.6	66.1	1.5
Female	74.7	72.4	2.3
All other persons	64.1	62.3	1.8
Male	61.1	59.5	1.6
Female	67.4	65.2	2.2
	Years at age 65		
All persons	14.6	13.5	1.1
Male	12.9	12.1	.8
Female	16.2	14.9	1.3
White	14.6	13.6	1.0
Male	12.9	12.1	.8
Female	16.3	15.0	1.3
All other persons	14.0	13.0	1.0
Male	12.6	11.7	.9
Female	15.5	14.3	1.2

tion of disability periods has a substantial effect on the expectation of life. Possibly more striking is the average amount of time lost to disability among members of the hypothetical life table population.

Although the conventional expectation of life in the United States now exceeds 70 years, the expected duration of disability-free life is not quite 65 years (Table 1). The difference between these two figures is the expectation of disability, approximately five years. Illness of the aged contributes heavily, as the expectation of more than three years of disability at age 65 indicates, but it is not the sole determinant. Younger age groups account for the difference of two years between expectation of disability at birth and that at age 65.

Using a less comprehensive definition of disability and discounting only the lifetime duration of days of bed disability changes the magnitude of these figures, but the results are still noteworthy. Expectation of life free of bed disability is about 68 years at birth, and the expectation of bed disability is approximately 2 years (Table 2). Again the relatively large cumulative impact of bed disability among younger persons can be detected by comparing the expectation of two years of bed disability at birth with the corresponding expectation of just over one year at age 65.

Although persons who survive to age 65 have a further life expectancy of almost 15 years, their prospects are somewhat dimmed by the fact that these 15 years can include more than 3 years of disability and more than a year of bed disability.

Sex differentials. Sex differentials in the expectation of life free of disability and the expectation of life free of bed disability are determined primarily by the large and well-known sex differences that exist in conventional life expectancies. Using any one of these three measures, the expectations for males are much shorter than those for females, both at birth and at age 65 (Tables 1, 2; Figure 1). Both white and other males face unfavorable prospects when compared with their female counterparts in terms of these life expectancies.

When the expectations of disability and of bed disability are considered, however, most of the sex differentials favor males (Tables 1, 2; Figure 2). Within both white and other groups, males have lower expectations of bed disability than females at birth and at age 65. White males also have lower expectations of all forms of disability at birth than do white females. Expectations of disability are equal at birth for all other males and females. Of the data given in this paper, only the expectations of disability at age 65 are consistently favorable for females.

These sex differentials need to be interpreted with considerable caution. In the surveys which

Figure 1. Approximate expectations of life free of disability and life free of bed disability for whites and other persons by sex, United States, mid-1960s.

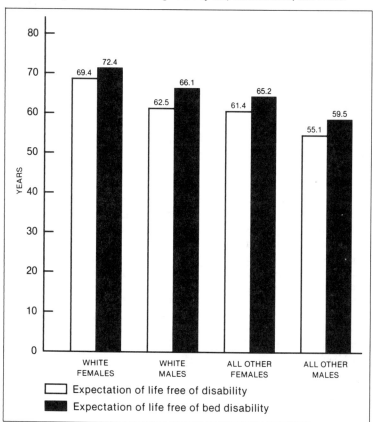

Figure 2. Approximate expectations of disability and of bed disability for whites and other persons by sex, United States, mid-1960s.

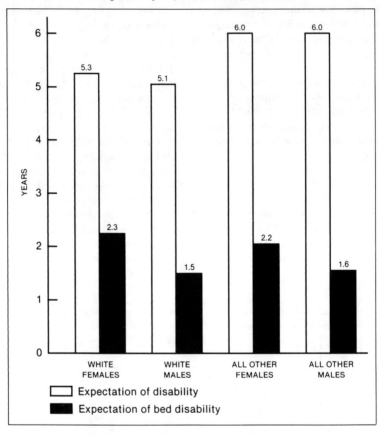

produced the data underlying these estimates, different definitions were used to determine the existence of chronic disability among men and among women. The nature of these differences and their possible consequences have been discussed extensively elsewhere (*4, 9*). In this paper, it seems sufficient to note the existence of these differences and to point out that they would affect the expectations of disability but not the expectations of bed disability. Expectations of bed disability favor males both at birth and at age 65. Pregnancy accounts for some but not all of the excess bed disability among females at younger ages. Consequently, it seems reasonable to conclude that bed disability, at least, imposes a heavier burden upon women throughout life.

Whites compared with other persons. Differences between whites and other persons in the expec-

tations of life free of disability and expectations of life free of bed disability are also largely a result of differences in conventional life expectancies. For each of these measures, expectations at birth for persons other than white are substantially less than for whites, and similar differences are observed among both males and females (Tables 1, 2).

At 65, differences between whites and other groups are numerically much smaller for each of these expectancies, although still favorable to whites. The difference is slightly more than one-half year for the expectation of life and for the expectation of life free of bed disability. It is more than two years, however, for the expectation of life free of disability.

Differences between whites and other persons in the expectation of disability and the expectation of bed disability correspond to these differences in life expectancies. Differences between whites and others in the expectation of bed disability, either at birth or at age 65, are only negligible. Consequently differences in the expectation of life free of bed disability are almost equal to differences in the conventional expectation of life.

There are noticeable differences in the expectation of disability between whites and other persons, however. At birth, whites have an expectation of disability of about one-half year shorter than the remainder of the population. This differential widens to more than 1½ years at age 65. At birth, the difference in expectation of disability (0.7 years) is a relatively small component of the difference in expectation of life free of disability (7.6 years). At age 65, however, the difference in expectation of disability (1.6 years) is the dominant component of the difference in expectation of life free of disability (2.2 years) and results in a difference between whites and other persons much larger than that shown by conventional life expectancies.

Thus, not only is the expectation of life shorter for persons who are not white, but the expected duration of disability of all types is greater—both absolutely and also proportionately in relation to length of life. When bed disability alone is considered, however, no substantial differentials between whites and other persons in expected duration are observed. Examination of the disability data underlying these measures confirms that the differences between whites and other persons in expectation of disability are primarily a result of differences in the prevalence of long-term disability that is neither bed disability nor institutional care. These episodes represent the experience of persons unable to carry on activities such as work, housework, or school attendance.

Methods

Data required to compute these indices are a current abridged life table and a set of current age-specific rates for disability days applicable to the population group of interest.

Computation of the indices. Computation of the expectation of life free of disability is illustrated in Table 3. Computations begin with the stationary population of the life table (L_x column). These figures can be interpreted as the number of life-years lived in successive age intervals among a cohort of births who experience during life the age-specific mortality rates observed during the current year. Within each age interval the number of life-years lived is multiplied by the average fraction of the year persons of that age group are free of disability. This factor (I_x) is calculated from current disability rates by the formula:

$$I_x = 1 - \frac{w_x}{365}$$

where w_x is the number of days of disability per person per year in the interval beginning at age x.

The result of these calculations is the set of $L_x\dagger$, interpreted as life-years free of disability in the given age interval. Values of $T_x\dagger$, and $\mathring{e}_x\dagger$ are then calculated in the conventional manner (10). (The dagger symbol, $\dagger$, is used in this paper to distinguish these weighted life table

Table 3. Computation of the approximate expectation of life free of disability ($\mathring{e}_x\dagger$) for white males, civilian resident population, United States, mid-1960s

Age group	Exact initial age x	1965 abridged life table values[a]		Disability weighting factor $I_x{}^b$	Life table values, weighted for disability[c]		
		l_x	L_x		$L_x\dagger$	$T_x\dagger$	$\mathring{e}_x\dagger$
Under 15	0	100 000	1 457 411	0.967	1 409 316	6 252 782	62.5
15–44	15	96 767	2 830 657	.964	2 728 753	4 843 466	50.1
45–64	45	90 639	1 623 962	.915	1 485 925	2 114 713	23.3
65–74	65	65 901	532 960	.802	427 434	628 788	9.5
75 and over	75	39 665	318 095	.633	201 354	201 354	5.1

[a] Reference (10).

[b] For each age group, the weighting factor is $I_x = 1 - \dfrac{w_x}{365}$ where w_z is the total number of disability days per person per year in the designated age group.

[c] The dagger symbol, $\dagger$, is used in this paper to distinguish weighted life table values from the corresponding values denoted by conventional notation.

values from the corresponding values denoted by the conventional notation.)

When expectation of life free of disability, $\mathring{e}_x$[†], has been obtained for a given age x, the corresponding expectation of disability can be calculated as:

$$\mathring{e}_x - \mathring{e}_x\,[†]$$

where $\mathring{e}_x$ is the conventional expectation of life. This expectation of disability can be interpreted as the number of years of disability a member of the life table cohort would experience if current age-specific rates of mortality and disability prevailed throughout the cohort's lifetime.

Measurement of disability. The disability rates (w_x) called for in the aforementioned general formula may be based upon any operational definition of disability for which adequate data are available. One could use, for example, any one of several disability variables measured by the National Health Interview Survey such as restricted-activity days, bed-disability days, or hospital days (*11*). In practice, choice is usually limited by the availability of data and the need to use a measure which is meaningful and technically adequate for the objectives in view.

In this paper results are presented and contrasted using two alternative definitions of disability. These definitions were selected because they are applicable to most members of the population and should provide comprehensive measures of the impact of disease and injury among the living. The disability data used were obtained almost exclusively from surveys conducted by the National Center for Health Statistics.

The disability measures used are based upon the concept of the total volume of disability, which is defined and discussed in greater detail in a forthcoming paper (*4*). This concept was developed to incorporate into a single figure the duration of all disability—both long-term and short-term—experienced by members of a population during a given year. The total volume of disability estimates used was calculated as the sum of three component estimates:

1. Days of health care in long-term institutions, obtained by allocating 365 days of disability per resident to the estimated annual average number of residents in institutions providing such care.
2. Days unable to carry on major activity

among members of the civilian noninstitutional population. These data were obtained by allocating 365 days of disability each to the estimated annual average number of persons having a chronic condition and also reported as usually unable to carry on appropriate activities such as work, housework, or school.

3. Days of restricted activity (not elsewhere included), derived from annual estimates for members of the civilian noninstitutional population not included in the categories previously mentioned. A day of restricted activity is one when the person cuts down on his usual activities because of illness or injury.

Bed disability measures are based upon a less comprehensive concept of disability. All days of bed disability are included in the total volume of disability, but days of disability are not necessarily days of bed disability. Computationally, the volume of bed disability is the sum of two component estimates:

1. Days of health care in long-term institutions. These are obtained as previously described.
2. Days of bed disability among the civilian noninstitutional population. These include all reported days of care in general service short-stay hospitals, whether or not the person is actually confined to bed on the day in question. Days of disability outside of hospitals and institutions are counted as days of bed disability only when the person is reported as confined to bed for more than half the daylight hours.

Total volume of disability estimates, upon which expectations of disability are based, include but greatly exceed the corresponding estimates of bed disability. Thus, the approximate lifetime expectation of disability is 5.3 years at birth while the corresponding expectation of bed disability is only 2.0 years (Tables 1, 2). The 5.3 year figure is so much larger because the underlying estimates of the total volume of days of disability include two large categories not counted in estimating the volume of bed disability days. These two categories are (*a*) days unable to carry on major activity excluding days of bed disability and (*b*) days of restricted activity excluding days of bed disability.

Estimates of the components of these disability measures were derived from data collected by the survey programs of the National Center for Health Statistics, supplemented by certain data from the U.S. Census of 1960. Since it was not possible to derive each component for the same year, the illustrative data shown are labeled mid-1960s to indicate they are synthetic estimates based on data for several different years. Nevertheless, it is felt that the results are reasonably accurate approximations applicable to the United States in mid-decade. Definitions of terms used in this paper, and a complete account of procedures used to estimate the total volume of disability are soon to be published (4).

Discussion

The objective of this mortality-morbidity index is to measure change over time in the health status of the nation as a whole. Reasons for using mortality and disability rates as components of a single index which may serve this purpose have been discussed elsewhere (1). If such a combination of rates for death and disability is desired, the techniques described have certain advantages.

Use of the life table model provides one solution to the problem of the relative weights to assign deaths and episodes of disability when attempting to measure both phenomena by a single index. The model is a familiar conceptual tool, conventionally used in weighting diverse schedules of mortality rates for comparison with each other. Its elaboration to permit comparison of disability rates as well may meet with fewer objections than would any other arbitrary equation of a death to some specific duration of disability.

The data in this paper only permit comparisons of whites and other persons and of sex, but the observed differences in expectation of disability are sizable enough to indicate the measure is sensitive to differentials in disability experience of a magnitude likely to occur in present-day populations. Since even fractional differences in this measure represent differences of months in the cumulative average experience of disability in the groups compared, the measure would seem to be a meaningful reflection of the impact of disease and injury among the living.

Although observed differences in the expectation of disability are fairly large in absolute terms, they make a relatively small contribution to differences cited here in expectation of life free of disability at birth. This fact may make it appear that mortality dominates comparisons based on the index. Where large differences in conventional expectations of life exist, as they do between the sexes and between whites and other persons in this country, they obviously will be a principal component of differences in expectations of life free of disability. But the disability rates also enter into computation of expectation of life free of disability and may widen or narrow the gap between populations for which the index is computed. In the event two populations approached equality in conventional expectation of life, they might still differ substantially in expectation of disability and this difference would be reflected in their expectations of life free of disability.

In this sense, the disability component emerges as a more prominent component in comparisons as mortality differences diminish. This tendency to enhance the role of disability in comparisons of health status between populations with similar mortality levels seems reasonably analogous to the relative weight frequently assigned to risks of death and disability when one is assessing the importance of a health problem (1).

A principal, and probably enduring, disadvantage of these indices is the heavy demands they make upon available data. Both conventional life tables and data on disability must be available for a population in order to calculate these measures. At the national level the required data can be obtained only for the total population and a few major population categories. Lack of data is likely to preclude application of the indices to states or local areas for the foreseeable future.

In addition to their data requirements, there are other problematical aspects of these measures. Problems in interpreting sex differences in disability resulting from the criteria of disability used have already been mentioned. Further studies are also needed to determine the sensitivity of the disability measures to changes over time. These problems and other limitations on the indices have been discussed more extensively (4).

References

(*1*) Sullivan, D.F. Conceptual problems in developing an index of health. PHS Publication No. 1000, Series 2, No. 17. U.S. Government Printing Office, Washington, D.C., May 1966.

(*2*) Chiang, C.L. An index of health: mathematical models. PHS Publication No. 1000, Series 2, No. 5. U.S. Government Printing Office, Washington, D.C., May 1965.

(*3*) Moriyama, I.M. Problems in the measurement of health status. In *Indicators of Social Change*, E.B. Sheldon and W.E. Moore, editors. Russell Sage Foundation, New York, 1968, ch. 11, pp. 573-600.

(*4*) Sullivan, D.F. Disability data components for an index of health. PHS Publication No. 1000, Series 2, No. 42. U.S. Government Printing Office, Washington, D.C. In press.

(*5*) U.S. Department of Health, Education, and Welfare. *Toward a Social Report*. U.S. Government Printing Office, Washington, D.C., 1969, pp. 3-4.

(*6*) Wolfbein, S.L. The length of working life. *Population Studies* 3:286-294, 1949.

(*7*) Stockwell, E.G., and C.B. Nam. Illustrative tables of school life. *J Amer Statist Assoc* 58:1113-1124, 1963.

(*8*) Sanders, B.S. Measuring community health levels. *Amer J Public Health* 54:1063-1070, 1964.

(*9*) Haber, L.D. Identifying the disabled: concepts and methods in the measurement of disability. *Soc Security Bull* 30:17-34, 1967.

(*10*) National Center for Health Statistics. *Vital statistics of the United States, 1965. Vol. II. pt. A, Mortality.* U.S. Government Printing Office, Washington, D.C., 1967.

(*11*) National Center for Health Statistics. *Health Survey Procedure.* PHS Publication No. 1000, Series 1, No. 2. U.S. Government Printing Office, Washington, D.C., May 1964.

POTENTIAL YEARS OF LIFE LOST BETWEEN AGES 1 AND 70: AN INDICATOR OF PREMATURE MORTALITY FOR HEALTH PLANNING[1]

J. M. Romeder[2] and J. R. McWhinnie[2]

The indicator of Potential Years of Life Lost between ages 1 and 70 (PYLL) is proposed with the primary objective of ranking major causes of premature mortality. This proposal is based on a review of existing mortality indicators and indices and of the history of the concept of potential years of life lost. The method of calculation along with the corresponding rate and the age-adjusted rate are discussed and presented with applications to Canadian data and interpretation. Several methodological aspects are discussed, particularly the comparison with more sophisticated approaches based on life tables which do not appear to alter the ranking of major causes of premature death. This indicator fits well into the category of Social Indicators and can help health planners define priorities for the prevention of premature deaths. Epidemiological studies could also make use of this indicator of premature mortality. The simplicity of calculation and ease of comprehension should facilitate its use.

INTRODUCTION

This paper addresses itself to the basic question of "How to compare the importance of major causes of death?" The indicator of "Potential Years of Life Lost between ages 1 and 70" is a concept which has been discussed by a number of authors over the past 30 years using various methods of calculation. This indicator is an attempt to incorporate both theoretical and practical aspects already discussed by others in the field of mortality analysis, with the primary objective of helping health planners define priorities, particularly with respect to prevention. Obviously untimely or premature death constitutes only one aspect of all health problems, and other dimensions such as morbidity and

disability have to be considered if one requires an overview of major health problems. However, in many jurisdictions routine data on these other dimensions are lacking.[3]

The objectives of this paper are to review existing or proposed mortality indicators and indices, demonstrate how to calculate Potential Years of Life Lost between ages 1 and 70[4] with associated rates, discuss alternative methodological approaches and underlying assumptions, and finally present some Canadian data and interpretation.

REVIEW OF MORTALITY INDICATORS AND INDICES

Most mortality indicators or indices have been proposed in order to compare mortality in different geographic areas, occupational groups or for different years. The concept of potential years of life lost, however, originated with the primary objective of comparing the relative importance of different causes of death for a particular population.

An excellent review of mortality indicators was made in 1943 by Woolsey (2) who described direct and indirect methods for standardizing death rates, with the resulting indices being called "Standardized Mortality Ratios." The life

Source: *International Journal of Epidemiology* 6(2):143-151, 1977. © Oxford University Press, 1977.

[1] This work was first presented at the Canadian Public Health Association, June 1974; a more detailed version is available in French and in English.

[2] Long Range Health Planning Branch, Department of National Health and Welfare, Jeanne Mance Building. Ottawa KIA OK9, Canada.

[3] In Canada, such data will be regularly collected by the Canada Health Survey which has been planned since early 1974 (1) and will provide the first annual data for the year 1978.

[4] The indicator of "Potential Years of Life Lost between ages 1 and 70" is referred to subsequently as the PYLL indicator.

table death rate, promoted by Brownlee (3) was reviewed and mention was made of the interesting debate which followed in 1922 in England on "The Value of Life-Tables in Statistical Research" (4). The question of "Standard Population" was discussed, followed by "The Method of Equivalent Average Death Rates" (5) which takes account of mortality before age 65 only. The last index reviewed by Woolsey, the "Relative Mortality Index," gives a decreasing importance to older age-groups, being a weighted average of age-specific rate ratios (ratios of given age-specific rates to standard age-specific rates) with weights equal to the population proportions of each age group.

In 1951, Yerushalmy (6) reviewed mortality indices and proposed a new "Mortality Index" similar to the Relative Mortality Index, where the weights are the relative lengths of the age intervals (such as five years for five-year age groups). His major criticism of the use of age-adjusted rates for comparing group mortalities was that "it puts relatively heavy premiums and penalties on minor proportionate changes in the older ages". A similar indicator called "An Objective Mortality Indicator" was proposed the same year by Kohn (7), with weights equal to the reciprocals of the age at which death occurs, which constitute "objective weights," constant for all countries and for all periods. Most of the previously proposed mortality indices have been reviewed subsequently in several papers (8-14) which also present new applications and methodological extensions.

Concept of Potential Years of Life Lost

The concept seems to have been introduced for the first time by Dempsey (15) in 1947, with the objective of comparing mortality due to tuberculosis with heart diseases and cancer. For each death, she calculated the years of life remaining up until the current life expectancy. In 1948 a paper entitled "What is the Leading Cause of Death," by Dickinson and Welker (16) proposed "life years lost" and "working years lost" which differed from Dempsey's method by using life expectancy at different ages instead of life expectancy at birth. This answered one of Greville's (17) criticisms of Dempsey's method.

In 1950, Haenszel (18) compared five different measures of years of life lost with corresponding standardized rates and showed that the ranking of different causes of death was unaltered whether or not one used life table values. As a result, he recommended the simple method of using the difference between age at death and age 75, chosen as an upper limit. This method was used by Doughty (19) in 1951 with an upper age limit of 70. In the same year Martin (20) proposed the use of life expectancy values restricted to the first 70 years of life.

In 1953 Logan and Benjamin (21) reviewed the subject to show changes in mortality patterns from 1848-1872 to 1952. They proposed two further variations on the years of life lost concept which was put into perspective more recently in a book by Benjamin in 1970 (22). Another proposal for "future working years lost" was made by Stocks (23) in 1953.

Rates of years of life lost per 10 000 total population for ages 15-64 and the total to age 85 are regularly published for England and Wales by the Office of Population Censuses and Surveys.

CALCULATION, RATE, AND STANDARDIZATION

Method of Calculation of PYLL[5]

The method of calculating PYLL for a particular cause or group of causes consists of a summation of the number of deaths at each age (between 1 and 70) multiplied by the remaining years of life up to age 70.

Let d_i = number of deaths between ages i and $i+1$

a_i = remaining years to live until age 70 when death occurs between ages i and $i+1 = 70 - (i+.5)$

assuming uniform distribution of deaths within age groups, where i represents age at last birthday

Therefore, PYLL is given by:

$$\text{PYLL} = \sum_{i=1}^{69} a_i d_i = \sum_{i=1}^{69} (70 - i - .5) \quad d_i \ (2.1)$$

It can be seen that PYLL is nothing but a function of the mean age at death, for deaths between ages 1 and 70.

An example of the calculation of PYLL for ischemic heart disease is given in Table 1, using

---

[5] PYLL refers to Potential Years of Life Lost between ages 1 and 70, calculated as indicated in this section.

Table 1. Calculation of potential years of life lost between ages 1 and 70 (PYLL), rate and age-adjusted rate, Ontario, ischemic heart disease, males, 1974.

Ages	Remaining years a_i	Number of deaths d_i	PYLL a_id_i	Correcting factor $\frac{Pir}{Nr} \div \frac{Pi}{N}$	Age-adjusted PYLL $a_i \times \frac{d_i}{P_i} \times \frac{Pir}{N_r} \times N$
				Standardized PYLL and rate (according to Canada age-structure)	
				PYLL and rate	
1-4	67.0	0	0	1.08	0
5-9	62.5	0	0	1.02	0
10-14	57.5	1	57.5	1.03	59.2
15-19	52.5	1	52.5	1.05	55.1
20-24	47.5	3	142.5	1.03	146.8
25-29	42.5	9	382.5	.97	371.0
30-34	37.5	26	975	.96	936.0
35-39	32.5	89	2892.5	.96	2776.8
40-44	27.5	198	5445	.95	5172.8
45-49	22.5	489	11 002.5	.94	10 342.4
50-54	17.5	772	13 510	.95	12 834.5
55-59	12.5	1015	12 687.5	1.00	12 687.5
60-64	7.5	1419	10 642.5	1.00	10 642.5
65-69	2.5	1630	4075	1.01	4115.8
Total (1-70)		5652	61 865.0		60 140.4

Rate of PYLL

$$\frac{61\ 865}{3\ 791\ 600} \times 1000 \qquad\qquad \frac{60\ 140.4}{3\ 791\ 600} \times 1000$$

$$= 16.3 \text{ per } 1000 \qquad\qquad = 15.9 \text{ per } 1000$$

N = 3 791 600 represents the Ontario male population between ages 1 and 70 in 1974.
N_f = 10 531 000 represents the Canadian male population between ages 1 and 70 in 1974.
Note: the corresponding rate of PYLL for Canada 1974 is 15.1 per 1000.

deaths by five-year age groups (with the exception of ages one to four) and the corresponding values of a_i. This shorter method for the calculation of PYLL is preferred as a good approximation of formula 2.1. When both calculations were made for several causes of death they differed by less than two percent for any one cause.

It should be noted that PYLL is additive for different causes of death.

If A and B are two causes of death, then:

$$PYLL(A + B) = PYLL(A) + PYLL(B) \qquad (2.2)$$

This facilitates the grouping or regrouping of causes of death without recalculation.

Rate of PYLL

If one wants to compare PYLL for two populations of different sizes then a rate must be used. A simple way is to express the rate of PYLL per 1000 population (Table 1), as is usually done for death rates. Hence,

$$\text{rate of PYLL} = \sum_{i=1}^{69} a_id_i \times \frac{1000}{N} \qquad (2.3)$$

where N = number of persons between ages 1 and 70 in the actual population.

Another method of calculating a rate of PYLL is to use the total potential years of life (TPYL) for persons between ages 1 and 70 as denominator (24). TPYL is calculated by summing the number of people at a certain age multiplied by the remaining years until age 70.

This second rate $\frac{PYLL}{TPYL}$ indicates the proportion of existing potential years of life which are lost during one year. However, the more simplistic rate per 1000 population is presented in this paper.

Age-Adjusted or Standardized Rate of PYLL

When mortality for specific causes is compared between two or more different populations it is usually done by using standardized death rates to eliminate the effect of different age structures among the different populations.

The proposed age-adjusted rate of PYLL corresponds to the direct method of standardization (*2, 14, 22*) and is given by:

Age-adjusted rate of PYLL =

$$\sum_{i=1}^{69} a_i \left(\frac{d_i}{P_i}\right) \left(\frac{P_{ir}}{Nr}\right) \times 1000 \qquad (2.4)$$

where

P_i = number of persons of age i in the actual population

P_{ir} = number of persons of age i in the reference population

N_r = number of persons between ages 1 and 70 in the reference population

Formula 2.3 can be written:

$$\sum_{i=1}^{69} a_i \left(\frac{d_i}{P_i}\right) \left(\frac{P_i}{N}\right) \times 1000$$

and formula 2.4 is then simply obtained by replacing $\dfrac{P_i}{N}$ (the proportion of persons in age group $(i, i+1)$ in the actual population) by the corresponding proportion $\dfrac{P_{ir}}{N_r}$ in the reference population. Therefore, the age-adjusted rate of PYLL corresponds to the number of potential years of life which would be lost in the actual population if it had the same age structure as that of the reference population. Table 1 gives the value of the age-adjusted or standardized rate of PYLL for ischemic heart disease in Ontario males, using Canadian males as reference population for 1974. The comparison of the age-adjusted rate and the crude rate for Ontario with the corresponding Canadian rate indicate that the difference between the Ontario crude rate and the Canadian rate is partially due to the older age structure of Ontario.

METHODOLOGICAL CONSIDERATIONS

The life table method is a very useful demographic technique which allows the calculation of life expectancies and has been successfully applied by numerous biostatisticians in a variety of research related to mortality or survival (*25, 26*). Public health authorities have often used life expectancy at birth as an overall indicator of progress. Similar to the PYLL indicator, life expectancy gives high weights to infant or early deaths, but the weights are not so readily noticeable. Three life table methods will be discussed and compared to the PYLL method which does not require life table values.

Three Life Table Methods

Method 1 can be referred to as *life expectancy with zero mortality for one cause* which involves the calculation of a life table assuming the complete elimination of a particular cause. The resulting hypothetical life expectancy can be compared with the actual life expectancy to indicate the relative importance of the cause. It should be noted that there is a non-additive effect of eliminating several causes of death. That is, the gain in life expectancy resulting from the elimination of two causes is greater than the sum of the gains resulting from their separate elimination.

Method 2 is described as *years of life lost according to life expectancy as age limit* and simply involves subtracting the age at death from life expectancy either at birth or at the given age at death. Use of life expectancy at the age of death would give a certain weight to all deaths, including those at very old ages. Another refinement would be to use expectations of life coming from a special life table calculated with the expectations of life coming from a special life table calculated with the assumption of zero mortality for the cause in question. This correction for the zero mortality assumption is also referred to as the *effect of competing risks*, implying that an individual dying from one cause at a certain age would have been exposed to risks of dying from other causes later in life, had he not died from that cause.

Method 3 involves the *use of life expectancy values with a fixed cut-off age* such that it only takes account of years of life below a certain fixed age. If age 65 were chosen as cut-off age then someone dying at age 40 would lose the average number of years to be lived up to age 65 derived from a current life table. Thus, one can calculate "the decrease, in years, in the expectancy of life (limited to a certain cut-off) caused by various diseases."

Comparison with the PYLL Method

The PYLL method corresponds to the very simple method of calculation indicated in the previous section, but where cut-off ages other than 1 and 70 could be used, and can best be compared to method 3 above. Table 2 compares the PYLL method with method 3 corrected to incorporate the effect of competing risks, and shows the corresponding results for all causes of death grouped in 10 categories.

Table 2. PYLLᵃ and corrected PYLL due to mortality before age 70 from other causes (competing risks) Canada, males, 1967, ten groups of causes.

ICDᵇ	Causes	PYLLᵃ (1-70)	%	Corrected PYLL (1-70)	%
I	Infectious diseases	10 200	1.29	9235.1	1.26
II	Neoplasms	124 290	15.69	11 4916.0	15.67
III & IV	Allergic, endocrine, & blood	14 310	1.81	12 980.9	1.77
VI	Nervous system	41 517	5.24	37 928.7	5.17
VII	Circulatory system	192 554.5	24.30	182 229.6	24.85
VIII	Respiratory system	33 139.5	4.18	30 259.5	4.13
IX	Digestive system	29 962.5	3.78	27 108.2	3.70
X	Genito-urinary system	8784	1.11	7953.7	1.08
XVII	Accidents	30 8147	38.89	283 457.5	38.66
V, XII, XIII, XIV, XV, XIV, XI	All other causes	29 429.5	3.71	27 125.7	3.70
	Total	792 334	100	733 194.9	100

ᵃ Potential Years of Life Lost between ages 1 and 70.
ᵇ International Classification of Diseases (chapters).

The calculations are for the year 1967, for which Canadian abridged life tables assuming total elimination of each of the 10 groups of causes of death (27) were available. The corrected PYLL was calculated as follows, for all years of life lost up to age 70. A person having just reached age 40 and dying from cancer was not considered to have lost 30 years of life, but a lesser amount corresponding to the average number of years he could live up to age 70, as derived from the life table assuming elimination of cancer. As can be seen in Table 2, the percentage distribution of PYLL did not change by more than 3 percent for any one cause as a result of this correction, which shows the negligible effect of the correction for competing risks. However, if one is interested in more than simply the ranking of major causes of premature death (such as cost-benefit analysis or expected disability-free life), the calculation of life table modifications might be preferable.

Why PYLL, and Why Between Ages 1 and 70?

According to the previous discussion, method 3 and the PYLL method are preferred since both concentrate on premature death defined by a cut-off age. Of these two methods, PYLL has the advantage of simplicity and is therefore more likely to be understood and used.

Having recognized the need for an arbitrary choice of a cut-off age, one needs to know the sensitivity of the method to the choice of cut-off age. Table 3 indicates the distribution, in percentage, of Potential Years of Life Lost before ages 65, 70, and 75 for five major causes.

In choosing a cut-off age above 70 one should consider that the determination of the underlying cause of death becomes difficult, particularly for very old people. On the other hand, age 65, proposed by several authors, appears rather young, since a great proportion of people are still productive at this age.

Recognizing the dependence of potential years of life lost on the choice of cut-off age,

Table 3. Potential years of life lost between age 1 and age 65, 70, 75: percentages for five major causes, Canada, 1974, Males.

Cause	Before age 65ᵃ	Before age 70	Before age 75
All causes	100.0	100.0	100.0
Motor vehicle accidents	25.2	18.2	17.2
Ischemic heart disease	12.2	15.1	21.0
Other accidents	18.2	12.6	13.0
Suicide	8.6	6.4	6.3
Malignant neoplasms of digestive organs	2.5	4.3	4.3

ᵃ The calculation of Potential Years of Life Lost before 65 differs from the one before 70 in two ways: deaths occurring before age 65 only are considered and the number of years lost for a death at age X is (65-X). Similar differences apply for age 75.

one should be flexible in using the corresponding rankings to define priorities but also keep in mind that all these rankings are quite different from the ranking based on number of deaths (Table 4).

Concerning the exclusion of infant deaths from the calculation of PYLL, two considerations should be kept in mind. Firstly, most cases of infant mortality are due to causes specific to this early period of life and often have a different etiology than death later on. Secondly, each infant death would account for almost 70 years lost, giving a weight double that of a death between ages 30 and 40. This appears to be an overestimation of the value accepted by society for such a loss in light of the fact that a "very early death is often replaced" (28) by another birth. Therefore, from the point of view of social criteria, infant mortality is less disrupting than mortality of older children and adults.

APPLICATION TO CANADIAN DATA AND INTERPRETATION

Distribution of PYLL in Canada

Figure 1 indicates the distribution of PYLL among major causes for each sex separately. It can be seen that the years of life lost by males are more than twice those lost by females. This is reflected by the difference of almost seven years in life expectancy at age one between the two sexes (69.8 for males and 76.6 for females in 1971). Motor vehicle accidents, ischemic heart disease, and other accidents are the three leading categories. It should be noted that the ranking of causes depends on how causes are grouped. For example, if all cancers were grouped together they would rank very high instead of being distributed throughout.

Table 4 indicates the number of deaths between ages 1 and 70 by cause, and the corresponding percentage contribution which can be compared with the contribution of PYLL for each cause.

Geographical Comparisons

Table 5 shows the distribution of PYLL for five major causes in Canadian provinces as well as the corresponding crude and age-adjusted rates. For motor vehicle accidents the age-adjusted rate of PYLL experienced by Manitoba or Ontario could serve as an achievable goal for other provinces such as New Brunswick.

British Columbia, which is one of the most economically developed provinces, has the highest rate of PYLL. Part of this higher premature mortality is attributable to the high mortality rate due to motor vehicle accidents and is related to the fact that British Columbia has the highest consumption of alcohol.

A striking example of the effect of age structure is the rate for ischemic heart disease in

Table 4. PYLL[a] and deaths between ages 1 and 70 by major causes[b], Canada, 1974.

Cause[b]	PYLL (1-70)		Deaths (1-70)	
	Total	%	%	Total
All Causes	1 312 675	100	100	77 440
Motor vehicle accidents (AE138)	239 283.5	18.2	8.0	5864
Ischemic heart disease (A83)	198 327.5	15.1	26.2	19 205
Other accidents (AE139-146)	165 264.5	12.6	6.5	4795
Suicide (AE147)	84 195	6.4	3.7	2716
Cancer of digestive organs (A46-49, 58A)	56 667	4.3	7 1	5186
Respiratory diseases (A89-96)	50 264	3.8	4.7	3425
Cancer of respiratory organs (A50, 51, 58B)	48 079.5	3.7	6.1	4444
Cerebrovascular diseases (A85)	45 418	3.5	5.5	4068
Cirrhosis of liver (A102)	34 954	2.7	3.0	2204
Breast cancer (A54)	30 919.5	2.4	2.9	2108
Diseases of nervous system & sense organs (A72-79)	29 634	2.3	1.5	1119

[a] Potential Years of Life Lost between ages 1 and 70.

[b] Causes responsible for more than two percent of total PYLL, with codes of the A list of the International Classification of Diseases, 8th revision (ICD-8).

Figure 1. Distribution of Potential Years of Life Lost between ages 1 and 70 (PYLL) by major causes, by sex, Canada, 1974.

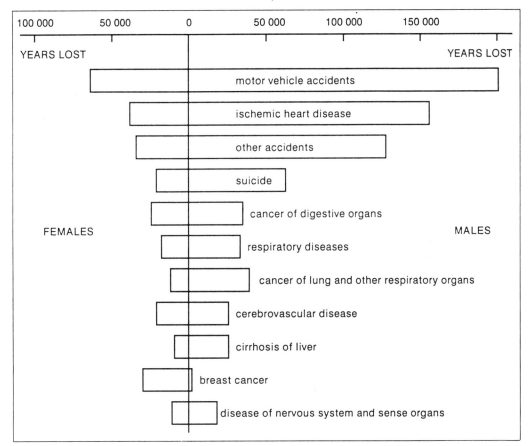

Newfoundland which appears much lower than the rate for Canada but standardization shows it to be slightly higher. This is because Newfoundland has a much younger population than Canada as a whole and because the incidence rates for ischemic heart disease are highest at middle and older ages.

CONCLUSION

After an extensive literature review, consideration of the basic issues and assumptions and experimentation with different techniques, it has been concluded that the indicator of Potential Years of Life Lost between ages 1 and 70 (PYLL) could be used in a variety of ways. The simplicity of calculation and ease of comprehension should facilitate its use but some of

the theoretical considerations should always be borne in mind.

Potential Years of Life Lost between ages 1 and 70 is essentially designed to give a broad view of the relative importance of major causes of premature mortality, leaving mortality before age one as a separate entity. The PYLL indicator is primarily designed for health planners who wish to define priorities and programs for the prevention of premature death. It could also be useful to evaluate priorities for health research activities.

Social indicators are considered useful for the general governmental interest in social policy, as well as for informing the public. PYLL summarizes most of the premature mortality, taking into account the number of deaths, the age at death, and incorporating the actual age struc-

Table 5. Rates[a] of PYLL[b] and percentage distribution for four major causes, Canada, and Provinces,[c] 1974.

Provinces	All Causes	%	Motor Vehicle Accidents	%	Ischemic Heart Disease	%	Other Accidents	%	Suicide	%
Canada	62.8	100	11.5	18.2	9.5	15.1	7.9	12.6	4.0	6.4
British Columbia	70.8		14.6		7.8		12.4		5.2	
	71.1	100	15.1	20.7	7.6	11.1	12.7	17.6	5.2	7.3
Alberta	63.3		12.8		7.0		9.8		5.5	
	64.6	100	12.7	20.2	7.5	11.1	9.8	15.5	5.6	8.7
Saskatchewan	64.2		13.6		6.7		9.9		3.9	
	63.5	100	13.8	21.2	6.1	10.4	10.0	15.4	4.2	6.0
Manitoba	62.9		8.1		9.1		10.2		4.5	
	61.9	100	8.2	12.9	8.7	14.4	10.3	16.2	4.6	7.2
Ontario	57.7		8.5		10.2		6.2		4.1	
	57.2	100	8.7	14.8	10.0	17.7	6.2	10.7	4.1	7.2
Quebec	64.9		13.0		10.4		6.5		3.4	
	65.3	100	12.7	20.0	10.6	16.0	6.5	10.1	3.3	5.2
New Brunswick	67.7		16.1		9.6		9.5		3.1	
	68.6	100	15.4	23.7	10.2	14.2	9.5	14.0	3.1	4.6
Nova Scotia	67.1		13.9		11.0		8.9		3.6	
	67.1	100	13.7	20.7	10.9	16.4	9.0	13.3	3.8	5.4
Newfoundland	53.8		11.2		7.7		8.5		.3d	
	57.6	100	10.4	20.8	9.6	14.3	7.8	15.8	.3	.5

[a] Under each crude rate per 1000 population between ages 1 and 70 is indicated in italics the age-adjusted rate, according to the Canadian population of 1974.
[b] Potential Years of Life Lost between ages 1 and 70.
[c] Only provinces with more than 500 000 population (Prince Edward Island excluded).
[d] Significance questionable (less than 50 deaths).

ture of the population considered. Further, the disaggregation of PYLL by causes is extremely simple, because it is additive by cause.

Most importantly, PYLL gives simple statistical expression to the harsh reality of death at younger ages. Because of the impact on society of premature death, Potential Years of Life Lost between ages 1 and 70 appears to be a particularly important social indicator.

ACKNOWLEDGEMENTS

We thank G. B. Hill and W. F. Taylor for their suggestions and encouragement in the development of this work. Several other colleagues gave us useful comments, particularly N. Collishaw, B. L. Ouellet, W. Saveland and S. D. Walter.

References

(1) Romeder, J.M. The need for a continuing national health survey in Canada. Unpublished note, Department of National Health and Welfare, Ottawa, 1973, p. 7.
(2) Woolsey, T. D. Adjusted death rates and other indices of mortality. Chapter IV of: *Techniques of Vital Statistics.* Reprint of chapters I-IV of: *Vital Statistics Rates in the United States 1900-1940,* by F.E. Linder, and P. Grove, National Office of Vital Statistics, US Government Printing Office, Washington, DC, 1959, (original 1943).
(3) Brownlee, J. *The Use of Death-Rates as a Measure of Hygienic Conditions.* Medical Research Council, Special Report Series, No. 60, HM Stationery Office, London, 1922.
(4) Greenwood, M., et al. Discussion on the value of life-tables in statistical research. *Journal of the Royal Statistical Society* 85:537, 1922.
(5) Yule, U.D. On some points relating to vital statistics, more especially statistics of occupational mortality. *Journal of the Royal Statistical Society* 97:1, 1934.
(6) Yerushalmy, J. A mortality index for use in place of the age-adjusted death rate. Am J *Public Health* 41:No. 8,907, 1951.
(7) Kohn, R: An objective mortality indicator. *Can J Public Health* 42:375, 1951.
(8) Liddell, F.D.K. The measurement of occupational mortality. *British J Indust Medicine* 17:228, 1960.
(9) Chiang, C.L. Standard error of the age-adjusted death rate, US Dept. of HEW, *Vital Statistics—Special Reports, Selected Studies,* Vol. 47, No. 9, 275, 1961.
(10) Kilpatrick, S.J. Occupational mortality indices. *Population Studies,* 1962, p. 175.
(11) Kilpatrick, S.J. Mortality comparisons in socioeconomic groups. *Applied Statistics,* Vol. XII, No. 2, 65, 1963.

12) Kitagawa, E.M. Theoretical considerations in the selection of a mortality index, and some empirical comparisons. *Human Biology* 38:No. 3, 293, 1966.

(*13*) Elveback, L.R. Discussion of 'Indexes of mortality and tests of their statistical significance'. *Human Biology* 38:No. 3, 322-324, 1966.

(*14*) Hill, G.B. The use of vital statistics and demographic information in the measurement of health and health care needs. Chapter 2 of: *Methods of Health Care Evaluation*, Sackett and Baskin (eds.), McMaster University, 1971.

(*15*) Dempsey, M. Decline in tuberculosis; the death rate fails to tell the entire story. *Am Rev Tuberculosis* 86:157, 1947.

(*16*) Dickinson, F.G. and E.L. Welker. What is the leading cause of death? Two new measures. Bureau of Medical Economic Research, American Medical Association, Bulletin 64, Chicago, 1948.

(*17*) Greville, T. N. E. Comments on Mary Dempsey's article on Decline in Tuberculosis: the death rate fails to tell the entire story. *Tuberculosis* 87:417, 1948.

(*18*) Haenszel, W. A standardized rate for mortality defined in units of lost years of life. *Am J Public Health* 40:17, 1950.

(*19*) Doughty, J.H. Mortality in terms of lost years of life. *Can. J Public Health* 42:134, 1951.

(*20*) Martin, W.J. Life table mortality as a measure of hygiene. *The Medical Officer*, 151, 1951.

(*21*) Logan, W.P.D. and B. Benjamin. Loss of expected years of life—a perspective view of changes between 1848-72 and 1952. *Monthly Bulletin of the Ministry of Health and Public Health Laboratory*, England, Vol. 12, 244, 1953.

(*22*) Benjamin, B. and H.W. Haycocks, *The Analysis of Mortality and Other Actuarial Statistics*. London, Cambridge University Press, 1970, pp. 392.

(*23*) Stocks, P. Cancer and the community. *Med J.* 847, 1953.

(*24*) Romeder, J.M. and J.R. McWhinnie. Health field indicators for policy planning. Canada and provinces, Part I: mortality and hospitalization. Department of National Health and Welfare, Ottawa, 1974, pp. 54.

(*25*) Dublin, L.I. and A.J. Lotloa. Uses of the life table in vital statistics. *Am Public Health* 27:481, 1937.

(*26*) Chiang, C.L. *Introduction to Stochastic Processes in Biostatistics* (chapter 9. The life table and its construction). New York, John Wiley, 1968, pp. 313.

(*27*) Gnansekaran, K. S. Background paper for the 1972-2001 population projections. Unpublished document, Statistics Canada, 1973.

(*28*) Lery, A. and J. Vallin. Un enfant qui meurt en bas âgo est souvent 'remplacé'. Economie et Statistique, Institut National de la Statistique et des Etudes Économiques, 63: 27, 1975.

AN EPIDEMIOLOGICAL STUDY OF ENDEMIC TYPHUS (BRILL'S DISEASE) IN THE SOUTHEASTERN UNITED STATES WITH SPECIAL REFERENCE TO ITS MODE OF TRANSMISSION

Kenneth F. Maxcy[1]

At the beginning of this century it was generally held that typhus fever had disappeared from the United States except for an occasional case imported from Europe or from Mexico.[2]

In 1910 Dr. Nathan E. Brill of New York, (1-3), called attention to a typhuslike disease occurring endemically in that city. He hesitated to identify it as typhus because of its generally milder course and its occurrence under circumstances different from those usually associated with that disease. He accordingly believed that he was dealing with a new clinical entity, "an infectious disease of unknown etiology." Cases of this type have since been known in the United States as Brill's disease.

In 1912 Anderson and Goldberger (4), who had previously reported on the experimental transmission of Mexican typhus ("tabardillo") to monkeys, were similarly successful in the inoculation of a Rhesus monkey with blood from a case of Brill's disease in New York. They found that, as in "tabardillo," one infection rendered monkeys immune to subsequent inoculations of the same passage virus. Furthermore, monkeys previously infected with Mexican typhus were thereafter found immune to Brill's disease, and vice versa. From these observations they concluded that Brill's disease was, in fact, identical with typhus fever, and this conclusion seems to have been quite promptly and generally accepted.

During the year or two following, stimulated by these publications, a considerable number of reports of the occurrence of cases similar to those described by Brill appeared in medical literature. In addition to these and since that time cases of clinical typhus have continued to be reported to the Surgeon General of the United States Public Health Service each year from various parts of the United States, but particularly from the Atlantic seaboard and the States near the Mexican border.

A certain portion of these have been imported, or traceable to infection recently imported from foreign sources. When this has been the case the epidemiological picture has been such as is usually associated with typhus as known in the Old World. For instance, in the fairly numerous instances when typhus has been introduced from Mexico in the last 10 years (5-9) the disease has been virulent, the mortality high, and the cases have been in persons obviously lousy or those in contact with them.

On the other hand, there remain a large number of sporadic cases of mild typhus which could not be traced to recent importation and occurring under circumstances which strongly suggested local origin of the infection. In regard to this so-called endemic typhus, Brill originally noted that the epidemiology presented points of difference from that which is

Source: *Public Health Reports* 41(52):2967-2995, 1926.
[1] Passed Assistant Surgeon, United States Public Health Service.

[2] August Hirsch, in his "Geographical and Historical Pathology" (Pub. by the New Sydenham Society, London, 1883), states that:

The proper era of typhus for the United States and Canada begins with the period when immigration from Ireland had set in on a large scale. We thus explain the fact that the ports on the east coast of North America have been the headquarters of the disease, and that the largest contingent of the sick has been supplied by the immigrants themselves, or their countrymen with whom they had come in contact. On the other hand, it is a noteworthy fact that the most careful search among the plentiful epidemiologic records in the literature of the United States fails to discover a single statement as to the occurrence of typhus in the Mississippi Valley or in the Western States, so that the greater part of the continent appears to enjoy absolute immunity from the disease, and in no part of the whole territory do endemic centers of typhus appear to have formed, notwithstanding importations on a large scale.

Besides the Irish, immigrants from other countries of Europe were from time to time responsible for small outbreaks in the cities of the eastern United States.

The endemic center of typhus (tabardillo) in Mexico has in like manner from time to time supplied the States of the southwest with infected immigrants who have given rise to small outbreaks.

generally assigned to typhus. He pointed out that the cases occurred sporadically, without traceable connection with each other, that they seldom, if ever, gave rise to new cases among those in contact with the sick person, that no localized outbreaks occurred, and finally, that their seasonal distribution differed from that of typhus. Later, accepting the identity of the virus with typhus as indicated by the work of Anderson and Goldberger, Brill (*10*) was led to raise the question whether some vector other than the louse might not be concerned in the transmission. The same question is raised by Allan (*11*) as a result of his observations upon a series of cases occurring in Charlotte, N.C.

In 1922, while detailed as acting State epidemiologist to the State Board of Health of Alabama, the writer had occasion to observe with Havens (*12*) a number of cases which were identified clinically as the endemic form of typhus described by Brill and which gave a positive Weil-Felix reaction. As the same question with regard to the mode of transmission arose in these cases, an epidemiological study was undertaken under instructions from the Surgeon General in cooperation with local health authorities, and has been continued up to the present. The opportunity for study has been especially favorable, since this section of the United States is little subject to immigration either from Europe or from Mexico; and with cases occurring in the smaller cities and towns one could exclude more surely the possibility of constant reintroduction of the virus from exotic sources and trace association between cases, if it existed.

EVIDENCE OF PREVALENCE IN SOUTHEASTERN UNITED STATES

Aside from the group of cases occurring in Alabama and in Savannah, Ga., which form the basis of this report, evidence has been collected of the existence of mild typhus in other cities and towns in North and South Carolina, Georgia, and Florida.

The first report from this section of the country was that by Paullin in 1913 (*13*), in which he described the clinical course of six cases seen by him in Atlanta, Ga.

In 1914 Newell and Allan (*14*) reported four cases from Charlotte, N. C. In a later report Allan (*11*) gave a detailed account of 24 cases which had occurred in that city, and no contact could be traced with recent arrivals, or, indeed, between any two cases.

In a personal communication (1925) Dr. William A. Smith, chairman of the City Board of Health and Welfare of Charleston, S. C., informed the author that cases of Brill's disease occurred in that city from time to time; that a considerable number, about 15 in all, had been reported within a short space of time two or three years previously. A rapid examination of the records of one of the city hospitals for 1923-1925 by the author revealed three typical clinical cases. Dr. H. Clay Foster (1925) submitted a typical clinical history of a case with a positive Weil-Felix reaction in a woman apparently infected in Beaufort, S.C. Dr. T. P. Waring (1925), of Savannah, made a similar clinical diagnosis on a little girl brought to him from Estill, S.C.

Since the report of Paullin (*13*) cases have continued to occur in Atlanta, Ga. Thus there were reported to the city health department in 1920, one case; in 1922, eight cases; and in 1923, six cases of typhus. Dr. T. F. Sellers informs me that in the State laboratory from August, 1923, up to November, 1925, 11 blood specimens from patients resident in Atlanta had been found positive by the Weil-Felix reaction. Sydenstricker (*15*) has reported six cases which have come under his observation at the university hospital, Augusta, and Dr. E. B. Murphey, 1925 (personal communication), of that city is authority for the statement that from one to five cases have occurred in that city each year since the disease was first recognized in 1915, and that he can recall having seen similar cases as far back as 1906. Information was also obtained through the State department of health of cases of mild typhus occurring during 1924 and 1925 at Waynesboro, Millen, Lagrange, West Point, Gainesville, and Albany, Ga.

For some years an occasional case of typhus has been reported from Jacksonville, Fla.; thus in 1924, three cases; in 1925, two cases; in 1926 (up to December), ten cases. The disease has also been reported in Tampa, Dunedin, Jensen, St. Petersburg, Callahan, and Lakeland, Fla.

DATA AVAILABLE FOR PRESENT STUDY

The cases which form the basis of this report are (1) those reported in the State of Alabama, 1922 to 1925, (2) those reported in the city of Savannah, Ga., 1923 to 1925.

A special effort was made by the author and associates in the Alabama State Board of Health to secure full information of the occurrence of the disease in that State. The matter was given some publicity through the medium of the full-time county health officers, having jurisdiction over 50 percent of the population, through papers read before the State medical society and through the press. It is thought, therefore, that so far as the disease was recognized, fairly complete information of its occurrence was obtained. This applies especially to the city of Montgomery, where, with the cooperation of the local physicians, the disease was intensively studied.

During the period of observation a total of 104 cases of clinical typhus were reported in Alabama, 62 of which were confirmed by the Weil-Felix reaction performed in the State laboratories. Forty-four of these cases, 28 of which were confirmed by the Weil-Felix, were in Montgomery. An epidemiological case history was made out for each case. Of the 44 Montgomery cases the author investigated personally 28; seven were investigated by Dr. C. H. Leach, acting State epidemiologist, and two by Dr. L. C. Havens, director of the State laboratories. The history form of the remaining seven was made out from information supplied by the attending physician. Of the 60 cases distributed in other cities and towns of the State only seven were personally investigated by the author, one by Doctor Leach, and one by Doctor Havens, information for the remaining 51 being obtained from the local health officer or the physician in attendance.

In Savannah, Brill's disease had first been brought to the attention of the medical profession by the report of a case before the local medical society in 1915 by Dr. Lawrence Lee. Beginning in 1923, an epidemiological study of the disease has been conducted by the author in collaboration with Dr. Victor C. Bassett, city health officer. The matter has been brought to the attention of the medical society, and cordial cooperation in the study given by the medical profession of the city.

Of the total of 93 cases reported, 32 have been confirmed by the Weil-Felix reaction. A history form has not been kept, as in the Alabama cases, but attempt has been made to secure certain items of information in each instance; viz, identification, including place of residence and place of business, occupation, recent travel, date of onset, clinical course, contact with preceding cases, secondary cases, presence of lice or other vermin. A majority of the cases have been seen personally by Doctor Bassett during the acute illness. When this was not done the information desired was obtained either by a personal visit to the patient himself after convalescence or from the physician in attendance, or a combination of these. The author has accompanied Doctor Bassett on many of these visits.

IDENTIFICATION AS TYPHUS

It has been tentatively accepted that the disease with which we are dealing in the southeastern United States is typhus, because of:

(1) Its clinical identification with Brill's disease (*16*).

(2) The Weil-Felix reaction.

(3) The work of Anderson and Goldberger (*4*), identifying the virus of Brill's disease with that of Mexican "tabardillo."

(4) The successful transmission of the disease to Rhesus monkeys and to guinea pigs from cases in Savannah and Montgomery by the author, and the character of the reaction in these animals. (Unpublished report.) Further studies of the activity of this virus in experimental animals and its relation to the European virus are in progress.

However, granting that the identification of this disease with typhus may be questioned, it may at least be said that the cases here referred to form a clinical group as distinct and as homologous as measles; that they resemble typhus fever much more closely than they resemble any other recognized specific infection, and that as yet they have not been differentiated from that disease. It is in this sense, then, that the designation "endemic typhus" is used in this paper.

EPIDEMIOLOGICAL CHARACTERISTICS

(a) *Distribution in Alabama.* The distribution of the Alabama cases by cities and towns for each of the four years of observation is given in Table 1. A majority of these cases occurred in the large cities, Birmingham, Mobile, and Montgomery, the remainder in the small towns. None have so far been reported from isolated

Table 1. Distribution of cases of endemic typhus in Alabama during four years of observation.

City or town	Population 1920	1922	1923	1924	1925	Total	Confirmed by Weil-Felix
Birmingham	178 806	1	3	2	1	7	4
Montgomery	43 464	6	6	8	24	44	28
Mobile	60 777	2	—	2	17	21	12
Atmore	1775	—	—	—	1	1	1
Brewton	2682	—	—	1	—	1	1
Red Level	385	—	—	—	1	1	1
Andalusia	4023	—	1	—	5	6	6
Opp	1556	—	—	—	1	1	1
Troy	5696	—	2	2	2	6	2
Sampson	1646	—	1	1	2	4	2
Hartford	1561	—	1	—	—	1	1
Dothan	10 034	—	—	—	6	6	1
Headland	1252	2	—	—	2	4	1
Kinston	163	—	—	—	1	1	1
Total		11	14	16	63	104	62

country districts, although three of the cases from Covington County during the past year lived on farms.[3]

The disease appears to be largely if not entirely confined to the southern part of the State. The city of Birmingham has three times the population of Mobile and four times that of Montgomery, and yet it has reported only seven cases as compared with 21 for Mobile and 44 for Montgomery. Inasmuch as the disease has been brought to the attention of the medical profession in Birmingham, and the reporting of communicable diseases is as good in this city as in the others, it is considered unlikely that the difference in incidence is attributable to undiscovered cases. Furthermore, diligent inquiry among physicians and health officers practicing in that part of the State which lies north of Birmingham has failed to reveal a single case during the four-year period.

The intermittent occurrence of cases in the small towns is notable. For example, in Troy, Ala., a town of 5696 population, case T2 became ill on November 18, 1923, case T3 on December 6, 1923, case T5 on March 25, and case T6 on March 26, 1924. No further cases occurred in this town so far as could be ascertained until November, 1925, a year and a half later, when a woman living next door to the house in which case T3 had resided came down

with the disease. In Sampson, population 1646, there was a case in 1923; after a period of 14 months another case occurred. In Headland, population 1252, there were two cases in 1922, and no more recognized or reported until 1925. The same characteristic is evident in the time distribution of the Montgomery cases, shown in Table 2. A period of three to six months sometimes elapsed before a new case was reported.

From the information available, therefore, the disease is not uniformly distributed in Alabama. It occurs in certain cities and towns of the southern part of the State. Its occurrence is scattered as regards place and time.

(b) Age. The series of cases is not sufficiently large to permit a detailed analysis of the age distribution in comparison with that of Old World typhus. By reference to the ages of the Montgomery and Savannah cases, given in Tables 3 and 4, however, it will be seen that only three of 137 cases here recorded were in children under 10 years of age. In the first 255 cases recorded by Brill his youngest case was 10 years of age, and there were relatively few under 20.

The mildness of typhus in children is a phenomenon well known to European observers. The consequently greater difficulty of clinical recognition may account in part for the low incidence recorded in this age group. It is also possible that differences in exposure may play a role.

(c) Sex. As indicated by Tables 5 and 6, *the incidence is almost twice as high in the male* as in the female in both the Montgomery and Savannah

---

[3] Dr. H. P. Rankin, county health officer, reports that during 1926 in Coffee County, adjoining Covington, there have been diagnosed 15 cases of Brill's disease. These cases were widely distributed in the rural areas of the county and without traceable association.

Table 2. Seasonal distribution of cases.

	Year	Jan.	Feb.	Mar.	Apr.	May	June	July	Aug.	Sept.	Oct.	Nov.	Dec.	Total
Savannah, Ga.	1923							7	8	6	11	5	1	38
	1924		1		2		1	1		4	2	2	1	14
	1925	2		1	3	3	0	9	7	1	8	4	3	41
		2		2	3	5	1	17	15	11	21	11	5	93
Montgomery, Ala.	1922						1				1	3	1	6
	1923	1	1							1		2	1	6
	1924			1					3			2	2	8
	1925		1	1	1	1	1	3	5	7	2	1	1	24
		1	2	1	2	1	2	3	8	8	3	8	5	44
Other cities and towns in Alabama	1922							4	1					5
	1923		1							2	1	2	2	8
	1924			2			1		2		1	1	1	8
	1925	2				3	2	5	7	4	4	6	6	39
		2	1	2		3	3	9	10	6	6	9	9	60
Grand total		5	3	5	5	9	6	29	33	25	30	28	19	197

cases, taken as a whole. Of the 24 cases reported by Allan (*11*) in Charlotte, N. C., 19 were men. Of 50 cases selected for analysis by Brill (*2*) 34 were males. The disproportionately high incidence of the endemic typhus of the United States among men may be due either to greater exposure in infection or to greater susceptibility.

(d) Race. In the eastern cities, Boston, New York, and Philadelphia, a large proportion of the cases of Brill's disease have been in persons born in Russia, and in southern Texas and California cases were chiefly among Mexicans; *but in the Southeastern States all the cases, with one or two possible exceptions, have occurred in native-born white Americans.* The negro for some unknown reason is almost exempt. For example, in Savannah, where negroes in 1920 constituted 47 percent of the population, only two of the 93 cases

recorded were in this race; in Alabama, where the population of the State is approximately one-third negro, only two of the 104 cases recorded were in negroes. Allan remarked upon the absence of cases among this race in Charlotte, N. C.

The question arises whether this apparent freedom of the colored race from the disease is a fact or whether it is simply due to lack of recognition and reporting of the disease in this race. The single case in a negro which I personally observed was typical in all respects, very severe, with a well-developed and plainly evident eruption as easily recognizable as in a white person. Practically all the physicians who recognized and reported cases among white people see in their routine practice a certain number of negroes. In Alabama a large propor-

Table 3. Cases of Brill's disease occurring in Montgomery, Ala. 1922-1925.

Case No.	Race	Sex	Age	Occupation	Date of onset	Weil-Felix day after onset	Reaction result	Remarks
					1922			
1	W	M	28	Waiter in cafeteria	June 5	5th	Neg	
						8th	Pos. 1-800	
2	W	F	35	Housewife	Oct. 8	14th	Pos. 1-640	
3	W	M	50	Proprietor, bottling works	Nov. 12	25th	Pos. 1-320	
4	W	F	38	Housewife	Nov. 20	16th	Pos. 1-160	Wife of No. 3
5	W	M	35	Clerk in pool room and lunch counter	Nov. 25	15th	Pos. 1-1280	

Table 3. (Continued.)

Case No.	Race	Sex	Age	Occupation	Date of onset	Weil-Felix day after onset	Reaction result	Remarks
6	W	F	60	Housewife	Dec. 19	8th	Neg. 1-80	
					1923			
7	W	M	38	Manager, clothing store	Jan. 7	8th	Neg.	
8	W	M	35	Stockyard employee	Feb. 15	6th	Neg. 1-80	
11	W	M	34	Machinist	Sept. 22	5th	Neg. 1-20	
						14th	Pos. 1-2560	
12	W	F	45	Housewife	Dec. 1	14th	Pos. 1-1280	Wife of No. 77.
13	W	M	22	Employee, wholesale shoe store	Nov. 30	9th	Pos. 1-320	
14	W	M	26	Employee, railroad yards	Dec. 10	19th	Pos. 1-1280	
					1924			
50	W	F	34	Housewife	Apr. 28	10th	Pos. 1-160	
51	W	M	15	Clerk, wholesale grocery	Aug. 6	5th	Neg.	
						14th	Pos. 1-5000	
52	W	M	45	Clerk, drug and seed store	Aug. 9	10th	Pos. 1-160	
53	W	M	54	Proprietor, clothing store	Aug. 24			Contact with No. 52?.
57	W	M	44	Manager, wholesale hardware store	Nov. 9	6th	Pos. 1-160	
58	W	F	38	Saleswoman, millinery store	Nov. 16	5th	Neg.	Guinea pigs.
						17th	Neg.	Positive.
59	W	F	11	Schoolgirl	Dec. 6	13th	Pos. 1-320	
60	W	F	36	Housewife	Dec. 7	8th	Neg.	
					1925			
61	W	M	52	Proprietor, furniture store	Mar. 20	11th	Pos. 1-320	
62	W	M	38	Sheriff	Feb. 28	7th	Neg. 1-20	
63	W	M	22	Clerk, drug store	Apr. 19	11th	Pos. 1-320	
64	W	F	24	Housewife	May 15	10th	Neg.	Typical clinically
65	W	F	20	Cashier, moving-picture theater	June 13	8th	Neg. 1-80	
66	W	M	25	Shoe salesman	July 7	10th	Neg.	
67	W	M	37	Butcher, meat market	July 28	9th	Pos. 1-320	
68	W	M	45	Probate judge	do	11th	Pos.	
69	W	M	46	Physician	Aug. 8			
70	W	M	56	Proprietor furniture store	Aug. 12			
71	W	M	17	Clerk, grocery store	Aug. 13	12th	Pos. 1-160	
72	W	M	43	Lawyer	Aug. 17	7th	Neg.	
						14th	Pos. 1-320	
73	W	F	45	Clerk, department store	Aug. 23	8th	Pos.	
74	W	M	32	Manager wholesale flour store	Sept. 12	14th	Pos. 1-640	
75	W	F	17	Schoolgirl	Sept. 17	7th	Pos. 1-160	
76	W	F	30	Housewife	Sept. 9	10th	Pos. 1-640	
77	W	M	63	Railroad engineer	Sept. 15	14th	Pos. 1-640	Husband of No. 12
78	W	F	11	Schoolgirl	Sept. 20	4th	Neg.	
						10th	Pos. 1-160	
79	W	M	22	Bank clerk	Sept. 30	12th	Pos. 1-1280	
80	W	M	35	Taxi driver	Sept. 27			
81	W	M	24	Produce salesman	Oct. 19	9th	Pos. 1-640	
82	Col.	M	58	Employee of restaurant	Oct. 30	3d	Neg.	
						15th	Pos. 1-1280	
83	W	M	31	Proprietor, wholesale flour and feed store	Nov. 4	9th	Pos. 1-640	
84	W	F	5	Child	Dec. 2	5th	Pos. 1-100	

Table 4. Cases of Brill's disease occurring in Savannah, Ga. 1923-1925.

Case No.	Race	Sex	Age	Occupation	Date of onset	Weil-Felix day after onset	Reaction result	Remarks
					1923			
1	W	M	23	Employee of restaurant	July 13			
2	W	M	45	Dealer in hay and grain	July 14			
3	W	F	30	Housewife	July 16			
4	W	M	52	Employee of restaurant	July 19			
5	W	M	38	Watchman, Salvation Army Industrial Home	July 21			
6	W	F	19	Housewife	July 27			
7	W	M	31	Salesman, meat packer	July 28			
9	W	M	60	Salesman, ship chandler	Aug. 3			
10	W	M	31	Salesman, tobacco warehouse	Aug. 4			
11	W	M	52	Salesman, wholesale candy	Aug. 6			
12	W	M	40	Tailor	Aug. 14			
13	W	M	49	Grocer	Aug. 16			
14	W	M	28	Butcher, store "H"	Aug. 27			
17	Col.	M	21	Dairy worker	Aug. 29			
8	W	M	21	Unemployed	Aug. 25			
16	W	F	51	Housewife	Sept. 1			
17	W	M	37	Clerk, wholesale warehouse	Sept. 2			
18	W	M	30	Clerk, grocery store	Sept. 17			
19	W	M	21	Employee, restaurant	Sept. 23			
20	W	F	35	Housewife	Sept. 24	7th	Pos. 1-160	
21	W	M	28	Fire department employee	Sept. 25	40th	Neg.	
22	W	F	32	Housewife	Oct. 1	11th	do	
23	W	F	25	do	Oct. 2	8th	do	
24	W	M	30	Clerk, grocery store	do	12th	Pos. 1-160	
25	W	F	17	Unemployed	Oct. 7	6th	Neg.	
26	W	F	35	Housewife, boarding house	Oct. 9			
27	W	F	14	Schoolgirl	Oct. 15			
28	W	F	40	Clerk, grocery store	Oct. 21	8th 17th	Neg.	
28	Col.	M	38	Painter	Nov. —			
29	W	M	38	Mechanic	Oct. 24	14th	Pos. 1-320	
29	W	F	38	Housewife	Oct. 25	10th	Neg.	
30	W	M	10	Child	do	do	Neg. 1-80	Son of No. 29.
31	W	F	5	do	do	do	Neg.	Daughter of No. 29.
32	W	M	32		Nov. 2			Husband of No. 29.
33	W	F	44	Housewife	Nov. 8	15th	Pos. 1-320	
34	W	F	26	do	Nov. 11	12th	do	
37	W	F	43	do	Nov. 14	do	do	
40	W	M	52	Convict guard	Dec. 10	9th 25th	Neg. Pos. 1-320	
					1924			
1	W	F	51	Housewife	Mar. 7	14th	Neg.	Guinea pigs.
2	W	F	40	do	May 1	8th	Neg. 1-80	
3	W	M	44	Railroad engineer	May 12			
4	W	F	14	Schoolgirl	June 11			
5	W	M	35	Shipping agent	July 9	14th	Neg.	
6	W	M	50	Foreman, railroad yards	Sept. 1			
7	W	M	48	Turpentine broker	Sept. 6			

Table 4. (Continued.)

Case No.	Race	Sex	Age	Occupation	Date of onset	Weil-Felix day after onset	Reaction result	Remarks
8	W	F	57	Housewife	Sept. 20			
9	W	F	19	Clerk, department store	do			
11	W	M	62	Farmer	Oct. 21			
13	W	M	19	Barber	do	15th	Pos. 1-60	
14	W	F	62	Housewife	Nov. 25		Pos. 1-160	
15	W	M	28	Employee, filling station	Nov. 18	14th	do	
16	W	F	50	Housewife, living over store	Dec. 18			
					1925			
17	W	F	18	Clerk, office	Jan. 30			
18	W	M	36	Foreman, transfer company	Mar. 28			
19	W	F	48	Housewife	Apr. 4	10th	Neg. 1-80	
						17th	Pos. 1-1280	
20	W	M	34	Proprietor, furniture store	Apr. 30	6th	Neg.	
21	W	M	56	Proprietor, hotel and taxi service	Apr. 18			
22	W	M	36	Superintendent, chemical works	May 16		Pos. 1-320	
38b	W	M	65	Butcher, store "A"	Jan. —			
23	W	F	35	Housewife, living next to bakery	May 7			
24	W	M	47	Mechanic	May 30			
25	W	F	52	Saleswoman, handicraft shop	July 9	16th	Pos. 1-640	
26	W	M	23	Printer, shop on water front	July 15	10th	Pos. 1-100	
27	W	M	29	Salesman, feed store "S"	July 5			
28	W	M	17	Employee, "X" dairy	June 25	22d	Pos. 1-320	
29	W	M	60	Farmer	July 22	10th	Neg. 1-40	
					1925			
30	W	F	30	Unemployed	July 28		Pos. 1-160	
31	W	M	30	Clerk, grocery	do	14th	do	
32	W	M	25	Employee, "X" dairy	July 9	12th	Neg.	
33	W	M	35	Employee, restaurant	Aug. 11	15th	Pos. 1-1280	
34	W	F	73	Housewife	Aug. 15		Pos. 1-320	
35	W	M	28	Clerk, feed store "S"	July 27	8th	Neg.	
36	W	M	17	Employee, "X" diary	Aug. 12			
38	W	F	33	Telephone operator, living over grocery store "A"	Aug. 16			
39	W	M	54	Clerk, feed store "S"	Aug. 7			
40	W	M	41	Carpenter	Aug. 26			
41	W	F	19	Schoolgirl	do			
42	W	M	16	Schoolboy	Sept. 17			
43	W	F	60	Housewife	Oct. 1		Pos. 1-100[a]	
44	W	M	10	Schoolboy	do	7th	do[a]	
45	W	M	27	Clerk, wholesale grocery	Oct. 2	11th	do[a]	
46	W	M	22	Clerk, wholesale tobacco warehouse	Oct. 5		Pos. 1-320	
47	W	F	20	Clerk, grocery store	Oct. 1	15th	do	
48	W	F	56	Housewife	Oct. 11	17th	Neg.	
50	W	F	7	School child	Oct. 19	8th	Pos. 1-160[a]	
51	W	M	50	Molder, living on water front	Oct. 16	20th	Pos. 1-320	
52	W	M	30	Manager, ice plant	Nov. 4	10th	Pos. 1-160	
53	W	M	57	Engineer	Nov. 9	5th	Pos. 1-320	
54	W	F	30	Clerk, physician's office	Nov. 7	10th	Pos. 1-160[a]	
55	W	M	52	Merchandise broker	Nov. 22	9th	Pos. 1-640	
56	W	M	14	School child	Dec. 13	8th	do	
57	W	M	26	Pipe fitter, railroad shop	Dec. 14	8th	Pos. 1-1280	
58	W	M	40	Painter	Dec. 15		Pos. 1-160	

[a] Microscopic agglutination with approximate dilution of dried blood.

Table 5. Number of cases and case rate of endemic typhus according to broad occupational groups in Montgomery, Ala., 1922–1925.

Group	Total persons in group		Number of cases in group		Case rate per 1000 exposed	
	Male	Female	Male	Female	Male	Female
Population 10 years of age and over	16 428	19 498	29	14	1.77	0.72
All occupations	13 242	7020	29	3	2.20	.39
Not gainfully employed	3186	11 878	0	11	0	.93
Agriculture, forestry, and animal husbandry	215	26	0	0	0	0
Extraction of minerals	24	1	0	0	0	0
Manufacturing and mechanical industries	4114	768	1	0	.250	0
Transportation	2608	131	3	0	1.15	0
Trade	3048	530	18	3	5.90	5.67
Public service	402	10	1	0	2.49	0
Professional service	650	571	3	0	4.62	0
Domestic and personal service	1102	4915	3	0	2.73	0
Clerical occupations	1079	668	0	0	0	0

Population figures from U. S. census, 1920

Table 6. Number of cases and case rate of endemic typhus according to broad occupational groups in Savannah, Ga., 1923–1925.

Group	Total persons in group		Number of cases in group		Case rate per 1000 exposed	
	Male	Female	Male	Female	Male	Female
Population 10 years of age and over	33 676	35 463	57	34	1.69	0.96
All occupations	28 986	12 880	52	7	1.79	.54
Not gainfully employed	4690	22 583	5	27	1.07	1.19
Agriculture, forestry, and animal husbandry	273	24	6	0	21.98	0
Extraction of minerals	13	0	0	0	0	0
Manufacturing and mechanical industries	10 816	1753	10	0	.92	0
Transportation	6573	245	5	1	.76	4.08
Trade	4810	878	23	4	4.78	4.56
Public service	940	9	2	0	2.13	0
Professional service	977	864	0	0	0	0
Domestic and personal service	1800	7710	6	0	3.33	0
Clerical occupations	2784	1397	0	2	0	1.43

Population figures from U. S. census, 1920

tion of the cases of continued fever, particularly where typhoid is suspected, are seen by the whole-time health officers. At Savannah, at Montgomery, and at Mobile a large number of the blood specimens which were submitted to the public health laboratories for the Widal test, as well as a considerable number of sera submitted for the Wassermann tests, were run against the Weil-Felix organism, with negative results so far as negroes are concerned, although by the same procedure a number of unrecognized cases among white persons were uncovered. With the available evidence, therefore, while the low incidence among the colored race may be in part accounted for by lack of recognition and reporting, this factor would seem not to account for all of the discrepancy. *The relative freedom of the negro from the disease is a fact which remains to be explained.*

(e) Seasonal distribution. A tabulation of the cases reported by months (see Table 2) shows that although the disease occurs in all months of the year, it reaches maximum incidence in the summer and fall. This characteristic has been constant through the four years of observation.

A similar seasonal distribution was found in New York City by Brill, who in his last report (*10*), based upon an experience of 500 cases over a period of some twenty-odd years, stated that 70 percent occurred from June to November.

The summer and fall maximum of the endemic typhus of the United States is in direct contrast with the high winter and spring incidence of typhus in the Old World. This is shown in [Figure 1], in which the curve given by seasonal distribution of the 197 cases of endemic typhus which are analyzed in this report is compared with the curve for typhus in Romania, 1922-1924 (*17*). The seasonal distribution of the disease in Russia, 1920-1924, and in Poland, 1922-1924, is similar to that of Romania. Typhus is generally accepted to be a disease of the colder months; but the endemic disease of the United States is at a minimum during the colder months.

(*f*) *Location by residence.* A study of the cases which occurred in Montgomery, located according to place of residence, . . . suggests a tendency toward focalization in the central portion of the city in and near the business district. The question arises whether this apparent concentration is merely the result of a greater density of population in that part of the city. The 39 cases living within the city limits were distributed among the seven city wards as follows:

Ward	Population, United States census 1920	Number of cases	Case rate per 1000 population
1	5636	4	0.71
2	9405	4	.43
3	4147	8	1.98
4	7035	10	1.42
5	5044	4	0.74
6	4075	4	.98
7	8122	5	.62

This division of the city is peculiarly unfavorable for the purposes in mind, inasmuch as the wards are arranged radially in such manner that all except one (ward 7) include portions of the central part of the city. Even though this be true, the tabulation indicates a slight excess of cases in wards 3 and 4, which include a large portion of the older residential section bordering upon the business district.

. . . the Savannah cases have in like manner been shown according to their places of residence. The distribution appears to be rather general, except perhaps for the newer residential portions and the outlying districts, where the incidence is apparently light. Population figures by wards for this city are not available in the United States census, and it is therefore not

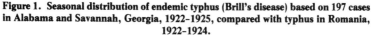

Figure 1. Seasonal distribution of endemic typhus (Brill's disease) based on 197 cases in Alabama and Savannah, Georgia, 1922–1925, compared with typhus in Romania, 1922–1924.

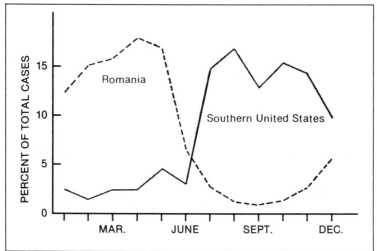

possible to compare rates for the different sections.

Summing up the data on location of cases by residence in both cities, one is impressed with the fact that the cases are scattered in the sense that *there are no sharply localized neighborhood outbreaks.* However, there seems to be a tendency for the cases to occur more frequently in the older, more centrally located residential districts.

(g) *Location by place of business.* Since an employed person is exposed to an even greater number of contacts at the place of business than in his home, the grouping of cases on this basis was also examined. . . . the Montgomery cases have been indicated according to place where employed, or if unemployed according to residence. *This . . . suggests a focal center of the disease in the heart of the business district.* A large proportion of the cases were employed (or lived, if unemployed) within four city squares of the corner of North Court and Monroe Streets. This section of the business district is largely made up of retail stores and markets, clothing stores, drug stores, grocery stores, butcher shops, fruit stands, seed and grain stores, etc.

. . . the Savannah cases have been spotted in like manner according to place where employed, or if unemployed within the city, according to residence. There is a similar grouping in the retail business section, but the disease is not so sharply focalized as in Montgomery. Attention is called particularly to . . . the location of the food-marketing center of the city.

(h) *Occupation.* The apparent focalization of the disease in the business district may be due to a concentration of employed persons in this area, or to a greater risk in certain occupations which are located in this part of the city. Evidence on this point has been obtained by an analysis of the cases according to the broad occupational groupings afforded by the United States census and presented in Tables 5 and 6.

In Montgomery 18 of the 29 cases in males (62 percent) were engaged in "trade" (clerks, proprietors, managers, salesmen, dealers, etc.), although only 23 percent of the total number of occupied males over 10 years of age are so engaged. Only one case occurred among the 4114 men employed in "manufacturing and mechanical industries"; three among the 2608 men in "transportation." The three cases charged to "domestic and personal service" were employed

in restaurants.

Similarly, in Savannah 23 of the 52 males (44 percent) were in "trade," although only 17 percent of the total number of occupied males are so engaged. The rates in "manufacturing and mechanical industries" and in "transportation" are comparatively low. In "agriculture, forestry, and animal husbandry" the cases consisted of four employed by dairies and two retired farmers; in "domestic and personal service" four employed in restaurants, one barber, and one hotel keeper.

Among employed females the distribution is much the same in both cities, though the groups are small. In both instances the highest incidence is found in "trade," the rate being approximately the same as for males in this group alone.

Using a different basis of classification, and the occupations as given in Tables 3 and 4, it is notable that in Montgomery 10 of the 32 employed persons (31 percent) who had typhus were engaged in handling foods, groceries, meat, produce, feed, flour, or were employed in feed stores and restaurants. In Savannah 20 of 59 employed persons (34 percent) having the disease were so engaged. The apparent excess of cases among food handlers is strikingly similar in the two cities, as are the rates for both males and females in "trade."

These analyses of the occupations of persons attacked by endemic typhus suggest very strongly that as compared with the rest of the population those engaged in "trade," and especially those employed in food depots, groceries, feed stores, and restaurants, are exposed to a distinctly increased risk of infection.

(i) *Social status.* The occupational analysis also brings out the fact that the disease attacked, for the most part, persons earning a reasonably good livelihood. There is a notable absence of cases among unskilled laborers and unemployed males.

From personal observation of the cases and their surroundings the author and his collaborators are convinced that the disease did not select the poor and uncleanly. It occurred among all classes. The cases so far as they were discovered present a fair cross section of the social strata of the average American community. This implies that a great majority of the cases were in persons cleanly in their homes and in their personal habits.

There were no cases among the inmates of

jails, prisons, or asylums. There was no particular association of the disease with cheap boarding or rooming houses. The time-honored characteristics of Old World typhus were entirely lacking in this respect.

(j) Contact between cases. One of the items of information on the case history form used in the Alabama series was, "History of Contact with Antecedent Case." In only one instance among the 44 cases in Montgomery was the patient or the physician in attendance or the investigator able to state that there was definite close association within three weeks prior to onset with a case of the same disease or a suspected case. The one exception was case No. 4, who came down eight days after her husband.

Of the 60 cases occurring in other parts of Alabama for whom a case history form was filed, in no instance was the patient or his physician aware of contact of the type described with a preceding case.

The same statement holds true for the Savannah cases with the following exceptions:

Case 32 came down about seven days after his wife and two children had become ill with the same disease.

Case 27, onset July 5; case 35, onset July 27; and case 39, onset August 7, were employed in a large wholesale grocery store. They were thus in casual contact at their place of business.

Case 28, onset June 25; case 32, onset July 9; and case 36 (fatal), onset August 12, worked on the same dairy farm and were in contact in their work. It will be noted that these cases occurred about the same time as those in the wholesale grocery store noted above. The dairy purchased feed from this store during the period involved, but personal contact of the men on the dairy farm with the men in the store could not be demonstrated. There were no known cases of typhus among the 100 or more patrons of the dairy.

It is thus seen that known contact with a preceding case is a very rare finding. It must be admitted, of course, that close contacts may have existed but were undiscovered, particularly in those cases in which dependence was placed entirely upon information supplied by the attending physician and his patient. On the other hand, it seems quite unlikely that any considerable number of actually traceable contacts with sick persons or convalescents should have been overlooked.

Moreover, there is evidence from another angle that the disease observed in this study was not readily communicable from person to person. For each case that occurred there were a number of persons in intimate contact with the patient, including other members of the family, physicians, nurses, and visitors. Notwithstanding the absence of prophylactic measures, infections among these known intimate contacts were rare.

Among the 197 cases on which this report is based there were only two instances, noted above, in which more than one case occurred in a family in such sequence as to suggest the possibility that the earlier case might have infected the later one.

Eighteen of the 93 Savannah cases and six of the 44 Montgomery cases were hospitalized. No effort was made to delouse the patient upon admission to the hospital; no precautions whatever were taken with regard to lice. Not a single case has occurred among nurses, attendants, physicians, or fellow patients. One physician had the disease in Montgomery, but he stated positively that he had not attended a case of known or suspected typhus for at least one month before the onset of his illness.

Brill (*10*) states that in over 500 cases of endemic typhus observed by him in New York City there have been only two instances in which more than one member of a family has been infected with the disease at the same time or nearly the same time. Many of the New York cases have been hospitalized, from 15 to 30 being reported in that city each year since 1912, but no contact cases among patients, nurses, or doctors have been reported.

Allan (*11*) was unable to trace any contact from case to case at Charlotte, N.C. In this connection mention should also be made of the numerous other cases reported in the literature and to the Surgeon General which have been sporadic and without secondary spread.

By way of contrast attention is called to Boyd's report (*6*) of a small outbreak of Mexican typhus ("tabardillo") in Iowa. During 1915-1918 a considerable epidemic of "tabardillo" raged in Mexico, and as a consequence sporadic outbreaks were originated in American territory by imported laborers. A Mexican laborer was admitted to the Santa Fe Railroad hospital, Fort Madison, Iowa. It was later discovered that he had typhus, and lice were found upon his clothes. Following the diagnosis of his case, the physician who examined him on admission, the nurse who took charge of his clothing, two male nurses who attended him, and two other hospital patients came down with the disease within 30 days.

The lack of a traceable relationship between cases and the extremely low secondary familial attack rate is a striking and constant characteristic of the endemic typhus of the United States.

Multiple cases on the same premises. Although cases have so rarely been observed in the same family in such close sequence as to suggest communication of the disease during its acute febrile stage, several instances have been noted in which cases recurred on the same premises separated by intervals of six months or more.

In Montgomery Mrs. R., living at _____ Columbus Street, had a typical attack of Brill's disease in December 1922. Three years later, in September 1925, while living at the same address, her husband had the disease.

In Savannah, at _____ Abercorn Street, there is an old frame building with a store on the first floor and a housekeeping flat on the second. In August 1923, a butcher who operated a meat market in the rear of the store had typhus. Eighteen months later, in January, 1925, his father-in-law, who lived with him and also assisted him in the meat shop, had the disease. In the flat above the store lived a family of nine persons; they had occupied these premises for eight years with the exception of six months in 1924. One of this family, Mrs. M., had the disease in August, 1925, seven months after the preceding case. Although treated at home, there were no other cases in the family, nor was it possible to obtain a history of any previous cases in this family.[4]

Louse infestation. In view of the evidence that the disease is typhus, and that typhus, as known

in the Old World, is transmitted from man to man by the louse, as careful inquiry as possible was made in each case to detect lice or any evidence suggesting prior infestation with them. This inquiry consisted in asking the physician in attendance and the patient, in all cases investigated, whether louse infestation had been noticed, or, indeed, whether the patient had noticed insect bites of any kind. In all cases investigated by the author in Alabama and in the few seen in Savannah search was made for nits or live insects on the hair of the head and body and on the bedclothes, and for scratch marks on the skin which might suggest infestation; at the same time other members of the family who were present were inspected and the environment was surveyed with the same purpose in view. Doctor Bassett has made the same search in all patients sick with this disease which he has seen in Savannah; in addition, in some few instances, he has carefully searched the clothing worn by the patient prior to his illness. Every physician who has attended a case of Brill's disease which came to the author's attention has been questioned with regard to the presence of lice on his patient.

In Alabama such inquiry has been uniformly negative, except that in one out of 104 cases there was a history of a young girl living in the same house with the patient having had head lice three months previous to the onset.

The inquiry in the 93 cases in Savannah was similarly negative with two exceptions; In case S12, 1923, proprietor of a cheap clothing store, a Jew, the attending physician made a positive statement that he had seen lice on the person and bed of the patient; in case S15, a negro, clinically positive for typhus, a health department inspector who had been sent to clean up the premises of the patient after his removal to the hospital stated that he had seen vermin on the bedclothes. In neither instance were there secondary cases in the household or among the known contacts of the patient.

While this evidence does not in any single case exclude the possibility that the patient may have been bitten by one or more lice prior to the onset of the disease, or may have had a light infestation which was not discovered, it does suffice to definitely establish that *the disease was not associated with lousiness.* This much is, indeed, sufficiently well established by the geographic and social distribution of the disease, a consid-

---

[4] In addition to these instances, two more have been noted in 1926. In the large wholesale grocery and feed store to which reference has been made under "Contact," in which three cases occurred during the summer of 1925, the manager became ill with the disease in August, 1926, no cases having occurred among other employees, so far as could be ascertained, in the meantime. A lunch room nearby, in which case No. 1 (July, 1923) was employed, recently changed owners, and the new owner, case S48, came down with the disease in August, 1926. In the same neighborhood D. K., a dealer in hides, furs, and chickens, was taken ill in June, 1926, followed by another worker in the same establishment six weeks later. There were no cases among the family contacts of either.

erable proportion of the cases having occurred in persons of such habits and living in such an environment that the harboring of lice is not to be suspected.

DISCUSSION

The evidence thus far adduced indicates that there is endemic in the southeastern United States a disease which is as yet indistinguishable from Old World typhus, clinically and serologically, except with regard to its relatively mild clinical course and low fatality rate. It appears to be identical with the disease described by Brill as endemic in New York City. On the other hand, the epidemiological characteristics of this disease present certain points of difference with Old World typhus which appear to be significant. They relate principally to the mode of transmission.

The louse (*P. humanus* var. *corporis* and *P. humanus* var. *capitis*) has been satisfactorily proven to be the usual—not necessarily the only—vector of Old World epidemic typhus. Transmission of the virus from man to man is accomplished by the agency of this insect. Reviewing the observations which have thus far been made upon the endemic typhus of the southeastern United States, consideration may be given to the evidence for and against transmission from man to man by the louse.

As regards positive evidence which would suggest association of this disease with lice, not a single circumstance has been discovered which suggests such a mode of transmission. In other words, if this disease had been considered as one of altogether unknown etiology, with no prior assumption as to its mode of transmission, the facts which have been brought out with respect to the cases observed in Alabama and Savannah, Ga., would not even give rise to the suspicion that infection was transmitted by the louse. Of positive evidence tending to incriminate the louse, then this study yields none.

Moreover, there are certain facts which weigh distinctly against the supposition that the disease, as observed in these areas, has been transmitted by lice. These are:

I. The seasonal distribution of the disease, reaching its maximum in the warm weather of summer and autumn, is the reverse of the seasonal distribution of diseases known to be louse-borne—Old World typhus, relapsing fever, trench fever, which characteristically reach their highest prevalence in the colder months of winter and spring.

II. The social and environmental distribution of the disease is not such as would be expected, and in a vast majority of cases (all but two in a series of 197) absolutely no evidence of louse infestation was discovered. It is in accordance with experience that cleanly persons upon whom lice cannot establish themselves may occasionally be bitten by lice accidentally picked up, and that people of this class may consequently become infected with a louse-borne disease, especially such as are in close contact with louse-infested patients. It is, however, contrary to all experience of Old World typhus and relapsing fever, known louse-borne diseases, that infection should be almost *exclusively confined* to persons who are not demonstrably infested, as has been the case here. It seems, indeed, almost inconceivable that in a louse-borne infection there should be such *absence* of association with lice.

III. As a corollary of the preceding, the lack of evidence of direct communicability, after a considerable period of observation, is not in accord with common experience in louse-borne diseases. The fact that contacts of the observed cases have rarely been infected is not by itself evidence against louse-borne infection, since these patients, being not lousy, would not be expected to spread the disease. On the other hand, it is a remarkable circumstance that the undiscovered cases which must have existed, if the disease be transmitted in this way, did not cause here and there small localized outbreaks in a labor gang, boarding house, or some equivalent group.

IV. Finally, reviewing the distribution of this disease and the circumstances existing in the communities studied, the facts seem to be incompatible with the assumption that the infection has been conveyed by lice under the conditions which are generally accepted as governing the transmission of Old World typhus (*18*) based upon the present status of epidemiological and experimental evidence in that disease.

These conditions may be briefly summarized as follows:

(1) That the virus exists in nature only (*a*) in the blood and tissues of infected human beings, and (*b*) in the bodies of lice which have fed upon such persons.

(2) That man is infective for the louse only for a brief period, namely, from the onset of the disease until defervescence has been established, a matter of two or three weeks.

(3) That one attack in man confers a definite, high, and durable immunity.

(4) That the louse, having bitten an infective man, after a period of five or six days is capable of conveying the infection to other persons by its bite.

(5) That the louse remains infective during the remainder of its life, a matter at most of two or three months (*19*).

(6) Almost all attempts to demonstrate the inheritance of infectivity in the louse have failed.[5]

To maintain the disease under these conditions of transmission, therefore, there must be available a supply of infective lice, renewed at frequent intervals by the occurrence of cases in lousy persons, either infected locally or imported. For *sustained endemic* prevalence, not tending to decline, the louse infestation of the population must be sufficient to establish on the average at least one new human infection for every one that is terminated by death or recovery. Otherwise the prevalence will decline. To meet these conditions a certain proportion of the cases, probably a majority of them, must occur in persons sufficiently infested with lice to serve as foci for the infection of others, since the cases which may occur in uninfested persons bitten casually by stray lice and living in a clean environment would not contribute to the further spread of the infection.

As to the communities considered in this study, it seems doubtful that the louse infestation of their population is sufficient to sustain an infection subject to these conditions of transmission. Obvious lousiness—heavy infestation with body lice—is an exceedingly rare condition

in the southern United States. The climate is mild; the winters are short; even the poorer population are relatively cleanly in person and surroundings. Lice are looked upon as a disgrace, and strenuous efforts are made to destroy them when they are found. They are occasionally encountered on beggars, vagabonds, or destitute and debilitated persons. Jails, institutions caring for the poor, and cheap lodging houses sometimes become infested. No outbreaks of this disease have been traced to such places.

Allan (*11*), commenting upon the absence of lice in the cases which he reported, stated that in 15 years of dispensary and office practice in Charlotte, N. C., he has never seen body lice on a patient. His experience in this regard is not different from that of a great many other physicians in this section of the country who have been questioned.

Head lice are not so very uncommon in school children; inspections sometimes reveal as high as 4 or 5 percent infestation in the poorer sections. In Montgomery head lice were found on a few children in three schools during 1924-1925, but less than one percent of the school population was affected. No relationship could be traced between these schools and the occurrence of cases.

With these observations in mind as regards the cases and the communities in which they have occurred, in order to account for the existence of a louse-borne person to person transmission in this disease in the southeastern United States one must assume the existence during at least three years of a *concealed* reservoir of infection in lousy persons, either (*a*) in the form of clinically recognizable cases which have somehow remained undiscovered by the investigation, or else (*b*) in a clinically unrecognizable form as larval cases (the "typhus exanthematique inapparent" of Charles Nicolle, *20*) or as passive carriers of the virus.

With regard to the first of these assumptions, it seems most improbable that clinically recognizable infections in louse-infested individuals should have been overlooked while such numbers of cases in vermin-free persons were discovered. Such a circumstance is the more unlikely because the cases in lousy individuals would, as has been pointed out already, give rise to household epidemics, which would attract attention.

---

[5] The above are given as the conditions of transmission which seem to be generally accepted for Old World typhus. It cannot be said that all these conditions have been rigidly proven. For instance, the possibility has not been excluded that the virus of typhus may have some mammalian host other than man, and in fact the existence of such a reservoir is suggested by the susceptibility of certain of the lower animals to experimental infection. Nor has it been proven that the louse is the only actual or potential insect vector, or that the infection is never transmitted to the progeny of infected lice. Likewise, while there is no positive evidence of long continued infectivity of man, the possibility of occasional prolonged latent infection has not been excluded.

Regarding the alternative assumption that the infection may have been spread from clinically unrecognizable cases which have occurred in lousy persons, it is undoubtedly true that mild atypical cases occur and that these may escape diagnosis, especially if the eruption is not well developed. As a result of having done a large number of Weil-Felix reactions on blood specimens from febrile cases suspected of being typhoid or typhus, it seems unlikely that abortive infections form a very appreciable proportion of the total number, and there is no particular reason why they should be more common in the lousy than in the nonlousy.

Concerning the existence among human beings of a large number of "inapparent infections" in the sense of Nicolle, there is little evidence to suppport his hypothesis. Nicolle reasons that they do exist by analogy with what occurs when certain rodents are inoculated with virus in the laboratory. The response of human beings to infection naturally acquired can hardly be compared with that of rodents artificially inoculated.

Human carriers of typhus virus have never been demonstrated, and from present knowledge it seems quite unlikely that they exist. The disease is apparently a blood-stream infection with localization in certain organs of the body, chiefly brain, spleen, and liver. It has been repeatedly shown experimentally that the virus disappears from the blood at the time of convalescence, or within a day or two after the temperature returns to normal. The virus has not yet been demonstrated in the discharges of the body. Upon recovery a sharp immunity is established.

In order to account for the transmission of the disease from man to man by the louse under the conditions which exist in the southeastern United States, it seems necessary to assume an entirely altered conception of this disease, a conception which does not appear to be in harmony with the established facts, experimental and epidemiological, so far as they have been ascertained. In fact, whatever the means of transmission from man to man, if it be assumed that it is an exclusively human infection, then it must exist largely in unrecognized form, since it is evident that the recognized cases do not link together. These considerations have led to a tentative rejection of the human louse as the principal vector and of man as the principal reservoir of the disease in this part of the United States and the search for some other mode of transmission.

It is generally accepted that typhus—and hence the disease with which we are dealing—belongs to that group of diseases known as the "rickettsiae." In addition to typhus, this group includes Rocky Mountain spotted fever, trench fever, Tsutsugamushi disease (including the variety described by Schuffner (*21*) and by Walch and Keukenschrijver (*22*) in Sumatra), and heartwater, a disease of sheep, goats, and cattle in South Africa described by Cowdry (*23*). These five diseases possess certain features in common. They are acute infections transmitted by blood-feeding insects or arachnids; they exhibit a fairly high fever, running a relatively definite short course; a single attack confers upon the survivors a comparatively high degree of immunity for a period of months or years, or even for life. There is invariably more or less involvement of the nervous system and there is a characteristic exanthem in all, with the single exception of heartwater. It seems reasonably well established that the etiologic agent of each belongs to the rickettsiae defined by Cowdry (*24*) as follows:

"Gram-negative, bacteriumlike organisms of small size, usually less than half a micron in diameter, which are found intracellularly in arthropods, which may be more or less pleomorphic and stain rather lightly with aniline dyes, but which resemble in most of their properties the type species, *R. prowazeki.*"

While the rickettsiae which have been described in these diseases typically inhabit arthropod tissues, it is questionable whether an arthropod reservoir of the parasites can exist indefinitely. In Rocky Mountain spotted fever, although hereditary transmission in the tick has been demonstrated, it is not yet known through how many generations the virus can be continued in its arthropod host. Wild rodents, such as rabbits and ground squirrels, probably play a role in maintaining the reservoir of the virus from which man becomes infected accidentally. In Japanese river fever the vector is a mite, *T. akamushi*, found in great numbers within the ears of the field mouse (*Microtus montebelli*), which probably acts as a reservoir of the virus. Walch has brought evidence to indicate that in Sumatra *T. deliensis*, likewise a parasite of the field rat, is responsible for the transmission of the pseudotyphus of Deli. Little is known of trench fever beyond its transmission from man to man by the louse. In heartwater Cowdry has found that hereditary transmission of the virus in ticks does not occur, hence some other reservoir of the virus is necessary for its maintenance; presumably the sheep, goats, and cattle sick with heartwater afford this, though the possibility of a reservoir existing among small rodents has not been excluded (25).

In typhus fever it has been shown by Nicolle and others that beside the chimpanzee and the monkey certain small rodents are susceptible to the virus; i.e., guinea pigs, rabbits, rats (white and gray), mice (white), the gerbil. In a recent publication Nicolle (26) reports a second series of passages of typhus virus through 12 generations of white rats.

In view of these considerations the question arises whether in the endemic typhus of the southeastern United States a reservoir of the disease may not exist other than in man, a rodent reservoir with accidental transmission to man through the bite of some parasitic bloodsucking insect or arachnid. Such a hypothesis is compatible with the epidemiological characteristics which have been presented, namely, (1) the uneven focal distribution of the disease; (2) its sporadic occurrence; (3) its apparent lack of direct communicability from an infected person; (4) its association with the place of business rather than with the home, particularly with those premises upon which foodstuffs are handled or stored; (5) the recurrence of cases on the same premises after considerable intervals of time; and (6) its seasonal incidence.

Obviously the rodents upon which suspicion immediately falls are rats and mice, and the parasitic intermediaries which are first suspected are fleas, mites, or possibly ticks.

Without desiring to emphasize the analogy, there is similarity between the epidemiology of this disease and that of plague as observed in the southern United States.

It is interesting to note also that the observations with regard to this typhuslike disease in the southeastern United States are not peculiar to this country. Many reports of a similar nature have appeared in medical literature in recent years from various parts of the world. Attention is called particularly to those from Australia and from the Federated Malay States.

Hone (27), in a series of papers, has described a situation in and around Adelaide strikingly similar to the one here reported for Savannah or Montgomery. The first 13 cases studied were in men who handled wheat, and later cases showed an apparent relationship to the handling of foodstuffs. More recently Wheatland (28) has reported a small epidemic of cases of mild typhus, giving a positive Weil-Felix, from a district surrounding Toowoomba, Australia. The occurrence of these cases seemed to be associated with a migration of mice, accompanied by an epizootic, and were at first called "mouse fever."

According to Fletcher and Lesslar (29) typhus was never recognized in the Federated Malay States until 1924. Between August, 1924, and January, 1925, a diagnosis of typhus was made in 18 cases, seven of which were in Europeans. The disease was sporadic in occurrence; there was no evidence of the direct infection from man to man, and apparently there was an association of the disease with cattle keepers and with a camping ground that was notorious for its rats.

In summary, despite the clinical, serological, and experimental evidence as to the identity of these cases in the southeastern United States with Old World typhus and "tabardillo," there are significant divergencies in the epidemiology. These lead to a tentative rejection of transmission from human to human through the louse as explaining the distribution of this endemic disease, and suggest the existence of some other mechanism for the propagation of the virus. From a consideration of what is known of this group of diseases, the "rickettsias," and specifically with regard to the susceptibility of rodents to typhus virus, it seems probable that a reservoir may exist apart from man. A reservoir in rats or mice, with accidental transmission to man through the bite of some parasitic blood-sucking arthropod, is compatible with the epidemiological characteristics which have been revealed by this study of the disease in Alabama and Savannah, Ga. Some experimental studies designed to test the theory of the existence of a rodent reservoir of the infection are now in progress in the hygienic laboratory of the Public Health Service, but have not yet progressed far enough for a report.

CONCLUSIONS

1. A disease giving a positive Weil-Felix reaction, and clinically indistinguishable from typhus fever except with regard to its relative mildness and low fatality rate, is endemic in the southeastern United States.

2. The epidemiology of this disease appears to differ significantly from that of Old World typhus.

3. The epidemiological characteristics afford no evidence suggesting louse transmission and are interpreted as being at variance with man-to-man transfer by lice, unless it be assumed at the same time that the disease occurs mostly in unrecognizable form.

4. It is suggested as an hypothesis which seems to afford a more probable explanation of the mode of transmission that a reservoir exists other than in man, and that this reservoir is in rodents, probably rats or mice, from which the disease is occasionally transmitted to man.[6]

ACKNOWLEDGMENTS

The author desires to express his grateful appreciation to Surg. W. H. Frost for many valued suggestions in the pursuance of this study and the preparation of the manuscripts; to Dr. Samuel J. Welch, State health officer, and associates in the Alabama State Board of Health; to Dr. Victor C. Bassett, city health officer of Savannah, Ga.; and to the many members of the medical profession who have generously aided in the collection of this data.

References

(1) Brill, Nathan E. A study of seventeen cases of a disease clinically resembling typhoid fever, but without the Widal reaction, etc. *NY Med J* 67:48-54; 77-82, 1898.

(2) Brill, Nathan E. An acute infectious disease of unknown origin. A clinical study based on 221 cases. *Am J Med Sci* 139:484-502, 1910.

(3) Brill, Nathan E. Pathological and experimental data derived from a further study of an acute infectious disease of unknown origin. *Ibid.* 142:196-218, 1911.

(4) Anderson, John F. and Joseph Goldberger. The relation of so-called Brill's disease to typhus fever. *Public Health Rep* 27(5):149-160, 1912.

(5) Pierce, C.C. Combating typhus fever on the Mexican border. *Public Health Rep* 32(12):426-429, 1917.

(6) Boyd, M.F. Recent appearance of typhus fever in Iowa; a report. *J Iowa State Med Soc* 7:45-51, 1917.

(7) Cumming, James G. and H.F. Senftner. The prevention of endemic typhus in California. *JAMA* 69:98-102, 1917.

(8) Armstrong, Charles. Typhus fever on the San Juan Indian Reservation, 1920 and 1921. *Public Health Rep* 37(12):685-693, 1922.

(9) Tappan, J.W. Protective health measures on the United States-Mexican border. *JAMA* 87:1022-1025, 1926.

(10) Brill Typhus. Nelson Loose-Leaf Medicine, v. 1:191-201.

(11) Allan, William. Endemic typhus fever in North Carolina. *South Med Surg* (Charlotte, N. C.) 85:65-68, 1923.

(12) Maxcy, Kenneth F. and Leon C. Havens. A series of cases giving a positive Weil-Felix reaction. *Am J Trop Med* 3:495-507, 1923.

(13) Paullin, James Edgar. Typhus fever, with a report of cases. *South Med J* 6:36-43, 1913.

(14) Newell, L.B. and William Allan. Typhus fever:A report of four cases. *South Med J* 7:564-568, 1914.

(15) Sydenstricker, V.P. Endemic typhus fever. (Abstract.) *JAMA* 87:124, 1926.

(16) Maxcy, Kenneth F. Clinical observations on endemic typhus (Brill's disease) in Southern United States. *Public Health Rep* 41(25):1213-1220, 1926.

(17) League of Nations. Statistics of notifiable diseases for the year 1924. *Epidemiological Intelligence* No. 9:31-33, 1925.

(18) Arkwright, J.A. Remarks on the virus of typhus fever and the means by which it is conveyed. *Proc Roy Soc Med* 13:87-95, 1920.

(19) Nuttall, George H.F. The biology of *Pediculus humanus*. *Parasitology* 10:80-185, 1917.

(20) Nicolle, Charles. Les infections inapparentes à propos du typhus exanthématique inapparent. *Presse méd* 33:1169-1170, 1925.

(21) Schüffner, W. and M. Wachsmuth. Ueber eine typhusartige Erkrankung. (Pseudotyphus von Deli.) *Ztschr f klin Med* (Berl.) 71:133-156, 1910.

(22) Walch, Eduard W. and Nicolaas C. Keukenschrijver. Ueber die Epidemiologie des Pseudotyphus von Deli. *Arch f Schiffs-u Tropen-Hyg* (Leipz.) 29:420-428, 1925.

(23) Cowdry, E.V. Studies on the etiology of heartwater, I. Observation of a Rickettsia, *Rickettsia ruminantium* (n. sp.) in the tissues of infected animals. *J Exp Med* 42:231-252, 1925.

(24) Cowdry, E.V. Studies on the etiology of heartwater, II. *Rickettsia ruminantium* (n. sp.) in the tissues of ticks transmitting the disease. 42:253-274, 1925.

(25) Cowdry, E.V. Rickettsiae and disease. *Arch Path Lab Med* 2:59-90, 1926.

(26) Nicolle, Charles. Contribution nouvelle a la

---

[6] This theory of the source and transmission of the "endemic typhus" referred to in this paper does not necessarily deny the identity of that disease with Old World typhus; for while it is satisfactorily proven that in its epidemic form typhus is transmitted from man to man by the agency of the louse, there remains the possibility—unsupported by positive evidence but not yet excluded—that the disease may exist also in rodents, and that in the intervals between epidemics the infection may be carried over in this reservoir.

connaissance du typhus expérimental chez les mer- idés. Arch de I'Inst Pasteur de Tunis 15:267-275, 1926.

(27) Hone, F.S. A series of cases resembling typhus fever. *Med J Aust* 1:1-13, 1922.

(28) Wheatland, F.T. A fever resembling a mild form of typhus fever. *Med J Aust* 1:261-266, 1926.

(29) Fletcher, William and J.E. Lesslar. Tropical ty- phus in the Federated Malay States. *Bull Inst Med Res Fed Malay States* (Kuala Lumpur) No 2:1-88, 1925.

ENDEMIC FLUOROSIS AND ITS RELATION TO DENTAL CARIES[1]

H. Trendley Dean[2]

INTRODUCTION

The first thorough study of mottled enamel, that of Black (1) and McKay (2) at Colorado Springs and including the Pike's Peak watershed, reported as early as 1916 that, in regard to caries, the teeth of these Colorado children compare favorably with those of other communities where endemic mottled enamel is unknown. Black also wrote of the difficulty of successfully filling carious mottled enamel teeth and stated that, though the percentage of carious teeth is less than in non-endemic areas, probably a greater proportion of filled teeth are eventually lost because of the difficulty of retaining fillings in the hypoplastic tooth structure.

Workers in other countries have also commented on the qualitative aspects of this phenomenon. Mottled enamel is endemic in the southwestern part of the Japanese Archipelago. Masaki (3) reported 18 endemic areas in the Prefectures of Hyogo, Fukuoka, Ehime, Hiroshima, and Aichi, 12 of the 18 being located in Hyogo and Fukuoka. In an English abstract of this original report, this investigator states that "It is also remarkable that the percentage of dental caries is comparatively small among those who suffer this abnormality." The number of observations upon which this generalization was based is not stated in the abstract.

Ainsworth has commented on the lessened prevalence of dental caries among children in the endemic areas of Maldon and Heybridge, Essex County, England. In connection with the studies of the Committee for the Investigation of Dental Diseases of the Medical Research Council, this investigator (4) examined approximately 4000 children in the public elementary schools in various parts of England and Wales. He states (5) that the condition of the teeth in the Council schools at Maldon and Heybridge[3] was generally good, being well above the average for Council schools. He specifically notes that "there was relatively little caries: 7.9 percent of the permanent teeth were carious, as compared with an average in all districts examined of 13.1 percent; and 12.9 percent of deciduous teeth were carious against 43.3 percent in all districts." The percentages just quoted are reported as corrected for age distribution (4) in the different schools.

Erausquin (6), who has studied mottled enamel extensively in the Argentine Republic, records that there appears to be an inverse variation between dental caries and "dientes veteados," the name by which endemic dental fluorosis is known in the Argentine. He stated, however, that the findings were not conclusive on the basis of the limited number of areas studied.

Probably the first attempt to study specifically the relationship of mottled enamel to dental caries was made by McKay (7) who, in 1929, attacked the hypothesis that dental decay might be superinduced by "defective" enamel structure, by citing as evidence the observation that mottled enamel teeth, which probably constitute "the most poorly constructed enamel of which there is any record in the literature of dentistry," do not appear to show any greater liability to dental caries than do normally calcified teeth.

His report refers to studies made at Bauxite (Ark.), Minonk (Ill.), Towner (Colo.), Bruneau (Idaho), and the Pima Indian School at Sacaton (Ariz.). Certain tabulated data from the last three named places are included in McKay's report. Table 1 has been compiled from certain of these data.

In 1933-34 a study was begun by the United States Public Health Service to determine the minimal threshold of toxicity of chronic endemic dental fluorosis. In this study (8, 9, 10)

Source: *Public Health Reports* 53(33):1443-1452, 1938.
[1] From the Division of Infectious Diseases, National Institute of Health, U.S.A.
[2] Dental surgeon, United States Public Health Service.

[3] A total of 214 children was examined in the two schools.

Table 1. Variation in prevalence of dental caries in normal and mottled enamel teeth of three endemic areas according to McKay.

Locality	Number of children examined	Total number of permanent teeth examined		Number of teeth examined and percentage with dental caries			
				All teeth		Molar teeth	
				Number examined	Percent carious	Number examined	Percent carious
Towner, Colo. (Pop. 154 in 1930)	55[a]	1264	Normal teeth	879	11	254	46
			Mottled enamel teeth	385	9	101	42
Bruneau, Idaho (Pop. 481 in 1930)	54[a]	1142	Normal teeth	356	16	126	64
			Mottled enamel teeth	797	8	213	33
Pima Indian School, Sacaton Ariz. (Pop. unstated)	78[a]	2178	Normal teeth	283	22	99	81
			Mottled enamel teeth	1895	14	529	58

[a] Age, sex, color, continuity of residence, and constancy of exposure to the mottled enamel-producing waters not recorded in the report.

consecutive monthly water samples were received from each of the cities surveyed, which permitted the computation of an arithmetic mean annual fluoride (F) content of the communal water supply. The clinical examinations in these cities were limited to those children who were born in the community, had always resided there, and had continuously used the common water supply for both drinking and cooking.

In certain of these cities, in addition to recording the degree of severity of mottled enamel, each child was examined for other defects of the enamel, such as present caries, past caries (fillings or extractions), pits and fissures, hypoplasias, etc. The examinations were made in a good light with the child seated facing a window. Mouth mirrors free from blemishes and new explorers were used. For each child examined in connection with the caries aspects of the study, the facts with respect to residence and continual use of the common water supply were verified by an interview with the child's parent or guardian.

The amount of caries recorded may appear somewhat higher than usual; for, in addition to definite cavitation, defects in the enamel on caries-susceptible surfaces showing either a discoloration or opacity around the edges and in which an explorer would cling, were counted as caries. All examinations were made, however, by one individual, the writer.

An analysis of these data indicates that a higher percentage of caries-free children is found in cities whose water supplies contain relatively toxic amounts of fluorides than in

those communities with water supplies not so affected. Since in certain cities only the nine-year-old children were examined, comparisons will be limited to children of this age. It was decided also to omit cities where less than 25 children were examined at this age. Table 2 presents the pertinent data.

The data shown in Table 2 indicate a greater freedom from dental caries in the 122 children exposed to domestic waters of higher fluoride (F) concentration, both with respect to permanent and deciduous teeth. It is a well-known fact that deciduous teeth are seldom affected with mottled enamel; in this particular group, only three children, all of Colorado Springs, showed even the mildest forms of mottled enamel in their deciduous teeth, generally in the second deciduous molars. Of the 122 children in the group, 60 were caries-free with respect to the permanent teeth. Of these 60, 33, or 55 percent, were affected with mottled enamel. In the whole group (122), the incidence of mottled enamel was 53 percent. These observations suggest that the limited-immunity-producing factor present in the water is operative whether or not the tooth is affected by mottled enamel. Whether this mechanism functions locally, systemically, or both ways, is not known.

RELATION OF ENDEMIC FLUOROSIS TO DENTAL CARIES IN LARGE POPULATION GROUPS

Source of data

The disclosure of an inverse relation between the prevalence of dental caries and the fluoride

Table 2. Percentages of caries-free children, 9 years of age, in 6 selected cities classified according to their continuous use of water of different fluoride (F) concentration.

Locality	Actual community mottled enamel index	Domestic water supply[a]		Number of children examined
		Fluoride (F) content	Total hardness	
		ppm	*ppm*	
Pueblo, Colo.	Negative	0.6	303	49
Junction City, Kans.	Negative	0.7	277	30
East Moline, Ill.	Borderline	1.5[b]	242	35
Monmouth, Ill.	Slight	1.7	288	29
Galesburg, Ill.	Slight	1.8	237	39
Colorado Springs, Colo.	Slight	2.5	20	54

Locality	Caries-free children					
	All teeth		Permanent		Deciduous	
	Number	Percent	Number	Percent	Number	Percent
Pueblo, Colo.	3	6	18	37	4	9
Junction City, Kans.	0	0	8	26	1	3
East Moline, Ill.	2	6	4	11	8	33
Monmouth, Ill.	6	21	16	55	6	21
Galesburg, Ill.	8	20	22	56	11	28
Colorado Springs, Colo.	13	24	22	41	21	40

Fluoride content in ppm.	Number examined	Composite sample of above 9-year-old children classified on the basis of exposure to domestic water of lower and higher fluoride (F) concentration.					
0.6-1.5	114[c]	5	4	30	26	13	11
1.7-2.5	122[d]	27	22	60	49	38	31

[a] For detailed mineral analyses of these waters, see refs. (8), (10).
[b] Subject to possible correction to 1.3 ppm.
[c] Of this group, 51 were boys and 63 girls; by color, 108 white and 6 colored.
[d] In this group 59 were boys and 63 girls; classified according to color, 116 white, 4 colored, and 2 Mexican.

concentration of the domestic water supply, as shown in Table 2, raises the question of the kind of relationship between these two variables in other and larger population groups. The requisite data on dental caries are provided by the dental survey of school children 6 to 14 years of age, made in 26 States in 1933-1934 (*11*) under the direction of the United States Public Health Service. This survey included a total of 34 283 examinations of white children in South Dakota, 15 465 in Colorado, and 48 628 in Wisconsin, made by dentists reported as using a mouth mirror and explorer in making the examinations. Furthermore, these examinations were made on a standard examination form and largely for the purpose of recording the amount of dental caries in the school population; the marked differences, therefore, in the amount of caries noted in groups using domes-

tic waters of different mineral composition take on an added significance.

Data on mottled enamel, on the other hand, are furnished by a recent (1938) survey of South Dakota made by the writer. During this survey (April-May 1938), approximately 3300 school children in 51 communities were examined for mottled enamel, and endemic mottled enamel was demonstrated in 35 communities, each having a common water supply. A comparable degree of mottled enamel was widely prevalent in the surrounding rural districts in certain of the counties, ascribable to the general custom of farmers of obtaining their domestic water supply from artesian wells in the Dakota sandstone. Moreover, the examination of school children with discontinuities in their residence pointed to 21 other places in the State, not as yet surveyed, but where, on the basis of clinical signs present in the children, mottled enamel is endemic.

Method of analysis

All South Dakota counties listed in [*Public Health*] *Bulletin* No. 226 (*11*) in which 35 percent or more of the estimated population of ages 6 to 14 years had been examined, were selected for study. On the basis of the mottled enamel data, these counties were divided into three groups: (*a*) Counties where mottled enamel is prevalent, (*b*) counties where mottled enamel distribution is uneven, and (*c*) counties which, so far as we know, are entirely free from mottled enamel. Both the 1933-34 dental needs survey and the 1938 mottled enamel studies were made in those South Dakota counties lying east of the Missouri River.

In computing an index which might point out differences in dental caries in the several counties, it was decided to express the amount of caries (severity) in terms of the number of carious permanent teeth per 100 children. In

order to study that age group with the maximum number of permanent teeth in the mouth, the 12 to 14 year group was selected for study. All children referred to in the tables to follow are white. The amount of caries was determined by combining the data associated with the following items: "Caries, permanent teeth," "Extraction indicated, permanent teeth," "Filled permanent teeth," and "Extracted permanent teeth." For each of these items, the bulletin gives the number of carious permanent teeth per 100 children. Adjustment was made for sex, and the amount of caries for each county was expressed in terms of the number of carious permanent teeth per 100 children. In *Public Health Bulletin* No. 226, examinations from communities with a population under 5000 were combined with examinations from the rural areas and designated "balance of county."

The South Dakota counties selected from the bulletin were classified solely on the basis of the prevalence of or freedom from endemic mottled enamel as shown by the mottled enamel study. The cities of Aberdeen, Huron, and

Figure 1. South Dakota, showing distribution of mottled enamel, with shaded areas indicating counties selected from *Public Health Bulletin* No. 226 for dental caries analyses.

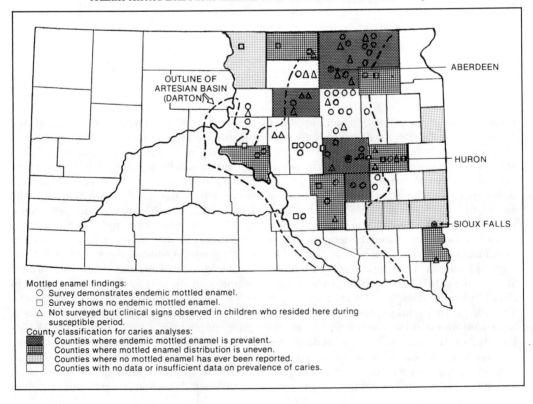

Mottled enamel findings:
○ Survey demonstrates endemic mottled enamel.
□ Survey shows no endemic mottled enamel.
△ Not surveyed but clinical signs observed in children who resided here during susceptible period.
County classification for caries analyses:
▓ Counties where endemic mottled enamel is prevalent.
▒ Counties where mottled enamel distribution is uneven.
░ Counties where no mottled enamel has ever been reported.
□ Counties with no data or insufficient data on prevalence of caries.

Sioux Falls were classified on the basis of whether or not the common water supply was producing mottled enamel. The results of these computations are contained in Table 3. Similar computations were also made for four Colorado cities and eight Wisconsin cities; the results are shown in Table 4.

DISCUSSION

This paper, after reviewing the findings of the earlier workers in the field, submits evi-

dence that furnishes support to the hypothesis that a limited immunity from dental caries is operative among school children residing in endemic mottled enamel areas. This evidence may be summarized as follows:

Prevalence

Observations made on a selected sample of 9-year-old children continuously exposed to waters of different fluoride concentrations, with the history of exposure personally verified in

Table 3. Dental caries attack rates in permanent teeth of 12 to 14-year-old white children in selected South Dakota counties and cities classified according to the prevalence of mottled enamel.

County	Number of children examined (12-14 years)	Number of carious permanent teeth per 100 children	Remarks
(a) Counties where mottled enamel generally is prevalent			
Beadle (less Huron)	332	256	Mottled enamel general throughout county. Areas include Hitchcock, Wolsey, Virgil, Yale, Cavour, and rural districts.
Brown (city, Aberdeen)	653	203	On basis of clinical examinations, old city deep well water contained fluorides in excess of minimal threshold.
Faulk	266	149	Mottled enamel general throughout county. Areas include Faulkton, Orient, Cresbard, Chelsea, and rural districts.
Marshall	391	251	Mottled enamel severe in western half of county, including Kidder, Britton, Langford, Newark, Amherst, and rural districts. No information on eastern half of county.
Sanborn	260	103[a]	Mottled enamel prevalent in county including Artesian and numerous rural districts.
Total	1902	201	
(b) Counties where mottled enamel distribution is uneven			
Jerauld	295	294	Alpena and Wessington Springs are negative; some mottled enamel in and around Lane.
Aurora	340	227	Mottled enamel around Stickney and rural districts in northern part of county.
Kingsbury	398	330	Distribution varied. Iroquois, Bancroft, Esmond, and Lake Preston are endemic. DeSmet and Arlington, two largest communities in county, are negative.
Day	666	309	Some mottled enamel in extreme western part of county around Pierpont. Bristol and Andover are negative by survey. No indications of mottled enamel in any other section of county.
Hughes	184	206	Blunt negative for mottled enamel; cases being developed in rural district around Harrold.
McPherson	340	394	Some mottled enamel in extreme eastern part of county around Leola. Eureka surveyed and negative. County generally free of mottled enamel.
Lincoln	536	284	Some mottled enamel observed from Beresford; no other record of mottled enamel in county.
Total	2765	314	

Table 3. (Continued.)

County	Number of children examined (12-14 years)	Number of carious permanent teeth per 100 children	Remarks
(c) Counties where no mottled enamel has ever been reported			
Beadle (city, Huron)	436	398	Negative for mottled enamel; obtains city water from James River with deep well as a reserve.
Campbell	264	368	No record of mottled enamel in this county. Herreid negative by survey.
Denel	212	218	No reports of mottled enamel in this county.
Hanson	271	382	Do.
McCook	344	407	Do.
Minnehaha:			
City, Sioux Falls	608	451	No reports of mottled enamel in this city; State chemist reports 0.4 ppm F in treated city water.
Balance of county	584	476	No reports of mottled enamel in this county.
Moody	433	498	Do.
Walworth	329	355	Do.
Total	3481	415	

[a] Only "caries and extractions indicated" of the permanent teeth are listed in Bulletin No. 226 for this county; adjusted for sex shows 68.6 per 100 children. This figure was raised to 103.1 per 100 children in order to compensate for the "unknown" filled and extracted permanent teeth per 100 children. The increase was based on the average ratio that these two missing items bear to the "caries and extraction indicated" reported in the 4 counties adjoining Sanborn County. The percentages that these items bear to the whole were as follows: Jerauld, 31; Kingsbury, 34; Beadle (less Huron) 34, and Aurora, 35.

Table 4. Dental caries attack rates in permanent teeth of 12 to 14-year-old white children of all Colorado and Wisconsin cities listed in Public Health Bulletin No. 226.

City	Number of children examined (12 to 14 years)	Number of carious permanent teeth per 100 children	Fluoride (F) content of common water supply (ppm)	Reference
Colorado				
Colorado Springs	203	162	2.5	(8)
Pueblo	411	194[a]	0.6	(8)
Denver	637	342	0.5	(12)
Fort Collins	207	296	None	(12)
Wisconsin				
Green Bay	687	275	2.3[b]	
Sheboygan	244	710	0.5	(13)
Manitowoc	661	682	0.35	(13)
Two Rivers	382	646	0.3	(13)
Milwaukee	2645	917	0.3	(13)
West Allis	160	831	0.3	(13)
Baraboo	119	733	0.2	(13)
La Crosse	47	731	0.12	(13)

[a] "Extraction indicated" for boys "Unknown"; 4.2 rate for girls used in this adjustment.—Author.
[b] Determination made by Senior Chemist E. Elvove, Division of Chemistry, National Institute of Health. Approximately the same amount has been reported by DeWitt and Nichols. *J Am Water Works Assoc* 29:980-984, 1937.

Note.—For the mineral constituents, other than fluorine, of these Wisconsin waters, see Public Water Supplies of Wisconsin, Wisconsin State Board of Health, July 1935.

each instance by an interview with the child's parent, indicate that a high percentage of children are caries-free in those places where the common water supply contains appreciable amounts of fluorides. For instance, of the 114 children who had continuously used a domestic water comparatively low in fluorides (0.6 to 1.5 ppm), only 5, or 4 percent, were caries-free. On the other hand, of the 122 children of comparable age who had continuously used domestic waters containing 1.7 to 2.5 ppm of fluorides, 27, or 22 percent, were caries-free. In other words, within the range of these observations, limited to a total of 236 nine-year-old children, the percentage of caries-free children in areas with domestic waters containing appreciable amounts of fluorides was over five times the corresponding percentage in areas with domestic water containing lower fluoride concentrations.

Severity, or amount of caries

To provide additional evidence of the relation of dental caries to endemic fluorosis, a computation of the dental caries attack rate on the permanent teeth of 12 to 14-year-old children was made with the use of data collected in 1933-1934 (*Public Health Bulletin* No. 226) and correlated with the data subsequently obtained on the geographical distribution of mottled enamel in South Dakota. Briefly, this study shows that, in the group of counties[4] where mottled enamel is generally prevalent, an examination of 1902 white children, 12 to 14 years of age, disclosed 201 carious permanent teeth per 100 children. In the intermediate group of seven counties where the mottled enamel distribution was uneven, and at times sporadic, the examination of 2765 children showed 314 permanent teeth affected per 100 children; and in the third group of counties and the cities of Huron and Sioux Falls, where no endemic mottled enamel areas are known to exist, an examination of 3481 children showed a dental caries attack rate of 415 permanent teeth per 100 children. These data indicate that the dental caries attack rate in this particular population is

inversely proportional to the prevalence of mottled enamel.

Similar comparisons made among four cities of Colorado show that in the non-endemic communities, Pueblo, Fort Collins, and Denver, the dental caries attack rate is 194, 296, and 343, respectively; on the other hand, in the endemic area, Colorado Springs, only 163 permanent teeth per 100 children were affected. Applying the same methods of study to eight Wisconsin cities, it was found that in the seven where no endemic mottled enamel is known to exist and where the fluoride (F) content of the communal water supplies ranges from 0.1 to 0.5 ppm, the severity of dental caries showed rates from 646 to 917 carious permanent teeth per 100 children. But in the city of Green Bay, where the city water contains 2.3 ppm of fluoride (F), only 275 carious permanent teeth per 100 children were recorded.

It is fully realized, of course, that the causes of dental caries are, as Rosenau states, "complex and perhaps multiple." Mill's recent analysis of *Public Health Bulletin* No. 226,[5] moreover, indicates that the dental caries attack rates (amount of dental caries) vary markedly in different geographical regions.

An inspection of the data included in this paper brings out the fact that, regardless of the dental caries attack rate of the region, the use of a domestic water which in itself is capable of producing mottled enamel is concomitant with a lower amount of dental caries.

Relation to dental caries research

The relationship of chronic endemic dental fluorosis (mottled enamel), a water-borne disease, to dental caries raises several questions, for example:

1. What role, if any, does the physical structure of a tooth play in either susceptibility to or immunity from dental caries?

2. Is the higher fluoride content of the enamel of a mottled-enamel tooth the immunity-producing factor?

3. Is the limited immunity due, directly or indirectly, to the well-known inhibitory action of fluorine on enzymatic processes?

4. While on the basis of our present knowledge it appears justifiable to associate the ob-

---

[4] The city of Aberdeen is included in this group of counties as this city was using a deep well water supply at the time of the dental caries survey. This water supply produced a mild degree of mottled enamel in about 20 percent of the children continuously using the water.

[5] *J Dent Res* 16: (Oct.), 1937.

served results with the presence of fluorides in the domestic water, the possibility should not be overlooked that other elements of comparatively rare occurrence in water or ordinary constituents of drinking water present in unusually large concentration may directly or through a synergistic action with the fluoride, produce the observed effects. For this reason, it appears essential to obtain as complete chemical analyses as possible of the domestic water of communities which are under investigation for dental caries.

SUMMARY

1. Examinations of 236 nine-year-old children with verified continuity of exposure showed that a higher percentage of children is caries-free in those communities where the domestic water supplies contain higher concentrations of fluorides (F) in comparison with communities using waters of lower fluoride concentrations. This limited immunity to dental caries seemed operative with respect to the deciduous teeth as well as the permanent teeth.

2. An analysis of dental caries attack rates in a relatively large number of children in the three States thus far studied (South Dakota, Colorado, and Wisconsin) indicates that the severity of dental caries is, in general, lower in mottled enamel areas as compared with normal areas in the same State.

3. Inasmuch as it appears that the mineral composition of the drinking water may have an important bearing on the incidence of dental caries in a community, the possibility of partially controlling dental caries through the domestic water supply warrants thorough epidemiological-chemical study.

ACKNOWLEDGMENT

The outline of the artesian basin in eastern South Dakota shown in Figure 1 was taken from plate LXIX, by N. H. Darton, in part 2 of the Seventeenth Annual Report of the United States Geological Survey, 1895-1896.

The writer desires to express his indebtedness to Senior Statistician Wm. M. Gafafer and Senior Chemist E. Elvove, National Institute of Health, for many helpful suggestions and criticisms in the preparation of this paper, to the Wisconsin State Board of Health for supplying information on the fluoride content of the water supplies of the seven Wisconsin cities with high dental caries attack rates, and to Principal Statistician Selwyn D. Collins, National Institute of Health, for a review of the paper.

References

(1) Black, G. V. (in collaboration with McKay, F. S.). Mottled teeth. An endemic developmental imperfection of the teeth, heretofore unknown in the literature of dentistry. *Dent Cosmos* 58:129-156, 1916.

(2) McKay, F. S. (in collaboration with Black, G. V.). An investigation of mottled teeth. *Dent Cosmos* 58:477-484, 1916.

(3) Masaki, T. Geographic distribution of "mottled teeth" in Japan. *Shikwa Gakuho* 36: October, 1931.

(4) Medical Research Council, Special Report Series No. 97, II, *The Incidence of Dental Disease in Children.* His Majesty's Stationery Office, London, 1925.

(5) Ainsworth, N. J. Mottled teeth. *Brit Dent J* 55:233-250 and 274-276, 1933.

(6) Erausquin, R.: Dientes vetados. *Rev Odont* (Buenos Aires) 23:296-313, 1935.

(7) McKay, F. S. The establishment of a definite relation between enamel that is defective in its structure, as mottled enamel, and the liability to decay, II. *Dent Cosmos* 71:747-755, 1929.

(8) Dean, H. T. and E. Elvove. Studies on the minimal threshold of the dental sign of chronic endemic fluorosis (mottled enamel). *Public Health Rep* 50:1719-1729, 1935.

(9) Dean, H. T. and E. Elvove. Some epidemiological aspects of chronic endemic dental fluorosis. *Am J Public Health* 26:567-575, 1936.

(10) Dean, H. T. and E. Elvove. Further studies on the minimal threshold of chronic endemic dental fluorosis. *Public Health Rep* 52:1249-1264, 1937.

(11) Dental survey of school children, ages 6 to 14 years, made in 1933-34, in 26 States. *Public Health Bulletin* No. 226. U.S. Public Health Service, Washington, D.C. 1936.

(12) Boissevain, C. H. The presence of fluorine in the water supply of Colorado and its relation to the occurrence of mottled enamel. *Colorado Med* 30:142-148, 1933.

(13) Wisconsin State Board of Health, Personal communication, June 21, 1938.

THE RACIAL AND SOCIAL INCIDENCE OF CANCER OF THE UTERUS

E. L. Kennaway[1]

FACTORS WHICH MAY AFFECT THE INCIDENCE OF CANCER OF THE UTERUS

Ritual Observances and Ablutions Associated with Menstruation and Childbirth

Jewish ritual

The earliest Jewish law prohibits intercourse during menstruation or any other discharge of blood from the uterus, and for a period of seven days after the cessation of any abnormal flow. The general prohibition is expressed as follows:

Leviticus, XVIII, 19: "And thou shalt not approach unto a woman to uncover her nakedness as long as she is impure by her uncleanness."

Leviticus, XX, 18: "And if a man shall lie with a woman having her sickness, and shall uncover her nakedness; he hath made naked her fountain, and she hath uncovered the fountain of her blood; and both of them shall be cut off from among their people."

The precautions to be taken are stated in an earlier chapter, which makes plain the abhorrence, which is, of course, by no means restricted to Jews[2], with which any contamination with genital blood was regarded.

Leviticus, XV, 19-28.—"19: And if a woman have an issue, and her issue in her flesh be blood, she shall be in her impurity seven days: and whosoever toucheth her shall be unclean until the even. 20: And everything that she lieth upon in her impurity shall be unclean; every thing also that she sitteth upon shall be unclean. 21: And whosoever toucheth her bed shall wash his clothes, and bathe himself in water, and be unclean until the even. 22: And whosoever toucheth any thing that she sitteth upon shall wash his clothes, and bathe himself in water, and be unclean until the even. 23: And if it be on the bed, or on any thing whereon she sitteth, when he toucheth it, he shall be unclean until the even. 24: And if any man lie with her, and her impurity be upon him, he shall be unclean seven days: and every bed whereon he lieth shall be unclean. 25: And if a woman have an issue of her blood many days not in the time of her impurity, or if she have an issue beyond the time of her impurity: all the days of the issue of her uncleanness she shall be as in the days of her impurity: she is unclean. 26: Every bed whereon she lieth all the days of her issue shall be unto her as the bed of her impurity: and every thing whereon she sitteth shall be unclean, as the uncleanness of her impurity. 27: And whosoever toucheth those things shall be unclean, and shall wash his clothes, and bathe himself in water, and be unclean until the even. 28: But if she be cleansed of her issue, then she shall number to herself seven days, and after that she shall be clean."

The law thus draws a distinction between normal menstruation (verses 19-24) and any other genital discharge of blood (verses 25-28). The normally menstruating woman ceases to be impure, if the flow has ceased, at the end of the seventh day from its commencement, but after any abnormal flow, a period of seven blood-free days is ordained, no doubt because there is greater danger of the recrudescence of any such bleeding. The law does not prescribe specifically for women any purification by washing such as is imposed upon men who have become contaminated. But subsequently, in Talmudic

---

Source: *British Journal of Cancer* 2(3):197-205, 1948.
[1] Pathological Department, St. Bartholomew's Hospital, London, E.C. 1.

[2] The supposed harmful influence of the menstruating woman upon men and children, and upon a great variety of objects (food and drink of every kind, cooking utensils, the domestic hearth, weapons, mirrors, crops, trees, livestock, and even upon roads and fisheries) is or has been the subject of stringent precautions and prohibitions among peoples all over the world, from Eskimos to Polynesians (for the immense literature on this subject see Ploss, Bartels and Bartels (*1*)). Hence there is nothing in principle peculiar to the Jewish people in the ordinances of Leviticus, but they are characterized, as are other parts of the Mosaic law, by great precision in detail, and have received the voluminous addition of Talmudic literature.

times[3] (about the third century A.D.), the law in regard to normal menstruation was altered in two respects, and these changes were set forth about 1000 years later in the Code Yoreh Deah: (1) The extension of the period of impurity until seven blood-free days had elapsed was applied to normal menstruation also. (2) The minimum first period, including the time of the actual flow, was laid down as five days. Hence the whole period of impurity is n + seven days, and n is never less than five, and under normal conditions will be five. Such a period of 12 days is nearly one-half of the normal menstrual cycle and will allow intercourse to be resumed near what is thought to be the usual time of ovulation, of which process those who laid down the rule of course knew nothing.

The modern practice follows these rules. "The law of Niddah is in full force to the present day" (2). The precautionary period of impurity begins 12 to 24 hours before the expected flow, and lasts for not less than five days from its commencement. The woman then examines herself and, if the flow has ceased, takes a bath. The second period, of seven days, during which she examines herself repeatedly, follows. If no blood has been found during this time, she takes another bath, followed by ritual immersion (Mikveh). The test for cessation of flow is made by inspection of a white cloth which has been pressed into the vulva.

Ritual immersion. The Talmudists developed the Mosaic law of Purification by ordaining that a woman after menstruation should wash her body, and then immerse herself completely (two or three times) either in a lake, river, or spring, or in a tank containing not less than the equivalent of 24 cubic feet of water, which must either come immediately from the earth as a spring, or be collected rain water. In medieval times one of the first cares of every Jewish community was to provide a suitable bath for this immersion. In these buildings a staircase leads to a dressing-room and then on beneath the water to the floor of the bath, which was generally below ground-level so that the ground

water, which could be regarded as spring water, could be utilized. Figures and architectural details of such baths are given by Ploss, Bartels and Bartels (1; figs. 460-463), and in the *Jewish Encyclopedia* (4; article "Andernach").[4] A suitable bath can be constructed in a private house (5).

Mere immersion in spring water, as an addition to an ordinary bath, could make little contribution to cleanliness and was not intended to do so; hence, from the present point of view this particular ritual is in itself of little importance; but its persistence affords valuable evidence of an obedience to the law which probably would extend to other ordinances, and especially to the abstention from sexual intercourse. The object of the preliminary bath was not cleanliness *per se*, but the removal of anything which would intervene between the skin and the water during the total immersion, and thus deprive this ritual of its efficacy.[5] Some medical writers have emphasized, in rather vague terms, the importance of the cleanliness enforced by the Mosaic law, hence it is important to note exactly what the law requires. The washing, in a normal woman, at the beginning and end of the seven days, adds two baths a month to whatever other ablutions she may carry out.

We have no data to show what proportion of Jewish women in any community carry out the whole procedure. One might form some estimate in London from the number of public ritual baths available, which are said to be not more than half a dozen; there are also some private ones. A new bath for this purpose was constructed in North London recently. But it

---

[3] A tractate (Niddah) of the Talmud, consisting of 10 chapters, deals with this subject. An English translation of Niddah is available (2). No translation of Yoreh Deah into a European language has been made; the relevant portions of it (chapters 183-200) have been summarized by Sorsby (3).

[4] This account of Jewish ritual immersion is taken from various articles in the Jewish *Encyclopedia* (4), from Ploss, Bartels and Bartels (1), and from Preuss (6). The Talmudic ordinances do not, of course, imply that women had not in earlier times purified themselves after menstruation by washing (see, for instance, the story of Bath-sheba, Sam. II, XI. 2-4).
[5] Chapter X of the tractate Niddah deals with numerous possible obstacles to the access of water to every part of the body. Thus the woman must not perform immersion in a harbor, because the passage of ships may stir up mud which would separate the skin from the water, and she must not raise her eyebrows unduly lest a wrinkle be produced into which the water does not penetrate. The ritual nature of the immersion is shown by the fact that, before it, all particles of food must be removed from between the teeth; although the mouth remains closed, there must be no potential obstacles to penetration. Such regulations are set forth in more accessible publications (7) for use at the present day.

seems probable that many women who do not go to the ritual bath may conform to the law in other respects, namely, the first and second bath, and abstention from intercourse, which are matters of purely private conduct.

The Mosaic law (Leviticus XII, 2, 5) relating to childbirth is important in view of the association of cancer of the cervix with parity. "If a woman conceive seed, and bear a man child, then she shall be unclean seven days; as in the days of the impurity of her sickness shall she be unclean. . . . And she shall continue in the blood of her purifying three and thirty days. . . . But if she bear a maid child, then shall she be unclean two weeks as in her impurity: and she shall continue in the blood of her impurity three score and six days." Thus the whole period of impurity was either 7 + 33 = 40, or 14 + 66 = 80 days. The practice in this country at the present time is said to be, to observe rather longer periods, of two and three months respectively.

Moslem law

The Koran (Sura 2) gives directions for the purification of women which are much less precise than those of the Jewish law. "They will ask thee also concerning the courses of women: Answer, they are a pollution: therefore separate yourselves from women in their courses, and go not near them, until they be cleansed. But when they are cleansed, go in unto them as God has commanded you." No periods of time are laid down, and no details of the method of washing are given. Obviously, immersion on the Jewish scale would be difficult in countries where water is scarce. Sale (8) in his commentary on the Koran, speaks of two degrees of purification from various contaminations, namely, immersion or bathing in water, and washing of the face, hands and feet in water or (Sura 4 and 5) in sand if water is not available; and he goes on to say that the former is incumbent upon women after menstruation, but this is not in the text of the Koran.

Parsee ritual

The Zend-Avesta (9) enacts that a woman having any normal or abnormal discharge of blood must be placed in a separate building as is done in many parts of the world (see footnote 2 on p. 279) and must be prevented as far as possible from defiling the elements of earth, water, and fire; she must be given very scanty food lest the evil power (Ahriman) within her be strengthened, and the person who brings this food must not approach within three paces of her, and must use a metal spoon to convey the food. "If she still see blood after three nights have passed, she shall sit in the place of infirmity until four nights have passed," and so on up to a flow lasting 8 nights, one day being added to the actual period. Then "they shall dig three holes in the earth" (magas) "and they shall wash the woman with gomez" (urine of cattle) "by two of those holes and with water by the third." Intercourse with a woman having a normal or abnormal issue of blood is a crime punishable with 200 stripes. A flow of blood lasting more than nine nights is the work of evil spirits.

Dr. Modi (10), a Parsee, quotes these laws and says: "At present also, most of the Parsee women generally observe the above practices. There are no separate Dastânistâns or houses for menses in Parsee towns or streets, but generally a sequestered part of one's own house is chosen for the purpose. The down-floor of the house was thought to be the proper place. But nowadays, in a crowded city like Bombay, the down-floor, instead of being a quiet and healthy place such as that contemplated by the early injunctions of the Vendidâd, is generally quite the contrary. So, most women in menses pass the period of menstruation on their upper floors, but in an isolated way. Every family has a separate iron cot for the occasion and a separate bedding, etc. They are supplied their meals from a distance by others and they neither come into contact with others, nor do they touch other things or do household work. The very rigorous isolation enjoined by the later books is not observed, but anyhow, some kind of isolation and separation is maintained by the generality of women. In the matter of taking food, very few use spoons now, though up to about 25 years ago, that was generally the case. In the matter of purification, they observe the bath enjoined by the early books, but the Vendidâd injunction of bathing over the three 'magas' is not observed at all. A separate place of bathing and for purposes of nature for women in this condition is generally provided in Parsee houses."

Hindu ritual

Dr. Khanolkar (personal communication) says that the Parsee laws regarding menstruation are almost identical with those practised by orthodox Hindus and probably both of them are derived from early Aryan ritual. The Abbé Dubois (11), writing about the beginning of the nineteenth century, quotes from the book *Padma-purama*, reputed to be the work of the hermit Vasishta, a rule for a three-day period of isolation for the menstruating woman, followed by a day of ceremonies and ablutions, including 36 total immersions in a river. During the three days " . . . the mere wish to cohabit with her husband would be a serious sin." Elsewhere he says, "The mother of the newly-born child lives entirely apart for a whole month or more, during which time she may touch neither the vessels nor the furniture of the house, nor any clothes, and still less any person whatsoever. The time of her seclusion being over, she is immersed in a bath, or else a great quantity of water is poured over her head and body. Women are similarly isolated during the time of their periodical uncleanness. In all decent houses there is a sort of small gynaeceum set apart for them; but amongst the poor, in whose huts there is no such accommodation, the women are turned into the street, under a sort of shed or outhouse, or else they are allowed a corner of the cowshed. . . . When the time of uncleanness is passed, all the garments that the woman has worn are given to the washerwoman. Her clothes are not allowed inside the house; in fact, no one would dare to look on them."

Jhaveri (12) says that in all Hindu religious books minute directions for baths on very many occasions are given. During the first four days of the first menstrual period everything which the girl touches must be washed and ". . . persons coming into contact with her have to take a bath." This author says nothing of subsequent periods. After childbirth a woman is impure for 10 days, even if given a daily bath by the midwife; ". . . no one dares to touch her."; after 40 days she is given a final bath, and is then pure (cf. the Jewish practice after the birth of a male child).

Ploss, Bartels and Bartels (1) state, without giving any original authority, that in Malabar the first three days are spent in a special room

of the house; on the fourth day the woman bathes and is then half-clean (i.e. can leave her room but not enter the temple), until the end of the seventh day. The three days of isolation, followed by ablutions on the fourth day, are obviously similar to the shortest procedure laid down for Parsees in the Zend-Avesta.

Dr. Khanolkar has very kindly sent me a translation from the Sanskrit of passages from the book *Dharmasindhu*, written about 1790 A.D. by Kashinath or Baba Padhye, which is the accepted basis of Hindu ritual and religious practices in the Bombay area. The menstrual woman must have no contact with other persons for three days and nights and is subject to numerous other prohibitions during this time. On the fourth day, after cleansing the body and after cleaning the mouth and teeth thoroughly, a full bath should be taken after sunrise at about the time when the cows are released to go to the pastures. This bath confers purification only for the purpose of touching ordinary household objects without polluting them, and for attending upon the husband. It is only on the fifth day that the woman is fit to participate in the worship of the gods and the ancestors. Dr. Khanolkar says that these regulations ". . . are still observed in the Hindu society, except by modern women in big towns, who work in schools, colleges, offices, etc., and cannot afford to remain in isolation every month."

The lenient Hindu view of intermenstrual bleeding is of interest in comparison with the Jewish law (p. 279). "If as a result of disease menses continue to appear continuously, the woman is not impure and remains as if she is not menstruating. But she is debarred from participating in any acts of worship of the gods or the ancestors, and despite continuous or infrequent discharges she shall carefully work out a monthly period and remain under the enjoined discipline for three nights and three days once every month."

Economic Conditions

The reference by Vineberg (13) to the conditions under which the majority of his hospital patients in New York lived is valuable in this connection. "When one stops to consider that of the total number of the Jewish women 1995 had badly lacerated cervices . . . and that they were living in the worst possible hygienic surroundings, amidst the greatest squalor and privation, such as obtain in the lower East Side of the Metropolis, it is truly remarkable that so few cases of cancer of the cervix were detected amongst them."

Childbearing

The association of cancer of the cervix with parity (*14*) makes the low incidence upon Jewesses all the more remarkable. (For references to literature on the incidence in nulliparous women see Donaldson, *15* and Smith, *16*). Sorsby (*3*) says, "Even a superficial acquaintance with the Jewish masses dispels the idea that Jewish women contain a large proportion of unmarried. The reverse is true; the number of unmarried is strikingly low—decidedly lower than among their neighbors. Nor do married women abstain from childbearing. Procreation is almost a matter of religious observance with the mass of Jewesses. . . . Uterine cancer ought to be, if anything, more common among Jewish women than among non-Jewish."

Various Talmudic writers (*17*, 29*b*-30*a*) laid down that a father should cause his sons to marry at 16 to 24, or 18 to 24, and that a daughter should "be dowered, clothed, and adorned, that men should eagerly desire her"; no age is stated at which a woman should marry. The general tendency was to give daughters rather early in marriage; this led to the Rabbinic ruling that a man must wait for his daughter to grow up before giving her in betrothal (*17*, p. 205). A modern compiler (*18*) states the law of Israel on this matter thus: "After a man has arrived at the age of 18 it is his duty to take unto himself a wife in order that he may be fruitful and multiply, at any rate he should not pass his 20th year without having taken a wife. "Having begotten a son and a daughter who are also generative, one has fulfilled the commandment "to be fruitful and multiply." . . . The command "to be fruitful and multiply" is not obligatory upon women; nevertheless a woman should not remain single lest she be liable to suspicion. . . . It is one of the mandates of the Sages that a man shall give his sons and daughters in marriage immediately they approach maturity. . . . " These Jewish practices thus laid down in the Law, and described by Sorsby as prevailing at the present day, should encourage early marriage.

The Abbé Dubois (*11*) says that " . . . A Hindu only marries to have children, and the more he has the richer and happier he feels. . . . No Hindu would ever dream of complaining that his family was too large, however poor he may be . . . barrenness in a wife is the most terrible curse that can possibly fall on a family."

Early Marriage

Lombard and Potter (personal communication) collected data from 549 cases of cancer of the cervix, and 550 cases of cancer of the breast, in state cancer hospitals of Massachusetts, and out of about 80 variables studied found 16 to be significant, and of these, marriage before the age of 20 was the most strongly associated with cancer of the cervix (Table 1). Thus 45 percent of women with cancer of the cervix, and only 16 percent of those with cancer of the breast, were married before that age. "Variables which might

Table 1. Cancer of the cervix and marital status. Massachusetts.
(Lombard and Potter.)

	Number in series	Married percent	Without children percent of married	Married under age of 20, percent of married
Cancer of cervix: 2 series	549	96.0–97.7	9.3–10.8	44.0–49.2
Cancer of uterus: 3 series	848	93.3–94.0	11.3–16.4	33.0–35.4
Cancer of breast: 5 series	1509	81.5–84.4	16.1–21.7	11.3–22.9
Cancer of other female organs: 1 series	234	83.3	20.5	21.0
First marriages of Massachusetts females, 1890–1939				18.6
Total female population; age-group 35–74.				
1940 census	—	83.2	17.2	—
1910 census	—	83.1	15.6	—

be considered are: Earlier childbirth, multiple children, poor obstetrical service, longer duration of married life, syphilis, immaturity of tissues at time of marriage, and excessive hormonal stimulation." Of these factors, longer married life could be eliminated by comparison with other groups. "One may surmise that a part, if not all, of the correlation between marriage under 20 and cancer of the cervix, which persists after elimination of the effect of the variables pertaining to pregnancy, economics, and syphilis may be due to either immaturity of tissue or to an oversupply of hormones. The latter may stimulate the individual to early marriage, and may also cause malignancy."

Modi (*10*) writing of Parsees says that "the marriageable age at present is generally after 21 for the males and after 16 for the females." "The average age of Hindu women at marriage is 16 years, and of Parsee women 25 years." (Khanolkar).

Genetic Factors

This factor is obviously a possible one, but its action is difficult to prove or disprove. A similar problem arises in the case of primary cancer of the liver in the African negro (*19, 20*). Data are required from other Semitic peoples most nearly related to the Jews.[6] Weir and Little (*21*) consider that the maximum incidence of uterine cancer one quinquennium later in Jewesses . . . compared with other women, suggests a genetic basis. Certainly the age at which some forms of cancer occur is affected by genetic differences; examples have been given in detail in another paper (*22;* xeroderma pigmentosum, familial polyposis intestini, cancer of the breast, gastro-intestinal tract, and corpus uteri in certain families). But a higher ratio of corpus to cervix cancer in Jewesses would have the same effect (Figure 1).

Circumcision.

Some authors (*23, 24*) consider that no explanation of the lower incidence of cervical cancer upon Jewesses need be sought beyond the (assumed) difference in the bacterial flora of the

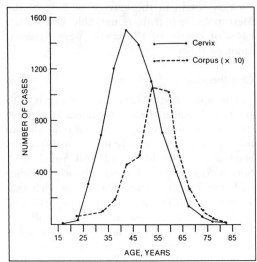

Figure 1. Cancer of cervix and corpus uteri (*14*).

female genital tract brought about by this factor, a matter which it would be possible to investigate. More data from Moslem populations who practise circumcision, and from Parsees, who do not, are obviously very desirable. Handley (*23*) has emphasized the value of statistics from Fiji, where the natives practice circumcision, in contrast to the Hindu immigrants, in whose native country phimosis and cancer of the penis are very common (*25*); certainly if these two races could receive equal medical attention interesting results might be obtained.[7]

Circumcision might act in another way, not dependent upon bacterial action. Phimosis, cancer of the penis, and cancer of the cervix appear to be common in certain areas (*25;* in China and among Hindus in India). If it be that material which accumulates under the prepuce contains carcinogenic compounds which can cause cancer of the penis, this material might, if conveyed in sufficient amount, cause cancer of the cervix. Plaut and Kohn-Speyer (*28*) have shown that smegma (horse), and its unsaponifiable fraction, are carcinogenic to mice. But such transmission does not seem very likely.

---

[6] See "The racial origins of jewish types," by Radcliffe N. Salaman, in "Wherein I Glory," London, 1948.

[7] The population of Fiji in 1945 included 115 724 Fijians and 117 256 Indians (*26*). Brewster (*27*) states that the majority of Indians were Hindus, " . . . although there was a fair proportion of Mohammedans."

Douching

Comparative data for the incidence of cancer of the cervix in countries where douching is more or less commonly performed would be of great interest. Dr. Denoix of the Ministère de la Santé Publique has been kind enough to inform me that no data are available from France for comparison with those from this country.

Smith (*16*) has described a positive correlation, of which there might of course be various explanations, between douching, and especially douching with lysol, and carcinoma of the cervix.

CANCER OF THE CORPUS UTERI

Cancer may affect either the cervix or corpus uteri, and in mass statistics, such as those based on death certificates, these two forms cannot be distinguished. This is very unfortunate because it is probable that they differ in etiology. We have no data which give directly the respective social incidence of cancer of the cervix, and of the corpus, but information should be available from hospitals which have separate accommodation for paying and other patients. The maximum incidence of cancer of the corpus falls about 10 years later than does that of cancer of the cervix (Figure 1 and Table 2), and this difference may suggest, when two batches of undifferentiated uterine cancers are compared, differences in the proportions of the two forms. For example: (1) The data from various parts of Bavaria given by Theilhaber (*29*) . . . show that the average age at death from cancer of the uterus is earlier in the poorer classes, and if

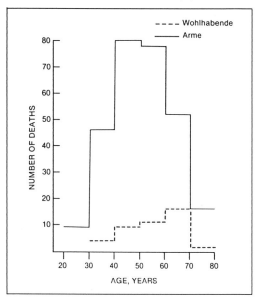

Figure 2. Age at death from cancer of uterus in Bamberg, Augsburg, Würzburg, Erlangen, Nürnberg, and the Province of Unterfranken, 1908, and in Munich, 1906, 1907, 1908 (*29*).

these figures, admittedly very few in number, are put in graphic form (Figure 2) they show a likeness to those for the two forms of cancer (Figure 1), which is compatible with a higher proportion of cervix cancers in the poorer women. (2) If one reckons the death rates of married women in England and Wales of the four lower social classes from cancer of the uterus . . . as percentages of the rate for Class I taken as 100, one obtains the result shown on

Table 2. Relation of civil state and age to cancer of cervix and corpus uteri in various countries (*14*).

	Total cases from literature	Cancer Cervix 7986	Cancer Corpus 389
	Of these, unmarried	170 = 2.1%	52 = 13.4%
	Mean age, years	45.75	53.3

Cervix	15—	20—	25—	30—	35—	40—	45—	50—	55—	60—	65—	70—	75—	80—
	3	33	269	667	1196	1474	1370	1084	691	395	134	49	13	3
Corpus	Under 30. 5		9	19	45	50	104	101	58	25	9	2	0	

Totals: Cervix, 7381; Corpus 427

Figure 3. Social incidence of cancer of uterus at early and late ages. Mean annual death rate per million. Married women, England and Wales, 1930–1932.

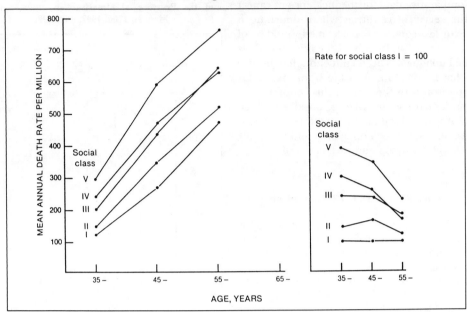

DISCUSSION

the right-hand side of Figure 3. The social difference becomes less as age advances from 35-45 to 55-65, which change is compatible with a decreasing proportion of cervical cancers, and suggests that it is this form which is affected by social factors.

The only authorities quoted in this paper who give any data for the incidence of cancer of the corpus upon Jewish and non-Jewish women are Smith (*30*) and Davidsohn (*31*). Smith's data . . . show that cancers of the corpus make up practically the same percentage of all gynecological conditions (7.1 and 7.8) in Jews and others, while the percentage of malignant gynecological tumors made up by cancers of the corpus is much higher (31.1) in Jews than in others (10.0), owing to the smaller incidence of cancer of the cervix in Jews. Davidsohn's figures . . . show much less difference between the percentages of specimens examined, made up by cancer of the corpus, and of the cervix, in Jewesses requiring gynecological treatment (0.83 and 0.93) than in other women (3.0 and 6.4). This difference is compatible with the idea that cancer of the cervix is the form of uterine cancer which occurs in Jewesses less than in other women.

1. Any comparison of the figures for Jews and non-Jews . . . with those from the various communities in Bombay . . . is possible only on the basis of cancers of the uterus, or of the cervix, reckoned as a percentage of all cancers in women. Obviously these data were obtained under varying conditions, but such as they are, they are summarized in Table 3.

2. The Jewish ritual has some unique features. More or less complete isolation of menstruating women is practiced by many other peoples and is laid down in the religious literature of some of these (Koran, Zend-Avesta, Dharmasindhu). Some quite primitive peoples (*1*; Aleuts, natives of the Congo, and of Australia) are stated to enforce isolation at the menstrual period for as long as 6 to 7 days. But the Jewish ritual appears to be the only one which imposes an exact test for the cessation, and possible recurrence, of the flow, and a post-menstrual isolation of 7 days. The 5 + 7 day rule of the Jews is of peculiar interest in regard to the time of ovulation.

The Jewish rule suggests the following calculation. Suppose that a Jewish woman is mar-

Table 3. Racial incidence of cancer of the uterus.

		Percentage of all cancers in women. Cancer of uterus	
		Minimum	Maximum
Europe and U.S.A.	Non-Jews	13.9	25–35
	Jews	3.9	10.5
		Cancer of cervix Mean	
Bombay	Hindus	44	
	Moslems	20.7	
	Parsees	14.8	
	Indian Christians	12.7	

ried at 17, and undergoes the menopause at 47, and that during 5 of these 30 years the menstrual cycle is affected by pregnancy and its sequels. This leaves 25 years of normal cycles; if the average duration of these is 28 days, there will be $\frac{9125}{28}$ = 326 periods, and 326 × 7 = 2282 days of abstention from intercourse after menstruation.

3. The low incidence of cancer of the cervix among Jews is the more remarkable because they tend to be exposed to factors (early marriage; childbearing; in some areas low economic status) which in other communities predispose to this form of cancer; by some means they are able in this respect to resemble the richer women of other races.

4. The scantiness of the data available for Hindu, Moslem, Parsee, and Indian Christian women does not allow one to draw any conclusions. In the Hindu community post-menstrual isolation of one day is combined with, in the male population, absence of circumcision and frequency of phimosis and cancer of the penis. The Parsees are of peculiar interest, as a one-day post-menstrual period is combined with absence of circumcision, but the only available data are those of the 25 cases of cervical cancer recorded by Khanolkar. These few cases are a very uncertain basis for any conclusions, but the much higher incidence upon Hindu women, who follow similar rules in regard to menstruation, suggest that these particular practices do not affect the matter, perhaps owing to the inadequate period of post-menstrual isolation. The four-day period of abstention possibly does not differ much from the practice of many persons whose action in this matter is not affected

by religion. We seem to have no information about the actual procedures of isolation and purification among Moslems. The vast area and population of China afford only a few indications that cancer of the cervix, and of the penis, and phimosis, are all prevalent.

5. The social incidence of cancer of the cervix is obviously of great interest, but seems not to arouse attention among gynecologists in this country. The social incidence upon married and single women illustrates the fundamental importance of Stevenson's work (*32, 33*) to students of human cancer. Perhaps the cervix-corpus junction resembles that between the stomach and intestine in being the limit of influence of external factors.

The term "Single Woman" is a definition of civil state which may include more than one physiological condition. But there can be no doubt that the social gradation shown by the 1294 cases of cancer of the uterus in single women . . . must depend upon factors less closely connected with sexual functions than are those discussed above under Jewish and other rituals. Possibly nutritional conditions are concerned here. These unique data are nearly 20 years old. After the next census it may be possible to learn whether any change has occurred which might be attributed to economic and dietetic differences.

6. One might make the following suggestions for further investigations: (*a*) An inquiry into the incidence of cancer of the cervix in Jewish women who observe the 12-day period, the ritual immersion being disregarded. A beginning might be made by collecting the personal histories in individual cases. (*b*) A comprehensive study by Indian workers of the unique material

which they have at hand in Hindu, Moslem, Parsee, and Christian populations. (*c*) Further, statistical study of the social gradation of uterine cancer in married and single women.

In all such investigations discrimination between cancers of the cervix and of the corpus should be attempted.

SUMMARY

1. The comparative incidence of cancer of the uterus in Jewish and non-Jewish women has been studied in material from London, Munich, Amsterdam, Rotterdam, Vienna, Budapest, Sweden, Palestine, New York, Chicago, Rochester, and Philadelphia.

2. All of the twenty collections of data which have been found in the literature show an incidence of uterine cancer which is greater on non-Jewish than on Jewish women. These data are calculated upon several different bases and hence are not all comparable. Seven authors express the figures for cancer of the uterus as a percentage of all cancers in women, which percentage ranges from 28 to 14 in non-Jews, and from 10 to 4 in Jews, the mean values being 20 and 7. A similar ratio of the order of 3 : 1 is given by death rates per 100 000 in all of five instances. Data based on admissions to hospitals show, as would be expected, much wider variations.

3. The low incidence of cancer of the uterus in Jews is the more remarkable in that they are subject to some conditions (early marriage and childbearing; in some communities low economic status) which in other peoples appear to increase the liability to this form of cancer.

4. Various degrees of isolation of the menstruating woman are, or have been, practised over a large part of the world. The Jewish ritual appears to be the only one which imposes an exact test for the cessation of the flow after 5 days, and for its possible recurrence during the following 7 days. This 12-day period of abstention from intercourse is of interest in regard to what is now known of the usual time of ovulation. The Jewish ritual immersion is probably of no direct significance in this matter.

5. The Hindu and Parsee women of the Bombay area follow rules, involving a menstrual isolation of 3 + 1 days only. The very scanty data available (25 cases only) show a much lower incidence of cancer of the cervix on Parsees. This might signify that so short a post-menstrual period does not affect the matter one way or the other, and this difference in liability to cancer must then be due to other factors. The similar social incidence in both married and single women in England and Wales shows that such factors exist.

6. Cancer of the uterus appears to be prevalent in some peoples (Hindus, Chinese) among whom phimosis and cancer of the penis are also common, while the Moslem women of India show a lower incidence. But any attribution of this difference to the practice of circumcision by Moslems is very doubtful in view of the similar low incidence on peoples (Parsees, Indian Christians, possibly some Dutch) in whom this factor is absent. But the numerical data on this matter are still quite inadequate.

7. The only numerical data on the social incidence of cancer of the uterus appear to be those from Bavaria 40 years ago, and from England and Wales, after the last census, in 1930–32. The liability to cancer of the uterus increases with descent in the social scale, and, in England and Wales, this is true of both married and single women.

8. The unavoidable mixture, in large-scale statistics, of cancers of the cervix and of the corpus uteri, is unfortunate, as these two forms probably differ in etiology. The difference of 8-10 years in the maximum age-incidence of the two sometimes enables suggestions to be made of the relative proportions of the two in numerical data.

9. The unique data of the Registrar-General upon the social incidence of cancer of the uterus in married and single women suggests a factor less closely connected with sexual functions than are those discussed above in connection with various rituals.

10. The data collected in this paper suggest the existence of two factors which may increase the incidence of cancer of the uterus, namely: (1) A factor which is opposed by the Jewish practice of abstention from intercourse during most of the first half of the ovulatory cycle; and (2) A factor which is intensified in both married and single women by descent in the economic scale.

I wish to express my thanks to the British Empire Cancer Campaign, the Anna Fuller Fund, and the Jane Coffin Childs Fund for grants. I am indebted to Rabbi Dr. I. Epstein, Principal, Jews' College, London, for information about Jewish literature, and for the loan of books. I wish to thank also Dr. V. R. Khanolkar, for unique unpublished data from Bombay, and for translations from Hindu literature. I am indebted also to Dr. Heyman and Dr. Karplus for data from Sweden, and from Palestine, respectively; to Dr. Hannah Billig, Dr. M. Landau, and Dr. Arnold Sorsby for information; to Mr. J. A. Heady, Statistician to this Hospital, for much help in calculations; and to my secretaries, Miss Fenning and Miss Atkin.

References

(1) Ploss, H., M. Bartels, and P. Bartels. *Das Weib in der Natur und Völkerkunde.* 11th edition. Berlin, 1927, Vol. 1, pp. 694-778.

(2) Epstein, I. *Niddah. The Babylonian Talmud. Seder Tohoroth Niddah.* (Ed. I. Epstein, Trans. I.W. Slotki.) London, 1948.

(3) Sorsby, M. *Cancer and Race.* London, 1931.

(4) *Jewish Encyclopedia.* Ablution; Andernach; Bath. New York and London, 1891.

(5) Miller, D. *The Secret of the Jew. His Life—His Family.* 6th edition. Oakland, California, 1930.

(6) Preuss, J. *Biblisch-talmudische Medizin.* Berlin, 1923.

(7) Hurwitz, H. *The Well of Purification.* Leeds, 1921.

(8) Sale, G. *The Koran, commonly called the Alcoran of Mohammed.* London, 1861.

(9) *Zend-Avesta.* Part 1. The Vendidad. Sacred Books of the East. (Ed. F. Max Müller, Trans. J. Darmesteter.) Oxford, 1880.

(10) Modi, J. J. *The Religious Ceremonies and Customs of the Parsees.* Bombay, 1922.

(11) Dubois, J. A. *Hindu Manners, Customs and Ceremonies.* (Trans. and ed. H. K. Beauchamp.) Oxford, 1906.

(12) Jhaveri, K. M. *J Anthrop Soc Bombay* 9:217, 1910.

(13) Vineberg, H. N. *Contributions to Medical and Biological Research dedicated to Dr. William Osler in honour of his 70th birthday.* New York, 1919, Vol. 2, p. 1217.

(14) Lane-Claypon, J. E. Reports on Public Health and Medical Subjects No. 40. H. M. Stationery Office, London, 1927.

(15) Donaldson, M. *Brit Med J* 1:291, 1946.

(16) Smith, F. R. *Am J Obstet Gynec* 21:18, 1931.

(17) Epstein, I. *Kiddushin, The Babylonian Talmud. Seder Nashim.* (Ed. I. Epstein, Trans. H. Freedman.) London, 1936, Vol. 1.

(18) Abramowitz, B. *The Law of Israel* (Trans. S. D. Aaronson.) New York, 1900.

(19) Berman, C. *S Afr J med Sci* 6:145, 1941.

(20) Kennaway, E. L. *Cancer Res* 4:571, 1944.

(21) Weir, P. and C. C. Little. *J Hered* 25:277, 1934.

(22) Kennaway, E. L. and N. M. Kennaway. *Yale J Biol Med* 7:139, 1944.

(23) Handley, W. S. *Lancet* 1:987, 1936.

(24) Handley, W. S. *Brit Med J* 2:841, 1947.

(25) Kennaway, E. L. *Brit J Cancer* 1:355, 1947.

(26) Statesman's Yearbook. Fiji. London, 1947.

(27) Brewster, A. B. *The Hill Tribes of Fiji.* London, 1922.

(28) Plaut, A. and A. C. Kohn-Speyer. *Science* 105:391, 1947.

(29) Theilhaber, F. Z. *Krebsforsch* 8:466, 1910.

(30) Smith, F. R. *Amer J Obstet Gynec* 41:424, 1941.

(31) Davidsohn, I. *Med Leaves* 2:19, 1939.

(32) Registrar General's Decennial Supplement. England and Wales, 1921. Part II. H. M. Stationery Office, London, 1927.

(33) Registrar General's Decennial Supplement. England and Wales, 1931. Part IIa. H. M. Stationery Office, London, 1938.

CONTRIBUTION TO THE STUDY OF THE ETIOLOGY AND PREVENTION OF CANCER OF THE CERVIX OF THE UTERUS[1]

Fabien Gagnon[2]

The aim and object of this presentation is the hope of broadening our knowledge concerning one of the factors long suspected of carcinogenetic action, affirmed by some and denied by others, and to show that prevention of carcinoma of the cervix is possible if the presence of this factor is really essential to its appearance and development.

Almost all publications mention the possibility that cervicitis is a basic cause of carcinoma of the cervix of the uterus.

Richard Te Linde, while agreeing with the opinion held by a number of gynecologists, based on actual clinical experience, namely, that chronic inflammation of the cervix predisposes to the development of cancer, declares textually "No one has ever proven conclusively that cervical lacerations and cervicitis predispose to the development of carcinoma." (1)

Norman Miller states: "While the causation of cancer of the cervix is unknown, much has been written concerning the common benign lesions of the cervix and cancer. Convincing evidence of such relationship is lacking, but even so the correction of all common cervical lesions is indicated on the grounds that cancer does not commonly appear in a healthy organ." (2)

Clinicians have reported the results of treatment of cervicitis and its relation to the development of carcinoma of the cervix. Craig writes that he did not observe a single case of cancer during a period of ten years and over in the 2895 cases of cervicitis which he treated and cured (3). Pemberton and Smith affirm that they did not discover a single case of cancer among the 1408 women whom they treated for and cured of chronic cervicitis. This is equally true of another 740 women on whom was performed an amputation of the cervix (4). Karnaky reports that at Jefferson Davis Hospital, where 5000 women underwent conization, not one case of cancer was observed (5).

On the other hand, Schiller and other authors have expressed the opinion that cervicitis, far from being the cause of the development of cancer, would, on the contrary, be but secondary to its appearance (6).

Novak declares: "There is still considerable difference of opinion among gynecologists as to the importance or unimportance of chronic cervical irritative lesions as predisposers to cancer and Miller has recently published a study in which this danger is minimized." And he adds, "Cancer can develop in cervices in which no evidence of previous chronic irritation can be demonstrated. In my own experience I have, as a matter of fact, been impressed with the fact that a considerable proportion of the early cancers which I have seen have been noted in cervices showing no noticeable evidence of previous chronic inflammation or irritation." (7)

In the presence of divergent, even contradictory opinions on the subject, it is not surprising that too often the treatment of cervicitis as a preventive measure be advised in listless, almost academic fashion, when it is perhaps of vital importance that it be advocated and generalized at all costs.

Two important questions therefore arise. The first is how to convince doctors, who do not specialize nor have any particular interest in gynecology, that they should not tolerate the presence of cervicitis among their patients. The second, how to launch a major educational campaign when many theories oppose one another and so much obscurity on the subject still exists.

Under these circumstances, it is absolutely necessary that the proof be established that cervicitis is one of the essential factors in the development of this cancer, if so it be. That is the crucial point, the key to the solution of the problem.

As previously stated, for some time gynecologists have remarked that they found no

Source: *American Journal of Obstetrics and Gynecology* 60(3):516-522, 1950.

[1] Presented, by invitation, at the Fifth Annual Meeting of the Society of Obstetricians and Gynaecologists of Canada at Jasper Park, Alberta, June 19 to 21, 1949.

[2] Department of Gynecology, Laval University, Quebec, Canada.

cancer among women who had been treated and cured of cervicitis. However, reports of observations of cancer developed in women so treated have or will be published. It would be difficult to imagine that all these patients were completely cured or that they never again will be exposed to the usual causes of cervicitis.

This approach to a vital problem would result only in endless discussions which would bring about the great disadvantage of delaying its solution. This is due to the fact that the preventive effects of such treatment cannot be judged until every patient has reached the age of at least 65 years, or until death has occurred. The proof could hardly come from this source. Because too many years of observation would be necessary before sufficient certainty could be acquired, it was decided to carry out the research work in another direction.

If, in reality, cervicitis is the basis of the cancer of the cervix, this cancer should not exist among women whose social state and mode of life protect them from the usual causes of cervicitis or chronic irritative lesions, namely nuns.

As a gynecologist, I have had, over a long period of years, the advantage of observing and studying a numerically important group of women living in the above-mentioned social state. This conviction gradually grew that this variety of cancer did not exist among them, or that, if it did, it existed only in very exceptional cases. To make sure that this was not an isolated fact, extensive research work in a number of similar groups dispersed over a wide area was carried out.

Purposely, unmarried women living in the ordinary outside world were omitted for research purposes, for reasons which it is not necessary to mention.

The investigation was concentrated exclusively on carcinoma of the cervix uteri and of the corpus uteri, the latter serving as basis of comparison.

A survey of the medical files of an annual average of 13 000 women, covering a twenty-year period, was carried out in the archives of many different convents of nuns. This figure of 13 000 adult women represents, in civilian life, a city with an unchanging population of approximately 65 000 inhabitants, calculation based on the last census taken in Canada.

This research, to be sure, covers a still longer period of time and a much wider range of subjects. Several of the groups concerned, as a matter of fact, furnished statistics extending over periods of 25, 30, 40, 60, and even 86 years, but these figures were not used despite the fact that the causes of death had been carefully recorded. Pathological reports evidently are absent, incomplete or obscured by too great a possibility of error, over such a long period of time, and dating so far back.

Although I had the privilege of consulting the medical files, compiled and well kept by the attendant physician of a convent for fifteen years, statistics covering a group of some 1500 women were set aside because, after their deaths, their files at the convent are destroyed.

In the case of another group, about 2000 women, it was also preferred not to use the information regarding them because the data, gathered from their Mother House over a period of twenty years, could not be verified completely. The reason for this was that the pathological reports of the district hospitals where they had been treated were not complete, although only a small fraction of these cases were not the subject of investigation.

The comparative frequency of carcinoma of the cervix uteri and the corpus uteri, according to the statistics of different authors, varies between 8 and 5 of the former for every single one of the latter. This proportion, according to Novak, is 7 to 1; to Meigs, 6.2 to 1; and to Norris and Vogt, 5.6 to 1 (*8*).

MATERIAL

In Table 1 are given the results of the research work carried out in the previously mentioned group.

Table 1. Annual average, 13 000 women, period of time: 20 years.

Carcinoma of corpus uteri		Carcinoma of cervix uteri
Histologically confirmed	12	—
Diagnosed in the course of operation	1	—
Diagnosed clinically	1	—
Total	14	—

By taking Meigs' index of frequency, 6 to 1, with 12 cases of cancer of the corpus uteri histologically confirmed, 72 cases of carcinoma of the cervix should have been found, but, I repeat, not a single one was discovered. The inverse ratio of frequency is evident in these statistical data.

The results in the groups set aside are identical to those which have just been given. If they were omitted, it was because the inquiries could cover only a period of fifteen years in one case, or could not be completed in the other.

It seems difficult to ignore the mathematical strength and power of these figures. To do so, it would be necessary to assume that the medical statistics on the subject, widely accepted and used for at least the past twenty years, were entirely wrong. This would mean that, if error there be, such statistics should have maintained that cancer of the corpus uteri is more frequent than cancer of the cervix uteri.

This would mean, too, that based on these results, in a city with an unchanging population of about 65 000 inhabitants, there would not have been a single case of carcinoma of the cervix uteri during a period of 20 years.

Intrigued by these observations, stupefied, not to say alarmed, it was decided to study and attack the problem from another angle. A survey of the archives of pathological laboratories and radium treatment centers was made, forgetting the archives of the convents which had heretofore been consulted.

The object in doing this was to verify, over a vast area in which there existed numerous identical groups but in which sphere no investigation had been made, whether or not the findings would contradict or confirm the results previously obtained. It was expedient to do this because the area was much too vast and the identical groups too numerous to be visited individually.

I therefore made a survey of the pathological archives of malignant tumors of the uterus in laboratories of two large hospitals in Montreal and also in the pathological diagnostic centers serving the hospitals of approximately the eastern two-thirds of the Province of Quebec, the Magdalen Islands, the French Islands of St. Pierre and Miquelon, and a few hospitals in New Brunswick. The statistical work in this connection covered periods of time varying from twelve to twenty years.

The archives of treatments given at Montreal's Radium Institute for the past twenty years and those of the Radium Institute of Quebec, since the latter's foundation twelve years ago, were the object of investigation.

Evidently, a large number of anatomical specimens which do not present any special diagnostic difficulties are not sent to diagnostic centers due to the considerable distance which exists between the latter and the various regional hospitals concerned. It is also likely that anatomical specimens are sent to laboratories in the metropolis not searched in the course of this investigation.

It is evident, of course, that a few of the tumors, once discovered in convents' archives by the first method of investigation, are duplicated among those found in the archives of pathological diagnostic centers where the anatomical specimens from these convents are sent for diagnosis.

Once again, would this research in hospital laboratories corroborate or come into conflict with the facts found in the archives of convents?

The verification of pathological reports resulted in the reclassification of two malignant tumors of the cervix uteri in the category of cancer of the corpus uteri. Actually, they were but the propagation of cancer of the corpus uteri to the cervix.

RESULTS

After taking these changes into consideration, the results obtained by the second method of investigation on malignant tumors found in nuns are shown in Table 2.

Table 2. Results obtained by the second method of investigation.

Carcinoma of the corpus uteri		Carcinoma of the cervix uteri
Histologically confirmed	19	3
Total	19	3

With the 6 to 1 ratio frequency, 114 cases of carcinoma of the cervix should have been discovered.

There is no necessity to comment on the surprising similarity of the results obtained by the research work carried out from two different angles.

It is possible, either inadvertently or as the result of clerical error, that a few cases of carcinoma of the cervix may have escaped attention. About 140 000-odd unclassified pathological reports were the object of survey in addition to those that were classified. There is certainly room for error.

However, the striking similarity of the data obtained by the two different methods of research leads one to believe that the errors, if any, would be so rare that they could in no way change the significance of the results.

Research work on such a large scale, covering so long a period of time, can hardly be done with absolute mathematical precision. It was therefore deemed advisable to narrow the field, but only to the extent the results obtained would be equally indicative and where, as far as possible, every nook and corner would be explored, namely, archives of the convents concerned, archives of pathological laboratories, and death certificates. In the course of this third investigation, a related study of cancer of all organs would now be made in relation to carcinoma of the cervix.

It is relatively easy to diagnose cancer of the breast and of the body and cervix of the uterus on account of their accessibility but it is much more difficult to do so with deep cancers. Because of this difficulty, it was necessary to choose carefully, with regard to medical supervision, the groups to be investigated. Each convent selected for special study is attended by a different staff of physicians, surgeons, and specialists, most of them university professors. The margin of error in diagnosis should therefore be acceptable.

This last investigation covered a yearly average of 3280 nuns over a period of twenty years. This number of 3280 nuns is the population of four different Religious Orders or four groups of convents of nuns. This number of adult women would represent in civilian life a city of an unchanging population of about 16 000 inhabitants. Results are shown in Table 3.

For several years, I have been in charge of Group I as gynecologist and have been in a particularly favorable position to study this group. The diagnosis of carcinoma of the corpus uteri observed in this group was first made clinically, then by exploratory curettage, and histopathologic examination. The two patients were operated upon and the diagnosis confirmed by macroscopic and histologic examination of the organ removed in the course of the surgical operation.

Since no carcinoma of the corpus uteri was observed in Groups II, III, and IV, there is

Table 3. Malignant tumors of all organs, annual average: 3280 women, period of time: 20 years.

Skin	3
Thyroid gland	1
Skeleton	1
Spleen	1
Urinary tract	5
Buccal cavity	3
Parotid gland	2
Greater omentum	1
Mesentery	1
Digestive tract	42
Liver	4
Pancreas	2
Breast	53
Ovary	9
Corpus uteri	2
Cervix uteri	0
Malignant tumors of all organs	130
Carcinoma of the cervix uteri	0

practically no likelihood of misinterpretation. Consequently, there are 130 malignant tumors of various organs on one hand and not a single one of carcinoma of the cervix uteri on the other.

Once again one might be amazed that in a city with an unchanging population of some 16 000 inhabitants over a period of twenty years, not a single case of carcinoma of the cervix would be observed. Then, why is it that cancer which strikes so savagely everywhere else in the human body stops short before the cervix of the uterus in these women?

COMMENT

What conclusions may one draw from these facts? In the field of cancer research, theories have given rise to so many disappointments that one must be prudent in the interpretation of facts. However, the significance of those submitted can hardly be overlooked.

In comparing two groups of women living in different social conditions, one frequently exposed to the cause of cervicitis and the other only exceptionally so, the immense importance of chronic cervicitis in the genesis of carcinoma of the cervix is clearly pointed out, and this without denying or minimizing the roles of heredity, acquired constitutional states, viruses, enzymes, deficiencies, and of biochemical and hormonal influences.

Ayre published recently an interesting study in which he claimed that vitamin B deficiency, thiamin and possibly riboflavin, in association with a local excess of estrogens and cervicitis, may indirectly cause carcinoma of the cervix. Since then, a few authors have done research work on the same subject.

It is commonly accepted that prolonged excessive estrogen stimulation causes hyperplasia of the endometrium. However, they have remarked that the hyperplasia of the endometrium was found only in a very few cases though it should frequently exist if really there is a prolonged stimulation by excessive estrogens due to vitamin B deficiency. So, if that is true, the importance of cervicitis may be still greater because probably the facts observed by Ayre would be secondary only (9).

It is true, however, that in very rare cases carcinoma of the cervix may be found in a virgin. How can one then reconcile this clinical fact with the hypothesis that cervicitis constitutes one of the essential factors in the development of carcinoma of the cervix?

It is necessary in my opinion that, exceptionally at least, this variety of cancer be found in virgin women. Otherwise, the previously mentioned facts might well serve to combat the theory of the carcinogenetic action of cervicitis. Authentic chronic cervicitis, most particularly inflammatory erosion, exists in virgin women even if this trouble is rare and pathological modifications superficial. This is a clinical truth observed by the attendant gynecologists of convents.

Consequently, it would be surprising were cancer never to develop in these women, if one accepts the premise that cervicitis really has carcinogenetic action.

Furthermore, from these statistical surveys it appears that, as far as the uterus is concerned, there exists no sole cause of cancer. Different factors are involved according to whether or not it is the corpus or the cervix which is affected.

If cervicitis is a necessary etiological agent, an obligatory one, its cure, theoretically, should also bring about the disappearance of cancer of the cervix. The clinical results brought forth by Douglas, Karnaky and Pemberton and Smith seem to confirm these theoretical views.

May I be permitted to add that in well over 4000 cases of cervicitis, treated systematically during the last 17 years, both at the hospital and in private practice, I have not yet come across a single carcinoma of the cervix. For the past decade, I have taught that the eradication of cervicitis equals the suppression of cancer and, up until now, not one single observation of carcinoma has been brought to my notice which would contradict such assertion.

"No one has ever proven conclusively that cervicitis predisposes to the development of carcinoma," says Richard Te Linde, previously quoted in this respect. At the risk of being accused of presumption, I believe that the results of this research may furnish a link leading to this long-needed proof.

References

(1) Te Linde, R.W. *Operative Gynecology*. Philadelphia, J. B. Lippincott Company, 1946, p. 360.

(2) Miller, N. *JAMA* 136:164, 1948.

(3) Crossen, H.S. and R.J. Crossen. *Operative Gynecology*, ed. 6. St. Louis, The C. V. Mosby Company, 1948, p. 149.

(4) Te Linde, R.W. *Operative Gynecology, Op. cit.*, p. 361.

(5) Karnaky, J. *Obst & Gynec Surv* 1:109, 1946.

(6) Greenhill, J.P. *Office Gynecology*, ed. 4. Chicago, The Year Book Publishers, Inc., 1945, p. 35.

(7) Novak, E. *Gynecological & Obstetrical Pathology*, ed. 2. Philadelphia, W. B. Saunders Company, 1947, p. 98.

(8) Novak, E. *Op. cit.*, p. 225.

(9) Greene, R.R. and E.E. Suckow. *Am J Obstet Gynecol* 58:401, 1949.

COMPARATIVE NEUTRALIZING ANTIBODY PATTERNS TO LANSING (TYPE 2) POLIOMYELITIS VIRUS IN DIFFERENT POPULATIONS[1]

John R. Paul, Joseph L. Melnick, and John T. Riordan[2]

The extent to which neutralizing antibody levels to type 2 (Lansing) strains of poliomyelitis virus, as determined in mice, may serve as an index of immunity to poliomyelitis in general, continues to be a matter of investigation (1-4). So far, the data indicate that the development of this antibody in man, although it represents but one type of the virus, seems to be a rough index of the development of immunity in general to poliomyelitis. Thus, most persons acquire Lansing neutralizing antibodies during childhood either rapidly or slowly, and maintain them during adulthood. Variables in this situation are many and it has not been clearly established what the exact relationships are between Lansing type neutralizing antibodies, as determined in mice and tissue cultures, and those of other (Brunhilde and Leon) types, as determined in monkeys and tissue cultures; or at what levels these antibodies, when once acquired, persist throughout life. Nor is it clear whether all strains of Lansing virus possess equal immunizing powers or equal powers of antibody production. To discuss the matter would take more space than this article can afford, but the reader can be referred to some of the literature, cited above, on this subject.

One approach to a better understanding of this problem is to compare within a given population the age distributional patterns of neutralizing antibodies to Lansing poliomyelitis virus with the past history of clinical poliomyelitis in that population. This we have attempted to do. In order to carry out such studies, it has been necessary to: (a) survey various populations with regard to their past history of, or experience with, poliomyelitis over recent (the previous 15) years; (b) determine the age of local patients who have contracted poliomyelitis

during that period; and (c) select a sample of the population for bleeding and determine from these serum specimens the age at which individuals within the community have acquired neutralizing antibodies to the Lansing (and occasionally to other) strains of poliomyelitis virus; and finally (d) seek for evidence of relationships between (a), (b) and (c).

We have selected for these surveys eight geographical areas, ranging from tropical to arctic zones, with living conditions which also differ as to crowding and sanitary standards. They include: (a) four tropical areas (Cairo, Egypt; Miami, Fla.; Hidalgo County, Texas; and Havana, Cuba); (b) two arctic areas (the island of Iceland and Barrow Village and other Eskimo villages on the north coast of Alaska); and (c) one temperate zone city in the United States (Winston-Salem, N. C.), and one in Europe (Munich, Germany).

METHODS

Morbidity Data. [These] were determined from existing records or reviewed first hand and usually on the spot, with local health departments or ministries of health.[3] In a few instances new information on attack rates was secured by personal investigations in hospitals or clinics within the area.

Collection of Blood for Serum Antibody Studies. These were secured on a voluntary basis from representatives of the local populations. In selecting representatives we have tried, not always with success, to meet the following criteria: (a) that the number of people bled for serum samples was of adequate size (preferably more than 200 people), and that there was sufficient repre-

Source: *American Journal of Hygiene* 56:232-251, 1952.

[1] Aided by a grant from the National Foundation for Infantile Paralysis.

[2] From the Section of Preventive Medicine, Yale University School of Medicine, New Haven, Conn.

[3] It is recognized that official morbidity data on poliomyelitis, particularly during years when the disease is not epidemic, leave much to be desired. Our incidence data, recorded in Figures 1, 2, 4, 5 and 6, suffer from certain deficiencies which the reader should recognize.

sentation of the more significant age groups (0 to 4 and 5 to 9 years) as well as the adult groups; *(b)* that these people were normal (i.e., not ill) unless they were suffering from noninfectious illness or injury; and *(c)* that there were included in the samples only those individuals who were truly representative of the local community and not newcomers or visitors.[4]

Classification of Populations on a Socioeconomic Basis. Our estimates as to whether a given population represented, in whole or in part, an isolated rural or urban group, or whether living (or sanitary) conditions were primitive (type A) or not (type B), are based on the judgment of the individual who visited the area for the collection of the blood or for the gathering of vital statistics. These designations of (A) or (B) are not made on the basis of statistical evidence but from a general impression.

Care of Serum. Precautions were taken to secure sterile samples of serum and to avoid deterioration either in holding the samples or while they were in transit to the testing laboratory. We have not added a preservative to the sera but have kept them either frozen or at refrigerator (4°C) temperature. Usually the tests were run within a year of the time when the sera were collected.

Technical Methods. All of the Lansing antibody determinations mentioned herein were carried out at the Laboratories of the Section of Preventive Medicine at New Haven. The technique of the Lansing neutralizing antibody test as used in our laboratory has been described in a previous communication *(5)*. Devised essentially for epidemiological survey work, it is a simple screening type of test which yields significant and reproducible results but should not be regarded as adequate for clinical diagnosis.[5] The designation of a serum as being positive when tested by this method is based on the arbitrary decision that the undiluted serum when mixed with an appropriate dose of virus and inoculated into eight mice should permit no more

than a quarter of the mice to succumb to infection.

For each test, a calculated dose of 10^2 ID_{50} was used. This was based on a series of titrations previously made on aliquot samples of the suspension of virus. Accompanying each test, a virus titration of the pool was carried out which, as a rule, showed that 10^2 ID_{50} doses were present in the test. Occasionally the titration carried out at the same time as the test would give a slightly higher or lower value than previous titrations on the virus pool, the range being $\pm 10^{0.4}$. Thus a virus pool giving a usual titration of $10^{-3.5}$ would occasionally give results as low as $10^{-3.1}$ and as high as $10^{-3.9}$. This means that in a particular test $10^{2.0} \pm 10^{0.4}$ ID_{50} doses of virus were present, as measured that day.

RESULTS

Tropical Areas

Recent work has indicated that the childhood development of immunity to a number of common infectious diseases may occur far more widely in the tropics than may have been suspected. This also applies to poliomyelitis and Sabin's observations in the Far East *(1)*, Gear's in South Africa *(7)* and Hammon's on the island of Guam *(2)* are examples of this.

Havana, Cuba, and Miami, Florida

A good opportunity for this type of study can be found in the two adjacent populations of Florida and Cuba. During 1946 both areas were involved in the same epidemic *(8)* and it was noted that poliomyelitis in Miami, Florida, was essentially a disease of children of school age, whereas contemporaneously in Havana, Cuba, poliomyelitis was essentially a disease of infants. The theory was put forward in 1949 *(8)* that this difference in the age incidence of the cases which occurred within the same epidemic area was not necessarily due to differences in the age composition of the two populations (Havana and Miami) but could be due, in part at least, to differences in the immune status of the two populations. In other words, the Miami school children might not have had the "benefit" of early infantile exposure to poliomyelitis virus to the same degree as had occurred among Havana children and, as such, the period of

---

[4] A review of criteria followed in selecting a sample of a given population for bleeding has been published previously by two of the authors (J. R. P. and J. T. R.) *(6)*.

[5] The actual technical procedures used here for carrying out the Lansing strain neutralization tests have been reviewed and are being given individual consideration by the Committee on Immunization of the National Foundation for Infantile Paralysis.

susceptibility for the Miami children extended to a later age than was the case with the Havana children. This would imply that infants in Havana had more ready access to sources of the virus than did infants in Miami and, therefore, had acquired their immunity earlier. A similar explanation has been brought forward to account for the difference in the average age which existed between rural and urban cases of poliomyelitis in this country *(9)* and elsewhere *(10)*, with rural cases, as a rule, occurring in older children than those found in adjacent urban children. This difference in age still exists in some parts of the United States, notably New York State *(11)*.

History of Poliomyelitis in Florida and Cuba.[6] Prior to 1930 it would appear that poliomyelitis had been uncommon and sporadic in both southern Florida and Cuba. Available data since 1935 have been charted in Figures 1 and 2. The record of the last 15 years in Florida, although incomplete, indicates that poliomyelitis was uncommon prior to 1941, but since that year the case rates have been steadily on the increase, and are now a little higher than those of other adjacent regions in the United States.[7] The 10-year average annual case rate in Miami, Florida (1941-1950), of 16.7 per 100 000, is also much higher than that of Havana, Cuba (3.3 per 100 000) (see Figure 2), a point which might be based on the fact that the diagnostic criteria for reporting cases in the two countries differ. For, in Cuba only paralytic cases are reported as cases of poliomyelitis, whereas in Florida both paralytic and nonparalytic cases are reported. This then would mean that according to United States standards there is "underreporting" of cases in Cuba and one might have to multiply the Cuban case rate by a factor of 1.5 or 2, perhaps, to make the rates from the two areas comparable; but even so, the Cuban case rates would still be far lower than the Miami rates.

Ages at Which Patients in Miami and Havana Acquired Poliomyelitis. As has already been mentioned in another communication *(8)*, patients from Havana proved to be much younger than those from Miami in the epidemic of 1946, which involved both populations. This difference in age has also persisted during the four years subsequent to 1946. In Cuba we still have, therefore, the infantile disease. As illustrated in Figures 1 and 2, the ages of the Miami patients have been progressively advancing since 1940, so that today 50 percent of them would be older than 9 years, whereas in Havana the infantile age of patients has remained more or less stationary. Fifty percent of them are younger than 3 years. When estimated on an age-specific basis in both areas, with data from the past five years included, the differences are still great and statistically of high significance. A simple demonstration of this difference appears in Table 1 where the ages of 163 poliomyelitis patients from Havana and 225 from Miami are listed for the period of 1946-1949, inclusive.

Collection of Sera. In Miami (Dade County), Florida, blood samples were obtained from the following sources: *(a)* individuals seen at a food handlers' clinic; *(b)* infantile and juvenile groups from the Well Baby Clinic of the Jackson Memorial Hospital; and *(c)* a small number obtained from other clinics in other hospitals.

The population of Miami from which the sample was taken has been designated as urban without undue crowding, and as type (B) in which living or sanitary conditions were not primitive.

In Havana Province, Cuba, sera were collected from individuals applying for antirabies treatment at a clinic devised for such a purpose, and also from the outpatient departments of local hospitals in which individuals were selected who were thought not to be suffering from infectious disease.

The population of Havana has been designated as urban without undue crowding and as type (A), i.e., primitive sanitary conditions.

Lansing Antibody Determinations. As stated in previous communications by Turner et al. *(4)*,

---

[6] We are indebted primarily to Dr. F. Ramirez Corria, former Director of the Finlay Institute, Havana, Cuba, for collecting, storing, and shipping the Cuban samples of serum to this laboratory, as well as securing data on poliomyelitis in Havana Province during visits by two of us (J. L. M. and J. R. P.) during 1949 and 1950, respectively.

In Miami we are primarily indebted to Dr. T. E. Cato, Health Commissioner, Dade County, Fla., and to members of his staff and also to Dr. F. Murray Sanders, Department of Bacteriology, Miami University, Miami, Fla., for assistance in making arrangements for collecting sera; and to Dr. (now Maj.) Horace T. Gardner (MC) and Dr. Lisbeth M. Kraft, for collecting the serum samples in that area.

[7] During the period 1932-1946 the average annual rate for northern counties in the United States was 7.60 per 100 000 and for southern counties 6.39. Recently the rate has been much higher.

Figure 1. The record of poliomyelitis case (attack) rates per 100 000 in Miami (Dade County), Florida, covering the period 1934-1951. The gradual increase in the median ages of the patients during the period 1940-1951 is also charted.

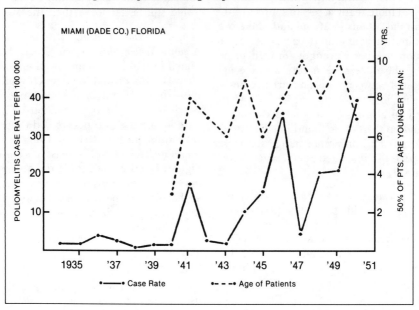

Figure 2. The record of paralytic poliomyelitis case (attack) rates per 100 000 in Havana Province, Cuba, covering the period 1934-1951. Rather crude estimates of the median age of the patients are charted for the period 1934-1944. There is little indication that the median age of patients is increasing in Havana.

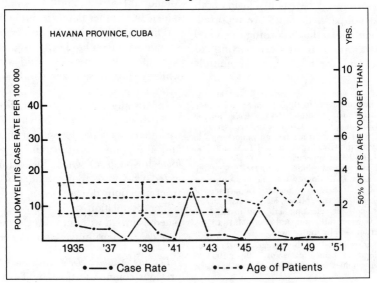

Table 1. Comparison of the age distribution of Lansing neutralizing antibody with clinical cases of poliomyelitis within four subtropical communities.

Age groups (years)	Havana Serol. tests No.[a]	Havana Serol. tests Per-cent +[b]	Havana Cases No.[c]	Havana Cases Cum. per-cent[d]	Miami Serol. tests No.[a]	Miami Serol. tests Per-cent +[b]	Miami Cases No.[c]	Miami Cases Cum. per-cent	Cairo Serol. tests No.[a]	Cairo Serol. tests Per-cent +[b]	Cairo Cases No.[e]	Cairo Cases Cum. per-cent	Texas Serol. tests No.[a]	Texas Serol. tests Per-cent +[b]	Texas Cases No.[f]	Texas Cases Cum. per-cent
<1	0		20	12	11	36	11	3	36	15	141	30.1	10	20	15	23
1-4	22	64	111	81	10	10	66	24	99	75	326	99.7	65	56	41	84
5-9	16	75	12	88	18	50	107	57	37	89	0	99.7	49	84	5	91
10-14	15	73	7	93	24	71	58	75	27	93	0	99.7	31	94	3	96
15-19	15	67	4	95	35	77	27	83	7	100	1	100.0	8	100	0	96
20-29	14	64	7	99	43	79	43	96	15	93	0	100.0	15	93	2	98
30-39			1	100	35	83	11	99	10	100	0	100.0	10	90	1	100
40-49			1	100	31	81	1	100	10	90	1	100.0	7	100	0	100
50+			0	100	18	83			7	100	0	100.0			0	100
Total	82		163		225		324		248		469		195		67	

[a] Number of sera collected in 1950 on which Lansing neutralization tests were run. The Texas sera were collected from Latin Americans living in the Rio Grande Valley, in the spring of 1948.
[b] Percentage of sera with Lansing neutralizing antibodies in each age group.
[c] Number of clinical cases of poliomyelitis reported in 1946-1949, inclusive.
[d] Cumulative percentage of cases.
[e] Number of new cases listed at the Electrotherapy Clinic, Children's Hospital, Cairo, 1948-1949.
[f] Number of cases among Latin Americans in Rio Grande Valley, Texas, during 1948.

and from this laboratory *(5, 12, 13)*, the age distributional pattern of Lansing antibodies within a given population can be readily expressed in terms of an antibody curve. Those illustrative of the patterns in Havana and Miami are charted amongst others in Figure 3. Data on which these curves are based are listed in Table 1.

It is unfortunate that sera from the youngest (under 2 years) age group were not obtained in Havana, but in spite of this defect it can be seen that in the 1-to-4-year age group, 64 percent of the Havana infants had acquired Lansing antibodies and at least this level is maintained through childhood and young adult life. In Miami, on the other hand, it is not until the age of about 12 years is reached that 64 percent have acquired the Lansing antibody. In other words, exposure to, or infection with, agents which give rise to this antibody occurs more slowly in Miami.

Age of Patients Cumulatively Expressed. In Figure 3 (see also Table 1), we have charted the ages at which clinical poliomyelitis is acquired and reported in Havana and in Miami in the form of cumulative percentages of cases in each age group. There seems to be a correlation between the age of local case acquisition and that

of local antibody acquisition within each of these two populations. A similar correlation appears when the comparison is made on an age specific basis.

Cairo, Egypt[8]

Reasons for selecting this site to study "tropical poliomyelitis" have been given in a previous paper *(13)*. Acute paralytic poliomyelitis in natives is endemic there and, as in Havana, it is essentially a disease of infants (i.e., true "infantile paralysis"). It is rare, or very uncommon, in native Egyptian adults; this is in striking contrast to its frequency in "immigrant" adults such as British and United States soldiers *(14)*. Unlike in Havana, however, local epidemics in Egyptian natives have not been reported. The infrequency of the reported disease may well be related to the fact that the native Egyptian population over the age of 5 years appears to be relatively, if not completely, immune to polio-

---

[8] We are indebted to Capt. J. J. Sapero, MC, U.S.N., Commanding Officer of Naval Medical Research Unit No. 3, in Cairo, for making this project possible and to Dr. W. A. McIntosh and Dr. J. M. Weir, representatives of the International Health Division of the Rockefeller Foundation in Cairo, for their invaluable assistance particularly during the visit by one of us (J. R. P.) to this area in 1950.

Figure 3. The age distribution of Lansing antibody curves compared with the age of the poliomyelitis cases in 8 different populations. The scale at the bottom denoting age has been arranged to give ample space for recording findings in those age groups which are usually most important (1–10 years) for the acquisition of this antibody and for clinical poliomyelitis. An insufficient number of patients in the Alaska series (lower right corner) is responsible for the omission of the case curve in that chart.

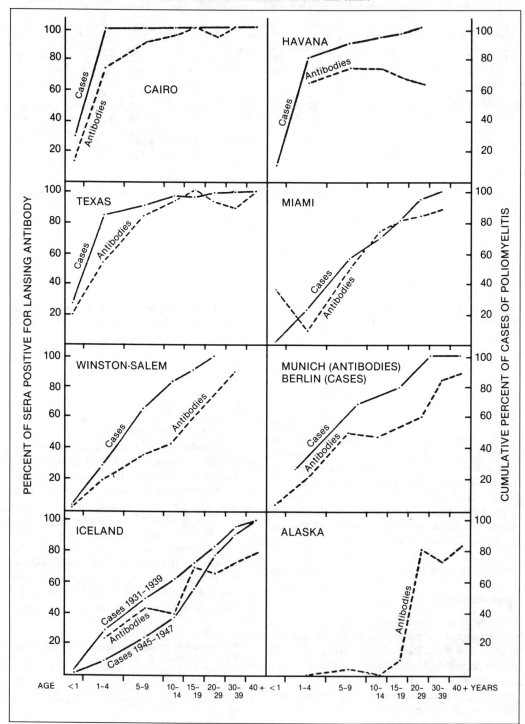

myelitis. On clinical grounds, therefore, one would suspect that such a high degree of childhood immunity might be reflected by a high level of Lansing antibodies which were acquired at an early age, and this turned out to be the case.

History of Poliomyelitis in Egypt. Officially the Egyptian Ministry of Health records do not indicate the incidence of poliomyelitis there, for recently only 2 to 11 cases per year are reported (notified) and most of these are fatal. To supplement the inadequate record of attack rate, based on reported cases, data have been included in Figure 4 which give crude and short-term estimates based on hospital outpatient department admissions. These estimates are based on a review of hospital records which indicated that between 210 and 260 new cases of paralytic disease in infants were listed as having been seen or treated in the dispensary of the Children's Hospital of Cairo in 1948 and 1949, respectively.[9] Our crude estimate of the attack rate for Cairo and its environs indicates, therefore, that it may lie in the range of 4 to 8 per 100 000 per annum. We have supplemented this estimate by inspection of a small number of actual patients in the clinic, and by the isolation of poliomyelitis virus from the stools of a patient with a typical case of paralytic poliomyelitis seen in the clinic *(13)*. With respect to the age of the patients, two-thirds of the cases occurred in infants under the age of 2 years, and 50 percent of these occurred before the infants were 18 months old! (See Figures 3 and 4, and Table 1.)

Collection of Sera.[10] These were obtained from the residents of a rural health district established and administered by the International Health Division of The Rockefeller Foundation and located some 30 kilometers north of the city limits of Cairo. The number of children bled whose sera was subsequently tested, and their age distribution, appear in Table 1.

Although the Cairo population in this health district is described as rural, actually the crowded villages simulate urban living with primitive sanitary conditions designated as (A).

Lansing Antibody Determinations. These are charted in Figure 3 (upper left). The trend indicates an early acquisition of this antibody, very shortly after the loss of the maternal antibody. By the time the children are 2 years old, 55 percent of them, and by 3 years of age, about 75 percent have acquired Lansing antibodies. In a previous paper *(13)* these Lansing antibody curves have been compared with those derived from neutralization tests, carried out in monkeys, with Brunhilde and Leon strains of poliomyelitis virus. The Lansing antibodies seemed to be acquired at a slightly earlier age by these Egyptian infants than were the antibodies to the other two strains.

Age of Patients Cumulatively Expressed. For purposes of comparison we have again charted the age at which poliomyelitis is acquired, together with the age at which the Lansing antibody is acquired in Cairo by natives. The curve is given in Figure 3. There is again a correlation here between the local age acquisition of paralytic poliomyelitis and the age of local Lansing antibody acquisition.

Comment. Our interpretation of these Lansing neutralizing antibody findings is that there is ample Lansing-type poliomyelitis virus present locally in Egypt to which the high attack rate of poliomyelitis cases (some of them due to the Lansing type of virus) in British and United States troops during World War II bore witness *(14)*. We would further presume that exposure of all age groups of natives to the Lansing and other types of poliomyelitis virus is heavy in Egypt, and that young infants not only share in this exposure but are the only natives who are susceptible. As the immunization of these infants proceeds at a much faster rate than is usually the case in this country, the number of susceptibles to whom the disease might spread never becomes large enough to allow a big epidemic to start. This heavy and continual seeding of the population with virus is perhaps responsible for the insignificant reporting of cases as shown in Figure 4, for it is well recognized

---

[9] We arrived at these figures as a result of personal reviews of the local situation in Cairo by one of us (J.R.P.) in 1944 *(14)*, and again in 1950 *(13)*.

We are indebted to Dr. A. Safwat of the Pediatric Department, Kasr-El-Aini Medical Faculty, for the privilege of examining patients and records at the Cairo Children's Hospital and the outpatient department; and to Dr. Abdul Aziz Zaky Hanna, Director of the Clinic for Electrotherapy at this institution.

[10] We are indebted to Mr. O. C. Dierkhising, HMC, U.S.N. NAMRU No. 3, for technical assistance in separating the sera.

Figure 4. The official rates of poliomyelitis are recorded for all Egypt as being almost nil for the years 1934–1951. Crude and limited estimates for the median ages of patients, based on a hospital outpatient department survey, for the years 1944 and for 1948–1949 are charted.

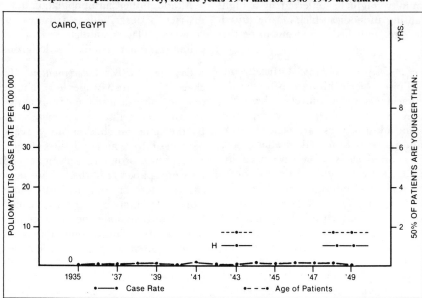

that the reporting of poliomyelitis cases in many countries during nonepidemic times is notoriously apt to be scanty.

Lower Rio Grande Valley (Hidalgo County), Texas[11]

This area is at a latitude of 26 degrees, north, the same as Miami, and close to our other two tropical areas (Havana, 23 degrees, and Cairo, 30 degrees). Investigations by the United States Public Health Service on dysentery in this area had been well under way when poliomyelitis appeared in an epidemic wave in 1948, reaching its peak in May. This epidemic, the first recorded in this area, will be described in detail by Watt and Paffenbarger who were instrumental in obtaining the sera for the present study. As serum samples in adequate number and data on age distribution were obtained only among the Latin-Americans of Hidalgo County, only this group will be considered here. Sixty-seven paralytic cases were observed in this population, which numbered 99 600 in 1948. In April of that year, serum was collected from healthy per-

sons in the towns of McAllen and Donna, and the results of neutralization tests on 195 samples are analyzed here.

The Lansing antibody pattern, shown in Figure 3, is strikingly similar to that shown in the curves for Havana and Cairo referred to above. In other words, antibodies were acquired early in life, with 56 percent of the children between 1 and 4 years of age yielding positive tests. This high rate of immunization was maintained, for 84 percent of those 5 to 9 years old had antibodies, and the level of positives was maintained at over 90 percent in those over 10 years of age. These data are presented in Table 1, together with the age distribution of paralytic cases in this population during the 1948 epidemic.

The population studied may be considered as a tropical one (even though there may be an occasional frost during the winter) and urban with low standards of hygiene designated as (A). The curves both for age distribution of cases and of antibodies are similar to those found in Havana and Cairo. Similarities in the curves for paralytic cases and Lansing antibodies in this Texas population, as measured at the starting phase of a poliomyelitis epidemic, suggest that exposure to the Lansing type of poliomyelitis virus had been of the same order, apparently, as

[11] We are indebted in particular to Dr. James Watt, United States Public Health Service, for assistance rendered to us in the study of this area, particularly during the visit of one of us (J. L. M.) to this area in 1948.

that for the strain or strains causing the epidemic. Other evidence available militates against the probability of a Lansing type virus being instrumental in the 1948 epidemic.[12]

Arctic Areas

Populations living in the Arctic and remote from civilization represent special groups of people among whom poliomyelitis penetrates seldom. Theoretically, then, the antibody pattern should reflect this fact and, indeed, previous studies *(5, 6, 15)* have shown this to be the case.

In such remote populations of relatively small size (as, for instance, under 25 000), whether they are located in the Arctic or not, the viruses of certain acute infectious diseases not only penetrate infrequently but, once there, fail to persist endemically for long within the population, in that they seem to die out after each outbreak. As a result, the periodicity of outbreaks of a given disease within a small isolated population is not dependent upon a build-up of susceptibles who become infected with a local strain of virus, but the outbreak depends rather upon a build-up of susceptible persons over a longer period of time who become infected only by the chance penetration of virus into the community from an outside source. The well-known experiences with severe epidemics of measles in remote populations, and with the common cold virus on the island of Spitsbergen during the pre-air-travel era are cases in point. Colds disappeared on that latter island during its long period of ice-bound winter isolation, to reappear again in the form of an explosive epidemic each spring with the arrival of the first boat *(16)*.

Thus one would suspect that the antibody patterns found in remote and partially isolated populations might be quite different from those of large urban populations. It is for these reasons that remote populations have significance for us here, and several of them exist in arctic areas.

Point Barrow, Alaska: History of Poliomyelitis[13]

Previous work from this laboratory *(5, 15)* has indicated that within certain Eskimo populations of the north coast of Alaska, and totaling about 1200 people, the recent periodic incidence of clinical poliomyelitis has been widely spaced. For example, the last recorded outbreak of poliomyelitis at Point Barrow occurred in 1930, or 19 years prior to the antibody survey *(5)*. Data on the severity of this outbreak and the age incidence of the cases are too scanty for analysis here. At least no fatal cases in adults were listed.

Antibody Pattern. In keeping with the history, the incidence of Lansing antibodies in the entire juvenile or adolescent population has been very low (see Figure 3, lower right corner). Thus in 1949, 95 percent of those Eskimos under 20 years of age did not have Lansing antibodies, whereas 85 percent of those over 20 years of age possessed these antibodies, giving a pattern, which for the first 20 years of life, is sharply divergent from any other curve that we have studied. It would appear that the absence of Lansing antibodies in childhood and adolescence followed by a sharp and sustained rise in Lansing antibodies at the age of 19 years, could be correlated in this population with the last recorded (1930) outbreak. In retrospect it would also appear that this 1930 outbreak presumably was due to a strain of the Lansing type of poliomyelitis virus. Neutralization tests indicating the age distribution of the Lansing antibody are listed in Table 2.

Other investigators have studied other small collections of Eskimo serum for antibodies. Dingle *(17)* has reported that among the population on Baffin Island there was a scarcity of positive tests for Lansing antibody in the sera of younger Baffin Island Eskimos. Clark and Rhodes *(18)* have collected sera from Eskimos at Chesterfield Inlet in the Canadian Arctic, and found that Lansing antibodies began to appear in serum of children from the age of 10 years

---

[12] Several strains isolated during the epidemic were inoculated into mice and cotton rats without producing disease in these rodents. Subsequently, 10 strains from the epidemic were proven by serological means to be related to the Brunhilde type.

[13] For facilities and the privileges of working in this area we are indebted to the Medical Science Division, Office of Naval Research, Washington, D.C., and to Dr. G. E. MacGinitie, Director (at that time) of the Arctic Research Laboratory, for many kindnesses shown during the visit of one of us (J. R. P.) in August and September, 1949.

Table 2. The age distribution of Lansing antibody levels within two Arctic communities.

Age groups (years)	Alaska Serol. tests 1949[a] No.[d]	Percent[e] +	Iceland — Serological tests[b] Urban and town No.[d]	Percent +	Rural No.[d]	Percent +	Total[c] No.[d]	Percent +	Clinical cases 1931-1939 incl. No.	Cum. percent[f]	1945-1947 incl. No.	Cum. percent
<1	0		0		0		0		12	2	8	1
1-4	5	0	8	37	5	0	14	29	144	28	93	10
5-9	49	4	21	60	6	0	33	49	110	48	158	24
10-14	45	0	19	47	8	25	31	41	78	62	141	38
15-19	30	10	16	62	3		21	71	61	73	196	56
20-29	47	85	26	69	3		29	69	74	86	228	77
30-39	31	74	17	73	1		21	67	42	94	139	91
40-49	16	87	12	83	2		17	82	} 33	} 100	} 95	} 100
50+	20	90	11	100	6	83	22	86				
Total	243		130		34		188		554		1058	

[a] Lansing neutralizing antibody determinations carried out on sera collected in 1949.
[b] Lansing neutralizing antibody determinations carried out on sera collected in 1950.
[c] Included in this total are 24 cases in which classification as to urban and rural was unknown. This accounts for the discrepancy in addition.
[d] Number of sera in each age group.
[e] Percentage with Lansing antibodies.
[f] Cumulative percentage of cases.

onwards and the serum of most adults proved positive. In brief, the findings from these areas have indicated that Lansing antibody acquisition has occurred more sporadically than elsewhere.

Iceland: Locale and History

Within this semi-arctic area the story of poliomyelitis has been well documented (since 1930 at least) and for this reason it was chosen for a serological survey.[14]

Situated close to the Arctic Circle the population of Iceland (totalling about 135 000) represents certain features common to insular groups where, if records of moderate to good accuracy are maintained, there are special opportunities for epidemiological observations. Iceland is not, however, an isolated community, i.e., exclusive of certain rural groups in remote parts of the island. In the city of Reykjavik, which accounts for about 40 percent of the local population, conditions are not very different from what one would find in a northern Scandinavian, Scottish, or Irish city. However, it is safe to say that in 1950 (the time of our survey) not more than 20 percent of the individuals questioned had been out of the country at one time or another and, epidemiologically speaking, some of the isolated districts from which blood samples were obtained do represent "remote populations." The island population has ranged in size from 94 000 in 1920 to about 132 750 in 1946, but it is not, or has not been, of sufficient size to support for long, measles as an endemic infection, or mumps, or pertussis, so that these children's diseases have recurred at perhaps longer intervals than one might have expected in a larger community with frequent outside contacts. With measles, for instance, the period between epidemics, since 1907, has usually been from 7 to 9 years, instead of the usual 3 to 6; with mumps, it has been 6 to 10 years.

Collection of Blood Samples.[15] Arrangements in Reykjavik (population 48 000) were made through the local Tuberculosis Clinic (which was attended by many individuals coming for

[14] We are greatly indebted to Dr. Bjorn Sigurdsson, Director of the Institute for Experimental Pathology, University of Iceland, Keldur, Reykjavik, for his tireless efforts to assist in this project, for his arrangements to have serum collected by various physicians and for many kindnesses shown during the visit by one of us (J. R. P.) to Iceland in August, 1950.

[15] We are indebted to Miss Anne G. Tryggradottir, of the Institute for Experimental Pathology at Keldur, for separating the sera from the whole blood specimens.

chest X rays as part of a mass survey), the State Hospital, and the Old Folks' Home. Through local health officers, blood samples were also obtained from two districts: *(a)* the town of Akureyri (population 6000), and *(b)* rural districts on the southeast coast of the island. The population was both urban and rural. Living conditions were for the most part not primitive and have been designated as (B).

The story of poliomyelitis on this island has been adequately covered in Sigurjónsson's paper *(19)*. The first recognized cases of the disease were recorded in 1904. In 1924 came a large epidemic, and since that date large epidemics have occurred with extraordinarily high rates (see Figure 5). The curves here show a record of periodic epidemics, with very high peaks for the years 1935 and 1936, 1938 and 1945 and 1946. The curve is quite out of line with that drawn for other areas. Furthermore, a confusing situation has arisen in that presumably recently a disease has appeared in Iceland which can be readily be mistaken for poliomyelitis (Sigurdsson et al, *20*). Primarily it was assumed

to be poliomyelitis, but its symptomatology, its seasonal distribution as a winter (September-February) disease, and the fact that it has tended to attack young adults rather than children, now indicate that it is probably something different. The story of poliomyelitis in Iceland has been, therefore, clouded during the years 1945-1948 and subsequently, by the fact that the status of this "poliomyelitis-like" disease has not been settled or its exact clinical limits defined. In any event the marked shift in the age distributions of "poliomyelitis" cases to the older age groups during the 1940s is probably due, in part at least, to the inclusion as poliomyelitis of cases of this as yet unnamed disease. This is illustrated in the bizarre and interrupted curve shown in Figure 5.

Age of Patients. In Figure 5 (upper left) there is also included a short line which indicates the "median age" of the Icelandic poliomyelitis cases for the years 1935-1939. This is again very high in that 50 percent of the cases for those years were younger (or older) than 11 years.

Figure 5. Case rates for "poliomyelitis" in Iceland covering the period 1934–1951. In 1945 the appearance of a disease which can be mistaken for poliomyelitis has rendered the incidence and median age figures for 1945–1951 sufficiently unreliable so that they are not recorded.

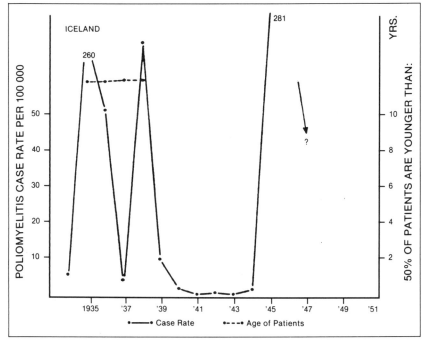

The number of cases which occurred in 1940-1944 are too few to warrant age estimates and those for the years 1945-1947 are probably not all poliomyelitis cases. These irregularities render a correlation between poliomyelitis age incidence and local Lansing strain antibody levels difficult, but they should not detract from the value of other aspects of the Lansing antibody determinations.

Antibody Patterns. It has been possible to divide our collection of serum samples from Iceland into two groups: *(a)* urban (including inhabitants of small towns) and *(b)* rural. The results of serological determinations have been listed accordingly in Table 2. Although the data from rural areas are scanty, no serum with Lansing antibodies was obtained from the 11 rural inhabitants tested under the age of 10 years. In charting these results (see Figure 3) rural and urban groups have been combined. Here the curve indicating the percentage of those Icelanders with Lansing antibodies rises slowly during childhood and adolescence, although not at a much slower rate than is the case with some other populations included in this survey and which are much closer to home. The "50 percent positive" point on this antibody curve occurs at about 15 years of age, the "70 percent positive" point is not reached until after the age of 30 years. One might have expected to find a low level of antibodies during childhood and adolescence in Iceland in the face of the relatively advanced age of the patients who have contracted poliomyelitis. As for the correlation between age of cases and antibody acquisition, this has been charted in Figure 3 according to two categories: *(a)* cases of poliomyelitis occurring during the 1930s and *(b)* those in 1945-1947. During the 1930s, when the diagnosis of poliomyelitis in Iceland was thought to be no more difficult than in other lands, the cumulative age curve for cases during that period (see Figure 3) lies *above* the Lansing antibody curve and shows a correlation comparable to that seen elsewhere. On the other hand, when the cumulative age curve for the cases from 1945 through 1947 is drawn, it lies *below* the antibody curve during the first 20 years of life. In no other area or population studied by us have we seen this latter situation. It would be another argument that during the years of 1945-1947, cases diagnosed as poliomyelitis in

Iceland may not all have been examples of that disease, but some other disease involving an age group older than that usually seen in poliomyelitis.

Temperate Zone Areas

Winston-Salem, N. C.

A previous study *(11)* has been reported from this laboratory dealing with the urban population in this North Carolina city of 88 000. In it Lansing antibody levels from two different socioeconomic groups (upper (B) and lower (A)) have been measured and compared. Details of the local situation will accordingly not be gone into here, except to mention that sera were collected from healthy children during the year (1948) of a poliomyelitis epidemic in that state.

History of Poliomyelitis in North Carolina.[16] Poliomyelitis case rates for the past 20 years are charted in Figure 6, indicating that periodic epidemics have been coming in shorter intervals since 1943 than before that year. During the entire 20-year period, the age of the patients has advanced but slightly with a median age of 3.5 years during the 1930s and nearer 5 years since 1943. This is still far below the median age of the Icelandic and Miami cases and one would hardly have expected that the Lansing antibody level would be about the same in these three populations, although this actually turns out to be the case.

Antibody Patterns. Two hundred and thirty-two samples were tested for Lansing antibody. Results are listed in Table 3 and charted in Figure 3. In the latter, one sees that the antibody curve rises slowly and it is not until the age of about 14 years that 50 percent of these children have acquired Lansing antibodies.

Age of Cases. This, too, is charted in Figure 3. Parallelism with the Lansing antibody curve is but approximate in that the antibody levels sag well below the case curve during the age period of 5 to 30 years. In other words, Lansing antibody levels do not seem to be a good index of poliomyelitis here. One might assume from this

---

[16] We are indebted to Dr. C. P. Stevick, Director, Division of Epidemiology, North Carolina State Board of Health, for supplying us with information relative to poliomyelitis in this state.

Figure 6. Case rates for poliomyelitis in North Carolina for the period 1931–1950. The median age of the patients has climbed somewhat during this period.

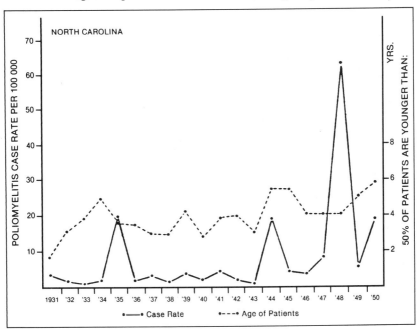

•—• Case Rate   •---• Age of Patients

that the Lansing strain of poliomyelitis has been playing less of a part in the general poliomyelitis situation in Winston-Salem than in some of the other areas studied and herein reported. We must admit, however, that we do not have an explanation for this situation.

Munich, Germany

This population was chosen as a representative large mid-European city even though the history of poliomyelitis in that city has not been too well documented. Nevertheless, samples of blood were obtained in 1951 from inmates of the Kinderklinik of the University of Munich hospital (service of Prof. Weiskott) and from other clinics associated with this university hospital.[17] The population has been classified as urban and the living conditions as not primitive (B). Subjects from whom blood was drawn were, for the most part, not suffering from infectious disease.

[17] We are greatly indebted to Dr. Luitgarde Bungards for collecting these serum specimens and to Lt. Col. H. Sprinz, MC, Director of Laboratories at the 98th General Hospital, European Command, for preparing the serum samples and holding them prior to shipment to the United States.

Antibody Patterns. A relatively delayed rise of antibody levels was found. Figures are listed in Table 3, and a graph is included in Figure 3. In general, the slope of this curve is quite comparable to that from Miami and Winston-Salem.

Age of Cases. We were unsuccessful in securing a list of poliomyelitis cases, which had occurred recently in Munich, and which was large enough for age analysis. Therefore, our comparison of the age at which Lansing antibodies were acquired with that at which clinical poliomyelitis was acquired, has been made with a Berlin series of 2475 poliomyelitis cases from their 1947 epidemic (21). The age of these cases, as designated by the slope of the curve, is again similar to that of several other temperate zone populations included in this report.

One could raise questions relative to the socioeconomic and sanitary conditions present in Munich and Berlin during the period in which we are particularly interested, i.e., 1936-1951. Obviously, from 1944 to about 1947 living conditions were not good. But from personal inspections by one of us (J.R.P.) during the period 1947-1951 it would appear that relatively good conditions were restored by about 1948.

Table 3. Age distribution of Lansing antibody levels compared with that of poliomyelitis cases in three temperate zone communities.

Age groups (years)	Winston-Salem, N.C. Serol. tests No.	Percent +	Cases^a No.	Cum. percent	Munich, Germany Serol. tests No.	Percent +	Cases^b No.	Cum. percent	Madagascar Serol. tests^c No.	Percent +
<1	22	0	3	4	19	3				
1-4	84	20	22	32	25	20	693	28	11	28
5-9	63	36	25	64	22	50			9	75
10-14	44	43	13	80	15	47	990	68		
15-19			9	92	4		297	80		
20-29			6	100	13	60				
30-39	19	90			11	83	421	97		
40-49					7	87				
50+					2		74	100		
Total	232		78		118		2475		20	

^a Cases of poliomyelitis occurring in 1948 in Winston-Salem only.
^b Cases of poliomyelitis occurring in 1947 in the City of Berlin. Actually the first two age groups here were: 0-5 = 28 percent; 6-14 = 68 percent.
^c Sera collected in 1951; all of those in the 5-9 age group were actually 5-6 years of age.

Madagascar[18]

A very small number of sera, 20 in all, are included in the report from Tananarive, Madagascar. We believe they are important in that they represent a population living under what might be called a temperate zone climate and primitive sanitary conditions but have not regarded this as a significant survey.

The sera were collected for us under the supervision of Dr. J. E. Smadel. They include young children and infants only. Antibody levels are listed in Table 3. Two points on a theoretical curve are all that is available from this small series but they suggest that the antibody response in this young age group falls in line with those of Cairo or Havana.

DISCUSSION

The Lansing type neutralizing antibody surveys herein reported give us a picture of the various rapidities with which infants, children and young adults acquire these antibodies in various parts of the world, and the eventual levels which are attained throughout adult life. A salient feature of the study is that we have not

found any geographical area or population in which the inhabitants lose this antibody. There are lag periods, lasting 10 or more years, in which the percentage of those who possess the antibody does not increase but never has the percentage fallen appreciably. One may conclude from this study, therefore, that according to the methods and criteria used and the populations studied, the Lansing antibody, once acquired, remains, at least at low titer. Of course, the extent to which the permanence of this antibody is dependent upon "booster doses" or multiple subclinical infections is not known but at least in the Alaskan population booster doses probably did not occur from 1930 to 1949.

Furthermore, within these different areas and populations we find that the age at which Lansing antibodies are acquired turns out in the majority of places tested to be more or less comparable to the age at which clinical poliomyelitis is acquired. Consequently, the degree to which a survey of Lansing antibodies becomes a measure or index of local immunity status to poliomyelitis, which was the question raised at the beginning of this study, is not completely answered. In certain areas such as Cairo, Egypt, and Miami, Florida, the index is quite good as of 1950, but the extent to which one can say that a local measure of Lansing neutralizing antibodies is a local measure of the immunity status of a given population is still unknown and might be further tested to advantage. It seems

[18] We are indebted for these sera to Dr. J. E. Smadel of the Army Medical Graduate Service School, Washington, D. C.; to Dr. Kenneth Goodner of Jefferson Medical College, Philadelphia, Pa., and to Dr. J. Robic, Director, Pasteur Institute, Tananarive, Madagascar.

clear that in future surveys more than one type of poliomyelitis antibody might well be included.

Another serious question which can be raised is whether the measure of the age of the reported cases of poliomyelitis within a community is really a good or true measure of poliomyelitis infection within that community. It is possible, as Sabin *(22)* has suggested, that population groups which live under conditions that are especially conducive to the continuous dissemination and consumption of small doses of virus may acquire poliomyelitis immunity without paralysis more frequently than is the case elsewhere. Under such circumstances the relative number of undiagnosed cases would be greater than would be the situation elsewhere. These questions can be answered better by future surveys than by speculation.

As for an evaluation of climate or environmental factors which might influence the spread of poliomyelitis and the speed of acquisition of Lansing antibodies, or the acquisition of the clinical disease, it would not appear that climate per se is a dominant feature. Two features stand out which seem to influence anti-body acquisition and case acquisition here. One of these is the self-evident fact that in populations remote from civilization one is apt to acquire poliomyelitis and immunity to it later in life than seems to be the case elsewhere. The other is that in the urban life where sanitary conditions are primitive and presumably facilities for the spread of this virus to young children are good, quite regardless of climate, both antibodies and the clinical disease are acquired very early in life. On this basis, rather than on the basis of climate, we can divide the antibody curves and the poliomyelitis case curves roughly into our two groups: (A) those in which the "sanitary" conditions are "more primitive" than usual in the United States and Europe; and (B) those in which they are not.

To this end we have prepared two final figures: one to designate the average antibody levels for groups (A) and (B) (Figure 7); and one to designate the average age distribution of the cases of poliomyelitis for groups (A) and (B) (Figure 8). The differences between groups (A) and (B) in each of these figures are apparent and the conclusions one might draw are quite in keeping with those of Hammon *(2, 3)* and

Figure 7. Lansing antibody levels charted on an age distributional basis for two population groups (A and B), divided more or less arbitrarily on the basis of: group A, crowding with primitive sanitary conditions; and group B, rural or urban with moderate crowding but with less primitive sanitary conditions.

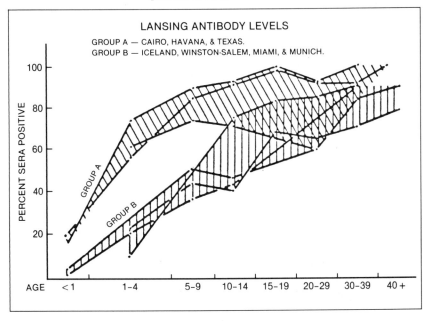

Figure 8. The cumulative age curves indicating when poliomyelitis is acquired in two population groups (A and B) divided as indicated in figure 7.

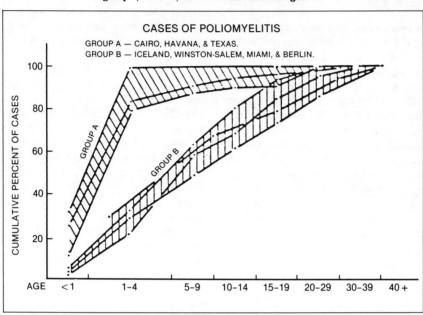

Melnick *(12)*; and in keeping with the historical situation in this country in which over a period of 50 or more years the disease has passed from one of infants to that of children of school age. No attempt is made here to designate what type of so-called social or sanitary conditions might be especially conducive for a special dissemination of the virus in certain population groups nor have we data on the effect of the size of the family in groups (A) and (B). The latter consideration must be included as a factor. It has been given some attention in Lansing antibody surveys *(2, 3, 12)* and should be the subject of future work.

SUMMARY

1. Neutralizing antibody levels to Lansing (type 2) poliomyelitis virus have been measured in individuals of various ages from eight different populations selected from subtropical, arctic and temperate zone localities.

2. The rates at which these antibodies are acquired in infancy, childhood, and adolescence, as well as the levels at which these antibodies are maintained in adult life, have been compared.

3. Regardless of geographic location, Lansing antibodies seem to be acquired at an earlier age by those populations which live under primitive sanitary conditions and particularly if crowding also exists.

4. In seven of these populations, the attempt has been made to compare the local ages at which clinical poliomyelitis has been acquired recently and the local ages at which the Lansing neutralizing antibody had been acquired. This correlation is quite close in at least four of the seven populations, a finding which suggests that Lansing neutralizing antibody surveys of this type may sometimes serve as an index of general immunity to poliomyelitis in certain populations but that the index does not hold universally.

References

(1) Sabin, A. B. The epidemiology of poliomyelitis: problems at home and among the armed forces abroad. *JAMA* 134:749-756, 1947.

(2) Hammon, W. McD. Immunity in poliomyelitis. *Bact Rev* 13:135-159, 1949.

(3) Hammon, W. McD., G. E. Sather, and N. Hollinger. Preliminary report of epidemiological studies on poliomyelitis and streptococcal infections. *Am J Pub Health* 40:293-306, 1950.

(4) Turner, T. B., D. H. Hollander, S. Buckley, U. P.

Kokko, and C. P. Winsor. Age incidence and seasonal development of neutralizing antibodies to Lansing poliomyelitis virus. *Am J Hyg* 52:323-347, 1950.

(5) Paul, J. R. and J. T. Riordan. Observations on serological epidemiology. Antibodies to the Lansing strain of poliomyelitis virus in sera from Alaskan Eskimos. *Am J Hyg* 52:202-212, 1950.

(6) Paul, J. R., J. T. Riordan, and L. M. Kraft. Serological epidemiology: antibody patterns in North Alaskan Eskimos. *J Immunol* 66:695-713, 1951.

(7) Gear, J. H. S. Poliomyelitis in Southern Africa. Proc. 4th Internat. Cong. Trop. Med. and Malaria. Dept. of State, Washington, D. C. 1:555-567, 1948. See also: Gear, J. H. S., V. Measroch, and J. Bradley. Poliomyelitis in South Africa. Studies in an urban native township during a non-epidemic year. *S Afr Med J* 25:297-301, 1951.

(8) Paul J. R., F. R. Corria, and D. M. Horstmann. Analyses from a tropical epidemic of poliomyelitis which occurred in Florida and Cuba in 1946. *Am J Trop Med* 29:543-554, 1949.

(9) Nicoll, M., Jr. Epidemiologic data in the poliomyelitis epidemic in New York State. *Am J Dis Child* 14:69-79, 1917.

(10) Olin, G. and N. O. Heinertz. Das Auftreten der Kinderlähmung in Schweden 1930-39. *Ztschr f Hyg u Infektionskrankheiten* 125:153-174, 1943. See also: Olin, G. and N. O. Heinertz. The epidemiological pattern of poliomyelitis in Sweden, 1925-1944. *Acta Pathol* suppl. 91:139-151, 1951.

(11) Paul, J. R. The peripheral spread of poliomyelitis through rural and urban areas: observations from a recent epidemic. *Yale J Biol Med* 19:521-536, 1947.

(12) Melnick, J. L., and N. Ledinko. Social serology: antibody levels in a normal young population during an epidemic of poliomyelitis. *Am J Hyg* 54:354-382, 1951.

(13) Paul, J. R., J. L. Melnick, V. H. Barnett, and N. Goldblum. A survey of neutralizing antibodies to poliomyelitis virus in Cairo, Egypt. *Am J Hyg* 55:402-413, 1952.

(14) Paul, J. R., W. P. Havens, and C. E. Van Rooyen. Poliomyelitis in British and American troops in the Middle East. The isolation of virus from human faeces. *Br Med J* 1:841-843, 1944.

(15) Paul J. R., J. T. Riordan and J. L. Melnick. Antibodies to three different antigenic types of poliomyelitis virus in sera from North Alaskan Eskimos. *Am J Hyg* 54:275-285, 1951.

(16) Paul, J. H. and H. L. Freese. An epidemiological and bacteriological study of the "common cold" in an isolated Arctic community (Spitsbergen). *Am J Hyg* 17:517-535, 1933.

(17) Personal communication from Dr. J. H. Dingle.

(18) Clark, F. M. and A. J. Rhodes. Poliomyelitis in Canadian Eskimos: Laboratory studies II. *Can J Med Sci* 29:216-235, 1951.

(19) Sigurjónsson, J. Epidemiologic characteristics of poliomyelitis in Iceland. *Am J Hyg* 51:109-125, 1950.

(20) Sigurdsson, B., J. Sigurjónsson, J. H. Sigurdsson, J. Thorkelsson, and K. R. Gudmundsson. A disease epidemic in Iceland simulating poliomyelitis. *Am J Hyg* 52:222-238, 1950.

(21) Anders, W. Epidemiologische Studien über die Poliomyelitis 1947-48 in Gross-Berlin. From: Die Poliomyelitis: bearbeitet nach den Erfahrungen bei den Berliner Epidemien 1947-49. *Aktuelle Fragen der inneren Medizin*, Berlin, W. De Gruyter and Co., 1949, pp. 12-40.

(22) Sabin, A. B. Paralytic consequences of poliomyelitis infection in different parts of the world and in different population groups. *Am J Pub Health* 41:1215-1230, 1951.

PREDICTION AND POSSIBLE PREVENTION OF CORONARY DISEASE[1]

Ancel Keys[2]

The problems of diagnosis and of management of coronary heart disease are so numerous and important that great efforts should be made toward their solution, but several limitations must be recognized. From all the available evidence there is no reason to hope that coronary heart disease can ever actually be cured in the sense that a cancer may be "cured" by surgical excision, or even that tuberculosis may be permanently arrested. Moreover, there is some reason to doubt whether, at present, early diagnosis of coronary heart disease will greatly change the eventual prognosis.

The basic lesion in almost all cases of coronary heart disease is the deposit of lipid materials in the walls of the coronary arteries. Once thoroughly established, these atherosclerotic deposits are nearly, or perhaps totally, irreversible. The real focus of attention for the control of coronary heart disease must be the problem of preventing these deposits from developing futher. An essential part of this problem is the question of predicting the threat of coronary disease, which is pretty much the same thing as recognizing the tendency of atherosclerosis to progress.

Not so long ago it was widely held that arteriosclerosis, and the particular variety called atherosclerosis, was an essential part of aging. The result was a defeatist attitude and a regrettable lack of research interest. Now, however, it is clear that age alone does not bring with it the cholesterol deposits in the arteries that currently constitute the basic cause of more deaths in the United States than any other disease category.

Atherosclerosis is a progressive development and it seems highly probable that the eventual appearance of clinical coronary disease usually represents the cumulative effect of a factor, or factors, operating over a period of years. Age, per se, is certainly not the cause, as is evident from the great variations between individuals of the same age in spite of a general *average* progression with age *(1, 2)*. Many factors are probably involved in the atherosclerotic development and in the clinical appearance of coronary heart disease, but there is no longer any doubt that one central item is the concentration, over time, of cholesterol and related lipids and lipoproteins in the blood serum *(3–7)*. No other etiological influence of comparable importance is as yet identified.

At this point, however, controversy begins about the particular substances in the blood that are most significant in this regard. Detailed arguments about the relative merits of different blood analyses for the recognition or prediction of coronary disease are not essential to the present discussion *(8–12)*. It is clear enough that total cholesterol, free cholesterol, phospholipids, beta lipoproteins, and the lipoproteins of various sizes and densities as they can be separated in the ultracentrifuge are all intimately interrelated and that none, by itself, affords a safe basis for prediction about the disease process in the individual. There is no doubt that of the several different analytical methods for recognizing these substances each may yield averages that differentiate, statistically, between *groups* of patients with clinical coronary disease and *groups* of clinically healthy persons who are otherwise comparable. From the evidence so far available, it is not possible to accept the claim of Gofman and his colleagues in California for the remarkable virtue of the ultracentrifuge in this regard. At this point a word of caution is appropriate to guard against the overinterpretation of any of these laboratory data for particular patients.

The argument for giving a prime place to the total blood serum cholesterol in any consideration of the public health aspects of these problems is simple. As a discriminator between coronary patients and their healthy counterparts,

Source: *American Journal of Public Health* 43:1399–1407, 1953.

[1] Address presented at the Annual Health Conference of New York at Lake Placid, N.Y., June 3, 1953.

[2] Director, Laboratory of Physiological Hygiene, and Professor, School of Public Health, University of Minnesota, Minneapolis, Minn.

the total cholesterol measurement seems to have much the same value as some other measurements (e.g., lipoprotein fractionation, ultracentrifugation); it is not claimed to be appreciably better. It has, however, a considerable practical advantage because the relatively simple cholesterol method is far more suitable for large-scale application and there is much more knowledge about it. Moreover, it should not be forgotten that cholesterol itself is the main intruder in the actual lesions of the coronary arteries. This cholesterol comes from the blood.

As will be seen, the cholesterol level in the blood (and the level of the related lipoproteins) can be influenced by the diet, both in man and in some animal species. However, the situation has been greatly confused by too much reliance on experiments with animal species differing from man in cholesterol metabolism. Adding equal amounts of cholesterol itself to the diet produces widely different results in the several species studied so far, the rabbit and the chicken being at one extreme, while man, the dog, and probably the monkey are at another and opposite extreme *(12)*. Atherosclerosis may be readily produced in the rabbit and in the chicken by feeding a diet containing large amounts of added cholesterol *(13)*. There is no doubt that the resulting arterial deposits of cholesterol are directly related to the concentration of cholesterol in the blood which rises to great heights in these species, while feeding cholesterol to man, or to the monkey, has very little effect on the blood even when enormous doses of cholesterol are given *(12–15)*.

The cholesterol-fortified diet commonly used to produce hypercholesterolemia and subsequent atherosclerosis in the rabbit contains 1–5 percent of added cholesterol. A 2 percent cholesterol diet for the rabbit, which is most commonly used, corresponds to about 15 gm. of cholesterol in a 3000-calorie diet for a man. Such an amount of cholesterol is fantastically far above anything that occurs in any natural human diet, the upper limit of the latter being of the order of 1 gm in 3000 calories. Even when concentrating on foods of naturally very high cholesterol content, it is difficult to devise a regular diet to provide, experimentally, as much as 2 gm of cholesterol in the daily diet *(16–18)*.

That dietary cholesterol is not important for man would be predicted from the fact that the biliary output of cholesterol from the human liver is from 10 to 20 times as much as the daily amount of cholesterol in any diet of natural foods. Repeated careful dietary surveys on large numbers of persons in whom blood cholesterol was measured consistently fail to disclose a relationship between the cholesterol in the diet and in the serum *(19–21)*. Infants and children, as well as adults, show this lack of dependence of serum content upon the exogenous supply of cholesterol *(22)*, but this does not mean that the diet is unimportant in regard to the blood cholesterol. Controlled experiments on men clearly show that serum cholesterol changes in direct relation to a change in the total amount of fat in the diet *(7, 23–25)*. Both animal and vegetable fats show this effect and the addition or removal of cholesterol in the diet does not change the result. The blood cholesterol may fall, however, if the diet is almost exclusively pure fat and is free of carbohydrate *(26)*; this highly artificial experiment would seem to have no relevance to natural situations.

Now this being the case in controlled experiments limited to a few months' duration, it is important to discover what may be the situation where there are lifelong differences in the amount of fat in the diet. Moreover, the controlled experiments so far have been limited to individuals who have previously always subsisted on a relatively high-fat diet.

The fact of the matter is that practically all Americans in modern times eat a relatively high-fat diet. Forty years ago the fat calories averaged slightly over 30 percent of the total and at present, on the average, fats provide over 40 percent of the total calories in the foods sold at the retail level in the United States *(27, 28)*.

No other country appears to match this level of fat consumption, the next highest values, with fats providing from 38 to 39 percent of the calories, being in Australia, New Zealand, and Canada. From 30 to 35 percent of the total calories come from fats in the United Kingdom, the Netherlands, and the Scandinavian countries. Far lower fat consumption is characteristic of Italy, Portugal, and Spain where, on the average, the total fats cover only some 19–23 percent of the total calories. Even lower values are found in parts of Latin America, while the smallest percentage of fat calories in the total, 10 percent or less, is found in Asia and Africa.

Before examining blood cholesterol data obtained in other countries, it is essential to consider the situation in the United States. Normative data for the urban "white collar" class have been provided by several thousand clinically healthy men in Minnesota (29), and the findings are in good agreement with other smaller series studied elsewhere in American cities (8, 30–32). The main features of these data are a marked curvilinear age trend and a considerable variation between individuals at any given age. The mean value for men aged 20 is about 180 mg of total cholesterol per 100 ml of serum and this tends to rise more or less linearly with age until around 50 years, the means from 50 to 60 years of age are about 260 mg; in very old persons low values predominate. This age trend in serum cholesterol is very similar to the findings on the incidence of marked atherosclerosis at autopsy (1, 33).

These characteristics of clinically healthy men in American cities are to be compared with recent findings in Italy, England, and Spain (12, 33–35). The first of these comparative studies was begun in Naples in 1952, where the general average of the diets, both of the whole population and of the particular men studied, was about 20 percent of calories from all fats.

The serum cholesterol values showed that the Minnesota and Neapolitan trends are not significantly different in youth but around age 30 they begin to diverge. In the fifties the Minnesota men average 40–50 mg. percent higher than the Neapolitans. In this respect, the Italian men are not aging like the Americans who have been studied. It might be asked whether this difference is related to relative obesity in the two countries. Actual measurements, however, showed that our Italian subjects were just about as fat as our Minnesotans as gauged both by relative body weights and by measurements of the thickness of subcutaneous fat.

The finding has extraordinarily interesting connotations and it is important to check it with other populations. Opportunity to do this was found in Spain. Our main series of Madrid subjects, in 105 poor families, was found to be characterized by subsistence on a diet low in both fats and total calories. These men were, on the average, much thinner than either the Minnesotans or the Italians, but in serum cholesterol they closely resembled the latter. Again, when comparison was made with the United States, the correspondence in youth and the divergence after age 30 was striking. In the fifties these Madrid men averaged over 50 mg. lower than the Minnesotans.

In Spain the great majority of the population is poor and subsists on a low-fat, low-calorie diet. The small wealthy and professional class, racially identical, lives on a diet at least as luxurious, and as high in fats and in calories, as in the United States. Study of a sample of clinically healthy men of this class in Madrid showed them to be very similar to the Minnesota men in regard both to body fatness and to serum cholesterol concentration. There was, then, a striking difference between the poor and the relatively rich Spaniards, as indicated in Tables 1 and 2.

Table 1. Mean serum total cholesterol concentration, in mg per 100 ml, in clinically healthy men in Naples, London, and two classes of Spaniards. All values here pertain to the nonbasal state and therefore are not precisely comparable to the basal norms for Minnesota.

Age	Naples	London	Spaniards Poor	Rich
20	135	187	181	202
30	216	205	215	217
40	231	248	223	243
50	229	255	210	264

Finally, it was possible to study a sample of clinically healthy men in the London area of England. These men were found to be, on the average, considerably thinner than the Minnesotans, the Neapolitans, or the rich Spaniards. Their diets, studied individually in a careful survey, averaged 35 percent of all calories in the form of fats—that is to say much more like the diets of the Minnesotans and rich Spaniards than the diets of the Neapolitans or poor Spaniards. The mean serum cholesterol values for these Englishmen are given in Table 1. The relative trends from age 30, given in Table 2,

Table 2. Mean serum total cholesterol concentrations at ages 30–55 in the several populations of clinically healthy men, expressed for each population as a percentage of the mean value at age 30.

Age	Minnesota	Naples	London	Madrid Poor	Rich
30	100	100	100	100	100
40	112	107	121	103	112
50	127	106	124	98	122
55	131	109	127	100	127

most precisely indicate the differences in the populations. Clearly, the whole series of data suggests that the serum cholesterol concentration and its age trend is primarily related to the fat content of the diet but not in the body fatness. So far, then, the picture is that the serum cholesterol is more or less independent of the diet in youth but that progressively after about 30 years of age the serum level is directly related to the total fats in the diet. The effect of obesity itself is apparently not so important, although in each population we found a small correlation between obesity and serum cholesterol. The next question is whether all this is related to the incidence and mortality from coronary and related heart disease.

For Spain we can only say that coronary heart disease is strikingly uncommon in the general population as surveyed in the hospitals and public clinics. There were, however, many cases among the wealthy patients of our friends, the fashionable practitioners. Unfortunately, Spanish vital statistics are either practically nonexistent or are relatively unreliable, so that it is impossible to cite valid figures for mortality specific for age and sex. For some other countries, however, comparable statistics are available, both for death rates and for national diets, and these prove to be extremely interesting.

Table 3 summarizes the death rates of men aged 40–44 and 50–54 ascribed to all circulatory diseases and to what may be termed "degenerative heart disease," predominately coronary heart disease, as computed from official statistics for 1948–1949 in several countries. Taken at face value, there is indicated a tremendous range from the figures for white men in the United States to Japanese men. For the age

range 50 through 54 years, these data indicate that the death rate from coronary heart disease and allied myocardial disorder in the United States is more than four times that of Italian men and over 10 times that of Japanese men of the same age.

Broadly speaking, death rates ascribed to specific causes are not very reliable under the best of circumstances. Certainly it would be difficult to insist that the values in Table 3 for "degenerative heart disease" in the different countries are strictly comparable nor would it be reasonable to suggest that the values listed for all circulatory diseases are actually precise. Yet we are not dealing here with the minutiae of differential diagnosis of relatively rare diseases. Can it be suggested seriously that in Canada a third of the deaths from circulatory disease are missed? Or, conversely, that in the United States many thousands of death certificates for relatively young men are each year falsely or erroneously labeled with one or another variety of circulatory disorder when the proper label should have been pneumonia or tuberculosis or some other cause in a completely unrelated category? It should be observed that in 1949 over one-third of all deaths of white men from 40 through 44 years of age were ascribed to circulatory diseases. To bring the rate down to the Italian or Japanese level would require either the assumption that the great majority of circulatory disease deaths reported in the United States actually were due to other causes or that in Italy and Japan only one-fourth to one-tenth of the true circulatory disease deaths were recognized as such.

It is useful to shift the focus to the total death rate from all causes, retaining, of course, the

Table 3. Deaths of men in 1948–1949, rates per 1000 of given age, ascribed to all circulatory diseases (International Category VII) and to degenerative heart diseases (myocardial diseases and coronary heart disease, Categories 93 and 94 in the International List of 1938).

Category	All circulatory diseases		Degenerative heart	
	40–44	50–54	40–44	50–54
U. S. Whites	1.66	5.65	1.19	4.44
Canada	1.10	4.03	0.89	3.43
" , % U. S.	66%	71%	75%	77%
England and Wales	0.70	2.73	0.27	2.04
" " " , % U.S.	42%	48%	22%	46%
Italy	0.63	1.86	0.25	1.02
" , % U. S.	38%	33%	21%	23%
Japan	0.55	1.25	0.14	0.37
" , % U. S.	33%	22%	12%	8%

essential specification of age and sex. Table 4 assembles such information for 17 countries for the period 1947–1949, expressed as percentages of the corresponding death rates in the United States in 1949. For the countries listed, these rates for deaths from all causes are, presumably, not subject to large errors.

The outstanding feature of Table 4 is that it shows the mortality from all causes to be surprisingly high in the United States, in comparison with other countries, for adults in this range of from 40 to 65 years of age. The relative inferiority of "health," as indicated by the death rate of the American male is particularly marked. Only Japan and Portugal have poorer records, and in these countries the high incidence of infective and parasitic diseases explains the high total mortality. The explanation of the high mortality among adult American males is, of course, ready at hand—excessive mortality from heart disease.

The improvement of vital statistics recording, and the accuracy of the death certificates on which they are based, has now reached the point in many countries where detailed analysis is rewarding. Such work is in progress in the Laboratory of Physiological Hygiene and the results are of much interest. For example, we find that when we compare the data for men of equal ages in the United States and in Italy we find

substantially the same values in the two countries for the ages 40–60 for all neoplasms, for cirrhosis of the liver, for nephritis and nephrosis, and for intracranial lesions of vascular origin. Among major causes of death, in fact, only the death rates ascribed to heart disease are grossly dissimilar. Why? Further analysis of the death rates from all circulatory disorders shows that when the degenerative group of coronary disease, angina pectoris, and myocardial disease are excluded, the death rates from the total of all *other* circulatory diseases are much alike in the two countries. Why? From every viewpoint the analysis brings us back to the conclusion that there is a major difference between these countries for the incidence and mortality of coronary heart disease. This problem is greatest among American men and tends to become progressively less as we pass to countries where fats contribute less and less to the total diet. As far as data have been made available, the blood cholesterol picture in the clinically healthy members of the populations are entirely in keeping with the dietary and the mortality data.

It should be recognized that, in addition to the character of the diet, another factor may possibly be involved. Differences in habitual physical activity cannot be ruled out of the picture since, in general, the population groups on

Table 4. Death rates, from all causes, in 17 countries with a total population of about 310 millions; all values are for the period 1947–1949 and are expressed as percentages of the corresponding rates in the United States in 1949.

Age	40–44		50–54		60–64	
Sex	M	F	M	F	M	F
Australia	75	91	87	96	94	94
Belgium	96	89	91	96	97	101
Canada	78	91	76	92	84	96
Denmark	59	83	63	88	70	100
England and Wales	68	78	76	83	93	88
France	96	100	91	91	93	91
Ireland	80	78	57	86	69	88
Italy	91	100	77	88	75	97
Japan	156	216	111	153	113	207
Netherlands	52	69	56	76	63	89
New Zealand	55	72	66	81	85	88
Norway	64	78	53	65	54	68
Portugal	139	125	99	96	99	103
Scotland	93	97	93	100	97	107
South Africa	93	108	102	115	94	104
Sweden	61	86	63	85	68	92
Switzerland	78	97	78	97	88	108
Mean	84.3	97.5	78.8	93.4	84.5	101.1

the lower fat diets are also characterized by a higher level of physical activity. Special studies on this point are already in progress.

Let us now return to the diet. There are enough good reasons to suspect that our present high-fat diet in the United States is scarcely favorable to the health of adult men, even though it is premature to blame it as the whole cause of our excessive mortality from heart disease. The changes in mortality in countries forced to alter their diets during the late World War cannot be ignored. These changes conform to the concept that the proportion of fat in the diet is closely related to the development of arteriosclerotic heart disease *(36–38)*. Changes in diabetes mortality among patients over 45 years of age, notoriously related to atherosclerosis, were equally marked during the war and the parallel with the dietary change is equally striking *(39, 40)*.

From the start of acceptable systematic records of the U.S. Department of Agriculture in 1909, the proportion of fats in the national food supply has steadily risen from roughly 30 percent of total calories to over 40 percent in 1950–1952. The same data indicate that the protein contribution to the total calories has remained substantially constant at around 12 percent, or a trifle less. Because of the uncertainties in regard to kitchen and plate waste, the actual intake of the several major nutrients cannot be specified with great precision; but there is no doubt that the per capita consumption of total fats in the United States is higher than anywhere else and it has been, and still is, steadily rising. In view of the facts and concepts expressed above, this constitutes a real problem for the public health.

Among other immediate questions that arise is that of the several sources of the fats in the present national dietary. In the classification of the U.S. Department of Agriculture, by far the largest proportion of the total fats, from 45 to 50 percent in recent years, is "fats and oils as such, excluding butter." This means cooking and salad fats and oils—lard, corn oil, cottonseed oil, hydrogenated vegetable oil shortening, margarine, mayonnaise, etc. Butter contributes only 5 percent of the total fat calories. It is evident that a large reduction in our present high-fat consumption could be achieved without affecting the fats associated with the more nutritionally valuable foodstuffs. In other words, it should not be difficult to reduce the total fat intake and still have a diet excellent in all other respects.

In this discussion I have attempted to present some salient features of a large and complex problem. The evidence is drawn from many fields but the whole provides, I believe, a consistent and important basis for futher studies and perhaps major public health attention. The focus is on men from age 30 to age 70. About women we know much less, but the coronary heart disease problem is apparently less important for them until later in life. Women, too, are eventually less than immortal, and their death rate from degenerative heart disease is high in the United States, the chief peculiarity being a later age of onset than that for men. From a study of vital statistics it appears that women are less prone to suffer from angina pectoris and sudden fatal coronary occlusion, a less spectacular, chronic development, leading to a diagnosis of chronic myocarditis or myocardial degeneration, being the rule. Finally, the effect of habitual differences in the level of physical activity has scarcely received any research attention. These and many other questions can and should be clarified by extensive and critical epidemiological studies.

References

(1) White, N. K., J. E. Edwards, and T. J. Dry. The relationship of the degree of coronary atherosclerosis with age, in men. *Circulation* 1:645, 1950.

(2) Ackerman, R. F., T. J. Dry, and J. E. Edwards. Relationship of various factors to the degree of coronary atherosclerosis in women. *Ibid.* 1:1345, 1950.

(3) Morrison, L. M., L. Hall, and A. L. Chaney. Cholesterol metabolism: Blood serum cholesterol and ester levels in 200 cases of acute coronary thrombosis. *Am J Med Sci* 216:32, 1948.

(4) Dock, W. Causes of Arteriosclerosis. *Bull NY Acad Med* 26:182, 1950.

(5) Gubner, R. and H. E. Ungerleider. Arteriosclerosis: A statement of the problem. *Am J Med* 6:60, 1949.

(6) Duff, G. L. and G. C. McMillan. Pathology of atherosclerosis. *Ibid.* 11:92, 1951.

(7) Allen, E. V., A. Keys, and J. W. Gofman. Atherosclerosis. A symposium. *Circulation* 5:98, 1952.

(8) Gertler, M. M., S. M. Garn, and H. B. Sprague. Cholesterol, cholesterol esters and phospholipids in health and in coronary artery disease. II. Morphology and serum lipids in man. *Ibid.* 2:380, 1950.

(9) Gofman, J. W., H. B. Jones, F. T. Lindgren, T. P. Lyon, H. A. Elliott, and B. Strisower. Blood lipids and human atherosclerosis, *Ibid.* 2:161, 1950.

(10) Keys, A. Cholesterol, "giant molecules," and atherosclerosis. *JAMA* 147:1514, 1951.

(11) Barr, D. P., E. M. Russ, and H. A. Eder. Pro-

tein-lipid relationships in human plasma. II. In Atherosclerosis and related conditions. *Am J Med* 11:480, 1951.

(12) Keys, A. Atherosclerosis: A problem in newer public health. *J Mt Sinai Hosp* 20:118, 1953.

(13) Katz, L. N. and J. Stamler. *Experimental Atherosclerosis.* Springfield, Ill., Thomas, 1953.

(14) Messinger, W. J., Y. Porosowska, and J. M. Steele. Effect of feeding egg yolk and cholesterol on serum cholesterol levels. *Arch Int Med* 86:189, 1950.

(15) Moses, C. Dietary cholesterol and atherosclerosis. *Am J Med Sci* 224:212, 1952.

(16) Okey, R. Cholesterol content of foods. *J Am Dietet Assoc* 21:341, 1945.

(17) Lange, W. Cholesterol, phytosterol, and tocopherol content of food products and animal tissues. *J Am Oil Chem Soc* 27:414, 1950.

(18) Pihl, A. Cholesterol studies. I. The cholesterol content of foods. *Scand J Clin Lab Investigation* 4:115, 1952.

(19) Keys, A. The physiology of the individual as an approach to a more quantitative biology of man. *Fed Proc* 8:523, 1949.

(20) Gertler, M. M., S. M. Garn, and P. D. White. Diet, serum cholesterol and coronary artery disease. *Circulation* 2:696, 1950.

(21) Wilkinson, C. F., Jr., E. Blecha, and A. Reimer. Is there a relation between diet and blood cholesterol? *Arch Int Med* 85:389, 1950.

(22) Heyman, W. and F. Rack. Independence of serum cholesterol from exogenous cholesterol in infants and in children. *Am J Dis Child* 65:235, 1943.

(23) Keys, A., O. Mickelsen, E. v.O. Miller, and C. B. Chapman. The relation in man between cholesterol levels in the diet and in the blood. *Science* 112:79, 1950.

(24) Hildreth, E. A., S. M. Mellinkoff, G. W. Blair, and D. M. Hildreth. The effect of vegetable fat ingestion on human serum cholesterol concentration. *Circulation* 3:641, 1951.

(25) Anderson, J. T. and A. Keys. Dietary fat and serum cholesterol. *Fed Proc* 12:169, 1953.

(26) Kinsell, L. W., G. Michaels, L. De Wind, J. Partridge, and L. Boling. Serum lipids in normal and abnormal subjects; observations on controlled experiments. *California Med* 78:5, 1953.

(27) *Consumption of Food in the United States 1909–1948* Misc. Publ. 691. Washington, D.C., U.S. Dept. of Agriculture, 1949.

(28) *Consumption of Food in the United States,* Misc. Publ. 691, Supp. for 1949. *Ibid.* Also data for subsequent years on file in the Bureau of Agricultural Economics, 1950.

(29) Keys, A., O. Mickelsen, E. v.O. Miller, E. R. Hayes, and R. I. Todd. The concentration of cholesterol in the blood serum of normal man and its relation to age. *J Clin Invest* 29:1347, 1950.

(30) Collen, M. F. Blood cholesterol studies in coronary artery disease. *Permanente M Found Bull* 7:55, 1949.

(31) McMahon, A., H. N. Allen, C. J. Weber, and W. C. Missey, Jr. Hypercholesterolemia. *Southern M J* 44:993, 1951.

(32) Schaefer, L. E., S. R. Drachman, A. G. Steinberg, and D. Adlersberg. Genetic studies on hypercholesteremia: Frequency in a hospital population and in families of hypercholesteremic index patients. *Am Heart J* 46:99, 1953.

(33) Keys, A. The cholesterol problem. *Voeding* 13:539, 1952.

(34) Keys, A., F. Fidanza, V. Scardi, and G. Bergami. The trend of serum-cholestrol levels with age. *Lancet* 263:209, 1952.

(35) Keys, A. Diet and the incidence of heart disease. *Bull Univ Minnesota Hosp, Minnesota M Found* 24:376, 1953.

(36) Malmros, H. The relation of nutrition to health. A statistical study of the effect of the war-time on arteriosclerosis, cardiosclerosis, tuberculosis and diabetes. *Acta med Scand* Supp. 245:137, 1950.

(37) Strøm, A. and A. R. Jensen. Mortality from circulatory diseases in Norway 1940–1945. *Lancet* 260:126, 1951.

(38) Pihl, A. Cholesterol studies. II. Dietary cholesterol and atherosclerosis. *Scand J Clin Lab Investigation* 4:122, 1952.

(39) Himsworth, H. P. Diet in the aetiology of human diabetes. *Proc Roy Soc Med* 42:323, 1949

(40) Keys, A., J. Brozek, A. Henschel, O. Mickelsen, and H. L. Taylor. *The Biology of Human Starvation* (Vol. II). Minneapolis, Minn., University of Minnesota Press, 1950. pp. 1040–1050.

A STUDY OF ENVIRONMENTAL FACTORS IN CARCINOMA OF THE CERVIX[1]

Ernest L. Wynder,[2] Jerome Cornfield,[3] P.D. Schroff,[4] and K.R. Doraiswami[5]

The present communication represents a study of the possible role of environmental factors in the production of cervical cancer. It is based upon a clinical-statistical study carried out jointly in the United States and in India.

The incidence of cervical cancer and the various suggested factors believed to have influenced these rates have served as a primary stimulus for the present investigation. We shall, therefore, briefly review the incidence of cervical cancer as encountered in various population groups and outline the factors suspected to have influenced this incidence pattern.

INCIDENCE

General. The uterine cervix is the second most frequent site of cancer in American women, accounting for approximately 10 percent of all newly diagnosed cases and for about the same percentage of total cancer deaths. In different American cities its annual incidence varies from 30 to 60 per 100 000 females (*1*). The incidence rates are about the same in Western Europe (*2*). Scattered reports from Asia suggest that in these countries the uterine cervix is the most important site and may account for 40 or more percent of all newly diagnosed cases of cancer (*3–6*).

Jews. The incidence of cervical cancer is far from uniform in different population groups. As early as 1906, Vineberg (*7*) was impressed with its infrequency among Jewish women. Since that time similar reports have emanated from Germany, Austria, England, Hungary, Holland, and various American centers (*8–17*). Some American data have been summarized in Table 1 (*18, 19*). This relatively low frequency of cancer of the cervix in Jewish women, which appears uniform, has been well summarized by Sorsby (*20*), Wolff (*21*), Davidsohn (*22*), Sugar and Levy (*23*), and more recently by Kennaway (*24*).

Fijis. Handley (*25*) calls attention to the relatively low frequency of cervical cancer among Fijis. A review of hospital records from the Fiji Islands, where 70 000 Indians and 90 000 Fijis live, shows 26 carcinomas of the cervix among the Indians and only 3 among the Fijis.

Moslems. Moslem women have a low frequency of cervical cancer as compared to other religious groups in their community. A report from the Institute of Pathology in Indonesia covering the period 1939 to 1949 shows 1.6 percent of Indonesian female patients and 4.9 percent of the Chinese female patients to have cancer of the cervix. In Indonesia, 90 percent of the Indonesians, but none of the Chinese, are Moslems (*26*). We show in Table 2 the frequency of cervical cancer in two hospital populations in India among different religious groups. In both hospitals cervical cancer is much less frequent among Moslem than among Hindu women.

Negroes. Recent incidence studies by the U.S. National Cancer Institute show a uniformly higher incidence of cervical cancer among Negroes than among whites (*1*) (Table 3), a finding supported by several hospital studies (*27–29*).

Low-Income Groups. Carcinoma of the cervix occurs more commonly in the lower income groups. The Registrar General of Great Britain (*30*) shows that the lower the social class, the higher the mortality of cervical cancer. Similarly, Clemmesen (*31*) shows that in Copenhagen carcinoma of the cervix occurs more commonly in the low-priced housing districts.

Source: *American Journal of Obstetrics and Gynecology* 68(4): 1016–1052, 1954.

[1] Presented at a meeting of the New York Obstetrical Society, Nov. 10, 1953.
[2] From the Division of Preventive Medicine of the Sloan Kettering Institute, Memorial Center, New York, New York.
[3] Office of Biometry of the National Institutes of Health, Public Health Service, Department of Health, Education and Welfare, Bethesda, Maryland.
[4] Department of Surgery of the Tata Memorial Hospital in Bombay, India.
[5] Department of Radiology of the Premier Radiological and Cancer Institute, Madras, India.

Table 1. Relative incidence of carcinoma of the cervix in Jews and non-Jews at three American hospitals.

Hospital	Years	Total cases of cervix cancer	Incidence of cancer of the cervix in non-Jews relative to that in Jews
Mt. Sinai, New York	1893-1906	18	17.0:1
	1909-1918	85	12.5:1
	1928-1948	323	5.3:1
Bellevue, New York	1925-1945	1317	5.9:1
Memorial Center, New York	1916-1937	3106	8.5:1

Table 2. Cervical cancer as a percentage of total female cancer admissions at the Tata Memorial Hospital, Bombay, 1941-1950, and the Premier Radiological Institute and Cancer Hospital, Madras, 1950-1952.

	Tata Memorial		Premier Radiological Institute	
	Total female cancer admissions	Percent cervix cancer	Total female cancer admissions	Percent cervix cancer
Hindus	3828	45	280	53
Christians	575	29	60	29
Moslems	818	16	67	18
Parsis	396	13	—	—

Table 3. Number of newly diagnosed cases of cervical cancer per 100 000 females, whites and nonwhites.[a]

City	White	Nonwhite
New Orleans	59	72
Chicago	28	65
Dallas	44	65
Birmingham	52	73
Detroit	37	54
Philadelphia	33	65

[a] Source: Federal Security Agency, Public Health Service, Cancer Morbidity Series, Nos. 1-10, 1950-1952.

Marital Status. Numerous authors have found a lower incidence of cervical cancer among single women. Stocks (*32*) finds that "Liability to cancer of the cervix uteri is greater at every age amongst married and widowed women than amongst single women, and especially between the ages of forty-five and sixty-five, when it is about seven times as great." Maliphant (*33*) points out that, "A woman who has reached the age of thirty-five or more has twice the risk of contracting cancer of the cervix if she is married." Similar results are reported by Dorn (*34*), Lombard and Potter (*35*) and Gilliam (*36*). Gagnon (*37*) points to the apparently very low inci-

dence of cervical cancer among nuns. Among one group of nuns studied in Canada, Gagnon found 12 cancers of the body of the uterus, but none in the cervix. In another group of 130 neoplasms among nuns, there were again no carcinomas of the cervix.

Prostitutes. A recent Danish survey by Rojel (*38*) shows prostitutes are four times as numerous among women with cancer of the cervix as among other women of comparable socio-economic groups.

SUGGESTED ETIOLOGICAL FACTORS

There have been numerous attempts to explain these variations among the different population groups by implicating possible etiological factors which vary in intensity in the same fashion from group to group.

Circumcision. One of the earliest to suggest lack of circumcision as a possible etiological factor was Handley, who points out that of those groups which have a low frequency of cervical cancer (Jews, Fijis, Moslems), all practice circumcision of their male population. In 1936, he (*25*) wrote, "There is evidence that the existence of phimosis, or in its absence carelessness as to subpreputial hygiene and cleanliness, is a menace even more serious to the female sex than to the sex in which they originate." Khanolkar (*39*) also draws attention to the fact that the Moslems in India, who do circumcise their males between the ages of 6 and 12, have a relatively low frequency of cervical cancer.

The Ritual of Abstinence. Kennaway, in an admirable review of carcinoma of the uterus in which he particularly stresses the low incidence of cervical cancer in Jewish women, states that the data suggest one cause for this low incidence to be "a factor that is opposed by the Jewish practice of abstinence from sexual intercourse during most of the first half of the ovulatory cycle." Kennaway (*24*) points out that the Parsis, who have a relatively low frequency of cervical cancer, are also supposed to have a period of abstinence after menses. Vineberg (*40*), as well as Sorsby (*20*) and Smith (*14*), also attributes significance to this factor. Weiner (*18*) and his associates suggest that the apparent greater frequency of cervical carcinoma in Jewish women today, as compared to the beginning of this century, might possibly be explained by a greater laxity of Jewish women in following the law of abstinence.

Other Racial Factors. Several authors believe that the low incidence of cervical cancer in Jews is based upon a genetic immunity of Jewish women to cervical cancer, as stressed by Maliphant (*33*). Clemmesen (*41*) also recently suggests that the rare incidence of cervical cancer in Jewish women may be based upon "a special hormonal status in these women."

Hormones. Animal experimentation has shown that estrogen administration can increase the incidence of cervical cancer in susceptible mice (*42*). Hofbauer (*43*) feels that excessive ovarian stimulation in multiparous women might be of etiological significance. Ayre (*44*) believes estrogen to be a growth-stimulating factor to cervical cancer. He found that 90 percent of 50 patients with cervix cancer had evidence of excessive tissue estrogens on the basis of vaginal and cervical cornification. Khanolkar (*39*) theorizes that women in the lower income groups with resulting inadequacy of diets might develop liver dysfunction and subsequently might have a higher hormonal blood level because the damaged liver is unable to detoxify the estrogens. On the basis of associated endometrial hyperplasia, Bainborough (*45*) proposes that excessive estrogen stimulation is a factor in the production of cervical cancer, a conclusion denied by Bayly and Greene (*46*), who find no significant degree of endometrial hyperplasia among patients with cancer of the cervix. Nieburgs (*47*) advances the contrasting idea that low estrogen levels might be of etiological significance. Lombard and Potter (*35*) propose that hormonal factors may account for earlier marriage and high divorce rates among patients with cervical cancer.

Low Economic Status. Kennaway (*24*) emphasizes a factor as responsible for a high incidence of cervical cancer, "a factor that is intensified in those married and single women by descent in economic scale." Lombard and Potter (*35*) suggest that low economic status has possible etiological significance, stating, "Concomitant with low economic status are such factors as: poor obstetrical care, improper housing, and poor nutrition." Smith (*14*) believes that "poor obstetrical care and post partum care and neglect of symptoms of the lacerated and ulcerated cervix account for the greater frequency of cervical cancer among the poorer classes." Clemmesen (*41*) also observes a higher incidence with low economic status, but emphasizes that rural areas in Denmark have a relatively low incidence of cervical cancer compared to the low-income city areas. He believes that sexual activity may be the common denominator to account for this observed incidence difference. Vineberg's (*40*) opinion, stated in 1919, is recalled with interest. "When one stops to consider that the total number of Jewish women, 1995, had badly lacerated cervices . . . and that they were living in the worst possible hygienic surrounding, amidst the greatest squalor and privation, such as obtained in the lower East Side of the Metropolis, it is truly remarkable that so few cases of cancer of the cervix were detected amongst them."

Diet. Khanolkar feels that cancer of the cervix is most common in Hindu women who have a badly balanced and deficient diet, especially during the childbearing stage, and considers this to have a possible effect upon the liver. Horwitz (*15*) considers ritual dietary laws among orthodox Jewish women to be of possible etiological significance. Ayre (*44*) proposes that deficiencies of thiamine and riboflavin might lead to a greater susceptibility of cervical tissues to cancer formation.

Chronic Cervicitis. Gagnon (37) places strong emphasis on chronic cervicitis as an etiological factor in cervical cancer. He states that in over 3000 cases of chronic cervicitis, systematically treated, no cervical carcinoma was seen, and that the rarity of chronic cervicitis in virgins accounts for the low incidence of cervical cancer among them. He states, "The eradication of cervicitis equals the suppression of cancer of the cervix." McKelvey (48) states that the factor of cervicitis could not account for the low incidence of epidermoid carcinoma of the cervix among Jewish women, who not uncommonly have chronic cervicitis.

Unrepaired Lacerations. Ewing (49) suggests unrepaired lacerations of the cervix to be of etiological significance in cervical cancer. Lombard and Potter (35) find 26 percent of their patients with cancer of the cervix and 13.2 percent of their matched controls to admit to cervical lacerations. They state that the "relationship between cancer of the cervix and unrepaired lacerations remained significant when partial correlations were computed."

Coal-Tar Douching. Lombard and Potter (35) find suggestive, though not conclusive, evidence that coal-tar derivatives are of etiological significance in cervical cancer. Smith (14) notes no significant difference in the type of douches used by Italians and Jews in his study.

Syphilis. Several authors have reported a positive association between syphilis and cervical cancer, a subject well summarized by Levin and his associates (50–52). Wallingford (53) suggests that the greater frequency of coitus suspected among women with syphilis may account for their greater chance of developing cervical cancer.

Pregnancy. A positive association between the number of pregnancies and cervical cancer has been reported by some and denied by others (33, 35, 36). Clemmesen (54) finds that the difference in the Danish incidence data from town and country cannot be explained by a simple direct relationship between birth rate and cervical cancer. Denoix (55) arrives at a similar conclusion on the basis of French data.

Vaginal Discharge. Hausdorff (56) suggests vaginal discharge as a causative factor in the production of cervical cancer.

THE PRESENT STUDY

In this investigation we have attempted to appraise those of the suggested factors that can be evaluated by an interview study. Some of these, such as circumcision, are well suited for study by means of an interview with a group of cervical cancer patients and suitable controls. Thus, if the difference in the incidence of cervical cancer between Jewish and non-Jewish women is in fact attributable solely to lack of circumcision in the latter group, the non-Jewish women with circumcised husbands should have as low an incidence as do Jewish women. Conversely, if early marriage is indeed an important etiological factor, then groups with a high incidence, such as Negroes, should have a high degree of early marriage. The present study was thus conceived as an attempt to determine by personal interview: (a) whether factors that could explain variations in the incidence of cervical cancer among the different population groups could also explain variations within each group, and (b) whether factors that explained variations within different population groups could also explain variations between them. Consequently, parallel studies among non-Jewish white women and Negro women were undertaken to determine whether the frequency of such factors as circumcision and early onset of first coitus varied between the cervix cancer and control groups separately for each population. In addition, studies of Jewish and Indian women were undertaken to see if the characteristics that occurred with greater frequency among the Indian women occurred with less frequency among Jewish women.

Other suspected etiological factors, such as genetic constitution and cervical lacerations, are not well suited to study by interview, and we were not able to explore them.

In view of the importance of economic level, which is, of course, an index to etiological factors rather than an etiological factor in itself, it seemed essential to draw controls from the same economic level as the cervical cancer cases. For this reason, we confined ourselves almost entirely to clinic populations, in which at least a rough equality in economic and social status may be assumed.

Hospitals. This study was a cooperative investigation, involving interviews at 12 different hospitals in the United States. The distribution of the cases interviewed by hospital and age is shown in Table 4.

Case Material. The control group was interviewed on gynecologic services. A breakdown of the various gynecologic conditions found among the controls is shown in Table 5. It will be noted that chronic cervicitis and polyps of the cervix were seen as frequently in the Jewish patients as in the white non-Jewish or the Negro patients.

In addition to the control and cervix cases shown in Tables 4 and 5, the following additional patients with cervical cancer were interviewed, but are not included in any of the analyses which follow:

	White		Negro
	Non-Jewish	Jewish	
Adenocarcinoma	14	4	15
Carcinoma in situ	18	3	13

The Interview. Regeena Goodwyn and Florence Moreno interviewed all patients at the Memorial Clinic and Memorial Wards,[6] and in Jersey City and Philadelphia. Dr. Charles Miller interviewed all the St. Louis patients. The pa-

---

[6] Some of the Jewish patients with cervical cancer seen on the Memorial Wards were interviewed by Miss E. Schwab and by E. L. Wynder.

Table 4. Number of patients with cancer of the cervix and controls by age and hospital of interview, White non-Jewish, Jewish, and Negro.

	White				Negro	
	Non-Jewish		Jewish			
Hospital	Cervix	Control	Cervix	Control	Cervix	Control
New York						
Memorial Gyn. Clinic	129	302	7	264	56	95
Memorial Hospital Wards	12	4	8	7	3	2
James Ewing	16	45	1	32	8	14
Bellevue Radiologic Clinic	26	41	1	13	13	12
Harlem Hospital	1	0	0	0	20	52
Jersey City						
Margaret Hague Med. Center	28	86	1	1	9	42
Philadelphia						
Univ. of Pennsylvania Hospital	33	31	1	6	45	66
Washington						
Georgetown	11	13	0	3	6	32
Walter Reed	28	9	0	0	3	2
Gallinger	3	1	0	0	16	39
Warwick Clinic of George						
Washington Hospital	15	2	0	0	19	11
St. Louis						
Barnes	24	28	1	0	9	15
Barnard	28	32	0	0	8	9
Total	354	594	20	326	215	391
Age at interview						
Less than 30 years	14	54	0	13	10	59
30-39	60	107	7	52	58	137
40-49	110	184	4	131	68	117
50-59	110	154	6	101	51	51
60 and over	60	95	3	29	28	27
Total	354	594	20	326	215	391

Table 5. Number of control patients by diagnosis: White non-Jewish, Jewish, and Negro, Memorial Clinic and all hospitals combined.

Condition	Memorial Clinic			All hospitals		
	White			White		
	Non-Jewish	Jewish	Negro	Non-Jewish	Jewish	Negro
Uterus, malignant	31	12	8	71	21	37
Uterus, benign	44	49	21	87	60	152
Cervicitis, chronic	71	60	26	111	63	43
Polyp of cervix	20	26	5	31	28	16
Carcinoma of ovary	13	2	4	26	4	17
Carcinoma of vulva	9	7	1	13	9	3
Malignant, misc.	7	14	5	25	17	15
Benign, misc.	69	59	17	120	64	73
No positive gyn. lesions	38	35	8	110	60	35
Total	302	264	95	594	326	391

tients seen in Washington, D.C., were interviewed by Drs. F. Ablondi, Tom Higgins, Mary Kiernan, James Leonard, Marion MacLean, and Ernest Wynder.

The interview approach was the same for all patients, since all had gynecologic complaints. The patient was told that this interview was necessary to complete her history and would assist in evaluating her particular problem. It was stressed that all of the questions had to be answered correctly, although some might seem personal, because they might be related to the development of her disease. The patient was assured that her replies would be kept absolutely confidential.

Special care was taken to assure accuracy in the question regarding circumcision. It was recognized that some women regard a loose and short foreskin as circumcision. The interviewers were therefore instructed not to accept a simple "yes" or "no" answer, but to probe for evidence of definite information. When such information was absent, the woman was asked to question her husband and then to give us her reply. If this was not possible, or the information was still inconclusive, the answer was left as "Don't Know." Identical procedures were followed for cervix and control cases.

After the interview was completed, the charts were reviewed for definitive diagnosis. In many of the cases the diagnosis was not available at that particular time and had to be added later. In all cases of cervical cancer, biopsy report was available.

Blind Interviewing. At the Memorial Gynecological Clinic the patients to be interviewed were selected on each clinic day from the clinic list of those present. The list gave no clue as to the patient's condition. The interviewing at the Memorial Clinic was thus completely blind. At other hospitals, however, it was not always possible to assure such automatic control on the objectivity of the interviewer. For this reason, the data obtained at the Memorial Clinic have been analyzed separately.

Age-Hospital Standardization. The distributions of cervical cancer and control patients by age at interview are not the same. Thus, only 2 out of 129 white non-Jewish cervix patients at Memorial Clinic were less than 30 years of age, while a considerably larger proportion of the controls—22 out of 302—were this young. Similarly, the distributions by hospital of interview were not the same. For example, one-third of the non-Jewish cervix cases studied were seen at the Memorial Clinic and one-half of the controls. To eliminate the effects of these differences in age and hospital distribution on the comparisons between cervix and control patients, we have uniformly adjusted the results for the control patients to the age-hospital distribution of the cervix cases.

The procedure used was designed to give each age-hospital group in the controls the same relative weight that it had in the cervix group. Thus if proportion w_i of all cervix cases fell in the ith age-hospital group and if proportion p_i of the control cases in this age-hospital group have some characteristic, i.e., being married, the age-hospital standardized estimate of the proportion married is $\Sigma w_i p_i$, the summation extending over all age-hospital groups. Routinely this adjustment was performed by assigning a multiplier to each age-hospital group in the controls and entering this multiplier on the punch card for each individual in that group. If w_i denotes the number of cases among the controls in the ith age-hospital group, the multiplier for this group was w_i/n_i. The age-hospital standardized estimate of the proportion of the controls having a certain characteristic, i.e., being married, is then obtained by (a) sorting out the cards for all control patients who were married, (b) obtaining on a tabulator the sum of the multipliers for all married controls. The 594 controls, age-hospital adjusted on this basis, give results of less precision, however, than would have been obtained with 594 controls matched on an age-hospital basis to the cervix patients. The 594 adjusted controls gave results of equivalent precision to what would have been obtained with 330 matched controls. For this reason, we have taken the control total as 330 and have referred to the number of cases resulting from this procedure in the various tables as the equivalent number of cases after age-hospital standardization.

The Negro controls were adjusted to the age-hospital distribution of the Negro cervix cancer cases. The 391 controls interviewed and adjusted were equivalent in precision to 287 matched and unadjusted controls. The white Jewish control cases were not adjusted to the white Jewish cervix group, which is too small to justify statistical analysis, but rather to the white non-Jewish cervix group. For the Indian data, the results were age-adjusted in the same fashion.

At some points in the following analysis we found it necessary to standardize out other factors, such as age at first marriage. The procedure employed in these cases is identical with that used for the age-hospital standardization.

RESULTS (AMERICAN)

In the following group of tables we compare the percentage distribution of patients with cancer of the cervix and controls separately for the white non-Jewish and Negro groups.

Results are shown separately for Memorial Clinic and for all hospitals combined for the one-way classifications. Memorial accounts for roughly one-third of all cases in all hospitals combined in both cervical cancer and control groups, both for the white non-Jewish and Negro groups after age-hospital standardization. For cross-classifications we show results only for all hospitals combined. All results are presented on an age-hospital standardized basis.

Comparable data are also shown for Jewish controls at Memorial Clinic, but discussion of these results is reserved for page 335. It would be misleading to present percentage distributions for the 20 Jewish cervical cancer cases. These cases are presented in Table 20.

Marital Status. There is a consistently smaller proportion of single women in the cervical cancer group as compared with the control group, both for whites and Negroes, in Memorial and all hospitals (Table 6). There is also a consistently higher proportion of divorced and separated women in the cervical cancer group. There is a higher proportion of widows in the cervical cancer group among the whites, but not among the Negroes.

Number of Marriages. There is a consistently larger proportion of women who have been married two or more times in the cervical cancer group (Table 7). In the white non-Jewish Memorial group, 29 percent of those with cancer of the cervix who had ever been married had been married twice or more. Among the controls the comparable figure is 12 percent, or less than half. For all hospitals combined the results are almost identical. In the Negro group in Memorial Clinic, multiple marriages had occurred among 35 percent of the ever-married cervix group, but among only 22 percent of the controls who had ever been married.

To what extent is this difference in the frequency of multiple marriages a consequence of the difference in marital status shown in Table 6? In Table 8 we show the frequency of multiple marriages separately for women who were married, divorced, or separated, or widowed at the time of interview. The differences persist for all three groups. There is a suggestion in the data that there is less difference in the frequency of multiple marriages between widowed cervical cancer patients and controls than for the other two groups. This difference is not statistically significant, however. We conclude that the difference in the frequency of multiple marriages between cervical cancer and control groups does not arise because of differences in marital status.

Table 6. Percent distribution of cervical cancer and control patients by marital status, White non-Jewish, Jewish, and Negro

Marital status at time of interview	White		Jewish	Negro	
	Non-Jewish				
	Cervix	Control	Control	Cervix	Control
Memorial Clinic					
Married	59	67	71	31	36
Never married	2	9	4	2	9
Divorced and separated	12	8	8	38	28
Widowed	27	16	17	29	27
Total	100	100	100	100	100
All Hospitals Combined					
Married	62	65		40	43
Never married	2	9		4	10
Divorced	14	11		33	27
Widowed	22	15		23	20
Total	100	100		100	100

Table 7. Percent distribution of cervical cancer and control patients who had ever been married, by number of marriages, White non-Jewish, Jewish, and Negro.

Number of marriages	White		Jewish	Negro	
	Non-Jewish				
	Cervix	Control	Control	Cervix	Control
Memorial Clinic					
1	71	88	89	65	78
2	28	11	11	31	18
3 or more	1	1	0	4	4
Total	100	100	100	100	100
All Hospitals Combined					
1	70	86		65	78
2	28	12		30	20
3 or more	2	2		5	2
Total	100	100		100	100

Table 8. Percent of cervical cancer and control patients who had ever been married, married two or more times, by marital status, White, non-Jewish, and Negro, all hospitals combined.

Marital status at time of interview	White, non-Jewish				Negro			
	Number of cases		Percent married two or more times		Number of cases		Percent married two or more times	
	Cervix	Control[a]	Cervix	Control	Cervix	Control[a]	Cervix	Control
Married	220	219	33	14	86	125	47	26
Divorced or separated	49	34	37	11	71	75	21	16
Widowed	76	49	19	16	49	59	35	19
Total	345	302	30	14	206	259	35	22

[a] Equivalent number of cases after age-hospital standardization.

Age at First Marriage and First Coitus. The cervix patients, both white and Negro, at Memorial Clinic and all hospitals, show a markedly earlier age of marriage than do the control patients (Table 9). Thus, 13 percent of the Memorial white non-Jewish cervical cancer group were married by age 16, as compared with 5 percent of the comparable controls. For Memorial Negroes, 32 percent of the cervical cancer group was married by age 16, and 13 percent of the controls. The differences for all hospitals combined are slightly smaller, but still pronounced.

No matter what the etiological significance of this difference, it is clear that age at first coitus may be a more crucial variable than age of first marriage, albeit one which may not be reported so accurately. It will be seen (Table 10) that the differences between cervical cancer and control groups in age at first coitus are somewhat larger than in age at first marriage. For Memorial white non-Jewish, the comparative percentages

Table 9. Percent distribution of cervical cancer and control patients who had ever been married by age at first marriage, White non-Jewish, Jewish, and Negro.

	White			Negro	
	Non-Jewish		Jewish		
Age at first marriage	Cervix	Control	Control	Cervix	Control
Memorial Clinic					
16 or less	13	5	4	32	13
17-19	38	26	15	39	38
20-24	31	38	46	19	25
25 or more	18	31	35	10	24
Total	100	100	100	100	100
All Hospitals Combined					
16 or less	14	8		32	19
17-19	40	25		36	34
20-24	29	39		21	29
25 or more	17	28		11	18
Total	100	100		100	100

Table 10. Percent distribution of cervical cancer and control patients by age at first coitus, White non-Jewish, Jewish, and Negro.

	White			Negro	
	Non-Jewish		Jewish		
Age at first coitus	Cervix	Control	Control	Cervix	Control
Memorial Clinic					
16 or less	17	6	4	45	28
17-19	38	27	15	41	44
20-24	32	34	43	13	16
25 or more	12	26	34	2	11
Never	1	7	4	0	1
Total	100	100	100	100	100
All Hospitals Combined					
16 or less	19	10		55	36
17-19	41	25		30	39
20-24	26	36		12	16
25 or more	12	22		2	7
Never	1	7		1	2
Total	100	100		100	100

for first coitus by age 16, are 17 for cervical cancer and 6 for control, as compared with 13 and 5 for first marriage by this age. Similarly, for age 25, the comparative percentages for first coitus by this age are 12 for cervical cancer and 26 for controls, as compared with 18 and 31 for first marriages by this age. It is also of interest to note that for both whites and Negroes 1 percent of all cervical cancer patients reported never having had coitus. Seven percent of the white controls and 2 percent of the Negro controls reported no such relations.

To what extent is this difference in age at first coitus simply a consequence of differences in the number of marriages shown in Table 7? In Table 11 we have classified cervical cancer and control patients both by age at first coitus and by number of marriages. It is clear from the table that these characteristics are correlated, in the sense that women with early coitus tend to marry more than once. From our present point of view, however, it is more important to note that differences between cervical cancer and control patients, in age at first coitus, persist even when the effect of number of marriages is eliminated. Thus, for the white non-Jewish group who had been married once, a considerably smaller proportion of the cervical cancer group than of the control group had their first

coitus after age 25, 14 percent for the former and 25 percent for the latter. Similarly, the differences between the cervix cancer group and control group in number of marriages persists even after the effect of age at first coitus is eliminated. For the white non-Jewish group which had their first sexual intercourse at age 20 to 24, a considerably larger proportion of the cervix than of the control group had been married two or more times, 20 percent for the former and 8 percent for the latter.

We show in Table 12 the percentage distribution by age at diagnosis of the white and Negro cervical cancer groups. It will be noted that for each group the patients with early coitus have cancer diagnosed at an earlier age. The median age of onset for white cervical cancer patients whose first sex relationship occurred before age 16 is 44; for those whose first coitus did not occur until after age 25, it is 54. For the Negro cervix patients much the same trend is evident, although the concentration of cases with early coitus makes the trend somewhat erratic and more doubtful. A roughly similar trend, however, is also found for the controls.

Number of Pregnancies. There is a small but consistent difference between the ever-married cervical cancer patients and control patients in

Table 11. Number of cervical cancer and control patients by age at first coitus and number of marriages, White non-Jewish, and Negro, all hospitals combined.

Age at first coitus	Cervix Number of marriages				Control[a] Number of marriages			
	Total	0	1	2+	Total	0	1	2+
White non-Jewish								
16 or less	66	1	35	30	34	1	25	8
17-19	143	1	93	49	83	1	60	22
20-24	98	1	77	20	117	1	107	9
25 or more	40	2	32	6	72	4	65	3
Never	3	3	0	0	22	22	0	0
No report	4	0	4	0	2	0	2	0
Total	354	8	241	105	330	29	259	42
Negro								
16 or less	119	4	70	45	103	5	71	27
17-19	64	3	42	19	112	9	82	21
20-24	25	1	17	7	48	5	35	8
25 or more	5	0	5	0	20	5	15	0
Never	0	0	0	0	5	5	0	0
No report	2	0	1	1	2	0	2	0
Total	215	8	135	72	290	29	205	56

[a] Equivalent number of cases after age-hospital standardization.

Table 12. Percent distribution of cervical cancer and control patients by age at diagnosis, age at first coitus, White non-Jewish, and Negro at all hospitals combined.

Age at diagnosis	Cervix Age at first coitus					Control Age at first coitus				
	16 or less	17-19	20-24	25 +	Never[a]	16 or less	17-19	20-24	25 +	Never[a]
White, non-Jewish										
30 or less	7	3	2	3	(0)	2	2	6	3	(6)
31-40	30	15	14	12	(0)	34	21	19	6	(11)
41-50	30	35	29	21	(67)	18	34	37	30	(23)
51-60	19	28	40	38	(0)	38	24	26	41	(20)
61 +	13	18	15	26	(33)	8	19	12	20	(41)
Total	100	100	100	100	100	100	100	100	100	100
Median age	44	49	51	54	(47)	48	48	47	54	(56)
Negro										
30 or less	6	5	(0)	(0)	—	5	5	4	(0)	(3)
31-40	31	18	(27)	(20)	—	34	22	28	(16)	(10)
41-50	28	37	(42)	(20)	—	29	40	24	(26)	(26)
51-60	25	25	(19)	(20)	—	24	22	27	(39)	(0)
61 +	10	15	(12)	(40)	—	8	11	17	(19)	(61)
Total	100	100	100	100	—	100	100	100	100	100
Median age	45	47	(45)	(55)		45	47	48	(53)	(51)

[a] Percent distributions based on fewer than 30 cases are shown in parentheses.

the proportion who have never been pregnant. In the white group, both at Memorial and in all hospitals, 9 percent of the cervical cancer group had never been pregnant, as compared with 12 percent in the control group (Table 13). Among the Negroes studied the difference is larger—11 percent in the cervical cancer group and 17 percent in the controls at Memorial and 11 and 18 percent in all hospitals. When the effect of number of pregnancies among those women who have ever been pregnant is considered, an additional difference appears between the two groups for the whites but not for the Negroes. Seventeen percent of the patients who had ever been pregnant in the white cervical cancer group at Memorial reported seven or more pregnancies, as compared with 11 percent in the controls. For all hospitals combined, the proportion with seven or more pregnancies is 20 in the cervix group and 11 in the controls. One would, of course, suspect some relation between age at first marriage and number of pregnancies, and it is of some importance to know the extent to which each of these characteristics is independently associated with the development of cervical cancer. In Table 14 we have classified cervical cancer and control pa-

tients simultaneously by number of pregnancies and age at first marriage. It is clear from this tabulation that these two factors are closely associated. Of the 49 white cervical cancer patients who had been married by age 16, only one had never been pregnant. Of the 58 who were not married until after age 25, 13 had never been pregnant. This association holds for both cervical cancer and control patients, white and Negro.

Do both factors exert independent effects, despite this association, as in the cases of age at first sexual intercourse and number of marriages (Table 11), or is only one of the factors truly independent? It is clear from inspection that even when the effect of number of pregnancies is held constant, cervix and control groups still differ in age at first marriage. Somewhat more than 10 percent of all white cervical patients who had been pregnant only once or twice were married by age 16, as compared with less than 3 percent among the controls. It is far from clear, however, when age at first marriage is held constant, that any difference remains in the frequency of pregnancies in the two groups. Thus, of the white cervical cancer patients who were married at age 17 to 19, 7 out of 138 had

Table 13. Percent distribution of cervical cancer and control patients who have ever been married by numbers of pregnancies, White non-Jewish, Jewish, and Negro.

Number of pregnancies	White			Negro	
	Non-Jewish		Jewish		
	Cervix	Control	Control	Cervix	Control
Memorial Clinic					
0	9	12	11	11	17
1 or more	91	88	89	89	83
Total	100	100	100	100	100
Pregnant					
1-2 times	35	41	42	50	38
3-4	32	29	38	18	28
5-6	16	19	13	14	19
7-8	10	7	4	14	6
9 or more	7	4	3	4	9
Total	100	100	100	100	100
All Hospitals Combined					
0	9	12		11	18
1 or more	91	88		89	82
Total	100	100		100	100
Pregnant					
1-2 times	37	44		46	46
3-4	27	29		25	25
5-6	16	16		14	16
7-8	10	6		8	5
9 or more	10	5		7	8
Total	100	100		100	100

Table 14. Number of cervical cancer control patients who had ever been married by number of pregnancies and age at first marriage, White non-Jewish, and Negro, all hospitals combined.

Number of pregnancies	Cervix Age at first marriage					Control[a] Age at first marriage				
	Total	16 or less	17-19	20-24	25 or more	Total	16 or less	17-19	20-24	25 or more
White, Non-Jewish										
0	30	1	7	9	13	37	1	3	8	25
1-2	116	13	37	38	28	114	3	22	50	39
3-4	87	12	39	27	9	78	6	23	35	14
5-6	53	10	28	10	5	41	5	14	17	5
7-8	30	7	8	13	2	17	4	8	4	1
9 or more	30	6	19	4	1	14	4	6	3	1
Total	346	49	138	101	58	301	23	76	117	85
Negro										
0	23	2	5	7	9	46	4	9	14	19
1-2	84	24	27	22	11	97	16	30	32	19
3-4	45	18	21	4	2	53	13	22	11	7
5-6	25	11	8	6	0	34	7	11	14	2
7-8	14	7	6	1	0	12	5	5	2	0
9 or more	14	4	7	3	0	17	5	10	2	0
Total	205	66	74	43	22	259	50	87	75	47

[a] Equivalent number of cases after age-hospital standardization.

never been pregnant. Three out of 76—or 4 percent—of the white control patients who were married at this age had never been pregnant. There appears to be no difference in pregnancy history when the comparison is confined to women who were married at the same age. To make certain that the impressions suggested by inspection are not misleading, we have in Table 15 standardized out the effect of age of marriage in the same way that the effects of age and hospital (page 324) were eliminated. The distributions of cervix and control groups by number of pregnancies shown in this table are essentially the same.

We conclude that these data provide no evidence of an association between the fact of pregnancy or of number of pregnancies and the development of cervical cancer. One will, of course, see fewer women who have never been pregnant in a cervical cancer group, but this occurs apparently because one will see fewer single women in such a group. Also, one will see somewhat more women with many pregnancies in a cervical cancer group, but only because this group contains more women who married early.

Age at First and Last Pregnancy. When cervix and control patients are compared with respect to age at first pregnancy and age at last pregnancy, marked differences appear, both in the

Table 15. Percent distribution of cervix and age at first marriage standardized[a] control patients by number of pregnancies, White non-Jewish and Negro, all hospitals combined.

Number of pregnancies	White non-Jewish		Negro	
	Cervix	Control	Cervix	Control
0	9	9	11	15
1-2	33	33	41	36
3-4	25	28	22	22
5-6	15	16	12	13
7-8	9	8	7	6
9 or more	9	6	7	8
Total	100	100	100	100

[a] Obtained from Table 14 by weighting the percent distribution by number of pregnancies for each age-at-first-marriage class in the control group by the number of cases in that class in the group with cancer of the cervix.

white non-Jewish, and in the Negro groups. Only 18 percent of the white non-Jewish cervix patients, but 34 percent of the controls had their first pregnancy at or after age 25 (Table 16). Similarly, 32 percent of the white non-Jewish cervix patients, but only 25 percent of the controls, had their last pregnancy at or before age 25.

One would, of course, expect age at both first and last pregnancies to depend on age at mar-

Table 16. Percent distribution of cervix and control patients who had ever been pregnant by age at first pregnancy and age at last pregnancy, White non-Jewish, and Negro, all hospitals combined.

Age at pregnancy	White non-Jewish control			Negro control		
	Cervix	Crude[a]	Standard-ized[b]	Cervix	Crude[a]	Standard-ized[b]
First						
16 or less	9	3	6	31	18	26
17-19	36	23	36	34	32	33
20-24	37	40	36	24	31	25
25 or more	18	34	22	11	19	16
Total	100	100	100	100	100	100
Last						
20 or less	12	7	10	30	20	23
21-25	20	18	18	27	24	24
26-30	26	25	25	17	24	21
31-35	25	24	24	14	15	15
36 or more	17	26	23	12	17	17
Total	100	100	100	100	100	100

[a] Standardized for age and hospital of interview, but not age at first marriage.
[b] Standardized for age at first marriage in addition.

riage. When the control groups are made comparable to the cervix patients in this respect, by standardizing with respect to age at first marriage, it will be noted that the differences are essentially eliminated. Therefore, the differences in age at first and last pregnancies do not appear to be independent variables, but merely reflect previous differences in age at marriage.

Miscarriages and Abortions. We have also investigated the distributions of the populations studied by number of miscarriages and abortions. No marked or consistent differences are apparent. This body of data has thus yielded no evidence that there are any differences between cervical cancer and control populations, in any characteristics associated with pregnancy, whether it be the number of such pregnancies, the age at which they occurred, or associated phenomena, such as abortions and miscarriages.

Syphilis. Previous studies have reported twice as many syphilitic patients among women with cervical cancer as in the general population (50-52). We found a similar difference between our cervical cancer non-Jewish white patients and the controls. Essentially no difference was found, however, between the Negro cervical

cancer and control patients. (Forty-one out of 215 of the former and 46 out of 290 of the latter reported a past history of syphilis.)

In view of the general unreliability of syphilis information obtained solely from personal interview, no great weight can be attached to our results. Of interest, however, is the fact that those reporting a past history of syphilis also reported, as one might expect, earlier age at first coitus. In fact, the relation between age at first coitus and prevalence of syphilis as reported is such as to lead one to expect a twofold difference between cervix and control patients solely because of their difference in age at first coitus. This result, although fragmentary, is consistent with Levin's (50) and Wallingford's (53) observation that the statistical association between syphilis and cervical cancer could arise from the greater frequency of coitus in the former group.

Circumcision Status of Partners. We present in Table 17 the distribution of cervix and control patients by circumcision status of partner. It will be noted that women with circumcised husbands and no other partners are found less frequently in the cervix than the control groups. Thus, in the white non-Jewish groups

Table 17. Percent distribution of cervix and control patients with sexual experience by circumcision status of partners, White non-Jewish, and Negro.

Circumcision status of partners	White		Jewish Controls	Negro	
	Non-Jewish				
	Cervix	Controls		Cervix	Controls
Memorial Clinic					
Circumcised husbands only:					
No other partners	3	9	93	0	8
Pre-, extra-, or postmarital partners	3	3	2	8	5
Circumcised and uncircumcised husbands	4	3	1	2	5
Uncircumcised husbands only	80	75	1	65	47
Circumcision status unknown	10	10	3	25	35
Total	100	100	100	100	100
All Hospitals Combined					
Circumcised husbands only:					
No other partners	5	14		< 1[a]	9
Pre-, extra-, or postmarital partners	3	4		7	9
Circumcised and uncircumcised husbands	6	3		5	4
Uncircumcised husbands only	75	69		66	49
Circumcision status unknown	11	10		22	29
Total	100	100		100	100

[a] Less than 0.5 percent (1 case out of 215).

at Memorial, 3 percent of the cervix patients, but 9 percent of the controls had relations with circumcised husbands only. At all other hospitals combined the comparable figures are 5 percent for the cervix groups and 14 for the controls. For the Negro patients the differences are even larger—0 percent and 9 percent at all hospitals.

There is an additional group of women with circumcised husbands who have had relations with other partners. In most cases the circumcision status of the additional male partner is unknown to the patient, although in view of the relatively low frequency of circumcision in the groups studied, it must be presumed that the bulk of these contacts involved at least one uncircumcised partner, particularly when there was more than one extramarital partner. Of the women with circumcised husbands, a considerably larger proportion in the cervix than in the control group reported additional exposures. The extent of this additional exposure is unknown to us. If it were infrequent, then presumably this group must also be treated as effectively exposed only to circumcised males. If it were extensive and involved many partners, it would be unrealistic to treat them in this way. In the absence of such knowledge, we can only say that between 5 and 8 percent of the white non-Jewish cervical cancer group were effectively exposed only to circumcised males, while the comparable figures for controls were between 14 and 18 percent. For Negro women the comparable figures are 0 to 7 percent for the cervical cancer group and 9 to 18 percent for the controls. The indeterminateness introduced by this group is not a doubt as to whether circumcision makes a difference, but how big the difference is.[7]

A considerable number of patients could not tell us the circumcision status of their partners. In many cases we were able to obtain this information from the partner himself, but even this was ineffective when the patient was widowed, divorced, or remarried. In consequence, 10 percent of the white non-Jewish patients and 20 to 30 percent of the Negro patients were

unable to report on circumcision status of partners. For patients who had been married only once, the proportion unknown was smaller, but still far from trivial—8 percent for the white and 20 percent for the Negroes. By making sufficiently unfavorable assumptions about the circumcision status of the unknowns, one could wipe out the difference in circumcision status between cervical cancer and control groups.

We have attempted to check on the circumcision results shown in Table 17 by using a different method of collecting the information—direct interviews with males in the wards of some of the hospitals where females were studied. Out of 489 white males, 80, or 16 percent, were circumcised; 37 out of 208, or 18 percent, of the Negro males were circumcised. These percentages agree with those reported by females. They also confirm the fact that in the ward and clinic population circumcision is equally common among whites and Negroes. This result is explained at least in part by the following facts: (1) at least twice as many native-born white males are circumcised as foreign-born males; Negro males are predominantly native-born, and (2) many Negroes are circumcised in their teens.

We show in Table 18 the simultaneous distribution of cervical cancer and control cases by circumcision status of partner and number of times married. For those married once, 10 percent of the cervix groups and approximately 20 percent of the controls reported a circumcised husband. This was true for both the white non-Jewish and Negro groups. For those married twice, the proportion with both husbands circumcised is, of course, smaller, but the difference between cervix and control groups is in the same direction and of approximately the same magnitude for both white non-Jewish and Negro groups, although only for the former groups is the difference statistically significant.

In Table 19 we show the simultaneous distribution of cervix and control cases by circumcision status of partner and age at first coitus for those married only once. This table shows that differences in frequency of circumcision between cervical cancer and control groups persist for both white non-Jewish and Negro groups, even after the effect of age at first sexual intercourse is held constant. There is also a suggestion that circumcised husbands are reported more frequently by those reporting late first coitus, although the effect is not large and can-

---

[7] This indeterminateness could have been avoided by obtaining information on pre-, extra-, or postmarital partners for women with uncircumcised husbands. At the time the survey was being planned, we were unwilling to ask such questions of more than the circumcised groups, for whom it was obviously necessary. We did not, of course, foresee the present difficulty.

not in any event account for the differences in circumcision status.

Menses. Age of onset of menses was the same in both cervix and control groups, both for whites and Negroes at Memorial and at all hospitals combined. In all cases the median age was 13 to 14. Comparison of length of flow showed also no essential differences between the two groups.

Table 18. Number of cervical cancer and control patients with sexual experience by circumcision status of partners and number of marriages, White non-Jewish, and Negro, all hospitals combined.

Circumcision status of partners	Cervix No. of marriages			Controls[a] No. of marriages		
	0	1	2+	0	1	2+
White non-Jewish						
Circumcised husbands only:						
No other partners	0	15	1	0	42	2
Pre-, extra-, or postmarital partners	0	9	2	0	10	4
Circumcised and uncircumcised husbands	0	0	21	0	0	8
Uncircumcised husbands only	0	197	67	0	188	26
Circumcision status unknown	5	20	14	6	21	2
Total	5	241	105	6	261	42
Negro						
Circumcised husbands only:						
No other partners	0	1	0	0	23	3
Pre-, extra-, or postmarital partners	0	12	3	0	22	4
Circumcised and uncircumcised husbands	0	0	10	0	0	10
Uncircumcised husbands only	0	96	45	1	113	25
Circumcision status unknown	8	26	14	23	46	13
Total	8	135	72	24	204	55

[a] Equivalent number of cases after age-hospital standardization.

Table 19. Number of cervical cancer and control patients who married once by circumcision status of partners and age at first coitus, White non-Jewish, and Negro, for all hospitals combined.

Circumcision status of partners	Cervix age at first coitus				Controls[a] age at first coitus			
	16 or less	17-19	20-24	25+	16 or less	17-19	20-24	25+
White non-Jewish								
Circumcised husbands only:								
No other partners	0	6	6	3	2	6	17	16
Pre-, extra-, or postmarital partners	2	4	1	2	2	1	2	5
Uncircumcised husbands only	30	76	64	24	20	48	80	39
Circumcision status unknown	3	7	6	3	2	4	10	6
Total	35	93	77	32	26	59	109	66
Negro								
Circumcised husbands only:								
No other partners	1	0	0	0	4	9	6	4
Pre-, extra-, or postmarital partners	5	6	1	0	12	6	3	1
Uncircumcised husbands only	48	31	12	4	42	44	20	5
Circumcision status unknown	16	5	4	1	14	22	4	5
Total	70	42	17	5	72	81	33	15

[a] Equivalent number of cases after age-hospital standardization.

Abstinence After Menses. About half the white non-Jewish and Negro patients reported some abstention after menses, both in the cervix and control groups. Of those who said they abstained, about 40 percent reported one or two days as the usual period of abstinence, but again this percentage was the same in cervix and control groups for both white non-Jewish and Negro patients. Of those abstaining in the white non-Jewish group, 16 percent of the controls and 11 percent of the cervix group reported abstention for seven or more days. Among the Negroes the comparable figures were 5 and 6 percent. Thus, there seems to be no difference in the practice of abstinence between cervix and control groups.

Only 30 percent of the Jewish controls reported no abstention, while of those abstaining, 40 percent reported abstinence for seven full days. There was a considerable difference by age groups. Eighty-three percent of those over 50 reported some abstention, but 62 percent of those under 50 abstained. Of those over 50 who abstained, 50 percent reported abstention for seven full days. For those under 50, the comparable figure was 28 percent. There is a considerable difference, therefore, in the practice of abstention between the Jewish and non-Jewish population, and an additional difference between younger and older Jewish women. The Jewish women presumably had the Talmudic proscription in mind while answering this question, whereas the non-Jewish women did not. Consequently, the answers may not have the same meanings for both groups. In particular, the Jewish women answering "yes" may have had a more habitual practice in mind than the non-Jewish women. In view of the lack of any reported difference between cervical cancer and control groups, however, it is difficult to draw any firm conclusion with respect to the significance of abstention in the etiology of cervical cancer.

Douching. No difference was found between cervix and control groups with respect to type or frequency of douching. One-fifth of the white non-Jewish patients in both cervical cancer and control groups reported never douching. Forty percent of both groups reported frequent douching. Practices among the Jewish controls were essentially the same. Negro patients, both cervical cancer and controls, reported somewhat more frequent douching than

the whites. Specifically, 52 percent of the controls reported frequent douching, while only 6 percent said they never douched. In the cervical cancer groups the comparable figures were 50 and 13. Of those that did douche, no differences were apparent between cervix and control groups, either in the frequency of douching, or in the types of douches used. In particular, the use and frequency of use of a brand-name coal-tar derivative was reported with equal frequency by both groups.

Contraception. No important differences were found between cervical cancer and control groups in contraceptive practice. One-third of the white non-Jewish patients reported no use of contraception, in both cervical cancer and control groups. About 40 percent of the Negro patients, both cervical cancer and control, reported no use of contraception. A slightly smaller proportion of white non-Jewish cervical cancer patients than of controls reported the use of condoms, both in Memorial and in all hospitals; but no such difference was found among Negro patients. It is to be noted that among those patients who used contraceptives no reliable data were obtained as to the relative frequency with which such contraceptives were used.

Other Factors. No significant differences were found between cervical cancer and control patients in comparing the history of irritative vaginal discharge, gonorrhea, hormone therapy, method of delivery, or abstinence after parturition.

Jewish Women. We list in Table 20 some of the characteristics of the 20 Jewish women with cervical cancer who were seen during the course of this study. Seventeen were seen at Memorial Hospital; 3 elsewhere. Of the 17 seen at Memorial, 7 cases were found during the course of blind interviewing at the Gynecological Clinic. During the same period, 264 Jewish controls were interviewed. At this clinic 431 white non-Jewish women were interviewed; 129 of these had cancer of the cervix. These results re-emphasize the relative infrequency of carcinoma of the cervix among the Jewish population. Ten additional Jewish patients with carcinoma of the cervix were interviewed after the bulk of the interviewing had stopped, in the hope of ob-

Table 20. Twenty cases of epidermoid carcinoma of the cervix among Jewish women, selected characteristics.

Age at diagnosis	Number of mar-riages	Age at first marriage	Age at first sexual inter-course	Age at first pregnancy	Number of preg-nancies	Absti-nence after menses, days	Circum-cision code[a]
53	1	22	22	23	3	0	1
61	1	19	19	20	3	0	1
67	1	20	20	21	7	7	1
59	1	24	24	26	2	4	1
54	1	24	24	—	0	3	1
43	1	21	21	21	1	5	1
52	1	19	19	19	2	0	1
46	1	24	24	25	4	7	1
50	1	27	27	—	—	7	1
46	1	24	24	25	3	7	1
58	1	25	25	26	3	7	1
39	2	25	15	33	1	0	2
32	1	23	18	24	1	0	2
39	1	23	18	24	2	0	2
36	1	18	16	18	3	0	2
45	1	18	18	19	3	0	2
32	1	25	25	25	2	0	2
66	3	16	16	16	2	2	3
36	1	27	19	20	5	3	4
34	2	22	22	24	2	0	4

[a] Circumcision code: 1. Circumcised husband and no other partners; 2. Circumcised husband but other partners; 3. Mixed circumcision in husbands; 4. Uncircumcised husbands.

taining further data on the characteristics of Jewish women with cervical cancer.

Firm conclusions can scarcely be drawn from 20 cases. Nevertheless, it is of interest to note that of the 20 patients, 9 reported coitus with uncircumcised men, a significantly higher number than would be expected on the basis of the Jewish controls. Of those 9, 6 had circumcised husbands and reported other exposures. Three of the 20 had uncircumcised husbands, however, and this is also significantly above expectation on the basis of the Jewish controls (5 uncircumcised husbands out of 246 married Jewish controls).

It will be noted that the age of onset of cervical cancer of the 11 exposed to circumcised men only is distinctly and significantly higher than that of the 9 with other exposures, but this may simply be due to the earlier age at first coitus of the latter group. All 20 have a somewhat earlier age at first coitus than the comparable controls. No other differences are manifest.

Estimated Relative Risks. The previous results have considered the extent to which cervix and

control patients differ with respect to certain characteristics. It is useful to invert the discussion and to consider the extent to which persons with certain characteristics differ with respect to their incidence of cervical cancer. Rather than asking how much more early coitus occurs in the cervical cancer group, we now ask how much more cervical cancer occurs among those with early coitus.

The assumptions necessary and the methods by which one can invert have been discussed by several authors (Cornfield—51, Sadowsky and co-workers—58, and Doll and Hill—59). All that needs repetition here is that even when all necessary assumptions are satisfied, the sampling error of the estimates is large. They are useful in showing the orders of magnitude of differences, not their precise values. In Table 21 we show the relative risk, estimated from the data in Table 11, as a function of number of marriages and age of first coitus. We have taken as unity the risk of women married once, with first coitus at ages 20 to 24.

On this basis, women married once with coitus at or before 16 have twice the risk, both in the white and Negro populations; those with

Table 21. Relative risk of developing epidermoid cervical cancer by number of marriages and age at first coitus, White non-Jewish and Negro women.

Category	White non-Jewish	Negro
Virgins	0.2	0
Other single	1.0	0.7
Married Once		
Age at first coitus:		
16 or less	1.9	2.0
17-19	2.2	1.0
20-24	1.0	1.0
25 or more	0.7	0.7
Married Twice or More		
Age at first coitus:		
16 or less	5.3	3.4
17-24	3.1	1.8
25 or more	2.8	—

Risk for women married once, with first coitus at age 20 to 24 = 1.0.

first coitus after 25, about 30 percent less. For those who were married twice or more the risks are approximately doubled.

In Table 22 (upper half) we show estimated relative risks, with the risk for women exposed only to uncircumcised males taken as unity. For those married only once, women with circumcised husbands have only 40 percent the risk of developing cervical cancer of those with uncircumcised husbands, both in the whites and Negroes. For those married twice, this risk is smaller, but not significantly so.

Table 22. Relative risk of developing epidermoid cervical cancer by circumcision status of partner, White non-Jewish and Negro.

	White non-Jewish	Negro
Married Once		
Circumcised husband	0.4	0.4
No other partners	0.3	0.1
Other partners	0.9	0.8
Uncircumcised husband	1.0	1.0
Married Twice or More		
Circumcised husband	0.2	0.2
No other partners	0.2	0.0
Other partners	0.2	0.4
Mixed circumcision	1.0	0.6
Uncircumcised husband	1.0	1.0

Risk for women with uncircumcised husbands = 1.0 separately for those married once and twice or more.

There are too few cases of cervical cancer among Jewish women to permit a similar calculation, but the differences are qualitatively the same.

Racial Differences. We consider here the extent to which differences among white non-Jewish, Jewish, and Negro women in the incidence of cervical cancer can be explained by the factors uncovered in the previous discussion: age at first coitus, number of times married, and circumcision status of partner.

The higher rate among Negro women is qualitatively consistent with their earlier age at first coitus and high remarriage rate and the lower rate among Jewish women is qualitatively consistent with their lower exposure to uncircumcised males and later age at first coitus. Quantitative, as well as qualitative, consistency is desirable, however. The incidence of cervical cancer is approximately 50 percent higher among Negro than among white non-Jewish women. Can a difference of this magnitude be deduced from the relative risks shown in Table 21 and the difference among white non-Jewish and Negro controls in age at first coitus and remarriage rate shown in Table 11? The estimating procedure is shown in detail in Table 23. On the basis of these calculations one would expect the incidence of cervical cancer to be about 40 percent higher among Negro women than among white non-Jewish. This is of the same order of magnitude as the actual difference of 50 to 60 percent (Table 3). We conclude that the differences between white and Negro women in the incidence of cervical cancer are quantitatively and qualitatively consistent with their differences in age at first coitus and remarriage rate.

The differences between Jewish and non-Jewish women in the incidence of cervical cancer are not known with the same precision as those between Negro and white non-Jewish. The data from Bellevue, Mount Sinai, and Memorial (Table 1) suggest that it is one-fifth to one-tenth as high in Jewish women, but a population survey is required to yield a reliable estimate. Because of the basic indeterminateness noted in our circumcision results, we are unable to say whether they are consistent with a difference of this magnitude.

If the appropriate group to use in measuring the relative risk due to lack of circumcision is that with circumcised husbands and no other

Table 23. Estimated risk of developing epidermoid cervical cancer for Negro women relative to White non-Jewish women on the basis of differences in age at first coitus and number of marriages.

Category	Percent distribution of controls — White non-Jewish (1)	Percent distribution of controls — Negro (2)	Relative risk — White non-Jewish (3)	Relative risk — Negro (4)	Estimated risk using white relative risks — White (1)×(3)	Estimated risk using white relative risks — Negro (2)×(3)	Estimated risk using Negro relative risks — White (1)×(4)	Estimated risk using Negro relative risks — Negro (2)×(4)
Virgins	6.7	1.7	0.2	0	1.34	0.34	0	0
Other single	2.1	8.3	1.0	0.7	2.10	8.30	1.47	5.81
Married Once								
Age at first coitus:								
16 or less	7.6	24.6	1.9	2.0	14.44	46.74	15.20	49.20
17-19	18.3	28.5	2.2	1.0	40.26	60.50	18.30	28.50
20-24	32.7	12.1	1.0	1.0	32.70	12.10	32.70	12.10
25 or more	19.7	5.2	0.7	0.7	13.79	3.64	13.79	3.64
Married Twice or More								
Age at first coitus:								
16 or less	2.4	9.4	5.3	3.4	12.72	49.82	8.16	31.96
17-24	9.4	10.1	3.1	1.8	29.14	31.31	16.92	18.08
25 or more	0.9	0	2.8	—	2.52	0	(2.52)	0
Total	99.8	99.9			149.01	212.75	109.06	149.29
Relative risk					100	143	100	137

partners, the relative risks due to lack of circumcision are consistent with a fivefold difference between Jewish and non-Jewish women. If the appropriate group is the entire group with circumcised husbands, without regard to other partners, the relative risk due to lack of circumcision is not consistent with a fivefold difference between the Jewish and non-Jewish population. Although difference in age at first coitus between the Jewish and non-Jewish population could account for part of the unexplained difference, it could not account for all of it.

RESULTS (INDIAN)

Concurrently with the American data results were obtained at Tata Memorial Hospital in Bombay. All data were obtained by personal interview. Three hundred four cervix cancer cases are histologically proved cases of epidermoid carcinoma. In addition, seven patients with adenocarcinoma were interviewed (four Hindus, two Christians, and one Moslem). Not all the controls were completely interviewed, since some of these were questioned only in respect to age of first marriage, age of first pregnancy, and number of pregnancies (Table 14). In most instances the interviewer (P. S.

Table 24. Number of cervix and control cases by religious group at Tata Memorial.

Groups	Cervix patients	Controls Complete	Controls Total
Hindu	255	146	238
Moslem	26	44	135
Indian Christians	22	29	80
Parsis	—	22	72
Jews	1		

Schroff) knew the diagnosis prior to the interview.

The Hindus, Moslems, and Indian Christians come essentially from the same racial stock (*60*), whereas the Parsis are of Persian descent.

Age Distribution. The distribution of the patients studied by age at which they were seen is shown in Table 25. The cervical cancer patients have a distinctly earlier age of onset than those in the United States. This is scarcely surprising in view of the fact that the Indian population in general is younger than that in the United States, a fact which is reflected in the age distribution of the controls as well. There is a suggestion that the Moslems have an earlier age of onset of cervical cancer and the Christians a later age, but since this is true of the controls as

Table 25. Number of cervix and control patients by age at interview, by religious groups, and by hospital, Tata Memorial Hospital.

Age at interview	Hindu		Moslem		Christian		Parsi	
	Cervix	Control	Cervix	Control	Cervix	Control	Cervix	Control
30 or less	17	54	5	22	1	12	—	7
31-40	86	66	6	54	3	16	—	16
41-50	97	74	9	42	8	24	—	22
51-60	39	36	3	7	8	18	—	13
61 or more	16	8	3	10	2	10	—	4
Total	255	238	26	135	22	80	—	62

well, no interpretation can be safely drawn. To complete the record for the Parsis, for whom no cervical cancer cases were interviewed, we give the age distribution of 45 cases of cervical cancer in this group, taken from the admission records of the Tata Memorial Hospital (1941–1950), as follows:

30 or less	0
31–40	2
41–50	7
51–60	14
61 or more	22
Total	45

Age at First Marriage and at First Coitus. First marriage occurs at a much earlier age in India than in the United States. First coitus, which may occur many years after marriage, is also much earlier. Of interest in Table 26 are the observations that: (1) first coitus and first marriage take place earlier in the Hindu cervical cancer group than in the controls, (2) Hindu and Moslem controls show no important difference in the age at first coitus or age at first marriage, and (3) both Indian Christians and Parsis show a distinctly later age at first marriage and first coitus than the Hindu and Moslem groups.

Number of Pregnancies. It is noteworthy that the distribution of Hindu cervical cancer and control patients by number of pregnancies is essentially the same (Table 27). It is also of interest to observe that the two groups with later

Table 26. Percent distribution of cervical cancer and control patients by age at marriage and by age at first coitus by religious groups, Tata Memorial Hospital.

	Hindu		Moslem		Indian Christian		Parsis	
	Cervix	Control	Cervix	Control	Cervix	Control	Cervix	Control
Age at Marriage								
13 or less	67	52	(58)	18	(5)	4		2
14	11	13	(8)	17	(5)	1		2
15	12	12	(0)	22	(13)	5		5
16	3	9	(15)	13	(9)	14		11
17-19	4	9	(15)	20	(32)	37		32
20 plus	3	5	(4)	10	(36)	38		48
Total	100	100	100	100	100	100		100
Age at First Coitus								
13 or less	40	23	(39)	13	(5)	0		
14	17	26	(15)	25	(5)	0		
15	20	22	(4)	22	(14)	10		
16	11	12	(19)	14	(10)	5		
17-19	8	12	(15)	15	(33)	55		20
20 plus	4	5	(8)	11	(33)	30		80
Total	100	100	100	100	100	100		100

age at marriage and first coitus, the Parsis and the Indian Christians, have a smaller number of pregnancies (Table 27).

Circumcision. In India, both Moslems and Jews practice universal circumcision. None of the other groups systematically circumcise their males.

The usual age at circumcision among Moslem males is between 6 and 12. No essential differences in age at circumcision were found between husbands of patients with cancer of the cervix and those of controls. In 11 cases of cancer of the cervix the husbands were examined for completeness of circumcision and the sulcus was found to be free in all cases.

The Tata material contains one case of cancer of the cervix in an Indian Jewish woman whose husband was circumcised at birth. She married at 12 and gave no history of extramarital coitus.

Onset of Menses. Onset of menses shows no significant difference between cervical cancer and control groups.

Miscellaneous. Douching was only rarely and sporadically practiced among the women studied. No differences were noted among the cancer and control groups. For a similar reason, contraceptives can be eliminated, since only one woman questioned had used them.

The factor of abstinence during and after menses was also negative, in view of the fact that only an occasional woman did not abstain during menses and only a few abstained after the menstrual period. In this respect, it must be emphasized that, contrary to a previously expressed theory, no abstention was found after menses among 62 Parsi women questioned.

Nearly all women interviewed abstained from coitus from one month to one year after each delivery, a measure employed chiefly as a means of birth control. However, no significant differences were noted in this respect between the cervical cancer and control groups.

Penile Hygiene. In view of the fact that circumcision showed up as a positive variable in this study, we have done some investigation on the extent of penile hygiene among American and Indian males. If one wanted to study this factor as a direct influence on the development of cervical cancer, it would require a study of the sexual partners of women with cervical cancer. Because of the obvious difficulty of such a study, we have merely sampled the general hospital population, breaking it down into private, clinic, non-Jewish white, Negro, and Jewish patients. In the non-Jewish groups only uncircumcised individuals were considered. The Indian data were broken down into the various religious groups. The Tata material was, in addition, separated into Deccani, Gujarati, and other Hindus, because of the fact that the Deccanis are of lower economic standing than the other two Hindu groups.

Hospital data are to be considered with caution, since many male patients may take a special bath before coming for examination. In general, the American data show a higher percentage of "smegma" formation among the clinic than among private patients. Of some interest was the observation that a rare Jewish

Table 27. Number of pregnancies of cervix and control patients by religion; the controls have been age adjusted to their respective cervix groups, Tata Memorial Hospital.

Number of pregnancies	Hindu		Moslem		Christian		Parsi Control
	Cervix	Control	Cervix	Control	Cervix	Control	
0	3	5	(4)	7	(0)	4	6
1 or more	97	95	(96)	93	(100)	96	94
If patient has ever been pregnant.							
1-2	16	20	(16)	27	(14)	17	24
3-4	17	19	(21)	18	(23)	31	31
5-6	23	26	(28)	24	(41)	28	18
7-8	22	17	(19)	17	(18)	7	14
9 or more	22	18	(16)	14	(4)	17	13
Total	100	100	100	100	100	100	100

Table 28. Percent distribution of "smegma" formation among American and Indian males.

	Number of cases	None (%)	Moderate (%)	Marked (%)
American				
Non-Jewish				
White (private)	580	92	7	1
White (clinic)	125	70	24	6
Jewish	980	99.4	0.6	0
Negro (clinic)	100	54	38	8
Indian (Bombay)				
Hindu (Deccani)	130	56	28	16
Hindu (Gujarati)	90	74	16	10
Hindu (Other)	70	70	29	1
Christian	50	56	30	14
Moslem	130	100	0	0
Parsi	50	94	4	2
Indian (Madras)				
Hindu (mixed)	61	16	66	18
Christian	48	27	63	10
Moslem	31	58	42 (slight)	0

patient, though circumcised, showed some evidence of "smegma" (Table 28).

The Indian data show the greatest extent of poor penile hygiene among the Deccanis, with the lowest extent among the Parsis and Moslems. The Moslem men, of course, are all circumcised. Two of the Moslem males at Tata had incomplete circumcisions, whereas among the group examined at Madras a considerable portion had a small part of foreskin left over the sulcus where slight "smegma" formation was noted.

Penile hygiene seems to be a consequence of economic status, as shown from both the American and Indian data. From these data, it cannot be concluded that poor penile hygiene is of etiological significance in cervical cancer, but in view of the circumcision data, such data are suggestive.

INTERPRETATION OF DATA

The body of data presented in the previous pages confirms certain statistical associations previously found and suggests others. Statistical associations, of course, do not by themselves necessarily establish the etiological significance of the associated factors. It is pertinent to inquire whether any pattern emerges from the associations found. The major associations which this study suggests or confirms are mar-

ital status, age at first marriage, age at first coitus, number of marriages, and circumcision status of the partner.

Circumcision. The circumcision data that we obtained are not ideal. The ideal would involve direct examination of each sexual partner of an interviewed female, and is scarcely attainable. The blind interviewing technique used at Memorial Clinic does eliminate the possibility of the differences between the cervical cancer and the control groups having arisen from the interviewer's preconception. We have been unable to visualize any other errors in the interview technique that could create an artificial difference. The fact that this difference is found separately for the white non-Jewish and the Negro populations and even in the small sample of Jewish women with cervical cancer, as well as in the Memorial Clinic and all clinics combined, reinforces the results of a purely statistical test of significance and indicates that this is not the kind of random difference that sometimes arises in the analysis of small bodies of data. The results are clearly consistent with the known differences in incidence of cervical cancer between Jewish and non-Jewish women and with the apparently large differences in frequency between Moslem and Hindu women.

It does not lie within the realm of this report to speculate on the reasons for circumcision being a positive variable. It should be noted, however, that the data are compatible with previous work on penile cancer, suggesting that a factor present under the male foreskin may be carcinogenic. It is perhaps of more than academic interest to note that many of the same population groups with a high incidence of cervical cancer also have a relatively high incidence of penile cancer. In this respect, our observation that patients of low-income levels have a poorer penile hygiene than those of high-income groups may be of significance. If lack of circumcision should prove to be of significance in the development of cervical cancer, a gradual reduction of this type of cancer may be expected in the United States. Among enlisted Navy personnel aged 20-29 Zullo (*61*) found 39 percent circumcised. Of these, 55 percent had been circumcised at birth; 33 percent between the ages of 1 and 9; and the remainder before the age of 20. Among the younger generation, the circumcision rate is even higher in the United States. A recent study of American hospitals showed that in all private hospitals and in many of the city hospitals surveyed the circumcision rate among non-Jewish males averages around 80 to 85 percent (*62*). This rate seems to have been in effect for 10 to 20 years in many of these hospitals. In evaluating the future effect of these circumcision data on the incidence of cervical cancer, the possible earlier age at first coitus among the younger as contrasted to the older generation must, of course, also be taken into consideration.

Marriage Factor. The positive effects of marriage, age at first marriage, and first coitus, and number of marriages are consistent with: (a) differences between white and Negro women in this country, and (b) the apparent differences in India between Parsis and Christians on the one hand and Hindus on the other; (c) the relative rarity of cervical cancer among nuns, and (d) the apparently higher incidence of cervical cancer among women with syphilis.

The early age at first marriage in the cervical cancer group is also consistent with the higher incidence of cervical cancer in the lower social and economic classes, where early marriage is more common. Thus, out of some 400 patients seen at the Strang Cancer Prevention Clinic, which draws patients from a higher social level than the Memorial Gynecological Clinic, only 12 percent were married before the age of 20.

This compares with more than twice this figure among the Memorial Gynecological controls.

The etiological significance of these differences is of course debatable. The association with early marriage could, as Lombard and Potter (*35*) suggest, be a result of greater sensitivity of young tissue and of excessive hormonal stimulation. It could be a measure of duration and intensity of exposure; it could be an index to more frequent coitus and with a larger number of partners. One might also argue that early marriage, early coitus, and remarriage all increase the exposure to males with poor penile hygiene. For this to be more than a plausible conjecture, however, more evidence is needed, particularly on the possible carcinogenic effects of "smegma" (*63, 64*).

Pregnancy. In comparing the number of pregnancies in the cervical cancer and control groups, we have been able to hold constant the effects of two associated variables, economic status and age at first marriage. The first was controlled approximately by confining interviews almost entirely to the clinic population; the second by direct cross tabulation against age at first marriage. When these two major variables are controlled, no difference in number of pregnancies between women with cervical cancer and a comparable group with other gynecological complaints is apparent. The strong association between age at first marriage and number of pregnancies is shown not only in our data, but also by the Milbank Memorial Fund's study of fertility (*65*). This association would appear to suggest the desirability of reexamination of previous results on the role of number of pregnancies in the light of possible disturbing effects introduced by differences in age at first marriage.

Effect of Abstinence. In view of the suggestion that the Jewish law of abstinence after menses might partially account for the lower incidence of cervical cancer among Jewish women, we studied this factor with special interest. The abstinence data show no uniform tendencies. It is true that Jewish patients with cancer of the cervix less frequently follow the Talmudic law of abstinence than control patients, but after allowing for the factor of extramarital relations and earlier onset of coitus among the patients with cervical cancer, no apparent differences remain. The remaining sample with cervical cancer is very small, however. If the abstinence data reported to us by non-Jewish women were completely accurate, the absence of any difference between cervix and control patients in this regard would be of great significance. The great difficulties involved in accurately reporting a practice, the importance of which may change with advancing age, suggest the necessity of evaluating this result with some reserve. More information on the abstinence question may become available when the young Jewish women who do not practice the law to the same extent reach the cancer age. Even here, however, earlier onset at first coitus, as well as possible greater exposure to uncircumcised males, presents an obvious complication.

Contraceptives. A proper evaluation of the factor of contraceptives is difficult because our data on the frequency of use are inadequate. The data suggest a slightly greater use of condoms among the control patients than in the cervical cancer group. There is also a suggestion that among cervical cancer patients there were more who never practiced contraception than were found among the respective control groups. In view of the absence of adequate frequency data on the use of contraceptives, no definitive conclusions can be drawn from these data.

Histologic Differences. The results of the study are based on the epidermoid type of cervical cancer. The data on the adenocarcinomas of the cervix are too few to permit evaluations similar to those made for epidermoid cancer of the cervix. The present frequency data on adenocarcinomas among Jewish women, however, suggest that the etiology of this type of cancer may be different from that of epidermoid cancers. The fact that adenocarcinomas predominate when cancer of the cervix occurs in the young also points to a different pattern of etiology of this type. It is of interest to note that one Jewish patient was reported to have a squamous-cell carcinoma on biopsy, but was later shown to have an adenocarcinoma on operation. This patient was included among the adenocarcinoma cases in this report.

Cancer of the cervix of the epidermoid type may occur in apparent virgins and in women with short duration of sexual exposures, though only relatively rarely. This appears evident also from Pollack and Taylor's (66) report which included four cases of epidermoid cancer of the cervix in patients under 20. The youngest patient with such a cancer in the literature is 16. Among these groups, adenocarcinomas seem more common. The present survey includes a 16-year-old girl, a virgin, with an adenocarcinoma of the cervix.

Data on carcinoma in situ are also too few to permit definitive conclusions. The rate of divorce and age at first coitus were in line with data for epidermoid cancers. There were three Jewish patients included in this report with carcinoma in situ, one of whom gave a history of multiple exposures to uncircumcised males. More data would have to be available in order that this particular type of research might contribute to the problem of determining what proportion of cancer in situ develops into invasive epidermoid cancer.

Other Factors. Some of the suggested etiological factors enumerated in the introduction of this report, such as diet, cervical lacerations, and chronic cervicitis, cannot be easily investigated by an interview and thus have not been covered. The frequency of chronic cervicitis, however, among our white non-Jewish, Jewish, and Negro controls is about the same, suggesting that, even if it is etiologically significant, other factors are required to explain the difference in incidence among these groups, as has been previously stressed by McKelvey (48).

Results Relative to Incidence Data. The effects of early coitus, remarriage, and circumcision are consistent with incidence differences between Jewish and non-Jewish women, white and Negroes, and the various religious groups in India. Thus, added significance is given to these factors. It is scarcely necessary to emphasize that if subsequent investigations confirm the role of circumcision, the preventive implications for many parts of the world will be far from trivial.

Multiple Etiological Factors. Carcinogenesis represents the effect of many factors, some of which may be endogenous and some exogenous. In the development of epidermoid cancer, exogenous factors seem to be of particular importance. Yet even this type of neoplasm is the result of multiple factors, many of which remain unknown in our current state of knowledge.

In our studies we can only throw light on some of these factors, hoping that, through them, we might advance our understanding of others. Yet, if our understanding of any given factor, however small, may lead to a possible reduction of such a cancer by practical preventive measures, then, though the total mechanism of cancer production may remain undetermined, our efforts must be pointed in that direction.

SUMMARY AND CONCLUSIONS

1. Environmental factors suspected to play a role in the development of cancer of the cervix were studied by the interview technique.

2. The patient material consists of patients with cancer of the cervix in several American and Indian hospitals. American control groups were represented by patients with pelvic diseases other than cancer of the cervix.

3. Due to basic differences in incidence rates, analysis of non-Jewish whites, Jewish whites, and Negroes was carried out independently. Similarly, Indian data were analyzed separately for Hindu, Moslem, Christian, and Parsi patients.

4. Cervical cancer patients had a significantly earlier age at first coitus and age at first marriage than the control groups.

5. The age at first coitus was earliest among Negro controls and latest among Jewish controls. In the Indian study, the age at first coitus was earliest among Hindu and Moslem women and latest among Christian and Parsi patients.

6. Multiple marriages were found to be very much more common among cervical cancer than among control patients.

7. Patients with cancer of the cervix were more frequently exposed to uncircumcised males than the corresponding control patients.

8. The use of contraceptives remains a questionable variable because of the difficulty associated with obtaining information on the frequency of use.

9. No statistical association between the number of pregnancies and cervical cancer could be obtained after eliminating the effects of age at first marriage, considering only married women and comparing groups of similar economic status.

10. Present evidence on the effect of abstinence suggests that abstinence after menses may not be as important a factor as has been supposed.

11. Data on syphilis suggest that the statistical association between this disease and cervical cancer could be accounted for by the earlier age at first coitus among cervical cancer patients with syphilis, as compared to patients with cervical cancer without syphilis.

12. Negative variables include onset and flow of menses, method of delivery, irritative discharge, frequency of douching, and history of gonorrhea.

13. Epidermoid cancer of the cervix has been noted in women exposed only to circumcised males and in virgins. Other etiological factors than those involving coitus and lack of circumcision must therefore exist.

14. Examination of penile hygiene among the various groups studied shows that males of population groups with a high incidence of cervical cancer have poor penile hygiene.

15. The present results are compatible with the concept that those population groups having a late age at first coitus and first marriage and a low remarriage rate, whose men are circumcised, have a lower rate of carcinoma of the cervix.

16. Possible interpretations of these results and their preventive implications have been discussed.

We wish to express our gratitude to the Chiefs of Staff of those various services, as listed in Table 4, who have permitted us to interview their patients. We also wish to thank Dr. Willard M. Allen and Dr. Rieva Rosh for their helpful advice and assistance in the incipiency of this investigation. We are grateful to the following who have critically reviewed the final draft: Clinical: Drs. Willard M. Allen, Alexander Brunschwig, Harold Burrows, M. Edward Davis, R. Gordon Douglas, Alfred Gellhorn, John B. Graham, E. H. Horning, and Ernest L. Vennaway. Statistical: Drs. Irwin Bross, J. Clemmesen, Richard Doll, Morton L. Levin, Herbert L. Lombard, and L. D. Sanghvi.

Finally, we feel greatly obliged to our senior interviewers, Regeena Goodwin and Florence Moreno, without whose careful interrogation this study would not have been possible, and to Marianne Bardeleben Vargish for her help in compiling the statistical data.

References

(1) National Cancer Institute. Cancer Illness. Cancer Morbidity Series, Number 1:10, 1950-1952. Bethesda, Md., National Institutes of Health, United States Public Health Service.

(2) World Health Organization. *Epidemiological*

and Vital Statistics Report, vol. 5, No. 1-2. Geneva, 1952.

(*3*) Bleich, A. R. *JAMA* 143:1054, 1950.

(*4*) Jefferys, W. H. and J. L. Maxwell. *The Diseases of China, Including Formosa and Korea*, ed. 2, Shanghai, China Medical Association, p. 479.

(*5*) Khanolkar, V. R. Personal communication.

(*6*) Cooray, G. H. *Indian J Med Res* 32:71, 1944.

(*7*) Vineberg, H. N. *Am J Obst* 53:410, 1906.

(*8*) Theilhaber, A. and S. Greischer. *Ztschr Krebsforsch* 9:530, 1910.

(*9*) Peller, S. *Ztschr Krebsforsch* 34:128, 1931.

(*10*) Theilhaber, A *Ztschr Krebsforsch* 8:466, 1910.

(*11*) Hoffman, F. L. *Am J Cancer* 17:142, 1933.

(*12*) Kennaway, E. L. Personal communication.

(*13*) Treusch, J. V., A. B. Hunt, and A. A. Rousuck. *Am J Obstet Gynecol* 52:162, 1946.

(*14*) Smith, F. R. *Am J Obstet Gynecol* 41:424, 1941.

(*15*) Horwitz, A. *Surg Gynecol Obstet* 44:355, 1927.

(*16*) Rothman, A., L. P. Rapoport, and I. Davidsohn. *Am J Obstet Gynecol* 62:160, 1951.

(*17*) Rubin, I. C. Cited by H. N. Vineberg. *J Mt Sinai Hosp* 10:33, 1943-44.

(*18*) Weiner, I., L. Burke, and M. A. Goldberger. *Am J Obstet Gynecol* 61:418, 1951.

(*19*) Kaplan, I. I. and R. Rosh. *Am J Roentgenol* 57:659, 1947.

(*20*) Sorsby, M. *Cancer and Race; A Study of the Incidence of Cancer Among Jews*, New York, N.Y., William Wood & Company, 1931.

(*21*) Wolff, G. *Am J Hyg* Sect. A 29:121, 1939.

(*22*) Davidsohn, I. *Medical Leaves*, 1939, p. 19.

(*23*) Sugar, M. and W. E. Levy. *New Orleans M & S J* 103:424, 1951.

(*24*) Kennaway, E. L. *Brit J Cancer* 2:177, 1948.

(*25*) Handley, W. S. *Lancet* 1:987, 1936.

(*26*) Tjokronegoro, S. Personal communication.

(*27*) Robinson, B. W. *Am J Roentgenol* 66:783, 1951.

(*28*) Quinland, W. S. and J. R. Cuff. *Arch Path* 30:393, 1940.

(*29*) Hynes, J. F. *Am J Roentgenol* 60:368, 1948.

(*30*) Registrar-General, Great Britain. *Statistical Review of England and Wales (1936)*. London, H. M. Stationery Office, 1937-1938.

(*31*) Clemmesen, J. and A. Nielsen. *Brit J Cancer* 5:159, 1951.

(*32*) Stocks, P., cited by W. L. Harnett. *Brit J Cancer* 3:433, 1949.

(*33*) Maliphant, R. G. *Brit M J* 1:978, 1949.

(*34*) Dorn, H. F. *Human Biol* 15:73, 1943.

(*35*) Lombard, H. L. and E. A. Potter. *Cancer* 3:960, 1950.

(*36*) Gilliam, A. G. *J Nat Cancer Inst* 12:287, 1951-1952.

(*37*) Gagnon, F. *Am J Obstet Gynecol* 60:516, 1950.

(*38*) Rojel, J. *The Interrelation Between Uterine Cancer and Syphilis.* Copenhagen, Nyt Nordisk, Forlag, 1953.

(*39*) Khanolkar, V. R. *Acta U Internat contra Cancrum* 6:881, 1948-1950.

(*40*) Vineberg, H. N. In *Contributions to Medical and Biological Research Dedicated to Sir William Osler.* New York, New York, Paul B. Hoeber, vol. 2, p. 1217, 1919.

(*41*) Clemmesen, J. *J Nat Cancer Inst* 12:1, 1951-1952.

(*42*) Gardner, W. U. *Surgery* 16:8, 1944.

(*43*) Hofbauer, J. *J Obstet Gynaecol Brit Emp* 46:232, 1939.

(*44*) Ayre, J. E. *Am J Obstet Gynecol* 54:363, 1947.

(*45*) Bainborough, A. R. *Am J Obstet Gynecol* 61:330, 1951.

(*46*) Bayly, M. A. and R. R. Greene. *Am J Obstet Gynecol* 64:660, 1952.

(*47*) Nieburgs, H. E. *Am J Obstet Gynecol* 62:93, 1951.

(*48*) McKelvey, J. L. In discussion of Gagnon (Ref. 37).

(*49*) Ewing J. *Surg Gynecol Obstet* (Supp. 2) 44:165, 1927.

(*50*) Levin, M. L., L.C. Kress, and H. Goldstein. *NY State J Med* 42:1737, 1942.

(*51*) Belote, G. H. *Am J Syph* 15:372, 1931.

(*52*) Harding, W. G., II *Cancer Res* 2:59, 1942.

(*53*) Wallingford, A. J. Cited by M. L. Levin, et al. (Ref. 50).

(*54*) Clemmesen, J. Personal communication.

(*55*) Denoix, P. F, M. P. Schützenberger, and G. Viollet. *Bull Inst Nat Hyg* 6:573, 1951.

(*56*) Hausdorff, H. *Zentralbl Gynäk* 72:1901, 1950.

(*57*) Cornfield, J. *J Nat Cancer Inst* 11:1269, 1950-1951.

(*58*) Sadowsky, D. A., A. G. Gilliam, and J. Cornfield. *J Nat Cancer Inst* 13:1237, 1952-1953.

(*59*) Doll, R., and A. B. Hill. *Brit M J* 2:1271, 1952.

(*60*) Sanghvi, L. D. and V. R. Khanolkar. *Ann Eugenics* 15:52, 1949.

(*61*) Zullo, R. J. Personal communication.

(*62*) Wynder, E. L. Unpublished data.

(*63*) Plaut, A. and A. C. Kohn-Speyer. *Science* 105:391, 1947.

(*64*) Fischer, R. *Obstet Gynecol Surv* 8:232, 1953.

(*65*) Kiser, C. V. and P. K. Whelpton. *Milbank Mem Fund Quart* 22:72, 1944.

(*66*) Pollack, R. S. and H. C. Taylor, Jr. *Am J Obstet Gynecol* 53:135, 1947.

DISCUSSION

DR. JOSEPH NATHANSON. In order to appreciate the tremendous work which these gentlemen have presented, especially from the standpoint of the adherence to ritual laws, I trust you will allow me to present a résumé of them. In the first place, in no religion in the history of the human race, have the laws, as they are known in the Hebrew, Nidah, which means separation from the husband, been so long existent. They were promulgated in Biblical times, certainly over 4000 years ago, and in spite of the very many Diasporas, they had been carried out with a great degree of adherence until about 100 years ago.

Now what are these laws? In the first place, the laws are that, whether a woman menstruates normally five days or one day, the minimum time during which she must call herself absolutely unclean is five days. In other words, if she menstruates only one day a month throughout her life, from the standpoint of the Mosaic laws, she is known to be unclean for five days plus a period of seven days beyond that.

Again, any woman who has any spotting larger in extent than three-quarters of an inch in diameter at any time in the month immediately is looked upon or regarded as an unclean woman. She is analogous to the menstruating woman, and is therefore subject to the Mosaic laws of menstruation. If a woman should menstruate for three days, she would necessarily have an unclean period of 12 days. If she spotted after the first coitus, again she would have to go through 12 more days. The implications of such episodes are at once apparent. It reduces the period of exposure to coitus, as the essayists have said, to a very considerable degree. As a matter of fact, this rationing puts to shame the rationing which was prevalent in the halcyon days of the New Deal. Some of these women were literally being placed in "sexual ostracism."

Although the question of contraception was not touched upon by the essayists, I think that it is important to discuss it. If smegma is irritating, and if the male wears a contraceptive device then the irritating factor should be reduced. If the male does not use it, but the female employs a contraceptive, is she preventing the smegma from irritating the cervix, or is she in turn irritating the cervix by the contraceptive? That point would be worth investigating.

It is important to note that in the Jewish race itself, if a couple adheres to the Mosaic laws of sexual practices, the male cannot use any device or contraceptive himself. On the other hand, the female is allowed to use a contraceptive.

With regard to how many women really observe the Mosaic laws of menstruation to the letter of the law, or even partially, at the present time, I should like to give you some figures which the late Dr. Hiram Vineberg presented in a paper about 30 years ago, on the same subject which is under discussion, namely, the differences in the racial incidence of carcinoma of the cervix. During these years, 1893–1903, he found cancer of the cervix in New York City was 20 times as frequent in non-Jews as in the Jews. That is significant, because you will remember that was the period in which the peak of immigration from Eastern Europe occurred. The majority of Jewish women during that period

observed the Mosaic laws of menstruation most faithfully. Then in the decade from 1909 to 1918 the rate had dropped to seven and one-half times as frequent in non-Jews as in the Jews. Even in Israel, there is now an appreciable incidence of carcinoma of the cervix. It may be of interest and quite surprising to you to know that, in my own 30 years of practice, I have never seen a case of primary carcinoma of the cervix in a private patient. I have seen a few cases of stump carcinoma at the Woman's Hospital in Jewish patients, and carcinoma of the cervix in a few Jewish women on another ward service.

I believe that no finality can be placed upon the Mosaic laws of menstruation as an explanation of the low incidence of cancer of the cervix in the Jewish race. At the present time they play rather an insignificant part I believe, and I feel, therefore, that another aspect deserves serious thought. The answer cannot come and will not come until at least two and perhaps three generations have passed, because few Jewish women are now adhering to the Mosaic laws of menstruation. It is my opinion that about 95 percent of the Jewish women in this city are not observing the laws of Nidah. This is not my own estimate; colleagues who have similar types of practice agree with me. Even rabbis have informed me in recent weeks that their impression is similar to ours. One rabbi told me recently that in a period of 18 years he had never been consulted by any Jewish woman in his congregation as to how to carry out the Mosaic laws of menstruation. Thus, at the present time, I do not believe that with the information at hand we are justified in stating that the Mosaic laws per se are the important factor in the prevention of carcinoma of the cervix in the Jewish race.

I believe Dr. Wynder said that one of the more definite observations was that if women married late and had coitus for the first time late in life the incidence of carcinoma is lower. Is that correct?

DR. WYNDER. That is correct.

DR. NATHANSON. If that is so, it is paradoxical to note that the Old Testament admonished the Jewish race to undertake early marriage. We should therefore have had a higher incidence of carcinoma in the Jews because they married earlier and they had coitus much earlier. How then can you account for the discrepancy? It is my belief, and of course it is only a belief, this will resolve itself into a question in which the geneticist will finally answer the problem. In other words, I believe, at least to a degree, that, for some reason or other, whether you call it biologic, or whether it is because for a period of over 4000 years Jewish females have observed the Mosaic laws of menstruation and have therefore been subjected to less irritation over generations, say a couple of hundred generations, the cervical epithelium in the Jewish woman has become endowed with the ability to resist neoplastic changes of a malignant type better than can that of her non-Jewish sister, who has not had the benefit of markedly reduced irritation of the lower genital tract.

DR. FRANK R. SMITH. Although I did not know that Dr. Wynder was doing this work in connection with the Gynecological Service at Memorial Hospital, I was interested to see that he has followed rather closely the pattern of study that I undertook at the same hospital in 1927.

In an effort to find out why some women developed cancer, we took a group of cancer patients and a group of controls and used a questionnaire.

The striking point that came from our study was the racial difference. After I found it appearing in the figures I began looking up the literature and found that the infrequency of cancer of the cervix in Jewish women was mentioned in a report from the Mayo Clinic about five years before. The other factor that came up was the use of Lysol douches. It was astonishing to note the number of women who used Lysol douches in the cancer group and the practical absence of their use in the control group. We noticed also in the cancer group that the time between marriage and the first pregnancy seemed to be greater than in the controls.

The observation about the Lysol douche illustrates one of the dangers in this type of analysis. The reason that women with cancer of the cervix used Lysol douches was because they had leukorrhea. The controls who were taken from another hospital did not have the necessity for douches.

I spent four and one-half years before the war chasing monkeys in pursuit of the answer to the Lysol problem. Every day one of us applied Lysol in different strengths to the vagina on tampons. Every three months we biopsied the cervices. It was pretty hard to get monkeys that had had young and were in good health, but we used about 18 in all. We were just beginning to get what looked like basal-layer changes in the cervix in the group in which the stronger solution of Lysol was used, when the war put an end to the work. So the experiment, except for the slides, which I still have, appears to have been worthless. It did not prove or disprove anything. Allen's group in New Haven used smegma in various dilutions for injection into the cervix, but without any positive results.

One must recognize the danger of using figures, and be very careful of interpretations. In our study we found that whereas Jewish women made up about 48 to 49 percent of the benign cases in Memorial Hospital, they comprised less than 4 percent of our cancer group. Italians, who are pretty prolific, made up only 8 percent of our cross section, yet they represented over 20 percent of our cases of cancer of the cervix.

I doubt that diet has much to do with the protection against cancer of the cervix, which brings us down to the question of circumcision as the explanation of the low incidence of cervix cancer in Jewish women. Circumcision is, of course, not peculiar to the Jewish people. In the Fiji Islands, where the population is made up of two groups, racially and culturally distinct, cancer of the cervix never appears in the group that practices circumcision.

DR. SAMUEL WOLFE. Immunity of Jewish women to cancer of the cervix may result from either racial resistance or from sexual practices different from those followed by other peoples. The factors involved in circumcision of the male and the practice of sexual abstinence for one week after menses have been considered by previous speakers.

The research as reported tonight suggests a natural resistance to cancer by Jewish women but for validity investigation along broader anthropological lines is required. The peoples of Europe and America are of Indo-Aryan stock while those of Jewish extraction are of Semitic derivation. Other peoples of Semitic origin, i.e., Arabs, should also be similarly investigated as a control group. If by such studies freedom from cancer of the cervix is shown in Jewish women only, conformity to their religious sexual regulations may be then inferred as the likely factor in freedom from cancer. If women of both Jewish and Arabic stock should show a low incidence of carcinoma, racial resistance would appear to be the answer.

DR. HOWARD C. TAYLOR, JR. I would like to draw attention to the general importance of the method which has been demonstrated to us for the study of cancer of the cervix. This method by which the patient's previous environment is surveyed in great detail may be applied to a good many types of chronic illness.

I doubt that there have been previous studies of cancer of the cervix made with such detail and with such a consideration for the validity of statistics, as has been presented tonight.

We do, however, as listeners, have to reach for some tangible conclusions from these statistics. The first efforts to find such a definite conclusion are perhaps a little disappointing. It seems to me that two rather contrasted theories have been offered. One view seems to be that extrinsic factors, in which various aspects of sex hygiene are important, play the principal role in the causation of cancer of the cervix. The other view seems to be that differences are intrinsic, constitutional, or perhaps genetic. I wonder whether the speaker in conclusion would address his remarks to these two rather divergent points of view.

DR. SAUL B. GUSBERG. I would like to ask a question: Does this same disparity exist between these groups in intra-epithelial carcinoma of the cervix? That is a question we have often been asked.

DR. WYNDER (Closing). First of all, I would like to state that we have learned a very great deal from the points the various discussers have raised. We are quite cognizant of the fact that the work done by Dr. Smith and others has given us many valuable leads to our studies. The studies presented tonight are just excerpts of a larger undertaking, which has gone into some detail on most of the points raised.

We have studied douching and found there was no statistical significance in Lysol douchings or in any type of douching. In India, hardly any of the patients, in either the control or the cervix cases, use douching.

The question of contraceptives is a most difficult one. We found a slightly greater use of condoms in the control group as compared to the cervix group, but because of the difficulty of obtaining data on contraceptives, we are not placing too much value on this. Diaphragms were used in less than 5 percent of the group of patients studied.

It should be emphasized that the control patients in this type of study are most important, a point frequently not recognized. Every control patient is as important as every patient with the type of cancer that we are studying. We have analyzed the control patients not only for age and economic standing, but also for religion, native background, and descent, as well as for hospitals of admission. Where differences existed, we have standardized for these differences, so that we believe that our controls are as comparable to the cervix cases as possible.

In regard to abstinence, we must consider the following: Certainly a woman who abstains for seven days and is truly religious is much less likely to have extramarital relationships, so that these two facts are most difficult to keep apart. We found that those Jewish women with cancer of the cervix who did have extramarital relationships did not practice abstinence. Therefore, these factors are very difficult to separate.

The factor of prostitution was mentioned. I had occasion on a visit to Denmark last month to see a study not yet published by Dr. Rojel in which he found that in Denmark prostitutes had as much as four times more cancer of the cervix than other women of the same economic standing.

Dr. Symeonidis pointed out a relatively high circumcision rate among Negroes. We initially found a similar fact, but as we became more careful in our question on circumcision, we found that Negroes do not circumcise more at birth, but they do practice a slightly greater amount of circumcision in their teens. However, we found a peculiar response among Negroes. For instance, if a Negro male patient was asked, "Were you circumcised?" he frequently said, "Yes," because he felt if he said he was not circumcised, we might perform the operation.

A point which interests me is the apparent lesser frequency or incidence of cancer of the cervix in Israel than in New York City. Might this possibly be explained on the basis of the fact that if a woman has extramarital relationships in New York City, she is more likely to have them with an uncircumcised male than in Israel where most men are circumcised?

A question was raised about the occurrence of cervical cancer in clinic and private patients. It is well known that cancer of the cervix occurs less commonly among private patients. As we have demonstrated there is certainly better penile hygiene among patients in the higher income group. It must also be considered that the age at first marriage is later in the private patients. We have conducted a survey of private patients at Memorial Hospital and found a significantly later age at first marriage among them as compared to our clinic patients.

There is one other point about the histologic variations that deserves comment. We separated our results into epidermoid cancer, carcinoma in situ, and adenocarcinoma. There were not enough data available on carcinoma in situ to analyze these statistically, but they appear to go in the same direction as the epidermoid cancer data. In adenocarcinoma, however, which we did not analyze statistically, we found, as has been pointed out previously, the incidence among Jewish women to be the same as among the non-Jewish. I think this reiterates the point that the etiology of epidermoid and adenocarcinoma is entirely different.

Another point I would like to stress refers to genetic factors and hormonal drive in respect to cancer of the cervix. Genetic factors have often been thought to be of etiological significance in many types of cancers, such as liver cancer among the Bantus, until it was shown that certain dietary factors could explain the high incidence of this cancer. Similarly, in cancer of the lung it was suggested that women have a genetic resistance until it was shown that the greater amount of smoking among males could explain this difference.

In India, we have similar genetic backgrounds in the Hindus, Moslems, and Christians, who are all from the same racial stock. Most of the Moslems and Christians are converts from the Hindu religion. The marked difference in frequency of cancer of the cervix can perhaps be best explained by the exogenous factors outlined.

What about the factor of hormonal drive influencing the sexual drive of a given woman? I believe that mores and social customs govern the onset and intensity of coitus rather than hormonal drive.

Finally, I should like to point to a factor which is becoming more and more accepted. Epidermoid cancer behaves quite differently from the other cancers. Epidermoid cancers rarely occur in sites not exposed to exogenous factors of irritation. Epidermoid cancer of the lung is a very uncommon occurrence in nonsmokers. Epidermoid cancer of the tongue, buccal mucosa, and larynx is very uncommon in patients not exposed to some exogenous factor of irritation. Epidermoid cancer of the cervix is very uncommon in virgins. So I think that, in view of the present evidence, the working hypothesis must be that extrinsic factors are operating here. We are quite aware that cancer is a concerted effort of many endogenous and exogenous factors, but we must strike at those factors which we can handle with the greatest degree of practical success.

DEATH BY LIVER CIRRHOSIS AND THE PRICE OF BEVERAGE ALCOHOL

John R. Seeley[1]

Any condition that causes death may well be of interest to physicians, no matter how relatively rare the prevalence. More particularly might they be interested if, simultaneously, prevalence were rising while measures, perhaps quite simple, to reduce these death rates appeared to be available. If, in addition, the measures suggested did not add to the workload of the already overburdened physician, they might well be as welcome as mosquito abatement in relation to yellow fever.

Liver cirrhosis as a cause of death may well be in this category. Its contribution to mortality is small, though not exactly trivial, in modern Western nations. In Canada, in the last 50 or 60 years we have seen rates (1) as low as 5.2 per 100 000 adults and as high as 11.4. Deaths so attributed have also ranged from about one-quarter of one percent to about two-thirds of one percent of all mortality (1). Such mortality is roughly comparable with suicide, or leukemia.

If we restrict interest to the years 1921-56 for which the data are relatively reliable, we get an impression of a rather dramatic rise in the proportion of the general mortality attributed to liver cirrhosis—and this at a time when nutritional deficiencies (which are commonly thought to be a contributing cause) have been widely and steadily diminishing. The average annual increase in the relative rate has been about 4 percent of each preceding year's rate, and the trend is so steady that statistically it "accounts for" 92 percent of the variance in mortality (2), as Figure 1 shows. Moreover, the picture is similar no matter whether we take all of Canada as the reporting unit, or Ontario alone, or even so small an area as Toronto (3).

Nor is this increase to be attributed in any important way to changes in the age-sex composition of the population. If the raw data are recomputed as age-sex specific mortality rates, and the then "expected" mortality is referred to a "standard million" of population, a linear fit of the data to time still accounts for 86 percent of all the variation found. In other words, only about 6 percent is attributable to age-sex changes (4) in the population.

A visual impression may be gained from Figure 2.

For a variety of reasons our interest in deaths from liver cirrhosis was led in the following directions.

RATIONALE OF STUDY

Some forms of liver cirrhosis, and more particularly some cirrhosis of sufficient severity to be a cause of death, have long been widely spoken of as a "complication of alcoholism" (5). Indeed, so close has the relation been held to be that liver cirrhosis death rates have provided the basis upon which nearly all alcoholism prevalence rates have been estimated (6, 7) even though it is not known what proportion, within very wide limits, of such deaths are due to or associated with alcoholism (8-10).

Given the fact, however, of a strong association between liver cirrhosis deaths and "alcoholism prevalence," we might well ask how close the association is between the death rate from cirrhosis and the consumption of beverage alcohol.

If, moreover, that association should prove to be close and positive, then an interest in economics or public health will prompt us to inquire further as to the dependence of alcohol consumption on the price of alcohol. It is into these two aspects that this paper is, more narrowly, to inquire.

Data. Readily available (1) for Ontario and Canada are (a) liver cirrhosis death rates, (b) dollar sales values of licit alcoholic beverages purchased, (c) gallonage by type of beverage (beer, wine, distilled spirits), (d) population 20 years of age and over, (e) disposable personal

Source: *Canadian Medical Association Journal* 83:1361-1366, 1960.
[1] From the Alcoholism Research Foundation of Ontario.

Figure 1. Deaths from liver cirrhosis per 1000 deaths from all causes in Canada, 1921-1956.

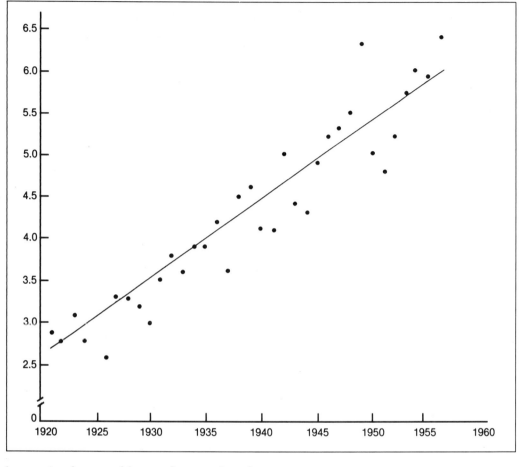

income (total personal income less taxes), and (f) consumer price indexes, if desired.

Price. From (b), (c), and (f) we may compute the average price each year of a gallon of absolute alcohol in standard dollars. From (d), (e), and (f) we may similarly compute disposable personal income per adult in standard dollars. And from these two, we may compute the price of an average gallon of absolute alcohol as a fraction of an average disposable income per adult. This "relative price" is what we shall use in what follows.

Consumption. From (c) and (d) we may compute the consumption of absolute alcohol per "adult" (person 20 years or more of age).

Mortality. We have the deaths from liver cirrhosis per 100 000 adults from (a).

These three sets of variables for Canada and Ontario, for the years for which data are available, respectively, are set out in Tables 1 and 2.

ANALYSIS

Alcohol Consumption and Liver Cirrhosis Death Rate

Three points are of major interest with regard to the relation between alcohol consumption and liver cirrhosis death rate: (a) How *close* is the correlation? (b) What is the seeming *form* of the relationship? (c) At what point of consumption might we expect liver cirrhosis deaths to be at a *minimum*?

The answer to the first question appears to be that the correlations are high and positive: the greater the consumption, the higher the death rate. For Canada, the correlation between alcohol consumption and the crude liver cirrhosis death rate is .960, which "accounts for" (statistically) 92 percent of the variation. The correlation between alcohol consumption and the age-

Figure 2. Alcohol price and consumption and liver cirrhosis death rate, Ontario, 1929–1958.

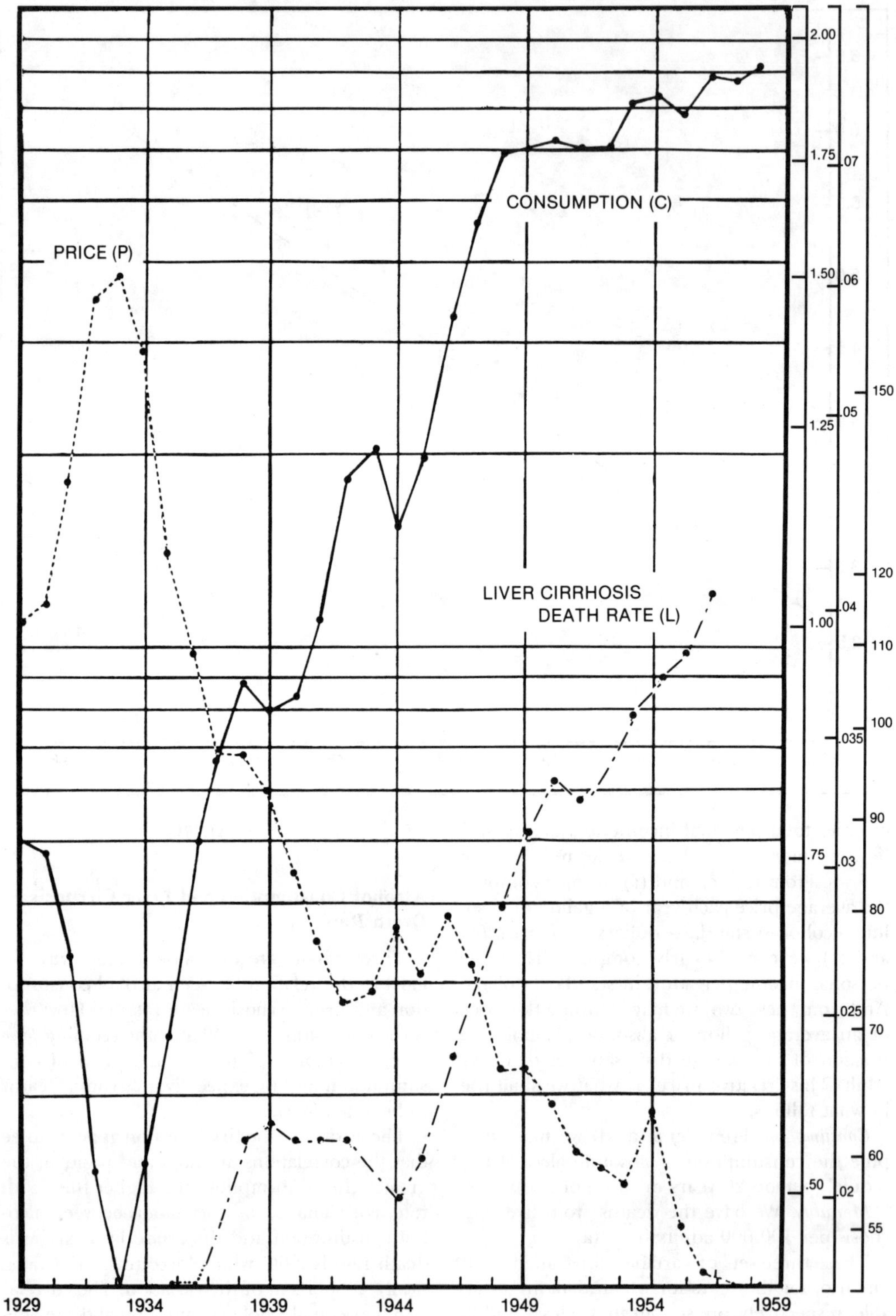

sex standardized death rate is lower but still considerable ($p = .910$) and it accounts for only a little less (83 percent) of the variance. The corresponding correlations for Ontario are very similar ($p = .969$ and .959, respectively).

The *fact* of a (statistical) relationship is hard to dispute. The *form* of that relationship is harder to establish. The question is essentially whether the basic relationship is linear—so that the death rate above a certain point is a simple multiple of the consumption rate, and deaths are at a minimum when consumption is at a minimum—or whether the relation is curvilinear, so that death rates tend to rise both above and below a certain consumption level. Statistical analysis favors (although it does not unequivocally establish) the second view. If we recall that the "consumption" we are speaking of is the "official" consumption (i.e., the consumption of alcohol from licit sources alone), the conclusion would run contrary neither to common sense nor to experience at other times and in other places, since it is credible that below a certain level of licit consumption enough

Table 1. Canada. Average standard relative price of alcohol, average consumption of alcohol, and average adult death rate by liver cirrhosis.[a]

Year	Price of alcohol[b]	Consumption of alcohol[c]	Unstandardized liver cirrhosis death rate[d]	Standardized liver cirrhosis death rate[e]
1926	.047	.62	—	—
1927	.049	.62	—	—
1928	.037	.77	—	—
1929	.041	.85	—	—
1930	.042	.87	—	—
1931	.046	.76	—	—
1932	.049	.65	—	—
1933	.065	.46	—	—
1934	.065	.46	—	—
1935	.052	.56	64.34	38.62
1936	.049	.63	65.17	38.75
1937	.046	.67	64.86	38.28
1938	.044	.74	68.38	40.05
1939	.044	.70	69.94	40.64
1940	.040	.74	67.08	38.68
1941	.037	.82	68.55	39.35
1942	.034	.91	72.60	41.44
1943	.035	.98	71.10	40.24
1944	.039	.82	69.13	38.98
1945	.037	.94	72.31	40.72
1946	.035	1.20	76.38	42.76
1947	.033	1.33	79.09	44.12
1948	.028	1.46	83.09	46.33
1949	.030	1.41	87.78	48.88
1950	.028	1.44	88.59	49.20
1951	.025	1.47	87.90	48.61
1952	.025	1.46	91.30	50.58
1953	.028	1.44	96.33	53.49
1954	.028	1.46	98.28	54.33
1955	.026	1.39	100.30	55.35
1956	.024	1.51	107.99	—

[a] The primary data upon which all rates shown in the table were based are to be found in *Statistics of Alcohol Use and Alcoholism in Canada, 1871-1956*. All liver cirrhosis death rates were corrected to allow for the effects of the Sixth Revision of the International Lists of Diseases and Causes of Death.

[b] Average price of an imperial gallon of absolute alcohol, shown as a fraction of average adult annual disposable personal income.

[c] Average consumption per "adult" (person 15 years of age or older) in imperial gallons of absolute alcohol.

[d] Deaths attributed to liver cirrhosis, per 1 000 000 "adults" (person 20 years of age and over); centered two-year moving averages.

[e] Expected deaths per standard million population.

Table 2. Ontario. Average standard relative price of alcohol, average consumption of alcohol, and average adult death rate by liver cirrhosis.[a]

Year	Price of alcohol[b]	Consumption of alcohol[c]	Unstandardized liver cirrhosis death rate[d]	Standardized liver cirrhosis death rate[e]
1929	.0400	.765	—	—
1930	.0409	.752	—	—
1931	.0471	.662	—	—
1932	.0589	.515	—	—
1933	.0605	.446	—	—
1934	.0555	.518	—	—
1935	.0434	.605	51.30	27.56
1936	.0386	.764	51.40	28.30
1937	.0342	.840	55.61	31.45
1938	.0342	.922	61.34	34.24
1939	.0327	.892	63.30	34.78
1940	.0298	.908	61.27	33.64
1941	.0273	.997	60.75	33.33
1942	.0254	1.175	61.51	33.46
1943	.0256	1.222	58.96	31.78
1944	.0278	1.107	57.18	30.88
1945	.0262	1.197	60.06	32.59
1946	.0280	1.435	66.70	36.07
1947	.0265	1.601	74.79	40.43
1948	.0234	1.737	80.99	43.96
1949	.0234	1.760	89.26	48.42
1950	.0225	1.766	94.63	51.49
1951	.0213	1.757	92.72	50.61
1952	.0209	1.775	94.99	51.99
1953	.0203	1.850	102.42	56.44
1954	.0222	1.876	106.69	58.84
1955	.0194	1.828	108.27	59.64
1956	.0183	1.917	115.49	—

[a] The primary data upon which all rates shown in this table were based are to be found in *Statistics of Alcohol Use and Alcoholism in Canada, 1871-1956*. All liver cirrhosis death rates were corrected to allow for the effects of the Sixth Revision of the International Lists of Diseases and Causes of Death.

[b] Average price of an imperial gallon of absolute alcohol, shown as a fraction of average adult annual disposable personal income.

[c] Average consumption per "adult" (person 20 years of age or older) in imperial gallons of absolute alcohol.

[d] Deaths attributed to liver cirrhosis, per 1 000 000 "adults" (person 20 years of age and over); centered two-year moving averages.

[e] Expected deaths per standard million population.

illicit alcohol is made available to raise the true total consumption, and perhaps to increase the physical damage per unit consumed.

If the hypothesis of a curvilinear relation is accepted, then it appears that:

(a) For Canada: (i) The unstandardized liver cirrhosis death rate would be at a minimum (66 deaths per million adults per annum) when consumption fell to an average of .60 gallon of absolute alcohol per adult per annum. Put another way, we should expect a 38 percent reduction in 1956 death rates if consumption fell by 60 percent. (ii) The standardized liver cirrhosis death rate would be at a minimum (39 deaths

per million standard population per annum) when consumption fell to an average of .65 gallon of absolute alcohol per adult per annum. This would mean about a 30 percent reduction in deaths, given a 57 percent fall in alcohol consumption.

(b) For Ontario: (i) The unstandardized liver cirrhosis death rate would be at a minimum (56 deaths per million adults per annum) when consumption fell to an average of .89 gallon of absolute alcohol per adult per annum. This means 48 percent of present deaths, with a fall of 54 percent in current consumption. (ii) The standardized liver cirrhosis death rate would be

4

at a minimum (31 deaths per million standard population per annum) when consumption fell to an average of .88 gallon of absolute alcohol per annum. This implies 52 percent of the deaths, given a 54 percent drop in consumption.

The foregoing relations may be presented synoptically in Table 3.

Greater consistency than this between the findings for Ontario and Canada, or, within each, for the standardized and unstandardized rates is hardly to be expected, given the heterogeneity across "Canada" and the different meanings of the questions answered by the standardized and unstandardized rates, respectively. What seems clear enough is that death rates of both kinds in both political units are closely related to alcohol consumption, and that reductions by about a third to a half might be "expected" if alcohol consumption were cut to a third or a half or somewhere in between.

The prediction takes it for granted that other alcohol "supply" conditions remain the same. It is for this reason that only the period 1935-56 was chosen to correlate alcohol consumption and liver cirrhosis death rates; before that date, alcohol supply conditions were sufficiently different that the stricture "all other conditions being equal" did not apply. (7).

From 1929-34, as a matter of fact, liver cirrhosis deaths did *not* vary intimately with price and consumption (which did vary inversely for the whole period). If, however, a longer time period were chosen—say from the beginning of prohibition, circa 1915, to the present, close covariation between alcohol consumption and liver cirrhosis death rate would be visually obvious, and statistically reflected in high correlations.

Alcohol Price and Alcohol Consumption

It remains to show the dependency of alcohol consumption on alcohol price.

Since the same questions were asked of these data as were asked about the relation of death rates to alcohol consumption, with similar results, it seems idle to restate the findings in the text, and preferable to summarize them in Table 4.

Again, the data seem to assert that the relation between price and consumption is very close, and that as price falls consumption rises.

They seem to assert, further, that consumption would be at a minimum of about half a gallon of absolute alcohol per adult per annum, whether in Ontario or Canada as a whole, when the price of a gallon of absolute alcohol was about one-twentieth of an average adult income. While such a price would represent a 137.5 percent increase in Canada, and nearly a 200 percent increase in Ontario, it needs to be recalled, to put the matter in perspective, that prices stood higher than this in Canada in 1933 and 1934, and in Ontario from 1932 to 1934. Consumption of less than half a gallon of absolute alcohol per adult also actually occurred in Canada in those two years, and in Ontario in 1933.

Alcohol Price and Cirrhosis Death Rates

If we omit consumption of alcohol as an "intervening variable"—even though common-sense may recommend it—and compute di-

Table 3. Canada and Ontario. Alcohol consumption and liver cirrhosis death rates, standardized and unstandardized.

Statistic	Liver cirrhosis death rate			
	Unstandardized		Standardized	
	Canada	Ontario	Canada	Ontario
Correlation between consumption and death rate	0.96	0.97	0.91	0.96
Percentage variance "accounted for"	92	94	83	92
Minimum death rate expected:				
(a) per million adults	66	56	39	31
(b) as percentage of 1955-6 death rate	62%	48%	70%	52%
Consumption point for minimum death rate:				
(a) in gallons absolute alcohol	0.60	0.89	0.65	0.88
(b) as percentage of 1956 consumption rate	40%	46%	43%	46%

Table 4. Canada and Ontario. Alcohol price and alcohol consumption.

	Region	
Statistic	Canada	Ontario
Correlation between price and consumption	−0.99	−0.96
Percentage variance "accounted for"	98%	92%
Minimum consumption expected:		
(a) in gallons absolute alcohol	0.51	0.49
(b) as percentage of 1956 consumption	34%	25%
Price at which minimum consumption expected:		
(a) as fraction of income[a]	.057	0.053
(b) as percentage of 1956 price	238%	293%

[a] Price stated as a fraction of average adult annual disposable personal income.

Table 5. Canada and Ontario. Alcohol price and liver cirrhosis death rates, standardized and unstandardized correlations.

		Liver cirrhosis death rate correlated with alcohol price	
Region	Statistic	Unstandardized	Standardized
Canada	p	−0.93	−0.91
	p^2	(0.86)	(0.83)
Ontario	p	−0.93	−0.90
	p^2	(0.86)	(0.81)

rectly the regression between alcohol price and the death rates, we get results very similar to those already presented. Space permits no more than a statement of the correlations found—as in Table 5 below; and those interested may be referred for further detail to the basic documents (*11*).

These seem to be rather striking direct relations.

[Figure 2], which shows for Ontario, from 1929 to 1958, the movements of alcohol prices, alcohol consumption, and the unstandardized cirrhosis death rate will, it is hoped, at least, avoid one too restricted interpretation of the correlations found: it is not the case simply that the price series has moved steadily down while the other series has moved steadily up. The covariation between all seems, on visual impression, as on statistical analysis, immediate, detailed and intimate.

DISCUSSION

It is one thing to establish the fact and nature of a relationship over a brief historical period,

and quite another to assume a causal relationship, and moreover, a causal relationship that can be extrapolated to the future.

There is only one way to test such a pair of assumptions and that is by way of an experiment. If an attempt were made by a suitable government to change (in either direction) to a sufficient degree (say 20 percent to 30 percent) the already, in effect, administered price of alcohol for a sufficient period (say three years), it could be determined whether indeed licit alcohol consumption and, therewith, the rate of death by cirrhosis of the liver changed in the expected direction and to the expected degree.

If the price were changed in the upward direction, we might reasonably expect some saving of life as well as a gain in scientific knowledge, and the opening up of a possibility of public health gains on the basis of precisely tailored economic measures. It can be shown (*11*) also that, by a curiously happy relationship among the variables, the increased taxation that would secure the higher price, and lowered consumption and death rates, would add sufficient additional revenue to government (even in the face of the diminished consumption) to pay for a very substantial increase in public health programs, or indeed, in any other desired governmental program. In Ontario, for instance, a doubling of price, despite its effect in reducing consumption, might be expected approximately to double the government's net revenue from alcohol. (We might also, incidentally, learn something as to how illicit alcohol supply and methods of tension management other than alcohol consumption vary with the price of licit alcohol supply.) In any case, the anticipated effect on revenue might also be regarded as a matter for experimental verification. Certainly, we have a situation here where the anticipated costs do not by any means, *prima facie*, stand in the way of experiment in a public health improvement measure.

The ethical problems involved in raising the price of a commodity to all, so that disaster may be avoided for some, merit extended discussion at another time and place. In effect, this is not far different from what happens when hospitals are supported in part out of any general tax, particularly an excise or sales tax. In the present case, the measures discussed would, if effective, relieve the taxpayer and the economy of an already existing expense, at least if it were assumed that when mortality rates fell, morbidity rates and public expense for hospitalization would fall with them. Moreover, the increased tax revenue could be used to make available additional general services, so that drinkers would be taxed not primarily for problem drinkers but for common services for all.

SUMMARY

It appears that deaths from liver cirrhosis, though small in number, are increasing rapidly, and rise and fall with average alcohol consumption. It also appears that alcohol consumption rises and falls inversely with alcohol price. It is sufficiently credible to justify a social experiment to determine whether an alcohol price increase would reduce liver cirrhosis mortality, while simultaneously furnishing a sizable increase in government revenue, and hence occasion an increase in government services or a reduction in other forms of taxation.

References

(*1*) Popham, R.E. and W. Schmidt. *Statistics of Alcohol Use and Alcoholism in Canada, 1871-1956.* Toronto, University of Toronto Press, 1959, p. 98.

(*2*) Seeley, J.R. and W. Schmidt. Substudy 1-1 and 4-58. Toronto, Alcoholism Research Foundation of Ontario. Unpublished material.

(*3*) Seeley, J.R and W. Schmidt. Substudy 1-1 and 4-58. Toronto, Alcoholism Research Foundation of Ontario, p. 3. Unpublished material.

(*4*) Seeley, J.R. and W. Schmidt. Substudy 1-1 and 4-60. Toronto, Alcoholism Research Foundation of Ontario. Unpublished material.

(*5*) Jolliffe, N. and E.M. Jellinek. Cirrhosis of the liver. In *Effects of Alcohol on the Individual.* Vol. 1. New Haven, Yale University Press, 1942, p. 273.

(*6*) World Health Organization Expert Committee on Mental Health. *Report on the First Session of the Alcoholism Subcommittee* Geneva, 1953. Technical Report Series No. 42

(*7*) Popham, R.E. *Q J Stud Alcohol* 17:553, 1956.

(*8*) Seeley, J.R. *Q J Stud Alcohol* 20:245, 1959.

(*9*) Jellinek, E.M. *Q J Stud Alcohol* 20:261, 1959.

(*10*) Brenner, B. *Q J Stud Alcohol* 20:255, 1959.

(*11*) Seeley, J.R. Substudy 23-1-60; 23.1-1-60; 23.1.1-1-60; 23.2-1-60; 23.3-1-60; 23.4-1-60; 23.4.1-1-60; 23.4.4-1-60; 23.5-1-60; 23.6-1.60. Toronto, Alcohol Research Foundation of Ontario. Unpublished material.

EPIDEMIOLOGICAL STUDIES OF CULTURE CHANGE

John Cassel[1] and Herman A. Tyroler[2]

Over the past four decades North Carolina has changed from a predominantly agricultural state to one that is rapidly becoming industrialized. While the population of the state has increased from 2 559 123 in 1920 to 4 556 155 in 1960, the proportion of the population engaged in farming has decreased during this period from 58.6 percent to about 27 percent. North Carolina thus presents an opportunity to study, in microcosm, some of the sweeping changes that, to a greater or lesser extent, are occurring throughout the world today. In particular, North Carolina offers numerous opportunities to study the impact of industrialization on health.

The process of rapid industrialization has afforded many opportunities to study the impact of a changing physical environment on health. Fewer attempts have been made, however, to study the health effects of the dramatic social and cultural changes that accompany industrialization, and it is this aspect of the process that we find most challenging and on which we are focusing a series of epidemiological studies.

Despite the growing body of theory postulating the significance of social and cultural factors in disease etiology (1-10), no unified series of concepts delineating these sociocultural processes has as yet been developed. While sociology and anthropology have provided structural schemes in abundance, there is little agreement as to which processes are relevant to health, how many crucial processes there are, and how these processes are linked to health states.

As a potential contribution to this field, we have presented elsewhere a generalized conceptual scheme outlining what we consider to be the nature of some of the social and cultural processes of relevance to health (11). We are now engaged in a series of studies designed to test the utility of this scheme.

The present investigation, which is the first of the series, is concerned with testing a general proposition derived from this scheme. According to this proposition, recent sociocultural change will raise the probability of incongruity between the culture of the migrant and the social situation in which he lives. Such incongruities as occur will place excessive adjustive burdens on the social groups in which the migrant interacts and on the personality system of individual migrants. Insofar as these stresses are not absorbed by the small group systems and/or the personality system, recent migrants to an industrial milieu are likely to manifest increased rates of psychological, somatic, and social ill health.

The study was conducted in a small industrial city of about 5000 people, situated in the western part of North Carolina. A little more than 50 years ago this city was a mountain village of no more than 100 people. At that time a large national corporation located a manufacturing plant in this village, and by deliberate management policy drew its labor force almost entirely from the surrounding area.

This policy continues to the present. The population from which the labor force is drawn is ethnically homogeneous, being predominantly of British stock and having lived in this area for well over a century. Practically no migration into this region has occurred during this period.

Within the factory it was possible to identify two groups according to the recency with which they had undergone the changes accompanying industrialization.

1. A group of "first generation" factory employees. This group, presently employed in the factory, are the children of farmers, and represent the people who have most recently undergone the change from a rural "folk" culture to an industrial social situation.

Source: *Archives of Environmental Health* 3:31-39, 1961.

[1] Professor of Epidemiology, Department of Epidemiology, The School of Public Health, The University of North Carolina, Chapel Hill, N.C., and Medical Director, Health Research Foundation.

[2] Associate Professor of Epidemiology, Department of Epidemiology, The School of Public Health, The University of North Carolina, Chapel Hill, N.C., and Research Director, Health Research Foundation.

2. A group of "second generation" factory employees. This group, also currently employed in the factory, differ from the preceding group in that they are the children of previous factory employees, and it is presumed that their cultural training is more congruent with the industrial situation in which they now live and work.

In terms of our general proposition the specific hypothesis to be tested is that the "first generation" factory employees will have higher indices of ill health than the "second generation" employees.

METHOD

The Sample

For this initial investigation the population studied was restricted to white male, hourly paid employees of the factory on the active company payroll for the 40-month period, January 1956 through May 1959. There were 968 employees satisfying these criteria, from whom a stratified random sample of 390 individuals was drawn for study. The stratification was made on the basis of age, absence experience, and medical examination status. This last was determined by comprehensive biennial examinations, for which all these individuals had been eligible.[3]

This study population of 390 individuals was then divided into "first generation" and "second generation" industrial workers. The "first generation" workers had had neither parent employed in the factory. As there were practically no other sources of employment other than farming available locally, the vast majority of the parents of these "first generation" workers were, thus, farmers. The "second generation" workers had had at least one parent employed in this factory.

It should be emphasized that the sample as chosen reflects known selective bias. All individuals either entering or leaving the population during the study period were excluded. Thus, all deaths, retirements, disability separations, and both voluntary and involuntary separations from employment were excluded from

the population at risk. The employee turnover for the period under study averaged 3-5 percent per year. Thus, for the 40-month study period an estimated 10-15 percent of the population were excluded for purposes of this study. In addition, as indicated above, the sample was restricted to hourly paid employees, excluding all foremen, management, and executive personnel. The latter will form the basis for a separate study.

Data Obtained

For each individual member of the sample, data were obtained on age, "generation status" (as defined above), length of service, marital status, and two general indices of health status. The first of these was a morbidity rate based on the number of absences of more than three consecutive days' duration attributed to illness, and the second the number of positive responses given on the Cornell Medical Index Health Questionnaire. It was recognized that these were two relatively crude indices of health status, but they were considered adequate as a first test of the hypothesis. Our confidence in the utility of absences as a general index of amount of illness was increased by the company policy requiring that all individuals having such absences present a certificate from their family doctor upon return to work and submit to an examination by the in-plant medical service.

RESULTS

Description of the Sample: Age and Length of Service in Each Generation Group[4]

The ages of the 390 men in the sample ranged from 20 to 50 years. As there were a greater proportion of first generation than of second generation workers in the older age groups, each generation group was stratified into a "young" group (20-34 years) and an "old" group (35-50 years) and separate analysis made on each age group. Table 1 shows the mean age and mean length of service of the "young" and "old" groups for each generation. It should be noted that each age group of first generation workers had the same mean length of service as

---

[3] Three categories of medical examination status were developed: those diagnosed as having any major or potentially serious medical abnormality, those with minor or no medical abnormalities, and those not examined.

[4] As less than 4 percent of the population were not married, marital status could not be included as one of the variables.

Table 1. Mean age and mean length of service by generation status.[a]

| | First generation (265) | | | | Second generation (125) | | | |
| | 20–34 Yr. (60) | | 35–50 Yr. (205) | | 20–34 Yr. (72) | | 35–50 Yr. (53) | |
	Mean	S.D.[b]	Mean	S.D.	Mean	S.D.	Mean	S.D.
Age	30.2	2.9	42.8	4.7	28.5	3.4	39.6	4.1
Length of service	5.8	4.3	16.3	7.1	6.4	4.3	16.4	6.8

[a] Numbers in parentheses indicate number of individuals in each category.
[b] Standard deviation.

the corresponding age groups of the second generation workers.

Morbidity Rates

As indicated above, morbidity rates in this study were based upon the number of absences of more than three consecutive days attributed to illness. From these data two rates were derived: (1) frequency rate (FR)—the number of such lost time episodes per 1000 population per year; and (2) disability rate (DR)—the mean number of days lost per person per year.

For the total sample the frequency rate was 570 lost-time episodes per 1000 population per year, while the disability rate was 13.6 work-loss days per person per year. These rates are considerably in excess of those found in the nation as a whole. For men over 17 years, the U.S. National Health Survey reports disability rates of only 7.2 work-loss days per person per year *(12)*. These rates, calculated for persons "usually working," include all absences of any duration, whereas in the present study only absences of longer than three days were included. If absences of three days or fewer had been included the rates in this population would thus have been higher. Not only are these rates higher than the national average, but they are higher in this Carolina division of the Company than in any of the other manufacturing divisions of the same Company. These other divisions, located in other states, are producing products similar to those of the Carolina division, and the workers are subjected to identical company policies and practices. Nevertheless, the disability rate in those divisions is approximately 10 work-loss days per person per year in comparison with 13.6 in the Carolina division.

Possible explanations for these high rates in terms of the findings of this study will be presented in the comment below.

Generational Differences

Table 2 shows the number of illness episodes and their duration in the two generation groups by length of service in five-year intervals for each of the two age groups. In Table 3 the frequency and disability rates of these illness episodes have been calculated for the same groups. To aid in the visualization of some of the relationships demonstrated in Table 3, Figure 1 presents the least squares lines of best fit of all such lost-time episodes for each group. In computing these lines every absence was considered for each year of length of service.

Frequency Rate

As can be seen from Table 3 and Figure 1, in the first generation factory workers, the frequency rate of illness episodes does not show any consistent change with increased length of service for either of the two age groups. By contrast, in second generation workers there is a marked decline in the frequency rate of illness episodes with increasing length of service, and this is manifested in both age groups.[5] Thus, first generation workers tend to have lower rates of illness episodes than do second generation workers in the early years of service but higher rates with increasing years of service.

---

[5] In the second generation, using a multiple linear regression model, age, length of service, and their interaction accounted for 10 percent of the variation in absence experience. The standardized partial regression coefficient indicated that the effect of length of service was approximately six times greater than the effect of age. Analysis of covariance demonstrated that the rate of change of absences with increasing length of service differed in the two generations, and the difference was statistically significant ($0.01 < p < 0.05$). The application of multiple linear regression showed no significant relationship between the variables under study (age and length of service) and absence experiences in the first generation.

Table 2. Number of illness episodes and their duration by generation status and length of service in two age groups (20–34 years and 35–50 years).

	Generation	All lengths of service	Length of service (yr.)		
			1–5	6–15	16–31
20–34 years					
No. in	1st	60	34	26	0
sample	2d	72	36	36	0
No. of illness	1st	113	62	51	—
episodes	2d	166	108	58	—
No. of days	1st	2787	1352	1435	—
of illness	2d	3333	2002	1331	—
35–50 years					
No. in	1st	205	13	91	101
sample	2d	53	5	24	24
No. of illness	1st	382	14	198	170
episodes	2d	83	19	33	31
No. of days	1st	9599	256	5298	4045
of illness	2d	1998	490	782	726

Table 3. Frequency and disability rates of illness episodes by generational status and length of service in two age groups (20–34 years and 35–50 years).

	Generation	All lengths of service	Length of service (yr.)		
			1–5	6–15	16–31
20–34 years					
Frequency rate	1st	565	547	588	
	2d	692	900	483	
Disability rate	1st	13.9	11.9	16.6	
	2d	13.9	16.7	11.1	
35–50 years					
Frequency rate	1st	599	323	653	505
	2d	470	1,140	413	388
Disability rate	1st	14.0	5.9	17.5	12.0
	2d	11.3	29.4	9.8	9.1

Disability Rate

This rate, a measurement of the amount of time lost due to illness, shows a similar pattern for the two generations as does the frequency rate. As demonstrated in Table 3, first generation workers in both age groups tend to lose less time than do second generation workers in the early years of service, but lose more time with increasing length of service.

Cornell Medical Index Scores

Three scores have been computed from responses to the Cornell Medical Index, based upon the total number of symptoms reported,

the number of organs involved, and the total number of positive responses to the "emotional component" of the index (Sections M-R).

These scores were chosen as previous work with the Cornell Medical Index has indicated that they are closely related to assessments of health status made independently by physicians *(13-21)*.

The scores as shown in Tables 4, 5, and 6 indicate that for the total sample those individuals with multiple absences had higher scores than those with no absences or one absence during the 40-month study period. Furthermore, both the total score and the number of organ systems involved increases with in-

Figure 1. Change in number of absences with length of service by generation status and age groups (least squares line of best fit).

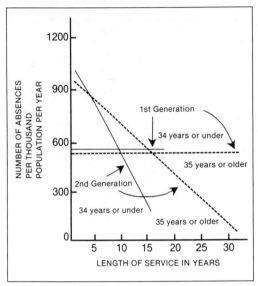

creasing age (a finding consistent with other reports) *(18)*. To compare differences between the two generations it was thus necessary to control for both age and absence experience. Furthermore, the scores were based upon tests performed at the end of the study period, that is, after all absences had occurred, and for those groups with many absences these scores might therefore be largely influenced by the absence experience that had previously prevailed. To eliminate the contaminating effect of such previous absences, our inferences as to genera-

tional differences have been restricted to the scores of individuals who had no absences or, at the most, one absence during the study period. The scores for these groups have been plotted in Figure 2.

References to Tables 4, 5, and 6 and to Figure 2 indicate that at all ages first generation workers who have had no absences or one absence during the study period have higher Cornell Medical Index scores than the second generation workers with the same absence experience. Thus, first generation workers complain of more total symptoms; these are distributed in more organ systems; and they have more symptoms relating to disorders of mood, feeling, and behavior than is the case in the second generation workers.

In an effort to gain further understanding of the increase in mean total score that occurs with increasing age in both generation and absence level groups (Table 4), the frequency distributions of these scores for the total sample were plotted and the results grouped into quartiles. In Figure 3 these distributions are presented for each generation in two age and absence level groups. It can be seen from this figure that in the first generation with no absences or one absence, 20 percent of the younger group, and an almost equal proportion (17 percent) of the older group, had scores in the highest quartile. In the first generation workers with two or more absences the proportions in the highest quartile were increased, but again were constant in the two age groups (39 percent and 40 percent respectively). Similarly, in the second gen-

Table 4. Mean total Cornell Medical Index scores by generational status, age, and absence levels.

		Age in years							
		All ages		21–30		31–40		41–50	
		N	Mean	N	Mean	N	Mean	N	Mean
All absence levels	Total	390	13.5	80	11.9	160	13.1	150	14.8
	1st gen.	265	14.4	31	12.8	103	14.0	131	15.0
	2d gen.	125	11.8	49	11.3	57	11.6	19	13.4
0 or 1 absence	Total	233	10.7	37	6.9	104	9.9	92	12.4
	1st gen.	162	11.4	16	9.3	70	10.6	76	12.6
	2d gen.	71	8.1	21	5.1	34	8.4	16	11.3
2 or more absences	Total	157	18.2	43	16.2	56	19.1	58	18.7
	1st gen.	103	19.0	15	16.5	33	21.1	55	18.4
	2d gen.	54	16.6	28	16.0	23	16.3	3	24.3

Table 5. Mean number of organ systems involved in Cornell Medical Index by generational status, age, and absence levels.

		Age in years			
		All ages	21–30	31–40	41–50
Total sample, all absence levels		6.3	5.5	6.3	6.8
0 or 1 absence	Total	5.5	4.0	5.3	6.3
	1st gen.	5.9	4.9	5.5	6.4
	2d gen.	4.7	3.4	5.0	5.9
2 or more absences	Total	7.6	6.8	8.2	7.6
	1st gen.	7.8	6.7	8.6	7.6
	2d gen.	7.2	6.8	7.6	7.8

Table 6. Mean score for "emotional component"[a] of Cornell Medical Index by generational status, age, and absence levels.

		Age in years			
		All ages	21–30	31–40	41–50
Total sample, all absence levels		2.9	2.8	3.2	2.9
0 or 1 absence	Total	2.1	1.6	2.0	2.5
	1st gen.	2.4	2.1	2.2	2.7
	2d gen.	1.4	1.3	1.5	1.5
2 or more absences	Total	4.0	3.8	4.7	3.5
	1st gen.	4.1	3.8	5.3	3.5
	2d gen.	3.8	3.8	3.8	3.8

[a] Positive responses to sections M-R of the Cornell Medical Index (symptoms relating to disorders of mood, feeling, and behavior).

Figure 2. Mean Cornell Medical Index scores by age and generation status for those people with no absences or one absence during the 40-month period.

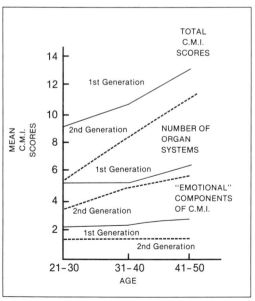

eration group the percentage of people with scores in the highest quartile was practically the same in the young as in the old group when absence level was controlled (0 percent and 4 percent in the 0-1 absence group, 32 percent and 31 percent in two or more absence group). The increase noted in Table 4 of mean total score with increasing age is therefore attained

Figure 3. Percentage distribution of total Cornell Medical Index scores at quartile positions for total population.

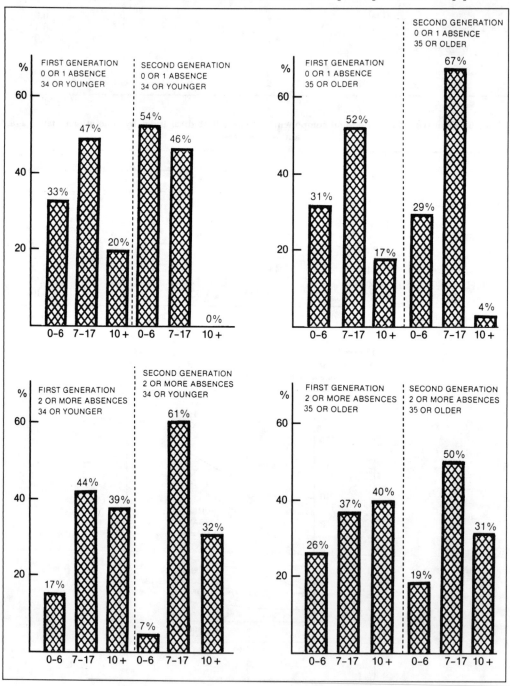

by a larger number of the old group scoring in the interquartile rather than the lowest quartile position, with the number in the upper quartile remaining relatively constant. These results would suggest that at all ages there are a relatively fixed small number of "sick" people who contribute most of the pathology experienced by that group, a finding in conformity with that of Hinkle *(22, 23)*.

If the distribution of scores in first generation workers is now compared with those of second generation workers it can be seen that at each absence and age level the proportion of first generation scores in the highest quartile is always greater than the proportion of second generation scores in this quartile. These findings suggest that at each absence level there are more of these "sick" people in the first than in the corresponding second generation.

COMMENT

It is not claimed that the results of this first study have "proved" our original hypothesis in any rigorous sense. The population from which this sample was drawn is a unique one, not necessarily representative of any other industrial population. Extensive replication of these findings in widely differing groups will therefore be necessary before any confidence can be placed in their generalization. What this study has demonstrated is that, in the sample drawn, the results are consistent with a hypothesis independently arrived at without any prior knowledge of the illness patterns in the two generations.

In this sample a greater proportion of first generation workers had poor health scores than was the case in second generation workers of comparable age working together in the same plant, subjected to the same company policies and practices, and derived from the same homogeneous ethnic stock. Insofar as absences attributable to illness are concerned, first generation workers when recently employed had fewer such episodes than did the second generation workers. With increasing length of service, however, they did not exhibit the decline in absences characteristic of the second generation, and their rates were consequently higher.

According to our general conceptual scheme these findings can be explained on the basis of postulated incongruity between the culture of the first generation workers and the social situation in which they now live. The assumption would be that their system of values, attitudes, and framework of knowledge with which they were equipped during their formative years was appropriate to the social situation in which they were reared, the "folk" society of a mountain cove. It is inappropriate to the industrial situation in which they now work. Consequently, increasing length of service does not increase adaptation to the factory situation as easily as it does in their second generation colleagues. For these the change from home to factory represents far less culture change in that their rearing has equipped them more adequately to anticipate and adjust to the demands made upon them by factory life.

The Carolina division, being situated in a rural area, is likely to have a greater preponderance of workers who have recently undergone this culture change than are the divisions of the Company which are situated in urban centers. The majority of industries in the country are also likely to have fewer "new industrial" workers on their payroll than is the case in this factory. In terms of the hypothesis developed in this paper these factors would account for the disability rates being higher in this population than in other divisions of the Company or the nation as a whole.

Despite the consistency of the findings of this study with our original conceptual scheme we recognize that they could be accounted for by various alternate hypotheses. Of these the possibility of selection factors is one of the more difficult to discount. By selection factors we mean the possibility that first generation workers differed from those in the second generation, not because of the recency of their culture change, but because they were sick or more predisposed to illness before seeking employment in the factory. This selection may have occurred either because first generation workers were representatives of a sicker population than were the second generation, or because those first generation individuals who left the farm to seek employment were the more maladjusted members of their group. To determine definitively whether such selection factors were accounting for our findings, it would be necessary to design a prospective study of the families of potential first and second generation employees and examine such employees before and after entering the factory. The probability that such selection factors accounted for a major portion of our findings is reduced though not eliminated by the Company policy requiring pre-employment medical examinations for each of its prospective employees. Thus any individuals with major medical abnormalities would not have been employed.

From our point of view, the major value of these findings lies in the direction they provide for further studies. One series of additional studies will need to be concerned with attempting to replicate these findings in widely differing groups. Such studies are needed not only to validate these findings but also to indicate the circumstances under which the postulated processes do and do not operate.

A second series will need to concentrate on developing instruments to test the general proposition in a more direct fashion. Such studies can address themselves to the following questions:

1. Are there in fact greater incongruities between the culture of first generation workers and their social situation than in the second generation?
2. Do the second generation "sick" group resemble the first generation "sick" group in terms of cultural incongruities more than they resemble other second generation workers?
3. Do the first generation "not sick" group resemble the second generation "not sick" group in terms of cultural incongruity more than they resemble the "sick" first generation group?

To carry out such studies it will be necessary to develop instruments to measure selected cultural attributes and to utilize more refined health indices than were used in the present study. We are currently in the process of developing these instruments.

If these further studies confirm the utility of our conceptual scheme, it will then be possible to ask the further question. Under what circumstances does rapid culture change lead to a poor state of health and high absenteeism? Is this equally true, for example, in workers who make this change together with their family as it is in single workers? Does company policy influence the effects of such change? Are the effects of such change in any way modified by neighborhood of living? These and similar questions

may provide clues as to what action is necessary and feasible if we wish to protect the health or increase the efficiency of workers in industry, without waiting until they become overtly ill or inefficient before taking action.

It is with great pleasure that we acknowledge our indebtedness to Dr. Logan T. Robertson, Consultant, Occupational Medicine, for making these data to readily available to us. We would also like to express our gratitude to Mr. Reuben Robertson, Sr., for his encouragement and financial support which made this study feasible.

References

(1) Simmons, L.W. and H.G. Wolff. *Social Science in Medicine.* New York, Russell Sage Foundation, 1954.

(2) Caudill, W. *Effects of Social and Cultural Systems in Reactions to Stress,* Social Science Research Council Pamphlet No. 14, June 1958.

(3) Galdston, I. (Ed). *Beyond the Germ Theory,* New York, Health Education Council, 1954.

(4) Epidemiology of cardiovascular disease: Cultural, societal, familial, psychological, and genetic influences. *Am J Public Health* (Supp.) 50:71-89, 1960.

(5) Slotkin, J.S. Culture and psychopathology. *J Abnorm Soc Psychol* 51:269-275, 1955.

(6) Hinkle, L.E. and H.G. Wolff. The nature of man's adaptation to his total environment and the relation of this to illness. *AMA Arch Intern Med* 99:442-460, 1957.

(7) Hinkle, L.E., et al. Ecologic investigations of the relationship between illness, life experiences, and social environment. *Ann Intern Med* 49:1373-1388, 1958.

(8) Mangus, A.R. Medical sociology: study of the social components of illness and health. *Sociol Soc Research* 39:158-164, 1955.

(9) Simmons, L.W. The relation between the decline of anxiety inducing and anxiety resolving factors in a deteriorating culture and its relevance to bodily disease. In *Life Stress and Bodily Disease,* (research publication of the Association for Research in Nervous and Mental Diseases). Baltimore, MD, Williams and Wilkins Company, 1950. Chap. 9, p. 29.

(10) *Interrelations Between the Social Environment and Psychiatric Disorders.* New York, Milbank Memorial Fund, 1953.

(11) Cassel, J., R. Patrick, and D. Jenkins. Epidemiological analysis of the health implications of culture change: A conceptual model. *Ann NY Acad Sci* 84:938-949, 1960.

(12) Health Statistics from *U.S. National Health Survey,* Series B10, May 1950.

(13) Brodman, K., A.J. Erdmann, Jr., I. Lorge, and H.G. Wolff. The Cornell Medical Index: An adjunct to medical interview. *JAMA* 140:530-534, 1949.

(14) Brodman, K., A.J. Erdmann, Jr., I. Lorge, and

H.G. Wolff. The Cornell Medical Index Health Questionnaire: II. As a diagnostic instrument. *JAMA* 145: 152-157, 1951.

(15) Brodman, K., A.J. Erdmann, Jr., I. Lorge, C. Gershenson, and H.G. Wolff. The Cornell Medical Index-Health Questionnaire: III. The evaluation of emotional disturbances in a general hospital. *J Clin Psychol* 8:289-293, 1952.

(16) Brodman, K., A.J. Erdmann, Jr., I. Lorge, C. Gershenson, and H.G. Wolff. The Cornell Medical Index-Health Questionnaire: IV. The recognition of emotional disturbances in a general hospital. *J Clin Psychol* 8:289-293, 1952.

(17) Erdmann, A.J., Jr., K. Brodman, I. Lorge, and H.G. Wolff. The Cornell Medical Index-Health Questionnaires: V. The outpatient admitting department of a general hospital. *JAMA* 149:550-551, 1952.

(18) Brodman, K., A.J. Erdmann, Jr., I. Lorge, and H.G. Wolff. The Cornell Medical Index-Health Questionnaire: VI. The relation of patients' complaints to age, sex, race, and education. *J Geront* 8:339-342, 1953.

(19) Brodman, K., A.J. Erdmann, Jr., I. Lorge, J. Deutschberger, and H.G. Wolff. The Cornell Medical Index-Health Questionnaire: VII. The prediction of psychosomatic and psychiatric disabilities in army training. *Am J Psychiat* 111:37-40, 1954.

(20) Erdmann, A.J., Jr., K. Brodman, J. Deutschberger, and H.G. Wolff. Health questionnaire use in an industrial medical department. *Industr Med Surg* 22:355-357, 1953.

(21) Brodman, K.J., Deutschberger, A.J. Erdmann, Jr., I. Lorge, and H.G. Wolff. Prediction of adequacy for military service. *U.S. Armed Forces Med J* 5:1802-1808, 1954.

(22) Hinkle, L.E., Jr. and N. Plummer. Life stress and industrial absenteeism: Concentration of illness and absenteeism in one segment of the working population. *Industr Med Surg* 21:363-375, 1952.

(23) Hinkle, L.E. et al. Studies in human ecology: factors relevant in the occurrence of bodily illness and disturbances in mood, thought, and behavior in 3 homogeneous population groups. *Am J Psychiatry* 114:212-220, 1957.

SCHIZOPHRENIA AND SOCIAL CLASS

E. M. Goldberg[1] and S. L. Morrison[2]

Since Faris and Dunham (1) found that the mental hospital admission rate for schizophrenia was higher in the central slum districts of Chicago than in the rest of the city, many studies have been carried out on the association between low social status and hospital admission with a diagnosis of schizophrenia. With few exceptions (2, 3) these studies have confirmed that those in the lowest social group (in this country class V in the Registrar-General's scheme) have the highest admission rates. Some of these investigations have been "ecological" or "indirect;" i.e., admission rates have been calculated for areas of a city defined, for example, as slum, working, or middle class areas, and the rates for these areas compared; other studies have been "individual" or "direct," where admission rates have been calculated for aggregates of individuals, defined as belonging to particular social classes, and the rates for the classes compared. An ecological study, like that of Faris and Dunham, may show that rates are higher in poor districts, but it does not necessarily follow that the patients admitted are themselves poor. Individual studies, however, do show that men in unskilled jobs have the highest admission rates.

To pursue the implications of the association between low social class and high admission rates for schizophrenia it is necessary to decide whether or not this association is due to the illness itself. Do men, before their first admission to mental hospital, drift down the occupation scale to unskilled jobs because of their premorbid personality or developing illness? The alternative explanation, that a high proportion of these patients are born into families with a lower social class distribution than normal, would suggest that socio-economic factors play a part in etiology. The "drift" hypothesis might also extend to the fathers of patients. Perhaps

genetic (or familial) elements in schizophrenia show themselves by a tendency for the parental generation to drift down in social class from the grandparents, and further drift by the patients themselves then leads to their known social class distribution.

We decided to carry out a clinical study of young men admitted to two mental hospitals and of their families, in an attempt to answer this and other questions. We planned to study all patients admitted, irrespective of diagnosis, in order (a) to obtain a group of patients where the diagnosis of schizophrenia had been specially assessed by psychiatrists, and (b) to compare our findings on schizophrenic patients with data on men suffering from other conditions. We investigated in detail the occupational histories of the patients themselves, of their fathers, and as far as possible of their grandfathers, uncles and siblings. (Other factors studied, including family attitudes and relationships, will be reported elsewhere.) We expected to find the usual excess of men in class V among the schizophrenic patients; we also wanted to find out whether their fathers showed this excess and, if so, whether the fathers had moved down from a more "normal" class distribution of grandfathers.

Soon after the study began we found that the patients showed the expected concentration in unskilled jobs, but their fathers appeared to represent a typical occupational sample of the population at the time of their sons' admission to a mental hospital. At this point we decided to carry out a large scale documentary study with the help of the General Register Office to complement the continuing clinical study of patients and their families. For clarity of exposition, the findings of the national documentary survey will be presented before those of the clinical study.

Source: *British Journal of Psychiatry* 109:785–802, 1963.
[1] Medical Research Council's Social Medicine Research Unit, London Hospital, London.
[2] Department of Public Health and Social Medicine, Usher Institute, Warrender Park Road, Edinburgh.

PART I. DOCUMENTARY STUDY

The object of this study was to test the hypothesis that young male patients on first admission to mental hospitals with a diagnosis of schizophrenia, while themselves having a marked excess of class V jobs immediately before their first admission, had been born into families with a similar social class composition to that of the general population.

Method

The General Register Office receives a card giving, *inter alia,* the name, date of birth, occupation and diagnosis of every patient admitted to a mental hospital in England and Wales. The Registrar General kindly agreed to draw a sample of these cards and then to search the birth records for the recorded details of each patient at birth. These include the occupation of the father at the time of the patient's birth. It would therefore be possible to establish the social class of the patient at the time of his admission to hospital and the social class of his father at the time of the patient's birth, and to compare the two distributions.

The sample was drawn from first admissions in 1956 of men aged 20–34 years at the time of admission. This age group was chosen to correspond with the age group of their fathers when the patients were born. It was intended to deal particularly with patients aged 25–34 years who could be presumed to have reached a reasonably "final" occupational status, the normal age of apprenticeship and studentship being well past.

Since the cards were filed alphabetically the sample was drawn by selecting all the cards for surnames beginning with the letters A to H, a total of 672 cards. It is therefore not a strictly random sample.[3]

The extraction of the cards and the tracing of the birth entries were carried out in the General Register Office by their own staff and the results were given to us only after names and addresses had been removed.

Of the 672 birth entries sought, 509 were found (75 percent); a large proportion of the patients whose entry could not be found had foreign names and were probably born abroad.

Results

In Table 1 the social class distribution of patients aged 25–34 years at the time of their first admission is compared with the 1951 Census distribution of all occupied men of the same age. The distribution shows the usual excess of patients in social class V (90 observed against 39 expected). The Table also compares the social class of the fathers at the time of the patients' birth with that of all occupied men aged 20–44 at the 1931 Census, i.e., it is assumed that the fathers were in that age group and that the patients were born around 1930. This comparison shows that the social class of the fathers is very similar indeed to that of the population as a whole and thus corroborates the hypothesis.

---

[3] The sample was drawn in two halves at different times. Results from the first half were reported earlier (*4*). Both halves gave very similar results and they are combined and treated as one sample in this paper.

Table 1. Social class distribution of schizophrenic patients and their fathers (male first admissions aged 25–34 years, England and Wales, 1956).

Social class	Patients at admission		Fathers at patients' birth	
	Observed	Expected[a]	Observed	Expected[b]
I	12	12	14	8
II	21	44	42	42
III	178	203	192	192
IV	52	55	66	68
V	90	39	55	59
Total	353	353	369	369
Not stated	18		2	

[a] From 1951 Census distribution of men aged 25–34.
[b] From 1931 Census distribution of men aged 20–44.

Table 2 illustrates the movements in social class between fathers and sons for the 351 patients for whom a social class could be allocated to both patients and fathers. There is both upward and downward mobility from father to son, but more down than up.

The results for men aged 20–24 are difficult to interpret and will not be dealt with. The patients show an excess in class V but the fathers do not resemble the general population as closely as do the fathers of patients aged 25–34. Numbers are much smaller and a further sample is needed.

Discussion

The results of this documentary study show that the patients aged 25–34 were born into families with a social class distribution very similar to that of the population as a whole. Thus the socio-economic environment in which these schizophrenic patients grew up seems unlikely to be grossly abnormal and it is unlikely therefore to be a major factor in the development of the disease. This finding is very different from that of Hollingshead and Redlich (5) and possible reasons for the difference are discussed later.

The documentary study leaves many questions unanswered. The clinical study, with fewer cases, attempts to answer some of these, and to clothe the skeleton of the documentary study. Thus it was designed to show whether, when a more rigorous diagnosis of schizophrenia was used than was possible in the documentary study, the families still showed a normal social class distribution; and to explore in detail the differences in kinds of occupation followed by fathers and sons. Moreover, the clinical study was designed to describe the occupational and educational history of the patients and to find

out at what stage of their careers they had fallen below the usual expectations of boys from a given social class; for example, had many of those in class V "drifted" down from better jobs, or had they never held better jobs?

PART II. CLINICAL STUDY

Part I demonstrated that the fathers of a national sample of young male schizophrenic patients had at the time of the patients' births an occupational distribution very similar to that of the general population, whereas the patients themselves showed an excess in social class V. This finding suggests that social "drift" occurs, since a considerable proportion of the schizophrenic patients in semi- and unskilled work were not born into social class V homes. However, the documentary study, based on two points only in a chain of events, cannot throw much light on the processes which may account for the drift. For example: are the fathers of schizophrenic patients somewhat inadequate and unstable people who tend to deteriorate in their own work performance later in life and drift into inferior neighborhoods, thus limiting the opportunities of their children? Is social inadequacy noticeable in other male relatives in the family, in the brothers, the grandfathers and uncles; or is the drift confined to the schizophrenic sons?

To learn more about the processes whereby schizophrenic patients are concentrated in the lower social classes, we made an intensive study of a series of consecutive admissions of men under 30 at two mental hospitals.

Hospital A receives patients from two contrasting boroughs. One is a rapidly expanding suburban community of increasing affluence in Greater London, the other a working-class dis-

Table 2. Social class of schizophrenic patients in relation to that of their fathers (male first admissions aged 25–34 years, England and Wales, 1956).

Social class of patients at admission	Social class of fathers at patients' birth					
	I	II	III	IV	V	Total
I	2	7	2	1	—	12
II	3	7	10	1	—	21
III	8	16	105	25	24	178
IV	—	4	23	19	4	50
V	—	4	43	19	24	90
Total	13	38	183	65	52	351

trict with a declining population adjoining the London docks. The hospital is situated within its catchment area, and we have reason to believe that few local patients are admitted to other mental hospitals. Hospital A thus offers good opportunities for studying occupational mobility, both because of the composition of its local population and because of its coverage.

Hospital B caters to a mainly working-class area in East London whose population has been declining for many years and whose successful citizens tend to "emigrate." The hospital, moreover, is situated 20 miles from its catchment area, and there is evidence that a proportion of patients suffering their first attack of mental illness are admitted to other hospitals. Studies of social mobility are therefore difficult in this area. For this reason we shall concentrate on the findings from the study carried out at Hospital A.

The Samples

In Hospital A we studied all males under 30 admitted between January, 1958 and December, 1960 whose parents lived in Great Britain. This sample will be called the A sample. Since we wanted to investigate inter-generation as well as personal social mobility, and to compare these findings with local census data, foreign-born patients, and also Irish patients whose families were resident in Eire, were excluded from intensive study. Severely subnormal patients and epileptics were also excluded. On all these "excluded" cases as much information as possible was gathered from hospital records and from the patients themselves, though not from the parents. (A detailed description of the patients excluded from the study is given in the Appendix.)

In Hospital B we studied all male patients under 30 admitted between March 1959 and April 1960, similarly excluding foreign-born and Irish and severely subnormal and epileptic patients. This sample will be called the B sample.

Diagnosis

Psychiatrists at the two hospitals kindly undertook to allocate the patients in the study, after a suitable period of observation, to three diagnostic categories: "definitely schizophrenic" (S), "possibly schizophrenic" (PS), and "definitely not schizophrenic" (NS). In 1961 a follow-up study was carried out on all the patients in the A and B samples and after its completion the Consultant Psychiatrist to this Unit, in collaboration with the hospital psychiatrists, reviewed the diagnoses in the light of all the information then available. Thus some patients classified initially as "possibly schizophrenic" had revealed themselves as "definitely schizophrenic;" and others as clearly "not schizophrenic." On the other hand the diagnosis of a few patients originally classified as "definitely schizophrenic" became doubtful in the light of subsequent developments and they were finally regarded as "possibly schizophrenic." The important point is that the group of *"definitely schizophrenic"* patients probably contained those who would generally be diagnosed as schizophrenic by psychiatrists in this country. They all showed, at some stage in their illness, delusions, hallucinations, ideas of reference and/or influence, incongruity and/or flattening of affect.

About half of the "possibly schizophrenic" patients had a short schizophrenia-like illness with an acute onset, returning quickly to normal life. Five had a long-drawn-out illness with vague schizoid symptoms and the rest showed a very mixed picture.

The "not schizophrenic" group contained a number of behavior disorders, various forms of anxiety neuroses and some cases of organic psychosis.[4]

The age distribution of the samples, and the numbers in the different diagnostic categories, are shown in Table 3.

It will be noticed that nearly half the schizophrenic patients in Hospital A were first admissions compared to less than a quarter in Hospital B. Only one-fifth of the schizophrenic patients in Hospital A had three or more previous admissions compared to nearly half in Hospital B. Furthermore, one-third of the Hospital B patients were admitted to other hospitals on their first attack compared to only three patients in the A sample. Thus the admissions to Hospital A probably represent a reasonable sample of all admissions from the catchment area while those in Hospital B are clearly an unrepresentative sample. This is an additional reason for concentrating our discussion on the findings of Hospital A.

---

[4] The final diagnoses of the 33 "not schizophrenic" patients in A were: anxiety states, 16; behavior disorder, 8; psychopathic personality, 5; organic psychosis, 4.

Table 3. Age distribution at sample admission according to "final" diagnosis[a] (clinical sample of consecutive male admissions to two mental hospitals).

	Hospital A				Hospital B			
Age	S	PS	NS	Total	S	PS	NS	Total
15–19	4	6	9	19	4	1	4	9
20–24	14	5	16	35	16	0	4	20
25–29	34	5	8	47	22	1	12	35
Total	52	16	33	101	42	2	20	64
Mean age	25	22	22		25	21	24	

[a] Diagnosis after review by Unit Psychiatrist, 1962.

Since we are mainly concerned with the problems of social mobility in schizophrenia, we shall disregard the "possibly schizophrenic" group as their diagnosis is uncertain.

Method of Study

The patients were seen in hospital soon after their admission and as much school and work history as possible was obtained from them. Relevant details from the patients' history were extracted from the hospital records. With the patients' and psychiatrists' permission the parents were then visited. The fathers' occupational histories were explored in considerable detail, and we also tried to get information on the main jobs of the paternal and maternal grandfathers, the paternal uncles, and the siblings of the patients. The patients' own school and work histories were discussed in detail. Follow-up visits were paid to parents or other key relatives during 1961 and special attention was again given to the employment situation of the patients. In addition to the information gathered in interviews, school reports were obtained on most patients, and the General Register Office kindly sought their birth records and found them in all but a few cases.

RESULTS

Social Class of Fathers and Sons

As in the documentary study, Part I, we compared the social class distribution of patients at the time of their first admission to hospital with that of occupied men in their areas of residence at the 1951 Census. We similarly compared the fathers at the time of the patients' birth with local men at the 1931 Census (Table 4).

Table 4. Social class distribution of schizophrenic patients on first admission and of their fathers at patients' birth (clinical sample of schizophrenic male admissions to two mental hospitals).

	Patients at admission				Fathers at patients' birth			
	Hospital A		Hospital B		Hospital A		Hospital B	
Social class	Observed	Expected	Observed	Expected[a]	Observed	Expected[b]	Observed	Expected[b]
I and II	2	8	—	4	7	8	1	4
III	21	23	16	21	28	26	15	19
IV and V	21	13	24	15	15	16	21	14
Total	44	44	40	40	50	50	37	37
Students	6		—					
School	—		1					
No occupation	2		1					
Not known	—				2		5	

[a] From 1951 Census distribution of all occupied males in their area of residence.
[b] From 1931 Census distribution of all occupied males in their area of residence.

In both hospitals there is an excess of patients in classes IV and V[5] compared with local men and a deficiency in classes I and II. These findings are similar to the national study. The social class distribution of the fathers in Hospital A at the time of their sons' birth was very close to that of other men in their areas of residence, again confirming the results of the documentary study. The picture is less clear in East London (Hospital B). Here there is an appreciable excess of fathers in classes IV and V and deficiency in classes I, II and III. However, when the jobs the East London fathers held around 1951 are compared with those of men residing in the same boroughs at the 1951 Census, the observed and expected figures are very close indeed (Table 5). This suggests that although the East London fathers possibly did not do as well as one might have expected at the time of their sons' birth, they were very similar to the ordinary run of local people at a later stage of their working lives.

The Work Careers of the Fathers

The first question that arises is whether the fathers were really as "normal" in their occupational achievements as the figures suggest. Perhaps the entries on the birth certificates conveyed an inflated notion of the actual jobs (although they tallied remarkably well with the

Table 5. Hospital B. The fathers' main jobs compared with all occupied males in their areas of residence in 1951 (clinical sample of schizophrenic male admissions to Hospital B).

Social class	Observed	Expected
I and II	3	4
III	22	21
IV and V	16	16
Total	41	41
N.K.	1	

information given to the investigators at the time of the interviews). Perhaps their performance deteriorated later on in life?

If three readings are taken of the fathers' work histories: (1) the job held when the patient was born, (2) their main job defined as the one held the longest, and (3) the last job, it can be seen (Table 6) that the job levels of the fathers of Hospital A patients rise appreciably during their career. Twenty-nine percent reach social classes I and II in their main job; there is then some expected decline in the last job and the proportion in social classes IV and V increases. The fathers of Hospital B patients also improved their work status. These figures reflect fairly solid and successful work careers, and this observation is confirmed by the steadiness with which most of the fathers worked. Thirty-eight in Sample A held their main jobs for 20 years or more, 29 of them remaining in the same firm or service throughout this period. Only four had many different jobs in short succession, and all these men were found to be unstable in other respects.

[5] Since the numbers in this clinical study are so small we decided to combine social classes I and II, and IV and V, for easier comparison, although in the documentary study the five classes have been kept separate.

Table 6. Social class distribution of fathers of schizophrenic patients; (1) at patient's birth, (2) main job, (3) present or last job (clinical sample of schizophrenic male admissions to two mental hospitals).

	Hospital A						Hospital B					
	Job at patient's birth (1)		Main job (2)		Present or last job (3)		Job at patient's birth (1)		Main job (2)		Present or last job (3)	
Social class	No.	%	No.	%	No.	%	No.	%	No.	%	No.	%
I and II	7	14	15	29	13	26	1	3	3	7	4	10
III	28	56	25	48	22	43	15	40	22	54	17	45
IV and V	15	30	12	23	16	31	21	57	16	39	17	45
Total	50	100	52	100	51	100	37	100	41	100	38	100
Not known	2				1		5		1		4	

Table 7. Social class mobility of fathers of schizophrenic patients in three areas (clinical sample of schizophrenic male admissions to two mental hospitals).

	Hospital A								Hospital B			
	Suburban borough				Working-class borough				East London			
	Father's job at patient's birth		Father's main job		Father's job at patient's birth		Father's main job		Father's job at patient's birth		Father's main job	
Social class	No.	%	No.	%	No.	%	No.	%	No.	%	No.	%
I and II	7	24	13	45	—	—	2	9	1	3	3	7
III	18	62	13	45	10	48	12	52	15	40	22	54
IV and V	4	14	3	10	11	52	9	39	21	57	16	39
Total	29	100	29	100	21	100	23	100	37	100	41	100
Not known	—		—		2		—		5		1	

Another way of testing the "normality" of the fathers' social class attributes is to enquire whether the careers of the fathers living in the more affluent borough are markedly different from those living in the working-class areas. They are, as Table 7 shows.

Ten percent of the fathers in the suburban borough are in social classes IV and V against 39 percent in the working-class area. Nearly half of the suburban fathers, most of whom where born in the borough, rise to positions in social classes I and II, whereas barely 10 percent do so in the other borough. It will be noticed that the social class distribution of the fathers in this borough is very similar to that of the fathers in East London. This is as expected since, according to the Registrar-General, the social class composition of these areas is very similar (see Table 8).

It may be objected that the Registrar-General's classifications are not a very sensitive index of social performance, but there is further evidence that these fathers are indeed successful workers, as suggested by this classification.

Table 9 shows that the careers of the fathers who reach social classes I and II in their main jobs are consistent in all but possibly one case. We thus have reason to believe that the entries on the patients' birth certificates correspond with the facts. If we take another index of the fathers' social circumstances, namely, the nature of their housing, we notice that all but three whose accommodation is related to their jobs, own their houses. (Two of three in tied accommodation, now nearing retirement, are looking for houses to buy; the third man died during the course of the study.)

The fathers in the B sample also reflect fairly accurately the general run of occupations prevalent in the district in which they live. For example, a number of them are tailors and dock workers. However, only one of the fathers reached social class II in his main job (a tailor with his own business), the other two fathers whose main jobs were in social class II have been living outside London for a long time.

Social Class of Other Male Relatives

We also enquired into the occupations of grandfathers, uncles and brothers of patients and found (Table 10) that they showed a similar class distribution to the fathers.

It seems then that the schizophrenic patients in the A sample came from families whose work performance and general social status were in accordance with the standards in their local communities. The poor work performance of

Table 8. Social class distribution of employed males (percentages) 1951 Census.

Social class	Working-class Borough	East London
I and II	9	9
III	49	52
IV and V	42	39
	100%	100%

Table 9. Work histories of fathers in social classes I and II (main job) and their housing conditions (clinical sample of schizophrenic male admissions to Hospital A).

Patient No.	Job at patient's birth	Main job	Housing conditions
S2	Estate Supt., County Council	Estate Supt., County Council	Council house
S3	Grocery Manager	Grocery Manager	Flat tied to shop
S9	Not known (Publican)[a]	Manager/Publican	Flat tied to off-license
S15	Manager/Wine Merchant	Manager Wine Shop	Own house
S20	Carpet Salesman	Buyer (carpets)	Own house
S21	Publisher's Clerk	Costing Clerk	Own house
S24	Plate Glass Merchant	Mirror Manufacturer	Own house
S26	Insurance Claims Supt.	Insurance Claims Supt.	Own house
S27	Schoolmaster	Head of Dept. of Languages	Own house
S28	Stoker	Senior Fuel Engineer	Own house
S35	Tailor (master)	Tailor (own workshop)	Own house
S38	Fishmonger	Fishmonger (own business)	Own house
S45	Grocer (own business)	Accountant	Own house
S48	Employment Clerk, M.O.L.	Superintendent, M.O.L.	Own house
S52	Meat Importer's Clerk	Manager, Shipping Firm	Own house

[a] Although the patient's birth certificate could not be found, the occupational history taken at the interview indicates that the father was the manager of a pub at the time of the patient's birth.

Table 10. Social class of fathers, paternal and maternal grandfathers, brothers and schizophrenic patients (clinical sample of schizophrenic male admissions to Hospital A).

	Father		Other male relatives								Patient	
	Main job		Paternal grandfather; main job		Maternal grandfather; main job		Paternal uncles;[a] main job		Brothers;[b] main job		Last job; 1st admission	
Social class	No.	%	No.	%	No.	%	No.	%	No.	%	No.	%
I and II	15	29	13	28	10	20	23	25	8	21	2	4
III	25	48	23	50	26	51	58	63	22	56	21	48
IV and V	12	23	10	22	15	29	11	12	9	23	21	48
Total	52	100	46	100	51	100	92	100	39	100	44	100
School	—		—		—		—		3		—	
Student	—		—		—		—		—		6	
Nil	—		1		—		7		3		2	
Not known	—		5		1		19		1		—	

[a] In two families no information was obtainable on the number and jobs of paternal uncles.
[b] 46 brothers were related to 30 patients.

the schizophrenic patients cannot thus be blamed on the occupational models and influences surrounding them in childhood and adolescence in the nuclear and extended family.

The Occupational Careers of the Patients

So far the results of the clinical study indicate that two possible explanations for the association between social class and schizophrenia are unlikely; namely, the artefacts resulting from faulty classification of either social class or diagnosis (6).

It must next be asked how it has come about that nearly half of the patients who came from families with reasonable standards of economic and social security are in semi- or unskilled occupations before their first admission to hospital. Has their performance been poor from the start, or is there a process of deterioration?

Eighteen of the 52 schizophrenic patients from Hospital A (37 percent) went to grammar and technical schools and one to a minor public school (Table 11). This is a good showing compared with the national average of around 20 percent of children born in the early and mid-

Table 11. Type of school attended by schizophrenic patients and their brothers (clinical sample of schizophrenic male admissions to two mental hospitals).

Type of school	Hospital A				Hospital B			
	No.	%	No.	%	No.	%	No.	%
Grammar	13	25	9	20	1	2	9	14[a]
Technical	5	10	2	4	2	5	3	5
Secondary modern or equivalent	30	58	34	74	32	76	32	50
ESN	2	4	1	2	2	5	—	—
Maladjusted	1	2	—	—	—	—	—	—
Other	1	2	—	—	4	10	5	8
Not known	—	—	—	—	1	2	15	23
Total	52	100	46	100	42	100	64	100

[a] 6 out of the 9 (9 percent) attenders at Grammar School belong to one family living outside London.

dle thirties attaining selected secondary education (7). Furthermore, the schizophrenic patients in the sample compare favorably with their brothers, of whom only 24 percent gained places in grammar and technical schools. Yet, as we saw before (Table 10), the brothers achieved better occupational status than the patients. In Hospital B there is no suggestion that the patients did better than the brothers at school.

Up to adolescence, then, there appears to be no indication that future schizophrenic patients lag behind in their achievement. However, for some of the boys the difficulties related to work and achievement seem to have started in adolescence, as the careers of the grammar school boys illustrate well (Table 12). Several were reported by their headmasters as having been below average. One boy obtained four "A" level passes, but even he failed to get into the University of his choice, slowly deteriorated during his course of study, and failed in his "finals." Another boy embarked on an academic course with great difficulty and eventually failed. Two attempted an Arts course, and one trained for the priesthood but had to abandon it in his fourth year. Only one patient qualified in a profession and is now practicing it. Thus with one exception, none of the grammar school boys in the sample completed any kind of professional or technical training and most of them ended up in routine clerical or laboring jobs. There is some evidence that these patients, despite their innate ability, seek routine jobs with strictly limited responsibility. Several were offered promotion; two refused, and two actually "tried to

be in charge"; but one broke down under the strain, the other went back to his routine job. The deterioration of performance among so many grammar school boys towards the latter years at school strongly suggests an insidious onset of the illness long before symptoms become apparent, since most of the boys were considered "well-adjusted" by their schoolteachers.

A feature worth noting is that most of the fathers of the grammar school boys and of those embarking on further training were in social classes I and II. Thus, to begin with, the boys fulfilled the normal expectations of their social environment, for there is still a strong relationship between social class of father and attainment of grammar school places (7, 8).

There were other boys who, though not attending grammar school, had shown promise in their pre-adolescent years and whose disturbances became marked around puberty. They, too, had jobs of an inferior type in comparison with their fathers. For example, one patient, whose father was an artist, went to a technical school, only worked for a short spell as a book packer and was admitted to hospital for the first time at the age of 16. Another boy, the son of a shop manager, became so disturbed at a boarding school that he had to leave. He completed his education at the local secondary modern school and was only able to work irregularly as a laborer before breaking down finally a few weeks after joining the forces at the age of 18.

In contrast, there were those patients who had worked in skilled trades for a considerable

Table 12. School and job history of grammar school boys (clinical sample of schizophrenic male admissions to Hospital A).

Patient No.	Father S.C.	School report	Further training	Job history
S3	II	Vth A stream; 2 "O" levels. Left 16-1/2.	Tried evening classes, draughtsman. Too much effort.	Routine clerical 3 years. Training course radio mechanic. Now radio repairer.
S4	V	Left 14. Homework difficult.	Nil.	Clerical jobs; little unemployment despite many admissions. Now shop assistant.
S5	(mother) II	Vth C stream; 3 "O" levels. Left 16½.	Nil.	Shop assistant, clerk. Helped in relative's shop. Much unemployment; many admissions. Suicide 1961.
S9	II	Below average. No G.C.E. Left 16.	RC Seminary 4 years. Failed.	Failed as clerk. Now messenger.
S12	III	Failed G.C.E. "A" level.	Now evening classes in chemistry.	Nil 4 years till admission. Started laboratory assistant job from hospital.
S13	III	Average Vth. Left 15½. Insisted on doing carpentry.	Apprenticed carpentry.	Carpentry with many gaps of unemployment.
S15	II	Had to repeat 3 subjects "A" level.	Dentistry.	Qualified aged 26 after 3 admissions. Practicing.
S24	I	VIth, below average. Passed mock matric. Left 16 (F. ill).	Crammers college. Failed matric. twice. Breakdown after first part finals.	In parents' business short while. No work or study for about 6 years. In hospital 4 years.
S26	I	Lower Vth. Above average. Exemption matric., distinction 4 subjects.	Nil; father could not afford.	Assistant in bookshop. 7 years at very low salary. Clerk after discharge. Now lorry driver's mate.
S27	I	Minor public school. School certificate.	Art Course Technical College. Interrupted by first illness.	Laboring jobs between many admissions. Now despatch porter.
S31	III	2 years VIa; above average; 8 "O" levels. Left 19.	Nil.	Odd clerical. Long gaps at home. Now porter British Railways.
S40	II	Vth 2 years. Below average. Failed 2 attempts G.C.E.	Nil.	Booking clerk 6 years. No work since discharge 2½ years ago.
S41	III	Below average; left 15½. Refused to return after summer holidays.	Royal Academy of Art. Excluded.	Intermittent laboring between admissions. Not worked for 3 years.
S48	II	4 "A" levels.	Science Course University. Failed finals.	Laboratory technician.

period until they sank to the level of a laboring job shortly before their first admission to hospital. A shipwright, whose father was a painter and decorator, became a laborer two months before his first admission, as he could not contain his delusions any longer while at sea; a capstan turner, the son of a ship's painter, became a laborer four months before going into hospital for the first time, as he could not concentrate on any precision work any longer; a qualified marine engineer, whose father was a buyer in a big firm, and who had emigrated to Canada as a youth, came home on board a ship as a greaser, already disturbed; and a young butcher, the son of a clerk, ended up as a chicken cleaner a few weeks before his first admission to hospital.

Another small group of patients had very different social class positions from their fathers mainly because they were subnormal as well as mentally ill and had no hope of achieving more than a laboring job.

Thus either prolonged illness, or in a few cases subnormality, is mainly responsible for the big social gap between father and son; in the remaining cases, the discrepancies can often be accounted for by the patient's deterioration in performance shortly before his first admission to hospital. These observations indicate that some factor associated with the disease results in the patient's low social class position.

How this occupational drift gathers momentum as the illness continues can be seen clearly if we compare the actual jobs in which the patients were mainly employed before their first admission with the jobs they were doing at the time of the follow-up visit, when over half of the patients had been re-admitted at least once.

Before their first admission we can still observe a full range of occupations (Table 13). There are students, skilled workers and clerks, as well as semi- and unskilled laborers. The 15 patients who were excluded from the intensive sample show a similar spread (see Appendix)—there were two students among them, a highly trained instrument maker, several belonging to less skilled trades and three laborers.

The Drift Towards Inactivity

The picture changes considerably as the patient's illness continues; it may become quiescent, erupt from time to time in acute episodes or be a long, drawn-out, continuous illness.

Slowly their occupational status worsens and the breadth and mixture of jobs shrink continually. The students have only produced one professional person. A mere handful of highly skilled workers are left and the latest information (August, 1962) indicates that there are even fewer now. (The painter has become a chronic patient, the trainee telephonist has committed suicide, and the clerk is now a driver's mate.)

The number of patients who have given up work more or less permanently is growing steadily. If we consider students as potential candidates for social classes I and II, then the drift has been most serious in the highest social classes and least in the middle grades. Nearly two-thirds of the patients in skilled and semi-skilled work have been able to maintain their position while only a third of the unskilled workers (three out of 14) continued as laborers[6] and the rest have ceased work altogether (Table 13). Comparing these findings with the similar study carried out in Bristol (9) there is broad agreement on the drift from social classes III, IV and V. However, in Bristol 75 percent of the social class I and II patients have maintained their position. One explanation may be that Cooper allocated students (whose number is not stated) to their father's social class; this may help to obscure the drift process, for if the young men at the end of the study were still in some ways regarded as students they would still retain their father's social class. Another partial explanation of the discrepancies may be that although both studies refer to the patients' last job before first admission, Cooper's sample consisted entirely of first admissions, while our sample includes first and subsequent admissions. Our small sample also does not bear out fully the conclusion drawn from the Bristol study that the majority of the patients who drop from their original social class become "not gainfully employed." This only applies to social classes IV and V from which no further downward drift is possible—if a person cannot maintain an unskilled job then he is virtually unemployable. Another point is relevant here: the histories of those who drop into unemployment from social classes IV and V reveal that only four out of these 15 had always been laborers;

---

[6] Only three of the five laborers working at the end of the survey period had been laborers in their main pre-admission job. The fourth was an ex-clerk and the fifth an ex-student.

Table 13. Main jobs held by the schizophrenic patients before first admission and at follow-up[a] (clinical sample of schizophrenic male admissions to Hospital A).

	Main job before first admission			Job at end of survey period		
Students	Art	1		Dentist	1	1
	Dentistry	1				
	Law	1	5			
	Theology	1				
	Science	1				
Apprenticed trades	Instrument maker	2		Shipwright	1	
	Marine engineer	2		Turner	1	3
	Mechanical engineer	1	7	Welder	1	
	Shipwright	1				
	Welder	1				
Other skilled trades	Painter	2		Radio repairer	1	
	Plumber	1		Laboratory technicians	2	5
	Lettering artist	1				
	Machine minder (printing)	1	8			
	Butcher's cutter	1				
	Carpenter	1		Painter	1	
	Electrician	1		Trainee telephonist	1	
Clerical and selling	Clerk	9		Clerk	1	
	Sales representative	1	12	Shop assistant	1	2
	Shop assistant	2				
Semi-skilled	Capstan turner	1		Glue spreader	1	
	Machiner (tailor)	1	3	Seaman	1	
	Lathe operator	1		Loader, British Railways	1	
				Presser	1	
				Machiner (tailor)	1	9
				Glass worker	2	
				Despatch checker	1	
				Platen feeder	1	
Laborers	Factory	6	14	Outdoor	5	5
	Outdoor	8				
No occupation	School	2	3	At home (over 2 months)	12	27[b]
	At home	1		In hospital	15	
		52			52	

[a] These jobs refer to the patient's main activities before 1st admission, i.e., that he held longest, and is not comparable with earlier social class data which referred to the last job held before 1st admission.

[b] Of the 15 patients in hospital at the time of follow-up, 10 had been in hospital more or less continuously since the sample admission and 5 had varying periods of employment since their sample discharge. Of the 12 who were unemployed at home, 2 had been working for a short time since discharge.

the remainder had drifted down the social scale before their admission to hospital, from technical and grammar schools or from skilled jobs.

The picture is still more dismal in Hospital B where 16, nearly half the patients in the sample, have done no work since their last discharge, three have been in hospital continuously, 13 are laboring and only five are doing skilled work. No information is available on five patients, three of whom are vagrants whose families do not know where they are.

The Work Histories in the "Not Schizophrenic" Group

The situation is very different among these patients, and there is little downward drift as a result of the illness (Table 14). Although none of the apprentices have finished their training and they have all instead become semi- or unskilled workers, the shop assistant has become a manager, the sales representative a sales manager, and the steward a hotel manager. With

Table 14. Main jobs held by non-schizophrenic patients before first admission and during follow-up period (clinical sample of "not schizophrenic" patients admitted to Hospital A).

Category	First admission			Follow-up		
Students	Art	1	1			
Apprentices	Electrical engineering	2	3	Training course instrument making	1	1
	Engineering	1				
Managerial Posts				Manager shoe shop	1	3
				Sales manager	1	
				Assistant hotel manager	1	
Skilled Trades	Welder	1	7	Welder	1	6
	Turner	1		Turner	1	
	Painter	1		Painter	1	
	Bricklayer	1		Bricklayer	1	
	French polisher	1		P.O. technician	1	
	Engraver	1		Lorry driver	1	
	Plumber	1				
Clerical and Selling Service	Steward	1	7	Waiter	1	3
	Waiter	1				
	Sales representative	1		Shop assistant	1	
	Shop assistant	1		Clerk	1	
	Clerk	3				
Semi-skilled	Machine minders	2	4	Electrician's mate	1	7
	Furniture sprayer	1		Guillotine operator	1	
	Driver's mate	1		Machine operator	1	
				Sprayers	2	
				Window cleaner	1	
				Mortuary assistant	1	
Laborers	Factory	6	10	Factory	6	9
	Outdoor	4		Outdoor	3	
No occupation			1			3
Not known				Not known		1
Total			33			33

one exception—the engraver is now a guillotine operator—the skilled men have retained their skills. The two additions to the "no work" category consist of a young man who sustained organic brain damage in an accident, and a psychopath addicted to drugs, who also displays many schizoid and paranoid symptoms.

On the whole those who have done well and retained their skills suffer from neurotic and depressive disorders, while the semi- and unskilled patients contain a high proportion of psychopaths.

DISCUSSION

This study illustrates the complementary nature of the extensive and intensive study. The "hunch" from the clinical pilot study that the fathers of schizophrenic patients were normally distributed by occupation was confirmed in a national sample of patients, using their birth certificates as a source of information. In turn, the processes involved in occupational drift (clearly demonstrated in both studies) could only be explored through a sample of actual case histories.

The "Drift" Hypothesis

The finding that the fathers of schizophrenic patients represent a typical occupational cross-section of the community in which they live and that they have, on the whole, steady and solid work careers, does not imply that they are particularly well adjusted in other respects; that family relationships were undisturbed or, in particular, that their relations with their sick sons were positive. In a subsequent paper on family organization and relationships it will be shown that the father's steady achievement can create a wide gap between him and a "lazy," unsuccessful and disorganized son. Often the son is protected by his mother against a rather critical father for whom achievement is important. This is illustrated dramatically in a family in which the father is an accomplished linguist, engaged also in intellectual leisure pursuits, and the son, after a checkered career at a public school and some attempt at music, has become a laborer. This patient is deeply aware of his failure and wants his father's approbation, but is unable to achieve communication with him. The father, irritated and ashamed of his son, seems often to be on the edge of mental illness himself. This young man is now pursuing his portering job in the more relaxed atmosphere of working-class lodgings.

This study demonstrates that the process of drift can only be seen clearly if the social class of the family is distinguished from the social class of the patient. The remarkable phenomenon is that although many of these young patients lived in semi-detached villas, had fathers in good positions and attended grammar schools, they themselves eventually became routine clerks or semi- or unskilled workers. If we had classified the patients on an index in which place of residence and education were included, as Hollingshead and Redlich (5) have done, the process of drift caused mainly by the illness would have been obscured.

Hollingshead and Redlich's "index of social position" was arrived at by weighting scores for area of residence, education and occupation; they then placed individuals in one of five social classes according to the weighted score. Using this index, Hollingshead and Redlich found in their study of treated mental illness in New Haven that 91 percent of the schizophrenic patients were in the same class as their families of orientation; of their class V patients, 89 percent came from class V families. They therefore discounted the possibility of downward social mobility as an explanation of the excess of patients in class V. It is clear both from the descriptions of typical members of each class and from the percentage distribution of the population of New Haven in these classes, that they do not

correspond to the Registrar-General's five classes.[7] However, there does appear to be some similarity between class V in New Haven and in England; the proportions are similar and they both include mainly unskilled workers. A comparison of the *patients* in class V in the two studies shows that in our national sample aged 25–34 years, 25 percent were in class V, while Hollingshead and Redlich found 45 percent of their schizophrenic patients in class V. No fewer than 89 percent of the New Haven patients in class V came from class V families, while only 27 percent of class V patients in our national sample came from families in that class; and the percentage was even lower in the clinical samples.

Our studies have dealt only with schizophrenic patients admitted to mental hospitals and a possible explanation of the different results (10) found in New Haven might be that Hollingshead and Redlich were considering all patients under treatment, irrespective of whether or not they were in hospital. In fact, however, 92 percent of their schizophrenic patients were found in State and Veterans Administration Hospitals, of their class V schizophrenic patients, 98 percent were in such hospitals.

The greatest difficulty in comparison arises from another aspect of patient selection. We considered *first* admissions of young men to hospital in the documentary study and all *current* admissions in the clinical study. Hollingshead and Redlich studied what was in effect the population of chronic schizophrenics of both sexes and all ages in mental hospitals in 1950. They base their refutation of the drift hypothesis on 872 schizophrenic patients of both sexes and all ages, the great majority of whom were in hospital, and whose mean number of years under treatment there ranged from about 10 years for classes I and II to about 15 years for class V. Their findings, therefore, refer mainly to chronic long-stay patients in mental

---

[7] Social class distribution of men aged 25–34 in New Haven and England and Wales.

Social class	New Haven (%)	England and Wales (%)
I and II	10.7	15.6
III	23.1	57.8
IV	53.8	15.6
V	12.4	11.0

hospitals and are not comparable with ours. It is just conceivable that a follow-up of the patients in our clinical study in 10 years' time might show that those patients who had remained in hospital all the time were the class V men from class V families; a finding of this kind would be interesting, but irrelevant to the main question.

Occupational Factors

The observation in the clinical study that the potential candidates for classes I and II have done as badly as the patients in classes IV and V, while the patients in class III carrying out jobs involving some degree of repetitive skill seem to manage better, raises some speculations.

1. Perhaps a job which gives the patient a framework within which he has to carry out certain operations demanding little initiative or control of others, and little intellectual or emotional effort, is peculiarly fitted to the needs and capacities of the potential or actual schizophrenic patient.

2. The failure of students and of the few who tried to "run" businesses suggests that the disciplined intellectual effort and application required in most academic studies, advanced apprenticeship courses or managerial jobs require more ego-strength, control and initiative than even the most intelligent and gifted young schizophrenic patients can command.

3. It seems that the unskilled worker, whether he is in this position from the beginning of his working life or as a result of occupational drift, has little margin for maneuver and is thus at much greater risk than a skilled worker of dropping out of the labor market altogether. It is also possible that the unstructured nature of most unskilled work gives minimal support to a patient who appears to need something in the nature of a repetitive stimulus. Many forms of unskilled work may thus be distressful and unhelpful to schizophrenic patients.

These considerations are of course additional to the many other factors which must influence the patient's capacity to work: for example, the level of his intellectual and personality development before he becomes ill, the severity of the illness itself, as well as the degree of residual disability and the nature of his immediate environment.

Further Studies

Certain pointers towards studies in secondary prevention of schizophrenia, i.e., by early detection and treatment, emerge.

1. Special attention might be devoted to adolescent schoolchildren and to students who deteriorate in their performance and/or who fail in examinations without any apparent reason.

2. Further retrospective and prospective studies of schizophrenic students and young men already established in professional or managerial jobs may throw light on the factors favoring survival or leading to downward drift. Such studies may also help to clarify the rather different findings in the Bristol and the present study regarding the fate of class I and II patients.

3. Studies of *schizophrenic patients at work in all classes* might be as useful as studies carried out among patients in their family settings. While these studies will not help with the problems of etiology, they might specify those conditions of work which are suited to the needs of schizophrenic patients and those which seem harmful.

SUMMARY AND CONCLUSION

A *documentary* survey of a national sample of males aged 25–34 on their first admission to a mental hospital in England and Wales for schizophrenia showed the usual excess of patients in social class V. However, the social class distribution of the fathers at the time of the patients' birth was very similar to that of the population as a whole. A *clinical* study of a representative series of consecutive admissions of male schizophrenics aged 15–30 living in a socially mixed area in outer London confirms these findings. It shows decline in occupational status both from father to son and in the patients' own history.

The main evidence of individual downward "drift" is the ability of schizophrenic patients to win places at grammar schools, though they end in semi- or unskilled jobs. The employment histories showed that in their adolescence many patients pursued varied careers, a considerable proportion aiming at professional or technical jobs; they still fitted broadly with the career expectations of their home environment.

The discrepancies in social performance between father and son could be mainly attributed to the disease process. Patients whose illness had an insidious onset at adolescence did not attain any professional or technical skill; those whose illness started acutely before admission dropped in social class shortly before admission; while those who were mentally subnormal as well as schizophrenic did not achieve any level of skill at all.

This social drift appears to affect the highest and lowest social classes most severely. Only one patient out of 13 grammar school boys attained social class I or II status, and over half of those in social class V had dropped out of the labor market by the end of the survey. On the other hand, two-thirds of the patients in social classes III and IV survived in jobs requiring a moderate degree of skill.

These findings suggest that gross socio-economic deprivation is unlikely to be of major etiological significance in schizophrenia. On the other hand, occupational factors, yet to be defined clearly, appear to exert some influence on the course of the disease.

ACKNOWLEDGMENTS

We wish to acknowledge gratefully the help of Miss S. Ini, who carried out the field work among the patients and relatives of Hospital B. We are greatly indebted to the Medical Superintendents and psychiatrists at both hospitals, and to our psychiatric colleague in the Unit, Dr. E.

Shoenberg, all of whom gave much time and thought to the problems of diagnosis and classification. We also received invaluable help from Miss E. M. Brooke, Mr. I. Murray and Mr. G. Rhodes of the General Register Office; and from the records staff at the two hospitals. We further wish to thank the Headmasters and teachers of the patients' schools for their co-operation.

We are grateful to Professor J. N. Morris and other colleagues in the Social Medicine Research Unit for much help and advice.

References

(1) Faris, R.E.L. and H.W. Dunham. *Mental Disorders in Urban Areas* (edited by B. Pasamanick) Chicago, 1939.

(2) Clausen, J.A. and M.L. Kohn. Relation of schizophrenia to the social structure of a small city. In *Epidemiology of Mental Disorders* (edited by B. Pasamanick) Washington, 1959.

(3) Jaco, E.G. *Am Soc Rev* 19:567–577, 1954.

(4) Morrison, S.L. *J Ment Sci* 105:999, 1959.

(5) Hollingshead, A.B. and F.C. Redlich. *Class and Mental Illness* New York, 1958.

(6) Wardle, C.J. *Society, Problems and Methods of Study* (edited by Welford et al.) London, 1962.

(7) Floud, J.E., A.H. Halsey, and F.M. Martin. *Social Class and Educational Opportunity* London, 1958.

(8) Logan, R.F.L. and E.M. Goldberg. *Br J Sociol* 4:323, 1953.

(9) Cooper, B. *Br J Prev Soc Med* 15:17–30, 1961.

(10) Susser, M.W. and W. Watson. *Sociology in Medicine* London, 1962.

APPENDIX: Patients excluded from clinical study.

	Hospital A			Hospital B			
	S	PS	NS	S	PS	NS	NK
Social class (on sample admission):							
I and II	—	—	1	—	—	1	—
III	7	1	8	10	1	7	1
IV and V	5	—	6	15	4	4	1
Students	—	—	2	—	1	1	1
No occupation	—	—	4	2	—	2	—
Total	14	1	20	28	6	14	2
Mean age (years)	25	24	25	24	24	22	26

Reasons for exclusion:	A	B
Refusal by patient or relatives or considered by psychiatrist	5	3
Severe subnormality and/or epilepsy	9	3
Foreign born, and/or parents abroad or inaccessible	15	29
In hospital less than one week	5	10
Omitted by error	1	5
	35	50

EPIDEMIOLOGY OF CHILDHOOD LEUKEMIA IN NORTHUMBERLAND AND DURHAM

George Knox[1]

Our understanding of the etiology of leukemia is progressing rapidly. Differentiation of chronic myeloid leukemia through an abnormal chromosome 21, a high risk of acute leukemia in mongols, again with anomalies of chromosome 21, a demonstrated association between the risk of leukemia and the dose of radiation received, and between therapeutic irradiation and chromosomal anomalies, indicate the importance of chromosomal changes in many instances of the disease. At least one poison, benzene, is also known to have caused leukemia in man. On the basis of animal experiments it is possible that other poisons may do the same.

Nevertheless the known specific effects have so far been shown to be responsible for only a small proportion of the leukemias of childhood, and other known facts indicate the presence of unidentified causal factors. The disease seems to have been increasing in frequency, the risk to adults varies according to their occupation, an urban-rural differential of risk has been reported, a systematic variation in incidence from the northwest to the southeast of England has been demonstrated, a variation between states in the U.S.A. has been found, a seasonal variation of onset in children has been claimed, the multimodal curve of risk according to age suggests a number of separate and superimposed causes each operating maximally at different ages, and the historical development of the age pattern suggests that some of these causes have become important only in the last 30 years.

Leukemia has also been stated, on several occasions, to occur in clusters in space and in time with undue frequency. Kellett (1) was perhaps the first to point out this apparent feature, and more recently Pinkel and Nefzger (2) in Buffalo, N.Y., and Wood (3) in Cornwall, have made similar suggestions. If this could be sub-

stantiated, it would clearly be a fact of the greatest importance, particularly although not exclusively with respect to theories of virus etiology. I have tried elsewhere (4) to analyze the methodological and conceptual problems of the space-time cluster, particularly when we are dealing with a low intensity of events, as we are in leukemia. Briefly, it is proposed that the examination of such events requires a separate examination for the three components of epidemicity: (a) concentrations in space, over the whole of the time of the study: (b) concentrations in time over the whole of the area of the study; (c) interactions between space and time concentrations. Examination for the last component amounts to a search for movements of high concentration areas and the method proposed is the examination of all possible pairs, or a selection of them, to see whether short geographical distances are positively correlated with short time intervals.

The present paper is an analysis, both in these terms and by more orthodox methods, of the space and time distribution of childhood leukemia in the North of England over a period of 10 years.

MATERIAL AND METHODS

The cases of leukemia accepted for analysis were those (a) with onset before the 15th birthday, (b) which occurred within the geographical limits of Northumberland, Durham, and that strip of the North Riding of Yorkshire between the Cleveland Hills and the River Tees, (c) with onset between January 1, 1951, and December 31, 1960, a total of 10 years.

The region covered measures approximately 90 × 45 miles, the area is approximately 3100 square miles, the total population at the 1951 census was 2.48 million, and the number of children at risk in 1956 approximately 599 500.

The ascertainment method included: (a) the examination of the diagnostic indexes or the ward admission books for the years concerned, and the following year, at the hospitals listed in

Source: *British Journal of Preventive and Social Medicine* 18:17-24, 1964.
[1]Department of Child Health, University of Newcastle upon Tyne.

the Appendix; *(b)* scrutiny of the records of the regional Cancer Registration Bureau with secondary reference to the hospitals which registered cases not already ascertained; *(c)* examination of certificates of death due to leukemia in the years 1951 to 1960 up to the 17th birthday, with secondary reference to the hospital notes. When death had occurred in hospital this last examination was done directly, and when death had occurred at home by telephoning the doctor who signed the certificate and finding out which hospital had undertaken investigation and treatment.

In this way we traced 185 cases, probably every case in the region. However, the details were not uniform. There were four coroner's cases for which there were no hospital notes and for these the day of death was accepted as the date of onset. There were also two cases whose notes were lost or destroyed but for whom we obtained from the admission index the date, age, and address at the time of the first admission for leukemia. In these cases we used the address given and accepted as the day of onset a date one month before admission. Finally, there was a small group of eight patients, who were treated in hospitals which did not reply to our requests, or who died at home and for whom we could not trace or could not read the name of the doctor signing the certificate and could find no record of a hospital admission despite a search of the alphabetical indexes at the likely places. For these few we accepted the diagnosis on the certificate, the home address as stated, and a date of onset six months before the date of death.

The date of the first symptom mentioned in the history taken at the first admission was accepted as the date of onset. This was usually reasonably precise, being related for example to the onset of pallor or bruising, or to a fairly abrupt onset of malaise and anorexia followed by other symptoms or failure to recover from infections such as otitis media. In a few cases it was more difficult as in one case when it was superimposed upon a pre-existing acholuric jaundice. In five children in whom the leukemia was a terminal phase of a lymphosarcoma, the onset of the primary illness was used as the date of onset.

In each case an exact if sometimes arbitrary date was chosen. If the first symptom was recorded "one month ago", exactly one month before the admission date was accepted. Ob-

viously we do not suggest that the nature of the symptoms permits a general accuracy of this order, but it is probable that the majority of dates of clinical onsets are correct to within say ±10 days and a large majority to within ±30 days.

The addresses in the larger towns were identified on large-scale street maps, usually taking the location as the center point of the street. A central point, such as a railway station or road junction, was accepted in small towns and villages for which we used a map of scale 1 inch to the mile. The National Grid is in kilometer squares and references were recorded using a least significant figure to the nearest 0.1 km. Accuracy is probably such that a substantial majority were positioned correctly to within 0.5 km. and almost all to within 1 km.

Besides the age and date and place of onset, any other readily available data were recorded, including details of cytology, the presence of malformations, the history of previous illness or of radiation exposure, the number of older siblings, mother's and father's ages at delivery, birth weight, and father's occupation.

RESULTS

The numbers of cases by sex and by age at onset are given in Table 1. This follows the well-recognized form of the age distribution of deaths from leukemia with an antimode at about 13 years separating the leukemias of childhood with the preschool peak from those of the adolescent peak *(5)* and the rising incidence of adult life. The 3:2 male:female ratio is also a well-recognized feature of the disease.

Table 1 also gives separately the age distributions of lymphoblastic and myeloblastic leukemias both in urban and in rural areas. For the purposes of this Table, "lymphoblastic" includes also undifferentiated acute leukemias and those following upon an initial diagnosis of lymphosarcoma. "Myeloblastic" includes those considered to be monocytic. "Urban" means addresses within the Tyneside conurbation or within towns of at least 50 000 inhabitants: Darlington, Middlesbrough, Stockton, Sunderland, and West Hartlepool. "Rural" means the remainder, but it should be understood that, particularly in County Durham, much of the "rural" population lives in Municipal Boroughs and Urban Districts of 10 000 to 50 000 people and that

Table 1. Sex, cytology, and place, by age at onset.

Age at last birthday (yrs)			0	1	2	3	4	5	6	7	8	9	10	11	12	13	14	Total
Cytology	Lymphoblastic	Urban	6	8	7	16	8	6	9	5	6	1	4	4	3	0	5	88
		Rural	5	5	11	7	4	6	2	2	1	3	4	0	0	1	0	51
	Myeloblastic	Urban	3	3	1	4	1	1	1	3	1	3	4	2	1	2	3	33
		Rural	0	0	0	2	2	1	0	0	1	4	1	0	0	0	2	13
Sex	Male		8	8	11	17	10	9	5	7	7	7	7	3	2	3	5	109
	Female		6	8	8	12	5	5	7	3	2	4	6	3	2	0	5	76
Total	(both sexes)		14	16	19	29	15	14	12	10	9	11	13	6	4	3	10	185

such groupings account for about 620 000 of the total population of that county.

Table 1 shows different age distributions for the lymphoblastic and myeloblastic varieties. This is a well-recognized phenomenon. However, the apparent difference in age distributions of lymphoblastic leukemias with urban and rural addresses has not been reported. The mean age at onset for the lymphoblastic leukemias in the large towns was 5.82 years and in the other areas 4.50 years. The significance level is close to but slightly greater than 0.05, the F-ratio being 3.7. For myeloblastic leukemias before the 15th birthday the mean age at onset was 7.70 years.

The different age distributions of urban and rural lymphoblastic leukemias results in a changing urban:rural ratio with age and the change is most evident if we compare children aged 5 years or less with those aged 6 years or more. For the younger children there were 51 urban and 38 rural addresses at onset and for the older children 37 urban and 13 rural. The urban:rural ratio for lymphoblastic leukemia with onset at 6 years or over is indistinguisable from that for the myeloblastic leukemias at all ages under 15.

When related to the population of children at risk, the rates by age and type of leukemia are as in Table 2. The actual distribution between years of age differed in different years as the post-war birthrate "bulge" moved up through the age groups considered, but as an approximation, over the whole period, the child population has been considered equally divided between years of age. The urban:rural distribution used is that for children aged 0–14 at the 1951 census and at that time 56.69 percent lived in urban areas as defined.

For leukemias of all kinds up to age 14 the rate was significantly higher in the urban than in the rural areas, 35.6 against 24.7 cases per million child years, $(\chi^2_{(1)} = 6.7)$. The lymphoblastic leukemias under about 6 years seem to differ from the other groups in that risk is the same in both urban and rural areas, the overall urban:rural difference being concentrated in the other types. The age demarcation has been chosen arbitrarily here and the justification for division depends as we have seen upon a difference of mean ages of borderline significance but further evidence, to be presented, tends to justify this presentation.

In Table 3 the lymphoblastic and myeloblastic leukemias are given according to the month of clinical onset. There is evidence here of a seasonal variation, maximized by comparing May to October with November to April. All cases together show 111 onsets in the summer against 74 in the winter and this is possibly concentrated in the lymphoblastic series with 84 summer and 55 winter onsets $(\chi^2 = 6.05)$ while the myeloblastic series has 27 and 19 respectively. The first ratio is significantly different from a 1:1 ratio, even if the χ^2 is allowed 2 degrees of freedom, the extra degree of freedom allowing

Table 2. Urban and rural incidence rates per million child-years.[a]

Cytology	Place	Age (yrs)	
		0-5	6-14
Lymphoblastic	Urban	37.5	18.1
	Rural	36.6	8.3
Myeloblastic	Urban	9.6	9.8
	Rural	4.8	5.1

[a] Populations at risk are estimated from a 1956 estimated population aged 0-14 years of 599 500, distributed equally between years of age and using the 1951 census estimate of 56-69 percent of such children living in the urban areas, as defined in the text.

Table 3. Type of leukemia by month of onset.

Cytology	Month of onset												Total
	1	2	3	4	5	6	7	8	9	10	11	12	
Lymphoblastic	12	10	8	7	13	23	10	10	14	14	8	10	139
Myeloblastic	4	3	3	4	3	4	3	5	5	7	1	4	46
Total	16	13	11	11	16	27	13	15	19	21	9	14	185

for arbitrary choice of phase. The second ratio does not differ significantly; nor however, is the difference between the two ratios significant. Table 4 shows the summer and winter onsets of lymphoblastic leukemia by age at onset, the seasonal variation being discernible up to about the 6th birthday but not thereafter. Before the 6th birthday there were 59 summer and 30 winter onsets and at later ages there were 25 of each. Thus the difference is greatest at the age which also shows best the change in the urban:rural ratio.

The group of cases associated with the seasonal factor seems to be capable of greater resolution through the exclusion of children who on prior grounds may be suffering from leukemias of etiologies different from the remainder.

There were, in the whole group of 185 cases of leukemia, nine children who were mongols and another in whom an exact diagnosis was not recorded but who was "slightly mongoloid," mentally defective with congenital heart disease, and whose mother was 42 years old at delivery. The ages at onset of these ten children were 11, 20, 22, 25, 25, 26, 41, 56, 56, and 66 months. Another child aged 63 months at onset suffered from Sturge-Weber's disease, a condition also sometimes stated to be associated with chromosomal anomalies (6) and so rare that the presence of a single case in a series of this size may be significant. Since all of these children were under 6 years old, we may say that about 11 percent of affected children in this age group probably had abnormal karyotypes.

Three of these eleven cases of leukemia were classified as myeloblastic and two as lymphoblastic, and the remainder were not classified.

Further possible exclusions are eleven children with lymphoblastic leukemia who had a history of irradiation either *in utero* or later. Omission both of these and of the group with abnormal karyotypes from the lymphoblastic leukemias under 6 years of age leaves a group of 68 children with 48 summer and 20 winter onsets, a ratio of 2:4:1.

The seasonal factor seems to be independent of the urban concentrating factor on the grounds of the different groups affected by each. In addition, however, the above 68 children included 37 with urban and 31 with rural addresses and the respective summer:winter ratios were 24:13 and 24:7. Within the appropriate age group and cytological type the seasonal factor operates equally in both the town and the country.

Table 5 presents the frequencies of summer and winter onsets of lymphoblastic leukemia in the above 68 children according to the year of onset. It shows that the seasonal variation has been present throughout the period examined, 8 of the 10 years showing the summer excess, and one of the remaining 2 years having equal numbers. Although total figures showed a rise compatible with the secular increase of the disease in recent years, it was not possible from our data to incriminate the seasonal or any other particular component. The children with abnormal karyotypes and those with a recorded

Table 4. Lymphoblastic leukemia by age at onset and season.

Age at onset (yrs.)	0	1	2	3	4	5	6	7	8	9	10	11	12	13	14	Total
Season of onset { May-October	9	8	12	16	6	8	5	3	4	3	3	2	1	1	3	84
{ November-April	2	5	6	7	6	4	6	4	3	1	5	2	2	0	2	55
Summer:Winter ratio			59:30 (5 yrs. and under)								25:25 (6 yrs. and over)					

Table 5. Season and year of onset in cases of lymphoblastic leukemia under age 6.

Year of onset		1951	'52	'53	'54	'55	'56	'57	'58	'59	1960	Total
Season of onset	May-October	8	5	5	2	3	5	3	6	8	3	48
	November-April	3	1	3	3	3	1	0	3	1	2	20

exposure to irradiation belonged mainly to the second half of the period, but this was probably due to improved recognition of these associations.

SPACE-TIME INTERACTIONS

Enough has been said now to establish the existence in these data of concentrations of incidence both in space and in time. If space and time are considered jointly as a three-dimensional block of space-time with coordinates of time, latitude, and longitude, and if incidence (occurrences related to the population at risk) is represented within the volume of the block, it follows that there must be some unevenness. The presence of these concentrations in space-time follows inevitably from what has already been demonstrated, even though the two concentrating factors appear to be independent of each other and to operate upon different groups of cases.

The further question arises whether the space and time concentrations show any interactions, in other words, whether spatial concentrations move about in the time dimension or, what amounts to the same thing, whether time concentrations exhibit out-of-phase patterns in different geographical areas. The apparent independence of the two factors so far demonstrated makes it unlikely that we shall find an interaction in cross-pairs from the groups separately affected by them, but there is still room for interactions within these groups.

First a computer analysis of the data for the total of 185 cases was carried out. There was no evidence of an interaction. However, this large number of pairs consists largely (approximately half) of noninformative cross-pairs between the two main groups already distinguished in terms of cytology, age, season, and address and it is quite possible that informative pairs could be difficult to distinguish against this background. We can use the language of communications and postulate an adversely affected signal:noise ratio. Separate analyses of different subgroups were therefore carried out.

Negative results were obtained for the following groups of pairs:

(a) Pairs within the group of myeloblastic leukemia, including monocytic, at all ages;

(b) Pairs within the group of lymphoblastic leukemias, including undifferentiated leukemia, of 6 years or older;

(c) Cross-pairs between the groups of lymphoblastic leukemia over and under 6 years old.

By contrast, positive results were obtained from various groupings of children affected before the 6th birthday. This consisted of an excessive number of pairs showing short distances and short times. The excess was evident over a range of times and distances up to about 2 months and 2 km. but was more evident as the upper limits of time and distance were reduced. Table 6 gives one of these tabulations showing an excess at distances less than 1 km. and less than 60 days. This Table does not represent too contrived a maximization. All but one of the ten children in the five close pairs had lymphoblastic leukemia, all were under 4 years old, all had summer onset, and none had been irradiated, thus affording scope for further maximization of the discrepancy through selection of the group examined and the upper limits accepted. Because of the differing mean distances between urban-urban, urban-rural, and rural-rural pairs, re-analysis of each kind of pair was carried out, but without challenging the general conclusion. The question of statistical significance is complex and has been discussed in general elsewhere *(4)*, but at this level of asymmetry of tabulation the five indepen-

Table 6. Ninety-six cases of leukemia under 6 years old, of any cell type, abnormal karyotypes excluded.

Distances apart (km)		0–1	Over 1	Total
Time apart (days)	0-59	5	147	152
	60-3651	20	4.388	4.408
Total		25	4.535	4.560

Expected: 1 km. and 60 days, 0.79
Poisson probability of 5 or more, 1/750

dent (in fact) pairs can probably be regarded as a Poissonian variable and the result is then highly significant.

The actual times and distances between these five close pairs in the under-6 age group were 53 days and 0.2 km.; 43 days and 0.8 km.; 5 days and 0.7 km.; 18 days and 0.4 km.; 36 days and 0.2 km. The months of onset were respectively May-June; July-August; September-September; October-October; September-October. In no case did the members of a pair have the same general practitioner, and indeed the ten children had ten different doctors. These five pairs, although a very small proportion of all possible pairs, involved ten children, a substantial proportion of the 96 in the affected group. Since the end of this investigation we have seen another close pair, a time of less than a month, a distance of about 0.2 km., both in young children with lymphoblastic leukemia and both with summer onset.

OTHER FACTORS

The whole group of leukemias was examined with respect to other factors recorded, particularly with a view to finding any confirmatory differentiations between the leukemia groups already separated, but little was found.

There was no clear differentiation in terms of the sex of affected children.

Maternal and paternal ages were respectively 27.9 and 30.9 at delivery for children under 6 years (excluding the mongols) and 26.2 and 28.8 for those over. These means differ neither between the groups nor from the population means.

Of 78 children under 6 (excluding mongols) with a record of birth rank, 29 (37.2 percent.) were first children. Of the 51 children of 6 or over with a record of birth rank, 21 (41.2 per cent.) were first children. These proportions differ significantly neither from each other nor from the population proportions. More detailed analysis by finer age groups revealed nothing significant.

Children under 6 years had birth weights recorded in 71 instances and the mean was 7 lb. 6.5 oz. Children affected after the 6th birthday (41 recorded) weighted 7 lb. 11.2 oz. The difference is largely accounted for by the four twins in the first group and is probably not significant.

Birth dates were examined for a seasonal variation. This was recorded precisely in 166 cases. There was no suggestion of a regular cycle and the maximizing dichotomy was June-November:December-May with 70 and 96 respectively, not a difference which can be considered significant. Interactions between the month of birth and month of onset, and between the month of birth and age at onset were sought and not found.

Fathers' occupations, which were recorded sufficiently well for classification in 125 cases, followed a social class distribution not grossly different from the regional distribution. There was, however, some difference in detail between the "5 and under" and the "6 and over" age groups. Eight of the 56 older children (14 percent) and 18 of the 73 younger ones (25 percent) had fathers who were miners or agricultural workers. This is probably a reflection of the different urban-rural distributions of the two groups.

DISCUSSION

The seasonal distribution demonstrated in this study corresponds well with the pattern demonstrated by Lee *(7)*. Lee's data were obtained from National Cancer Registrations, which achieve only a partial ascertainment, and the results were therefore suspect in that completeness might, for some reason, have varied with the season. The present data are largely independent of Lee's. Although some cases were registered under the Cancer Registration Scheme, local registrations of leukemia were in fact very incomplete during the period of the study. As well as affording mutual confirmation of the cycle, the two sets of data agree remarkably in detail, with June the highest month in both distributions and July showing a concordant dip in the middle of the summer excess.

Steinberg *(8)* gives recent figures for seasonal distributions of onset in New England, U.S.A. He uses χ^2 with 11 degrees of freedom to assess significance and his negative conclusion is due partly to the statistical inefficiency of this method. Dichotomy of the year as in the present study (May-October; November-April) gives 242 and 207 cases respectively. This is not in itself significant, but the pattern is sufficiently like the present one, and like Lee's, to have made subdivision by cell type and age group of some interest.

A difference of the present study from Lee's analysis is that age as well as type of leukemia appears to be correlated with the presence of the cycle. In the northern data the cycle was evident up to about the 6th birthday and not beyond. Lee does not give a detailed breakdown by month and age, but quarterly percentages of onsets seem to indicate a more widespread age distribution of the cycle in the national data. The failure to demonstrate the pattern in our own older patients may be in part a question of small numbers, but variations of diagnostic criteria and their interaction with age may play some part.

Both the national and regional data agree in showing that the seasonal variation has been evident at least since 1951 in a fairly regular annual pattern.

Calculation of rates for the large towns of 50 000 population and over, together with those in the conurbation of Tyneside, showed an excess of cases compared with the other areas. Again this showed differences according to age and the type of leukemia, and it was especially evident in those groups not subject, in our data, to the seasonal cycle.

An urban-rural difference has been noted before. Stewart, Webb, and Hewitt (9) found it in England and Wales in the years 1953-55, although within this pattern the rates (deaths) in towns of 50 000 to 100 000 inhabitants were greater than in the very large towns and conurbations. Meadors (10) found it in death rates in the U.S.A. in 1944-48. His result is of particular interest because, among the childhood cases, the urban-rural ratio of rates per million changed with age; in the successive age groups 0-4, 5-9, and 10-14, the ratios were 1.28, 1.44, and 1.59. This pattern is analogous with our own results and confirms differentiation in terms of geographical distribution between younger and older children. Stewart and others (9) did not analyze their results in terms of age

at death or at onset, and neither they nor Meadors analyzed them according to the cytological type of leukemia.

The search for interactions produced one positive result. In the children under 6 years old, those especially affected by lymphoblastic leukemia and by the seasonal cycle, there were five very close pairs, closer than 60 days in their dates of onset and closer than 1 km. on the map. As the proportionate expected value was 0.79 pairs, the observed figure, which is seven times this, may probably be considered statistically significant. Nine of the ten children had lymphoblastic leukemia, they were all young children of 4 years or less, and all had summer onset. It is probable that the clustering factor is a genuine one and is due to a factor closely associated or identical with that responsible for the seasonal factor.

Pinkel and Nefzger (11) also described space-time clusters in childhood leukemia in Buffalo, N.Y., but did not separate space-clustering from time-clustering from space-time interactions. Their tests of significance were negative and it is doubtful whether their definition of a close pair as one within 2 years and one-third of a mile is accurately justified. In their paper they give positions on a map and serial numbers, although not dates. Some re-analysis has proved possible. A centimeter grid was placed over the map as published, references calculated on this basis, and a standardized form of dating achieved simply by successive labelling of the 95 cases in Buffalo as dates 1 to 95. The results are presented in Table 7; the main suggestive finding was the occurrence of eight time-adjacent pairs (i.e., a serial difference of one) closer than 1 cm. on the map approximately two-thirds of a mile on the ground) against an expected value of 4.6. Sub-analysis of particular age groups and cell types would be worthwhile in this series.

Specific interpretation of the nature of the clustering is not yet possible. The seasonal fac-

Table 7. **Analysis of data of 95 cases in Buffalo, N.Y.** (*11*).

Map distance (cm.)	<1	−2	−4	−8	>8	Total
Adjacent cases	8(4.6)	5	28	47	6	94
1 to 4 Intervening cases	20(18.1)	35	118	170	23	366
5 to 8 " "	14(17.3)	34	101	182	19	350
All possible pairs	221	445	1423	2094	282	4465

Expected numbers in parentheses.   1 cm. on map is approximately 2/3 of a mile.

tor, the clustering effect, the known virus etiology of leukemia in animals (e.g. see *12*), and the production of leukemia in mice by injection of filtered extracts of tissues and blood from leukemic patients together suggest very strongly that a virus infection may operate in the acute lymphoblastic leukemias of the younger children. However, there are several other possible interpretations and there is no real suggestion from our results that leukemia was transmitted from one case to another, only that two cases may sometimes have a common source. This could be interpreted variously as a toxic rather than an infective agency, spread through atmospheric pollution, or contamination of food or water supplies, or as a result of direct contact with toxic weed killers, paints, solvents, and other poisonous materials, and so on. Moreover, the risk of exposure to many of these hypothetical factors might also be seasonal.

If the factor were an infective or toxic agent, effective following a short exposure, we must consider the likely length of the latent interval before the appearance of the first symptom. We can infer, because the seasonal variation is discernible in children of less than 1 year old, and certainly of less than 2 years, that the latent period may be less than one year. This is less than the latent period following large doses of radiation in adults, namely 3 to 5 years (*14*). On the other hand, the nature of the disease makes a very short interval unlikely, and a possible range of, say, 6 to 18 months is perhaps as accurate a guess as is possible. The exact season of operation and therefore the nature of the seasonal factor are quite uncertain.

The effect could of course represent simply a seasonally correlated effect upon the rate of development of the pathological process in the pre-symptomatic phase, or even an artefact related to recognition or parental memory, rather than an event of etiological significance. However, the interaction effect is less easily explained in this way and the suggestion that both the interaction and the seasonal variation are common manifestations of a single factor has a bearing on the interpretation of the latter. A seasonally distributed and clustered event of short duration, that is a trigger mechanism, seems a more likely explanation.

This point may be important in relation to either of two recently demonstrated features of childhood malignant disease. The first is the recently described geographical concentration of malignant lymphoma in African children and the suggestion that its distribution corresponds with that of the tsetse fly or some other biting arthropod, and therefore that the tumor may be infective in origin. The question of an insect vector in England is interesting, but would be very difficult to investigate until we have some idea of the seasonal phasing of the supposed trigger event.

The second is the demonstration by Stewart and others (*9*) that severe respiratory infections are unduly frequent in the 2 years preceding the onset of leukemia, particularly those infections for which antibiotics were given. Stewart and her colleagues interpreted this association in an indirect manner, but the possibility of a direct effect of an infective organism, or of anoxia, or of the drugs used is not disproved.

The question of social class differences in the leukemias of childhood is a vexed one and different studies have produced different results. Stewart and others (*9*) found none. On the other hand, Pinkel and Nefzger (*2*) found an interesting difference in the U.S.A. between the social groups of older and younger affected children. Our own data are inconclusive in terms of the overall social class distribution, but showed differences in detail between older and younger children analogous with the American data; both results could be secondary to different geographical distributions at different ages.

The maternal age effect reported by Stewart and others (*9*) was not present in our data. A possible explanation of the difference might be underreporting of mongolism in their series. Their reported incidence of sixteen mongols among 677 leukemias is considerably less than our own—nine, or possibly ten, among 185.

SUMMARY

There were 185 clinical onsets of leukemia in children under 15, in Northumberland, Durham, and on Tees-side, in the 10 years 1951 to 1960. Their distribution in space and time showed evidence of (*a*) a seasonal variation with a summer peak, and (*b*) a high risk in children living in the larger towns. These two factors appeared to affect different groups of cases and to be independent of each other, the seasonal variation affecting especially the lymphoblastic leukemias in younger children, the large-town concentration being evident only in the myeloblastic leukemias and in the lymphoblastic leukemias of children over 6 years old. There was, in addition, evidence of a clustering factor, a space-time interaction, affecting the lymphoblastic leukemias of young children, such that pairs of cases occurring within 60 days and within 1 km. of each other were unduly frequent. The data suggest that the seasonal variation and the clustering effect may be common properties of a single factor.

The series showed a high incidence of leukemia in mongols. There was a variation between the occupational groups of younger and older affected children which was probably secondary to the urban-rural distributions. Apart from the association with mongolism there was no evidence of maternal age or birth rank variations of risk.

The findings suggest further heterogeneity in the epidemiology and possibly the etiology of childhood leukemias and, particularly in the case of younger children, suggest exposure to a seasonally variable factor which tends to be localized both in space and in time.

Acknowledgements are due to the Eugenics Society and the Tyneside Leukemia Research Fund for supporting this investigation. Thanks are also due to The Registrar General and to Dr. W. M. Court-Brown for access to and preparation of death certificate data, to the National Cancer Registration Bureau for access to their records, and to all the Pediatricians and Hospital Records Officers who cooperated.

References

(1) Kellett, C. E. *Arch Dis Child* 12:239, 1937.
(2) Pinkel, D. and D. Nefzger. *Cancer* 13:102, 1960.
(3) Wood, E. E. *Br Med J* 1:1760, 1960.
(4) Knox, G. *Br J Prev Soc Med* 17:121, 1963.
(5) Lee, J. A. H. *Br Med J* 1:988, 1961.
(6) Patau, K., E. Therman, D. W. Smith, S. L. Inhorn, and B. F. Picken. *Am J Hum Genet* 13:287, 1961.
(7) Lee, J. A. H. *Br Med J* 1:1737, 1962.
(8) Steinberg, A. G. *Cancer* 13:985, 1960.
(9) Stewart, A., J. Webb, and D. Hewitt. *Br Med J* 1:1495, 1958.
(10) Meadors, G. F. *Public Health Rep* 71:103, 1956.
(11) Pinkel, D. and D. Nefzger. *Cancer* 12:351, 1959.
(12) Syverton, J. T. and J. D. Ross *Am J Med* 28:683, 1960.
(13) Bergol'ts, V. M. Problems of Virology 4:2. Abstracted in English. *Year Book of Cancer 1960-61*, ed. R. L. Clark and R. W. Cumley, Chicago, 1959, p. 229.
(14) Court-Brown, W. M. and R. Doll. Leukemia and aplastic anemia in patients irradiated for ankylosing spondylitis. *Med Res Counc Spec Rep Ser* No. 295, H.M.S.O., London, 1957.

APPENDIX

List of Hospitals: Bishop Auckland General Hospital, Dryburn Hospital, Fleming Memorial Hospital, Ingham Infirmary, Middlesbrough General Hospital, Newcastle General Hospital, Preston Hospital, Queen Elizabeth Hospital, Royal Victoria Infirmary, Shotley Bridge General Hospital, South Shields General Hospital, Stockton Children's Hospital, Sunderland Children's Hospital, Walkergate Hospital, West Hartlepool General Hospital.

GEOGRAPHIC AND CLIMATIC ASPECTS OF MULTIPLE SCLEROSIS: A REVIEW OF CURRENT HYPOTHESES[1]

Leonard T. Kurland and Dwayne Reed[2]

Multiple sclerosis is a neurological disease of unknown cause and is often progressive and fatal. It has an unusual geographic distribution which has defied an explanation that might elucidate its cause or lead to effective treatment or prevention. The disease has been the subject of numerous intensive mortality and morbidity analyses which provide excellent illustrations of survey technics in chronic disease epidemiology.

An essential preceding step to effective field studies is the clear description of the clinical syndrome. Unfortunately, in multiple sclerosis there is no specific laboratory or clinical procedure to confirm the diagnosis of multiple sclerosis cases, nor do we have assurance that what we count as cases are the same disease entity. Because there are many neurological diseases of genetic and unknown etiology which resemble multiple sclerosis, the diagnosis is often reached only after the patient has had more than one episode and other possibilities have been excluded. The error of diagnosis is greatest early in the disease; yet the early cases are the very ones which might facilitate identification of some predisposing or disease precipitating experience. Since early symptoms often develop insidiously and may remit and recur, the precise season or even the year of onset may be uncertain. Furthermore, a delay of months or even years from onset to diagnosis is not uncommon and further complicates the recognition of significant events which may have preceded the onset of the disease.

Since incidence rates are relatively small and difficult to obtain accurately, most geographic comparisons have been limited to prevalence rates. These are statistically more stable but may be biased if severity of the illness or longevity of the patients differs geographically or if there is appreciable migration of patients into or out of the community under study. In spite of these difficulties, many epidemiological surveys have been undertaken to clarify the basic issue of whether genetics or environment is the major causative influence.

In view of the early clinical impression that multiple sclerosis selectively occurred in people of northern European origin or extraction (1), a first step in the series of epidemiologic investigations was to examine the geographic pattern of multiple sclerosis mortality. Figure 1, based on Limburg's study in 1948 (2), reveals an inverse relation between crude mortality rates for multiple sclerosis and the mean annual temperature of the major city of each country. Mortality studies with age-adjusted rates showed a similar pattern. Although it appears that the colder the climate the higher the crude death rate, alternate explanations such as the relative amount of neurological diagnostic services cannot be ignored.

Because of the nonuniformity of many international mortality reporting sources, it seemed more profitable to map the geographic pattern over a wide area which had similar coding, classification systems, language, and medical standards. Figure 2 shows the distribution of the average annual age-adjusted multiple sclerosis mortality rates per 100 000 population for the United States and Canada. The high rates are associated with the northern United States and Canada.

The next step was to determine the morbidity and mortality of multiple sclerosis in detail in several large, widely separated communitites in which the standards of medical practice were high. These studies were completed in Boston, Winnipeg, New Orleans, Denver, and San Francisco (3).

All available diagnostic sources, including hospitals, clinics, and practitioners serving the respective communities, were studied to dis-

Source: *Multiple Sclerosis* 54(4):588:597.
[1] This paper was presented before the Epidemiology Section of the American Public Health Association at the Ninetieth Annual Meeting in Miami Beach, Fla., October 18, 1962.
[2] The authors are associated with the Epidemiology Branch, National Institute of Neurological Diseases and Blindness, National Institutes of Health, Bethesda, Md.

Figure 1. Crude death rate for multiple sclerosis for selected countries by annual mean temperature.[a]

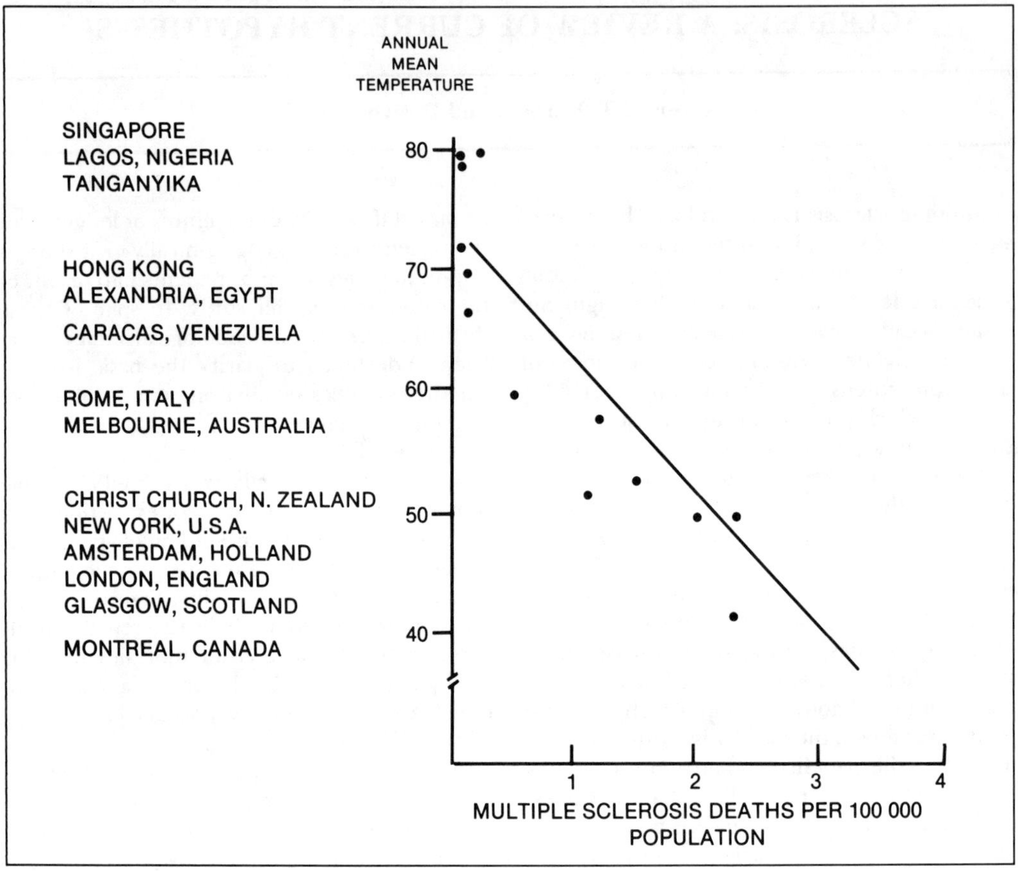

[a]Modified from Limburg, C. *Multiple Sclerosis and the Demyelinating Diseases.* Williams and Wilkins, 1950, Chapter II.

cover cases of multiple sclerosis and allied disorders. Duplicates were consolidated, the latest diagnosis and living or dead status was determined, and the prevalence rates were computed for a date about one year prior to the study to partially compensate for the long delay from onset to diagnosis. Table 1 shows that multiple sclerosis prevalence was much greater in the northern cities than in New Orleans. Although there appears to be a north to south gradient, there was no obvious focalization of cases within these cities. There were so few conjugal or familial cases that ordinary transmissibility or a common source of exposure seemed unlikely. In spite of the differences in prevalence, the clinical features of the disease were similar in all cities; however, the mean age of onset appeared to progressively decrease as the prevalence rate

increased. In New Orleans and Winnipeg (4), the two cities whose latitude and multiple sclerosis prevalence differed the most, a particularly intensive reevaluation was made, including an additional examination of the patients.

All patients uncovered by the earlier study, plus those found by a review of all sources, were interviewed and examined by a neurologist. The numbers in parenthesis in Table 1 show that the agreement with the overall result of the earlier survey was good, but that the previous estimate of a 3.6 to 1 ratio between Winnipeg and New Orleans was conservative. The review following neurologic examination revealed a ratio of 6.6 to 1. The discrepancy occurred because many cases in New Orleans which had been counted were not acceptable when examined.

Figure 2. Average mortality rates/100,000 population, Canada and the United States, for white population, 1949–1951.

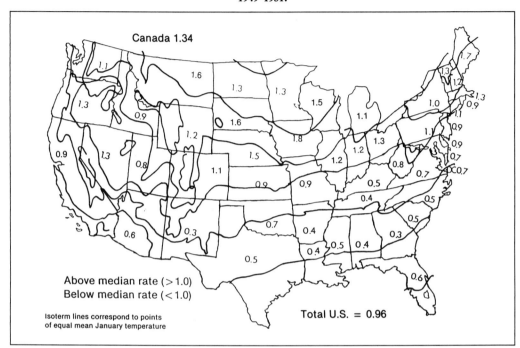

Table 1. M. S. prevalence ratio for white population, U. S. and Canadian communities (NINDB Study).

Community	Latitude °N	Temp. mean Jan. °F	Prevalence ratio per 100 000 population
Winnipeg	50	−3.5	42[a] (40)[b]
Boston	42	28	41
Denver	40	31	38
San Francisco	37	50	30
New Orleans	30	55	13[a] (6)[b]

[a] Preliminary result.
[b] Final result after detailed neurological examination of patients.

Figure 3 shows multiple sclerosis prevalence rates by age in Winnipeg and by age and race in New Orleans. This is a graphic illustration of the difference in the rates, at all ages, between the two cities. There was no statistically significant difference between Caucasians and Negroes in New Orleans.

A further follow-up study in Winnipeg by Stazio is now in progress and preliminary results

are available (5). There was no indication of any change in the annual incidence rates for the 20 years prior to 1961. About 30 percent of the 1951 cases were no longer acceptable as multiple sclerosis and an additional 20 percent, mostly cases which had been symptomatic but undiagnosed in 1951, were now included. The overall result in prevalence was not appreciably affected, but there is a discrepancy in a sizable proportion of the individual cases. Inaccuracies of about 40 percent underreporting and 18 percent overreporting for multiple sclerosis as the primary cause of death were also noted.

In order to elucidate any etiological or associated factors, numerous characteristics of the Winnipeg patients prior to the onset of the disease were compared with a representative, matched sample of the Winnipeg population (4).

No statistically significant difference was found in the comparison in regard to: areas of Europe from which the individuals or their ancestors had migrated, place of birth, birth order, education, occupation, urban or rural residence, source of food and water, exposure

Figure 3. **Multiple sclerosis prevalance[a] ratios per 100 000 population.[b] Winnipeg, by age, New Orleans, by age and color, January 1, 1949.**

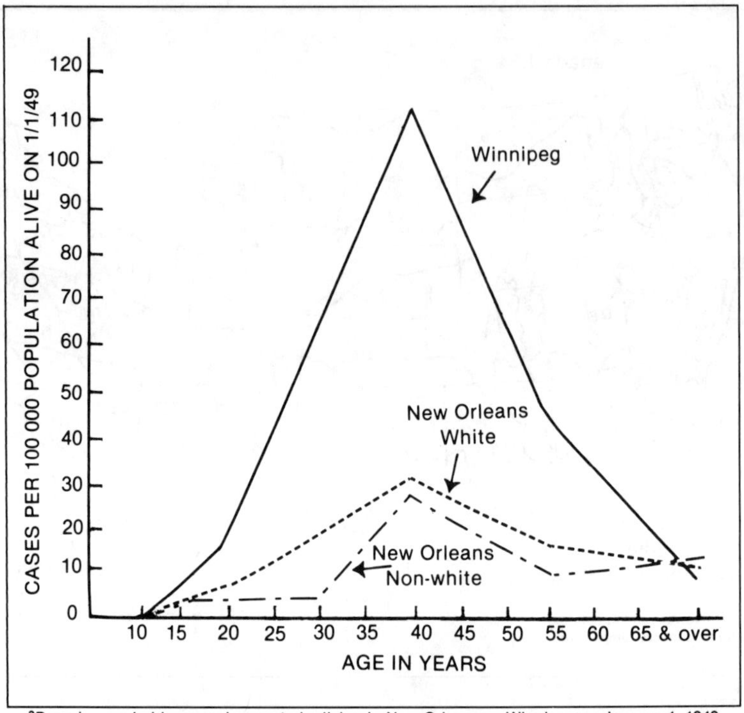

[a]Based on probable cases known to be living in New Orleans or Winnipeg on January 1, 1949.
[b]New Orleans population estimated, 1947: Winnipeg population from 1946 census.

to animals, vaccinations and inoculations received prior to onset, previous illness, back injuries, and head injuries.

Ethnological differences appeared to be of little significance. In Winnipeg there was no difference in prevalence for persons of English, French, or Ukrainian descent. In the earlier study in Boston, the rate among Caucasians and Negroes was similar and was considerably higher than the corresponding rates among Caucasians and Negroes in New Orleans.

In recent years, other population surveys have been completed in Ireland, Scotland, Denmark, Canada, and the United States (*1, 6-8*). These surveys also attempted to enumerate all the living, medically attended multiple sclerosis patients in a specified population. In most instances, patients were examined by the investigator or a neurologic consultant and the diagnostic criteria of multiple sclerosis which were expressed or inferred are believed to be sufficiently alike to justify a comparison.

The results of these and many other investigations could be summarized as follows: multiple sclerosis is found in many parts of the world and among all major racial groups. In the Northern Hemisphere it is more prevalent among the people of northern Europe, Great Britain, Canada, and the northern United States where the rates range from about 35 to 65 per 100 000 population. In these areas the rates are in the high to moderately high range, and it is difficult to see any pattern which would suggest a difference in risk for the northern Europeans as compared to those in Canada and the northern United States. The rates are generally higher (within the same geographic latitude) in the smaller communities, but this is probably due to the greater intensity of the study which is possible in such homogeneous populations. Among the people of the tropics and subtropics, the rates are considerably lower than in the temperate zones.

The one area in the Northern Hemisphere

which does not show the north to south gradient is Japan (*9*). An effort was made to conduct a survey, using the same techniques as used in the United States, in two Japanese communities of over 300 000 population separated by 10° latitude. The results failed to show a variation in multiple sclerosis prevalence rates which were approximately two per 100 000 in each city. This may be an accurate picture, but the low rates may also be due to a number of limitations and difficulties inherent in the study. Neurology has only recently developed as a separate medical discipline in Japan and case finding is always influenced by the mode of medical diagnosis and the differences in neurologic training of physicians. We prefer to consider these rates as minimal values until further surveys now in progress are completed.

Data on the Southern Hemisphere are limited but Acheson (*10*) has studied mortality rates of multiple sclerosis in Australia, New Zealand, and South Africa and found a relationship to latitude similar to that in the Northern Hemisphere. Dean (*11*) had first observed that multiple sclerosis is far more common among European immigrants to South Africa than among persons of European stock born and raised in South Africa.

Dean's more recent studies (*12*) show that multiple sclerosis does occur in South African born persons who have not been overseas, but the rate is very low—about two per 100 000. This area is about the same distance from the equator as New Orleans and the rates compare quite well with those of similar latitudes in the Northern Hemisphere. Among the immigrants from European countries the prevalence of multiple sclerosis is nearly as high as in the country of their origin. Dean's most interesting finding is that the prevalence of multiple sclerosis in South African born persons who visit Europe is about seven and a half times greater than in South African born persons who do not leave Africa.

The phenomenon of mass migration offers unique opportunities for investigating the question of geographic influence on multiple sclerosis. First Rozanski (*13*) and later Alter (*14*) took advantage of the unusual population composition of Israel to study this question.

A large segment of the Jewish population of Israel has been exposed to the influences of diverse climatological and geographic conditions. They have gathered as one population in Israel where immigration is not limited by any medical restrictions, and where the doctor-patient ratio is the highest in the world.

The findings are far more suggestive of an association with a geographic factor than a racial one. The prevalence rate among northern European immigrants was five to ten times higher than among Jews of Oriental, southern European, and Mediterranean origin. Among those persons born in Israel, the rates were low, regardless of the national origin of their parents. Both Alter, et al. (*14*), and Dean (*12*) have computed a minimum latent period (from presumed exposure in the "high risk" temperate areas to the onset of symptoms after migration) of about 9 to 12 years among immigrants to Israel and South Africa. Although this procedure introduces several gross assumptions, it is the first reasonable effort to approach the question of an "incubation period" in such a chronic disease. The present mechanism does not enable one to determine the upper limit of such a latent interval.

The geographic pattern showing a more frequent distribution of multiple sclerosis further away from the equator has been accepted by most investigators. It is still uncertain, however, which of the many possible factors related to latitude may be relevant to the etiology of multiple sclerosis. Various meteorological and climatological influences such as "colder" winter temperatures or diminished sunshine appear to correlate with multiple sclerosis distribution. Whether these act directly on the patient or indirectly through plants, animals, or vectors in his environment is a purely speculative matter at this time.

Dietary deficiencies and excesses, including fat, lead, and copper, which may vary in different regions, have been investigated. There is no convincing evidence that any of these play a direct role even though Swank (*15*), a proponent of the theory that a high-fat diet causes multiple sclerosis, claims to have "astonishing results" with his low-fat regimen. Viruses and allergic-hyperallergic reactions have been suggested in the continuing research efforts, but clear, reproducible evidence has not followed theory. Ichelson's (*16*) report of "successful" culture of spirochetes from the spinal fluid of multiple sclerosis patients has once again stimulated the search for a microorganism, but others have demonstrated that Ichelson's spirochetes were contaminants in her culture medium.

A more recent attempt to identify meaningful variables correlated with latitude was made by Acheson, Bachrach, and Wright (*17*). They studied the distribution of multiple sclerosis in men discharged from Veterans Administration Hospitals with a diagnosis of this disease, between 1954-1958. This study was concerned with the birthplace of the patients whereas previous studies have been concerned with the residence of the patients either at death or following the onset of the disease.

A multiple-regression analysis was done using the following variables: multiple sclerosis rate per million for the mean year of birth of the patients (1920), degrees north latitude of birthplace, average hours of sunshine, average annual degree day (an index of severity of winter), and average daily December solar radiation. The highest correlations of multiple sclerosis prevalence were with average total annual hours of sunshine and with average daily December solar radiation. The fact that the correlation between multiple sclerosis and sunshine was a negative one indicates that if sunshine exerts an effect it must be preventive or protective rather than harmful.

The best illustration of the possible importance of sunshine is shown in Table 2, selected from Acheson's data. The rates of multiple sclerosis per million (by birthplace) decrease from north to south in three principal cities on the Pacific coast. The main difference in climate along this coast lies in sunshine (and precipitation) rather than in severity of winter.

Table 2. Rates of multiple sclerosis per million population in three principal cities on the Pacific Coast.[a]

City	Degrees north latitude	Multiple sclerosis cases per million population	Average annual sunshine hours
Seattle	48	31	2049
San Francisco	38	12	2935
Los Angeles	34	4	3217

[a] From Acheson, Bachrach and Wright (*17*). Some comments on the relationship of the distribution of multiple sclerosis to latitude, solar radiation and other variables. *Acta Psychiat Neurol Scand* 35:132-147, 1960.

Further speculation concerning the direct protective qualitites of solar radiation comes from the work of Schneider (*18*). He identified a strain of mice which are, genetically, 100 percent susceptible to the development of experimental allergic encephalomyelitis (EAE), when inoculated with a suspension of brain tissue and adjuvant. When such animals were subjected to a flux of approximately 3000 foot candle from a bank of high output fluorescent lamps, EAE was reduced 50-75 percent. Schneider thinks the near infrared wave length is responsible for this phenomenon. One drawback is that other investigators have noted that heat and stress may also have a similar effect. This relationship between multiple sclerosis and solar radiation remains uncertain. If one assumed that the latent period from "exposure" to onset or exacerbation were constant, a seasonal variation in incidence would be expected. However, several investigations have not revealed any such variation (*19*).

In view of the difficulties in explaining the geographic distribution of multiple sclerosis, Barlow (*20*) has sought a new association. He plotted several sets of mortality and morbidity data for multiple sclerosis against the geomagnetic latitude of the location from which the data were obtained. The geomagnetic latitudes relate to the earth's magnetic field and are skewed with respect to parallels of geographic latitude.

The plotted rates versus geomagnetic latitude showed a consistent rapid rise in multiple sclerosis between the geomagnetic latitudes of 40° and 50°, and a leveling off above 50°. According to Barlow, the distribution of multiple sclerosis and particularly the low rate area of Japan are better correlated with geomagnetic than geographic latitudes. One of the phenomenena known to be related to geomagnetic latitude is cosmic radiation, and Barlow thought it appropriate to examine the various cosmic ray parameters. He found that altitude was a more important parameter of cosmic ray intensity than latitude. At sea level the latitude change between 0° and 50° is only 14 percent, while from sea level to 6500 feet there is a 70 percent increase. The present difficulty with the cosmic ray hypothesis is that, while the number of high energy particles observed at very high altitudes varies with latitude, these particles appear to be filtered out by the atmosphere and no material increase in their effects can be observed at sea level.

The epidemiological approach with its emphasis on the host-environment relationship does not mean we have satisfied ourselves that no genetic factor is involved. The results of studies in Great Britain, Ireland, Scandinavia, Germany, and the United States (6-8) have been interpreted as showing that familial incidence is higher than would be expected by chance.

In Sutherland's (8) series, seven out of 545 sibs (1.3 percent) of 127 patients were said to be affected; while in Hyllested's (6) series, 44 of 11 924 sibs (0.4 percent) were considered affected. The difficulty is that these findings do not differentiate between the effects of an environmental exposure common to members of the same family and a genetic disease (21). Concordance with respect to multiple sclerosis has been studied in identical twins and found to be low (22). This is one of the most serious arguments against a purely hereditary basis for multiple sclerosis. Aside from the tendency to a slightly higher rate in females and a slight tendency to a familial aggregation of cases, the occurrence of multiple sclerosis in a community appears to be on an almost random basis within the young adult group.

A very practical question which is often asked is: Should patients with early multiple sclerosis be advised to migrate to a warmer latitude where the prevalence is low? Multiple sclerosis is a disease marked by remissions and exacerbations; in general, the more frequent the exacerbation, the more rapid the progression. The cause of the exacerbation is no better understood than the etiology of the disease. Longstanding clinical attitude has been to recommend that patients move to a low prevalence area in the hope that exacerbations would be fewer; however, there is no evidence that such a change has a beneficent effect. No patient group which has migrated from one area to another has been carefully evaluated. The only comparative study was on life expectancy in New Orleans and Winnipeg (4). Although the life expectancy of patients who could be identified in the two communities seemed to be equal, the data were limited and the results thus indecisive. In the absence of any specific treatment, and until a decisive study is made, it seems that migration to a warm latitude might be worth trying if it would cause no economic or emotional hardship, and if the patient recognizes that the benefits are uncertain.

There are many other areas yet to be explored. The similarity of the geographic distribution of multiple sclerosis to that of rheumatic fever remains a point of interest and speculation. The cause of rheumatic fever is unknown, but a hypersensitive reaction to streptococci is suspected. It has been suggested that multiple sclerosis may also be a manifestation of an allergic hypersensitivity possibly triggered by a virus infection. The analogy between the tissue-specific type of hypersensitivity reactions reported in various animals inoculated with kidney and heart tissue and that of demyelination produced in animals inoculated with brain substance might also be cited as evidence of an isoallergic factor in multiple sclerosis. However, the sequence of events that could initiate such an allergic reaction in humans (liberation of tissue antigen from the CNS stimulating antibody formation, which in turn react with the original tissue) is as yet completely unknown.

Multiple sclerosis may be a syndrome in which a specific agent prevalent in the temperate zones is rare or absent in the subtropics and tropics, accounting for the differential incidence geographically. Another possibility is that clinically recognized cases of multiple sclerosis represent only a small segment of the total spectrum of the disease process and that, for reasons still unknown, the proportion of subclinical cases is less in the temperate than in the other zones.

Efforts continue to be made to isolate a virus from multiple sclerosis patients. A new area in this field has been opened by the studies on scrapie, a chronic neurological wasting disease of sheep (23). Under natural conditions this disease seems to be genetically determined. Experimentally the disease has been successfully transmitted after an incubation period of months or even years to sheep, goats, and mice by the inoculation of brain homoginate from affected animals. This possible dual mechanism of a genetic and an infective agent (so-called provirus) could provide better understanding of etiologic mechanisms of human disease.

Summary and Conclusions

Multiple sclerosis has a remarkable geographic pattern with the highest prevalence and mortality rates in the temperate zones of both hemispheres and with decreasing rates in the subtropics and tropics. This difference is associated with geography rather than with race or national origin. No specific exogenous or genetic basis for the geographic pattern has been identified, but it is speculated that some climatologic condition influences the frequency of the disease. It is unknown whether this effect is a direct one on the patient or an indirect effect on the animal or plant life in his environment. Migratory populations have been especially useful in this research and indicate that the rate among those migrating from a high to a low risk area exceeds that of the population into which they have immigrated. In the studies of migrating populations, the average minimal latent period from presumed exposure in their prior home to the onset of symptoms has been estimated to be about 9 to 12 years.

It will be essential to clarify many of the features referred to above. Communities on the same latitude, but having different climates with respect to temperature and sunshine, should be compared. Similarly, investigation of communities having different altitudes could be rewarding.

It may well be that the causes of multiple sclerosis are determined by several factors, including a genetic predisposition, and the importance of each factor may vary in different geographic areas. It is still reasonable to expect that future etiologic hypotheses should be consistent with the known geographic distribution.

References

(1) McAlpine, D., N. Compston, and C. Lumsden. *Multiple Sclerosis and the Demyelinating Diseases*. Baltimore, Williams and Wilkins, 1955.

(2) Limsburg, C. The Geographic Distribution of Multiple Sclerosis and Its Estimated Prevalence in the United States. Chap. II in *Multiple Sclerosis and the Demyelinating Diseases*. Baltimore, Williams and Wilkins, 1950.

(3) Kurland, L. T. and K. Westlund. Epidemiological factors in the etiology and prognosis of multiple sclerosis. *Ann NY Acad Sci* 58:682-701, 1954.

(4) Westlund, K. and L. T. Kurland. Studies on multiple sclerosis in Winnipeg, Manitoba and New Orleans, Louisiana. *Am J Hyg* 57:380-407, 1953.

(5) Stazio, A. Personal communication.

(6) Hyllested, K. *Disseminated Sclerosis in Denmark. Prevalence and Geographical Distribution.* Copenhagen, J. Jorgenson, 1956.

(7) Millar, J. and R. Allison. Familial incidence of disseminated sclerosis in Northern Ireland. *Ulster M J* 23:29-91, 1954.

(8) Sutherland, J. Observation on the prevalence of multiple sclerosis in Northern Scotland. *Brain* 75:635-654, 1956.

(9) Okinaka, S., D. McAlpine, D., K. Miyagawa, N. Suwa, Y. Kuroiwa, H. Shiraki, S. Araki, and L. T. Kurland. Multiple sclerosis in Northern and Southern Japan. *World Neurology* 1:22-42, 1960.

(10) Acheson, E. Multiple sclerosis in British Commonwealth countries in the Southern Hemisphere. *Br J Prev Soc Med* 15:118-125, 1961.

(11) Dean, G. Disseminated sclerosis in South Africa. *Br M J* 1:842-845, 1949.

(12) Dean, G. Personal communication.

(13) Rozanski, J. Contribution to the incidence of multiple sclerosis among Jews in Israel. *Mon Rev Psychiat Neurol* 123:65-72, 1952.

(14) Alter, M., L. Halpern, B. Bornstein, J. Silberstein, and L. T. Kurland. Multiple Sclerosis in Israel. *AMA Arch Neurol Psychiat* 7:253, 1962.

(15) Swank, R., O. Lerstad, A. Strom, and J. Backer, Multiple sclerosis in rural Norway. *New England J Med* 246:721-728, 1952.

(16) Ichelson, R. Cultivation of spirochete from spinal fluid of multiple sclerosis cases and normal controls. *Proc Soc Exp Biol Med* 95:57, 1957.

(17) Acheson, E., C. Bachrach, and F. Wright. Some comments on the relationship of the distribution of multiple sclerosis to latitude, solar radiation and other variables. *Acta Psychiat Neurol Scand* 35:132-147, 1960.

(18) Schneider, H. and J. Lee. The effect of high intensity fluorescent illumination on experimental allergic encephalomyelitis. *Fed Proc* 46th Ann. Meeting 21:270, Mar.-Apr., 1962.

(19) Kurland, L., D. Mulder, and K. Westlund. Multiple sclerosis and amyotrophic lateral sclerosis—etiologic significance of recent epidemiologic and genetic studies. *New England J Med* 252:649-653, 1955.

(20) Barlow, J. S. Correlation of the geographic distribution of multiple sclerosis with cosmic ray intensities. *Acta Psychiat Neurol Scand* 35:108-131, 1960.

(21) Reese, H. and L. T. Kurland. Multiple sclerosis—an unsolved problem in medicine: A review of present investigation into etiologic factors and pathogenic mechanisms. *Medicine in Japan* 5:741-748, 1959.

(22) Muller, R. Genetic aspects of multiple sclerosis. *AMA Arch Neurol Psychiat* 70:733-740, 1953.

(23) Parry, H. Scrapie: A transmissible and hereditary disease of sheep. *Heredity* 17:75-105, 1962.

NATURAL NIDALITY OF TRANSMISSIBLE DISEASES IN RELATION TO LANDSCAPE EPIDEMIOLOGY OF ZOOANTHROPONOSES

E. Pavlovsky

THE BASIC PRINCIPLES OF THE THEORY OF NATURAL NIDALITY OF DISEASES

Zoonoses, Anthroponoses, Zooanthroponoses, Transmissible Diseases

There are a great many diseases of man, animals, and plants on Earth. The diseases of animals are grouped under the term *zoonoses* (derived from the Greek *zoion*—animal and *nozos*—disease). Many zoonoses are common *only* to animals and do not occur in man (for example, plague in cattle, pigs, etc.). Some zoonoses, however, can under certain circumstances be transmitted from sick animals to man directly or by a vector. The vectors are various invertebrate animals, mainly bloodsucking ticks and insects which, on biting a sick man or animal (or a healthy parasite host) ingest a disease-producing agent. When they subsequently bite a healthy man or animal, this agent is transmitted to the latter. Such diseases are known as *transmissible* diseases.

By this mode of transmission of a disease-producing agent by vectors, certain zoonoses, for example, rabies, etc., are communicated to man. Also listed among such zoonoses are cases of asymptomatic invasion by microbes which, when transmitted to humans, exhibit obvious virulence.

The diseases in this group are called *zooanthroponoses* or *anthropozoonoses*, i.e., diseases common to animals and man (from the Greek *anthropos*—man, *zoion*—animal, *nozos*—disease) irrespective of their route of transmission to man.

But there are also certain diseases which at the present stage of evolution of the animal kingdom occur exclusively in man. They are few, however; for example, measles, scarlet fever and diptheria among *non-transmissible* diseases, and human malaria among transmissible ones. Such diseases occurring only in man are grouped under the name of *anthroponoses*.

Hereafter these terms will be used without further explanation of the general meaning of the names of disease groups. This, however, does not rule out the need for a detailed description of the features peculiar to the process of transmission of disease-producing agents by vectors or of acquiring such agents through other routes and from other sources.

Prerequisites for the Theory of Natural Nidality of Diseases

Cases of various diseases affecting humans in diverse regions—the taiga, the steppes, and deserts—have been known for a long time.

We have in mind not those diseases which may affect man in any locality but diseases typical of a particular place, to which people are susceptible in certain (undeveloped or under-developed) areas. These diseases are known as *endemic*.[1]

Such diseases depending on particular circumstances were isolated or spread among whole communities of people. For example, in the last century in the Central Asian semidesert along the river Murgab in Turkmenistan, whole regiments, almost to a man, were afflicted with oriental sore otherwise known as Penjdeh sore. The cause of this mysterious phenomenon remained unknown until the thirties of this century.

Oriental sore, or cutaneous leishmaniasis, takes its name from the British surgeon W. Leishman who gave a scientific description of the causative agent of this disease. But even

---

Source: Excerpted from E. Pavlovsky, *Natural Nidality of Transmissible Diseases in Relation to Landscape Epidemiology of Zooanthroponoses*. Urbana, University of Illinois Press, 1965. © 1965 by the Board of Trustees of the University of Illinois.

[1] Derived from ancient Greek: *en*—in, inside and *demos*—country, place; *endemic*—characteristic of a certain place, territory, country.

before Leishman this parasite had been identified in Tashkent by Prof. P. F. Borovsky, who published a paper on his discovery in the *Journal of Military Medicine* (1898). Therefore, cutaneous leishmaniasis began to be called Borovsky's disease.

It owes its name, Penjdeh sore, to the Turkmenian oasis of Penjdeh, where this disease was frequent. It is also widespread in the tropical countries of the East (India, Iraq, etc.).

After the Great October Socialist Revolution, reports began to arrive about severe and apparently infectious diseases involving the brain in people who had stayed in wild taiga regions. These diseases affected woodcutters, topographers, road-builders, and residents of new villages which sprang up close to the taiga in cleared spaces. Some cases proved fatal. Many survivors were found to have paralyses of various groups of muscles—of the arms, neck, etc.—these lesions disabled them for the rest of their lives.

These examples of human diseases in natural surroundings have the following characteristics: *connection of a disease with a definite geographical landscape* and *seasonal outbreaks of a disease* (in the warm season of the year, in spring, and early summer, etc., Figure 1).

The circumstances contributing to the occurrence of diseases in natural surroundings needed an explanation, even if preliminary, which was based on certain assumptions or working hypotheses.

In uninhabited localities, infection of man by man is out of the question; therefore, the source of a disease should be sought among the local fauna. Various geographical landscapes must apparently have the following inhabitants:

(1) causative agents of transmissible diseases, i.e., diseases spread by the agency of *vectors*, mainly bloodsucking insects and ticks. By biting an animal or man with a disease-producing agent in their peripheral blood, a vector also becomes infective, receiving the pathogen in the ingested blood; within the vector the disease-producing agent may either multiply directly or pass through a part of its complex life-cycle, at the end of which the vector becomes *infective* and capable of transmitting the pathogen (i.e., of infecting healthy susceptible humans or animals) through a bite;

(2) animals which may be *the donors* of the causative agents of these diseases to vectors;

Figure 1. Changes in disease incidence according to decades in a transmissible outbreak of tularemia. From the monograph *Tularemia* by N. G. Olsufyev and G. P. Rudnev (1960).

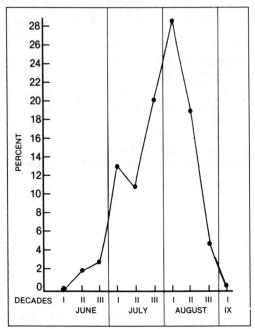

(3) vectors themselves, specifically those species of bloodsucking ticks or insects, which transmit the pathogen they receive from a donor to susceptible animals called *recipients*. Under certain conditions, man can also be a recipient of a causative agent.

The study of the mysterious diseases people are likely to be infected with in natural surroundings made it necessary to send expeditions to corresponding localities to carry out surveys on the spot.

The basic centers of such research carried out by the author and his associates were successively the S. M. Kirov Academy of Military Medicine, the former A. M. Gorky All-Union Institute of Experimental Medicine, the Department of Parasitology and Medical Zoology at the Academician N. F. Gamaleya Institute of Epidemiology and Microbiology under the U.S.S.R. Academy of Medical Sciences, the Institute of Zoology under the U.S.S.R. Academy of Sciences, the Tadjik branch of the U.S.S.R. Academy of Sciences, now the Academy of Sciences of the Tadjik Republic, and other institutions within the system of the U.S.S.R. Ministry of Health and the Academies of Union Republics, particularly of the Kazakh Republic, etc.

Guided by the above prerequisites, personal investigations, field and experimental studies were carried out by the author and many other research workers during numerous scientific expeditions. The results of this research, together with an analysis of the available scientific literature on medicine, veterinary medicine, and biology, led the author to summarize his views of *the natural nidality of transmissible diseases* in the form of a theory, which is basically applicable to parasitic diseases also. Moreover, the problems of studying the focal character of certain non-transmissible infections have also been raised of late.

Non-transmissible diseases is the collective name given to those infections whose agents are not vector-borne, for instance, smallpox, diphtheria, scarlet fever, etc. Their agents may be communicable directly from a sick to a healthy person by contact, by inhaling air contaminated with a disease-producing agent when talking, coughing, or sneezing, (*respiratory route of infection*), etc.

The agents of certain diseases are spread with and without the aid of vectors. For example, the plague-like disease tularemia is transmitted not only by at least 40 species of vectors but also in the process of skinning tularemia-affected water rats, and from contact with water containing dead water rats; anthrax may be communicated by wearing felt boots and coats made from the wool and skins of animals killed by anthrax, etc.

It is characteristic that the agents of most transmissible diseases are spread *only by vectors* (yellow fever by mosquitoes, malaria by *Anopheles* mosquitoes, tick-borne encephalitis by the *Ixodes persulcatus* and other *Ixodes* ticks, etc.). Such diseases are known as *specific obligato-transmissible* diseases. The pathogens of other diseases are transmitted by various routes, including vectors. Such diseases, the so-called *facultative* or *potentially transmissible diseases* are, for example, enteric fever, cholera, tularemia, plague, etc.

A number of transmissible diseases are characterized by their foci being confined to an environment untouched by man or modified by man, intentionally or unintentionally, in the past or at present. The foci of such diseases are known as natural foci and the corresponding diseases as *diseases with natural foci.*

What we call the natural nidality of transmissible diseases is characterized by the following features:

(a) The existence of any transmissible disease depends on *the successive transit of its causative agent from the body of the animal donor* (sick animal, asymptomatic virus carrier, or parasite host) *to the vector body. This transmission usually takes place when the vector draws blood from the donor and subsequently transmits the causative agent to the animal recipient, commonly when drawing its blood also; the infected recipient may* in its turn *become a donor for another group of vectors*, etc. In this manner, there occurs, as we say, *circulation* (spiral-type circulation, Figure 2) of the causative agent from organism to organism in one and the same or another population of the natural focus of a disease. The circulation of a pathogen, beginning from its reception by a vector from an animal donor and including the time required for the vector to become infective and infect the animal recipient which in its turn becomes a donor of the pathogen for a fresh vector, is called the complete cycle or tour of the pathogen during its circulation. But such a cycle is not a complete round, since the next time the pathogen is transmitted by a vector it goes not to the animal from which it came originally but to another animal of the same population or an animal of another systematic position (from another specific population). This consecutive transmission of the pathogen occurs as though in a spiral form. The vector which has received the pathogen from a wild donor may transmit it also to man who then becomes infected and develops the corresponding disease.

(b) This circulation *takes place only when the environmental conditions are favorable* (for instance, at a definite temperature) *or at any rate do not obstruct any of the stages.*

A natural focus of disease exists when there are a specific climate, vegetation, soil, and favorable microclimate in the places where vectors, donors, and recipients of infection take shelter. In other words, *a natural focus of disease is related to a specific geographical landscape*, such as the taiga of a certain botanical composition, a hot sand desert, the steppe, etc., i.e., *a biogeocoenosis.*

Man falls victim to an animal disease with natural foci only when he stays in the territory of its natural focus at a definite season of the year, and is attacked as prey *by hungry bloodsucking vectors* which have already acquired infection from biting wild animals—the carriers and donors of this disease. This accounts for the seasonal occurrence of

Figure 2. Diagram showing the "spiral" transition (circulation) of tick-borne encephalitis virus from organism to organism (D,RD) in a natural focus of disease by the agency of tick vectors (TV). Drawing by E. N. Pavlovsky. (M—infection of man from ticks (T) having acquired the virus from a wild animal, the virus donor (D); (RD)—one and the same animal: (R) as a virus recipient, (D) as a virus donor in the period of virusemia; (M) cul-de-sac in subsequent virus circulation (man); (TV) one and the same tick individual: (T) as a virus recipient, (V) as a virus vector; I, II, III, tours of circulation.)

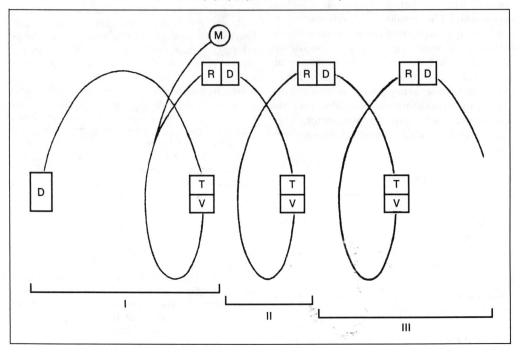

such diseases; indeed, vectors in natural surroundings are not, as a rule, active round the year, but only in a fairly warm season.

Not every individual of a given vector species transmits infection but only those which have acquired it from an animal donor and, under the influence of environmental factors, have reached an infective stage, i.e., have become capable of infecting other animals and man. In such cases, a vector acquires *natural* or *spontaneous* infectivity and *an infective power*.

A natural focus of disease harboring hungry, naturally infected vectors is said to be in *a latent state*, i.e., capable of infecting both animals and man.

The natural foci of certain diseases may occur in geographical landscapes of varied character, in which they are connected with specific biotopes, otherwise called habitats. In mountainous areas, important features are the elevation above sea level, and whether the mountain slopes face north or south; the disease foci are associated with burrows, cervices, overhanging rocks, caves, spaces under stones, and mountain streams. In the plains, disease foci are associated with river creeks, flooding rivers, and lakes; on the sea coast, with small residual reservoirs, etc.

Other diseases with natural foci are more markedly linked with definite landscapes; the foci of the Penjdeh sore of the desert (rural) type are linked with the semidesert zone.

One and the same geographical landscape may simultaneously have natural foci of two or three diseases, and one and the same specific focus may harbor causative agents of different diseases. A focus is said to be *polyvector* if it is inhabited by *several types of vectors* sometimes even belonging to widely different systematic categories. One example is the rodent burrow in Central Asia (Figure 3).

Such foci of two or three diseases existing simultaneously are known as *conjugate*, for instance, the foci of tularemia and plague, Penjdeh sore, and tick-borne relapsing fever, etc.

Figure 3. Diagram showing summary epidemiological significance of the rodent burrow biocoenosis as a natural focus of various diseases of man and animals (anthropozoonoses). Drawing by E. N. Pavlovsky. Arrows indicate members of biocoenosis, venomous (scorpions and spiders) or harmless to man; oval lines show the route of transmission of pathogenic agents from rodents to man.

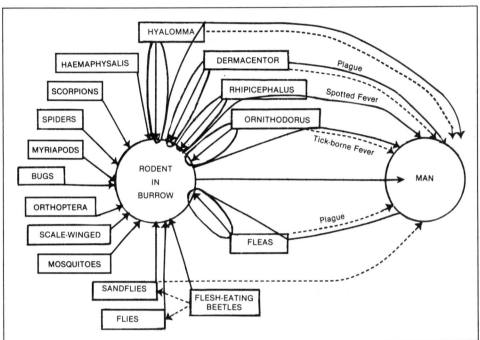

When inhabited by several species of animals—donors of a causative agent—a natural focus of disease is said to be *polyhostal* in regard to the disease-producing agent.

The following diseases are at present known to have natural foci: tick-borne spirochetosis, tick-borne and Japanese encephalitides, highly virulent infections (tularemia, plague), lymphocytic choriomeningitis, equine encephalomyelitis, tick-borne rickettsioses, desert-type cutaneous leishmaniasis, listerellosis, erysipeloid, hemorrhagic fevers, nephroso-nephritis, and apparently brucellosis, rabies, ornithoses, etc.; among the helminthiases—opisthorchiasis and diphyllobothriasis, trichinellosis, bilharziasis, etc. It is quite probable that a viral disease such as pappataci fever as well as psittacosis, leptospiroses, and other diseases also have natural foci. Outside the Soviet Union, diseases originating in natural foci are jungle yellow fever, kala-azar in Africa, trypanosomiases (African sleeping sickness), and others. The isolation of the causative agent of pseudotuberculosis of rodents along with plague cultures in the Tsagan-Nur district of the Mongolian People's Republic from the narrow-skulled vole gives one reason for attributing pseudotuberculosis to diseases with natural foci also.

The number of known diseases with natural foci is steadily growing and will continue to grow as research advances, particularly in the tropical countries. There are frequent cases of the discovery of new viruses transmitted by *Arthropoda*—ticks or mosquitoes (arboviruses).

Animals which are donors and recipients of the causative agent of a transmissible or parasitic disease, the agent itself (of whatever nature), and infection vectors are all members of a pathobiocoenosis (E. N. Pavlovsky) associated with a specific biotope (or several biotopes) of a particular geographical landscape, or of a biogeocoenosis (as defined by Academician V. N. Sukachev).

OBSERVATIONS ON RECENT INCREASE IN MORTALITY FROM ASTHMA

F. E. Speizer,[1] R. Doll,[2] and P. Heaf[3]

An increase in the mortality from asthma, particularly in children, has been reported from Australia (1), the United States (2), and Britain (3), and suggestions have been made that the increase is due to the introduction of new methods of treatment (4, 5, 6). We have therefore examined the trends in mortality from asthma throughout the world and have sought evidence to account for the increase in England and Wales.

TRENDS IN MORTALITY AT ALL AGES

Before 1948 deaths classified as asthma ranged from various forms of bronchitis and influenza to deaths associated with a variety of cardiovascular, renal, and allergic diseases. In 1948, with the sixth revision of the *International Classification of Diseases,* asthma was given a more specific category (List No. 241), but it was still classified with several conditions in which asthma may have played only a subsidiary part. These included "asthmatic bronchitis" and other forms of bronchitis where asthma was mentioned without specifying that it was allergic. When the seventh revision of the *Classification* was undertaken in 1955 these types of "bronchitis" were removed and the asthma category began to correspond to a single disease entity (Table 1).

These changes reflect, in part, changes in the clinical concept of the disease, and further revisions may be expected as diagnostic precision and knowledge of causation improve. Meanwhile the available statistics can be used only as initial guides to trends in mortality.

In England and Wales the number of deaths decreased progressively from 1879 in 1952 to 1507 in 1957, dropped with the new classification to 1214 in 1959, and rose subsequently to 2040 in 1966. Between 1959 and 1966 the death rate increased by 56 percent, from 2.7 to 4.2 per 100 000 persons.

The trends in 19 countries between 1951 and 1964 have been summarized by the World Health Organization (7). These show that:

(1) In virtually every country there was a sharp decline in the crude mortality rate between 1957 and 1959 which presumably reflected the change from use of the sixth revision of the *International Classification* to the seventh revision.

(2) With the exception of Venezuela, every country with data available before 1958 showed an excess mortality in males, and since 1958 this excess has been reduced. Before 1958 the excess is likely to have been due to the inclusion of a high proportion of deaths from bronchitis, a condition which is appreciably commoner in males.

(3) In 1964 the crude mortality varied between the countries from 1.1 to 9.7 per 100 000 persons, a variation which is likely to be due, in part, to variation in diagnostic criteria.

(4) Between 1959 and 1964 several countries showed sporadic increases in mortality, but the general picture is of a constant rate with a slight tendency to decrease.

(5) England and Wales alone showed a steady increase.

TRENDS IN AGE-SPECIFIC MORTALITY

Not all the deaths attributed to asthma are likely to have been due to asthma, and this is particularly true for deaths that occurred in infancy and old age. Under five years of age asthma may be confused with bronchiolitis or bronchitis which has led to airway obstruction and presented as overinflation with wheezing. Over 65 years of age asthma is commonly com-

Source: *British Medical Journal* 1:335-339, 1968.
[1] U.S. Public Health Service Special Fellow, Medical Research Council's Statistical Research Unit.
[2] Director, Medical Research Council's Statistical Research Unit.
[3] Chest Physician, University College Hospital, London W.C.1.

plicated by bronchitis and heart failure, which may be the result of the underlying respiratory disease or of independent heart disease. In both these age groups the selection of asthma as the underlying cause of death is partly subjective, and many deaths attributed to asthma could more properly be attributed to other causes.

A more accurate picture of the trend in mortality attributable to the disease may therefore be obtained by confining the comparison to ages 5 to 64 years. At these ages the increase in mortality in England and Wales is even more pronounced; the annual number of deaths increased from 720 in 1959 to 1401 in 1966, and the corresponding death rate nearly doubled (from 2.0 to 3.7 per 100 000 persons).

Figures 1 and 2 show that the rates have been approximately equal in both sexes in three age groups—10 to 14 years, 5 to 34 years, and 35 to 64 years. Between 1957 and 1960 the rates fell at ages 35 to 64 years, due largely to the change in the method of classification, but there was little consistent change at younger ages. Since 1960–61 the rates have increased.

Figure 1. Asthma mortality in males aged 10 to 14 years, 5 to 34 years, and 35 to 64 years in England and Wales from 1952 to 1966.

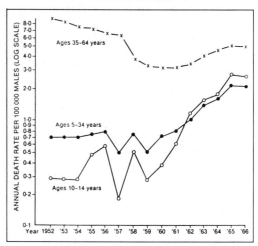

Table 2 shows the changes since 1959 in greater detail. Since the male and female rates have been approximately equal the figures for both sexes have been combined to reduce the effect of random fluctuation due to small num-

Table 1. International Classification of Causes of Death: Description of deaths attributed to asthma between 1938 and 1966.

1938-1947—5th Revision of I.C.D.

112	Asthma

	Asthmatic bronchitis	Hay asthma
	Bronchial asthma	Hay fever
	Bronchitic asthma	Spasmodic asthma
	Catarrhal asthma	

112.1	With influenza as a contributory or secondary cause
112.2	With chronic endocarditis as a contributory or secondary cause
112.3	With myocardial disease as a contributory or secondary cause
112.4	With arteriosclerosis as a contributory or secondary cause
112.5	With chronic nephritis as a contributory or secondary cause
112.6	Without any of the complications here specified (1-5)

1948-1957—6th Revision of I.C.D.

241	Asthma (bronchial)

	Allergic (any cause)	Bronchitis, allergic
	Sporadic	Hay asthma
	Asthmatic bronchitis	Hay fever with asthma

This title excludes cardiac asthma (434.2) and pneumoconiotic asthma (523-524)

1958-   —7th Revision of I.C.D.

241	Asthma (bronchial)

	Allergic (any cause)	Bronchitis, allergic
	Sporadic	Hay asthma
		Hay fever with asthma

This title excludes cardiac asthma (434.2) and pneumoconiotic asthma (523-524.) It also excludes asthma not indicated as allergic with mention of bronchitis (acute) (chronic) (500-502).

bers. From Table 2 it is evident that an increase in mortality began to occur in about 1961 and

Figure 2. Asthma mortality in females aged 10 to 14 years, 5 to 34 years, and 35 to 64 years in England and Wales from 1952 to 1966.

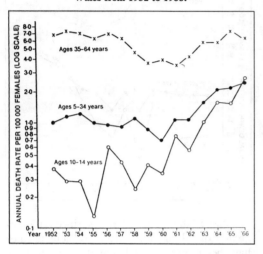

that all ages between 5 and 64 years of age have been affected. The greatest increase in mortality has taken place at ages 10 to 14 years, at which ages the rate has increased eight times, from 0.3 to 2.5 per 100 000 persons. The increase has, however, been substantial at all ages from 5 to 34 years, and at these ages the annual number of deaths increased by 308 and the death rate trebled from 0.7 to 2.2 per 100 000 persons.

In the rest of this paper we have confined our observations to mortality at ages 5 to 34 years, partly because this age group has shown a large increase in mortality, partly because asthma which develops under 35 years of age is usually classed as "allergic" and can be distinguished clinically from the disease which develops at a later age, and partly because the mortality from bronchitis begins to exceed that from asthma at about 35 years of age and the possibility of confusing these conditions as the cause of death increases rapidly with advancing years.

Table 2. Number of deaths and death rates from asthma per 100 000 persons, by age: England and Wales, 1959 to 1969.[a]

Age in years	Deaths	1959	1960	1961	1962	1963	1964	1965	1966
5-9	No.	6	12	6	6	9	23	18	17
	Rate	0.18	0.37	0.18	0.18	0.27	0.67	0.51	0.47
10-14	No.	12	13	24	29	41	53	66	80
	Rate	0.33	0.35	0.65	0.84	1.21	1.60	2.02	2.46
15-19	No.	19	17	24	39	36	62	73	91
	Rate	0.64	0.55	0.77	1.11	0.99	1.67	1.96	2.45
20-24	No.	24	27	28	32	56	51	79	83
	Rate	0.85	0.94	0.97	1.09	1.87	1.66	2.49	2.52
25-29	No.	32	28	39	38	45	69	90	79
	Rate	1.12	0.98	1.37	1.31	1.53	2.33	3.00	2.64
30-34	No.	30	31	48	47	83	84	77	81
	Rate	0.99	1.04	1.61	1.57	2.79	2.85	2.63	2.78
5-34	No.	123	128	169	191	270	342	403	431
	Rate	0.66	0.68	0.89	1.00	1.40	1.76	2.05	2.18
35-64	No.	597	594	568	655	845	903	1072	970
	Rate	3.32	3.29	3.13	3.60	4.64	4.96	5.89	5.34
5-64	No.	720	722	737	846	1115	1245	1475	1401
	Rate	1.96	1.96	1.99	2.26	2.97	3.30	3.90	369
All ages	No.	1214	1188	1269	1352	1655	1800	2080	2040
	Rate	2.67	2.60	2.75	2.89	3.52	3.80	4.35	4.24

[a] From the *Registrar General's Statistical Reviews of England and Wales* for 1959 to 1965, the *Quarterly Return for England and Wales*, 3rd Quarter 1966, and personal communication.

The relative importance of the increase in mortality between 1959 and 1966 is indicated by the change in the proportion of all deaths attributed to asthma over the same period. In 1959 and 1960 approximately 1 percent of all deaths at ages 5 to 34 years were attributed to asthma; in 1966 the proportion was 3.4 percent. At ages 10 to 14 years the proportional mortality increased from 1 percent to 7.2 percent.

Data are not yet available for the numbers of deaths due to other causes in 1966; but in 1965, when asthma accounted for 5.7 percent of all deaths at ages 10 to 14 years, it ranked sixth in the list of causes of death (Table 3). The only categories with substantially higher rates were motor accidents (I.C.D. List Nos. E810 to E825), malignant neoplasms other than leukemia (List Nos. 140–203, 205), congenital malformations (List Nos. 750–759), and diseases of the nervous system and sense organs (List Nos. 330–398). Other diseases whose rates were of the same order as asthma were leukemia (List No. 204) and pneumonia (List Nos. 490–493).

TRENDS IN OTHER COUNTRIES

Mortality rates and trends in mortality in other countries fall into two fairly distinct groups. Those countries whose death rate for asthma at ages 5 to 34 was less than 0.5 per 100 000 persons in 1959 to 1960 and those whose rate ranged between 0.5 and 1 per 100 000 persons. The United States and virtually all western European countries apart from Britain (including Belgium, France, Italy, Netherlands, Spain, West Germany, Denmark, and Sweden) fall into the first group, and none of these showed any appreciable increase in mortality up to 1964, irrespective of whether or not they showed any change in total asthma mortality at all ages.

The remaining countries need to be considered individually. *Scotland's* death rate for asthma at ages 5 to 34 years was generally lower than in England and Wales. After 1962, however, the increase in the number of deaths was similar. The increase became appreciable in 1963, and in 1964 the rate was approximately three times the average for 1961 and 1962. At ages 35 to 64 years there has also been some increase, but less pronounced.

Before 1964 *Australian* death rates at ages 5 to 34 years were higher than in England and Wales; and until then they were relatively stable. A substantial increase took place from 1963 to 1964 (from 0.9 to 1.8 per 100 000 persons), but

Table 3. Ten major causes of death in England and Wales in children aged 10-14 years for the year 1965.[a]

Cause of death (I.C.D.)	No.			Percentage of total deaths in age group
	Male	Female	Total	
1. All motor accidents (E810-E825)	127	66	193	16.6
2. Malignant neoplasms other than leukemia (*I.C.D.* 140-203, 205)	85	39	124	10.7
3. All congenital malformations (*I.C.D.* 750-759)	50	51	101	8.7
4. All diseases of nervous system (*I.C.D.* 330-398)	53	37	90	7.8
5. Leukemia and aleukemia (*I.C.D.* 204)	39	35	74	6.4
6. Asthma (*I.C.D.* 241)	43	23	66	5.7
7. All pneumonia (*I.C.D.* 490-493)	27	36	63	5.4
8. Drowning (E929)	44	9	53	4.6
9. All gastrointestinal diseases (*I.C.D.* 530-587)	31	19	50	4.3
10. All genito-urinary diseases (*I.C.D.* 590-637)	14	33	47	4.1
All other diseases	190	109	299	25.8
Total all diseases	703	457	1160	100.0

[a] *Registrar General's Statistical Review of England and Wales for the Year 1965.*

there was no further increase in 1965. In contrast to England and Wales and Scotland, comparable increases also occurred at ages 10 to 14 years and at ages 35 to 64 years.

In *Japan* the rates have shown a somewhat different trend. At ages 5 to 34 years there has been a steady but rather slow increase in mortality, which in 1964 had risen by about 40 percent, in contrast to the rise of over 250 percent in England and Wales. This, however, was accompanied by a decrease in mortality at ages 35 to 64 years.

New Zealand alone had an asthma death rate at ages 5 to 34 years of over 0.5 per 100 000 persons in 1959 and showed no increase in mortality in the next six years.

Different results are obtained when the comparison is limited to ages 10 to 19 years—the decade in which the largest increase was recorded in England and Wales. Five-year age-specific rates are available for the whole period 1959 to 1964 for only 11 countries, and these are shown in Table 4. The individual results are irregular, but when the countries are grouped regionally, to reduce the effect of random fluctuation of small numbers, it is found that there

has been an increase in mortality rates from 1959–1961 to 1962–1964 in each region. The increase has been largest in Britain—162 percent at ages 10 to 14 years and 84 percent at ages 15 to 19 years. In Western Europe, Japan, and Australasia increases have occurred in the range of 85 to 103 percent at ages 10 to 14 years and in the range of 23 to 45 percent at ages 15 to 19 years. In the United States the increases have been small, but they still show the same trend. Small increases were again observed in 1965 (to 0.30 and 0.40 per 100 000), but provisional data for 1966, for which we are indebted to the Division of Vital Statistics of the Department of Health, Education, and Welfare of the U.S. Public Health Service, suggest that a substantial increase may now have occurred. From 1965 to 1966 the number of deaths attributed to asthma at ages 1 to 14 years increased by 64 percent, from 146 to 240.

REASONS FOR INCREASED DEATH RATE

One possible explanation of the increase in England and Wales is that it is an artifact brought about by changes in the diagnostic cri-

Table 4. International death rates from asthma for ages 10-14 and 15-19 years: 1959-61 and 1962-1964.[a]

Country	Age in years	1959-1961		1962-1964		Percent increase 1959-1961 to 1962-1964
		No. of deaths	Average yearly death rate per 100 000	No. of deaths	Average yearly death rate per 100 000	
Britain:						
England and Wales	10-14	59	0.48	143	1.26	162.5
Scotland	15-19	69	0.67	151	1.23	83.6
Australasia:						
Australia[b]	10-14	21	0.56	44	1.14	103.6
New Zealand	15-19	30	0.94	40	1.16	23.4
Europe:						
Germany						
Sweden						
Denmark	10-14	29	0.21	54	0.39	85.7
Netherlands	15-19	31	0.24	47	0.35	45.8
Belgium						
Japan	10-14	87	0.26	147	0.50	92.3
	15-19	107	0.38	172	0.55	44.7
U.S.A.	10-14	104	0.21	140	0.26	23.8
	15-19	124	0.30	153	0.33	10.0

[a] Data compiled from the Official National Vital Statistics Record for each country for the years 1959-1964, with the exception of Australia.

[b] Data from Dr. B. Gandevia (personal communication).

teria used by physicians certifying the cause of death. This possibility has been investigated by comparing the trends in mortality attributed to asthma and a variety of other respiratory diseases; that is, from all forms of bronchitis (*I.C.D.* List Nos. 500–502), bronchiectasis (List No. 526), emphysema without mention of bronchitis (List No. 527.1), pneumonia (List Nos. 490–493), and other chronic interstitial pneumonias (List No. 525). The annual numbers of deaths and the death rates attributed to these causes are summarized in Table 5. Some decrease occurred in the number of deaths attributed to pneumonia, but the reduction (107 deaths between 1959 and 1965) is less than a half of the increase in asthma deaths (280 over the same period) and the pneumonia death rate oscillated while the asthma mortality increased steadily. No appreciable change took place in the death rates attributed to bronchitis or other chronic respiratory diseases, and changes in the use of these categories cannot by themselves have led to an increase in the number of deaths attributed to asthma. Moreover, the number of deaths attributed to bronchitis for which asthma was mentioned on the death certificate did not decrease at these ages—as would be expected if there had been a tendency for doctors to attribute the underlying cause to asthma alone rather than to asthma and bronchitis—but increased from 24 in 1959 to 49 in 1966.

Further evidence is provided by the fact that the number of asthma deaths that were certified by coroners after necropsy examination increased even more rapidly than the total (from 43 at ages 5 to 34 years in 1959 to 237 in 1966). If the increase were an artifact we should have to postulate that there had been an even greater change in the diagnostic criteria used by pathologists than in those used by clinicians, or that there had been a change in the type of case referred to coroners.

We conclude, therefore, that the increase in mortality attributed to asthma at ages 5 to 34 years is, in large part, real and represents a true increase in the annual number of deaths from the disease.

TWO EXPLANATIONS

One explanation of a true increase in mortality could be that the number of patients suffering from asthma had risen. This cannot be tested directly, but an indication of its validity can be obtained by comparing the frequency with which patients have consulted their general practitioners. In 1955 to 1956 the Royal College of General Practitioners in cooperation with the Registrar General collected figures on morbidity from a variety of diseases, including asthma *(8)*, and similar data have been made available to us for the years 1961 to 1966 for a selected group of practices covering approximately 20 000 patients (Table 6). Over this 10-year period there has, in fact, been a tendency

Table 5. Death rate per 100 000 persons aged 5-34 years from selected respiratory diseases: England and Wales 1959-1965.[a]

Diagnostic category	Deaths	1959	1960	1961	1962	1963	1964	1965
Acute and chronic bronchitis	No.	121	107	124	128	126	121	131
	Rate	0.65	0.57	0.66	0.67	0.65	0.62	0.66
(*I.C.D.* 500-502)								
Chronic respiratory[b] diseases	No.	84	92	73	76	73	76	78
(*I.C.D.* 525, 526, 527.1)	Rate	0.45	0.49	0.39	0.40	0.38	0.39	0.40
Pneumonias	No.	486	403	423	474	416	398	379
(*I.C.D.* 490-493)	Rate	2.61	2.15	2.24	2.47	2.15	2.04	1.93
Asthma	No.	123	128	169	191	270	342	403
(*I.C.D.* 241)	Rate	0.66	0.68	0.89	1.00	1.40	1.76	2.05

[a] From the *Registrar General's Statistical Review of England and Wales* for each year 1959-1965.
[b] See text for definition.

Table 6. Morbidity from asthma recorded in general practice.

Episodes per year per 1000 persons aged (in years):	1955-1956[a]	1961[b]	1962	1963	1964	1965	1966
5-14	10	9.2	4.9	6.8	3.9	4.9	4.3
15-44	7	6.6	3.6	3.0	5.1	6.4	6.6
45-65	10	5.2	9.3	5.1	5.2	4.5	9.6
All ages	9	5.8	3.8	5.6	5.2	5.3	4.6

[a] Fry (8).
[b] 1961 to 1966, Dr. D. L. Crombie, Royal College of General Practitioners (personal communication).

for the number of episodes of asthma leading to consultation to decrease at ages 5 to 14 years and to stay approximately the same at ages 15 to 44 years. A reduction in the number of episodes at young ages could be due to a decrease in the incidence of the disease or to some change in therapy keeping the patients away from the doctor; but even in the latter case it would seem most unlikely that the incidence of the disease could have increased appreciably.

Another explanation could be that there has been an increase in the case fatality rate. We have again not been able to test this directly, but it is notable that the proportion of asthma deaths at ages 5 to 34 years that were certified by coroners increased from 35 percent in 1959 to 55 percent in 1966. The proportion of deaths from all causes certified by coroners over this period is not available separately for different age groups, but there is no reason to suppose that the proportion has increased differentially in this age group, and for all ages it has remained approximately 10 percent. It appears probable, therefore, that the mode of death from asthma at young ages has changed. In the absence of evidence to the contrary, it would seem that an increase in the case fatality rate is the most likely explanation of the increased mortality rate, and we have accepted this as a working hypothesis.

ENVIRONMENTAL HAZARDS

Several factors could be responsible. Changes in the prevalence of environmental hazards could cause patients with asthma to be more severely affected and so could result in an increased mortality. Alternatively, new methods of management of asthmatic patients might

produce temporary symptomatic relief, but increase the hazards of dying from the disease later.

Morbidity studies in New Orleans, U.S.A., have suggested that asthma can reach epidemic levels under particular conditions of atmospheric pollution (9), but it is difficult to believe that this could be a factor in England. Certainly the increase could not be due to smoke pollution, which has decreased in English towns over the last decade, nor could it be attributed to pollution with sulphur gases, which has remained approximately constant (10). Motor traffic has increased considerably, and one of the contituents of motor fumes could perhaps have had a harmful effect. If this were the case, however, a substantial difference in mortality would be expected between urban and rural areas, and we have failed to find any evidence of this in the national mortality data for 1966. The death rate was 2.0 per 100 000 persons aged 5 to 34 years in conurbations, 3.0 in urban areas of more than 100 000 population, 2.2 in urban areas of under 50 000 population, and 1.9 in rural districts.

Other environmental hazards are associated with smoking and occupation, but these cannot be responsible for changes that have been observed characteristically at ages 10 to 14 years in both sexes.

NEW METHODS OF TREATMENT

Substantial advances in the management of respiratory failure from a variety of chronic pulmonary diseases have been made in the last 15 years (11), and new methods of both emergency and long-term therapy have been introduced for the treatment of asthma. Corticosteroids were introduced into the management of the disease in 1952, but the increase in mortality did not begin until nine years later. This discrepancy, however, is not sufficient to exculpate them entirely. The frequent and prolonged use of corticosteroids spread slowly, and the risk of harmful effects may be at a maximum only after patients have been under treatment for several years. A much closer correlation obtains with the use of pressurized aerosols containing sympathomimetics. These were introduced in England and Wales in 1960 and began to gain wide acceptance in 1961; and in the next five years their consumption is estimated to have increased more than fourfold (Ministry of Health, unpublished data). The closeness of the correlation justifies inquiry into the possibly harmful effect of the preparations, but a temporal correlation of this sort, taken by itself, is a poor basis for drawing conclusions about cause and effect.

If either of these forms of therapy is to be considered as a possible cause of an increased fatality rate, it will be necessary to inquire why a similar effect has not been recorded in other countries where they have also been widely used. It may be, however, that a large increase in mortality has not been recorded in some of those countries where the mortality from asthma was initially much lower than in Britain, because similar deaths have been, and currently still are, attributed to other causes. In New Zealand the size of the population is so small that chance factors might obscure the evidence of even a substantial increase in risk. It is notable, however, that since 1959 an increase in the mortality has been recorded at ages 10 to 19 years widely throughout the world. At these ages children have begun to act independently and may be particularly prone to misuse a self-administered form of treatment.

SUMMARY

The mortality attributed to asthma has increased annually in England and Wales from 1960 to 1965. The increase is more pronounced at ages 5 to 34 years than at older ages and is most pronounced at ages 10 to 14 years. In this last age group the mortality increased nearly eight times in seven years, and in 1966 asthma accounted for 7 percent of all deaths.

No comparable increase has been observed in any other country, but smaller increases at ages 10 to 19 years have been observed in Australasia, Japan, western Europe, and the United States.

There is no evidence to suggest that there has been any change in diagnostic habits, certification of deaths, or methods of classification which could account for the increase in Great Britain, and it is concluded that the increase is real.

General practitioners' records provide no evidence of an increase in prevalence and it seems probable that there has been an increase in case fatality.

No environmental hazards are known which could have increased the severity of the disease, and the possibility has to be considered that the increase may be due to new methods of treatment. Corticosteroids have been used increasingly since 1952, and in Great Britain the use of pressurized aerosols containing sympathomimetics has increased rapidly since 1960.

Addendum. Since this paper was submitted figures for 1966 in New Zealand supplied by the Public Health Statistician for New Zealand have been made available to us by Dr. Gandevia. These reveal an apparent increase in deaths attributed to asthma for the age group 9–54 years. Age-specific death rates are not yet available, but Dr. Gandevia suggests that an upward trend in mortality may now be occurring (Gandevia, personal communication).

We are grateful to the Registrar General of England and Wales for supplying many of the data, and for supplying them with minimal delay. We are grateful also to the Ministry of Health for information about the sale of aerosol bronchodilators; and to Miss A.M. Hetzel, Chief of the Statistical Resources Section of the Division of Vital Statistics, U.S. Public Health Service, Dr. B. Gandevia, Associate Professor in Thoracic Medicine, the Prince Henry Hospital, Little Bay, New South Wales, Professor S. Koller, Professor of Medical Statistics, University of Mainz, and Dr. D. L. Crombie, Director of the Records and Statistics Unit of the Royal College of General Practitioners, for information about the mortality from asthma in the United States, Australia, and the German Federal Republic, and for morbidity data in Britain.

Dr. F. E. Speizer was supported by the National Center for Air Pollution, Bureau of Disease Prevention and Environmental Control, U.S. Public Health Service.

References

(1) Gandevia, B. *Br Med J* 2:441, 1967.

(2) Richards, W. and J.R. Patrick. *Am J Dis Child* 110:4, 1965.

(3) Smith, J.M. *Lancet* 1:1042, 1966.

(4) Ford, R.M. *Med J Aust* 2:196, 1966.

(5) Kessler, A. and C. Geller-Bernstein *JAMA* 196:458, 1966.

(6) Greenberg, M.J. and A. Pines. *Br Med J* 1:563, 1967.

(7) World Health Organization. *Epidemiol Vital Statis Rep* 19:525, 1966.

(8) Fry, J. *Morbidity Statistics from General Practice,* Vol. 3. London, H.M.S.O., 1962, pp. 15–33.

(9) Weill, H., M.M. Ziskirdj, V.J. Derbes, R.J.M. Horton, R.O. McCaldin, and R.C. Dickerson. *Arch Environm Health* 10:148, 1965.

(10) Ministry of Technology. *The Investigation of Atmospheric Pollution, 1958–1966. 32nd Report.* London, H.M.S.O., 1967.

(11) Detty, T.L. *Management of Chronic Obstructive Lung Diseases.* Washington, D.C., Public Health Service Publication No. 1457, 1966.

THE CHOLERA NEAR GOLDEN SQUARE

John Snow

The most terrible outbreak of cholera which ever occurred in this kingdom, is probably that which took place in Broad Street, Golden Square, and the adjoining streets, a few weeks ago. Within two hundred and fifty yards of the spot where Cambridge Street joins Broad Street, there were upwards of five hundred fatal attacks of cholera in ten days. The mortality in this limited area probably equals any that was ever caused in this country, even by the plague; and it was much more sudden, as the greater number of cases terminated in a few hours. The mortality would undoubtedly have been much greater had it not been for the flight of the population. Persons in furnished lodgings left first, then other lodgers went away, leaving their furniture to be sent for when they could meet with a place to put it in. Many houses were closed altogether, owing to the death of the proprietors; and, in a great number of instances, the tradesmen who remained had sent away their families: so that in less than six days from the commencement of the outbreak, the most afflicted streets were deserted by more than three-quarters of their inhabitants.

There were a few cases of cholera in the neighborhood of Broad Street, Golden Square, in the latter part of August; and the so-called outbreak, which commenced in the night between the 31st August and the 1st September, was, as in all similar instances, only a violent increase of the malady. As soon as I became acquainted with the situation and the extent of this irruption of cholera, I suspected some contamination of the water of the much-frequented street-pump in Broad Street, near the end of Cambridge Street; but on examining the water, on the evening of the 3rd September, I found so little impurity in it of an organic nature, that I hesitated to come to a conclusion. Further inquiry, however, showed me that there was no other circumstance or agent common to the circumscribed locality in which this sudden increase of cholera occurred, and not extending beyond it, except the water of the above-mentioned pump. I found, moreover, that the water varied, during the next two days, in the amount of organic impurity, visible to the naked eye, on close inspection, in the form of small white, flocculent particles; and I concluded that, at the commencement of the outbreak, it might possibly have been still more impure. I requested permission, therefore, to take a list, at the General Register Office, of the deaths from cholera, registered during the week ending 2nd September, in the sub-districts of Golden Square, Berwick Street, and St. Ann's, Soho, which was kindly granted. Eighty-nine deaths from cholera were registered, during the week, in the three subdistricts. Of these, only six occurred in the four first days of the week; four occurred on Thursday, the 31st August; and the remaining seventy-nine on Friday and Saturday. I considered, therefore, that the outbreak commenced on the Thursday; and I made inquiry, in detail, respecting the eighty-three deaths registered as having taken place during the last three days of the week.

On proceeding to the spot, I found that nearly all the deaths had taken place within a short distance of the pump. There were only ten deaths in houses situated decidedly nearer to another street pump. In five of these cases the families of the deceased persons informed me that they always sent to the pump in Broad Street, as they preferred the water to that of the pump which was nearer. In three other cases, the deceased were children who went to school near the pump in Broad Street. Two of them were known to drink the water; and the parents of the third think it probable that it did so. The other two deaths, beyond the district which this pump supplies, represent only the amount of mortality from cholera that was occurring before the irruption took place.

With regard to the deaths occurring in the locality belonging to the pump, there were sixty-one instances in which I was informed that the deceased persons used to drink the pump-water from Broad Street, either constantly or occa-

Source: Excerpted from *Snow on Cholera*. Cambridge, Harvard University Press, 1949. By permission of the publisher.

sionally. In six instances I could get no information, owing to the death or departure of every one connected with the deceased individuals; and in six cases I was informed that the deceased persons did not drink the pump-water before their illness.

The result of the inquiry, then, was that there had been no particular outbreak or increase of cholera, in this part of London, except among the persons who were in the habit of drinking the water of the above-mentioned pump-well.

I had an interview with the Board of Guardians of St. James's parish, on the evening of Thursday, 7th September, and represented the above circumstances to them. In consequence of what I said, the handle of the pump was removed on the following day. . . .

The additional facts that I have been able to ascertain are in accordance with those above related; and as regards the small number of those attacked, who were believed not to have drunk the water from Broad Street pump, it must be obvious that there are various ways in which the deceased persons may have taken it without the knowledge of their friends. The water was used for mixing with spirits in all the public houses around. It was used likewise at dining-rooms and coffee-shops. The keeper of a coffee-shop in the neighborhood, which was frequented by mechanics, and where the pump-water was supplied at dinner time, informed me (on 6th September) that she was already aware of nine of her customers who were dead. The pump-water was also sold in various little shops, with a teaspoonful of effervescing powder in it, under the name of sherbet; and it may have been distributed in various other ways with which I am unacquainted. The pump was frequented much more than is usual, even for a London pump in a populous neighborhood.

There are certain circumstances bearing on the subject of this outbreak of cholera which require to be mentioned. The Workhouse in Poland Street is more than three-fourths surrounded by houses in which deaths from cholera occurred, yet out of five hundred and thirty-five inmates only five died of cholera, the other deaths which took place being those of persons admitted after they were attacked. The workhouse has a pump-well on the premises, in addition to the supply from the Grand Junction Water Works, and the inmates never sent to Broad Street for water. If the mortality in the workhouse had been equal to that in the streets

immediately surrounding it on three sides, upwards of one hundred persons would have died.

There is a brewery in Broad Street, near to the pump, and on perceiving that no brewer's men were registered as having died of cholera, I called on Mr. Huggins, the proprietor. He informed me that there were above seventy workmen employed in the brewery, and that none of them had suffered from cholera—at least in a severe form—only two having been indisposed, and that not seriously, at the time the disease prevailed. The men are allowed a certain quantity of malt liquor, and Mr. Huggins believes they do not drink water at all; and he is quite certain that the workmen never obtained water from the pump in the street. There is a deep well in the brewery, in addition to the New River water.

At the percussion-cap manufactory, 37 Broad Street, where, I understand, about two hundred workpeople were employed, two tubs were kept on the premises always supplied with water from the pump in the street, for those to drink who wished; and eighteen of these workpeople died of cholera at their own homes, sixteen men and two women. . . .

Dr. Fraser also first called my attention to the following circumstances, which are perhaps the most conclusive of all in proving the connection between the Broad Street pump and the outbreak of cholera. In the "Weekly Return of Births and Deaths" of 9th September, the following death is recorded as occurring in the Hampstead district: "At West End, on 2nd September, the widow of a percussion-cap maker, aged 59 years, [suffered] diarrhea two hours, cholera epidemica sixteen hours."

I was informed by this lady's son that she had not been in the neighborhood of Broad Street for many months. A cart went from Broad Street to West End every day, and it was the custom to take out a large bottle of the water from the pump in Broad Street, as she preferred it. The water was taken on Thursday, 31st August, and she drank of it in the evening, and also on Friday. She was seized with cholera on the evening of the latter day, and died on Saturday, as the above quotation from the register shows. A niece, who was on a visit to this lady, also drank of the water; she returned to her residence, in a high and healthy part of Islington, was attacked with cholera, and died also. There was no cholera at the time, either at West End or in the neighborhood where the niece died. Besides these two persons, only one servant partook of the water at Hampstead West End, and she did not suffer, or, at least, not severely. There were many persons who drank the water from Broad Street pump about the time of the outbreak, without being attacked with cholera; but this does not diminish the evidence respecting the influence of the water, for reasons that will be fully stated in another part of this work. . . .

The limited district in which this outbreak of cholera occurred contains a great variety in the quality of the streets and houses; Poland Street and Great Pulteney Street consisting in a great measure of private houses occupied by one family, whilst Husband Street and Peter Street are occupied chiefly by the poor Irish. The remaining streets are intermediate in point of respectability. The mortality appears to have fallen pretty equally amongst all classes, in proportion to their numbers. . . .

Table 1 exhibits the chronological features of this terrible outbreak of cholera.

It is pretty certain that very few of the fifty-six attacks placed in the table to the 31st August occurred till late in the evening of that day. The irruption was extremely sudden, as I learn from the medical men living in the midst of the district, and commenced in the night between the 31st August and 1st September. There was hardly any premonitory diarrhea in the cases which occurred during the first three days of the outbreak; and I have been informed by several medical men that very few of the cases which they attended on those days ended in recovery.

The greatest number of attacks in any one day occurred on the 1st of September, immediately after the outbreak commenced. The following day the attacks fell from one hundred and forty-three to one hundred and sixteen, and the day afterwards to fifty-four. A glance at Table 1 will show that the fresh attacks continued to become less numerous every day. On September the 8th—the day when the handle of the pump was removed—there were twelve attacks; on the 9th, eleven; on the 10th, five; on the 11th, five; on the 12th, only one; and after this time, there were never more than four attacks on one day. During the decline of the epidemic the deaths were more numerous than the attacks, owing to the decease of many persons who had lingered for several days in consecutive fever.

Table 1. Chronology of cholera outbreak.

Date	No. of fatal attacks	Deaths
August 19	1	1
August 20	1	0
August 21	1	2
August 22	0	0
August 23	1	0
August 24	1	2
August 25	0	0
August 26	1	0
August 27	1	1
August 28	1	0
August 29	1	1
August 30	8	2
August 31	56	3
September 1	143	70
September 2	116	127
September 3	54	76
September 4	46	71
September 5	36	45
September 6	20	37
September 7	28	32
September 8	12	30
September 9	11	24
September 10	5	18
September 11	5	15
September 12	1	6
September 13	3	13
September 14	0	6
September 15	1	8
September 16	4	6
September 17	2	5
September 18	3	2
September 19	0	3
September 20	0	0
September 21	2	0
September 22	1	2
September 23	1	3
September 24	1	0
September 25	1	0
September 26	1	2
September 27	1	0
September 28	0	2
September 29	0	1
September 30	0	0
Date unknown	45	0
Total	616	616

There is no doubt that the mortality was much diminished, as I said before, by the flight of the population, which commenced soon after the outbreak; but the attacks had so far diminished before the use of the water was stopped, that it is impossible to decide whether the well still contained the cholera poison in an active state, or whether, from some cause, the water had become free from it. The pump-well has been opened, and I was informed by Mr. Farrell, the superintendent of the works, that there was no hole or crevice in the brickwork of the well, by which any impurity might enter; consequently in this respect the contamination of the water is not made out by the kind of physical evidence detailed in some of the instances previously related. I understand that the well is from twenty-eight to thirty feet in depth, and goes through the gravel to the surface of the clay beneath. The sewer, which passes within a few yards of the well, is twenty-two feet below the surface. The water at the time of the cholera contained impurities of an organic nature, in the form of minute whitish flocculi visible on close inspection to the naked eye, as I before stated. Dr. Hassall, who was good enough to examine some of this water with the microscope, informed me that these particles had no organised structure, and that he thought they probably resulted from decomposition of other matter. He found a great number of very minute oval animalcules in the water, which are of no importance, except as an additional proof that the water contained organic matter on which they lived. The water also contained a large quantity of chlorides, indicating, no doubt, the impure sources from which the spring is supplied. Mr. Eley, the percussion-cap manufacturer of 37 Broad Street, informed me that he had long noticed that the water became offensive, both to the smell and taste, after it had been kept about two days. This, as I noticed before, is a character of water contaminated with sewage. Another person had noticed for months that a film formed on the surface of the water when it had been kept a few hours.

I inquired of many persons whether they had observed any change in the character of the water, about the time of the outbreak of cholera, and was answered in the negative. I afterwards, however, met with the following important information on this point. Mr. Gould, the eminent ornithologist, lives near the pump in Broad Street, and was in the habit of drinking the water. He was out of town at the commencement of the outbreak of cholera, but came home on Saturday morning, 2nd September, and sent for some of the water almost immedi-

ately, when he was much surprised to find that it had an offensive smell, although perfectly transparent and fresh from the pump. He did not drink any of it. Mr. Gould's assistant, Mr. Prince, had his attention drawn to the water, and perceived its offensive smell. A servant of Mr. Gould who drank the pump water daily, and drank a good deal of it on August 31st, was seized with cholera at an early hour on September 1st. She ultimately recovered.

Whether the impurities of the water were derived from the sewers, the drains, or the cesspools, of which latter there are a number in the neighborhood, I cannot tell. I have been informed by an eminent engineer, that whilst a cesspool in a clay soil requires to be emptied every six or eight months, one sunk in the gravel will often go for twenty years without being emptied, owing to the soluble matters passing away into the land-springs by percolation. As there had been deaths from cholera just before the great outbreak not far from this pump-well, and in a situation elevated a few feet above it, the evacuations from the patients might of course be amongst the impurities finding their way into the water, and judging the matter by the light derived from other facts and considerations previously detailed, we must conclude that such was the case. A very important point in respect to this pump-well is that the water passed with almost everybody as being perfectly pure, and it did in fact contain a less quantity of impurity than the water of some other pumps in the same parish, which had no share in the propagation of cholera. We must conclude from this outbreak that the quantity of morbid mater which is sufficient to produce cholera is inconceivably small, and that the shallow pump-wells in a town cannot be looked on with too much suspicion, whatever their local reputation may be.

Whilst the presumed contamination of the water of the Broad Street pump with the evacuations of cholera patients affords an exact explanation of the fearful outbreak of cholera in St. James's parish, there is no other circumstance which offers any explanation at all, whatever hypothesis of the nature and cause of the malady be adopted.

MILK-BORNE STREPTOCOCCIC INFECTIONS[1]

Ernest L. Stebbins, Hollis S. Ingraham, and Elizabeth A. Reed[2]

Detailed clinical and epidemiological observations were made by members of the staff of the Division of Communicable Diseases of the New York State Department of Health in 7 milk-borne epidemics of streptococcus infection comprising 1529 cases and 24 deaths occurring in the 3 year period 1934-1936. Three of the epidemics studied, consisting of 806 cases and 16 deaths, were classified clinically as scarlet fever, and 4 epidemics, consisting of 723 cases and 8 deaths, were classified as septic sore throat. An analysis was made of data obtained during the investigation of these seven epidemics, with special reference to the clinical and immunological characteristics of the streptococcus infections observed.

All the epidemics occurred in villages of less than 6000 population, and in each instance the incriminated milk supply was one of raw milk or cream. The generally accepted identifying characteristics of milk-borne epidemics were observed in each outbreak. All the epidemics were explosive in character; in each outbreak elimination or pasteurization of the incriminated milk supply was followed by a marked decline in case incidence. As shown in Table 1, each epidemic was characterized by an age distribution typical of milk-borne outbreaks, a higher proportion of cases occurring among adults than among children. An overwhelming majority of the cases in each epidemic occurred among patrons of a single dairy as shown in Table 1 by case rates per 100 quarts of milk among customers of the implicated dairy and among customers of all other dairies.

Efforts to determine the source of contamination of the milk supply resulted in the discovery of acute mastitis in members of the producing herds in six of the seven epidemics. The organism isolated from milk produced by the cows suffering from mastitis in each instance was found to be a hemolytic streptococcus of the type usually associated with human infection (Lancefield's Group A) (1, 2) and was indistinguishable from the organism isolated from throat cultures obtained from typical cases observed in the same epidemic. In five of the seven outbreaks, acute cases, or recent illnesses, strongly suggestive of hemolytic streptococcus infection were found to have occurred among the milkers or milk handlers associated with the producing herds, the date of onset of the infection in the milk handler always preceding the development of acute mastitis in the cow. In the one epidemic where examination of the producing herd revealed no acute mastitis, it was found that the milk had been bottled and capped by hand by a person suffering from an acute sore throat.

Evidence of transmission of streptococcus infection by personal contact in milk-borne outbreaks is frequently obscure. This lack of evidence is probably due to the almost universal exposure of members of households in which the contaminated milk supply is used, resulting in the simultaneous infection of nearly all susceptible persons in the household. In two of the epidemics studied, one of scarlet fever and one of septic sore throat, there was a considerable number of instances in which the original case in the family was a worker in a factory where the incriminated milk was regularly served but whose household contacts had no known exposure to this milk supply. In these families there was evidence of transmission of infection by direct personal contact similar to that observed in epidemics of scarlet fever in which dissemination appeared to be solely by personal contact. A comparison of the secondary attack rates in such a group in the Owego scarlet fever epidemic, with the attack rates observed in a contact epidemic of scarlet fever in Binghamton, New York, is shown in Table 2. A secondary attack rate of 20 percent was observed among 50 such household contacts in the Baldwinsville

Source: *American Journal of Public Health*, 27:1259-1266, 1937.

[1] Read before the Epidemiology Section of the American Public Health Association at the Sixty-sixth Annual Meeting in New York, N.Y., October 6, 1937.

[2] Division of Communicable Diseases, State Department of Health, Albany, N.Y.

Table 1. Summaries of three milk-borne scarlet fever epidemics and four milk-borne septic sore throat epidemics, New York State, 1934-1936.

Type and location of epidemic	Number of cases	Number of deaths	Percent of cases 15 years of age or over	Cases per 100 quarts of milk sold daily by incriminated dairy	Cases per 100 quarts of milk sold daily by all other dairies
Scarlet fever					
Owego	532	8	71.4	145.0	5.9
Wellsville	201	6	68.8	27.2	1.1
Red Creek	73	2	69.8	45.0	2.5
Septic sore throat					
Baldwinsville	500	7	75.3	107.1	4.3
Corfu	112	0	75.0	88.7	8.2
Dryden	56	1	87.5	62.4	1.9
Waterloo	55	0	70.7	51.0	0.3

epidemic of septic sore throat. These findings suggest that streptococcus infections occurring in milk-borne epidemics are as readily transmitted by direct contact as are similar infections seen as sporadic cases or in epidemics in which there is no evidence of a common source of infection.

CLINICAL CHARACTERISTICS

The clinical manifestations of the illnesses observed in the various outbreaks were strikingly similar with the exception of the presence or absence of a characteristic scarlet fever rash and desquamation. Almost without exception the patients suffered from sore throat with fever of from 100°F. to 104°F., general malaise, and varying degrees of prostration. The throat was almost invariably red and frequently edematous. A punctate rash was frequently seen on the palate both in epidemics classified as scarlet fever and as septic sore throat. The tonsils were red and swollen and frequently covered with exudate. The anterior cervical lymph glands were almost invariably enlarged and tender. In the three epidemics classified as scarlet fever, a typical scarlet fever rash was observed in approximately 60 percent of the cases, but a significantly higher incidence of the rash was noted in children than in adults. Eighty percent of the scarlet fever patients under 15 years of age developed a rash as compared with 50 percent of those 15 years of age or over. In almost all cases the rash was followed by desquamation. Those patients developing a rash were clinically indistinguishable from sporadic cases of scarlet fever or cases of scarlet fever observed in contact epidemics. Cases in which no rash was observed occurring in epidemics classified as scarlet fever were clinically indistinguishable from cases occurring in the epidemics of septic sore

Table 2. Secondary attack rates by age among household contacts (1) in a contact epidemic of scarlet fever and (2) in a milk-borne epidemic of scarlet fever where the primary case occurred in a consumer of the incriminated milk supply but where the members of the household had not consumed the incriminated milk.

Age group	Contact epidemic Binghamton		Milk-borne epidemic Owego		Secondary attack rate percent	
	Persons exposed	Number of cases	Persons exposed	Number of cases	Contact epidemic	Milk-borne epidemic
0-14	465	93	73	10	20.0	13.7
15 and over	773	41	192	14	5.3	7.3
Total	1238	134	265	24	10.8	9.0

throat. Scarlet fever cases without rash and cases of septic sore throat were also clinically indistinguishable from the type of case frequently seen in the absence of any epidemic and usually diagnosed as severe tonsillitis.

COMPLICATIONS

Approximately 25 percent of the patients seen during each epidemic developed one or more serious complications. The complications most frequently encountered were: arthritis and rheumatism, otitis media, mastoiditis, quinsy, cervical abscess, nephritis, pneumonia, sinusitis, and erysipelas. The same complications were observed in all seven epidemics and, as shown in Table 3, these complications occurred with approximately the same frequency in scarlet fever and septic sore throat outbreaks.

There were 16 deaths among the 806 cases of scarlet fever, and 8 deaths among the 723 cases of septic sore throat. Eleven of the 16 deaths in scarlet fever epidemics occurred during the 1st week of the illness, 1 in the 2nd week and 4, 4 weeks or more after the onset of the original infection. Of the eight deaths in septic sore throat outbreaks, only two occurred in the first week of the illness, one in the second, one in the third, and four occurred four weeks or more after the onset of the primary infection. Complications were given as contributory causes of death in 12 of the 16 deaths occurring in scarlet fever outbreaks. Of the eight deaths occurring in septic sore throat epidemics, all were among individuals suffering from a complication of the original infection.

SUSCEPTIBILITY

The occurrence of relatively large numbers of cases of streptococcus infection within short periods of time and in limited areas presented unusual opportunities to study the various factors which might be expected to influence susceptibility to infection. There was no evidence of difference in susceptibility to infection by sex. The age distribution of cases corresponded closely to the age distribution of the population of the community in which the particular epidemic occurred, indicating no difference in susceptibility according to age, either in scarlet fever or in septic sore throat epidemics.

The quantity of infectious material consumed, however, did influence the probability of infection. In four epidemics, a milk census was taken, either of the entire village in which the epidemic occurred or in a random sample of the population of that village, and data were obtained concerning the regular and supplementary milk supplies of the family, together with information as to the amount of milk consumed per day by each individual. Table 4 shows attack rates according to quantity of milk consumed among patrons of the incriminated dairy in the Owego scarlet fever epidemic. The attack rates varied directly with the amount of milk consumed, irrespective of age of the persons exposed. Milk census data in the other epidemics studied, both those of scarlet fever and of septic sore throat, showed the same increased probability of infection with increased milk consumption.

It has been generally assumed that scarlet fever produces subsequent immunity to infec-

Table 3. Complications observed in milk-borne epidemics of septic sore throat in Baldwinsville and Dryden and of scarlet fever in Owego and Wellsville.

Complications	Scarlet fever		Septic sore throat	
	Number of cases	Percent	Number of cases	Percent
Arthritis and rheumatism	59	8.2	69	13.1
Otitis media and mastoiditis	48	6.6	50	9.5
Quinsy	26	3.6	48	9.1
Cervical abscess	2	0.3	15	2.8
Nephritis	11	1.5	6	1.1
Pneumonia	6	0.8	5	1.0
Sinusitis	24	3.3	4	0.8
Erysipelas	11	1.5	6	1.1
Number of cases observed	723		526	
Cases with one or more complications	180	24.9	130	24.7

Table 4. Attack rates according to age and quantity of milk consumed per day among regular consumers of the incriminated milk—Owego scarlet fever epidemic.

Average daily milk consumption	0-14		15 and over		Attack rate, percent	
	Persons exposed	Cases	Persons exposed	Cases	0-14	15 and over
None	17	2	90	15	11.8	16.7
1-7 oz.	29	8	227	57	27.6	25.1
8 oz. and over	203	84	230	95	41.4	41.3
Total	249	94	547	167	37.8	30.5

tion in a considerable proportion of those attacked, but it has not been thought likely that scarlet fever produces immunity to septic sore throat. The effect of a previous attack of scarlet fever upon susceptibility to scarlet fever or septic sore throat was studied by means of household attack rates. Attack rates among persons living in households in which one or more cases occurred are given in Table 5 by age and according to history of previous scarlet fever for three epidemics of scarlet fever and two of septic sore throat. A previous attack of a streptococcus infection, diagnosed scarlet fever, apparently produced little or no immunity to subsequent infection with the hemolytic streptococcus associated with either milk-borne scarlet fever or septic sore throat epidemics. Scarlet fever patients who gave a history of a previous attack were apparently as severely ill as were those who denied having previously suffered from scarlet fever, case fatality rates and the incidence of complications being the same in the two groups. The only difference between these two groups appeared to be the proportion

of cases in which a rash was observed. Less than 30 percent of the patients previously attacked developed a rash, while nearly 65 percent of those with no history of scarlet fever developed a rash.

It has been repeatedly demonstrated that an attack of scarlet fever usually results in reduced skin sensitivity to the toxin produced by the infecting hemolytic streptococcus. From four to eight weeks after the peak of two of the scarlet fever and two of the septic sore throat outbreaks, tests of skin sensitivity to a standard hemolytic streptococcus toxin (Strain New York 5) were made, both in individuals who had suffered an attack during the epidemic and in a comparable group who had not been ill. The results of these tests according to history of illness are given in Table 6.

The proportion of negative skin tests in the group who had recently recovered from scarlet fever was approximately twice that observed in the group tested in the same community who had not been ill during the epidemic. Among scarlet fever patients equally high percentages

Table 5. Attack rates among persons living in households where one or more cases occurred according to age and history of previous scarlet fever in milk-borne epidemics of scarlet fever in Owego, Wellsville, and Red Creek and of septic sore throat in Dryden and Waterloo.

Age group	Scarlet fever epidemics						Septic sore throat epidemics					
	Previous scarlet fever		No previous scarlet fever		Attack rate percent		Previous scarlet fever		No previous scarlet fever		Attack rate percent	
	Number of persons	Cases	Number of persons	Cases	Previous scarlet fever	No previous scarlet fever	Number of persons	Cases	Number of persons	Cases	Previous scarlet fever	No previous scarlet fever
0-14	36	9	459	223	25.0	48.6	9	5	43	16	55.5	37.2
15 and over	263	101	1000	434	38.4	43.4	45	20	129	59	44.4	45.7
Total	299	110	1459	657	36.8	45.0	54	25	172	75	46.3	43.6

Table 6. Percent negative skin sensitivity tests[a] according to age and history of attack during the milk-borne epidemics of scarlet fever in Owego and Wellsville and of septic sore throat in Baldwinsville and Corfu.

| Age group | Scarlet fever epidemics | | | | | | Septic sore throat epidemics | | | | | |
| | Ill | | Not ill | | Percent negative | | Ill | | Not ill | | Percent negative | |
	Number tested	Number negative	Number tested	Number negative	Ill	Not ill	Number tested	Number negative	Number tested	Number negative	Ill	Not ill
0-14	112	82	1052	361	73.2	34.3	121	50	412	145	41.3	35.2
15 and over	164	142	410	193	86.6	47.1	116	61	190	100	52.6	52.6
Total	276	224	1462	554	81.2	37.9	237	111	602	245	46.8	40.7

[a] Strain New York 5.

of negative tests were observed in those who did not develop a rash and in those who had a typical scarlet fever rash. Among those tested following an epidemic of septic sore throat, there was no difference between the percentage of negative skin tests among persons who had recently suffered an attack of the infection and those who had not. These observations indicate the development of an immunity to the skin manifestations produced by the toxin of the standard strain of streptococcus in individuals recovered from scarlet fever, but show no evidence of immunity, as measured by skin test, following septic sore throat.

It has frequently been observed that the proportion of persons with negative skin tests increases with increasing age in the general population. During the past two years a considerable number of skin tests have been performed in New York State communities where the incidence of scarlet fever was not, and had not, recently been high. As seen in Table 7, the proportion of negative skin tests was distinctly higher among persons giving a history of scarlet fever but increased with age regardless of such a history. In the milk-borne epidemics of scarlet fever under consideration, a decreased incidence of rash with increasing age was observed which closely paralleled the decrease in skin sensitivity as measured by the skin test in the general population (Table 8). Figure 1 shows graphically the percentage of cases with a rash by age in the milk-borne epidemics of scarlet fever studied and the percentage of positive

Table 7. Percent negative skin sensitivity tests[a] according to age and history of scarlet fever in various New York State communities, 1934-1937.

| Age group | History of scarlet fever[b] | | No history of scarlet fever | | Percent negative | |
	Number tested	Number negative	Number tested	Number negative	History of scarlet fever	No history of scarlet fever
0- 4	—	—	132	30	——	22.7
5- 9	232	162	2816	882	69.8	31.3
10-14	284	216	2713	1194	76.0	44.0
15-19	83	66	751	351	79.5	46.7
20-29	23	20	139	62	87.0	44.6
30-39	16	14	62	30	87.5	48.4
40-49	13	13	32	21	100.0	65.6
50 and over	17	15	31	24	88.2	77.4
Total	668	506	6676	2594	75.7	38.8

[a] Strain New York 5.
[b] Exclusive of cases of milk-borne epidemics.

Table 8. Percent positive skin sensitivity tests[a] by age among persons tested in New York State, 1934-1937, and percent of cases with rash among scarlet fever patients in milk-borne epidemics in Owego, Wellsville, and Red Creek.

Age group	Skin sensitivity tests[b] New York State, 1934-1937			Scarlet fever cases in milk-borne epidemics according to rash		
	Number tested	Number positive	Percent positive	Number of cases	Number with rash	Percent with rash
0- 4	135	104	77.0	61	53	86.9
5- 9	3080	2030	65.9	97	76	78.4
10-14	3046	1611	52.9	75	53	70.7
15-19	842	422	50.1	93	55	59.1
20-29	167	82	49.1	199	105	52.8
30-39	82	36	43.9	111	63	56.8
40-49	48	11	22.9	79	35	44.3
50 and over	51	9	17.6	72	16	22.2
Total	7451	4305	57.8	787	456	57.9

[a] Strain New York 5.
[b] Exclusive of cases of milk-borne epidemics.

skin tests by age observed in the general population, indicating a positive correlation between sensitivity as measured by the skin test and the development of a rash.

SUMMARY AND CONCLUSIONS

An analysis was made of 1529 cases of streptococcus infection occurring in seven epidemics in New York State during the period 1934-1936. That each outbreak was milk-borne was established beyond a reasonable doubt. The source of contamination of the milk supply in six of the seven epidemics was shown to be a cow suffering from an acute mastitis caused by a hemolytic streptococcus of the type usually associated with human infection (Lancefield's Group A) (*1, 2*) and there was at least suggestive evidence of a human source of the bovine infection in each instance.

Figure 1. Percent positive skin sensitivity tests by age among 7451 persons tested in New York State, 1934-1937, and percent of cases with rash by age among 787 scarlet fever patients in milk-borne epidemics in Owego, Wellsville, and Red Creek.

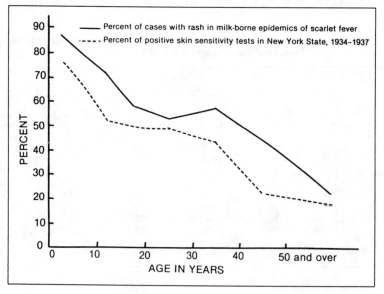

There was evidence in epidemics both of scarlet fever and septic sore throat of transmission by personal contact comparable to that observed in contact epidemics of scarlet fever.

The appearance of a rash was the only distinguishing characteristic between cases in epidemics classified as scarlet fever or as septic sore throat. All other clinical characteristics, including frequency and type of complicating condition, were practically the same.

The effect of various factors which might be expected to influence susceptibility to infection were studied. No evidence of age or sex selection was found. Dosage of the infectious material seemed to be an important factor in determining whether or not a given individual became ill.

A previous attack of scarlet fever seemed to produce little or no immunity to an attack of milk-borne streptococcus infection but did materially lessen the probability of the development of a scarlet fever rash.

The effect of an attack of milk-borne scarlet fever or septic sore throat upon skin sensitivity to standard streptococcus toxin was tested in communities in which epidemics occurred, and a reduced skin sensitivity was observed following milk-borne scarlet fever comparable to that observed after scarlet fever transmitted by contact but no reduction of skin sensitivity was observed following septic sore throat.

Since a previous attack of scarlet fever did not prevent subsequent attacks, but did reduce the incidence of rash, and inasmuch as those persons recovered from scarlet fever showed an increased proportion of negative skin tests, it seems likely that an intradermal test with a standard streptococcus toxin measures susceptibility to the skin manifestations of scarlet fever but fails to indicate susceptibility to other and more important manifestations of the disease. This observation is further supported by the positive correlation between skin sensitivity and incidence of rash by age.

References

(1) Lancefield. R.C. A serological differentiation of human and other groups of haemolytic streptococci. *J Exper Med* 57:571-595, 1933.

(2) Swift, H.F., R.C. Lancefield, and K. Goodner. The serologic classification of haemolytic streptococci in relation to epidemiologic problems. *Am J Med Sci* 190:445, 1935.

ACKNOWLEDGMENT

The authors wish to acknowledge gratefully the advice and assistance of Dr. George H. Ramsey during the study and his helpful suggestions and criticism during the preparation of the manuscript.

CONGENITAL CATARACT FOLLOWING GERMAN MEASLES IN THE MOTHER

N. McAlister Gregg

In the first half of the year 1941, an unusual number of cases of congenital cataract made their appearance in Sydney. Cases of similar type, which appeared during the same period, have since been reported from widely separated parts of Australia. Their frequency, unusual characteristics and wide distribution warranted closer investigation, and this report is an attempt to bring to notice some of the more important features of what might almost be regarded as a mild epidemic.

I am indebted to many of my colleagues in New South Wales, Victoria and Queensland for particulars of very many of the cases reviewed. These, for the most part, conform very closely to the general features noted in my own series of cases on which the following description is based. The total number of cases included in this review is seventy-eight. My own cases total thirteen, and in addition I have seen seven others included in my colleagues' lists.

GENERAL DESCRIPTION AND SPECIAL FEATURES

The first striking factor is that the cataracts, usually bilateral, were obvious from birth as dense white opacities completely occupying the pupillary area. Most of the babies were of small size, ill-nourished and difficult to feed, with the result that many of them came under the care of the pediatrician before being seen by the ophthalmic surgeon. Many of them were found to be suffering from a congenital defect of the heart—a fact which, as will be explained later, has adversely affected full investigation of the condition of the lens and in some cases the treatment. The pupillary reaction to light was weak and sluggish; in some cases the irides had a somewhat atrophic appearance. This was more noticeable after mydriasis when the pupillary border appeared as a flat dark band seemingly devoid of any iris stroma.

Source: *Transactions of the Ophthalmological Society of Australia* 3:35-46,1941.

Full mydriasis was difficult to obtain; in my experience it varied from one-half to three-quarters of the normal; moreover, an unusual number of the patients showed intolerance to atropine. In a large proportion of the cases one was forced to rely upon repeated installations of homatropine to maintain the mydriasis.

Cataract. In the undilated condition of the pupil the opacities filled the entire area. After dilatation the opacities appeared densely white—sometimes quite pearly—in the central area with a small, apparently clear, zone between this and the pupillary border of the iris. Closer examination revealed in this zone a less dense opacity of smoky appearance, and, outside this, only a narrow ring through which a red reflex could be obtained.

The cataractous process seemed to have involved all but the outermost layers of the lens, and was considered to have begun early in the life of the embryo. Generally the cataract was symmetrically situated, but in a few cases it was somewhat excentric—in these there was some sparing of more of the fibers in the lower portion of the peripheral zone. Although the general appearance was much the same in all cases, two main types were noticed in the character of the cataract. In one the contrast between the larger, dense white central area and the smaller, cloudy more peripheral zone was very marked. In the other, the density of the cataract was more uniform throughout and occupied an intermediate stage between that of the two portions of the other type. This distinction has been confirmed by the immediate results of operation. When needling was undertaken in cases of the first group, the dense white central portion was difficult to divide and sometimes separated off as a firm white disk. In others the whole lens seemed to be pushed away by the needle. Subsequent absorption in this group was delayed.

In the second type, discission was easier to perform and absorption regular and uniformly progressive. In one case under my care both these types were present. The first type in the right eye and the second type in the left eye. In my opinion these variations and those described by other observers are not essentially different from each other, and the apparent differences are due merely to a variation in intensity and duration of action of the same noxious factor.

The appearance of the cataract does not, in my opinion, exactly correspond to any of the large number of morphological types of congenital and developmental lenticular opacities that have been described. I do not wish to add to what Duke Elder (*1*) has described as "the confusion which has arisen from the enthusiasm of various observers in the multiplication of types which differ but little in their essential pathology and vary only in their shape and position." I shall, therefore, merely describe the cataract as subtotal. Other descriptions by my colleagues in notes on their cases have been: central nuclear, complete, discoid, nuclear plus, anterior polar, dense central with riders, complete pearly, mature, and total lamellar. In sixteen cases of the whole series reviewed, the cataract was unilateral.

Vision. In all cases the response to light was good; the babies appeared to follow readily any movement of the light stimulus.

Nystagmus. In the very young patients nystagmus was not noted, but in older babies or in cases in which treatment had to be delayed it was present. The movements were of a coarse, jerky, purposeless nature rather than a true nystagmus. It was a searching movement of the eyeballs and indicated the absence of any development of fixation. In my own cases it was always present if treatment had been delayed beyond the age of three months. In one case, in which the parents deferred operation in order to try some other form of treatment of which they had been informed, it developed before they consented to operation. In another case it developed after operation during the process of absorption. This development during the waiting period before operation has been noticed by other observers.

Variations. One case in my series was particularly interesting. The baby was referred to me at the age of three weeks with a diagnosis of bilateral keratitis. The corneas were quite white at birth and both parents had been subjected to a Wassermann test with negative results. At examination I noted a peculiar corneal haze, denser in the center than in the periphery. The iris was just visible through this haze in the peripheral zone. The tension was normal and there was no inflammation. I advised reexamination under anesthesia. This was done two weeks later. By this time the corneas had cleared and the typical white cataracts were seen in the pupillary areas. This baby subsequently became very ill and it was only a few weeks ago that I was able to operate. At operation mydriasis was fuller than usual in these cases and the cataracts were the largest observed in this series.

Two other cases with similar corneal involvement have been noted—namely, by A. Odillo Maher and H.E. Robinson. Involvement was unilateral in Maher's and bilateral in Robinson's case. In these cases there had apparently been some temporary interference with the nutrition of the cornea. Maher's case is also interesting in that the mother developed cataract during pregnancy at the age of twenty-seven. This is the only instance throughout the series of any familial history of cataract.

In another case, reported by S.R. Gerstman, there was "bilateral subluxation of the lenses, mature cataracts, accompanied by arachnodactyly and large fontanelle. Hip regions appeared normal."

Other complications reported have been cleft palate, one; congenital stenosis of naso-lachrymal duct, three; *calcaneus varus*, one; although it is not certain whether these are above the average incidence in any group of infants of similar numbers.

Monocular Cases. The monocular cases merit special consideration. Sixteen of these have been reported, and in ten of them definite microphthalmia has been described.

In one of my cases—there were three in all—the cataract was noted by the mother only when the child was seven weeks old, though she stated that it may have been present before that date. The affected eye was definitely microphthalmic, and examination of the other eye under mydriasis revealed a large pale area with some scattered pigmentation in the lower half of the fundus suggestive of a coloboma.

In another case the mother gave a history that both eyes were said to have had conjunctivitis at birth. This inflammation, she stated, cleared up under treatment in three weeks, and then two weeks later she noticed a white mass in the left pupil. Conceding the accuracy of these histories, I have no doubt that the cataracts were present at birth in the central portion of the lens and that it was the final opacification of the more peripheral fibers which made them apparent. In all other cases the cataracts have been apparent from birth.

Reporting her case of left-sided monocular cataract, Dr. Aileen Mitchell wrote:

No difference was noticed in the size of the eyes when the child was seven weeks old; when the child was aged four months there was microphthalmia of the left eye. The mother said the eye had got small. Diameter of the right cornea was about 11 millimeters, of the left cornea 8.5 millimeters. Nystagmus, which was not present at the first examination, had developed and was coarse in nature with roving movements of the eyeballs. The fundus of the right eye appeared pale, and some scattered irregular-shaped spots of pigment were observed.

L. Stanton Cook described one case, monocular central opacity of the lens, and writes: "It would appear that this cataract is a developmental defect rather than a toxic type." As the baby also had the typical congenital defect of the heart, I feel that this is open to question.

The accompanying microphthalmia, definitely noted in 66 percent of cases, suggests an inhibitory effect on the development of the eye generally. In an autopsy performed in a monocular case at the Royal Alexandra Hospital for Children the following measurements were recorded: Left eye (affected), antero-posterior diameter, 1.6 centimeters; transverse diameter, 1.5 centimeters. Right eye (unaffected), these measurements were, respectively, 1.8 centimeters and 1.9 centimeters. It was also noted that the left cornea was smaller than the right in proportion to the general variation in size of the eyes.

Microphthalmia. Microphthalmia is present so frequently (66 percent) in the cases of monocular cataract that closer attention to the size of the eyes in the binocular cases is advisable. Is it not possible that both eyes may be smaller than normal, and that this feature may be unnoticed because it is bilateral? Further information on this aspect can be obtained from measurements at autopsies and by observation of the subsequent growth of the eyes in the living infants. In

this respect the following measurements obtained at autopsies in other cases at Royal Alexandra Hospital for Children are interesting:

B.S., *aetatis* five months. Right eye: antero-posterior diameter, 1.5 centimeters; transverse, 1.7 centimeters. Left eye: antero-posterior diameter, 1.4 centimeters; transverse, 1.7 centimeters.

M.M., *aetatis* three months. Right eye: antero-posterior diamter, 1.5 centimeters; transverse, 1.5 centimeters. Left eye: antero-posterior diameter, 1.6 centimeters; transverse, 1.6 centimeters.

M.O.S., *aetatis* five and a half months. Both eyes: antero-posterior diameter, 1.6 centimeters; transverse, 1.8 centimeters.

J. Maude described one case as "bilateral microphthalmos, right eye smaller." According to Scammon and Armstrong (2), the average measurements of the eyeball at birth are: sagittal diameter, 17.6 millimeters; transverse diameter, 17.1 millimeters; vertical diameter, 16.5 millimeters. Postnatal growth is very small in the first six months, but they stated that it is most probable that the figures for this period are too low because of the inclusion of premature cases.

By comparison with these average measurements of the normal eye at birth the figures quoted above show a definite diminution in the antero-posterior diameter and a reversal of the normal relationship between the respective lengths of the antero-posterior and transverse diameters.

In the cases under consideration here it must be remembered that many of the babies are generally undersized, so that any estimation of the size of the eyes must be considered in relation to the general size and body weight of the baby.

Heart. As previously mentioned, an extremely high percentage of these babies had a congenital defect of the heart. I am indebted to Dr. Margaret Harper for the following description of eight cases seen by her:

All these babies were seen because of difficulty in feeding and failure to thrive. They all had symptoms suggesting a cardiac defect such as difficulty in taking the breast; they had to be fed in their cots by bottle and some by gavage. They were all in the acyanotic or potentially cyanotic groups of cardiac defects. None was cyanotic. There was a harsh systolic murmur over the base of the heart and down the sternum in all. Some had a thrill. All had signs suggesting the continuance of a fetal condition or of a malformation of the heart.

In my own series this condition was present in all but one case. In the whole series it has been present in forty-four cases; in eleven cases there is no record of the cardiac condition; in ten cases it has been recorded as normal or apparently normal; in four cases in which the condition was not reported upon, the babies died and death was sudden; in another the baby was "ill-nourished"; and in three cases the report was "no defect noted."

Autopsy in three cases at the Royal Alexandra Hospital for Children revealed a wide patency of the *ductus arteriosus*, and I understand that in autopsies performed elsewhere a similar condition has been found. The reports on the cardiac condition from autopsies in three cases at the Royal Alexandra Hospital for Children are as follows:

M.O.S.: There was hypertrophy of the ventricular muscle; the left measured 0.9 centimeters and the right 0.5 centimeters. A few petechial hemorrhages were detected on the surface of the myocardium. The endocardium and valves were normal and all the septa intact. The *ductus arteriosus*, however, was widely patent.

B.S.: There was no free fluid in the pericardial sac. The heart was enlarged, with particular hypertrophy of the right ventricle. Right ventricle measured 0.7 centimeters and the left 0.8 centimeters. There were a few petechial hemorrhages visible on the surface of the myocardium and one fairly large "milk spot." The membranous portion of the interventricular septum was patent. The *foramen ovale* was not completely occluded, although it appeared to have been functionally closed. The heart valves and great vessels were normal, but the *ductus arteriosus* was widely patent.

P.F.: The right heart was somewhat dilated. The right ventricle wall was 0.35 centimeters in its thickest part. The left ventricle wall was 0.5 centimeters in its thickest part. All valves were normal. No septal defect was present. Vessels were normal except for a wide patency of the *ductus arteriosus*.

Additional Findings. In one case at the Royal Alexandra Hospital for Children there were several additional findings worth record here.

Both lungs had a considerable degree of hypostatic congestion at the bases. Throughout the remainder of the lungs there were a very large number of hemorrhagic spots, some of which were confluent and covered considerable areas. Hemorrhagic spots were detected on the inner surface of the pericardium and on the surface of the myocardium. In addition, the visceral pericardium over the upper anterior aspect of the left ventricle bore a "milk spot." The right kidney was situated in such a position that the ureter entered the pelvis on the lateral side of the kidney after coursing across its anterior surface. The right kidney consisted of two distinct lobes, the upper one about twice as large as the lower. Each lobe had its own separate pelvis, and the ureter divided outside the kidney into two branches, one to each lobe. Both ovaries were cystic. The uterus was bicornuate in type.

Another complication noted in a few cases was the development of a dry, scaly eczematous condition, involving the face, scalp and limbs, which was very resistant to treatment.

Sex. Thirty-three of the patients were males, thirty-five were females. In the remaining ten cases the reports did not specify the sex of the child.

Deaths. In this series of cases fifteen deaths have been recorded. Details are not available in all cases of the mode or cause of death, but bronchopneumonia has been noted in several. In three cases within my own knowledge there has been a sudden rise of temperature up to 105° F. or even 106° F., accompanied by extreme distress, and death has followed within twenty-four hours.

Intolerance to Atropine. Intolerance to atropine has been a noticeable feature of the cases in my own series and in no single instance has it been possible to continue its administration throughout the treatment. In most cases, even after one or two instillations, the baby has exhibited considerable constitutional disturbance with pyrexia, restlessness, and irritability, and the difficulty of feeding has been intensified. In one case in which two instillations were made over a period of twenty-four hours, the temperature rose to 105° F. Homatropine, 2 percent, was substituted and the temperature returned to normal, and was not subsequently elevated. Other observers have noted the same intolerance to atropine.

ETIOLOGY

Although one was struck with the unusual appearance of the cataracts in the first few cases, it was only when other similar cases continued to appear that serious thought was given to their causation.

The remarkable similarity of the opacities in the lens, the frequency of an accompanying affection of the heart, and the widespread geographical incidence of the cases suggested that there was some common factor in the production of the diseased condition, and suggested it was the result of some constitutional condition of toxic or infective nature rather than of a purely development defect.

The question arose whether this factor could have been some disease or infection occurring in the mother during pregnancy which had then interfered with the developing cells of the lens. By a calculation from the date of the birth of the baby, it was estimated that the early period of pregnancy corresponded with the period of maximum intensity of the very widespread and severe epidemic in 1940 of the so-called German measles.

Special attention was accordingly paid to the history of the health of the mothers during pregnancy, and in each new case it was found that the mother had suffered from that disease early in her pregnancy, most frequently in the first or second month. In some cases she had not at that time yet realized that she was pregnant.

The investigation was then repeated in the early cases in which such a history had not been sought, and again the history of early "German measles" infection was definite. Moreover, in all these cases the health of the mother during the remainder of the pregnancy was described as good.

As the constant involvement of the central nuclear fibers in the cataractous process suggested an early incidence of the noxious factor, it was considered that a possible solution of the problem had been obtained. Confirmation for this theory was therefore sought from any of my colleagues who had seen lesions of this type, and they kindly agreed to assist me by inquiry into the health of the mothers during pregnancy. The result of their inquiries confirmed the amazing frequency of the "German measles" infection.

"Congenital cataract may be due to a mal-

development, a physical or chemical element acting on the developing lens, or inflammation during the embryonic or fetal period" (3).

Duke Elder (4) stated: "The etiology of these opacities depends upon some disturbances of the development of the lens, but what the actual disturbance may be, or the precise method of its action, is a matter of considerable doubt in most cases."

From his anatomical studies, Jaensch (5) concluded that an intrauterine inflammation was a frequent cause of a total opacity of the lens. Toxic influences also may play a part in the production of opacities, and it is conceivable, writes Duke Elder (6), that toxic or infective processes in the mother may cause a derangement in the lens of fetus, or that similar causes, error of feeding and nutrition or acute exanthemata in the infant, may have a similar effect.

Ida Mann (7) has stated that the exanthemata, measles, mumps, smallpox, chickenpox, scarlet fever etcetera, are all known to be transmissible transplacentally.

Whatever the disturbing factor may be, it is fair to assume that the earlier it acts, the more will the central portion of the lens be likely to suffer.

In the developing lens, in the 26 millimeter stage of the embryo, the original central primitive fibers, elongations of the cells of the posterior wall, have completed their growth. Then begins the development of the secondary lens fibers from the cells in the equatorial region. All subsequent growth in the lens is from these equatorial cells, which give rise to successive layers of new lens fibers, these fibers enveloping and compressing the central fibers. With the development of these fibers comes the appearance of the suturing which eventually takes on the typical "Y" pattern of the fetal nucleus.

In the cases under review the cataractous process has involved these early fibers. Can we not fairly assume that the morbid influence began early? As successive layers of fibers were also affected, until the greater part of the lens became involved, this noxious factor must also have persisted in diminishing strength until finally with its disappearance some normal fibers were formed.

Just how and where this disturbance took place I cannot say. Much more histological evidence than is at present available will have to be obtained before any suggestions can be made. However, if we allow the possibility that the lens may be affected by infective processes in the mother, and if we find the same infection occurring at approximately the same early period in the pregnancy in almost all the cases, and if we then find that the babies of these mothers have cataracts of a more or less uniform type which involve the fibers formed at that period, then I think it is reasonable to assume that the occurrence cannot be a mere coincidence, but that there must be some definite connection between that infection and the morbid condition of the lens.

Although it is rare, cases of the exanthemata have been seen in the newborn baby. Ballantyne (8) noted twenty recorded examples of fetal measles up to 1893; whilst up to 1902 not more than twenty well-authenticated cases of scarlet fever in the fetus had been recorded, varicella *in utero* was not unknown.

The remarkable frequency of the accompanying congenital defect of the heart and the apparent constancy in type of this defect seem to me to indicate a common causative factor. Could this not be some toxic or infective process resulting in a partial arrest of development?

INCIDENCE OF GERMAN MEASLES IN THIS SERIES

In all but ten cases in this series the history of "German measles" infection is present. In two of these ten cases the report is negative for measles; in one there was "history of kidney trouble"; in two others the report is definitely "history not asked for"; in the remaining five cases the report is "no history of measles" or "not known." It is interesting to note that the majority of these were cases occurring in 1940 or early in 1941 before the theory of a possible association between "German measles" and the congenital cataracts was promulgated.

Among the cases that have come under my own notice, in only one is the history negative. In this case the mother stated that she was kept so busy looking after her ten children that she could not recollect any details of her own health beyond the fact that she was ill at about the sixth week of pregnancy when one of the other children died suddenly from whooping cough. Even though she was ill, she was unable to go to bed during the last month before the baby was born one month before full term. In the vast majority of the cases infection occurred either in the first or second month of pregnancy. In a few cases it was during the third month, and in one it is reported as a severe attack occurring three months before pregnancy.

This maternal infection occurred in July or August 1940 in the majority of cases; in the minority of cases outside this period the date of infection ranged from December 1939 to January 1941.

Out of thirty-five cases in which the record is available, the affected baby was the first child in twenty-six instances; in three others it was a second child; whilst in the six remaining cases the baby was the third, fourth, fifth, seventh, eighth and tenth child, respectively. I believe that these figures, with the noticeably high incidence in the children of *primiparas*, afford confirmatory evidence of the close association between congenital cataract in the baby and the maternal infection. For it was this young adult group, to which these *primiparas* belong, which was particularly affected by this epidemic of "German measles."

GEOGRAPHICAL DISTRIBUTION

Although the majority of the cases reported came from the suburban districts of Sydney and Melbourne, others were from widely separated country towns in New South Wales and Victoria, and eight were from Queensland distributed between Brisbane, Rockhampton, and Ipswich.

NATURE OF EPIDEMIC

Within my own experience I have not previously seen German measles of such severity and accompanied by such severe complications as occurred during this epidemic in 1940. The swelling of the glands of the neck, the sore throat, the involvement of the wrist and ankle joints, and the general constitutional disturbance were all very pronounced. The average stay in hospital of patients treated at the Prince Henry Hospital was eight days as against four days in previous years.

The peak period of the epidemic from returns at this hospital was from mid-June to early August.

Running concurrently with this epidemic were the epidemics of sore throat known as the Ingleburn throat or Puckapunyal throat etcetera, deriving its name from the military camp with which it was associated. These epidemics started in the camps and spread to the civilian population. Could they not have been streptococcal in origin and is it not possible that the rash diagnosed as "German measles" may have been, in some cases, a toxic erythema accompanying a streptococcal infection?

In this respect it is interesting to note that the rash occuring in this so-called "German measles" epidemic has been described to me by physicians as macular, morbilliform, scarlatiniform, and toxic erythematous; in other words, it was pleomorphic. I have also been informed by two physicians that they have at present an unusual number of young adult patients suffering from arthritis and other rheumatic conditions, and these patients all have a history of "German measles" last year. Because "German measles" is not a notifiable disease it is impossible to obtain any details of the epidemic from the health authorities, but from my own observations and inquiries I have formed the opinion that the 1940 "German measles" epidemic differed greatly from the ordinary virus infection bearing that name.

MANAGEMENT

From the purely ocular standpoint the essential consideration is the same as in cases of the ordinary lamellar type of cataract—to permit sufficient light stimulus to reach the retina so that fixation may be developed. In this respect the time factor is of the utmost importance. If the stimulus is insufficient or delayed, nystagmus will result.

The special considerations in this series are: (a) the marked density and large size of the opacity; (b) the difficulty in obtaining mydriasis, so that the transparent area for entrance of light is minimal; (c) the high frequency of intolerance to atropine.

These factors compel us to operate at the earliest possible moment. In my opinion the only contraindication to early interference is the general state of health of the baby. In many cases this has been so bad that physicians have refused to give an anesthetic until some improvement has been obtained in the general condition. So frequently has nystagmus been observed to develop during this waiting period that I am convinced that some risk is later justified in order to operate at the earliest possible moment, particularly as later experience has shown that the babies take the short anesthetic required more easily than had been anticipated.

When operation has to be deferred it is essential to maintain the fullest possible degree of mydriasis, by atropine if tolerated. If atropine cannot be employed, then repeated instillation of homatropine must be substituted for it.

The value of early operation is well illustrated by one case reported by E. Temple Smith in which he performed discission on a baby aged three weeks. Clear pupils resulted and there has been no sign of nystagmus developing.

Operation

Discission has frequently proved more difficult than usual. The anterior chamber is particularly shallow, and in many cases the very dense central portion of the lens has proved very resistant to the needle. Sometimes it has separated off as a firm disk, in others the whole lens has tended to move away from the point of the needle and one has obtained the impression that it would have been possible to perform an ordinary extraction. In other cases, on the other hand, discission has been straightforward and easy.

Results of Operation. Absorption has been slower than that of the ordinary lamellar cataracts. I have not yet had an opportunity to examine the fundi of any patient after absorption of the lens matter, but I propose to do so in as many cases as possible under general anesthesia. Careful search will be made for any other defects. The unhealthy appearance of the iris in some cases suggests that there may be possibly some changes in the choroid, particularly since the patients in the monocular cases are so frequently microphthalmic.

PROGNOSIS

It is difficult to forecast the future for these unfortunate babies. We cannot at this stage be sure that there are not other defects present which are not evident now but which may show up as development proceeds. The cardiac condition also tends to make the prognosis doubtful. One baby which had survived two operations some months ago, suddenly died quite recently at the age of seven months. The possibility of the appearance of neurotropic manifestations at a later date will be kept in mind. The prognosis for vision depends on the presence or absence of nystagmus and, of course, on the condition of the retina and choroid.

I look forward to further improvements in contact glass development, for herein lies the greatest possibility for help in the future.

If we agree that these cases are the result of infection of the mother by "German measles," what can we do to prevent a repetition of the tragedy in any future epidemic? Is the mass of modern research into the causation of senile cataract going to be helpful by the discovery of some remedy whch could be given to the mother to inhibit the formation of opacity in the developing lens of the embryo?

In the present state of our knowledge the only sure treatment available is that of prophylaxis. We must recognize and teach the potential dangers of such an epidemic or, I think, any other exanthem, and do all in our power to prevent its spread and particularly to guard the young married woman from the risk of infection.

As to confirmation of the theory of causation put forward in this paper, I suggest that the following line of investigation may be helpful. In all prenatal clinics and maternity hospitals very careful histories should be taken and recorded of exposure of the mother to infection of any kind during the entire period of pregnancy.

ACKNOWLEDGMENTS

I wish to thank all those colleagues, too numerous to mention, for the reports they have furnished me of their cases and for their permission to include them in this review.

I am also indebted to Dr. J. Ringland Anderson for his help with the literature on the subject; to Dr. Margaret Harper for her report on the cardiac condition; to Dr. B. Van Someren, of the New South Wales Government Health Department, for placing the records of his department at my disposal, and particularly to the sisters in charge of several of the baby health centers for the excellent reports they so kindly furnished; to Dr. Douglas Reye for his reports on the autopsies; and to Professor Harold Dew for his timely and helpful criticism on the presentation of this paper.

References

(1) Duke Elder, W. Stewart. *Text Book of Ophthalmology*, vol. ii, p. 1364.
(2) Scammon, Richard E. and Ellery N. Armstrong. "On the growth of the human eyeball and optic nerve." *Comp Neurol* 38:165, 1924-1925.
(3) Kirby, Daniel B. *The Eye and its Diseases.* (Ed. C. Berens.) 1936, p. 577.
(4) Duke Elder, W. Stewart. *Op. cit.*, p. 1365.
(5) Jaensch, P.A. Anatomische Untersuchungen eines angeborenen Totalstars. *Archiv für Ophthalmologie* 115:81, 1924.
(6) Duke Elder, W. Stewart. *Op. cit.*, p. 1366.
(7) Mann, Ida. *Developmental Abnormalities of the Eye.* 1937. p. 18.
(8) Ballantyne, J.W. *Manual of Antenatal Pathology and Hygiene.* 1902, part 1, p. 196.

* * *

D.R. GAWLER (Perth) referred to a child with this disease. It was seen when four months old and was ill-nourished and suffering from impetigo. It showed intolerance to atropine and mydriasis was poor. The cataracts were nuclear and bilateral. The irides were blue and atrophic around the pupil. The Wassermann test applied to blood and cerebro-spinal fluid produced no reaction. No inquiry was made regarding maternal German measles. D.R. Gawler needled one eye and found the cortex and nucleus resistant. The cortex flaked off the anterior surface. There was little reaction to the needling. There was no epidemic of German measles in the district during the early months of pregnancy, but the mother said that there was another child in the town similarly affected. D.R. Gawler had no particular theories, but there might have been an endocrine deficiency, possibly involving the parathyroids.

ARCHIE S. ANDERSON (Melbourne) had seen a few cases of this type and in every instance the mother had had German measles during the second month of pregnancy. He congratulated N. McA. Gregg on his striking and original inquiry.

G.H. BARHAM BLACK (Adelaide) said that he had seen one case in which monocular cataract and nystagmus were present. The mother had German measles six weeks after the last menstrual period. No inquiry had been made into the child's heart condition. The epidemic of German measles had occurred about the same time as in other states. There had been a number of severe cases. A soldier had died of encephalitis at Renmark. In South Australia an investigation had been made of streptococcal infections of the throat, but no streptococci had been found. Volunteers had submitted to inoculations from "camp" throat infections, but the results were inconclusive.

A.W. D'OMBRAIN (Newcastle) had seen four patients, two of whom had heart disease. He asked why the infection was described as "so-called German measles." One mother had German measles three months before pregnancy.

A.L. TOSTEVIN (Adelaide) spoke of a case he had seen. The mother, aged twenty-eight years, had had good health during pregnancy except for German measles at three months. There was no evidence of any abnormality of the child's heart. The mother noticed, when the child was six weeks old, that it could not see. He needled the eyes at three months. One cataract absorbed quickly, but the other, which was difficult, did not absorb well and the eye converged. Nystagmus did not develop. He prescribed + 10 diopter spheres and the child could apparently see reasonably well. The pupil did not dilate sufficiently well to allow of fundus examination. The eyes looked small and the irides were atrophic. He considered that N. McA. Gregg's contribution was very important and offered his congratulations.

W.M.C. MACDONALD (Sydney) added his compliments and stated that he had performed needling in some cases. One patient so treated had obtained a good result, but yet had developed nystagmus. In some of the others needling was difficult and the results were indifferent. It would be interesting to watch further developments. In all his cases there were heart conditions, and this showed how widespread was the involvement. The patients were all weakly.

LEONARD J.C. MITCHELL (Melbourne) asked whether there was more in the new syndrome than a mysterious association with German measles. He considered it a matter for continued research by internists in order to discover the unknown factor at work in this most remarkable series of cases. He congratulated Dr. Gregg, and said he thought that this series of cases would be epoch-making.

N. McA. GREGG, in reply, said he did not want to be dogmatic by claiming that it had been established the cataracts were due solely to the "German measles." However, the evidence afforded by the cases under review was so striking that he was convinced that there was a very close relationship between the two conditions, particularly because in the very large majority of cases the pregnancy had been normal except for the "German measles" infection. He considered that it was quite likely that similar cases may have been missed in previous years either from casual history-taking or from failure to ascribe any importance to an exanthem affecting the mother so early in her pregnancy. He quoted the case of one mother with an affected child who was informed by another mother that her boy, who was born with cataracts, had died suddenly from disease of the heart at the age of seven, and that during this pregnancy she had had German measles. For the past five months he had asked the mother of every healthy young baby he had contacted whether she had been affected by "German measles" during the pregnancy and in no single case had there been any infection.

In regard to the few cases in the series in which there was no history of "German measles," he considered it quite likely that the infection had been slight and overlooked. He quoted Professor Dew as saying that in every virus epidemic some cases were subclinical. In reply to A.W. D'Ombrain, he said he had used the term "so-called German measles" because he believed this epidemic was different from the usual mild epidemics of this infection. The severity of the symptoms, the variability in the character of the rash, and the frequency of rheumatic sequelae in the victims seemed to him to support this view. He felt it was virus *plus*. He congratulated A.L. Tostevin on prescribing glasses for his patient at such an early age. He regretted he had been unable to make a slit lamp examination in his cases, but considered he was not justified in subjecting the babies to an anesthetic for the length of time necessary to make such examination. In answer to L.J.C. Mitchell he said that in the more recent cases he had operated on both eyes at once, as this involved only one anesthetic.

He informed G.H. Barham Black that he had operated on one child with a monocular cataract. He mentioned that in those cases in which the weight of the baby at birth was known, the average weight was five pounds.

RICKETTSIALPOX—A NEWLY RECOGNIZED RICKETTSIAL DISEASE[1]

Morris Greenberg,[2] Ottavio J. Pellitteri,[3] and William L. Jellison[4]

During the summer of 1946, an outbreak of an unclassified disease occurred in a housing development in one of the boroughs of New York City. A clinical, epidemiological, and laboratory study was undertaken by the New York City Department of Health in cooperation with the U.S. Public Health Service in July and was completed in October. This report will deal with the epidemiological features of the epidemic.

LOCATION OF OUTBREAK

The outbreak was localized to a development consisting of a group of 69 houses in the Borough of Queens in New York City, about 15 miles from the center of the city. The houses occupy three oblong blocks, each block consisting of 23 connected houses arranged so that some face wide courts and others face the street. They are three stories in height, two or three families living on each story, and each family occupying three or four rooms. The general arrangement of the houses is the same in each of the blocks. There are small houses in the immediate vicinity, but no cases of the disease were reported in residents of these. The neighborhood is suburban in type with wide streets, many trees and bushes, well-kept lawns, but surrounded at a distance by large lots of unkept grass, weeds, and scrub forest. Close to the development are several highways on which considerable traffic passes between New York and Long Island. A total of 483 families occupied the apartments in the development at the time of investigation. The total number of residents was about 2000, of whom 600 were children under age 15.

Cases were first seen by physicians in the neighborhood at the beginning of the year 1946.[5] Some of the physicians thought they were dealing with atypical chickenpox; others were unable to make a diagnosis. By early summer it became evident that the disease was occurring in a sharply localized epidemic. Intensive investigation was started in July. Doctors practicing in the vicinity were canvassed and histories were obtained of earlier cases. All newly reported cases were visited by one of us. Patients and other residents were questioned about the occurrence of similar cases in other residents and friends. A canvass was made of about half of the 69 buildings in the three-block area and a systematic visit was made to each resident in these buildings.

Records of 124 cases who had become ill between January and October were obtained. These are arranged in Figure 1 according to week of onset. The sex distribution was approximately equal: 63 males and 61 females were affected. Table 1 shows the distribution of cases by age. Cases occurred among all age groups; the youngest was an infant of 3 months, the oldest a woman of 71. The incidence in children under 15 was 5.3 percent, in adults, 6.5 percent. In the entire group it was 6.2 percent. All residents of the buildings and most of the employees were white. There were, however, some Negro porters. No cases were seen among the Negroes.

CLINICAL FEATURES

The clinical features have already been described elsewhere (3). In brief, there occurred an initial lesion at the presumed site of bite by a mite, a papule, which when fully developed measured ½ to 1½ cm in diameter. The papule became vesicular in the center and dried, leav-

Source: *American Journal of Public Health* 37:860–868, 1947.
[1] From the Bureau of Preventable Diseases, New York City Department of Health and the Rocky Mountain Laboratory of the Division of Infectious Diseases, National Institute of Health, Hamilton, Montana.
[2] Acting Director, Bureau of Preventable Diseases, New York City Department of Health.
[3] Epidemiologist, New York City Department of Health.
[4] Parasitologist, U.S. Public Health Service, Hamilton, Montana.
[5] Dr. Leon N. Sussman of Manhattan; Drs. Benjamin Shankman, Harry N. Zeller, and Joan Daly of Queens. We are indebted to these physicians for their cooperation. Dr. Sussman and Dr. Shankman have published reports of their cases (1, 2).

Figure 1. Onset of Rickettsialpox cases by week, from January to October 1946.

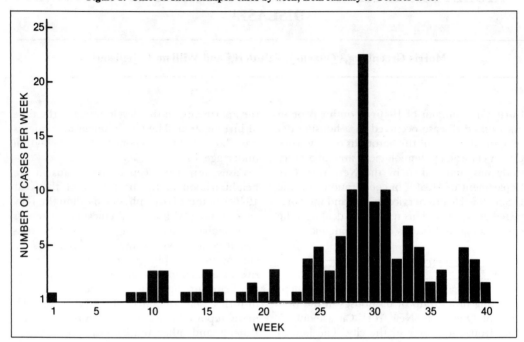

Table 1. Rickettsialpox distribution of cases by age.

Age	Number of cases	Population	Incidence per hundred
0-1	2		
1-4	16		
5-9	11		
10-14	3		
0-14	32	600	5.3
15-19			
20-24	3		
25-29	9		
30-39	42		
40-49	23		
50 and over	15		
15 and over	92	1400	6.5
Total	124	2000	6.2

ing a black eschar. This eschar ultimately sloughed leaving a small scar. The regional lymph glands usually became enlarged. About a week after the occurrence of the initial lesion, there was an acute onset of illness with fever, chills, sweats, backache, and headache, followed in from two to four days by a maculopapular and papulovesicular rash. The duration of ill-

ness from initial lesion to complete recovery was about three weeks; the duration of the acute symptoms and of the rash was about one week to 10 days. There were no complications and no deaths. Laboratory findings were generally negative except for leucopenia. The usual bacterial agglutination tests were uniformly negative in the convalescent as well as the acute stage of the disease.

EPIDEMIOLOGICAL FEATURES

There appeared to be no relationship between disease incidence and occupation. Many of the adult female cases were housewives. Cases also occurred among both men and women who worked in various occupations in different parts of the city. There were among them salesmen, manufacturers, office workers, teachers, foremen, etc. No one occupation predominated. The children of primary school age attended public schools in the vicinity; those of high school age traveled to one of several schools in the city.

The possibility that the disease was imported was investigated. Of the total number of 124 cases, 112 were born in this country. The remainder had been born in European countries but had lived in the United States for a number of years. The median length of residence in the same apartment was between three and four years. Only three patients had lived there less than one month. Except for a few whose cases will be discussed later, none had been out of the city in the month preceding the onset of illness. None of the cases occurred in returned veterans.

Although few of the patients manifested even mild gastrointestinal symptoms, the possibility of a source of infection through a common food article was investigated. Morning and evening meals were almost always eaten at home. Lunch was eaten at home by the housewives and the small children. The older children ate at the schools they attended and the employed adults ate in various restaurants near their places of employment. Provisions, including meats, groceries, and cakes, were purchased from one of several markets in the immediate vicinity. The same markets supplied families where cases occurred and those where no cases occurred. Furthermore, residents in the surrounding areas purchased their supplies from the same markets that were patronized by the residents of the development.

Milk was also obtained at the provision markets. It came in sealed glass or cardboard containers, pasteurized, and approved by the Department of Health. The milk was supplied to the markets by ten different wholesale distributors. The same brands of milk in similar containers were sold to other residents of the Borough.

Water was supplied to the development from the regular New York City system through six three-inch brass service lines. All the piping was brass, Flush tubes of water closets were provided with vacuum breakers. All washstands, bathtubs, and kitchen sinks were provided with over-rim water supply fixtures. Water pressure was adequate. No breakdowns, defects, or other emergencies had occurred for many months. Samples of water were taken at two different units; analysis indicated water of good, potable quality.

Sanitary inspections of the immediate neighborhood yielded negative results. Two vacant lots adjacent to the development were inspected. They were covered by vegetation. There had been heavy precipitation in the days prior to the inspection, but only one mosquito breeding impoundment was found. This was in the basement of an unfinished building about 200 yards from the apartment houses. Mosquito larvae were abundant in this water, and numerous adults collected from the ceiling of the basement were identified as *Culex pipiens* L. by Dr. Alan Stone of the U.S. National Museum. Adults of this same species were found to be fairly abundant in dark basement corners in the affected apartment houses. Specimens collected in the apartment basements were tested for infection, with negative results. The shrubbery was carefully searched but no ticks were found. The lots were sanitary, and although dog droppings were seen and field mice were in evidence, no garbage or bulk of other offensive material was found. The seeded area and the shrubbery along the highways near the development were also inspected. Here, too, no insanitary conditions were found, nor were ticks observed in the shrubbery. The seeded areas in the immediate vicinity of the apartments were mowed regularly.

There were two dog kennels near the development and these were inspected and their owners interviewed. The dogs were clean and free of fleas and ticks. The shrubbery at the kennels was likewise free of ticks. Two nearby riding stables, occasionally patronized by residents of the development, were also inspected. No mosquitoes were seen on the walls and ceilings and no ticks were found on the horses.

Although the management of the development did not permit animals in the apartments, some of the tenants did keep dogs. A number of these tenants were interviewed. None had noted ticks on the dogs. Examination of dogs seen near the houses did not reveal ticks or insects on any of them. In almost all instances the animals were quite clean.

The buildings were new and modern in design. The apartments were generally found to be clean and spacious in relation to the size of the families concerned, and the standard of living was high. Most of the windows were screened. The tenants were specifically asked about the presence of insects. They rarely saw mosquitoes; flies were not bothersome; and ticks were never seen. All the tenants interviewed were certain, however, that rodents were abundant. These were house or field mice and were seen in the basements of the buildings, in the courtyards, and in some of the apartments. Mice were particularly in evidence in the basements, which were used as storage places, and which also housed the incinerators of the buildings. Living and dead mice were seen in the basements, in the incinerators, and in the courtyards, and mouse droppings were also in evidence.

The possibility that the rodents played a part in the transmission of the disease was considered and a temporary laboratory was established in one of the buildings in order to trap numbers of them for study, and also to examine them for ectoparasites. A clue to the possible vector was furnished late in July 1946 by Charles Pomerantz, who discovered small mites on the basement walls. These were identified as *Allodermanyssus sanguineus* (Hirst).[6]

At this stage of our investigation a strain of rickettsia had been isolated from the blood of a patient (4). Antigens prepared from it (MK strain) gave positive complement-fixation reactions when tested with sera of recovered cases, but gave negative reactions when tested with the serum of normal human beings and of recovered cases of syphilis, endemic typhus, tsutsugamushi fever, and Q fever. There was some serologic relationship to Rocky Mountain spotted fever; about 80 percent of the sera from recovered cases also gave a positive reaction with the antigen of Rocky Mountain spotted fever, but in lower dilutions than with the MK antigen. The name rickettsialpox was proposed for the disease. Later, an identical strain of rickettsia was isolated from the blood of another patient.

Systematic trapping of rodents and collection of mites from walls and mouse nests in the different buildings of the development were carried out. Several types of suction apparatus were used for drawing the mites into vials. While some of the mites were found on freshly trapped house mice (*Mus musculus*), most of them were recovered from the external walls of the incinerators in the basement. Some were flat and colorless and had apparently not recently fed, while others were engorged and bright red in color. Smears made from the latter showed typical mammalian erythrocytes. The numbers

found varied in the different buildings. On the incinerator walls of some of the buildings no mites were found, on the walls of others they were found in small numbers, and on the walls of still other houses they were found in abundance, as many as 100 being collected from the walls of a single incinerator. It must be pointed out that differences in the temperature of the walls and other factors may have influenced the number of mites found at one time. No other rodents and no other rodent parasites were found in the development during our investigation. Rickettsial strains were isolated from each of two lots of mites. The isolation of these strains and the establishment of their identity with the MK strain isolated from a rickettsialpox patient were discussed in an earlier paper (5) of this series and the name *Rickettsia akari* was proposed for the organism.

There was an incinerator in each building serving the needs of the six to nine families living in the building—a total of 69 incinerators. Openings to a chute leading down to each incinerator were provided on the respective floors of each building; the openings were closed by a hinged, metal door when not in use. Each incinerator was located in the basement and was composed of two brick-lined compartments, the openings of which were protected by hinged iron doors. The upper and lower compartments were separated from each other by an iron gate. Both compartments were part of and continuous with the chute leading to the upper floors. Garbage, paper, and refuse thrown down the chute by the tenants landed on the fire grate of the incinerator in the basement. Once or twice daily an attendant was supposed to set fire to the material. As it burnt itself out, the ashes and small debris would fall through the grate into the lower compartment, whence it could be removed into large cans for disposal by the Department of Sanitation. All objects not reduced by fire were picked out of the upper compartment by the attendant. Even the debris falling through the coarse fire grate contained much food for mice.

This method of garbage and waste disposal might have worked out well under normal conditions. During the four or five years preceding the outbreak, however, the services of laborers had been at a premium. In this group of houses, as elsewhere, the necessary complement of handymen was lacking; as a result the build-

[6] Identification of original specimens was made by E.W. Baker, of the Bureau of Entomology and Plant Quarantine, U.S. Department of Agriculture.

ings were not cleaned as well as formerly; basements were dirty and cluttered up, and the incinerators were not regularly fired. Combustible material was not sufficient to complete incineration of the garbage. The accumulation of garbage in the upper compartments of the incinerators and even the debris in the lower compartment furnished an excellent food supply for mice. Both living and dead mice were found by us on our inspections. When disturbed by the opening of the door to the compartment, the mice would scamper about and disappear in the crevices between the bricks.

Many of the tenants interviewed complained of the presence of mice. Some had seen them only in the basement, others complained in addition of hearing them at night in the walls. Some found mice in their apartments. In two instances, mice were actually found by the tenants in the beds used by patients. In one apartment, mouse droppings were observed in a patient's bed between the sheet and mattress, and mice were caught in traps laid in this apartment. Not all houses were equally afflicted nor were the three blocks of houses equally infested. Block I was apparently the greatest sufferer. Whether this was due to less adequate and conscientious janitorial service in this block compared to the others, we are not prepared to state. It should be mentioned that there was no regular exterminating service in the houses at the time of our investigation.

Complement-fixing antibodies of rickettsialpox were demonstrated in sera from trapped mice. Such antibodies could not be demonstrated in laboratory mice nor in mice trapped in the Washington area. An organism identical with the MK strain of rickettsialpox was recovered from one of the mice trapped in the infested apartments (6).

A routine search for mites was made in the houses of the development, particular attention being paid to the basements and especially the incinerator walls. Some of the houses were visited more than once, but repeated visits were not made to all the houses. In 9 of the 69 houses no search was made because the basements were locked and the attendants could not be located at the time of visit. In Table 2, the total number of reported cases is arranged according to the block of residence and the presence of mites in the building. It will be noted that 67 cases were reported from 19 houses in which mites were found, an incidence of 3.5 cases per house, as compared with 42 cases observed in 41 houses where no mites were found, an incidence of one case per house. Stated differently, mites were found in 19 or approximately one-fourth of the houses; from these houses came 67, or more than half of the known cases. It is also interesting to observe that in each of two buildings in which mites were found in great abundance, one in Block I and the other in Block III, 8 cases were found as compared with an average of 3.5 cases per building in which mites were found, but not in abundance.

Another point of interest was the occurrence of multiple cases in families. The 124 cases investigated were reported from 78 families. Single cases were reported from 47 families, 2 cases each from 20, 3 cases each from 7, and 4 cases each from 4 families.

Although many of the patients referred to the initial lesion as an insect bite, none actually recalled being bitten and none saw a mite or insect at the site of the initial lesion. However, three housewives in whose families cases occurred had noticed tiny blood spots on the bed sheets.

After the investigation at the development was terminated, we examined two patients with rickettsialpox in other parts of the city, both of whom volunteered the information that they had been bitten. One was a boy of 17 who re-

Table 2. Rickettsialpox cases distributed according to residence and presence of mites in building.

Building	Block I Number of		Block II Number of		Block III Number of		Total Number of	
	Buildings	Cases	Buildings	Cases	Buildings	Cases	Buildings	Cases
Mites found	12	47	3	4	4	16	19	67
No mites found	6	13	19	20	16	9	41	42
No search made	5	15	1	0	3	0	9	15
Total	23	75	23	24	23	25	69	124

called being bitten on his arm while in a stable, and scratching the site vigorously. The other was a nurse who said she was bitten on her right hand. Both later developed an initial lesion of rickettsialpox at the site of the bite, one on the same day and the other two days after being bitten. Neither had seen a mite or insect on the skin.

OTHER CASES IN NEW YORK CITY

As information about the clinical aspects of the cases began to reach physicians, we were called upon to see suspected cases in various parts of the city. By the time our investigation had ended we had seen 20 additional cases in four of the five city boroughs. Particular interest is attached to a group of cases in an apartment house in the Bronx at some distance from the site of the above outbreak and, as far as we were able to determine, completely unrelated to it. The house is an 11-story brick and stone building and has 102 apartments. There are two self-service elevators and two incinerators. A physician (Dr. Victor Stern), who has his office in the building, informed us that he had seen many cases in residents of the building in the past few years, which he had diagnosed as atypical chickenpox. He had records of 10 cases. His description of the clinical findings was typical of our cases. Blood counts in all of his cases showed a moderate leukopenia, but other usual laboratory tests were negative. We were able to interview two of the patients who had recently recovered and to obtain blood specimens from them. The sera gave positive complement-fixation reactions with the MK antigen (strain of rickettsialpox) in high dilutions; they did not agglutinate the antigens of Proteus OX 19, OX 2, or OX K.

The tenants and the physician stated that they were not bothered by mosquitoes, ticks, flies, or other insects, but mice had been seen. We visited the basement, which is on a lower level than the main entrance. Many of the tenants use the basement entrance when leaving and returning. We inspected the incinerators and found garbage in the upper compartments. On the walls of one of the incinerators were many mites, both flat and engorged, which we collected. These were identified as *Allodermanyssus sanguineus*. Three mice were trapped, one in the incinerator and two in the storage room. The serum of one of these gave a positive complement-fixation reaction with the MK antigen of rickettsialpox in a dilution of 1:64.

INCUBATION PERIOD

Since the patients had lived continuously in the development and since none recalled being bitten, the incubation period could not be definitely determined in most cases. In one instance, however, it was found to be 10 days. In this case a woman living in Manhattan visited her daughter and son-in-law, both of whom were ill, on one day only. She developed acute symptoms 10 days later; she observed an initial lesion 3 days before onset. In two cases outer limits could be determined: one of us (W.L.J.) became acutely ill 23 days after arriving at the development to set up a laboratory: an initial lesion was first noted 8 days before onset of illness. Another patient became ill 24 days after returning to her home from a vacation; she noted an initial lesion 9 days before onset of symptoms. In the case of two members of a family, the lower limit of incubation was determined. Both became ill out of town, one, 9 days after leaving home, and the other, 11 days; only one of them had observed a primary lesion 5 days before onset of symptoms.

CONTROL MEASURES

Methods of control are under study. The elimination of mouse harborages appears to be an important factor in such control. The landlord was ordered to clean up the basements, take adequate measures to kill mice in the buildings, and to see to it that the incinerators were properly fired at least once daily.

COMMENT

The results of the investigation of the epidemic in Queens indicated that we were dealing with a hitherto undescribed disease, rickettsialpox, caused by an organism, *R. akari*, which was recovered from the blood of two patients early in the disease. The concomitant finding of bloodsucking mites, *A. sanguineus*, in the group of buildings where the patients lived, and the recovery of *R. akari* from two pools of these mites justified the belief that the mites were the vectors of this disease. The only other parasites or hematophagus insects found in the buildings were adult mosquitoes. Several hundred were collected from dark basement corners. Some were tested for infection, with negative results. Specimens sent to the National Museum were identified as *Culex pipiens* L. by Dr. Alan Stone. The only rodents found in the housing development were house mice, which were present in large numbers. The finding of mites as ectoparasites of mice, the presence of mammalian erythrocytes in smears made from engorged mites, the laboratory determination of the presence of complement-fixing antibodies of rickettsialpox in the blood of trapped mice, and the isolation of *R. akari* from one of them, indicated that the mice acted as the animal reservoirs. The occurrence of a significantly greater number of cases in buildings where mites were readily found and the finding of multiple cases in families strengthened the hypothesis that the mites were the vectors of the disease.

The initial lesion probably represents a reaction to the bite of an infected mite. That no patient remembered being bitten is not surprising in view of the small size of the mite and the fact that no itching or pain was caused. It is not unusual for persons to be bitten by ticks and to be unaware of the fact until the acarid is discovered adhering to the skin or scalp by another person.

It is interesting to observe that rickettsialpox, as here observed, is a domiciliary disease. In the epidemic described, incinerators played an important role in maintaining the infection. This was not due to anything inherent in incinerators but to the fact that if not fired frequently and regularly they become excellent harborages for mice due to the accumulation of garbage. Also, they are warm and the particular mites identified as vectors of rickettsialpox thrive well in warm places. However, cases of rickettsialpox may occur in homes where there is no incinerator service. We have observed several such in other parts of the city. In all instances, however, mice harborages existed.

The eradication of the disease where it exists and prevention of its spread depend on the eradication of mouse harborages. Where incinerators are used in a building, they should be fired frequently and thoroughly.

SUMMARY

The epidemiologic features of an outbreak of rickettsialpox in a housing development in New York City are discussed. Evidence is presented that the disease is caused by *Rickettsia akari*; that it is transmitted by a rodent mite, *Allodermanyssus sanguineus*; and that the house mouse, *Mus musculus*, acts as a reservoir. The presence of mouse harborages in the basements was responsible for maintenance of the infection. Incinerators, especially since they were not fired nor cleaned frequently, served as sources of food for the mice and must be considered as a factor in the maintenance of the animal reservoir of the disease.

References

(1) Sussman, L.N. Kew Gardens' spotted fever. *NY Med* 2:27–28, 1946.

(2) Shankman, B. Report on an outbreak of endemic febrile illness, not yet identified, occurring in New York City. *NY State J Med* 96:2156–2159, 1946.

(3) Greenberg, M., O. Pellitteri, I.S. Klein, and R.J. Huebner. Rickettsialpox—a newly recognized rickettsial disease. II. Clinical findings. *JAMA* 133:901–906, 1947.

(4) Huebner, R.J., P. Stamps, and C. Armstrong. Rickettsialpox—a newly recognized rickettsial disease. I. Isolation of the etiological agent. *Public Health Rep* 61:1605–1614, 1946.

(5) Huebner, R.J., W.L. Jellison, and C. Pomerantz. Rickettsialpox—a newly recognized rickettsial disease. IV. Isolation of a rickettsia apparently identical with the causative agent of rickettsialpox from *Allodermanyssus sanguineus*, a rodent mite. *Public Health Rep* 61:1677–1682, 1946.

(6) Huebner, R.J., W.L. Jellison, and C. Armstrong. Rickettsialpox—V. Recovery of *Rickettsia akari* from a wild house mouse (*Mus musculus*). *Public Health Rep* (in press).

OUTBREAK OF PARALYSIS IN MOROCCO DUE TO *ORTHO-*CRESYL PHOSPHATE POISONING

Honor V. Smith[1] and J. M. K. Spalding[2]

We went to Morocco on September 25, 1959, as "temporary advisers to the World Health Organization in order to advise the Moroccan health authorities in investigating an outbreak of a paralyzing disease of unknown origin." A full account of the outbreak is in preparation in association with colleagues in Morocco, but in view of recent newspaper reports a short account of our personal experience may be of interest. Moreover, cresyl phosphates, which commonly include *ortho*-cresyl phosphate (O.C.P.), have many industrial uses, because they are very heat-stable and are also important plasticizers. Although O.C.P. is notorious among industrial users for its toxicity, and it is used only with strict precautions, the possibility of poisoning must not be forgotten.

When we reached Morocco, a large amount of epidemiological and statistical information had already been collected by the Moroccan health authorities, and was made available to us in Rabat, the administrative capital of Morocco, where we had our headquarters.

EPIDEMIOLOGY

To summarize the information we were given:

1. The first cases occurred between Aug. 31 and Sept. 2. The incidence then rose until between Sept. 18 and 24, 200-300 new cases were being reported daily. By Oct. 2, when we left Morocco, more than 2000 cases were already known and it was clear that more were to be expected.

2. The outbreak was centered on Meknes and the towns in the vicinity, notably Sidi Slimane, Sidi Kacem, and Khemisset. Of the few patients seen elsewhere, almost all had recently been in Meknes. One man developed the disease in Marrakesh fourteen days after leaving Meknes.

3. Within Meknes itself the distribution of cases varied sharply from district to district. With one exception (a man who had adopted the Moslem way of life), no cases were seen among the Europeans, among the Jews, or among the better-to-do Moslems. The cases were grouped in distinct areas on the periphery of the town where the poorest of the Moslem population live. Even in these areas, however, the distribution was uneven in that the poorest of the poor were largely spared.

4. Both sexes and all ages were liable to the disease, but the chief incidence was in adult women, adult men, and older children—in that order. When there was more than one case in the same family they tended to follow one another at intervals of four to five days.

5. From Sept. 14 to 18 over a quarter of a million people visited Meknes and its neighborhood to celebrate the feast of the birth of the Prophet. So far as was known, not one of the visitors had developed the disease either in Meknes or after leaving it. It is usual for such visitors to bring their own food with them.

6. A company of 100 soldiers was stationed at Meknes during the outbreak. Only two of these developed the disease, and both were unusual in being accustomed to eat in the town, not in barracks. Similarly no cases were seen in the prison in Meknes, but a few prisoners developed the disease within a few days of their release.

CLINICAL PICTURE

In the typical case, the illness began with aching pain and tenderness in the calf, followed by paresthesia and loss of superficial sensation of stocking-and-glove distribution. After a day or two the disturbance of sensation decreased and might disappear, and at about the same time motor weakness appeared, involving first the muscles of dorsiflexion and eversion of the foot and a little later the calf muscles. Later still the muscles of the hand were commonly affected also. Only the more severe cases were admitted to hospital, and victims of the disease who were

Source: *Lancet* II: 1019-1021, 1959.

[1] M.D. London, M.R.C.P., Department of Neurology, Oxford Hospitals.

[2] D.M. Oxon., M.R.C.P., Department of Neurology, Oxford Hospitals.

Note: We have omitted the map of the affected area which appeared in the original. Ed.

not in hospital could easily be identified at a distance by their ungainly high-stepping gait.

On examination all voluntary movements below the knee were found to be lost, and although in exceptionally severe cases the muscles of the thigh and even of the pelvic girdle might be affected, it was often surprising how abruptly the weakness stopped at the level of the knee-joint. The hands might be spared, but more commonly there was obvious weakness of the intrinsic muscles of the hand, which developed a few days after the weakness in the lower limbs. Muscular wasting was not conspicuous, but no patient had been paralyzed for more than three weeks by the time we saw them. The tendon reflexes in the upper limbs were commonly preserved; and although, as might be expected, ankle-jerks were usually diminished or absent, it was sometimes surprising that even in cases with severe weakness the ankle-jerks were nevertheless obtainable. The knee-jerks were usually exaggerated, in contrast to the predominantly lower-motor-neurone type of weakness distally. The superficial reflexes were normal, with the exception of the plantar reflexes which were necessarily absent when movement of the toes was paralyzed.

Signs of general ill health were uncommon. About one-third of the patients, however, had a history of recent diarrhea. Some patients had had a little transient fever and some a short-lived bradycardia, noticed within a few days of their admission to hospital. All routine investigations were negative, including analysis of the cerebrospinal fluid and of the blood.

The picture, therefore, was essentially one of acute peripheral neuritis in which the distribution of the weakness was overwhelmingly distal. In addition there were less striking signs of an upper-motor-neurone lesion.

ETIOLOGY

Opinion was divided whether the disease was due to an infection or to poisoning.

Infection. There was a strong *a-priori* case to suggest infection, probably by a virus. In favor of this was the appearance of a few cases followed in two to three weeks by an explosive outbreak; the fact that it attacked the poor, whose mode of life favors dissemination of infection by feces, nasopharyngeal secretions, or insect vectors; and its occurrence in one subject

as much as fourteen days after he left Meknes. If, however, this was an infection, it must be one not hitherto described, and moreover it must carry a high clinical attack rate among the susceptible population. These considerations made it difficult to account for the distribution described.

Poisoning. In favor of the toxic theory was the fact that a number of poisons can produce peripheral neuritis. Against it was the disseminated distribution and the evolution of the epidemic over weeks. Moreover, so far as was known, no essential change had taken place recently in the way of life of the people of Meknes, nor did this differ essentially from that of the inhabitants of other towns.

FINDINGS

A visit to Meknes convinced us that the infective theory was untenable.

In Borj Moulay Omar, a suburb of Meknes where the standard of living is low, both the poor and very poorest sections of the population were so closely intermingled that it was impossible to conceive of an infection attacking one section and sparing the other. It was equally impossible to imagine that one section could react to an infection as "a virgin population" while the other section reacted as an immune community. Finally, those conditions favoring the spread of infection enumerated above bore more heavily on the poorest of the poor, among whom the incidence was lower. This opinion was confirmed by the lack of infection among the visitors to Meknes for the festival. These visitors had returned to their homes in all parts of the country, and had they been exposed to a highly infectious illness they must have contracted the disease or acted as carriers. Whether the incubation period was four to five days (the shortest possible) or fourteen days (the longest), new cases must have appeared by then in different parts of the country. No such cases had been seen.

By contrast the toxic theory received overwhelming support.

The doctor in charge of the dispensaries at Meknes told us that he had recently seen samples of cooking oil which were as dark as old motor oil and that some patients believed that this oil was responsible for the illness. One family had been so suspicious that they gave some food cooked in this oil to their dog. As the dog showed no immediate sign of illness they ate the food themselves. Within a few days both the family and the dog were affected.

After leaving Borj Moulay Omar we visited a certain quarter of the medina—the old Arab town, occupied largely by Arabs of the artisan class—where there had been a severe but sharply circumscribed outbreak. In a grocer's shop in this area we found and bought a colored bottle three-quarters full of very dark oil, bearing a trade name of a cheap brand of olive oil. Other bottles, of colorless glass, bearing the same trade name were seen in the same and neighboring shops containing oil of the normal yellow colour. In the meantime, the health authorities had investigated the manufacture and distribution of cooking oils in Meknes and discovered that the same wholesaler supplied oil to all affected areas. Finally, those questioned declared that the dark oil had been offered for sale only during the past month.

There was thus strong evidence that at least one consignment of cooking oil had been contaminated and was the cause of the outbreak. The contaminant was, we then supposed, a mineral oil. In the first place, the clinical picture corresponded closely to that described in outbreaks of o.c.p. poisoning seen in Germany and Switzerland since 1939 and in the U.S.A. before the war, and o.c.p. is added to certain oils for special purposes. Secondly, this hypothesis accounted for the pattern of the outbreak; the well-to-do people could afford to buy better brands of oil, while the very poor could hardly afford to buy any oil at all. It explained the absolute immunity of the Jews, who have their own market. It also accounted for the extraordinary immunity of visitors to Meknes for the festival, since such visitors ordinarily bring their own food. Finally, the period during which the dark oil had been on sale corresponded precisely to the period of the outbreak.

The oil bought at the grocer's shop in the medina of Meknes, and other samples of "olive" oil bought both in affected and unaffected areas, were analyzed. Before we left, the Institute of Hygiene at Rabat had demonstrated the presence of phosphates and cresols. In this country a well-known industrial company with a highly specialized knowledge of oils very kindly undertook further examination of the samples. This firm demonstrated that the "olive" oil obtained in the medina at Meknes contained about 33 percent of vegetable oil and, much to our surprise, no mineral oil. The firm then showed that the toxic oil was a man-made lubricating oil containing nearly 3 percent of mixed cresyl phosphates, mainly the *meta-* and *para-* compounds. These oils are synthesized in order to withstand the very high temperatures to which oils used to lubricate turbo-jet engines are exposed. They are very expensive, but as engine design alters and the science of lubrication progresses the oils periodically become out of date, and are then of little value. The firm was able to identify the specification to which the oil was made, and it was one that is no longer current. Cresyl phosphates occur as a mixture of *ortho-*, *meta-*, and *para-* compounds; but, as the dangers of the *ortho-* compounds are well known in the industry, manufacturers remove as much of them as possible.

DISCUSSION

*Ortho-*cresyl phosphates are highly toxic to the nervous system. Tri-ortho-cresyl phosphate, though by no means the most toxic member of the group, is nevertheless the best-known, and was held responsible for the great outbreak of paralysis in the U.S.A. in the early 1930s. The disease then earned the name of Jake paralysis because the o.c.p. was present in a soft drink called "Ginger Jake" or "Jamaica Ginger".

The clinical picture is well documented (*1-3*), but less is known of the pathology, at any rate in man, because even in severe poisoning the mortality is remarkably low. In the Moroccan outbreak the clinical picture was characteristic, and we agree with Burley that it must be virtually pathognomonic. At the time of our visit no one had died of the disease, nor has any death been reported since.

The prognosis depends on the severity of the paralysis. Those with distal weakness alone recover well, but commonly take at least a year to do so. Those with weakness of proximal muscles in addition recover less completely, and those with marked signs of damage to the spinal cord are usually left permanently disabled. In the Swiss outbreak (*2*) very severe poisoning followed ingestion of a single large dose, and 25 percent of the patients were left permanently disabled. In the Moroccan outbreak, however, traces of o.c.p. were consumed over many days, and fortunately the great majority of cases that we saw were mild. In all probability, therefore, in a year's time the great majority will be well on the way to recovery.

SUMMARY

A personal account is given of a visit to Morocco to assist in investigating an outbreak of paralysis. Two thousand cases had occurred before we left Morocco and the outbreak continues. It proved to be due to poisoning by *ortho*-cresyl phosphate, present in lubricating oil sold as "olive oil." The lubricating oil was man-made and was synthesized to withstand the very high temperatures pertaining in turbo-jet aircraft engines.

We wish to thank our medical colleagues in the administrative and clinical services in Morocco for their unreserved cooperation during our visit. The industrial firm in this country which conducted the analysis wishes to remain anonymous, but we are grateful to its research staff for their invaluable work.

References

(*1*) Burley, B.D. *JAMA* 98:298, 1932.
(*2*) Hunter, D. *The Diseases of Occupations.* London, 1955.
(*3*) Jordi, A.U. *J Aviation Med* **23**, 623, 1952.

ADENOCARCINOMA OF THE VAGINA[1]: ASSOCIATION OF MATERNAL STILBESTROL THERAPY WITH TUMOR APPEARANCE IN YOUNG WOMEN

Arthur L. Herbst, Howard Ulfelder, and David C. Poskanzer

ABSTRACT

Adenocarcinoma of the vagina in young women had been recorded rarely before the report of several cases treated at the Vincent Memorial Hospital between 1966 and 1969. The unusual occurrence of this tumor in eight patients born in New England hospitals between 1946 and 1951 led us to conduct a retrospective investigation in search of factors that might be associated with tumor appearance. Four matched controls were established for each patient; data were obtained by personal interview. Results show maternal bleeding during the current pregnancy and previous pregnancy loss were more common in the study group. Most significantly, seven of the eight mothers of patients with carcinoma had been treated with diethylstilbestrol started during the first trimester. None in the control group were so treated (p less than 0.00001). Maternal ingestion of stilbestrol during early pregnancy appears to have enhanced the risk of vaginal adenocarcinoma developing years later in the offspring exposed.

Cancer of the vagina is rare, occurring usually as epidermoid carcinoma in women over the age of 50 years (1). Between 1966 and 1969, however, seven girls 15 to 22 years of age with adenocarcinoma of the vagina (clear-cell or endometrial type) were seen at the Vincent Memorial Hospital (2). Although isolated case reports of histologically similar adenocarcinomas of the vagina had previously been published (3-8), these carcinomas, too, were usually in older patients. No such case in the younger age group had been seen at this institution before 1966.

The tumor typically caused prolonged vaginal bleeding that, occurring in young women, was mistaken for anovulatory bleeding and delayed the correct diagnosis. Routine vaginal cytology was often negative, and the tumor was not palpated on rectal examination. The correct diagnosis was arrived at only after vaginal examination had been performed.

Histologically, one of the tumors resembled endometrial carcinoma, but the remainder were characterized by tubules and glands lined by clear cells containing glycogen or "hobnail" cells. The clear cells also appeared in solid nests. There was a high prevalence of benign adenosis of the vagina in this group of patients. Although these tumors with clear cells and hobnail cells have been termed "mesonephroma," there is evidence that they are of Müllerian origin (2).

Because of the apparent clustering of these cases, which appeared within four years, attention was focused on possible other similarities among them. However, they did not uniformly use any intravaginal irritant, douches, or tampon. Only one patient had had sexual exposure. Before the onset of the present illness, none had been given birth-control pills. We then decided to conduct a case-control, retrospective study that would compare in detail these patients and their families with an appropriate control group to uncover factors that might be associated with the sudden appearance of these tumors.

METHODS

Four matched controls for each patient with vaginal carcinoma were selected by examination of the birth records of the hospital in which each patient was born. Females born within five days and on the same type of service (ward or private) as the eight propositae were identified. Women who gave birth to daughters closest in time to each patient with carcinoma were first

Source: *New England Journal of Medicine* 284(16): 878-881, 1971.

[1] From the Vincent Memorial Hospital (Gynecological Service of the Massachusetts General Hospital. Supported by a grant (1393-C-1) from the American Cancer Society (Massachusetts Division), Inc.

considered. Interviewing of all mothers was done from a standard questionnaire by personal interview carried out by a trained interviewer.

In addition to the seven cases cited above, an eighth identical case of clear-cell adenocarcinoma of the vagina occurred in 1969 in a 20-year-old patient, who was treated at another Boston hospital.[2] Because she and her family with their matched controls were as available as our own cases, this patient has been included with the original group, and these eight cases form the basis of this study.

Comparison of the data obtained from patients and controls was carried out with the use of the paired t-test for parametric data and the matched control method suggested by Pike and Morrow *(9)* for nonparametric data. Unpaired t-tests and chi-square tests with Yates correction were also carried out but were not significantly different from the results obtained with the paired methodologies.

RESULTS

Table 1 summarizes chronologic details of each patient with her therapy and results. The table demonstrates the clustering of patients for time of birth and occurrence of tumor. In Table 2 the data for seven pertinent areas of inquiry for each patient and her matched controls are displayed, including maternal age at the birth of the child, maternal smoking (at least 10 cigarettes per day before the birth of the child),

---

[2] We are indebted to Dr. Donald P. Goldstein, of Boston, for permission to include his case in this study.

bleeding during study pregnancy, any prior pregnancy loss, maternal estrogen therapy during study pregnancy, breast feeding of infant and intrauterine x-ray exposure.

There is a highly significant association between the treatment of the mothers with estrogen diethylstilbestrol during pregnancy and the subsequent development of adenocarcinoma of the vagina in their daughters (p = less than 0.00001). Other factors found to be different between propositae and controls but at lower levels of significance are maternal bleeding in the study pregnancy (p = less than 0.05) and any prior pregnancy loss (p = less than 0.01). No significant differences between the populations were found for maternal age at time of birth of patient, smoking in parents, intrauterine X-ray exposure and breast feeding. Other topics covered in the questionnaire that also were not statistically significant are listed in Table 3.

All the mothers who took stilbestrol began therapy in the first trimester of pregnancy. They received either a constant dose administered throughout the pregnancy, or a continually increasing dose given almost to term. Six of the seven mothers volunteered the information that stilbestrol had been prescribed for them. The seventh was uncertain, but her obstetrician identified the drug as diethystilbestrol. Bleeding during this pregnancy or previous pregnancy loss (or both) led to the administration of stilbestrol in all seven cases. The programs of management for these pregnancies occasionally included vitamins, iron or calcium.

Table 1. Summary of cases with carcinoma.

Case no.	Age at first symptoms (year)	Year of birth	Year of treatment	Therapy	Status 1971
1	20	1949	1969	Posterior exenteration & vaginectomy	Living & well
2	15	1951	1967	Radical hysterectomy & vaginectomy, with vaginal replacement	Living & well
3	14	1950	1968	Exploratory laparotomy	Died (1968)
4	15	1950	1966	Wide local excision	Living & well
5	19	1949	1969	Radical hysterectomy & vaginectomy, with vaginal replacement	Living & well
6	16	1951	1967	Radical hysterectomy & vaginectomy, with vaginal replacement	Living & well
7	18	1949	1968	Anterior exenteration, with bowel substitution of vagina	Living & well
8	22	1946	1968	Anterior exenteration, with bowel substitution of vagina	Living & well

Table 2. Summary of data comparing patients with matched controls.

Case No.	Maternal age (year)		Maternal smoking		Bleeding in this pregnancy		Any prior pregnancy loss		Estrogen given in this pregnancy		Breast feeding		Intra uterine X-ray exposure	
	Case	Mean of 4 Controls	Case	Control	Case	Control	Case	Control	Case	Control	Case	Control	Case	Control
1	25	32	Yes	2/4	No	0/4	Yes	1/4	Yes	0/4	No	0/4	No	1/4
2	30	30	Yes	3/4	No	0/4	Yes	1/4	Yes	0/4	No	1/4	No	0/4
3	22	31	Yes	1/4	Yes	0/4	No	1/4	Yes	0/4	Yes	0/4	No	0/4
4	33	30	Yes	3/4	Yes	0/4	Yes	0/4	Yes	0/4	Yes	2/4	No	0/4
5	22	27	Yes	3/4	No	1/4	No	1/4	No	0/4	No	0/4	No	0/4
6	21	29	Yes	3/4	Yes	0/4	Yes	0/4	Yes	0/4	No	0/4	No	1/4
7	30	27	No	3/4	No	0/4	Yes	1/4	Yes	0/4	Yes	0/4	No	1/4
8	26	28	Yes	3/4	No	0/4	Yes	0/4	Yes	0/4	No	0/4	Yes	1/4
Total			7/8	21/32	3/8	1/32	6/8	5/32	7/8	0/32	3/8	3/32	1/8	4/32
Mean	26.1	29.3												
Chi square (1 df)[a]			0.53		4.52		7.16		23.22		2.35		0	
p value			0.50		<0.05		<0.01		<0.00001		0.20			
		(N.S.)[b]	(N.S.)								(N.S.)		(N.S.)	

[a] Matched control chi-square test used as described by Pike & Morrow (9).
[b] Standard error of difference 1.7 yr (paired t-test); N.S. = Not statistically significant.

Table 3. Additional factors compared in patients and controls not found to be significantly different.[a]

Birth weight
Age at onset of menses
Complications & outcome of study pregnancy
Ingestion of other medications during pregnancy
Childhood diseases of mothers & patients
History of tonsillectomy
Childhood ingestions
Household pets
Noteworthy illnesses of patients & parents
Cosmetic use in patients & mothers
Cigarette smoking in patients
Alcohol consumption in parents
Occupation & year of education of parents

[a] Events compared before date of onset of present illness for each study patient & her matched controls.

DISCUSSION

By the choice of a control group consisting of females born within five days of the birth of the propositae in the same hospital and on the same type of service, socioeconomic differences are reduced. Of the candidates for the control group found on hospital birth lists 25 percent could not be located. A selection bias is therefore possible because only the families remaining in the same area could be reached for comparison. However, all eight of the families of our patients are still living in or near the community where the patients were born. Control subjects still living in the community may be a more suitably matched study population. One potential control family was excluded because the birth record indicated that the offspring had Down's syndrome. It was necessary to locate only 34 women to obtain 32 control families who would collaborate with this study.

It should be emphasized that among the eight study mothers there was a total of 10 prior pregnancy losses and only six among the 32 controls. As can be seen from Table 2, bleeding during pregnancy was also more frequent in the study group. The fact that these were truly high-risk pregnancies was the indication for stilbestrol administration. The associations observed with bleeding in the study pregnancy and with previous pregnancy loss may reflect the characteristics of the population that was selected for estrogen treatment. In one of the eight mothers whose daughter had clear-cell adenocarcinoma, there was no evidence that estrogens were administered during pregnancy, nor had she experienced prior pregnancy loss or bleeding during the study pregnancy. Furthermore, these tumors were known to occur, though rarely, in women born before the availability of oral estrogens. Thus, factors other than maternal stilbestrol ingestion appear to be operative in their development. Moreover, the stilbestrol pills prescribed for these mothers were those available between 1946 and 1951. The ingredients of these tablets, the estrogenic potency of stilbestrol and its other chemical properties must all be recognized as possible elements in the association observed. Finally, among four of the eight families there are five female siblings, ranging in age from 18 to 22 years, who are also products of pregnancies during which their mothers took diethylstilbestrol. Up to the present, a vaginal tumor has not developed in any of these girls.

To try to estimate the frequency of stilbestrol administration and the risk of development of these tumors in female offspring whose mothers took stilbestrol during pregnancy, we have examined the files of one of the hospitals in this study for the years 1946 through 1951. During this interval there was a special high-risk pregnancy clinic at the Boston Lying-in Hospital in which stilbestrol was prescribed to 675 ward patients. There were approximately 14 500 ward deliveries, indicating that at that time roughly one in 21 ward patients at the Boston Lying-in Hospital were treated during pregnancy with stilbestrol. Thus, it appears to be well within the range of statistical expectation to have a control group in which the frequency of stilbestrol use was 0 in 32. In the interval 1946 to 1951 the private service at the Boston Lying-in Hospital had more deliveries than the ward service. We have knowledge of only one case of clear-cell adenocarcinoma developing in a patient born at the Boston Lying-in Hospital, and she was delivered on the private service. Whatever the risk of tumor development in the exposed offspring, it appears to be small.

The high concurrence of benign vaginal adenosis with these adenocarcinomas suggests that an anomaly of vaginal epithelial development may be a predisposing condition. Previous reports have described an association between adenosis and this tumor in older women *(3,8)*, and their concurrence in younger patients was initially noted in the present cases *(2)*. It may be that an increase in adenosis occurs at menarche in these patients and results in greater quantities of benign tissue at risk for malignant change. It is also possible that stilbestrol alters fetal vaginal cells in utero, with changes that do not become manifest in a malignant form until years later. Animal experiments as well as further follow-up data on patients who were exposed to estrogens in utero may provide some answers. Regardless of the ultimate explanation, histologic observations of associated adenosis combined with the known estrogenic effect of stilbestrol further support a Müllerian and not a mesonephric origin for these adenocarcinomas.

The time of birth of these patients (1946 to 1951) coincides with the beginning of the widespread use of estrogens in support of high-risk pregnancy. *(10)*. It is likely that more patients with this tumor will appear as girls who were exposed in utero come to maturity. Furthermore, although our oldest patient was discovered at the age of 22 years, it is possible that these tumors will appear in even older women as the "at-risk" population matures. Although the chance of development of these tumors appears to be very small, the results of this study suggest that it is unwise to administer stilbestrol to women early in pregnancy. Furthermore, abnormal bleeding in adolescent girls can no longer be assumed to be due to anovulation, and the possibility of vaginal tumor should be excluded by a physician's examination.

ACKNOWLEDGMENTS

We are indebted to Miss Jean Sheridan, who carried out the interviews and helped with analyses and preparation of the manuscript, to Dr. Theodore Colton, of the Department of Preventive Medicine, Harvard Medical School, for helpful suggestions with statistical analysis, to Dr. Robert E. Scully, of the Department of Pathology, Massachusetts General Hospital and Harvard Medical School, for assistance, and to the directors and record librarians of the participating hospitals for co-operation.

References

(1) Herbst, A.L., T.H. Green, Jr., and H. Ulfelder. Primary carcinoma of the vagina: an analysis of 68 cases. *Am J Obstet Gynecol* 106:210-218, 1970.

(2) Herbst, A.L. and R.E. Scully. Adenocarcinoma of the vagina in adolescence: a report of 7 cases including 6 clear-cell carcinomas (so-called mesonephromas). *Cancer* 25:745-757, 1970.

(3) Plaut, A. and M.L. Dreyfus. Adenosis of vagina and its relation to primary adenocarcinoma of vagina. *Surg Gynecol Obstet* 71:756-765, 1940.

(4) Novak, E., J.D. Woodruff, and E.R. Novak. Probable mesonephric origin of certain female genital tumors. *Am J Obstet Gynecol* 68:1222-1242, 1954.

(5) Studdiford, W.E. Vaginal lesions of adenomatous origin. *Am J Obstet Gynecol* 73:641-656, 1957.

(6) Nix, H.G. and H.L. Wright. Mesonephric adenocarcinoma of the vagina. *Am J Obstet Gynecol* 99:893-899, 1967.

(7) Droegemueller, W., E.L. Makowski, and E.S. Taylor. Vaginal mesonephric adenocarcinoma in two prepubertal children. *Am J Dis Child* 119:168-170, 1970.

(8) Sandberg, E.C., R.W. Danielson, R.W. Cauwet, *et al.* Adenosis vaginae. *Am J Obstet Gynecol* 93:209-222, 1965.

(9) Pike, M.C. and R.H. Morrow. Statistical analysis of patient-control studies in epidemiology: factor under investigation on all-or-none variable. *Br J Prev Soc Med* 24:42-44, 1970.

(10) Smith, O.W. Diethylstilbestrol in the prevention and treatment of complications of pregnancy. *Am J Obstet Gynecol* 56:821-834, 1948.

SALMONELLOSIS ASSOCIATED WITH MARIJUANA: A MULTISTATE OUTBREAK TRACED BY PLASMID FINGERPRINTING[1]

David N. Taylor, I. Kaye Wachsmuth, Yung-Hui Shangkuan, Emmett V. Schmidt, Timothy J. Barrett, Janice S. Schrader, Charlene S. Scherach, Harry B. McGee, Roger A. Feldman, and Don J. Brenner[2]

ABSTRACT

In January and February of 1981, 85 cases of enteritis caused by *Salmonella muenchen* were reported from Ohio, Michigan, Georgia, and Alabama. Initial investigation failed to implicate a food source as a common vehicle, but in Michigan 76 percent of the patients, in contrast to 21 percent of the control subjects, admitted personal or household exposure to marijuana ($P<0.001$, relative risk $= 20$). Marijuana samples obtained from patients' households contained as many as 10^7 *S. muenchen* per gram.

The outbreak-related isolates of *S. muenchen* were sensitive to all antibiotics and were phenotypically indistinguishable from other *S. muenchen*. Plasmid fingerprinting, however, revealed that all isolates related to marijuana exposure contained two low-molecular-weight plasmids (3.1 and 7.4 megadaltons), which were absent in control strains. Plasmid analysis of the isolates showed that the outbreaks in Ohio, Michigan, Georgia, and Alabama were related, and analysis of isolates submitted from various other states demonstrated that cases associated with marijuana may have been dispersed as far as California and Massachusetts.

Salmonella is considered one of the most common foodborne pathogens. Over 50 outbreaks caused by this organism are reported annually to the Centers for Disease Control. Although there are more than 1800 different salmonella serotypes, 10 serotypes account for more than two thirds of the total isolates in the United States (*1*). Most outbreaks result from group exposure to a contaminated food item or meal, but exposure to products that are contaminated at the time of production and have a wide distribution may lead to multistate outbreaks. Such multistate outbreaks have been most successfully traced when they have been caused by uncommon serotypes or common serotypes with an unusual antibiotic-sensitivity pattern or phagelysis pattern. These outbreaks have involved chocolate contaminated with *S. eastbourne* (*2*), carmine dye capsules with *S. cubana* (*3*), hamburger and precooked roast beef with *S. newport* (*4,5*), and powdered milk with *S. newbrunswick* (*6*).

In January 1981 we investigated two outbreaks of salmonellosis caused by multiply sensitive *S. muenchen* strains that occurred in Ohio and Michigan. The simultaneous occurrence of two outbreaks due to the same serotype in adjacent states suggested a common vehicle. The outbreaks were traced to contaminated marijuana, which had not previously been reported as a vehicle for the transmission of bacterial pathogens. By analyzing plasmid profiles (fingerprinting), we were able to distinguish the epidemic strain from commonly occurring *S. muenchen* and to demonstrate the extent of the outbreak. Before the outbreak, the use of plasmid fingerprinting had been restricted to investigation of nonenteric, nosocomial infections (*7*).

Source: *New England Journal of Medicine* 306(21): 1249-1253, 1982.

Note: We have omitted figures 2 and 3 which appeared in the original.

[1] Presented at the 21st Interscience Conference of Antimicrobial Agents and Chemotherapy, Chicago, November 6, 1981.

[2] From the Enteric Bacteriology and Epidemiology Branch, Bacterial Diseases Division, Center for Infectious Diseases, Centers for Disease Control, Atlanta, Georgia 30333.

451

METHODS

Epidemiology

We identified patients with *S. muenchen* infection and obtained case histories by reviewing hospital and health-department records and by interviewing patients in Ohio and Michigan. We defined a case as the isolation of *S. muenchen* from blood or stool during December 1980 through February 1981, from the first person in a household to become ill. These initial studies led to a case-control study in which a questionnaire on foods, restaurants, recreation, and contact with animals was administered by telephone to 32 case and control households in Ohio. Control households were randomly selected from case neighborhoods by means of a street directory. Control households were excluded if any family member had been ill with a diarrheal illness lasting for more than two days in the past two months. The initial case-control study led to a second survey of case households, in which specific information on interactions with other case patients and the use of illicit drugs was obtained.

To determine whether marijuana was more frequently used in case households than in control households, we conducted a case-control study of 17 cases in Michigan and 34 control subjects matched for age and neighborhood. Statistical testing of the responses from case and control patients was performed according to the method of Miettinen (cases matched with a variable number of controls) (8). Samples of marijuana (less than 5 g) were requested from case households in Ohio, Michigan, Georgia, and Alabama and were submitted for microbiologic testing.

Laboratory Investigations

Salmonellae were isolated from fecal and blood specimens by hospital laboratories using standard isolation techniques and were serotyped by state health departments (9). Biochemical reactions (9) and antibiotic susceptibilities (10) were determined for all isolates, including control strains of *S. muenchen* not related to the epidemics or to marijuana use. A quantitative estimate of salmonella contamination in the marijuana samples was made by plate counts of *S. muenchen* isolates. To confirm that the samples were marijuana and to determine the quantities of the various cannabinoids present in each sample, samples contaminated with salmonella were sent to the Research Institute of Pharmaceutical Sciences (University of Mississippi) for gas-chromatographic analysis (11).

The plasmid profile of 116 isolates of *S. muenchen* was determined by agarose-gel electrophoresis of plasmid DNA. Strains of *S. muenchen* and antigenically related salmonellae previously isolated from diverse areas of the United States were also analyzed by agarose-gel electrophoresis and served as controls. Broth cultures were lysed by sodium dodecyl sulfate with high salt (12) or by the nonionic detergent Triton X-100 (13) and then cleared by centrifugation (14).

All plasmid DNA was analyzed by electrophoresis with vertical-slab agarose (15). Plasmid DNA from *Escherichia coli* strain V517 served as a control for molecular weight (16). Purified plasmid DNA from selected strains was prepared for digestion with the restriction endonuclease Hpa II (Miles Laboratories) (17). Bacteriophage lambda DNA with a known Hpa II cleavage pattern was used as a control for complete enzyme digestion of DNA.

RESULTS

Cases in Ohio and Michigan

The National Salmonella Surveillance System receives 300 to 400 reports per year of isolation of *S. muenchen* from human beings (1). Like isolations of many other salmonella serotypes, isolations of this serotype are most frequently reported during the summer months. In 1981, in contrast to previous years, there was a sharp increase in the number of isolates reported (Figure 1). There were 63 isolates of this serotype reported in January 1981 and 87 in February 1981; 70 percent of the isolates in January and 35 percent of those in February were reported from Ohio and Michigan.

The age distributions of cases were similar in the two states. The median age overall was 10 years; in patients under one year old it was five months. The age distribution of cases in this outbreak was compared with the age distribution reported for 1980. In these two outbreaks 14 of 62 persons (23 percent) were 20 to 29 years old, as compared with 33 of 268 (12 per-

Figure 1. Isolates of *Salmonella muenchen* from cases of infection, in the United States, January 1978 through August 1981.

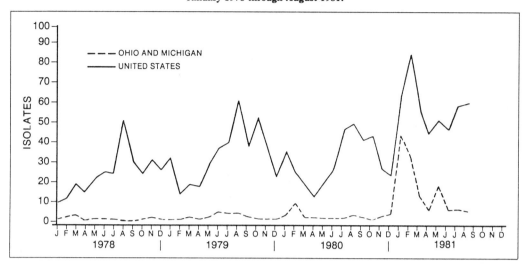

cent) from whom *S. muenchen* was isolated in 1980. This increase was significant (P = 0.04, Fisher's exact test, two-tailed) and was associated with a decrease in the proportion of persons 50 years old or older, from 20 percent to 8 percent. The predominant symptoms were diarrhea (90 percent), fever (81 percent), abdominal pain (73 percent), bloody diarrhea (54 percent), and nausea and vomiting (44 percent). Thirty-nine of the cases (62 percent) were hospitalized. The median duration of illness was eight days.

The case-control study in Ohio failed to correlate a place (such as a supermarket, restaurant, bar, or recreational center) or a food (such as a meat product, cheese, dressing, spice, or holiday food—chocolate or fruitcake) with the outbreak. However, we found that 44 percent of the case households, but none of the control households, had children under one year of age (P<0.001), and that all the case households, but only 41 percent of the control households, included persons 15 to 35 years old (P<0.001).

Because of the association with young adults, the lack of association with a food, restaurant, or activity, and some anecdotal information, we asked about the use of illicit drugs in a second interview with members of case households. None of the household members admitted using any drug except marijuana, but exposure to marijuana appeared to be high. In Ohio and Michigan 49 patients (78 percent) had been ex-

posed to marijuana: 13 patients (21 percent) admitted to personal use of marijuana, 22 (35 percent) had been exposed to marijuana in the household but had not smoked it, and 14 (22 percent) had been exposed to marijuana outside the household but denied smoking it. Fourteen (22 percent) had no known exposure to marijuana.

We conducted the second case-control study in Michigan soon after the association in Ohio was discovered. Seventy-six percent of the patients, as compared with 21 percent of the control subjects, reported personal or household exposure to marijuana (Table 1). Patients were 20 times as likely as their matched control subjects to have been exposed to marijuana in the two weeks before the patient's illness (P<0.001). The patients firmly denied ingestion of marijuana in foods.

Table 1. Personal or household exposure to marijuana among cases and controls in Michigan, January through February 1981.[a]

		Controls		
		Both Yes	1 Yes 1 No	Both No	Total Triplets
Cases {	Yes	1	4	8	13
	No	0	1	3	4
	Total triplets	1	5	11	17

[a] There was a significant difference between cases and controls (P = 0.0006, relative risk = 20).

Cases in Other States

As a result of the studies in Michigan and Ohio, two cases of enteritis caused by *S. muenchen* were reported from Alabama and 21 cases were reported from Georgia (*18,19*). Both patients in Alabama were under six months of age and had diarrhea; one was hospitalized. The mothers of both children smoked marijuana in the household. In Georgia, information could be obtained about 15 of the patients. Ten of the patients were under seven years old, and five were 20 to 27. All the young adults smoked marijuana, and the parents of seven of 10 of the affected children smoked it in the household.

Laboratory Investigations

S. muenchen was isolated from marijuana samples from three of four case households in Ohio and from one case household each in Michigan, Alabama, and Georgia. The plate-count estimate of salmonella organisms per gram of marijuana indicated extremely high levels of contamination (Table 2). The microorganisms isolated in the three other samples were similar. Biochemical analysis of the suspected marijuana samples confirmed that they were marijuana, but the pattern did not suggest their country of origin.

The *S. muenchen* strains isolated from the patients and the marijuana in Ohio and Michigan were sensitive to all antibiotics tested and were biochemically indistinguishable from control *S. muenchen* (in a battery of 36 test reactions). Ini-

tially, the strains from the Ohio epidemic were analyzed and found to contain two plasmids with molecular weights of 3.1 and 7.4 megadaltons. . . . These plasmids were subsequently found in every strain, regardless of antibiotic sensitivity, that was isolated from patients involved in outbreaks traced to contaminated marijuana. None of the control strains isolated in previous years or isolated recently from known negative sources (i.e., sources unrelated to marijuana) contained the same two plasmids. Further plasmid analysis of *S. muenchen* strains isolated from patients during December 1980 through February 1981 in nine states identified this plasmid pattern in residents of California, Arizona, and Massachusetts (Table 3). Similar restriction-endonuclease digests of plasmid DNA from *S. muenchen* from Ohio, Georgia, and California confirmed that they were related by Hpa II recognition sites (CCGG [cytosine-cytosine-guanine-guanine] nucleotide sequence) and size. . . .

DISCUSSION

In this investigation we concluded that two simultaneous outbreaks of *S. muenchen* gastroenteritis in Ohio and Michigan were caused by exposure to contaminated marijuana, after demonstrating that the use of marijuana was significantly more prevalent in case households than control households and after isolating *S. muenchen* from marijuana samples from case households in both states.

Table 2. Characteristics of salmonella isolated from marijuana samples obtained from case households, February 1981.

Sample	State	Serotype	Colony count per gram[a]	Other microorganisms found[b]	Antibiotic sensitivity[c]
A	Ohio	*S. muenchen*	8×10^5	1,2,3,4	S
B	Ohio	*S. muenchen*	4×10^7	1,2,3,4	S
		S. oslo	4×10^6	NT	S
C	Ohio	*S. muenchen*	5×10^7	1,2,3,4,5	S
D	Michigan	*S. muenchen*	QNS	NT	S
E	Georgia	*S. muenchen*	QNS	NT	S
F	Alabama	*S. muenchen*	QNS	NT	R

[a] QNS denotes quantity not sufficient for determination.

[b] 1 denotes *Staphylococcus epidermidis*, 2 *Escherichia coli*, 3 *Klebsiella pneumoniae*, 4 Group D streptococci, and 5 *Pseudomonas aeruginosa*. NT denotes not tested.

[c] S denotes sensitivity to all antibiotics tested, and R resistance to ampicillin.

Table 3. *Salmonella muenchen* plasmid profiles.

Origin of organism	Characteristic plasmids[a]	None or other plasmids
	No. of strains	
Alabama	4[b]	—
Arizona	4	—
Georgia	4	—
West Virginia	4	—
Ohio	12[b]	1
Michigan	26[b]	2
Massachusetts	9	11
California	3	12
Wisconsin	1	5
New Hampshire	—	1
Washington (state)	—	4
Pennsylvania	—	3
Texas	—	7
Vermont	—	3
C2 controls	—	10[c]
Controls with *S. muenchen*	—	16[c]
	67	75

[a] The sizes of characteristic plasmids are approximately 3×10^6 and 7×10^6 daltons.
[b] This number includes *S. muenchen* strains isolated directly from marijuana.
[c] Control strains obtained from stock collection of Centers for Disease Control.

When marijuana is ready to be sold, it is stored at room temperature in a dry atmosphere. Under these conditions salmonellae can remain viable but will not grow. The quantitative studies performed on these specimens indicated that the degree of contamination (10^6 to 10^7 salmonellae per gram of marijuana) was unlikely to have occurred through simple inoculation from users' hands contaminated by other sources. The similarities of the accompanying microflora in the three specimens also suggested contamination with direct mixing of marijuana with animal feces, which might occur as a result of fertilization with untreated animal manure, inadvertent contamination during drying or storage, or simply direct adulteration with dried animal manure to increase the weight of the product.

The United States Drug Enforcement Agency estimates that in 1980 the marijuana used in this country was grown in Colombia (75 percent), Mexico (11 percent), Jamaica (7 percent), and the United States (7 percent) (20). The Agency suggests that most of the marijuana brought in from Mexico remains in the southwestern United States, whereas marijuana grown in the United States is not distributed outside the state where it was grown. The coast-to-coast distribution of this marijuana leads us to suspect that Colombia or Jamaica was the country of origin.

Investigation of this outbreak revealed a new vehicle for salmonella infection capable of causing a multistate outbreak; it also increased our understanding of the infection by showing that a vehicle that is not ingested can cause salmonellosis. Marijuana can contaminate the fingers during preparation of a marijuana cigarette or contaminate the lips during smoking. In this outbreak the number of salmonellae ingested by hand-to-mouth or cigarette-to-mouth contamination was sufficient to cause infection in young adults. The cases in children may have occurred through direct contact with flecks of marijuana, contact with infected persons, or secondary contamination of foods.

The high degree of contamination and the prolonged use or exposure may suffice to explain the infection, but other host factors may be involved as well. In another study, long-term users of cannabis were found to have little or no gastric acid and could have been infected with lower numbers of *Vibrio cholerae* 01 than were required to infect other volunteers (21). Since gastric acidity acts as an important barrier to ingested microorganisms, this decreased acidity could have predisposed this group to infection after they had ingested smaller inocula. In the persons smoking contaminated marijuana it is possible that some salmonella organisms were inhaled into the lungs.

The proportion of cases in young children (50 percent of whom were under 10 years of age) in this outbreak was similar to that reported to the Salmonella Surveillance System (40 percent) (1). In this outbreak children certainly had less exposure to the vehicle than did adults. This suggests that in an outbreak of salmonellosis, even though a large proportion of the cases may have occurred in infants and young children, investigation to determine the vehicle of transmission should include examination of exposures common to the adults of the households.

The plasmid DNA analysis of these epidemiologically related strains identified two small plasmids that were unique to the strains associated with and isolated from marijuana. Although small cryptic plasmids are commonly seen in enteric organisms, other *S. muenchen* that are known to be unrelated to marijuana use did not contain either of these plasmids. Comparison with other, previously assayed salmonellae also revealed no similar pattern. The additional evidence for a single plasmid profile was the identical Hpa II-enzyme-digestion patterns. . . .

It was not expected that the two small plasmids would be unique to epidemic-associated or marijuana-associated strains or that they would remain as stable as they did. There is no known function for these plasmids and consequently no known natural or laboratory pressure selective for them. It is possible that any *S. muenchen* strain with one or neither of these bands may have lost the DNA that by definition is not essential to the survival of the bacterial cell. It is also possible that epidemic-related *S. muenchen* strains may acquire a plasmid; this did occur without affecting the two small plasmids or any known culture characteristic. . . . The intestine provides such a rich source of potential donors and recipients of plasmid DNA that it is quite interesting that the marijuana-associated *S. muenchen* fingerprint remained essentially unaltered over a broad geographic area and after passage through several human hosts. Thus, plasmid fingerprinting is a useful method to identify community-acquired organisms that cannot be typed by other techniques.

We are indebted to Drs. William Hall, James Alexander, and Richard Goodman and to Mr. Robert Campbell for their assistance in the epidemiologic investigation of this outbreak; to Ms. Mardi Russell and Dr. Carlton Turner for the biochemical analysis of the marijuana samples; to Mrs. Joy Wells and Dr. Earl Renshaw for their assistance in the laboratory investigation of this outbreak; to Mrs. Dot Anderson for the preparation of the manuscript; and to Ms. Charlotte Turner and Drs. Mitchell Cohen and Paul Blake for their review of the manuscript.

References

(1) *Salmonella Surveillance: Annual Summary.* Atlanta, Centers for Disease Control, 1981.

(2) Craven, P.C., D.C. Mackel, W.B. Baine, et al. International outbreak of *Salmonella eastbourne* infec-tion traced to contaminated chocolate. *Lancet* 1:788-793, 1975.

(3) Lang, D.J., L.J. Kunz, A.R. Martin, S.A. Schroeder, and L.A. Thomson. Carmine as a source of nosocomial salmonellosis. *N Engl J Med* 276:829-832, 1967.

(4) Fontaine, R.E., S. Arnon, W.T. Martin, et al. Raw hamburger: an interstate common source of human salmonellosis. *Am J Epidemiol* 107:36-45, 1978.

(5) Multi-state outbreak of *Salmonella newport* transmitted by precooked roasts of beef. *Morbid Mortal Weekly Rep* 26:277-278, 1977.

(6) Collins, R.N., M.D. Treger, J.B. Boring III, D.B. Coohon, and R.N. Barr. Interstate outbreak of *Salmonella newbrunswick* infection traced to powdered milk. *JAMA* 203:838-844, 1968.

(7) Schaberg, D.R., L.S. Tompkins, and S. Falkow. Use of agarose gel electrophoresis of plasmid deoxyribonucleic acid to fingerprint gram-negative bacilli. *J Clin Microbiol* 13:1105-1108, 1981.

(8) Miettinen, O.S. Individual matching with multiple controls in the case of all-or-none responses. *Biometrics* 25:339-355, 1969.

(9) Edwards, P.R., and W.H. Ewing. *Identification of Enterobacteriaceae.* 3d edition. Minneapolis, Burgess, 1972.

(10) Bauer, A.W., W.M.M. Kirby, J.C. Sherris, and M. Turck. Antibiotic susceptibility testing by a standardized single-disk method. *Am J Clin Pathol* 45:493-496, 1966.

(11) Fetterman, P.S., N.J. Doorenbos, E.S. Deith, and M.W. Quimby. A simple gas liquid chromatography procedure for determination of cannabinoidic acids in *Cannabis sativa* L. *Experientia* 27:988-990, 1971.

(12) Guerry, P., D.J. LeBlanc, and S. Falkow. General method for the isolation of plasmid deoxyribonucleic acid. *J Bacteriol* 116:1064-1066, 1973.

(13) Humphreys, G.O., G.A. Willshaw, and E.S. Anderson. A simple method for the preparation of large quantities of pure plasmic DNA. *Biochim Biophys Acta* 383:457-463, 1975.

(14) Elwell, L.P., J. deGraaff, D. Seibert, and S. Falkow. Plasmid-linked ampicillin resistance in *Haemophilus influenza* type b. *Infect Immun* 12:404-410, 1975.

(15) Meyers, J.A., D. Sanchez, L.P. Elwell, and S. Falkow. Simple agarose gel electrophoretic method for the identification and characterization of plasmic deoxyribonucleic acid. *J Bacteriol* 127:1529-1537, 1976.

(16) Macrina, F.L., D.J. Kopecko, K.R. Jones, D.J. Ayers, and S.M. McCowen. A multiple plasmid-containing *Escherichia coli* strain: convenient source of size reference plasmid molecules. *Plasmid* 1:417-420, 1978.

(17) Radloff, R., W. Bauer, and J. Vinograd. A dye-buoyant density method for the detection and isolation of closed circular duplex DNA: the closed circular DNA in HeLa cells. *Proc Natl Acad Sci USA* 57:1514-1521, 1967.

(18) *Salmonellosis Traced to Marijuana* (Communicable Disease Report no. 9.) Alabama Department of Public Health, March 1981, p. 2.

(19) Salmonellosis and Marijuana: Unexpected Transmission (Georgia Epidemiology Report). Atlanta: Georgia Department of Human Resources, February 1981, p. 1.

(20) The National Narcotics Intelligence Consumers Committee. *Narcotics Intelligence Estimate: The Supply of Drugs to the U.S. Illicit Market from Foreign and Domestic Sources in 1979.* Washington, D.C., Drug Enforcement Administration, 1979.

(21) Nalin, D.R., M.M. Levine, J. Rhead, et al. Cannabis, hypochlorhydria, and cholera. *Lancet* 2:859-862, 1978.

TOBACCO SMOKING AS A POSSIBLE ETIOLOGIC FACTOR IN BRONCHIOGENIC CARCINOMA: A STUDY OF SIX HUNDRED AND EIGHTY-FOUR PROVED CASES[1]

Ernest L. Wynder and Evarts A. Graham[2]

General Increase. There is rather general agreement that the incidence of bronchiogenic carcinoma has greatly increased in the last half-century. Statistical studies at the Charity Hospital of New Orleans (*1*), the St. Louis City Hospital (*2*), and the Veterans Administration Hospital of Hines, Illinois (*3*) have revealed that at these hospitals cancer of the lung is now the most frequent visceral cancer in men.

Autopsy statistics throughout the world show a great increase in the incidence of bronchiogenic carcinoma in relation to cancer in general. Kennaway and Kennaway (*4,5*), in a careful statistical study of death certificates in England and Wales from 1928 to 1945, have presented undoubted evidence of a great increase in deaths from cancer of the lung. In this country statistics compiled by the American Cancer Society show a similar trend during the past two decades (*6*).

Tobacco as a Possible Cause of Increase. The suggestion that smoking, and in particular cigarette smoking, may be important in the production of bronchiogenic carcinoma has been made by many writers on the subject even though well controlled and large scale clinical studies are lacking. Adler (*7*) in 1912 was one of the first to think that tobacco might play some role in this regard. Tylecote (*8*), Hoffman (*9*), McNally (*10*), Lickint (*11*), Arkin and Wagner (*12*), Roffo (*13*), and Maier (*14*) were just a few of the workers who thought that there was some evidence that tobacco was an important factor in the increase of cancer of the lungs. Müller (*15*) in 1939,

from a careful but limited clinical statistical study, offered good evidence that heavy smoking is an important etiologic factor. In 1941 Ochsner and DeBakey (*16*) called attention to the similarity of the curve of increased sales of cigarettes in this country to the greater prevalence of primary cancer of the lung. They emphasized the possible etiologic relationship of cigarette smoking to this condition. In a recent paper Schrek (*17*) concluded that there is strong circumstantial evidence that cigarette smoking is an etiologic factor in cancer of the respiratory tract and finds that his data are in agreement with the results of a preliminary report presented by Wynder and Graham at the National Cancer Conference in February 1949 (*18*).

Purpose of Study. The purpose of the present study was to attempt to determine, so far as possible by clinical investigations, statistical methods, and experimental studies, the importance of various exogenous factors that might play a role in the induction of bronchiogenic carcinoma. In this regard we intended to learn the relative importance of previous diseases of the lungs, rural and urban distribution of patients, various occupations, and hereditary background as well as smoking habits. By obtaining all this information, we hoped to determine whether any of these factors, either singly or in combination, have had an effect in increasing the incidence of bronchiogenic carcinoma.

In the present paper the chief emphasis will be placed on our findings in regard to smoking.

METHOD OF STUDY

The results of this study are based on 684 cases of proved bronchiogenic carcinoma. It should be emphasized that the results in this report have not been obtained from hospital records since we learned at the outset of our

Source: *Journal of the American Medical Association* 143(4):329-336, 1950.
[1] This study has been aided by a grant from the American Cancer Society. Other phases of it will be presented in subsequent publications.
[2] From the Department of Surgery, Washington University School of Medicine and Barnes Hospital.

study that the routine records did not supply satisfactory answers to our questions. It was therefore decided to seek the desired information by special interviews. Six hundred and thirty-four patients reported on in this paper have been personally interviewed, and in 33 cases we obtained the information by mailing a questionnaire.[3] In the remaining 17 cases information for the questionnaire was obtained from a person who had been intimately acquainted with the patient throughout his adult life.

Through the cooperation of many hospitals and physicians throughout all parts of the country who permitted us to interview their patients, it is felt that a fairly good cross-section of the entire United States has been obtained. The list of cooperating institutions and physicians is presented below.[4]

In order to make this survey as uniform as possible, each interviewer used the questionnaire shown in Table 1.

In regard to smoking habits, we considered it particularly essential to learn how much a patient had smoked formerly, even though he might not smoke at all or smoke little at the time

[3] The questionnaires were sent to male and female patients with cancer of the lungs from Dr. W. L. Watson's Thoracic Surgery Service at Memorial Hospital, New York.

[4] CALIFORNIA: Private patients of Drs. L. Brewer, Daniels, F. Dolley, D. Dugan, H. Garland, E. Holman, J. Jones, W. Rogers, P. Samson, B. Stephens. Hospitals: Birmingham General, French, Good Samaritan, Letterman General, Los Angeles County, Southern Pacific General, Stanford, United States Marine, United States Naval University of California, Wadsworth General. COLORADO: Private patients of Drs. A. Brown, F. Condon, J. Grow, F. Harper, M. Peck. Hospitals: Colorado General, Denver General, Fitzsimmons, Fort Logan Veterans, General Rose, St. Lukes. DISTRICT OF COLUMBIA: Private patients of Drs. B. Blades, E. Davis. Hospitals: Georgetown, George Washington, Walter Reed. ILLINOIS: Hospitals: Cook County, Veterans Administration, Hines, Ill. MARYLAND: Hospitals: Johns Hopkins, United States Naval. MASSACHUSETTS: Private patients of Drs. D. Harken, R. Overholt. Hospitals: Boston City, Massachusetts General, New England Deaconess. MICHIGAN: Hospitals: Dearborn Veterans, MISSOURI: Private patients of Drs. J. Flance, A. Goldman, R. Smith. Hospitals: Jefferson Barracks Veterans, Jewish, St. Louis City, St. Louis County. NEW JERSEY: Hospitals: Berthold S. Pollack, Newark City. NEW YORK: Private patients of Drs. W. Cahan, H. Maier, J. Pool, W. Watson. Hospitals: Bellevue, Veterans Administration, Brooklyn Cancer Institute, Kings County Memorial, Montefiore, New York City Cancer Institute, New York Hospital, Presbyterian, Roswell Park Memorial Institute. OHIO: Hospitals: Veterans Administration. PENNSYLVANIA: Private patients of Dr. J. Johnson. Hospitals: Jefferson Medical College, Temple University, University of Pennsylvania. UTAH: Private patients of Drs. W. Rumel, Cutler. Hospitals: Holy Cross, St. Marks, Salt Lake County General, Veterans Administration, Dr. W. H. Groves, Latter-Day Saints.

of the interview. The reason for this is the well-known existence of a time lag between the exposure to a carcinogenic substance and the appearance of cancer. Many patients coming into the hospital with chronic disease of the lungs had stopped smoking months, or even years, previously. We therefore asked the patients to estimate the average use of tobacco during the last twenty years of their smoking period. The control patients were questioned in an identical manner; thus any possible error lying in this method of estimating smoking habits was balanced.

In questioning patients about occupations, we attempted to learn all the occupations of a given patient, the years during which he had held these jobs and to what type of dusts or fumes he had been exposed. Similar details were obtained in regard to other possible exposures, such as those a patient might have had in connection with certain hobbies.

Classification of Smoking. In order to facilitate a statistical analysis of the results, the arbitrary classification of smoking habits given in Table 2 was established. If a patient smoked for less than twenty years, his amount of smoking was adjusted to a twenty-year period. Thus a patient smoking 20 cigarettes for ten years only was classified as smoking 10 cigarettes daily (class 2). Such adjustments were rarely necessary, since only a few patients had smoked for less than twenty years.

If a man smoked habitually more than one type of tobacco during the last twenty years, the various types were added together to make up his classification. Thus a man who smoked one package of cigarettes daily, as well as two cigars, was classified as a class 4, or an excessive, smoker.

Histologic Types. To insure an undoubted diagnosis, microscopic confirmation of the presence of carcinoma was obtained in all cases. Some difficulty arose in the histologic classification because of the variation of terms employed by pathologists in the different hospitals who examined the specimens. For example, what some pathologists would designate as an adenocarcinoma others would classify as an undifferentiated carcinoma. Likewise, the term oat cell or round cell carcinoma was at times used, a designation which is not recognized by some pathologists. In some cases pathologists called a lesion, from biopsy section, merely a carcinoma, unclassified. It may be said, however, that in general by far the most prevalent histologic types were the epidermoid or squamous carcinoma and its variant the undifferentiated carcinoma. These are the most common types found in males. In females the adenocarcinoma has so

Table 1. Etiologic Survey.

Name: .... Age: ....

1. Have you ever had a lung disease? If so, state time, duration, and site of disease:

   Pneumonia   Asthma   Tuberculosis   Bronchiectasis
   Influenza   Lung Abscess   Chest Injuries   Others

2. Do you or did you ever smoke?   Yes ☐ No ☐

3. At what age did you begin to smoke?

4. At what age did you stop smoking?

5. How much tobacco did you average per day during the past 20 years of your smoking?
   Cigarettes .... Cigars .... Pipes ....

6. Do you inhale the smoke?   Yes ☐ No ☐

7. Do you have a chronic cough which you attribute to your smoking, especially upon first smoking in the morning? If so, for how long?
   Yes ☐   No ☐

8. Do you smoke before or after breakfast?   Before ☐ After ☐

9. Name the brand or brands, and dates, if any given brand has been smoked exclusively for more than five years.

   Change frequently? ☐

   First brand—from 19.... to 19....

   Second brand—from 19.... to 19....

10. What kind of jobs have you held? Have you been exposed to dust or fumes while working there? (Use back of page for detailed description of possible exposure)

From	To	Position	Dust or Fumes

11. Have you ever been exposed to irritative dusts or fumes outside of your job? In particular have you ever used insecticide spray excessively? If so, state time and duration.
    Yes ☐ No ☐ Type .... Duration ....

12. How much alcohol do you or have you averaged per day? State time and duration in years.
    Whiskey .... Beer .... Wine ....

13. Where were you born and where have you lived most of you life? State the approximate time span you have lived in a certain locality. Up to what grade did you attend school?
    Birthplace .... Home .... Educational Level ....

14. State the cause of death of your parents, and of brothers and sisters if any.

15. *Site of Lesion*   *Microscopic Diagnosis*   *Papanicolaou Class*   *Etiological Class*

Interviewer ....

Table 2. Classification of smoking habits.

Group 0	Nonsmokers (Less than 1 cigarette per day for more than 20 years)[a]
1	Light smokers (From 1 to 9 cigarettes per day for more than 20 years)[a,b]
2	Moderately heavy smokers (From 10 to 15 cigarettes per day for more than 20 years)[a]
3	Heavy smokers (From 16 to 20 cigarettes per day for more than 20 years)[a]
4	Excessive smokers (From 21 to 24 cigarettes per day for more than 20 years)[a]
5	Chain smokers (35 cigarettes or more per day for at least 20 years)[a]

[a] Pipe and cigar smokers have been included by arbitrarily counting 1 cigar as 3 cigarettes and 1 pipeful as 2½ cigarettes.
[b] Includes minimal smokers (from 1 to 4 cigarettes a day, or the equivalent in pipes or cigars for more than 20 years).

far been nearly as common as the other types. It is unquestionably the epidermoid and undifferentiated carcinomas which have shown the greatest increase in recent years. For this reason we were particularly interested in studying these types separately from the adenocarcinomas. The present report includes 605 male and 25 female patients with epidermoid, undifferentiated, and unclassified carcinomas and 39 male and 15 female patients with adenocarcinoma. In order to determine possible sex variations in the etiology of cancer of the lung, results in men and women are reported separately.

Control Study I. To check all possible bias on the part of the interviewers who saw only patients believed to have bronchiogenic carcinoma, it was deemed advisable to conduct a control study in which a nonmedical investigator would interview every patient admitted to the Chest Service of Barnes Hospital without knowing the diagnosis in advance. Two interviewers[5] were used for this purpose. When the final diagnosis was determined, all cases of cancer of the lungs (75 men) were separated from the other cases (132). Control patients under the age of 30 were excluded since there were no cases of cancer in this age group. Seventeen male patients for whom no definitive diagnosis could be made were also omitted.

In addition, these interviewers interrogated patients with cancer of the lung at other St. Louis hospitals,[6] also without previous knowledge of diagnosis. Here the interviewers were given the names of several patients with diseases of the chest in a comparable age group, of whom at least one was suspected to have bronchiogenic carcinoma. The patients with proved cancer of the lung (25 men) and the other patients (54 men) were added to the Barnes Hospital groups, thus collectively making up control study I.

To determine the smoking habits, as well as the other data contained in the questionnaire of our study of other hospital patients, the nonmedical investigators also questioned patients without cancer of the lungs on the general surgical and medical services at Barnes Hospital, the Jefferson Barracks Veterans Hospital, and the St. Louis City Hospital. This group, called "general hospital population," consists of 780 patients. Also, a total of 552 female patients without cancer of the lungs have been interviewed as control patients on our surgical and medical services.

Two objects were to be realized by this control study. One was to learn of possible exposures to exogenous irritants of a large group of patients without cancer of the lung and the other to test the validity of the interviews made by those who knew the suspected diagnosis in a given case in advance.

Age Distribution in Control Cases: For proper statistical evaluation of a study of this kind it is obvious that the age distribution should be the same in the control cases as in the cases of cancer of the lungs. Since no patients with cancer of the lungs below 30 or above 80 years of age were seen, no controls beyond these ages have been included. The controls comprised the unselected patients as they entered the Barnes Hospital and other St. Louis hospitals. For that reason their age distribution is not identical with that of the patients with cancer.

[5] Betty G. Proctor, A.B., and Adele B. Croninger, M.A.

[6] City Hospital, Jewish Hospital, and Veterans Administration Hospital.

In order to be able to evaluate the cases without cancer on the basis of the same age distribution as that found in the cases of cancer, the following adjustments were made:

The combined results include data on 780 cases without cancer. Among these there is the following age distribution: 30 to 39, 18.7 percent; 40 to 49, 21 percent; 50 to 59, 26.9 percent; 60 to 69, 20.5 percent, and 70 to 79, 12.8 percent. (For the age distribution in the 605 cases of cancer see Table 5.)

The smoking classifications of the control cases have been made proportional to the age distribution among the cases of cancer by multiplying the percentage value of each smoking classification for each age group of the controls by the proportion of cases of cancer in that age group. For example, in the age group 30 to 39 of the controls there were 146 (18.7 percent) patients, of whom 20 (13.6 percent) were nonsmokers. However, since of the patients with cancer only 2.3 percent fell into this age group, the value of 13.6 percent was made proportional to the age distribution in the cases of cancer (2.3 per cent).[7] In a similar manner the smoking values for the control group aged 40 to 49 were made proportional to 17.4 percent. Finally, the quotients of the smoking classifications in each age group were added to make the percentage values shown in Figure 1. The detailed data which compare the smoking classifications of the two groups according to age are shown in Table 6. It was from those data that the proportional values were obtained.

The 100 cases of cancer and the 186 cases of control study I were made proportional in the same manner.

Control Study II. In addition to the control study just cited, it was thought to be valuable to have other physicians carry out similar interviews using our questionnaire. It was thought that the results would serve as an effective control for the cases collected under our own supervision.

At this time we are reporting preliminary results based on 83 patients interviewed at the Bellevue Hospital, Columbia University Division (New York), by Dr. H. G. Turner[8]; at the Boston City Hospital by Dr. G. W. Ware[9]; at the Crile Veterans Hospital (Cleveland, Ohio) by Dr. C. T. Surington, and at the Veterans Administration Hospital, Hines, Illinois, by Dr. E. J. Shabart.

RESULTS

The first data to be presented are based on 605 proved cases of bronchiogenic carcinoma in men, other than adenocarcinoma. Five hundred and ninety-five of these cases have been diagnosed on the basis of tissue biopsy, nine on the basis of examination of sputum and one on the basis of study of the pleural fluid.[10]

Comparison of Independent Studies. Before the smoking habits of the 605 patients with cancer of the lungs are compared with those of the general hospital population, it might be well to compare the results in the two control studies and the group of 422 patients (study III) interviewed and collected by one of us (E.L.W.) to determine any possible bias in cases in which the suspected diagnosis was known in advance and whether the data are sufficiently similar to warrant their discussion as a group.

Control Study I: This group consists of 100 patients with cancer of the lungs and 186 with diseases of the chest other than cancer interviewed by two nonmedical investigators who had no previous knowledge of the diagnosis in a given case. The data show no nonsmokers (Figure 2) among the cancer group, while there are 14.1 percent nonsmokers among the patients with other thoracic diseases. Ninety-five percent of the patients with cancer are in the classification of moderately heavy to chain smokers and 53 percent are excessive and chain smokers, while among the patients without cancer, 75.3 and 23 percent, respectively, fell among these smoking groups.

Control Study II: The data in Table 3 cover 83 male patients with cancer of the lungs interviewed independently by physicians in other cities. Among each small group of cases some

---

[7] $\dfrac{13.6 \times 2.3}{100} = 0.312.$ This is the quotient which, added to the others determined in the same manner, makes the data shown in figure 1.

[8] Of the service of Dr. James B. Amberson.

[9] Of the service of Dr. John W. Strieder.

[10] Eight of these cases were diagnosed in Dr. Papanicolaou's laboratory on conclusive evidence of carcinoma. One sputum and one pleural fluid examination were made at the Boston City Hospital.

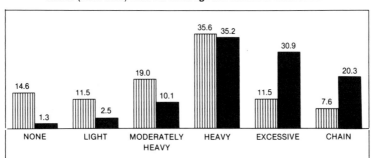

Figure 1. Percentages for amount of smoking among 605 male patients with cancer of the lungs (solid bars) and 780 men in the general hospital population without cancer (lined bars) with the same age and economic distribution.

variation is, of course, to be expected. In each of the individual groups nearly half or more of the patients are excessive or chain smokers. Grouping the data of the four independent investigators together, we find 2.4 percent nonsmokers and 93.9 percent moderately heavy to chain smokers (Figure 3), while 59 percent are excessive and chain smokers. The results of the two control studies correspond closely to one another as well as to the results of study III (Table 4).

The results in relation to the areas or hospitals where the cases were observed show uniformity. Small differences between the groups may well be explained on the basis of the small size of each series. The mountain state series includes 13 patients of Mormon faith. Mormons in general were found to smoke much less than our general hospital population. Among the Mormon patients with cancer of the lung, how-

ever, there was only one nonsmoker (72 years old). The others were long-time users of tobacco.

Comparing the three studies, we note little difference. For example, nonsmokers account for 0.0 percent in control study I, 2.4 percent in control study II, and 1.4 percent in study III. The percentage of heavy to chain smokers in these three groups is 88, 86.7, and 85.2 respectively, while the percentage of excessive and chain smokers totals 53, 59, and 49 respectively.

Since we thus have not been able to determine any essential difference in the amount of smoking in the three studies, we shall from here on refer to the total results of 605 cases.

Age Distribution. The age distribution of cancer of the lungs in the present series shows 2.3 percent of the patients to be under 40 years of age, while 79.3 percent were 50 years or

Table 3. Control Study II: amount of smoking in 83 cases of proved cancer of the lung as determined by investigators using the same questionnaire as that used in the cases of this study.

	Bellevue Hospital (Turner)	Boston City Hospital (Ware)	Crile Veterans Hospital (Surington)	Hines Veterans Hospital (Shabart)
Cases	22	16	15	30
Amount of Smoking:				
None	1	0	1	0
Light	2	0	0	1[a]
Moderately heavy	2	3	1	0
Heavy	6	2	6	9
Excessive	8	5	7	6
Chain	3	6	0	14

[1] Minimal smoker. (For definition see previous classification of smokers.)

Figure 2. Control study I: amount of smoking in percentage among 100 male patients with cancer of the lungs (solid bars) and 186 male patients with other chest diseases (lined bars) having the same age and economic distribution.

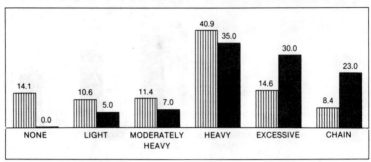

older (Table 5). This distribution readily shows that it would be of little value to study the smoking habits of the younger age groups for the purpose of control studies, since in them, for reasons still unknown to us, cancer of the lungs is a rare phenomenon.

Combined Data on Amount of Smoking. The data on the amount of smoking among 605 patients with cancer of the lungs and 780 male patients with other diseases reflect the results of the individual studies reported. It may also be noted that there is no essential difference in the amount of smoking between the general hospital population and patients with diseases of the chest who do not have cancer. The total results show that whereas there are 14.6 percent non-smokers among the male general population there are 1.3 percent nonsmokers among the

male patients with cancer of the lungs; and while there are 54.7 percent heavy to chain smokers and 19.1 percent excessive and chain smokers among the general hospital group there are 86.4 and 51.2 percent, respectively, among the patients with cancer. All these differences seem highly significant.

The results on the amount of smoking according to age groups (Table 6) show that in general the patients with cancer of the lungs in their forties and early fifties have smoked more heavily than the older patients with this disease. This observation does not seem to apply to the few patients in their thirties. The age group 70 to 79 has the greatest percentage of light and moderately heavy smokers.

The frequency of nonsmokers in the age groups shown for the patients without cancer is significantly different from that among patients

Table 4. Study III: Amount of smoking among male patients with cancer of the lung in relation to area or hospital where cases were observed (Wynder)[a].

Areas or hospitals	Smoking classification, %						Average Age
	V	IV	III	II	I	0	
Barnes (76)	18.4	31.5	43.4	5.3	0.0	1.3	54.8
Los Angeles (50)	12.0	32.0	12.0	12.0	0.0	4.0	59.5
San Francisco (50)	20.0	28.0	36.0	14.0	2.0	0.0	54.9
Mountain states (50)	14.0	26.0	36.0	18.0	4.0[b]	2.0	60.1
St. Louis (25)	20.0	36.0	32.0	12.0	0.0	0.0	58.2
Eastern and northern states (50)	16.3	23.6	40.0	20.0	0.0	0.0	56.1
New York City (66)	20.0	40.0	32.3	7.7	0.0	0.0	55.8
Memorial Hospital (55)	23.6	27.3	29.1	10.9	5.5[b]	3.6	57.6
Total (422)	18.2	30.8	36.7	11.4	1.4	1.4	56.7

[a] This Table does not include any cases represented in control studies I and II.
[b] Includes one minimal smoker.

Table 5. Age distribution in 605 cases of cancer of the lung in men.

Age groups	Percentage of cases
30-39	2.3
40-49	17.4
50-59	42.6
60-69	30.9
70-79	6.8

with cancer in the same age groups. However, in the 30 to 39 age group the smoking habits of the patient with cancer are difficult to evaluate since too few patients of this age have been seen.

In comparing the amount of smoking among the various age groups, one must also consider the type of tobacco used, which has undergone a marked shift particularly when the youngest and oldest age groups are considered.

Statistical Analysis of Data. The statistical analysis of these data has been carried out by

Dr. Paul R. Rider, professor of mathematics at Washington University, and H. David Hartstein, M.A., instructor of statistics at Washington University.

On the assumption that smoking has no effect on the induction of cancer of the lungs, the probability (p) of a deviation from expectation as great or greater than that observed is as follows:

Control Study I: Class 0, p is 0.0002; class 0 plus class I, p is 0.0002; classes 3 to 5 inclusive, p is 0.0226, class 4 plus class 5, p is 0.0002; class 4, p is 0.0046, and class 5, p is 0.0016.

Combined Results: The values for the combined results of 605 patients with cancer of the lung as compared with 780 men in the general hospital population are as follows: class 0, class 0 plus class 1, classes 3 to 5 inclusive, class 4 plus class 5. Class 4 and class 5 have p values which are in all cases less than 0.0001.

Their conclusion is as follows: "On the basis of the statistical data for both the control study I and the combined results, when the non-

Figure 3. Control study II: percentages for amount of smoking in 83 cases of cancer of the lungs collected independently by Dr. E. J. Shabart (Chicago), Dr. C. T. Surington (Cleveland), Dr. H. G. Turner (New York), and Dr. G. W. Ware (Boston).

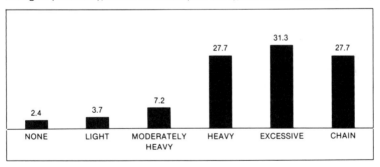

Table 6. Percentage distribution of amount of smoking in respect to age groups among 780 men in the general hospital population and 605 men with cancer of the lungs.[a]

	Age Groups									
	30-39		40-49		50-59		60-69		70-79	
No. of cases	(146)	(14)	(164)	(105)	(210)	(258)	(160)	(187)	(100)	(41)
				Amount of smoking,						
class: 0	13.6	7.1	9.7	0.0	14.8	1.6	14.3	1.1	25.0	2.4
1	5.5	7.1	9.7	1.9	7.1	1.6	18.7	1.1	13.0	12.2
2	17.1	14.3	18.9	3.8	17.6	7.4	20.6	13.6	21.0	24.4
3	41.0	42.9	37.1	29.5	43.3	36.0	28.7	38.0	16.0	29.3
4	14.3	28.6	14.0	28.6	10.5	34.1	10.6	30.5	15.0	17.1
5	8.2	0.0	10.3	36.2	6.7	19.4	6.8	15.5	10.0	14.6

[a] The percentages for the general male hospital population are given in the left-hand columns.

smokers and the total of the high smoking classes of patients with lung cancer are compared with patients who have other diseases, we can reject the null hypothesis that smoking has no effect on the induction of cancer of the lungs. If smoking does not have anything to do with the induction of cancer of the lungs, then the observed deviation could occur only with the probability (p) as shown above."

Miscellaneous Data. Nearly all (98.7 percent) the cigarette smokers of the cancer group, but fewer pipe (62.5 percent) and cigar (18 percent) smokers, stated that they inhaled consciously. Seventy-eight and a half percent of cancer patients interviewed stated that they usually began to smoke before breakfast.

Type of Tobacco: Among the general hospital population pipes and cigars were smoked most prominently in the older age groups. For example, only 4.3 percent of the smokers in the age group 30 to 39 used chiefly pipes or cigars, 11 percent in the age group 40 to 49, 12.9 percent in the age group 50 to 59, 30 percent in the age group 60 to 69, and 38 percent in the age group 70 to 79. Only those patients were tabulated as either pipe or cigar smokers who smoked a given type of tobacco predominantly over the last twenty years of their smoking period. Among the age-adjusted general hospital population we find 12.4 percent pipe smokers and 7.8 percent cigar smokers and among the patients with cancer 4.0 percent and 3.5 percent respectively (Figure 4).

The average age of the pipe smokers with cancer of the lung was 60.5, with a range of 52 to 78, and the average age of the cigar smokers with cancer of the lung was 63.1, the range being from 53 to 76. The average number of pipes smoked by the cancer patients was 15.6 and the average number of cigars 6.8 per day for the last twenty years of their smoking history. This amount of smoking is decidedly higher than that found among the general cigar and pipe smokers.

Duration of Smoking: The duration of smoking in years dates to the first time the patient began smoking habitually to any degree. Of 605 patients with cancer in our series, 96.1 percent had smoked for twenty years or more, 85.4 percent for thirty years or more, 68.2 percent for thirty-five years or more, and 50.2 percent for forty years or more. One patient with epider-

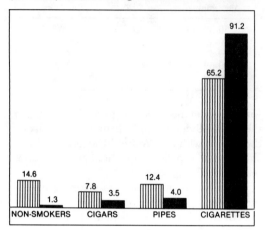

Figure 4. Smoking habits and type of tobacco smoked (in percentages) in 605 cases of cancer of the lungs (solid bars) and 780 men in the general hospital population (lined bars) with a similar age and economic distribution.

moid cancer began to smoke at 45 (20 cigarettes a day), and clinical symptoms of cancer of the lungs developed at 50 (class I smoker). He had no other exposure to irritants. Only three of the patients with bronchiogenic cancer began to smoke after the age of 25 (Figure 5).

Adenocarcinoma in Men: Among 39 men[11] with adenocarcinoma there were four nonsmokers (10.3 percent), a percentage higher than that found for the other types of bronchiogenic carcinoma. There were seven chain smokers (18 percent), significantly more than in the general male hospital population. Ten and three-tenths percent were excessive, 38.5 percent heavy, 15.4 percent moderately heavy, and 7.7 percent light smokers. Among the latter there were two minimal smokers.

Data on Women:[12] Among 13 women with adenocarcinoma and two designated as having terminal bronchiolar carcinoma there was not one heavy smoker. Thirteen were nonsmokers and two light smokers. Among 25 patients with epidermoid and undifferentiated carcinoma, however, there were 15 smokers of many years duration as well as 10 nonsmokers. Among those who smoked there were one light, four

[11] Includes three cases of Dr. C. T. Surington and one case of Dr. H. G. Turner.
[12] Includes four cases of Dr. H. G. Turner and three cases of Dr. G. W. Ware.

Figure 5. Percentages for duration of smoking in years, starting with the time when the patient first began to smoke habitually, in 605 cases of cancer of the lungs.

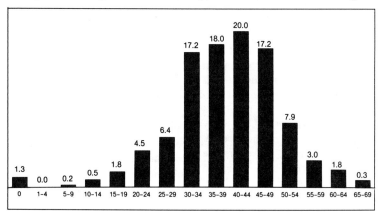

moderately heavy, six heavy, two excessive, and two chain smokers.

To determine the smoking habits among women in the general hospital population, 552 patients without cancer of the lung have been interviewed at this hospital. The data resulting from this study show that but few women in the cancer age have been heavy smokers for many years and that most of the heavy smokers are young women. On the basis of our arbitrary smoking classification, we found 79.6 percent of the women to be nonsmokers while 11.3 percent were moderately heavy to chain smokers,

and only 1.2 percent of the controls in the cancer age[13] were excessive or chain smokers for at least twenty years (Figure 6).

COMMENT

Universal Increase. If one feels that the greatly increased incidence of cancer of the lungs is real and that this increase is most marked in men, one may theorize that the

---

[13] See Table 5.

Figure 6. Amount of smoking in percentage among 780 male patients (lined bars) and 552 female patients (solid bars) of the general hospital population with the same age and economic distribution as found among cases of cancer of the lungs.

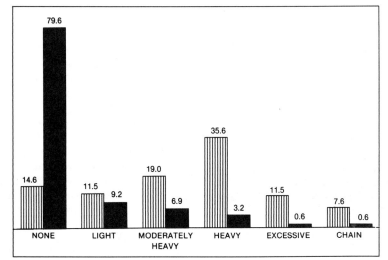

change has been due to an external factor, or group of factors, nationally prevalent but applicable to men more and over a longer period than to women.

Influence of Tobacco. Since in a small percentage of cases cancer of the lungs occurs in nonsmokers and minimal smokers and since it obviously does not develop in every person who has been a heavy smoker for a long time, it is apparent that smoking cannot be the only etiologic factor in the induction of the disease. From the evidence presented, however, the temptation is strong to incriminate excessive smoking, and in particular cigarette smoking, over a long period as at least one important factor in the striking increase of bronchiogenic carcinoma for the following reasons: (1) it is rare to find a case of epidermoid or undifferentiated carcinoma in a male patient who has not been at least a moderately heavy smoker for many years; (2) the use of cigarettes is much greater among patients with cancer of the lungs than among other patients of the same age and economic groups; (3) the sex distribution of cancer of the lungs roughly corresponds to the ratio of long-term smoking habits of the two sexes (see section on "Duration of Smoking"); (4) the enormous increase in the sale of cigarettes in this country approximately parallels the increase of bronchiogenic carcinoma.[14]

Amount of Smoking. The data have clearly shown that the average patient with cancer of the lungs smokes much more heavily than the average patient of the same age and economic group with some other disease. This contrast becomes even greater if our observation of Mormons is considered, who as a group smoke far less than the general hospital population; Mormons with cancer of the lung were, with one exception, considerable smokers.

The fact that patients with bronchiogenic cancer in their forties and fifties had smoked more heavily than those in whom the cancer developed at a later age may indicate that the greater the irritation the sooner will cancer develop in a susceptible person. Such an observation obviously does not apply to the individual case but rather to the age groups taken collect-

ively. Too few patients below the age of 40 have been seen in order to evaluate this age group.

In general it appears that the less a person smokes the less are the chances of cancer of the lung developing and, conversely, the more heavily a person smokes the greater are his chances of becoming affected with this disease.

Type of Tobacco. The majority of patients with cancer of the lungs are cigarette smokers rather than pipe or cigar smokers, the ratio being over and above that found in the general population. This fact may be due to one of the following reasons:

1. Cigarette smoke is more frequently inhaled than is that of either pipes or cigars. Obviously the lungs of an inhaler are exposed to a greater concentration of smoke than those of a person who does not consciously inhale.

2. Because of the greater physical and economic convenience, more persons are heavy smokers of cigarettes than of either pipes or cigars. Among the latter one finds more minimal and light smokers than among the former.

3. Certain irritative substances may be present in cigarettes in greater amounts than in pipes or cigars. The role of paper, the use of insecticides during the growth of the tobacco and other ingredients warrant further research in this regard.

Duration of Smoking. One of the chief reasons many investigators have thought that tobacco has no effect on the development of cancer of the lungs has been their belief that women today smoke as much as men and that if tobacco plays a role the sex ratio of the disease should be about equal. The data presented demonstrate that it makes little difference how many women smoke today or have smoked for the past ten years, since results have shown that over 96 percent of patients with cancer of the lungs have smoked for more than twenty years and that over 80 percent have smoked for more than thirty years.

It is, of course, difficult to tell whether the important point in this regard is the fact that these persons have smoked for many years or that they have been heavy smokers for a brief period, because we have noted that also among the general male hospital population nearly all smokers have been smoking since their youth. For this reason it is difficult to evaluate the one

[14] It is taken for granted, of course, that by itself such parallelism would mean little since similar curves could be drawn for many other commodities.

case in our study in which the patient smoked only from his forty-fifth to his fiftieth year, at which time clinical signs of cancer developed. If one may judge from control data on women, it would appear that a long duration of smoking is at least one important factor in the induction of cancer of the lungs. The relatively low incidence of the condition in women might be explained by the fact that few women in the cancer age have smoked for an extensive period.

On the basis of a twenty-year period of smoking, it may be of interest to note that, while only 1.2 percent of the women were excessive or chain smokers, by contrast 19.1 percent of the male controls were in those smoking groups, a ratio which points in the same direction as the sex ratio of lung cancer.

Lag Period. If smoking is to be regarded as an important etiologic factor in the development of cancer of the lungs, apparently a time lag exists for this disease as well as for carcinoma of the bladder, known to occur years after cessation of exposure to aniline. We have now seen three cases in which clinical signs of cancer of the lung appeared ten years or more after the patient stopped smoking. The three patients had smoked for thirty years or more, and none gave a history of occupational or other irritative exposures. Two of them had stopped smoking because of a bothersome chronic cough and one because of concomitant heart disease. In one of the patients, a 67-year-old warehouse clerk, clinical symptoms of cancer developed thirteen years after the cessation of smoking. The phenomenon of the lag period is, of course, well known in cancer research.

Adenocarcinoma in Men. Since the great increase in cancer of the lungs has mostly involved the epidermoid and undifferentiated carcinomas, it would appear that the exogenous factors possibly affecting these types of cancer play a lesser role, if any, in the induction of adenocarcinomas of the lung in men. As yet we have not seen a sufficient number of cases of this type of cancer to warrant definitive conclusions. It appears, however, that on the basis of present data one is more likely to find nonsmokers or minimal smokers with this type of cancer than with the other types. At the same time, however, the percentage of chain smokers among men with adenocarcinomas of the lung

is greater than among the general hospital population. It seems, therefore, that tobacco smoke has also some influence on the induction of adenocarcinoma in men, even though, as judged from the incidence, the influence on this type is much less marked than on the other types of bronchiogenic carcinoma.

Cancer of the Lungs in Women. Many observers have commented on the fact that bronchiogenic carcinoma, while on the increase among men and women, is increasing more rapidly among men. In 100 consecutive cases collected by Lindskog (*19*) in 1938 to 1943 the ratio was 4.5 to 1, and in another series collected in 1947 and 1948 the ratio had reached 24 to 1 (*20*). At Barnes Hospital the ratio in our last 150 cases has been 18.5 to 1. This shift in ratio has been noted in varying proportions throughout the country. Such a radical change warrants a careful analysis.

The insufficient number of cases of cancer of the lungs in women in our survey does not allow definite conclusions at this time. So far, however, smoking seems to have had no apparent effect on the incidence of adenocarcinoma in women. It is of great interest that we have observed 10 cases of epidermoid and undifferentiated carcinoma of the lungs of women who were nonsmokers with no history of occupational or other irritative exposure. This percentage of nonsmokers in women with cancer of the lung is much higher than that found among men. Proper explanations for this finding remain to be advanced. At the same time it appears strongly suggestive that heavy smoking plays a significant role in the induction of epidermoid and undifferentiated carcinoma of the lungs in women, since the percentage of heavy smokers is considerably higher in the cancer group than in the general hospital control group.

CONCLUSION AND SUMMARY

1. Excessive and prolonged use of tobacco, especially cigarettes, seems to be an important factor in the induction of bronchiogenic carcinoma.

2. Among 605 men with bronchiogenic carcinoma, other than adenocarcinoma, 96.5 percent were moderately heavy to chain smokers for many years, compared with 73.7 percent among the general male hospital population

without cancer. Among the cancer group 51.2 percent were excessive or chain smokers compared to 19.1 percent in the general hospital group without cancer.

3. The occurrence of carcinoma of the lung in a male nonsmoker or minimal smoker is a rare phenomenon (2.0 percent).

4. Tobacco seems at this time to play a similar but somewhat less evident role in the induction of epidermoid and undifferentiated carcinoma in women. Among this group a greater percentage of nonsmokers will be found than among the men, with 10 of 25 being nonsmokers.

5. Ninety-six and one-tenth percent of patients with cancer of the lungs who had a history of smoking had smoked for over twenty years. Few women have smoked for such a length of time, and this is believed to be one of the reasons for the greater incidence of the disease among men today.

6. There may be a lag period of ten years or more between the cessation of smoking tobacco and the occurrence of clinical symptoms of cancer.

7. Ninety-four and one-tenth percent of male patients with cancer of the lungs were found to be cigarette smokers, 4.0 percent pipe smokers, and 3.5 percent cigar smokers. This prevalence of cigarette smoking is greater than among the general hospital population of the same age group. The greater practice of inhalation among cigarette smokers is believed to be a factor in the increased incidence of the disease.

8. The influence of tobacco on the development of adenocarcinoma seems much less than on the other types of bronchiogenic carcinoma.

9. Three independent studies have resulted in data so uniform that one may deduce the same conclusions from each of them.

ADDENDUM

Since the data presented in this paper were tabulated, 45 additional interviews of male patients with epidermoid or undifferentiated cancer of the lung have been obtained. Eight of these patients have been interviewed by Dr. J. L. Ehrenhaft from the University of Iowa Hospital, nine were given our questionnaire by Lt. Col. J. M. Salyer from Fitzsimmons General Hospital, and seven were reported on by Dr. E. J. Shabart from the Veterans Administration Hospital, Hines, Illinois. Among these 24 cases

there were no nonsmokers or light smokers, seven heavy smokers, 13 excessive smokers, and four chain smokers. Twenty-one additional patients have been interviewed by Miss Croninger on the Barnes Hospital Chest Service. Among these there were one nonsmoker (a 72 year old blacksmith), 10 heavy smokers, six excessive smokers, and four chain smokers. These 45 cases, which include reports independently made at two additional centers (University of Iowa and Fitzsimmons General Hospital), show the same trend noted in the larger series.

References

(1) Ochsner, A., and M. DeBakey. Surgical considerations of primary carcinoma of the lung, *Surgery* 8:992-1023, 1940.

(2) Wheeler, R. Personal communication to the authors.

(3) Avery, E. E. Personal communication to the authors.

(4) Kennaway, N. M., and E. L. Kennaway. A study of the incidence of cancer of the lung and larynx. *J Hyg* 36:236-267, 1936.

(5) Kennaway, E. L., and N. M. Kennaway, A further study of the incidence of cancer of the lung and larynx. *Brit J Cancer* 1:260-298, 1947.

(6) Statistics on Cancer, New York, American Cancer Society, Statistical Research Division, 1949, p. 19.

(7) Adler, I. *Primary Malignant Growths of the Lungs, and Bronchi*. New York, Longmans, Green and Co., 1912.

(8) Tylecote, F. E. Cancer of the lung. *Lancet* 2:256-257, 1927.

(9) Hoffman, F. L. Cancer of the lung. *Am Rev Tuberc* 19:392-406, 1929.

(10) McNally, W. D. The tar in cigarette smoke and its possible effects. *Am J Cancer* 16:1502-1514, 1932.

(11) Lickint, F. Der Bronchialkrebs der Raucher. *München Med Wochenschr* 82:1232-1234, 1935.

(12) Arkin, A. and D. H. Wagner: Primary carcinoma of the lung. *JAMA* 106:587-591, 1936.

(13) Roffo, A. H. Der Tabak als Krebserzeugende Agens. *Deutsche Med Wochenschr* 63:1267-1271, 1937.

(14) Maier, H. C. Personal communication to the authors.

(15) Müller, F. H. Tabakmissbrauch und Lungencarczinom. *Ztschr f Krebsforsch* 49:57-85, 1939.

(16) Ochsner, A. and M. DeBakey. Carcinoma of the lung. *Arch Surg* 42:209-258, 1941.

(17) Schrek, R., C. H. Baker, G. P. Ballard, and S. Dolgoff. Tobacco smoking as an etiological factor in disease. *J Cancer, Cancer Research* 10:49-58, 1950.

(18) Wynder, E. L. and E. A. Graham. Tobacco and Bronchiogenic Carcinoma: Preliminary report to the National Cancer Conference, Memphis, February 1949.

(19) Lindskog, G. F. Bronchiogenic carcinoma. *Ann Surg* 124:667-674, 1946.

(20) Lindskog, G. F. and W. D. Bloomer. Bronchiogenic carcinoma. *Cancer* 1:234-237, 1948.

CANCER AND TOBACCO SMOKING:
A PRELIMINARY REPORT[1]

Morton L. Levin,[2] Hyman Goldstein,[2] and Paul R. Gerhardt[2]

The published literature on use of tobacco and its possible association with human cancer fails to show clear-cut consistent observations. Reviews of the literature for the past twenty years reveals that it is often conflicting and that it consists for the most part of studies which are inconclusive because of lack of adequate samples, lack of random selection, lack of proper controls or failure to age-standardize the data. Potter and Tully (1) have reported a higher proportion of smokers in patients with cancer of the "buccal cavity" and "respiratory tract" among males "over the age of 40" who were seen at Massachusetts cancer clinics.

Since 1938 a history of tobacco usage has been obtained routinely from all patients admitted to the Roswell Park Memorial Institute, Buffalo. These histories are part of the regular clinical history and are taken before the final diagnosis has been established. This procedure is considered especially important from the standpoint of excluding bias. Approximately half the patients admitted to the institute are subsequently found not to have cancer. Special attention with respect to the history of smoking has not been paid to any single group of conditions, so that these records may be presumed to be free from bias which might result from preconceived ideas as to relation between smoking and a particular form of cancer.

The histories record the date smoking began, duration, type of smoking, and amount per day. The reliability of the quantitative aspects of smoking obtained by a history is of course highly variable. It is presumed, however, that such errors are not selective with respect to

presence or absence of cancer, especially since only patients suspected by their physicians of having cancer are admitted to the Institute.

This report is based on a study of 1045 male cancer patients and 605 male noncancer patients. The cancer sites selected were lung, lip, pharynx, esophagus, colon, rectum, and a scattered number of other sites. The noncancer patients were those with symptoms referable to the same sites but which proved not to be due to cancer. Only the users of cigarettes, pipes, and cigars are considered here, since the number of patients who used snuff or chewing tobacco was negligible. Smokers engaging in more than one form of smoking entered into separate analysis for each such form, so that the sum of smokers is less than the sum of smokers of each type. The factor studied was whether or not the patient had ever smoked, regardless of whether he was a smoker at the time of admission.

Over 80 percent of all patients were smokers (Table 1). Prevalence of smokers, regardless of type, did not vary strikingly with age past the age of 25 (see Figure 1). Prevalence of cigarette smokers, however, decreased with age, and that of pipe smokers and cigar smokers increased with age. Obviously, comparison of groups with differing age composition would show different proportions of cigarette, pipe, and cigar smokers because of this factor alone. Accordingly, comparisons should be made of age-specific prevalence rates or of prevalence rates standardized for age by applying the age-specific rates to a standard population. The latter device was adopted, using the entire series of 1650 patients as the standard population.

The significant observations are summarized in Tables 1, 2, 3, 4, and 5. There were more smokers among cancer patients than noncancer patients, because of an excess of cigarette and pipe smokers among the former (Table 1). This excess was due entirely to the increased percentage of cigarette smokers among patients with cancer of the lung and the increased percentage of pipe smokers among patients with

Source: *Journal of the American Medical Association* 143(4):336-338, 1950.
[1] With technical assistance of Elizabeth Brezee and David Robbins. Dr. Louis C. Kress, Dr. Joseph G. Hoffman, and Miss Olive C. Ralston, of the staff of the Roswell Park Memorial Institute, assisted by making available the records of the institute and by making suggestions as to the planning of the study.
[2] From the Bureau of Cancer Control, Division of Medical Services, New York State Department of Health.

Table 1. Prevalence of smokers among male cancer and noncancer patients by type of smoking.

	No. of cases	Percentage of smokers[a]			
		All types	Cigarettes	Pipes	Cigars
Cancer	1045	84.8	56.0	30.3	22.4
Noncancer	605	77.8	46.0	24.3	20.8
P[b]		0.01	0.01	0.01	0.47

[a] Age standardized.
[b] P denotes probability here and in Tables 2 and 3.

cancer of the lip (Table 2). These differences, in turn, were confined to those who had smoked cigarettes or pipes for twenty-five years or longer (Table 3).

It should be noted that the prevalence rates of smokers in columns 2 and 4 of Table 3 are age-standardized rates, obtained by applying the age-specific rates for each subgroup to the age distribution of the total group of 1650 male patients. Since length of smoking is related to age, this statistical procedure was necessary to exclude the possibility that the greater percentage of "25 years or more" smokers in the cancer groups was due solely to the greater proportion of older persons in these groups. The failure to find comparable differences in smokers of less than twenty-five years' duration may be due to the relatively small percentage of such smokers which may be expected in an older population. Further study of large numbers of younger patients may alter this observation.

In Tables 4 and 5 the data are presented to show the relative prevalence of lung and lip cancer among nonsmokers and among cigarette, pipe, and cigar smokers in the patient population. There were more than twice as many cases of lung cancer among cigarette smokers as among any other group. Pipe smokers and cigar smokers had no more cancer of the lung than did nonsmokers. Lip cancer was significantly increased among pipe smokers but not among cigarette smokers. Cases of lip cancer were increased also among cigar smokers.

In Table 4, persons who smoked more than one type of tobacco are counted in each category. In Table 5, only those who smoked but one type of tobacco are considered. The observations in Table 4 with respect to lung cancer are the same as in Table 5, i.e., only cigarette smokers show any significant increase of lung cancer over nonsmokers. For lip cancer, only

Figure 1. Percentage of patients who had ever smoked by type of smoking.

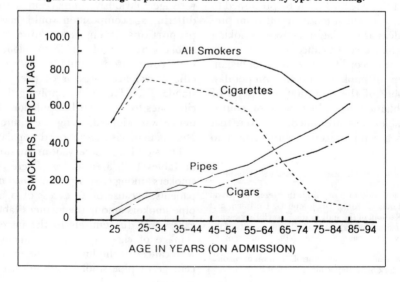

Table 2. Prevalence of smokers among male patients by type of smoking and diagnostic group.

Diagnosis	No. of cases	Percentage of smokers[a]							
		Any type (1)		Cigarettes (2)		Pipes (3)		Cigars (4)	
		%	P	%	P	%	P	%	P
Lung cancer compared with:	236	84.7	—	66.1	—	13.5	—	11.2	—
Other cancer (except lip)	666	82.9	0.53	48.0	0.01	25.8	0.01	20.3	0.01
Lung nontumors	124	81.1	0.39	53.1	0.02	25.5	0.09	13.4	0.64
Other noncancer	481	78.3	0.03	44.1	0.01	25.3	0.01	22.7	0.01
Lip cancer compared with:	143	84.5	—	45.3	—	48.1	—	26.5	—
Other cancer (except lung)	666	82.9	0.58	48.0	0.48	25.8	0.01	20.3	0.11
Lip nontumors	51	74.0	0.09	43.0	0.78	30.7	0.02	34.9	0.22
Other noncancer	554	78.1	0.23	46.4	0.81	23.8	0.01	19.6	0.08

[a] Age standardized.

Table 3. Prevalence[a] of cigarette and pipe smokers among male patients by duration of smoking and diagnostic group.

Diagnosis	No. of cases	Duration of smoking					
		Under 25 yr.			25 yr. and over		
		(1) No.	(2) %[a]	P	(3) No.	(4) %[a]	P
				Cigarette smokers			
Lung cancer compared with:	236	25	11.7	—	148	54.1	—
Other cancer (except lung and lip)	666	74	13.0	0.62	233	34.9	0.01
Lung nontumors	124	19	16.3	0.23	54	36.9	0.01
Other noncancer	481	92	14.3	0.34	128	29.8	0.01
				Pipe smokers			
Lip cancer compared with:	143	8	7.8	—	60	35.7	—
Other cancer (except lung and lip)	666	26	3.9	0.02	162	22.9	0.01
Lip nontumors	51	5	10.6	0.35	11	21.5	0.04
Other noncancer	554	35	5.8	0.24	87	17.9	0.01

[a] Age standardized.

Table 4. Comparison of the proportion[a] of cases of lung and lip cancer among male nonsmokers and smokers of 25 years' duration or more at Roswell Park Memorial Institute, 1938-1948.

	No. of persons	Lung Cancer			Lip Cancer		
		Cases	Rate[a]	P[b]	Cases	Rate[a]	P[b]
Nonsmokers compared with:	293	23	8.6	—	20	6.9	—
Cigarette smokers[c]	600	148	20.7	0.01	37	5.9	0.55
Pipe smokers[c]	353	33	8.6	1.00	60	13.4	0.01
Cigar smokers[c]	263	22	8.5	0.97	39	12.5	0.03

[a] Standardized for age against age distribution of total males.
[b] Probability of the observed difference between smokers and non-smokers occurring by chance alone.
[c] Multiple smokers, e.g., persons smoking more than one type of tobacco plus those smoking only one type.

Table 5. Comparison of the proportion[a] of cases of lung and lip cancer among male nonsmokers and smokers of 25 years' duration or more at Roswell Park Memorial Institute, 1938-1948.

	No. of persons	Lung cancer			Lip cancer		
		Cases	Rate[a]	P[b]	Cases	Rate[a]	P[b]
Nonsmokers compared with:	293	23	8.6	—	20	6.9	—
All smokers[c]	761	148	17.1	0.01	73	8.9	0.29
Cigarette smokers[c]	479	115	20.9	0.01	22	5.1	0.29
Pipe smokers[c]	166	19	10.6	0.48	34	15.7	0.01
Cigar smokers[c]	116	14	12.8	0.18	17	11.6	0.13

[a] Standardized for age against age distribution of total males.
[b] Probability of the observed difference between smokers and non-smokers occurring by chance alone.
[c] Persons smoking only one type of tobacco.

pipe smokers show a significant increase over nonsmokers.

No other site of cancer that was included in this study was found to be associated with any particular type of smoking. However, not all sites of cancer were studied. It is planned to continue analysis of the records of the Roswell Park Memorial Institute to provide data regarding all types of malignant tumors.

These data indicate that, in a hospital population, cancer of the lung occurs more than twice as frequently among those who have smoked cigarettes for twenty-five years than among other smokers or nonsmokers of comparable age. Pipe smokers apparently experience an almost equal increase in the incidence of lip cancer, compared with other smokers or nonsmokers. It is somewhat surprising to find that the type of smoking, i.e., cigarettes for lung cancer, pipe for lip cancer, is the associated factor, rather than the actual use of tobacco.

The data suggest, although they do not establish, a causal relation between cigarette and pipe smoking and cancer of the lung and lip, respectively. The statistical association may, of course, be due to some other unidentified common

factor between these types of smoking and lung and lip cancer. Cancer is now generally considered a disease attributable to multiple causative factors. Among these are "irritants." The generalization has been advanced (2,3) that, although not all irritants are carcinogenic, all carcinogens are irritants, that is, capable of inducing chronic reparative hyperplasia. Berenblum (3) has shown also that an irritant (croton resin; basic tar fraction) which is noncarcinogenic alone may nevertheless increase the percentage of tumors produced when its action is combined with that of a carcinogen. Thus, some experimental basis exists for explaining the apparent effect of cigarette and pipe smoking, although the true nature of the association with lung and lip cancer remains to be determined.

References

(1) Potter, E.A. and M.R. Tully. The statistical approach to the cancer problem in Massachusetts. *Am J Public Health* 35:485-490, 1945.

(2) Berenblum, I. Irritation and carcinogenesis. *Arch Pathol* 38:233-44, 1944.

(3) Pullinger, B.D. First effect on mouse skin of some polycyclic hydrocarbons. *J Pathol Bacteriol* 50:463-471, 1940.

SMOKING AND CARCINOMA OF THE LUNG: PRELIMINARY REPORT

Richard Doll[1] and A. Bradford Hill[2]

In England and Wales the phenomenal increase in the number of deaths attributed to cancer of the lung provides one of the most striking changes in the pattern of mortality recorded by the Registrar-General. For example, in the quarter of a century between 1922 and 1947 the annual number of deaths recorded increased from 612 to 9287, or roughly fifteenfold. This remarkable increase is, of course, out of all proportion to the increase of population—both in total and, particularly, in its older age groups. Stocks (1), using standardized death rates to allow for these population changes, shows the following trend: rate per 100 000 in 1901-1920, males 1.1, females 0.7; rate per 100 000 in 1936-1939, males 10.6, females 2.5. The rise seems to have been particularly rapid since the end of the First World War: between 1921-1930 and 1940-1944 the death rate of men at ages 45 and over increased sixfold and of women of the same ages approximately threefold. This increase is still continuing. It has occurred, too, in Switzerland, Denmark, the U.S.A., Canada, and Australia, and has been reported from Turkey and Japan.

Many writers have studied these changes, considering whether they denote a real increase in the incidence of the disease or are due merely to improved standards of diagnosis. Some believe that the latter factor can be regarded as wholly, or at least mainly, responsible—for example, Willis (2), Clemmesen and Busk (3), and Steiner (4). On the other hand, Kennaway and Kennaway (5) and Stocks (1) have given good reasons for believing that the rise is at least partly real. The latter, for instance, has pointed out that "the increase of certified respiratory cancer mortality during the past 20 years has been as rapid in country districts as in the cities with the best diagnostic facilities, a fact which does not support the view that such increase merely reflects improved diagnosis of cases previously certified as bronchitis or other respiratory affections." He also draws attention to differences in mortality between some of the large cities of England and Wales, differences which it is difficult to explain in terms of diagnostic standards.

The large and continued increase in the recorded deaths even within the last five years, both in the national figures and in those from teaching hospitals, also makes it hard to believe that improved diagnosis is entirely responsible. In short, there is sufficient reason to reject that factor as the whole explanation, although no one would deny that it may well have been contributory. As a corollary, it is right and proper to seek for other causes.

POSSIBLE CAUSES OF THE INCREASE

Two main causes have from time to time been put forward: (1) a general atmospheric pollution from the exhaust fumes of cars, from the surface dust of tarred roads, and from gasworks, industrial plants, and coal fires; and (2) the smoking of tobacco. Some characteristics of the former have certainly become more prevalent in the last 50 years, and there is also no doubt that the smoking of cigarettes has greatly increased. Such associated changes in time can, however, be no more than suggestive, and until recently there has been singularly little more direct evidence. That evidence, based upon clinical experience and records, relates mainly to the use of tobacco. For instance, in Germany, Müller (6) found that only 3 out of 86 male patients with cancer of the lung were nonsmokers, while 56 were heavy smokers, and, in contrast, among 86 "healthy men of the same age groups" there were 14 nonsmokers and only 31 heavy smokers. Similarly, in America, Schrek and his co-workers (7) reported that 14.6 per-

Source: *British Medical Journal*, September 30, 1950, pp. 739-748.
[1] Member of the Statistical Research Unit of the Medical Research Council.
[2] Professor of Medical Statistics. London School of Hygiene and Tropical Medicine; Honorary Director of the Statistical Research Unit of the Medical Research Council.

cent of 82 male patients with cancer of the lung were non-smokers, against 23.9 percent of 522 male patients admitted with cancer of sites other than the upper respiratory and digestive tracts. In this country, Thelwall Jones (8) found 8 non-smokers in 82 patients with proved carcinoma of the lung, compared with 11 in a corresponding group of patients with diseases other than cancer; this difference is slight, but it is more striking that there were 28 heavy smokers in the cancer group, against 14 in the comparative group.

Clearly, none of these small-scale inquiries can be accepted as conclusive, but they all point in the same direction. Their evidence has now been borne out by the results of a large-scale inquiry undertaken in the U.S.A. by Wynder and Graham (9).

Wynder and Graham found that of 605 men with epidermoid, undifferentiated, or histologically unclassified types of bronchial carcinoma only 1.3 percent were "non-smokers"— that is, had averaged less than one cigarette a day for the last 20 years—whereas 51.2 percent of them had smoked more than 20 cigarettes a day over the same period. In contrast, they estimated from the experience of 882 other male patients that 14.6 percent of general hospital patients of the same age composition as the bronchial carcinoma cases are "non-smokers" and only 19.1 percent smoke more than 20 cigarettes a day. They found a similar contrast between the 25 women with epidermoid and undifferentiated bronchial carcinoma and the other female patients, but no such association with smoking could be found in the small group of patients with adenocarcinoma.

PRESENT INVESTIGATION

The present investigation was planned in 1947, to be carried out on a sufficiently large scale to determine whether patients with carcinoma of the lung differed materially from other persons in respect of their smoking habits or in some other way which might be related to the atmospheric pollution theory. Patients with carcinoma of the stomach, colon, or rectum were also incorporated in the inquiry, as one of the contrasting groups, and special attention was therefore given at the same time to factors which might bear upon the etiology of these forms of malignant disease. A separate report will be made upon these inquiries. The present study is confined to the question of smoking in relation to carcinoma of the lung.

The method of the investigation was as follows: Twenty London hospitals were asked to cooperate by notifying all patients admitted to them with carcinoma of the lung, stomach, colon, or rectum. For the most part these hospitals were initially confined to one region of London (the northwest), to allow ease of traveling, but others were subsequently added to increase the scope of the inquiry. A list of those taking part is given at the end of the paper. The method of notification varied; in some it was made by the admitting clerk on the basis of the admission diagnosis, in others by the house-physician when a reasonably confident clinical diagnosis had been made, and in yet others by the cancer registrar or the radiotherapy department. None of these methods is likely to have resulted in complete notification, but there is no reason to suppose that those who escaped notification were a selected group—that is, selected in such a way as to bias the inquiry—as the points of interest in the investigation were either not known or known only in broad outline by those responsible for notifying.

On receipt of the notification an almoner, engaged wholly on research, visited the hospital to interview the patient, using a set questionary. During the inquiry four almoners were employed and all the patients were interviewed by one or other of them. As well, however, as interviewing the notified patients with cancer of one of the four specified sites, the almoners were required to make similar inquiries of a group of "non-cancer control" patients. These patients were not notified, but for each lung-carcinoma patient visited at a hospital the almoners were instructed to interview a patient of the same sex, within the same five-year age group, and in the same hospital at or about the same time. (Where more than one suitable patient was available the choice fell upon the first one in the ward lists considered by the ward sister to be fit for interview.)

At two specialized hospitals (Brompton Hospital and Harefield Hospital) it was not always possible to secure a control patient by this method, and in such cases a control patient was taken from one of the two neighboring hospitals, the Royal Cancer and Mount Vernon Hospitals. Even with this relaxation of the rule control cases were deficient at the Brompton Hospital and the numbers had to be made up by using the records of patients who had been interviewed as cancer patients, either there or at the Royal Cancer Hospital, but in whom cancer was finally excluded. Because of these differences in technique the records obtained from these hospitals were analyzed separately. As, however, the results were in accordance with those found at the other hospitals, all the records are presented here as a single series.

In view of the method of notification used it could not be expected that the diagnosis then given would invariably be accurate. The diagnosis of each patient was checked, therefore, after discharge from or death in hospital, and this check was made in all but nine instances (0.4 percent of the total). In these few cases (three of carcinoma of the lung, two of carcinoma of the stomach, two of carcinoma of the rectum, and two non-cancer) no records of any sort could be traced, and they have had to be classified according to the information available at the time of their interview. As a general rule the hospital diagnosis on discharge was accepted as the final diagnosis, but occasionally later evidence became available—for example, by histological examination at necropsy—which contradicted that diagnosis. In these instances a change was made and the diagnosis based upon the best evidence.

THE DATA

Between April 1948, and October 1949, the notifications of cancer cases numbered 2370. It was not, however, possible to interview all these patients. To begin with, it had been decided beforehand that no one of 75 years of age or more should be included in the inquiry, since it was unlikely that reliable histories could be obtained from the very old. There were 150 such patients. In a further 80 cases the diagnosis was incorrect and had been changed before the almoner paid her visit. Deducting these two groups leaves 2140 patients who should have been interviewed. Of these, 408 could not be interviewed for the following reasons: already discharged 189, too ill 116, dead 67, too deaf 24, unable to speak English clearly 11, while in one case the almoner abandoned the interview as the patient's replies appeared wholly unrelia-

ble. No patient refused to be interviewed.

The proportion not seen is high, but there is no apparent reason why it should bias the results. It was in the main due to the time that inevitably elapsed between the date of notification and the date of the almoner's visit. The remaining 1732 patients, presumed at the interview to be suffering from carcinoma of the lung, stomach, or large bowel, and the 743 general medical and surgical patients originally interviewed as controls, constitute the subjects of the investigation. The numbers falling in each disease group—that is, after consulting the hospital discharge diagnoses—are shown in Table 1. The carcinoma cases are here divided into two groups: Group A consisting of cases in which the diagnoses were confirmed by necropsy, biopsy, or exploratory operation, and Group B of the remainder.

The 81 patients classified in Table 1 as having "other malignant diseases" were interviewed as cases of carcinoma of the lung, stomach, or large bowel, or as non-cancer controls. On the subsequent checking of the diagnosis either they were found to have primary carcinoma on some site other than one of those under special investigation or histological examination showed that the growth was not, in fact, carcinoma—for example, sarcoma, reticulo-endothelioma, etc. The 355 "other cases" either were interviewed as cases of carcinoma of the lung, stomach, or large bowel and were subsequently found not to be cases of malignant disease or, having been interviewed as non-cancer controls, they became redundant when the cases of carcinoma of the lung with which they were paired were found not to be carcinoma of the lung. The four "excluded" cases were excluded on grounds of doubt about their true category. Two were diagnosed at hospital as primary carcinoma of the lung, but there was reason to suppose that the growths might have been secondary to carcinoma of the breast and to carcinoma of the cervix uteri respectively; the other two showed evidence of primary carcinoma in two of the sites under special investigation— that is, lung and colon, and stomach and colon.

The 709 control patients with diseases other than cancer form a group which was, as previously stated, deliberately selected to be closely comparable in age and sex with the carcinoma of the lung patients. Comparisons between these two groups are shown in Table 2.

Table 1. Number of patients interviewed in each disease group. Subdivided according to certainty of diagnosis.

| | No. of cases | | |
| | Group A. Diagnosis confirmed at necropsy, etc. | Group B. Other criteria of diagnosis | |
Disease group			Total
Carcinoma of lung	489	220	709
Carcinoma of stomach	178	28	206
Carcinoma of colon and rectum	412	19	431
Other malignant diseases	—	—	81
Diseases other than cancer (controls)	—	—	709
Other cases	—	—	335
Excluded	—	—	4
All cases	—	—	2475

It will be seen that the lung-carcinoma patients and the control group of non-cancer patients are exactly comparable with regard to sex and age, but that there are some differences with regard to social class and place of residence. The difference in social class distribution is small and is no more than might easily be due to chance ($X^2 = 1.61$; n = 2; $0.30 < P < 0.50$). The difference in place of residence is, however, large ($X^2 = 31.49$; n = 5; P < 0.001), and Table 2 shows that a higher proportion of the lung patients were resident outside London at the time of their admission to hospital. This difference can be explained on the grounds that people with cancer came to London from other parts of the country for treatment at special centers. When a comparison is made between the 98 lung-carcinoma patients and the 98 controls who were seen at district hospitals in London— that is, those regional board hospitals which do not have special surgical thoracic or radiotherapeutic centers—the difference disappears. Of these 98 patients with carcinoma of the lung, 56 lived in the County of London, 42 in outer

Table 2. Comparison between lung-carcinoma patients and non-cancer patients selected as controls, with regard to sex, age, social class, and place of residence.

Age	No. of lung-carcinoma patients M	F	No. of noncancer control patients M	F	Social class (Registrar-General's categories, men only)	No. of lung-carcinoma patients	No. of non-cancer patients
25-	2	1	2	1	I and II	77	87
30-	6	0	6	0	III	388	396
35-	18	3	18	3	IV and V	184	166
40-	36	4	36	4			
45-	87	10	87	10	All classes	649	649
50-	130	11	130	11	*Place of residence*		
55-	145	9	145	9	County of London	330	377
60-	109	9	109	9	Outer London	203	231
65-	88	9	89[a]	9	Other county borough	23	16
70-74	28	4	27[a]	4	Urban district	95	54
					Rural district	43	27
					Abroad or in services	15	4
All ages	649	60	649	60	Total (M + F)	709	709

[a] One control patient was selected, in error, from the wrong age group.

London, and none elsewhere; of their non-cancer controls the corresponding numbers were 60, 38, and 0, clearly an insignificant difference.

It is evident, therefore, that the control group of patients with diseases other than cancer is strictly comparable with the group of lung-carcinoma patients in important respects but differs slightly with regard to the parts of England from which the patients were drawn. It is unlikely that this difference will invalidate comparisons, but it must be kept in mind; fortunately, it can be eliminated, if necessary, by confining comparisons to the smaller group of patients seen in the district hospitals.

ASSESSMENT OF SMOKING HABITS

The assessment of the relation between tobacco-smoking and disease is complicated by the fact that smoking habits change. A man who has been a light smoker for years may become a heavy smoker; a heavy smoker may cut down his consumption or give up smoking—and, indeed, may do so repeatedly. An acute respiratory disease may force the sufferer to stop smoking, or he may be advised to stop for one of many pathological conditions. In 1947 a further complication was introduced by the Chancellor of the Exchequer, the duty on tobacco being raised to such an extent that many people made large cuts in the amount of tobacco they smoked—often to restore them partially or completely in the succeeding months. Fortunately the interviewing of patients was not begun till a year after the last major change was made in the tobacco duty; in any case the effect was minimized by interviewing the control patients *pari passu* with the lung-carcinoma patients, so that the change in price is likely to have affected all groups similarly.

The difficulties of a varying consumption can be largely overcome if a more detailed smoking history is taken than is customary in the course of an ordinary medical examination—for example, one man who was described in the hospital notes as being a non-smoker admitted to the almoner that he had been a very heavy smoker until a few years previously. In this investigation, therefore, the patients were closely questioned and asked (*a*) if they had smoked at any period of their lives; (*b*) the ages at which they had started and stopped; (*c*) the amount

they were in the habit of smoking before the onset of the illness which had brought them into hospital; (*d*) the main changes in their smoking history and the maximum they had ever been in the habit of smoking; (*e*) the varying proportions smoked in pipes and cigarettes; and (*f*) whether or not they inhaled.

To record and subsequently to tabulate these details it was necessary to define what was meant by a smoker. Did the term, for example, include the woman who took one cigarette annually after her Christmas dinner, or the man of 50 who as a youth smoked a couple of cigarettes to see whether he liked it and decided he did not? If so, it is doubtful whether anyone at all could be described as a nonsmoker. A smoker was therefore defined in this inquiry as a person who had smoked as much as one cigarette a day for as long as one year, and any less consistent amount was ignored. The histories obtained were, of course, a function of the patient's memory and veracity. To assess their reliability 50 unselected control patients with diseases other than cancer were interviewed a second time six months or more after their initial interview. Table 3 shows the comparison between the two answers obtained to the question "How much did you smoke before the onset of your present illness?"

The answers to the other questions on smoking habits showed a variability comparable to that shown in Table 3. It may be concluded, therefore, that while the detailed smoking histories obtained by this investigation are not, as would be expected, strictly accurate, they are reliable enough to indicate general trends and to substantiate material differences between groups.

SMOKERS AND NONSMOKERS

The simplest comparison that can be made to show whether there is any association at all between smoking and carcinoma of the lung is that between the proportion of lung-carcinoma patients who have been smokers and the proportion of smokers in the comparable group of subjects without carcinoma of the lung. Such a comparison is shown in Table 4.

It will be seen that the vast majority of men have been smokers at some period of their lives, but also that the very small proportion of those with carcinoma of the lung who have been non-

Table 3. Amount of tobacco smoked daily before present illness as recorded at two interviews with the same patients at an interval of six months or more.

First interview; no. of persons smoking	Second interview, no. of persons smoking						
	0	1 cig. −	5 cigs. −	15 cigs. −	25 cigs. −	50 cigs. +	Total
0	8	1					9
1 cig. −		4	1				5
5 cigs. −		1	13	3			17
15 cigs. −			4	9	1		14
25 cigs. −				1	3	0	4
50 cigs. or more					1	0	1
Total	8	6	18	13	5	0	50

Table 4. Proportion of smokers and non-smokers in lung-carcinoma patients and in control patients with diseases other than cancer.

Disease group	No. of nonsmokers	No. of smokers	Probability test
Males:			
Lung-carcinoma patients (649)	2 (0.3%)	647	P (exact method) = (0.00000064
Control patients with diseases other than cancer (649)	27 (4.2%)	622	
Females:			
Lung-carcinoma patients (60)	19 (31.7%)	41	$X^2 = 5.76; n = 1$ $0.01 < P < 0.02$
Control patients with diseases other than cancer (60)	32 (53.3%)	28	

smokers (0.3 percent) is most significantly less than the corresponding proportion in the control group of other patients (4.2 percent). As was to be expected, smoking is shown to be a much less common habit among women; but here again the habit was significantly more frequent among those with carcinoma of the lung. Only 31.7 percent of the lung-carcinoma group were non-smokers, compared with 53.3 percent in the control group.

AMOUNT OF SMOKING

In the simple comparison of Table 4 all smokers have been classified together, irrespective of the amount they smoked. In Table 5 they have been subdivided according to the amount they smoked immediately before the onset of the illness which brought them into hospital. (If they had given up smoking before then, they

have been classified according to the amount smoked immediately prior to giving it up.) This classification is described subsequently as "the most recent amount smoked."

From Table 5 it will be seen that, apart from the general excess of smokers found (in Table 4) in lung-carcinoma patients, there is in this group a significantly higher proportion of heavier smokers and a correspondingly lower proportion of lighter smokers than in the comparative group of other patients. For instance, in the lung-carcinoma group 26.0 percent of the male patients fall in the two groups of highest consumption (25 cigarettes a day or more), while in the control group of other male patients only 13.5 percent are found there. The same trend is observable for women, but the numbers involved are small and the difference here between the carcinoma group and their control patients is not quite technically significant. If,

Table 5. Most recent amount of tobacco[a] consumed regularly by smokers before the onset of present illness: lung-carcinoma patients and control patients with diseases other than cancer.

Disease group	No. smoking daily					Probability test
	1 cig. – [a]	5 cigs. –	15 cigs. –	25 cigs. –	50 cigs. +	
Males:						
Lung-carcinoma patients (647)	33 (5.1%)	250 (38.6%)	196 (30.3%)	136 (21.0%)	32 (5.0%)	$X^2 = 36.95$; n = 4; P<0.001
Control patients with diseases other than cancer (622)	55 (8.8%)	293 (47.1%)	190 (30.5%)	71 (11.4%)	13 (2.1%)	
Females:						
Lung-carcinoma patients (41)	7 (17.1%)	19 (46.3%)	9 (22.0%)	6 (14.6%)	0 (0.0%)	$X^2 = 5.72$; n = 2; 0.05<P<0.10 (Women smoking
Control patients with diseases other than cancer (28)	12 (42.9%)	10 (35.7%)	6 (21.4%)	0 (0.0%)	0 (0.0%)	15 or more cigarettes a day grouped together)

[a] Ounces of tobacco have been expressed as being equivalent to so many cigarettes. There is 1 oz of tobacco in 26.5 normal-size cigarettes, so that the conversion factor has been taken as: 1 oz of tobacco a week = 4 cigarettes a day.

however, the female lung-carcinoma patients are compared with the total number of women interviewed—that is, bringing in the other cancer groups interviewed and making appropriate allowance for age differences between them—then the significance of the trend in their case also is established ($X^2 = 13.23$; n = 2: P approximately 0.001).

The results given in Tables 4 and 5 are shown together graphically in Figure 1. (The percentages in the figure are not all exactly the same as those in the tables. In the figure the percentages are based on the total number of patients in each disease group, smokers and non-smokers alike; in Table 5 they are percentages of smokers alone.)

SMOKING HISTORY

Going one stage further, it has been noted earlier that the amount smoked daily at any one period does not, of course, necessarily give a fair representation of the individual's smoking history. This has been overcome to some extent in the previous tables by classifying a patient as a non-smoker only if he has never smoked regularly, by classifying him according to the amount he last smoked regularly if he had given up smoking, and by ignoring changes in smoking habits which had taken place subse-

quent to the illness which brought the patient into the hospital. Other methods of analysis have also been adopted. Thus Table 6 shows the results in the two main groups when a comparison is made between the maximum amounts ever smoked regularly, and Table 7 shows a comparison between the estimated total amounts of tobacco smoked throughout the patients' whole lives. The estimates of the total amount smoked (expressed as cigarettes) have been made by multiplying the daily amount of tobacco smoked by the number of days that the patient has been in the habit of smoking and making allowance for the major recorded changes in the smoking history. Such estimates may, needless to say, be only very rough approximations to the truth, but they are, it is thought, accurate enough to reveal broad differences between the groups.

The results in Tables 5, 6, and 7 are, it will be seen, closely similar. Whichever measure of smoking is taken, the same result is obtained—namely, a significant and clear relationship between smoking and carcinoma of the lung. It might perhaps have been expected that the more refined concepts—the maximum amount ever smoked and the total amount ever smoked—would have shown a closer relationship than the most recent amount smoked before the onset of the present illness. It must be

Figure 1. Percentage of patients smoking different amounts of tobacco daily.

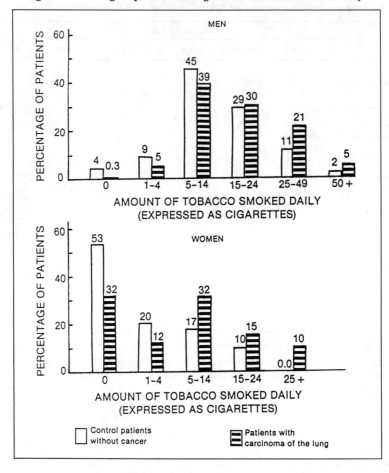

Table 6. Maximum amount of tobacco ever consumed regularly by smokers: lung-carcinoma patients and control patients with diseases other than cancer.

Disease group	No. smoking as a daily maximum					Probability test
	1 cig. −	5 cigs. −	15 cigs. −	25 cigs. −	50 cigs. +	
Males:						
Lung-carcinoma patients (647)	24 (3.7%)	208 (32.1%)	196 (30.3%)	174 (26.9%)	45 (7.0%)	$X^2 = 23.16$; n = 4; P<0.001
Control patients with diseases other than cancer (622)	38 (6.1%)	242 (38.9%)	201 (32.3%)	118 (19.0%)	23 (3.7%)	
Females:						
Lung-carcinoma patients (41)	6 (14.6%)	15 (36.6%)	12 (29.3%)	8 (19.5%)	0 (0.0%)	$X^2 = 7.58$; n = 2;
Control patients with diseases other than cancer (28)	12 (42.9%)	9 (32.1%)	6 (21.4%)	0 (0.0%)	1 (3.6%)	0.02<P<0.05 (Women smoking 15 or more cigarettes a day grouped together)

Table 7. Estimate of total amount of tobacco ever consumed by smokers: lung-carcinoma patients and control patients with diseases other than cancer.

Disease Group	No. who have smoked altogether					Probability test
	365 cigs. −	50 000 cigs. −	150 000 cigs. −	250 000 cigs. −	500 000 cigs. +	
Males:						
Lung-carcinoma patients (647)	19 (2.9%)	145 (22.4%)	183 (28.3%)	225 (34.8%)	75 (11.6%)	$X^2 = 30.60$; n=4; P<0.001
Control patients with diseases other than cancer (622)	36 (5.8%)	190 (30.5%)	182 (29.3%)	179 (28.9%)	35 (5.6%)	
Females:						
Lung-carcinoma patients (41)	10 (24.4%)	19 (46.3%)	5 (12.2%)	7 (17.1%)	0 (0.0%)	$X^2 = 12.97$; n=2; 0.0001<P<0.01 (Women smoking
Control patients with diseases other than cancer (28)	19 (67.9%)	5 (17.9%)	3 (10.7%)	1 (3.6%)	0 (0.0%)	15 or more cigarettes a day grouped together)

supposed, however, that any greater efficiency that might be introduced by the use of these measures is counterbalanced by the inaccuracy which results from requiring the patient to remember habits of many years past. It seems, therefore, that we may reasonably adopt "the most recent amount smoked" in subsequent tables as the simplest characteristic to describe a patient's smoking experience.

Comparisons of the age at which patients began to smoke, the number of years they have smoked, and the number of years they have given up smoking are shown in Table 8.

It will be seen that the lung-carcinoma patients showed a slight tendency to start smoking earlier in life, to continue longer, and to be less inclined to stop, but the differentiation is certainly not sharp and the difference is technically significant only with respect to length of time stopped.

CIGARETTES AND PIPES

So far no distinction has been made between cigarette and pipe smokers, and it is natural to ask whether both methods of smoking tobacco are equally related to carcinoma of the lung. Again the difficulty arises that a man who describes himself as a pipe smoker may have smoked cigarettes until shortly before inter-

Table 8. Age of starting to smoke, number of years smoked, and number of years stopped smoking in lung-carcinoma patients and control patients with diseases other than cancer (male and female).

Age at starting	Lung-carcinoma patients No.	%	Control patients No.	%	No. of years smoking	Lung-carcinoma patients No.	%	Control patients No.	%	No. of years stopped	Lung-carcinoma patients No.	%	Control patients No.	%
Under 20	541	78.6	488	75.1	1 −	14 } 5.1		18 } 7.7		0	649	94.3	590	90.8
20 −	118	17.2	129	19.8	10 −	21		32		1 −	30	4.4	37	5.7
30 −	17 } 4.2		22 } 5.1		20 −	351	51.0	338	52.0	10 −	4 } 1.3		14 } 3.5	
40 +	12		11		40 +	302	43.9	262	40.3	20 +	5		9	
All ages	688		650		Total	688		650		Total	688		650	

$X^2 = 2.40$; n=2; 0.30<P<0.50 $X^2 = 4.65$; n=2; 0.05<P<0.10 $X^2 = 8.59$; n=2; 0.01<P<0.02

rogation, or, alternatively, he may have had his teeth extracted and substituted cigarettes for his pipe. To overcome this, we have excluded all the men who gave a history of having ever consistently smoked both pipes and cigarettes and have compared the proportions of "pure pipe" and "pure cigarette" smokers among the lung-carcinoma and non-cancer control patients. The results are as follows: of the 525 lung-carcinoma patients who had smoked either pipes or cigarettes, but not both, 5.7 percent were pipe smokers and 94.3 percent were cigarette smokers; of 507 control patients with other diseases, 9.7 percent were pipe smokers and 90.3 percent were cigarette smokers. The lower proportion of pipe smokers, and the corresponding excess of cigarette smokers, in the lung-carcinoma group is unlikely to be due to chance ($X^2 = 5.70$; $n = 1$; $0.01 < P < 0.02$).

It therefore seems that pipe smoking is less closely related to carcinoma of the lung than cigarette smoking. On the other hand, it has been shown in Table 5 that light smoking is less closely related to carcinoma of the lung than heavy smoking, so that the result might be explained merely on the grounds that pipe smokers tend to smoke less tobacco.

In fact, pipe smokers do consume, on the average, less tobacco than cigarette smokers, but this is unlikely to be the whole explanation of the relative deficiency of pipe smokers observed in the carcinoma group. We find a higher proportion of cigarette smokers and a lower proportion of pipe smokers among the lung-carcinoma patients than among the control group of non-cancer patients at each level of consumption of tobacco—that is, at 1-4, 5-14, 15-24, and 25+ cigarettes or their equivalent a day. On the other hand, if we consider the "pure pipe" smokers by themselves and subdivide them according to the amount smoked, then we find a higher proportion of the carcinoma patients than of the control group in the higher smoking categories—that is, smoking more than 6 oz of tobacco a week. In short, the results of this subdivision are similar to those shown in Table 5 for all smokers. It seems that the method by which the tobacco is smoked is of importance and that smoking a pipe, though also related to carcinoma of the lung, carries a smaller risk than smoking cigarettes. With the data at our disposal we are unable to determine how great the difference in risk may be.

INHALING

Another difference between smokers is that some inhale and others do not. All patients who smoked were asked whether or not they inhaled, and the answers given by the lung-carcinoma and non-cancer control patients were as follows: of the 688 lung-carcinoma patients who smoked (men and women) 61.6 percent said they inhaled and 38.4 percent said they did not; the corresponding figures for the 650 patients with other diseases were 67.2 percent inhalers and 32.8 percent non-inhalers. It would appear that lung-carcinoma patients inhale slightly less often than other patients ($X^2 = 4.58$; $n = 1$; $0.02 < P < 0.05$). However, the difference is not large, and if the lung-carcinoma patients are compared with all the other patients interviewed, and the necessary allowance is made for sex and age, the difference becomes insignificant ($X^2 = 0.19$; $n = 1$; $0.50 < P < 0.70$).

INTERPRETATION OF RESULTS

Though from the previous tables there seems to be no doubt that there is a direct association between smoking and carcinoma of the lung it is necessary to consider alternative explanations of the results. Could they be due to an unrepresentative sample of patients with carcinoma of the lung or to a choice of a control series which was not truly comparable? Could they have been produced by an exaggeration of their smoking habits by patients who thought they had an illness which could be attributed to smoking? Could they be produced by bias on the part of the interviewers in taking and interpreting the histories?

SELECTION OF PATIENTS FOR INTERVIEW

The method by which the patients with carcinoma of the lung were obtained has been discussed earlier; there is no reason to suppose that they were anything other than a representative sample of the lung-carcinoma patients attending the selected London hospitals. The control patients, as was shown in Table 2, were exactly comparable so far as sex and age were concerned and they were sufficiently comparable with regard to social class for the difference between the two series to be ignored. They were not wholly comparable from the point of view

Table 9. Most recent amount smoked by lung-carcinoma and control patients seen in district hospitals (male and female).

Disease group	No. smoking daily				
	0	1 cig. −	5 cigs. −	15 cigs. −	25 cigs. +
Lung-carcinoma patients (98)	2	12	36	27	21
Control patients with diseases other than cancer (98)	9	9	50	19	11

$$X^2 = 11.68; \ n = 4; \ 0.01 < P < 0.02$$

of place of residence. The difference in this respect, however, was that more of the lung-carcinoma patients came from small towns and rural districts, and the figures in this inquiry show that consumption of tobacco per head in these areas is less than in London. Clearly this feature cannot have accounted for the observation that the lung-carcinoma patients smoked more. Further, if the comparison is confined to patients seen in district hospitals—and all of these resided in Greater London—the results are the same (Table 9).

It might possibly be argued that the choice of a control group of patients with various medical and surgical conditions has, of itself, resulted in the selection of subjects with a smoking history less than the average. This would seem very unlikely, as we know of no evidence to suggest that less than average smoking is a characteristic of persons with any one group of diseases, and it certainly could not be held that it is equally a characteristic of persons suffering from all diseases other than carcinoma of the lung. Yet in Table 10 the smoking habits of the patients in five main groups of diseases are compared, allowing for their sex and age composition, and no significant difference can be demonstrated between them. (We have brought into this table all the patients with diseases other than carcinoma of the lung.)

As in other tables where sex and age differences between groups have had to be taken into account, the "expected" numbers have been obtained by taking the actual numbers of patients with each type of disease in each age and sex subgroup, and calculating what proportion of them would fall in each smoking category if they had had exactly the same habits as all the patients included in the Table. In other words, we have computed what ought to be the smoking habits of each disease group if it behaved in each sex and at each age like the total popula-

Table 10. Most recent amount smoked by all patients other than those with carcinoma of lung, divided according to type of disease (male and female).

Disease group	No. smoking daily				
	0	1 cig. −	5 cigs. −	15 cigs. −	25 cigs. +
Cancer, other than carcinoma of lung (718)	236[a]	78	237	110	57
	220.0	*85.3*	*236.9*	*122.8*	*53.0*
Respiratory disease, other than cancer (335)	42	33	128	98	34
	47.0	*29.7*	*136.1*	*84.1*	*38.1*
Cardiovascular disease (166)	22	19	64	38	23
	17.7	*16.7*	*73.8*	*39.5*	*18.3*
Gastro-intestinal disease (328)	39	31	143	81	34
	55.7	*32.3*	*130.2*	*75.8*	*34.5*
Other diseases (215)	38	24	91	44	18
	36.6	*21.1*	*86.0*	*48.9*	*22.1*

$$X^2 = 20.14; \ n = 16; \ 0.20 < P < 0.30.$$

[a] The roman figures show the actual numbers observed, those in italics are the numbers that would have occurred if the disease group in question had had in each sex and at each age exactly the same smoking habits as all the patients included in the table.

Table 11. Most recent amount smoked by all patients other than those with carcinoma of lung, divided according to whether they were notified or selected for interview (male and female).

Method of selection of patient	No. smoking daily				
	0	1 cig. −	5 cigs. −	15 cigs. −	25 cigs. +
Notified by hospital (1032)	307[a]	114	354	179	78
	301.8	*119.0*	*345.2*	*186.1*	*80.0*
Selection by interviewer (730)	70	71	309	192	88
	75.2	*66.0*	*317.8*	*184.9*	*86.0*

$X^2 = 2.14$; n = 4; 0.70<P<0.80.

[a] See footnote to Table 10.

tion of patients, and compared them with what, in fact, they were. The relatively large numbers of non-smokers in some of the groups are due to the fact that these disease groups included many old women.

There remains the possibility that the interviewers, in selecting the control patients, took for interview from among the patients available for selection a disproportionate number of light smokers. It is difficult to see how they could have done so, but the point can be tested indirectly by comparing the smoking habits of the patients whom they did select for interview with the habits of the other patients, other than those with carcinoma of the lung, whose names were notified by the hospitals. The comparison is made in Table 11 and reveals no appreciable difference between the two groups.

It can therefore be concluded that there is no evidence of any special bias in favor of light smokers in the selection of the control series of patients. In other words, the group of patients interviewed forms, we believe, a satisfactory control series for the lung-carcinoma patients from the point of view of comparison of smoking habits.

PATIENT'S SMOKING HISTORY

Another possibility to consider is that the lung-carcinoma patients tended to exaggerate their smoking habits. Most of these patients cannot have known that they were suffering from cancer, but they would have known that they had respiratory symptoms, and such knowledge might have influenced their replies to questions about the amount they smoked. However, Table 10 has already shown that patients with the other respiratory diseases did not give smoking histories appreciably different from those given by the patients with non-respiratory illnesses. There is no reason, therefore, to suppose that exaggeration on the part of the lung-carcinoma patients has been responsible for the results.

THE INTERVIEWERS

When the investigation was planned it was hoped that the interviewers would know only that they were interviewing patients with cancer of one of several sites (lung, stomach, or large bowel) but not, at the time, the actual site. This, unfortunately, was impracticable; the site would be written on the notification form, or the nurse would refer to the diagnosis in pointing out the patient, or it would become known that only patients with cancer of one of the sites under investigation would be found in one particular ward. Out of 1732 patients notified and interviewed as cases of cancer, the site of the growth was known to the interviewer at the time of interview in all but 61. Serious consideration must therefore be given to the possibility of interviewers' bias affecting the results (by the interviewers tending to scale up the smoking habits of the lung-carcinoma cases).

Fortunately the material provides a simple method of testing this point. A number of patients were interviewed who, at that time, were thought to have carcinoma of the lung but in whom the diagnosis was subsequently disproved. The smoking habits of these patients, believed by the interviewers to have carcinoma of the lung, can be compared with the habits of the patients who in fact had carcinoma of the lung and also with the habits of all the other patients. The result of making these com-

Table 12. Most recent amount smoked by patients with carcinoma of lung and by patients thought incorrectly by the interviewers to be suffering from carcinoma of lung (male and female).

Disease group	No. smoking daily				
	0	1 cig. −	5 cigs. −	15 cigs. −	25 cigs. +
Patients with carcinoma of lung (709)	21[a]	40	269	205	174
	31.7	*48.0*	*276.0*	*201.0*	*152.7*
Patients incorrectly thought to have carcinoma of lung (209)[b]	35	25	83	50	16
	24.3	*17.0*	*76.0*	*54.0*	*37.3*

$X^2 = 29.76$; n = 4; P<0.001.

[a] See footnote to Table 10.

[b] There is a large number of cases in this group because one hospital notified all cases admitted for bronchoscopy; 147 out of the 209 incorrectly thought to have carcinoma of the lung were interviewed at this hospital.

parisons is shown in Tables 12 and 13, and it will be seen that the smoking habits of the patients who were incorrectly thought to have carcinoma of the lung at the time of interview are sharply distinguished from the habits of those patients who did in fact have carcinoma of the lung (Table 12), but they do not differ significantly from the habits of the other patients interviewed (Table 13).

It is therefore clearly not possible to attribute the results of this inquiry to bias on the part of the interviewers, as, had there been any appreciable bias, the smoking habits of the patients thought incorrectly to have carcinoma of the lung would have been recorded as being like those of the true lung-carcinoma subjects and not the same as those without carcinoma of the lung.

We may add that the results cannot be due to different workers interviewing different numbers of patients in the cancer and control groups, for, while the four interviewers did not

see exactly the same proportions of patients in all the groups, the proportions were very close. Moreover, if the patients seen by each of the interviewers are treated as four separate investigations, highly significant differences are found between the lung-carcinoma patients and the other patients interviewed in three instances. In the fourth the difference is in the same direction, but, owing to the small number of patients seen, the results are not technically significant (P lies between 0.10 and 0.05; in this instance the almoner had to stop work because of illness, having seen only 46 patients with carcinoma of the lung).

DISCUSSION

To summarize, it is not reasonable, in our view, to attribute the results to any special selection of cases or to bias in recording. In other words, it must be concluded that there is a real

Table 13. Most recent amount smoked by patients incorrectly thought by the interviewers to be suffering from carcinoma of lung and all other patients not suffering from carcinoma of lung (male and female).

Disease group	No. smoking daily				
	0	1 cig. −	5 cigs. −	15 cigs. −	25 cigs. +
Patients incorrectly thought to have carcinoma of lung (209)[b]	35[a]	25	83	50	16
	36.8	*20.4*	*82.0*	*48.8*	*20.8*
All other patients not suffering from carcinoma of lung (1553)	342	160	580	321	150
	340.2	*164.6*	*581.0*	*322.2*	*145.2*

$X^2 = 2.58$; n = 4; 0.50<P<0.70.

[a] See footnote to Table 10.

[b] See footnote to Table 12.

association between carcinoma of the lung and smoking. Further, the comparison of the smoking habits of patients in different disease groups, shown in Table 10, revealed no association between smoking and other respiratory diseases or between smoking and cancer of the other sites (mainly stomach and large bowel). The association therefore seems to be specific to carcinoma of the lung. This is not necessarily to say that smoking causes carcinoma of the lung. The association would occur if carcinoma of the lung caused people to smoke or if both attributes were end-effects of a common cause. The habit of smoking was, however, invariably formed before the onset of the disease (as revealed by the production of symptoms), so that the disease cannot be held to have caused the habit; nor can we ourselves envisage any common cause likely to lead both to the development of the habit and to the development of the disease 20 to 50 years later. We therefore conclude that smoking is a factor, and an important factor, in the production of carcinoma of the lung.

The effect of smoking varies, as would be expected, with the amount smoked. The extent of the variation could be estimated by comparing the numbers of patients interviewed who had carcinoma of the lung with the corresponding numbers of people in the population, in the same age groups, who smoke the same amounts of tobacco. Our figures, however, are not representative of the whole country, and this may be of some importance, as countrymen smoke, on the average, less than city dwellers. Moreover, as was shown earlier, the carcinoma and the control patients were not comparable with regard to their places of residence. The difficulty can

be overcome by confining the comparison to the inhabitants of Greater London.

If it be assumed that the patients without carcinoma of the lung who lived in Greater London at the time of their interview are typical of the inhabitants of Greater London with regard to their smoking habits, then the number of people in London smoking different amounts of tobacco can be estimated. Ratios can then be obtained between the numbers of patients seen with carcinoma of the lung and the estimated populations at risk who have smoked comparable amounts of tobacco. This has been done for each age group, and the results are shown in Table 14. It must be stressed that the ratios shown in this table are not measures of the actual risks of developing carcinoma of the lung, but are put forward very tentatively as proportional to these risks.

Thus Table 14 shows clearly, and for each age group, the conclusion previously reached—that the risk of developing carcinoma of the lung increases steadily as the amount smoked increases. If the risk among non-smokers is taken as unity and the resulting ratios in the three age groups in which a large number of patients were interviewed (ages 45 to 74) are averaged, the relative risks become 6, 19, 26, 49, and 65 when the number of cigarettes smoked a day are 3, 10, 20, 35, and, say, 60—that is, the midpoints of each smoking group. In other words, on the admittedly speculative assumptions we have made, the risk seems to vary in approximately simple proportion with the amount smoked.

One anomalous result of our inquiry appears to relate to inhaling. It would be natural to suppose that if smoking were harmful it would

Table 14. Ratios of patients interviewed with carcinoma of lung and with a given daily consumption of tobacco to the estimated populations in Greater London smoking the same amounts (male and female combined; ratios per million).

Age	Daily consumption of tobacco						
	0	1-4 cigs.	5-14 cigs.	15-24 cigs.	25-49 cigs.	50 cigs. +	Total
25 –	0[a]	11	2	6	28	—	4
35 –	2	9	43	41	67	77	29
45 –	12	34	178	241	429	667	147
55 –	14	133	380	463	844	600	244
65-74	21	110	300	510	1063	2000	186

[a] Ratios based on less than 5 cases of carcinoma of the lung are given in italics.

be more harmful if the smoke were inhaled. In fact, whether the patient inhaled or not did not seem to make any difference. It is possible that the patients were not fully aware of the meaning of the term and answered incorrectly, but the interviewers were not of that opinion. In the present state of knowledge it is more reasonable to accept the finding and wait until the size of the smoke particle which carries the carcinogen is determined. Until this is known nothing can be stated about the effect which any alteration in the rate and depth of respiration may have on the extent and site of deposition of the carcinogen (*10*).

How, in conclusion, do these results fit in with other known facts about smoking and carcinoma of the lung? Both the consumption of tobacco and the number of deaths attributed to cancer of the lung are known to have increased, and to have increased largely, in many countries this century. The trends in this country are given in Figure 2, and show that over the last 25 years the increase in deaths attributed to cancer of the lung has been much greater than the increase in tobacco consumption. This might well be because the increased number of deaths in the latter years is partly an apparent increase, due to improved diagnosis; in other words, it is not wholly a reflection of increased prevalence of cancer of the lung. On the other hand, it is possible that the carcinogenic agent is introduced during the cultivation or preparation of tobacco for consumption and that changes in the methods of cultivation and preparation have occurred as well as changes in consumption. However that may be, it is clearly not possible to deduce a simple time relationship in this country between the consumption of tobacco and the number of deaths attributed to cancer of the lung.

The greater prevalence of carcinoma of the lung in men compared with women leads naturally to the suggestion that smoking may be a cause, since smoking is predominantly a male habit. Although increasing numbers of women are beginning to smoke, the great majority of women now of the cancer age have either never smoked or have only recently started to do so. It

Figure 2. Death rate from cancer of the lung and rate of consumption of tobacco and cigarettes.

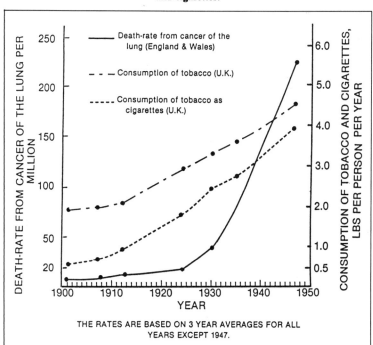

THE RATES ARE BASED ON 3 YEAR AVERAGES FOR ALL YEARS EXCEPT 1947.

is therefore tempting to ascribe the high sex ratio to the greater consumption of tobacco by men. If this were true it would be expected that the incidence of carcinoma of the lung would be the same among non-smokers in both sexes. In this series, 2 out of 649 men and 19 out of 60 women with carcinoma of the lung were non-smokers.

To calculate the incidence rates among non-smokers of either sex it is necessary to estimate the number of nonsmokers in the population from which the patients were drawn. For reasons given earlier this cannot be done, but an estimate can be obtained of the expected sex ratio of cases occurring among nonsmokers in the Greater London area. From the experience of the patients without carcinoma of the lung who lived in Greater London at the time of their interview it can be calculated that there were, in 1948, 175 000 men and 1 582 000 women in London between the ages of 25 and 75 who had never been smokers according to our definition of the term. Taking these figures, subdivided by age, in association with the age distribution of the 16 cases of carcinoma of the lung observed among nonsmokers living in Greater London, it can be calculated that, if the incidence of the disease were equal among non-smokers of both sexes, one case should have occurred in a man and 15 in women. In fact, the observed ratio was 0 to 16.

This finding is consistent with the theory that the risk of developing carcinoma of the lung is the same in both men and women, apart from the influence of smoking. It is not, however, possible to demonstrate with the data at our disposal that different amounts of smoking are sufficient to account for the overall sex ratio.

As to the nature of the carcinogen we have no evidence. The only carcinogenic substance which has been found in tobacco smoke is arsenic (*11*), but the evidence that arsenic can produce carcinoma of the lung is suggestive rather than conclusive (*12*). Should arsenic prove to be the carcinogen, the possibility arises that it is not the tobacco itself which is dangerous. Insecticides containing arsenic have been used for the protection of the growing crop since the end of the last century and might conceivably be the source of the responsible factor. This, too, might account for the observation that deaths from cancer of the lung have increased more rapidly than the consumption of tobacco.

SUMMARY

The great increase in the number of deaths attributed to cancer of the lung in the last 25 years justifies the search for a cause in the environment. An investigation was therefore carried out into the possible association of carcinoma of the lung with smoking, exposure to car and fuel fumes, occupation, etc. The preliminary findings with regard to smoking are reported.

The material for the investigation was obtained from twenty hospitals in the London region which notified patients with cancer of the lung, stomach, and large bowel. Almoners then visited and interviewed each patient. The patients with carcinoma of the stomach and large bowel served for comparison and, in addition, the almoners interviewed a noncancer control group of general hospital patients, chosen so as to be of the same sex and age as the lung-carcinoma patients.

Altogether 649 men and 60 women with carcinoma of the lung were interviewed. Of the men 0.3 percent and of the women 31.7 percent were nonsmokers (as defined in the text). The corresponding figures for the noncancer control groups were: men 4.2 percent, women 53.3 percent.

Among the smokers a relatively high proportion of the patients with carcinoma of the lung fell in the heavier smoking categories. For example, 26.0 percent of the male and 14.6 percent of the female lung-carcinoma patients who smoked gave as their most recent smoking habits prior to their illness the equivalent of 25 or more cigarettes a day, while only 13.5 percent of the male and none of the female noncancer control patients smoked as much. Similar differences were found when comparisons were made between the maximum amounts ever smoked and the estimated total amounts ever smoked.

Cigarette smoking was more closely related to carcinoma of the lung than pipe smoking. No distinct association was found with inhaling.

Taken as a whole, the lung-carcinoma patients had begun to smoke earlier and had continued for longer than the controls, but the differences were very small and not statistically significant. Rather fewer lung-carcinoma patients had given up smoking.

Consideration has been given to the possibility that the results could have been produced by the selection of an unsuitable group of control patients, by patients with respiratory disease exaggerating their smoking habits, or by bias on the part of the interviewers. Reasons are given for excluding all these possibilities, and it is concluded that smoking is an important factor in the cause of carcinoma of the lung.

From consideration of the smoking histories given by the patients without cancer of the lung a tentative estimate was made of the number of people who smoked different amounts of tobacco in Greater London, and hence the relative risks of developing the disease among different grades of smokers were calculated. The figures obtained are admittedly speculative, but suggest that, above the age of 45, the risk of developing the disease increases in simple proportion with the amount smoked, and that it may be approximately 50 times as great among those who smoke 25 or more cigarettes a day as among nonsmokers.

The observed sex ratio among non-smokers (based, it must be stressed, on very few cases) can be readily accounted for if the true incidence among nonsmokers is equal in both sexes.

It is not possible to deduce a simple time relationship between the increased consumption of tobacco and the increased number of deaths attributed to cancer of the lung. This may be because part of the increase is apparent—that is, due to improved diagnosis—but it may also be because the carcinogen in tobacco smoke is introduced into the tobacco during its cultivation or preparation. Greater changes may have taken place in the methods involved in these processes than in the actual amount of tobacco consumed.

Cooperating Hospitals: Brompton, Central Middlesex, Fulham, Hackney, Hammersmith, Harefield, Lambeth, Lewisham, Middlesex, Mount Vernon and the Radium Institute, New End, Royal Cancer, Royal Free, St. Bartholomew's, St. Charles's, St. James's, St. Mary's, St. Thomas's, University College, Whittington.

We are indebted to the staffs of the above-named hospitals for having allowed us to interview their patients and to have access to the hospital notes; also to the individual members of the staffs, both medical and lay, who notified the cases and collected the notes for examination. The work could not have been carried out without their cooperation. Sir Ernest Kennaway and Dr. Percy Stocks took part in a conference called by the Medical Research Council, at which this investigation was initiated, and we have been fortunate in having their helpful advice throughout its course. Professor W. D. Newcomb has advised us on individual problems of pathology. We are most grateful for this assistance. Finally, we wish to thank Miss Marna Buckatzsch, Miss Beryl Iago, Miss Keena Jones, and Miss Rosemary Thomson, who interviewed the patients and helped with the analysis of the results; and Dr. J. T. Boyd for assistance in the calculations.

References

(1) Stocks, P. Studies on medical and population subjects. No. 1. Regional and Local Differences in Cancer Death Rates. H.M.S.O., London, 1947.

(2) Willis, R.A. *Pathology of Tumours*. London, Butterworths, 1948.

(3) Clemmesen, J. and T. Busk. *Br J Cancer* 1:253, 1947.

(4) Steiner, P.E. *Arch Path* 37:185, 1944.

(5) Kennaway, E.L. and N.M. Kennaway. *Br J Cancer* 1:260, 1947.

(6) Muller, F.H. *Z Krebsforsch* 49:57, 1939.

(7) Schrek, R., L.A. Baker, G.P. Ballard, and S. Dolgoff. *Cancer Res* 10:49, 1950.

(8) Jones, T. Personal communication, 1949.

(9) Wynder, E.L. and E.A. Graham. *JAMA* 143:329, 1950.

(10) Davies, C.N. *Br J Industr Med* 6:245, 1949.

(11) Daff, M. and E.L. Kennaway. *Br J Cancer*. In press, 1950.

(12) Hill, A. Bradford and E.L. Faning. *Br J Industr Med* 6:245, 1949.

THE INTERRELATION BETWEEN UTERINE CANCER AND SYPHILIS: A PATHO-DEMOGRAPHIC STUDY

Jørgen Røjel

SOCIAL FACTORS IN THE PATIENT AND CONTROL SERIES

Social Factors

It is an old clinical experience that cancer of the cervix uteri is most common in the lower strata of society, whereas cancer of the body is more common on a higher social level.

Theilhaber (1) was among the first to study the social distribution of cervical cancer. His series comprised 5848 women, 133 of whom had cervical cancer. Patients with cancer of the body were ruled out. After dividing this series into 11 social groups, Theilhaber found 3.7 percent in the highest three groups and 96.3 percent in the remaining groups.

In 1910, Theilhaber and Greischer (2) studied the death certificates for women over 25 years of age dying in Munich during the period 1907-09. The number of women dying from cervical carcinoma proved to increase down the social scale, while the reverse applied to breast cancer. They found also that poor patients with cervical cancer died sooner than the well-to-do ones.

An objection which may be raised against Theilhaber and Greischer's investigation is the absence of any account of the social distribution of the entire population in Munich. Moreover, they do not give the age distribution in their own material.

The relation of social factors to uterine carcinoma in England and Wales was first dealt with in the Report of the Registrar General for 1930-32 (3). This series, comprising 7831 cases of uterine carcinoma among married and 1294 among unmarried women, is divided into five occupational groups (the husband's as far as the married women are concerned). The mortality from uterine cancer proved to be higher in the lower classes of society. Hurdon (4) has re-

ported a higher incidence of cervical carcinoma among the lower classes of society, but she attributes it to the higher fertility among these classes. The above-mentioned report from the Registrar General for England and Wales, however, showed a higher mortality from cancer in the lower classes of society among married as well as among unmarried women. For instance, the mortality of married women in the lowest social group was twice that of social group I; moreover, single women in groups 4-5 had a mortality exceeding that of the single women in groups 1-2 by 44 percent. This led to the following conclusion: "There must exist factors closely bound up with the social class differentiation, either relative or environmental or both, which are productive of uterine cancer quite apart from the parturient histories of the women concerned."

This report of the Registrar General for 1930-32 suffers from serious shortcomings, as no distinction is made between carcinoma of the cervix and of the body, and as it deals with mortality, not incidence.

In New York City, Smith (5) found cervical carcinoma almost exclusively among the poorer classes of society. He states: "Cancer of the cervix is found almost exclusively in the ward or clinic type of patients, rarely being seen in the type of patients who can afford private care."

Kennaway (6) studied the incidence of cervical carcinoma among Jewesses in Munich, Amsterdam, Rotterdam, Vienna, Budapest, Sweden, Palestine, New York, Chicago, Rochester, and Philadelphia. On the average, he found cervical cancer to be three times as common among non-Jewish as among Jewish women. The low incidence of cervical cancer among Jewesses is all the more remarkable as they are exposed to factors which among other races appear to increase the tendency to cervical cancer, such as poor social circumstances, early marriage, and numerous childbirths. In Kennaway's opinion, the low incidence of cervical carcinoma among Jewesses is due in part to

Source: Excerpted from Jørgen Røjel, *The Interrelation Between Uterine Cancer and Syphilis: A Patho-Demographic Study.* Copenhagen, NYT Nordisk Forlag Arnold Busck, 1953.

Niddah's law which forbids orthodox Jewesses coitus for seven days after the termination of each menstrual period; during this period she is considered unclean. After the cessation of the menstruation which the woman had to ascertain by pressing a white cloth into the vulva, she had a bath and a vaginal irrigation before she could celebrate coitus. Moreover, Niddah's law enjoined sexual abstinence after childbirth—after the birth of a boy for 7 plus 33 days, and after the birth of a girl for 14 plus 66 days. Kennaway concludes that in his opinion there are two factors which may increase the incidence of cervical carcinoma: (1) A factor which is counteracted in Jewesses by sexual abstinence during the menstrual period and for seven days after its cessation, (2) a social factor operative in the case of married as well as unmarried women, as the incidence increases down the social scale.

Handley (7, 8) believes that the low incidence of cervical cancer in Jewesses is due to an alteration in the bacterial flora of the genital tract due to the Jewish men's circumcision.

In Plant and Kohn-Speyer's opinion (9), circumcision relieves Jewish men of an accumulation of smegma which causes a lower incidence of penile carcinoma. They believe that smegma in sufficient quantities may induce cervical carcinoma. They are of the opinion that horse smegma and an unsaponifiable fraction thereof is carcinogenic when administered to mice.

Clemmesen and Nielsen (10) studied the incidence of cervical carcinoma in various parts of Copenhagen. Their series comprises all cases of cervical carcinoma in Greater Copenhagen during the period 1943-47. The social level was expressed by the annual house rent in the different districts. The authors found a parallelism between the level of the rent and the incidence of cervical carcinoma, the latter increasing in frequency with a decreasing rent. In the poorest areas with the lowest rent, they found an incidence 183 percent of the average as compared with 50 percent in the wealthy borough of Gentofte.

The present study was not designed to investigate the influence of social factors on uterine cancer, but since uterine cancer and syphilis must be presumed to occur with varying frequency in the different classes of society, a detailed social analysis of the patient and control series proved necessary to find out whether social factors have any perceptible influence on the conclusions drawn. . . .

The occupational grouping of the married women was according to the husband's occupation, of widows according to the deceased husband's occupation except when the widow still had her own occupation. Single, separated, and divorced women were grouped according to their own occupation.

The patient and control series were divided into four social groups comprising the following occupations:

Group A: Managing directors, factory owners, wholesale merchants, superior civil servants, physicians, lawyers, architects, and superior persons in the liberal professions.

Group B: Master artisans, businessmen, subordinate civil servants, and employees.

Group C: Skilled workmen, shop assistants, and clerks.

Group D: Unskilled workmen, housemaids, charwomen, seamstresses, and persons whose occupation is not stated.

Table 1 shows the distribution of the patient and control series in the four social groups and

Table 1. Social distribution of 1262 patients with cervical cancer, 176 patients with cancer of the body, and 1392 controls. The incidence of syphilis is given for each social group.

Social group	A. Absolute number of patients with cervical cancer	B. Syphilitic patients with cervical cancer	B % of A	C. Absolute number of pts. with cancer of the body	D. Syphilitic patients with cancer of the body	D % of C	E. Absolute number of controls	F. Syphilitic controls	F % of E
A	101	14	13.8	38	0	—	100	2	2.0
B	263	28	10.6	59	1	1.6	389	10	2.5
C	278	43	15.4	30	5	16.6	319	14	4.3
D	620	82	13.2	49	4	8.0	584	31	5.3
Total	1262	167	—	176	10	—	1392	57	—

moreover the incidence of syphilis in the various groups. In a more detailed investigation of the social status—to which I shall revert—the series were divided into age groups. In this analysis, however, no regard was paid to age, as it does not purport to be any more than a preliminary orientation to find whether the poorer classes of society show an accumulation of syphilitics among the women with cervical carcinoma. If this had shown a massive accumulation of syphilitics in the lowest social groups, the preponderance of syphilis found in the series with cervical cancer might have been due to a chance coincidence.

Such an accumulation, however, is not apparent. On the contrary, the incidence of syphilis among the patients with cervical carcinoma is higher in social group A than B. It is, therefore, evident that syphilitics are not accumulated among the patients with cervical carcinoma in the lowest social strata, but are diffusely distributed in all four social groups. In the control series the syphilitics are also diffusely distributed in all four social groups.

Loose Women in the Patient and Control Series

It seemed reasonable to investigate the patient and control series with respect to special occupations in which syphilis is known to be common. I was particularly interested in restaurant staff and sailors. These two categories, however, proved so small that the analysis had to be given up.

Then I tried to find the number of prostitutes in the patient and control series in order to ascertain to what extent the two materials are tainted with syphilitic scorti. *A priori*, it could not be ruled out, that, for instance, the cases of cervical carcinoma contained so many prostitutes that this alone could explain the preponderance of syphilis, as syphilis in their case is an "occupational disease." Both patient and control series were, therefore, checked with the police file on prostitutes in Copenhagen.

By an act of October 11, 1906, prostitution is not a legalized occupation in Denmark. Women who try to make a living by prostitution may be prosecuted under the Penal Code of April 15, 1930, section 199, sub-section I: "Should anyone live in idleness under circumstances which give reason to presume that he is not trying to

earn his living in a legal manner, the police *enjoin* him to seek a legal occupation within a given, reasonable notice and, if possible, refer him to such occupation. If the person concerned fails to comply with this enjoinder, he is punished for loitering under section 198 (imprisonment for up to one year). Sub-section 2: "Gambling, prostitution, or support from women earning their living by prostitution are not considered legal occupations."

Section 200, sub-section I says: "When anyone has been convicted according to section 198 or 199, the police may, within a period of five years from his final discharge, issue an *injunction* commanding him to appear at certain intervals to report where he is living or staying and how he is earning his living." Sub-section 2: "Violation of such injunction is punished by imprisonment for up to four months, and under particularly mitigating circumstances with a fine."

The Third Police Chamber is charged with combatting prostitution in Copenhagen, in part by supervising certain parts of the town and in part by raiding foreign ships in the harbor. Since, according to the law, it is loitering without legal occupation which is punishable, a semiprostitution has developed in the course of time, i.e., the women also have a legal occupation to avoid getting into conflict with the police.

In addition to the supervision of prostitutes, the Third Police Chamber has the task of tracing venereal patients who have failed to appear for medical treatment.

This category of my control and cancer series was then divided into (1) prostitutes, i.e., women known to have earned their living exclusively by prostitution, (2) semiprostitutes, i.e., women who earned their living partly by prostitution, (3) women who were presumably guilty of prostitution, (4) women involved in infection proceedings, and (5) "delinquents," i.e., women who have been ordered to undergo treatment for venereal diseases, but who have failed to appear.

Table 2 shows how the persons from the police file are distributed on the patient and control series. Although one gains some idea of the sexual habits of women entered on the file as "delinquents" or as involved in infection proceedings, the prostitutes and semiprostitutes are of primary interest. And it is evident from

Table 2. Number of persons among the patients with cervical carcinoma and the controls who were found on the files of the Third Police Chamber.

	Patients			Controls		
	Absolute numbers of pts. with cervical carcinoma	% of 1262 patients with cervical carcinoma	Number of syphilitics	Absolute number of controls	% of 1392 controls	Number of syphilitics
Prostitutes	40	3.1	15	11	0.8	4
Semiprostitutes	6	0.4	0	0	0	0
Presumed prostitutes (not proved)	5	0.3	3	0	0	0
Involved in infection proceedings	11	0.8	5	1	0.07	0
"Delinquents"	15	1.1	3	5	0.03	2.
Total	77	—	26	17	—	6

the Table that the number of prostitutes among the patients with cervical carcinoma is about four times that among the controls. This figure increases to five times, if it is extended to include also semiprostitutes and women presumed to be guilty of prostitution.

It will be seen from Table 2 that among 77 patients with cervical carcinoma known to the Third Police Chamber, 26, or 35 percent, were syphilitic, and among the 17 control persons 6, or 35 percent. Among the 51 patients with cervical carcinoma who had carried on prostitution, there were 18 syphilitics, i.e., 35 percent; among the 11 prostitutes of the control material there were 4 syphilitics, or 36 percent.

As might be expected, all the prostitutes belong to social group D, in the patient as well as the control material. But even if group D of both series were cleared of prostitutes, there would still be a significant preponderance of syphilitics among the patients with cervical carcinoma (cf. Table 4).

As stated above, the incidence of syphilis was the same among the prostitutes in the patient and control series. On the other hand, there is a striking number of prostitutes in the series of cervical cancer. Since the social level of both materials is the same, it is reasonable to relate the high incidence of prostitutes among the patients with cervical carcinoma to their sexual habits. From hearings in the Third Police Chamber it is known that in "busy periods" some of these women may have coitus with different "customers" up to 10-15 times in the 24-hours. It might, therefore, be imagined that

direct mechanical irritation was a contributory etiological factor. It is striking that the group of patients with cancer of the body did not contain any prostitutes.

Age and Social Conditions in the Patient and Control Series

For practical reasons I left the age distribution in the patient and control series out of account in the preliminary analysis. Since age is a factor relevant to syphilis as well as to cancer, I divided the material into age groups, showing the incidence of syphilis in the various age ranges among the patients with cervical carcinoma, carcinoma of the body and the controls. The result of this analysis is presented in Table 3. It could not be ruled out *a priori* that the age analysis might give age groups in which the incidence of syphilis in the control series would exceed that of the patient series. This did not, however, occur in any case.

As might be expected, the incidence of syphilis depends on age. A comparison of the incidence of syphilis in the cases of cervical carcinoma and in the control series shows in all age groups a marked preponderance of syphilitics in the former.

Lastly, the cases were analyzed from the point of view of age as well as social distribution. All three series were first divided into the above-mentioned social groups A, B, C, and D; each social group was then sub-divided into age groups, and the incidence of syphilis is stated for each age group. Thereafter, social group A

Table 3. Age distribution of 1262 patients with cervical cancer, 176 patients with cancer of the body, and 1392 controls; the incidence of syphilis is stated in percent for each age group.

Age	A. Absolute number of patients with cervical cancer	B. Absolute number of syphilitic pts. with cervical cancer	B % of A	C. Absolute number of pts. with cancer of the body	D. Absolute no. of syphilitic pts. with cancer of the body	D % of C	E. Absolute number of controls	F. Absolute number of syphilitic controls	F % of E
-40	129	7	5.4	0	0	—	136	3	2.2
41-50	361	61	16.9	10	3	30	357	20	5.6
51-60	362	51	14.1	39	2	5.1	414	25	6.0
61-70	266	36	13.5	71	3	4.2	299	5	1.7
71-	144	12	8.3	56	2	3.6	186	4	2.2
Total	1262	167	—	176	10	—	1392	57	—

was combined with B and group C with D to obtain larger and socially more representative groups.

As previously stated, the cases of cervical carcinoma contained 40 prostitutes and 6 semi-prostitutes, 15 of whom were syphilitic. The controls contained 11 prostitutes, 4 of whom were syphilitic (see Table 2). To be on the safe side, I excluded the prostitutes owing to their high incidence of syphilis, to see whether this would affect the preponderance of syphilis among the cervix cancer patients.

The results of this analysis are set out in Table 4. A comparison of the incidence of syphilis in the series with cervical carcinoma and in the control series reveals in all social groups a significant difference between the incidence of syphilis among the patients with cervical carcinoma

Table 4. Age and social distribution in the patient and control series; incidence of syphilis stated in percent for each age group.

Social group	Age	Absolute number of patients with cervical cancer	Absolute number of syphilitic patients with cervical cancer	%	Absolute number of pts. with cancer of the body	Absolute number of syphilitic patients with cancer of the body	%	Absolute number of controls	Absolute number of syphilitic controls	%
A + B	-40	19	2	10	0	0	—	25	0	—
	41-50	65	10	15	4	0	—	73	4	5
	51-60	52	14	26	24	0	—	129	5	4
	61-70	183	11	6	32	1	3	186	3	2
	71-	45	5	11	37	0	—	76	0	—
	Total:	364	42	11.5	97	1	1.0	489	12	2.5
C + D less prostitutes	-40	105	5	4	0	0	—	109	3	2
	41-50	277	45	16	6	3	50	282	15	5
	51-60	296	30	10	15	2	13	280	17	6
	61-70	75	23	30	39	2	5	111	2	1
	71-	99	7	7	19	2	10	110	4	3
	Total:	852	110	12.9	79	9	11.4	892	41	4.5
prostitutes	-40	5	0	—				2	0	—
	41-50	19	6	—				2	1	—
	51-60	14	7	—				5	3	—
	61-70	8	2	—				2	0	—
	71-	0	0	—				0	0	—
	Total:	46	15	33				11	4	36

and the controls. This difference is present in all age groups, and in most of them it is highly significant.

The exclusion of prostitutes from social groups C and D does not affect the preponderance of syphilis in the series of cervical cancer. The analysis shows, moreover, that there is no question of an accumulation of syphilitics in the lowest classes of society, but that they are equally distributed on all four social groups.

This must be tantamount to a relationship between syphilis and cervical carcinoma which cannot be explained by the social conditions recorded.

It is strange that in the age range 51-60 there are 26 percent syphilitics as compared with 10 percent in groups C and D (less the prostitutes). In the age range 61-70, the reverse applies, i.e., 6 percent syphilitics in social groups A and B as against 30 percent in groups C and D (less the prostitutes).

A comparison of the incidence of syphilis in the series with carcinoma of the body and in the control material had to be abandoned as far as social group A + B was concerned, as there

were practically no syphilitics in this group of patients with cancer of the body. In social group C + D, there is a preponderance of syphilitics among the patients with cancer of the body but this preponderance can hardly be attributed with any significance.

Economic Status in the Patient and Control Series

It must be admitted that occupational grouping reflects the social status only to a certain extent. It was, therefore, supplemented by investigating the assessable incomes of the cancer patients and controls. It was previously mentioned that as far as the cancer patients were concerned, the assessable income for the year prior to their admission to the Radium Centre was chosen as the most suitable one. In the case of the controls, the assessable income was ascertained for the same year as that of the cancer patient to whom the individual control acted as a pendant.

Owing to the relation which earning capacity bears to age, Table 5 was set up to show the income in the different age groups of the con-

Table 5. Annual assessable income of 1392 controls and 1438 patients with uterine cancer.

Age	Controls Assessable income					Patients with uterine cancer Assessable income				
	Income not known	<1000 kr.	1-4000 kr.	4-9000 kr.	>9000 kr.	Income not known	<1000 kr.	1-4000 kr.	4-9000 kr.	>9000 kr.
21–25	0	0	1	0	0	0	0	1	0	0
26–30	0	0	3	2	0	0	1	1	0	0
31–35	4	4	20	11	1	0	7	16	12	1
36–40	2	7	50	27	4	5	13	40	31	1
41–45	4	11	62	53	8	10	19	75	41	7
46–50	6	26	95	87	5	18	19	110	62	10
51–55	5	22	109	64	14	9	24	101	64	8
56–60	3	31	96	61	9	2	32	91	65	5
61–65	1	31	75	47	10	5	41	104	40	11
66–70	4	22	76	25	8	4	25	75	24	8
71–	5	42	110	20	9	15	60	95	18	12
Total	34	196	697	397	68	68	241	709	357	63
% of 1392 controls	2.4	14	50	28.5	4.8					
% of 1438 patients with uterine cancer						4-7	16.7	49.3	24.8	4.3

trols and patients. It is evident from this table that the controls are most amply represented in the income group exceeding 9000 kroner, while in the occupational grouping the cancer patients made up the greater part of social group A. This divergence is due to the fact that in the occupational grouping, the widows were grouped according to the occupation of their deceased husbands, and this has assigned them to a higher social position than their income would have done.

There is also a slight preponderance of controls in the income group 4 – 9000 kroner; this accords quite well with the preponderance in social group B in the occupational grouping. The group 1 – 4000 kroner is equally large in both series, whereas the group below 1000 kroner is somewhat larger in the patient material than among the controls. This last-mentioned finding also accords with what social group D had previously shown.

This analysis appears to show that also in respect to economical status, the patients and controls are uniform.

Figure 1 presents graphically the economic status in the patient and control series. It will be seen that the curves are parallel in each income group in both.

Lastly, I investigated how many of the cancer patients and of the controls had received poor relief, had been convicted or had otherwise forfeited their civil rights. The result of this analysis will be seen from Table 6.

It will be seen from this Table that poor relief had been received by a slightly larger number of husbands and wives in the control than in the patient series. In return, a slightly larger number of cancer patients had forfeited their civil rights. The criminality appears to have been approximately the same in both series.

The investigation of matrimonial status in the patient and control series showed that in this

Figure 1. Graphic representation of the annual assessable income of 1392 controls and 1438 patients with uterine cancer.

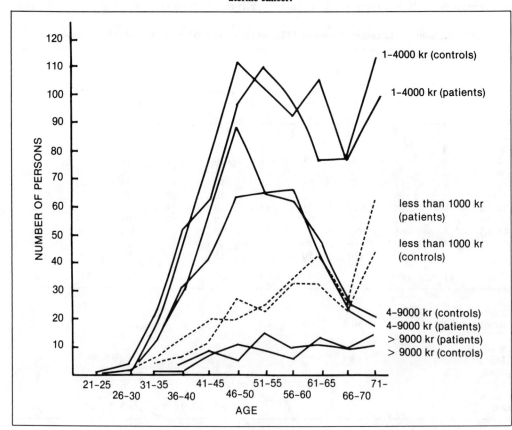

Table 6. Number of controls and patients who had received poor relief, been convicted or had otherwise forfeited their civil rights.

Controls	Absolute number of husbands	% of 902 husbands	Absolute number of women	% of 1392 controls
Received poor relief	55	6	87	6.2
Convicted	31	3.4	13	—
Forfeited civil rights	9	—	22	1.5
Patients	Absolute number of husbands	% of 780 husbands	Absolute number of women	% of 1438 patients with uterine cancer
Received poor relief	39	5	59	4.1
Convicted	24	3	12	—
Forfeited civil rights	7	—	37	2.5

respect too the two series were uniform. There was, however, a significant predominance of divorced women among the patients with cervical carcinoma. The data regarding the number of children were not reliable enough to be used.

Conclusion

The occupational and economical analyses of the patient and control series showed the two to be uniform from the social point of view. Comparing the incidence of syphilis among the patients with cancer of the cervix uteri with that among the controls, we find a preponderance of syphilis in the former in all social groups. This preponderance is apparent in all age groups, and in most of them it is highly significant. At the same time, the syphilitics proved to be evenly distributed on the four social groups. This must indicate a relationship between syphilis and cervical carcinoma, a relationship which cannot be explained by the social findings.

An exclusion of prostitutes from both series does not eliminate the preponderance of syphilitics among the patients with cervical carcinoma.

References

(1) Theilhaber, A. Zur lehre von der enststehung der Uterustumoren. *Münch Med Wsch* 58:1272, 1909.

(2) Theilhaber, A. and S. Grcichcr. Zur aetiology der carcinome. *Z Krebsforsch* 9:530, 1910.

(3) Registrar General's Decennial Supplement. England and Wales, 1931. Part II. London, 1938.

(4) Hurdon, E. *Cancer of the Uterus.* London, 1942.

(5) Smith, F.R. Nationality and carcinoma of the cervix. *Am J Obstet Gynecol* 41:424, 1941.

(6) Kennaway, E.L. The racial and social incidence of cancer. *Br J Cancer* 2:177, 1948.

(7) Handley, W.S. The prevention of cancer. *Lancet* 987, 1936.

(8) Handley, W.S. Penile carcinoma. *Br Med J* 11:841, 1947.

(9) Plaut, A. and A.C. Kohn-Speyer. The carcinogenic action of smegma. *Science* vol. 105, April 11, 1947.

(10) Clemmesen, J. and A. Nielsen. The incidence of malignant diseases in Denmark 1943 to 1947. Copenhagen, 1952.

RELATIONSHIP BETWEEN PREGNANCY EXPERIENCE AND THE DEVELOPMENT OF CERTAIN NEUROPSYCHIATRIC DISORDERS IN CHILDHOOD[1]

Abraham M. Lilienfeld[2], Benjamin Pasamanick,[3] and Martha Rogers[4]

A continuum of reproductive casualty is postulated, extending from fetal deaths—abortion, stillbirth, and neonatal—through a descending gradient of brain damage manifested in neuropsychiatric disorders. The research and administrative public health implications of these findings and the concept of the continuum are briefly but provocatively discussed.

During the past few years we have been engaged in a series of studies concerning the association of maternal and fetal factors with the development of cerebral palsy, epilepsy, mental deficiency, behavior disorders in childhood, and speech defects. A detailed description of the methods and results with regard to specific disease entities either has been or will be reported elsewhere (1-4). Here, we would like to discuss these studies in a general way with particular regard to the methods used and the implications of the results.

The method of study was generally the same with a slight variation for each condition. It consisted of first selecting a series of cases that had been born in a given period within a particular geographic area. A record of events that had occurred during the mother's pregnancy was then obtained. The frequencies of complications of pregnancy, prematurity, obstetric and neonatal difficulties were then compared with a suitable control group.

The first study concerning cerebral palsy was carried out in the New York State Department of Health. The Crippled Children's case register maintained for administering the department's crippled children's program was

searched for those children who had been born between 1940 and 1947, and the birth register maintained by the Health Department's Office of Vital Statistics was searched for the birth certificates of these individuals. Since 1940 in upstate New York, the complications of pregnancy and labor, operative procedures, and birth weight have been voluntarily reported by physicians on the birth certificate in addition to such routine data as age of mother and order of birth. Comparisons of the frequency of complications, prematurity, etc., were made with the total births of children who had survived the first month of life. It was thought that the surviving group was more suitable for comparison than the total birth group, since an infant who had not survived the neonatal period had no chance of developing cerebral palsy.

The investigations of epilepsy, mental deficiency, and speech defects were carried out in Baltimore. The cases selected were those of children registered in various clinics, hospitals, schools, and institutions in the city who had been born between 1935 and 1952 and whose birth certificates were located in the files of the Baltimore City Health Department. Certain information, such as maternal age, birth order, place of birth, etc., was obtained from the birth certificate. As a control series, the next child in the birth register who had survived the neonatal period from the same place of birth matched by race and maternal age group was selected. In those instances where the case and the matched control were born in a hospital, information concerning pregnancy and delivery was abstracted from the hospital record. This was necessary since the reporting of complications, etc., on birth certificates was not instituted in Baltimore until 1949. The person

Source: *American Journal of Public Health*, 45:637-643, 1955.
[1] This paper was presented before a joint session of the Maternal and Child Health and Statistics Sections of the American Public Health Association at the Eighty-Second Annual Meeting in Buffalo, N.Y., October 15, 1954.
This work was aided by grants from the Foundation for Mentally Retarded and Handicapped Children of Baltimore, Md.
[2] Chief, Department of Statistics and Epidemiological Research, Roswell Park Memorial Institute, Buffalo, N.Y.
[3] Associate Professor of Public Health Administration, Division of Mental Hygiene, Johns Hopkins School of Hygiene and Public Health, Baltimore, MD.
[4] Professor of Nursing Education, New York University, New York, NY.

obtaining this information from the hospital record was not informed which birth was a case or control.

The behavior problem children were those who had been referred by public school teachers or principals in Baltimore to the Division of Special Services of the Department of Education and who had been born during the period 1940-1945 *(5)*. (The psychological consultation service is located in this division.) A child of the same sex in the same class as the child with the behavior problem and who had not been referred to the Division of Special Services was selected as a control. This selection of a control resulted in automatic matching by race, economic status, and age due to segregation and school districting. Controls were chosen in this manner in order to be certain that they were without behavior problems as defined in the study. Birth certificates and hospital records were reviewed and the necessary information was obtained. The methods of selection of the groups in these studies are summarized in Table 1.

RESULTS

Space does not permit a detailed report of the findings in all of the studies. As a prototype of these findings, we would like to review the results with regard to cerebral palsy in slightly more detail and then review the other findings more generally. The results are briefly summarized in Table 2.

The mothers of about 38 percent of the cerebral palsied group had had complicated pregnancies as compared with 21 percent of mothers with children who had survived the first month of life. With regard to specific complications of pregnancy, the data suggested that those complications resulting in higher stillbirth and neonatal death rates had a greater degree of association with cerebral palsy. Those complications which are more prone to produce nonmechanical injury to the fetus, such as placenta previa, were more highly associated with cerebral palsy than those complications such as dystocia which usually result in mechanical trauma.

Table 1. Summary of sources of information for each type of neuropsychiatric disorder studied.

Type of neuropsychiatric disorder	No. of cases studied	Geographic area of study	Years of birth of cases	Source of cases	Source of control group	Source of record of mother's pregnancy experience
Cerebral palsy	561	Upstate New York	1940–1947	Crippled Children's Register, New York State Department of Health	Total population of births in same area over same period of time	Reporting on birth certificate
Epilepsy	564					
Mental deficiency	1081	Baltimore	1935–1952	Clinics, hospitals, institutions, schools	Next birth certificate in Birth Register matched by place of birth, maternal age, and race	Birth certificates and hospital obstetrical records
Speech defects	424					
Behavior problems in children	1151	Baltimore	1940–1945	Referral by public school teachers and principals to Division of Special Services, Baltimore City Department of Education	Child in same classroom not referred to Division of Special Services	Birth certificates and hospital obstetrical records

Table 2. Summary of the association of maternal and fetal factors with certain neuropsychiatric disorders of childhood.

Type of neuropsychiatric disorder		One or more complications (percent)	Prematurity (percent)	Abnormal neonatal conditions (percent)	Total abnormalities (percent)	Maternal age and birth order	Maternal history of previous infant loss	Operative procedures
				Frequency of				
Cerebral palsy								
	Cases	38	22	Not studied		+?[a]	+[b]	−[c]
	Controls	21	5					
Epilepsy								
White	Cases	27	13	17	34	−	+	−
	Controls	19	4	6	25			
Nonwhite	Cases	47	15	14	55	−	+	−
	Controls	43	12	3	50			
Mental deficiency								
White	Cases	35	12	16	46	+	−	−
	Controls	25	7	8	31			
Nonwhite	Cases	59	18	7	65	+	−	−
	Controls	55	12	6	60			
Behavior disorders								
White	Cases	33	6	10	39	−	−	−
	Controls	25	2	7	31			
Nonwhite	Cases	64	17	14	73	−	−	−
	Controls	51	5	15	54			
Speech defects								
White only	Cases	25	5	9	29	−	−	−
	Controls	19	8	11	26			

[a] +? = Suggestive association
[b] + = Definite association
[c] − = No association

It was found that 22 percent of the cerebral palsied group had been prematurely born as compared with 5 percent of the total births. This association existed both when prematurity did and did not result from complications of pregnancy. A possible influence of maternal age and birth order was suggested in that there appeared to be an excess of older mothers with first births in the cerebral palsied group. Further investigation, with a larger series of cases, would be required to substantiate this observation. No association was found with operative obstetric procedures. An observation of considerable interest was that 35 percent more of the mothers of the cerebral palsied children had a history of one or more previous stillbirths or infant deaths than the control group.

In the other neuropsychiatric disorders, the necessity of obtaining the required information from hospital records made it possible to collect data on the neonatal condition of the infant. In view of the associations between complications, prematurity, and abnormal neonatal conditions, it was considered necessary to summarize these factors by disregarding the overlapping that occurs between these conditions. Thus, we considered only those children who were exposed to one or more complications, prematurity without complications, and neonatal abnormalities without either complications or prematurity. This net result is expressed in Table 2 as total abnormalities. It was also necessary to take into consideration the fact that a given case might have one or more of the neuropsychiatric disorders. The data presented in Table 2 refer to cases with only one disorder.

The findings with regard to epilepsy and mental deficiency are in general similar to those observed in the case of cerebral palsy. There exists an association of these two conditions with complications of pregnancy and abnormal neonatal conditions and prematurity. In addition, those complications which were actually significant were those associated with non-mechanical fetal injury. In the case of mental deficiency, there was an association with maternal age and birth order which was not present in epilepsy. On the other hand, mothers of the epileptics had had more previous infant loss than the control group. This was not observed among mothers of the mental defectives.

The frequencies of the abnormalities that were studied were not significantly greater among the nonwhite cases as compared to their controls, although they were all in the same direction as was found among the white cases. It is not completely clear why the nonwhite differences were not significant. It is possible that the much smaller number of cases was not sufficient to demonstrate a difference. In addition, the nonwhites have a smaller percentage of hospitalized births leading to some selection for abnormal pregnancies and deliveries which would tend to diminish differences between the cases and controls. In neither of these disorders was an association with operative procedures found.

In the behavior disorder group, an increased frequency of complications of pregnancy and prematurity was observed. The specific complications that were excessive were those productive of nonmechanical fetal injury. No association was found with regard to operative procedures, maternal age, birth order, and mother's history of previous infant loss. Of considerable interest was the fact that when the various types of behavior disorders were studied individually only a specific type was found to be associated with maternal and fetal factors. The behavior disorders so incriminated were those classified as the "confused, disorganized and/or hyperactive" group.

In the case of speech defects where there exists an impression that there is a relationship with pregnancy experience, no associations with the factors studied were found. Frankly, we must admit that such a completely negative re-

sult was comforting since it eliminates the possible existence of a constant bias that may have been inadvertently introduced into the routine processing of the material.

Several considerations must be taken into account in interpreting these results. Of prime importance is the fact that in cerebral palsy, mental deficiency, and epilepsy the association is not with a single set of factors. There appears to exist a pattern of relationship which provides additional support to the findings. This is not true in the case of behavior disorders where the association would appear to be more limited in scope. However, in this instance, some weight must be given to the fact that the association appears to exist with a particular type of behavior disorder which has been suspected on clinical grounds as being the result of organic brain damage.

DISCUSSION

Prior to considering some of the implications of these results, it is important to keep in mind the limitations on interpretation imposed by the type of material utilized. The question of possible bias due to the selection of cases from case registers of a health department and from clinics must be borne in mind. This would be particularly true with regard to socioeconomic selection of the cases. In the studies carried out in Baltimore, a comparison of the cases and controls with regard to socioeconomic status, using census tract data, indicated that they were alike in this respect. Serious consideration must be given to underreporting of the maternal and fetal factors on both birth certificates and hospital records. However, it seems to us that this would tend to diminish the degree of association rather than strengthen it. An important limitation results from the fact that each of the neuropsychiatric conditions studied probably represents a heterogeneous group of conditions caused by multiple factors. Consequently, these results should not be interpreted as implying that maternal and fetal factors are the only etiologic ones. Nonetheless, they would appear to be rather influential and a quantitative estimate of their relative importance must await more refined methods of investigation.

In interpreting these results in terms of specific causal effects, a reasonable hypothesis would appear to be that the various maternal and fetal factors either produce, or influence the production of injury to the brain of the fetus. The fact that those complications which are incriminated are those that result in anoxia or nonmechanical injury, rather than those that result in mechanical injury is in agreement with pathological observations reported by other investigators (6, 7). Of course, any extrapolation from statistical associations to biological causes and effects must at this stage be considered speculative.

Of considerable interest is the fact that the pattern of factors, such as pregnancy complications and prematurity, which are associated with the neurospsychiatric disorders studied are those which influence infant loss. This has led us to postulate the existence of a "continuum of reproductive casualty" with a lethal component consisting of abortions, stillbirths, and neonatal deaths and a sublethal component consisting of cerebral palsy, epilepsy, mental deficiency, and certain behavior disorders of childhood. This implies that certain conditions occurring in utero may result in lethal damage to the infant. A certain proportion of the fetuses are able to withstand the lethal effect and survive with varying degrees of sublethal injury which would be manifested as organic damage to the brain. Indirect support for this hypothesis is obtained from the fact that the strength of association with the factors studied is greatest in the case of stillbirths and neonatal deaths, but is successively less in cerebral palsy, epilepsy, and mental deficiency and least in the case of behavior disorders. Thus, the gradient of the degree of association parallels what might be considered a gradient of clinical severity of the disease entities studied which in turn reflects the amount of organic brain damage present.

The findings indicate that hope for the prevention of these disorders, at least in part, must be based on attaining knowledge sufficient to prevent the various complications of pregnancy and other abnormalities. This knowledge is not available at present. The hypothesis of the "continuum of reproductive casualty" provides a conceptual framework for further research. It emphasizes the need for a concurrent longitudinal study starting as soon after conception as possible and continuing through the prenatal and natal periods until the child is several years of age. Detailed information of events occurring during the prenatal, natal, and postnatal course could be obtained and related to fetal deaths, malformations, and congenital diseases and disabilities. Since the state of the mother prior to conception may also have an influence on the outcome of pregnancy, this also should be included in such a study. Thus, a fruitful area of research would be a study of the relationships of intrauterine and endocrine abnormalities to maternal complications and of these abnormalities to the fetal and postnatal development of the child.

In addition, these results have a bearing on the selection of indexes for the evaluation of programs or services. During a period of high mortality, the prime objective of medical care and public health programs is the reduction of mortality. In the case of maternal health programs, maternal and infant mortality have diminished to unexpected levels. It appears that maternal and fetal morbidity in addition to producing death are also related to certain neuropsychiatric disorders which are in themselves important public health problems. Therefore, in this period of low mortality, should not our emphasis be shifted to maternal and fetal morbidity and should not indexes of such morbidity be developed? Admittedly, this is a difficult problem, but it appears to be basic to the next phase in maternal health program planning. This would also prevent the development of an attitude of complacency which results from noting the marked mortality changes that have occurred during the past 20 years.

Before concluding, there are two points of a methodological nature that appear worthy of mention. In epidemiologic research we are accustomed to study the distribution of a disease by certain population parameters, such as age and sex. In the studies that we have discussed, the characteristics of the individuals studied relate to the time prior to their birth and to the period of their fetal existence. That such characteristics might have importance for other types of diseases is suggested by the recent work of Strong and other investigators (8). In mice, they have obtained evidence that suggested an influence of maternal age on the incidence of mouse leukemia and other types of malignancies. A second point of interest relates to the fact that these studies resulted from a collation of data routinely obtained by health departments and hospitals. We are certain that greater use can be made of such records in other areas of research, perhaps not for the investigation with conclusive results, but for one that provides hypotheses and serves as the necessary basis for further research.

In summary, significant relationships exist between certain abnormal experiences during pregnancy and parturition and such neuropsychiatric disorders of childhood as cerebral palsy, epilepsy, mental deficiency, and behavior disorders. This relationship is not present in speech disorders when the other conditions are absent.

References

(1) Lilienfeld, A.M. and E.A. Parkhurst. A study of the association of factors of pregnancy and parturition with the development of cerebral palsy: Preliminary report. *Am J Hyg* 53:262, 1951.

(2) Lilienfeld, A.M. and B. Pasmanick. Association of maternal and fetal factors with the development of epilepsy 1. Abnormalities in the prenatal and paranatal periods. *J A M A* 155:719, 1954.

(3) Pasamanick, B. and A.M. Lilienfeld. Association of maternal and fetal factors with the development of epilepsy 2. Relationships to some clinical features of epilepsy. *Neurology* 5:77, 1955.

(4) Lilienfeld, A.M. and B. Pasmanick. Association of maternal and fetal factors with the development of cerebral palsy and epilepsy. *Am J Obst Gynecol* In press.

(5) Rogers, M. Association of Maternal and Fetal Factors with the Development of Behavior Disorder in Elementary School Children. Unpublished doctoral dissertation. Johns Hopkins University School of Hygiene and Public Health, Division of Mental Hygiene.

(6) Anderson, G.W. Obstetrical factors in cerebral palsy. *J Pediat* 40:340, 1952.

(7) Courville, C.B. *Contributions to the Study of Cerebral Anoxia.* Los Angeles, San Lucas Press, 1953.

(8) Miner, R.W. Parental age and characteristics of the offspring. *Ann Acad Sci NY* 57:451, 1954.

A SURVEY OF CHILDHOOD MALIGNANCIES

Alice Stewart, Josefine Webb,[1] and David Hewitt[2]

SECTION I. BACKGROUND TO THE SURVEY

The present survey is based on an earlier study of the vital statistics relating to leukemia (1). This had revealed an unusual peak of mortality in the third and fourth years of life which indicated that the subsequent survey should, in the first instance, be restricted to children. The earlier investigation had also led to the suggestion that it might be particularly worthwhile to study modern innovations, such as radiology.

Method

An attempt was made to trace all children in England and Wales who had died of leukemia or cancer before their tenth birthday during the years 1953 to 1955 (case group) and to compare their prenatal and postnatal experiences with those of healthy children (control group). Details of control selection and method of recording data are given later, but the basic idea was to obtain the necessary facts from the mothers by sending a specially appointed "survey doctor" to interview, first, the mother of a dead child, and, secondly, the mother of a live child matched for age, sex, and locality but otherwise picked at random from the local birth register.

Available Cases. The total number of deaths in the category required was 1694, of which 792 were ascribed to leukemia and 902 to other cancers (2). By May, 1957, the mothers of 1416 of these children had been interviewed (677 leukemia and 739 other cancers). The lost cases represented 16.4 percent of the total, and included 6.8 percent who belonged to families that had moved abroad or to an unknown address and 3.1 percent where the interview could not be arranged in time. The remainder represented refusals to cooperate, 4.5 percent by parents and 2.0 percent by doctors.

Appointment of Survey Doctors. It was a basic principle of the survey that the same doctor

should interview both mothers of a given case/control pair, but that pairs in different local authority areas might be seen by different doctors. The 90 pairs belonging to the London County Council area were seen by one of us (J.W.) and the remaining 1326 pairs by "survey doctors" appointed by the principal medical officer of health to the areas. All local authorities cooperated, so that all parts of the country are represented in the survey. To ensure uniformity in the recording of data and the selection of controls one of us (A.S.) visited each one of the health departments to give detailed instructions about field-work procedures.

Collecting of Data

Each survey doctor was given a list of the cases in his area. If the mothers or foster mothers were still living in the area he was to see them and the corresponding control mothers: if a mother had left the area he was to find and interview a control, but return the case papers to Oxford. These were eventually sent on to the new area, but in this way a central record was kept of all "transfers." No case/control pairs seen by different doctors have been included in the analyses making direct comparison between cases and controls, but they may feature in other analyses—for example, incidence of mongolism. Since the records obtained from foster mothers contained no information about the prenatal environment they too have been excluded from the case/control comparisons.

The questionaries for recording the interviews were the same for cases and controls, and were distributed in pairs bearing the same serial number and a so-called final date. This was the date of death of the case, and was a reminder that the medical history of the control child should cease at the so-called onset date—that is, the date when the corresponding child fell ill. The first half of the questionary described the children's medical experiences before the onset date—that is, illnesses, X-ray exposures, and antibiotics—their feeding habits, and their ex-

Source: *British Medical Journal* 1:1495–1508, 1958.
[1] In receipt of a grant from the Medical Research Council.
[2] All from the Department of Social Medicine, Oxford University.

posures to nonmedical ionizing radiations (television, luminous toys, and pedoscopes) during this period. The second half described the mother and other relatives. The mother's illness and X-ray histories ceased at the date of birth of the survey child, but the family histories continued to the date of the interview (this allowed the total number of children in the family, and the number of relatives dying from cancer, to be the number up to the time of the interview). The mother's illness and X-ray histories were recorded separately for three periods of her life: (1) the first period, before marriage; (2) the middle period, between marriage and the relevant conception; and (3) the final period, during the relevant pregnancy. If the child was illegitimate the first period extended to the relevant conception.

Control Selection

It was clear that some "matching" of the live and dead children was needed, but it was decided to restrict this to three features of cancer deaths which it was not intended to study—namely, age, sex, and locality. The distribution of the dead children in respect of these three influences could be readily obtained from official mortality statistics, but as yet nothing was known about, for example, their parity or social class distribution.

Accompanying the papers of each case/control pair was a so-called control selection list. On this was entered the name of the dead child, its sex, when it was born, and the home address at the time of death. Space was provided for half a dozen names of mothers who, in the stated locality, gave birth to a child of the same sex in the same month or half-year. These names were to be obtained from the official registers of births. When completed, the list might be passed to a health visitor with instruction to visit the houses in the order in which they were listed. If it proved impossible to arrange an interview with the first mother the reason was to be entered on the list and the second house visited. In this way a record was kept of all first and later choices, also the reasons for not obtaining the control of choice.

Survey Objectives

The survey doctors were told that the purpose of the survey was to compare the medical and social histories of the children before and after birth, and that the promoters were interested both in the nature of all "previous" illnesses and in the investigations and treatments associated with them (the schedules had separate headings for diagnoses, antibiotics, and X-ray histories).

Interviewing began in December, 1955, and by the following August 547 case/control records had been completed and returned to Oxford. These formed the basis of a preliminary report, which showed that abdominal X-ray films in the relevant pregnancy—that is, direct fetal irradiation—had been reported in 85 cases and 45 controls (*3*). For records completed after this date the corresponding numbers were 107 and 58. There is therefore nothing to indicate that awareness of an important finding has affected these records.

Preliminary Findings. The 1416 case/control pairs completed by May, 1957, included 89 transfers and 28 adoptions. After removing these 117 pairs the remaining 1299 (on which most of the findings are based) included 619 leukemias and 680 other cancers. The controls were represented by 775 first choices and 524 later choices. Only 60 percent of first choices may seem a low proportion, but the birth registers from which the names were taken had been compiled, on average, six or seven years before the survey began. With the use of a register which is revised annually the Survey of Sickness obtained 84 percent of their first choices (*4*). A quarter of the children wanted as controls had definitely left the district and a further 5 percent (marked "no reply") may have done so. Only 6 percent of the mothers either refused to cooperate or were dead, and 3 percent were deliberately rejected because the child was dead or had always lived away from its mother. However desirable it may be in theory to include such children in the sample, in practice the records would have been so defective that they would have been of very little use for case/control comparisons.

Failure to obtain 100 percent of first choices has led to deficits in the control group of three types of children—namely, first-born children, migrants, and twins.

First-Born Children and Migrants. The cases included 510 first-born children and the 427 controls. By national standards the first figure is nearer expectation (approximately 500) than the second; it is therefore reasonable to suppose that there is a genuine deficit on the control side and that it is related to the fact that one-child families tend to move house more often than larger families. Because of this deficiency we have, wherever indicated, done separate analyses of the first- and later-born children of primiparae and multiparae, and of migrant and static families.

Twins. The birth registers from which the controls were taken were, in effect, lists of maternities; hence the control group should contain approximately half the normal proportion of twins. The actual number of control twins was 15 and the "expected" number in the region of 28. By this calculation the number of twins in the case group, 33, is higher, but not significantly higher, than the expected number. Though numerically small, the twins are from the point of view of fetal irradiation important. For this reason they are considered separately in Section II.

In spite of the larger number of first-born children in the case group there was no excess of small families. By the time of the survey most of these children had acquired younger brothers and sisters, and the average family size was the same in both groups (see Section VI).

Demographic Characteristics

The following information about the age, sex, and locality distribution of the cases is based not on the survey findings but on death certificate data.

Age and Sex. The death rates were higher for males than for females and for children under 5 than for children aged 5 to 10. In the leukemia series the early peak of mortality was shown by a higher death rate for children between 2 and 4 years of age than for younger or older children.

Locality. Only two regions—Surrey and Manchester—had a suggestive excess of leukemia deaths, but in general these and the other cancer deaths showed a remarkably even geographical distribution. Classification by size of town revealed greater contrasts, but the highest death rates were in medium-sized towns, not in the largest (see Table 1).

Birth-Rank Distribution. Since the control group was deficient in first-born children the birth-rank distribution of the cases has been compared with national figures for the years which corresponded to the births of these children—that is, 1943–55 (5). According to these statistics, the birth-rank distribution of childhood cancers, other than leukemia, is typical of the population at large, but among leukemic children there appears to be a 10 percent excess of first-born children. Division of these children into two groups—(1) lymphatic and blast-cell leukemias, and (2) other leukemias—revealed further peculiarities (see Figure 1). Thus, between the ages of two and four years the distribution of lymphatic and blast-cell leukemias indicates a 70 percent higher risk for first-born children than for other children. Whether this risk is related to the antenatal or postnatal peculiarities of first-born children we do not know. It is, however, deaths in this narrow age group which are largely responsible for the remarkable post-war increase in childhood deaths from leukemia both in this country and in the U.S.A. (1). Our own data on postnatal X-ray exposures

Table 1. Comparative mortality ratios for age group 0-14 in five density aggregates, 1953–1955 (England and Wales = 100).

	Leukemia	Other malignant disease
Conurbations	108	100
Towns with over 100 000 inhabitants	98	100
Towns with 50 000 to 100 000 inhabitants	124	110
Towns with under 50 000 inhabitants	92	96
Rural areas	86	100
$X^3(4)$	12.372	1.451
Value of P	<0.02	>0.80

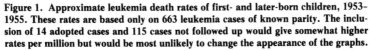

Figure 1. Approximate leukemia death rates of first- and later-born children, 1953–1955. These rates are based only on 663 leukemia cases of known parity. The inclusion of 14 adopted cases and 115 cases not followed up would give somewhat higher rates per million but would be most unlikely to change the appearance of the graphs.

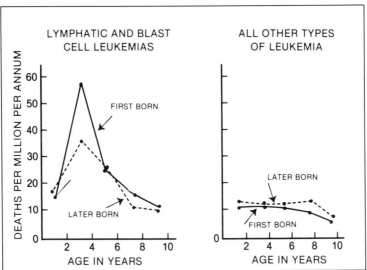

(see Section IV) also suggest that some of the children who survive to the age of two, but are dead of leukemia before the age of four, belong to a separate etiological group.

Maternal Age. The average age of the mothers at the date of birth of the survey children was 28.91 years for the leukemia series and 28.43 for the other cancer series—that is to say, the group which contained the higher proportion of primiparae was, on average, 25 weeks *older* than the other group. Further examination of the maternal ages showed that this greater average age was determined by a small group of mothers who were over the age of 40 when the leukemic child was born. These mothers represented 6.9 percent of the leukemic series and only 3.5 percent of the other cancer series. To avoid confusion with the high incidence of mongolism in the leukemia series (see Section IV) the mothers of mongols were excluded from the next analysis and primiparae were separated from multiparae. In the latter group (which contained the bulk of women over 40) the average age was 52 weeks higher for the leukemia than for the other cancer series, a difference which is statistically significant (P<0.01). Assuming that age of the mother has not affected the prevalence of other childhood

cancers, this suggests that the risk of dying of leukemia before the age of 10 years is twice as great as usual if the mother is over 40 years of age at the date of birth (this estimate is in no way dependent on the slightly higher incidence of obstetric X-ray examinations in elderly women). The independent findings, first, of a large number of mongols in the leukemia series, and, secondly, of a relatively large number of "old" mothers in the leukemia series suggest that childhood leukemia and mongolism are influenced by a common factor, rather than that one disease predisposes to the other (see also Section IV). In a recent American survey the ages of the mothers in a smaller group of children with leukemia and other cancers also show these contrasts (6).

Social-Class Distribution. The basis of the social-class distribution was the father's occupation. A statement of family-income was also obtained for 87 percent of cases and 88 percent of controls. Since it is common knowledge that professional families move house more often than working-class families, the social and economic distributions have been calculated separately for children who moved house after they were born (migrant series) and children who did not (static series). On this basis there are virtually no social-class or economic distinctions as between cases and controls or between cases of leukemia and cases of other cancer. (National mortality rates suggest that leukemia deaths at later ages tend to have an upward social gradient, and other cancer deaths a slight downward gradient.)

SECTION II. MOTHERS' X-RAY HISTORIES

Although the mothers were questioned first about their children and only later about their own health, we shall deal first with the mothers' X-ray histories and illnesses. These were recorded separately for (1) the first period, before marriage; (2) the middle period, between marriage and the relevant conception; and (3) the final period, during the relevant pregnancy. Three categories of exposure were distinguished—therapeutic, occupational, and diagnostic. The first two need not detain us. Only 16 mothers (7 cases, 9 controls) reported any radiotherapy and the treatments never coincided with the relevant pregnancy. A further 19 mothers (12 cases, 7 controls) may have been exposed to X rays in the course of their work, and for three—all mothers of cases—the work was continued during the final period. The occupations in question were: nurse in a radiotherapy department, nurse in a radiological department, and a metal-tester.

Diagnostic X-Ray Histories

A summary of the mothers' diagnostic X-ray histories is given in Table 2. Figures are given for the three periods, separately and jointly, and for two main types of X-ray examination (abdominal and other). The figures are numbers of *mothers,* not numbers of films or examinations—that is to say, no woman has been counted more than once in any cell of the Table (consequently the figures for "any period" and "any X-ray exposure" are rather lower than the sum of the figures for separate periods and separate types of examination). The figures in italics give the ratios between the numbers of case mothers and the corresponding numbers of control mothers.

It will be seen that 692 mothers of cases reported at least one diagnostic X-ray exposure compared with only 593 mothers of controls, a case/control ratio of 1.17. Though this case excess is significant, it is not very large, and might perhaps be attributed to relative underreporting of X-ray exposures on the control side. If, however, underreporting by control mothers was the only reason for the case excess one would expect to find similar case/control ratios for each type of examination and for each period of life. In fact, the ratio is higher for abdominal (1.38) than for other types of examination (1.16), and higher for all examinations during the relevant pregnancy (1.48) than during earlier periods (1.22 and 1.07). In particular, the ratio for abdominal X-ray examinations during the relevant pregnancy is outstandingly high (1.91). The chance probability of obtaining so high a ratio is less than one in ten million. Moreover, as the footnote to Table 2 shows, this ratio is significantly higher than the ratio for X-ray examinations of other sites in this period,

Table 2. Number of mothers reporting X-ray examination of different sites (abdomen and other) in three periods (see text).

Period	X-ray examinations		
	Abdominal	Other	Any
Before marriage	44/26[a] = *1.69*	335/275 = *1.22*	361/296 = *1.22*
Between marriage and relevant conception	109/121 = *0.90*	213/184 = *1.16*	304/285 = *1.07*
During relevant pregnancy	178/93 = *1.91*	117/100 = *1.17*	273/184 = *1.48*
Any period	296/215 = *1.38*	531/456 = *1.16*	692/593 = *1.17*

The case/control ratio of 1.91 for abdominal x-ray exposures during the relevant pregnancy (1) differs from the "expected" ratio (1.00) at the level of $P<10^{-1}$; (2) differs from the contemporary ratio for other x-ray exposures (1.17) at the level $P\simeq0.011$ and from the ratio for other X-ray exposures in any period (1.16) at the level $P<0.001$; and (3) differs from the ratio for abdominal X-ray exposures in any period (1.38) at the level $P\simeq0.012$.

[a] 44/26, etc., represent ratio of case mothers to control mothers.

and than the ratio for abdominal X-ray examinations as a whole. Hence there is prima facie evidence that abdominal X-ray examinations during pregnancy—the only type of examination involving direct exposure of the fetus—can contribute to the etiology of malignant disease in children.

Most of the remainder of this section is devoted to further analysis of the apparent association between fetal irradiation and malignant disease in childhood, but it is necessary first to say something about the figures for the other maternal X-ray histories.

One group of maternal X-ray histories—those relating to X-ray exposures of the abdomen during the middle period—shows a small excess on the *control* side. This was at first thought to be due to the fact that on the control side there were more previous children, and hence more occasions for obstetric X-ray exposures in the middle period. However, when the obstetric X-ray examinations were separated from the other abdominal X-ray examinations belonging to this period and related to the number of pregnancies at risk (see Table 3) there was still a slight excess on the control side. This strengthens the view that the control mothers were as efficient as the mothers of cases in recalling their abdominal X-ray examinations.

In the pre-marriage period there was a case excess for abdominal X-ray exposures which has to be accepted as technically significant (P<0.05). The possibility has therefore to be considered that damage to the maternal gonads may increase the risk of childhood malignancy. But even if this is the correct explanation such damage is of minor interest, for, as judged by the numbers involved, its importance can only be one-quarter of that of direct fetal irradiation.

Unlike the case excess for abdominal X-ray examinations, that for other X-ray examinations showed no tendency to concentrate in the period of the relevant pregnancy. This seems to dispose of the notion that scatter from X-ray exposure of sites other than the abdomen had been harmful to the cases. The meaning of the steady case excess in all periods is not clear. To be on the safe side we will assume (see Table 7) that it is an average measure of the relative underreporting of X-ray exposure by control mothers compared with the case mothers. However, even this group is not completely homogeneous as regards case/control comparisons. On further breakdown it was found that mothers reporting chest X-ray examinations were in substantial excess on the case side (ratio of 1.20), but that the numbers reporting skull or limb exposures were virtually identical (133 and 132).

The first step in pursuing the association between fetal irradiation and malignant diseases was to check all reports of abdominal X-ray examinations during the relevant pregnancy against hospital records. This revealed a few inaccuracies. Five mothers of cases and five of controls were found to have reported an examination which in fact had been performed during a different pregnancy. In a further 14 instances (9 cases and 5 controls) no hospital record of the alleged examination could be found. The figures shown in Table 2 do not include any of these faulty records (the effect of removing them was to alter the case/control ratio from 1.86 to 1.91).

Twins. As already explained there are only 15 twins in the control group compared with an expected number of 28 (see Section I). Since seven of these 15 children had been X-rayed *in utero* it is reasonable to suppose that with a full quota of twins there might have been six more control mothers reporting abdominal X-ray examinations in the final period.

First-Born Children. Separate analysis of the maternal X-ray histories in groups defined by

Table 3. Comparison between cases and controls in respect of obstetric X-ray examinations in the middle period (i.e., between marriage and the relevant conception).

	Cases	Controls
Total No. of previous pregnancies	1623	1742
No. of women reporting obstetric (abdominal) X-ray examinations between marriage and relevant conception:		
(*a*) Actual	79	96
(*b*) Expected	84.41	90.59

Table 4. Histories of direct fetal irradiation distinguishing three birth-rank groups of cases and controls.

Position in family of child (birth rank)	Cases		Controls		
	No.	%	No.	%	Ratio
First	85/510	16.7	36/427	8.4	1.99
Second	47/393	12.0	28/448	6.3	1.90
Later	46/396	11.6	29/424	6.8	1.71
All	178/1299	13.7	93/1299	7.2	1.91

parity (Table 4) showed that the proportion of first-born children who were X-rayed *in utero* was approximately 2 percent higher than the proportion for other children. This slight difference is equivalent to about two "extra" records of direct fetal irradiation on the case side.

Migration (see Table 5). Independent case/control comparisons based on the "migrant" and "static" series (see Section I) showed no significant differences between these two groups.

The last point to be considered is whether the high case/control ratio for abdominal X-ray examinations in the relevant pregnancy could be due to the existence in the case group of a condition or conditions which only incidentally caused the child to be X-rayed *in utero*. In this connection it is clearly appropriate to draw a distinction between X rays taken for purely obstetric reasons and other abdominal X rays which happened to coincide with the pregnancy (see Table 6). According to this analysis over 90 percent of the X-ray examinations were taken for obstetric reasons, other abdominal X-ray examinations representing 9 percent of cases and 6 percent of controls. Inasmuch as these other abdominal X-ray examinations tended to take place earlier and to involve heavier exposures

than the obstetric X rays, they might be expected to concentrate on the case side if there were a causal relationship between direct fetal irradiation and childhood malignancies. Hence the slight excess of other abdominal X-ray exposures on the case side in no way disturbs this hypothesis.[3]

We are now in a position to judge the effect of all the factors which might possibly have contributed a spurious element to the case/control ratio for abdominal X-ray examinations in the relevent pregnancy. To do this we have made three assumptions which are unfavorable to an explanation in terms of a causal link between fetal irradiation and childhood malignancies. These are: (1) that the excess of twins in the case group is wholly spurious; (2) that ill health during pregnancy is of such overruling importance that any associated X-ray exposure should be ignored; and (3) that the case mothers were 16 percent more efficient than the control mothers in reporting X-ray exposures (on the grounds that the case/control ratio for other X-

---

[3] Judging by the number of deaths among the children of case and control mothers, the older and the younger children of the case mothers were just as healthy as the older and younger children of the control mothers, nor was there any difference in the stillbirth rates for the case and control groups (see Section VII).

Table 5. Frequency of direct fetal irradiation of cases belonging to "migrant" and "static" families and of corresponding controls.

Fetal irradiation	Migrant series		Static series	
	Cases	Controls	Cases	Controls
Yes	57	23	121	70
No	325	359	796	847
Total	382	382	917	917
X^2	15.205		14.610	
P	<0.001		<0.001	

Table 6. Numbers of mothers reporting obstetric and other abdominal X-ray examinations during the relevant pregnancy.

X-ray category and reasons for X-ray examinations	Cases		Controls	
	No.	%	No.	%
Obstetric:				
Position	61	36.3	29	34.5
Size (? twins)	53	31.5	29	34.5
Routine pelvimetry	35	20.8	20	23.8
Diagnosis of pregnancy	4	2.4	1	1.2
Total	153	91.0	79	94.0
Other abdominal:				
Barium meal	6	3.6	1	1.2
Intravenous pyelogram	3	1.8	—	—
Injury	4	2.4	1	1.2
Other	2	1.2	3	3.6
Total	15	9.0	5	6.0
Total of all known indications	168	100.0	84	100.0
Indication for X-ray examination unknown	10	—	9	—

ray examinations was 1.16) (see Table 2). These three assumptions have been worked into Table 7, which excludes all twins, counts all abdominal X-ray examinations in the final period, other than purely obstetric X-ray examinations among the non-irradiated totals, and gives "expected" numbers which are calculated not on the basis of equality but on an "expected" case/control ratio of 1.16 to 1.00. In spite of these drastic modifications there is still an excess of abdominal X-ray examinations on the case side which is so large that it would occur by chance in less than one of 500 repeated trials.

In the remainder of this section it is assumed that there is a causal relationship between irradiation *in utero* and childhood malignancies, and four aspects of the risk involved are considered: (1) its relationship to X-ray dose, (2) its relationship to the maturity of the fetus at the time of exposure, (3) its relationship to the type of malignant disease, and (4) its absolute size.

Dose-Response Relationship

Court-Brown and Doll (7) have studied the incidence of leukemia and aplastic anemia in adults given deep X-ray therapy to the spine. Although they had only 37 cases at their disposal they were able to demonstrate a strong relation between dose and risk of disease. The present series of children includes no fewer than 178 in whom malignant disease had been preceded by antenatal irradiation, and therefore appears to offer ample material for studying dosage effects. There is, however, an important difference which nullifies the advantage of larger numbers. Court-Brown and Doll had an almost "pure" series of radiation-leukemias, since they gave evidence that over 90 percent of them would not have occurred but for the preceding X-ray exposures. In the present series a high proportion of the cases X-rayed *in utero* developed the fatal disease for *other* reasons. The existence of these cases is bound to hinder recognition of a dose-response relationship.

Attempts to collect data for the study of dosage effects met with great difficulties. Over 200

Table 7. Actual (and expected) numbers of cases and controls with and without a history of direct fetal irradiation. Revised basis of comparison (see text).

	Cases	Controls	Total
Irradiated	141(118.44)	81(103.56)	222
Not irradiated	1125(1147.56)	1204(1181.44)	2328
Total	1266	1284	2550

$\chi^2_{(1)}$ with continuity correction is 9.644, equivalent to a normal deviate of 3·10; $P<0.002$.

different hospitals had to be asked for records, many of which related to events of more than five years previously. Radiologists supplied all the technical details available, but these were rarely sufficient to support a calculation of dose. Finally, we were reduced to using, as an extremely crude index of dose, the number of films believed to have been taken, though even this was often no more than a reasoned guess on the part of the radiologist and did not include films discarded by the radiographer. Table 8 shows a classification of the cases and controls on this basis. Except in the group with no films the numbers are small and therefore the sampling errors of the case-control ratios are large. The group representing three films breaks the rising sequence of ratios, but at least the lowest and highest ratios (0.93 and 3.20) correspond to the lowest and highest number of films (nil and four or more films). A small group of mothers, not distinguished in the table, who had five or more abdominal X-ray examinations during the relevant pregnancy, included 15 cases and only

2 controls. Thus the figures are consistent with, though they do not establish, a relationship between increasing dose and increasing risk.

Timing Effects

The precise date of exposure was ascertained in most cases, and on this basis each mother was classified according to the month of the first exposure (see Table 9). The dated series did not include a single mother examined within 28 days of conception, and only 20 mothers were certainly X-rayed in the first half of pregnancy. However, in this small group there were 18 cases and only 2 controls, which represents a much higher case/control ratio than the one for exposures in the second half of pregnancy (148 cases, 83 controls). The variations in the second half of pregnancy all lie within the accepted range of chance variation.

Tissue Sensitivity

Previous work suggests that, in adults, leukemia is more likely to be produced by ionizing radiations than other malignant diseases (7, 8). But our own data suggest that in a fetus there may be other tissues which are at least as sensitive to X rays as the reticulo-endothelial system (see Table 10). In this table the cases have been divided into eight diagnostic groups, and the number of irradiated cases in each of these is compared with the number which would be expected if the X-ray exposures were evenly distributed among the cases. In calculating these expected numbers, we have standardized them in ten-yearly age groups, in order to allow for changes in X-ray habits during the years in which the survey children were born. On this

Table 8. Distribution of cases and controls irradiated *in utero*. According to the numbers of abdominal films reported taken during the relevant pregnancy.

No. of films	Cases	Controls	Ratio
0	1121	1206	0.93
1	37	27	1.37
2	60	26	2.31
3	23	18	1.28
4 or more	32	10	3.20
(Unknown number)	(26)	(12)	(2.17)
Total	1299	1299	1.00

Table 9. Distribution of cases and controls irradiated *in utero* according to month of pregnancy.

Gestation period in months	Cases	Controls	Case/control ratio
1st to 5th	18	2	(9.00)
6th, 7th	15	9	1.67
8th	20	19	1.05
9th	55	30	1.83
10th	58	25	2.32
Total known	166	85	1.95
Unknown	12	8	(1.50)
Total	178	93	1.91

A statistical comparison of the cases and controls in the five "known" categories above yields $\chi^2_{(4)} = 9.656$, for which $P < 0.05$.

Table 10. Comparative incidence of direct fetal irradiation in eight diagnostic groups.

| Diagnosis | No. of cases | Irradiation *in utero* | | |
		%	Actual no.	Expected no.
Lymphatic leukemia	292	14.4	42	40.31
Myeloblastic	124	7.3	9	16.24
Blast-cell and other leukemias	203	13.8	28	27.93
Lymphosarcoma, other reticuloses	109	7.3	8	14.24
Malignant tumors of C.N.S.	212	12.7	27	28.75
” ” kidney	120	15.8	19	16.68
” ” suprarenals (incl. *all* neuroblastomas)	87	18.4	16	12.68
Malignant tumors of other sites	152	19.1	29	21.16
Total	1299	13.7	178	177.99

In an 8×2 table the comparison of actual and expected numbers irradiated and not irradiated $\chi^2_{(y)} = 11.832$, compared with 12.017 at the level $P = 0.10$.

basis the differences between the actual and expected numbers are of a magnitude which, under chance conditions, would be expected to occur in about one out of ten samples. The group labeled "other sites" had the highest percentage (19.1 percent). This included three retinoblastomas with three X-ray exposures, and 12 teratomas with seven X-ray exposures. We hesitate to draw any conclusion about the retinoblastomas, because in an independent series of 39 children who were said to have survived surgical removal of a retinoblastoma we found there had been only seven prenatal X-ray examinations, which is no more than average for all forms of cancer. However, the chance of obtaining as many as seven X-ray exposures in 12 cases is only one in a thousand, so it may be that the nests of embryonic tissue contained in teratomas are exceptionally radiosensitive.

Delayed Effects of Fetal Irradiation

The survey was deliberately restricted to children under 10 years of age because it was thought that this was a convenient limit to the time that mothers might be expected to recollect events. But by so doing we may have missed some of the consequences of direct fetal irradiation. If the effects of prenatal irradiation are exhausted by the age of 10 years one would expect the case/control ratio for fetal irradiation to be higher for children who were under 5 years of age at the onset date than for children who were 5 or over. But, as Table 11 shows, this ratio is 1.73 for the younger children and 2.50 for the older children.

Table 11. Case/control ratio for direct fetal irradiation, comparison of cases and controls defined by age at the "final date."

	Cases	Controls	Ratio
Deaths at ages 0 to 4	123	71	1.73
” ” 5 to 9	55	22	2.50
” ” 0 to 9	178	93	1.91

Estimates of Risk

The following estimates are based on the figures shown in Table 2 and necessarily represent a rough appraisal of the situation. In the case group 13.7 percent of the children were X-rayed before birth and 86.3 percent were not. The corresponding percentages for control children were 7.2 and 92.8. On this showing children who have been X-rayed *in utero* are $\frac{(13.7 \times 92.8)}{(7.2 \times 86.3)}$ times, or twice as likely to die of a malignant disease before their tenth birthday as other children. Since at the present time about one in every 1200 children in Britain die in this way, it follows that less than one in a thousand of the prenatal X-ray examinations performed in recent years have led to death from malignant disease before the age of 10 years. An alternative way of expressing this estimate is to say that abdominal X-ray examinations of pregnant women have in recent years been responsible for (13.7–7.2) percent or between 6 and 7 percent of all deaths from malignant disease before the age of 10 years.

To sum up: there appears to be no doubt that there is a causal relationship between prenatal

exposure to X rays and the subsequent development of malignant disease, and there are indications that the risk is related both to the dose
of X rays and to the date of exposure. There is
nothing to suggest that irradiation *in utero* explains the early peak of leukemia mortality (see
Section IV for data on postnatal X-ray exposures) and it may even cause deaths from
malignant disease after the age of 10 years.
Thorough estimates of risk which are given
here apply only to one period of time and to the
X-ray doses in use at that time. Evidently radiotherapy of pregnant women is an extremely
rare event in this country, and contributed
nothing to the cases we have considered.

Addendum. After this report had been written
we received the results of an independent study
(9) which had been designed specifically to test
the conclusion announced in our preliminary
communication. This study concerned children
who had died under the age of 10 in the State
of Louisiana during the years 1951–5. Although conducted on a rather small scale it had
one important advantage over our own inquiry:
all the information was obtained direct from
professional sources, thus minimizing the risk
from emotional bias or selective memory in the
informants. The incidence of irradiation *in
utero* discovered by Paterson was as follows:
among 77 children who died of leukemia, 27.3
percent; among 70 children who died of other

cancers, 28.6 percent; and among 293 control
children who died of other causes, 18.4 percent.
These percentages are much higher than those
found in England and Wales, but show two
important resemblances: (1) the significantly
higher incidence of fetal irradiation among
children with malignant disease than among
controls, and (2) similar figures obtained for
children with leukemia and those with other
forms of malignant disease. Using Paterson's
figures in the same way as our own to derive an
estimate of the relative risk of malignant disease
associated with irradiation *in utero*, we have
$\frac{27.9}{18.4} \times \frac{81.6}{72.1} = 1.72$, which is in reasonable
agreement with our own estimate.

SECTION III. MOTHERS' ILLNESSES

The mothers were asked whether they had
ever had a serious illness or injury before the
survey child was born. Although these events
were actually recorded separately in the three
periods (see Section II), only two periods are
distinguished in the following analysis–namely,
before and during the relevant pregnancy. Only
information of a reasonably objective and definite type has been considered, and unless a
common childhood infection—for example,
measles—coincided with the relevant pregnancy it has been omitted from the following

Table 12. Illnesses of mothers arising before and during the relevant pregnancy.

International classification main category	Arising before relevant pregnancy		Arising during relevant pregnancy	
	Cases	Controls	Cases	Controls
I. Infective	86	82	13	1
II. Neoplasms	9	11	2	2
III. Allergic, etc.	24	22	1	3
VI. Nervous system	32	37	1	0
VII. Circulatory	53	44	0	4
VIII. Respiratory	219	207	12	13
IX. Digestive	74	91	12	4
X. Genitourinary	62	44	0	0
XI. Pregnancy	32	32	113	77
XII. Skin	33	43	5	5
XIII. Bones and muscles	15	20	3	0
XIV. Congenital	5	7	—	—
XVII. Accidents	48	57	0	0
Total no. of illnesses	692	697	162	109
Total no. of women	565	554	155	104

analyses. After omission of these items and such vague conditions as nervous breakdowns, influenza, anemia, and injuries other than fractures, approximately half the mothers were left with no diseases before the birth of the survey child. The remaining records were classified according to the *International Classification of Diseases (10)*, and the results are shown in Table 12.

Illnesses Originating Before the Relevant Pregnancy. The total number of illnesses in this category was 1389 (cases 692 and controls 697) and the number of mothers affected was 1119 (cases 565 and controls 554). Unlike the series reported by Manning and Carroll (6) there were no case/control differences for allergic conditions (category III), but compared with this American series the incidence of these conditions was low. The only group of illnesses with a substantial difference between cases and controls was category X (diseases of the genitourinary system) with 62 records for cases and 44 for controls. The difference was confined to disease of the renal tract as such (49 cases and 30 controls), which represents a significant case excess (P approx. 0.04).

Illnesses Arising During the Relevant Pregnancy. The total number of illnesses recorded in this period was 271 (162 cases, 109 controls) with 259 mothers affected (155 cases, 104 controls). Further analysis of the records showed that this case excess, which is statistically significant, was restricted to two categories—namely, infective disease (13 cases, 1 control) and direct complications of pregnancy (113 cases, 77 controls). The latter group (see Table 13) is dominated by toxemias of pregnancy (67 cases, 57 controls), but there were also 29 urinary infections (19 cases, 10 controls) and 37 threatened abortions (27 cases, 10 controls). The difference between cases and controls is not significant for toxemia of pregnancy, and the difference for urinary infections is complicated by the fact that six of the mothers on the case side had also had an abdominal X-ray examination during the relevant pregnancy (mostly intravenous pyelograms). This leaves threatened abortions and

Table 13. Illnesses of mothers specifically associated with the relevant pregnancy.

I.C.D. numbers	Illness	Leukemia		Other cancers		Total	
		Cases	Controls	Cases	Controls	Cases	Controls
642	Toxomias of pregnancy	29	31	38	26	67	57
640-641	Infections of genitourinary tract during pregnancy	8	3	11	7	19	10
648.0	Threatened abortion	14	4	13	6	27	10
	Total	51	38	62	39	113	77

Table 14. Infections during the relevant pregnancy.

Maternal infection	No. of cases	Corresponding children
Rubella	3	Congenital sarcoma of mediastinum Neuroblastoma at 12 months Lymphoblastoma at 15 months
Mumps	2	Congenital sarcoma of the meninges Leukemia at 5 years
Herpes zoster	4	Healthy control Leukemia at 7 years Leukemia at 8 years Cerebral tumor at 6 years
Infective hepatitis	2	Leukemia at 4 years Cerebral tumor at 6 years

infective diseases as the only ones with a significant and unambiguous excess on the case side. The infective disease group included 10 virus infections on the case side and one on the control side. These undated infections were associated with the childhood diseases shown in Table 14.

To summarize: there is nothing in the illness records to suggest that the case mothers were, before the relevant pregnancy, less healthy than the control mothers. During the relevant pregnancy they appear to have suffered more from threatened abortions and virus infections than the control mothers, but the numbers involved are small.

SECTION IV. CHILDREN'S X-RAY HISTORIES

As already stated, the survey doctors had been told to record the illnesses of the children up to but not beyond the onset dates, these being defined as the dates on which the corresponding children first showed signs of the fatal disease. (In the following analyses the years before this date are referred to as the *pre-onset* period.) Since it was more likely that the mothers of the living children would mistakenly include events after this date than the mothers of dead children, we have in the following analyses discriminated carefully between accurately dated X-ray exposures and illnesses and those in which there was a margin of error. We will deal first with nonmedical X-ray and then with medical X-ray exposures, but pedoscope exposures will be mentioned in both parts.

Nonmedical X-Ray Exposure. Three non-medical sources of ionizing radiations were considered—television sets, luminous clocks or toys, and pedoscopes. Only one fact relating to these (undated) exposures has been analyzed—

namely, whether the child was ever exposed during the pre-onset period. For each of the three sources there was a slight excess on the control side. In the case of television sets (278 cases and 301 controls) and luminous objects (328 cases and 333 controls) the differences were negligible, and even for pedoscopes (212 cases and 242 controls) they were not significant (P approximately 1 in 7). As, however, the exposures were undated, it is possible that the few extra cases in the control side represent exposures which occurred after the onset date. The possible effects of this type of mistake on the pedoscope records are considered again at the end of this section.

Medical X-Ray Exposure. Records of diagnostic and therapeutic X-ray exposures were comparatively uncommon, but a slight excess was shown on the case side (see Table 15). The excess was confined to 11 children having radiotherapy (8 cases, 3 controls) and 167 children who had been radiographed on more than one occasion (90/77). For single radiographic examinations there was a slight deficiency of cases (88/100).

Tissue Sensitivity. When a child is X-rayed *in utero* it is safe to assume that the whole body has been exposed; but after birth this rarely happens. It was therefore appropriate to examine the records for an association between the parts of the body X-rayed after birth and subsequent developments. We have, however, searched the records in vain for any sign of this.

Estimate of Dose. No attempt was made to discover the number of films taken at each X-ray examination or to check the dose used in radiotherapy. The latter were all of the type to treat minor skin conditions, and no examples of deep X-ray treatments of the kind recently fol-

Table 15. Numbers of children with postnatal medical X-ray exposure.

Type of exposure	Leukemia		Other cancers		Total	
	Cases	Controls	Cases	Controls	Cases	Controls
Diagnostic:						
Once[a]	43	42	45	58	88	100
More than once	47	38	43	39	90	77
Therapeutic	5	1	3	2	8	3
Total	95	81	91	99	186	180

[a] Includes some children for whom the number of examinations was not ascertained.

lowed up by Simpson and Hempelmann (*11*) were recorded. The 11 children with histories of radiotherapy were all girls treated for naevi. The cases included five leukemias, one glioma, one neuroblastoma, and one sarcoma of the umbilicus (not the site exposed to X rays). At least eight of these children (possibly nine) were treated before their first birthday, and two (both cases) had already been X-rayed *in utero*.

Time Relationship

In view of the evidence already presented that a fetus may be specially radiosensitive, the postnatal X-ray exposures (diagnostic and therapeutic combined) were analyzed by age at first exposure (see Table 16) to discover whether there were any time relationships. Included in this Table are 67 children (27 cases, 40 controls) who have been classified as "age at first exposure unknown." These children were definitely X-rayed before the onset date, but the possible dates covered a period of more than 12 months. The remaining children included 128 where the month and year of the first X-ray exposure was known, and 171 where the date was given to within 12 months. In the latter group we have assumed that the actual date of exposure was midway between the two possible extremes and have placed the child accordingly. The last two columns of the Table (where all cases and all controls are compared) show a significant excess on the case side of children exposed before their third birthdays. This ex-

cess is greater for the leukemic children than for the children with other cancers. For first exposures between fourth and tenth birthdays the balance is on the control side, but the absolute and relative difference is small and may well be due to chance. In the interpretation of these figures much depends on the 67 children whose first exposures were inadequately dated. If the first exposure dates for these children were distributed in roughly the same way as in the dated series it would strengthen the impression of a genuine difference between early and later exposures, but if the distribution were markedly different it might have the opposite effect.

No such reservations need apply to the figures in Table 17. Here the children have been placed according to their age in years at the onset date, and only three children have had to be relegated to the "age unknown" category. In three of the five age groups there were more cases than controls, and in two there were more controls than cases, but the most striking case/control difference relates to children who were aged between 2 and 3 years at the onset date (58 cases, 27 controls).

A similar arrangement by age at the final date (which was usually within a few weeks or months of the onset date) also picked out children who died between the second and fourth birthdays (51 cases, 24 controls), and again the difference was more marked for leukemia than for other cancers. This is particularly interesting, since it is precisely this age group which has

Table 16. Distribution of children with postnatal medical X-ray exposure according to age at first X-ray exposure.

Age at first exposure	Leukemia				Other Malignant				Total			
	Cases		Controls		Cases		Controls		Cases		Controls	
0	19		12		23		13		42		25	
1	21	57	10	31	12	50	15	43	33	107	25	74
2	17		9		15		15		32		24	
3	6		4		10		13		16		17	
4	5		14		9		8		14		22	
5	5		9		5		6		10		15	
6	5	25	3	33	2	27	3	33	7	52	6	66
7	3		2		1		3		4		5	
8	1		1		0		0		1		1	
9	0		0		0		0		0		0	
Not known	13		17		14		23		27		40	
Total	95		81		91		99		186		180	

Table 17. Distribution of children with postnatal medical X-ray exposure according to age of the child at the onset date.

Age at onset date (years)	Leukemia		Other malignant		Total	
	Cases	Controls	Cases	Controls	Cases	Controls
0, 1	6	7	14	10	20	17
2, 3	35	11	23	16	58	27
4, 5	23	25	21	32	44	57
6, 7	17	22	17	27	34	49
8, 9	14	15	15	13	29	28
Not known	0	1	1	1	1	2
Total	95	81	91	99	186	180

[a] The onset date is defined as either the date of onset of the fatal illness (case children) or the date when the corresponding case developed its fatal illness (control children).

borne the brunt of the recent increase in childhood leukemia mortality both in this country and in the U.S.A.

Thus far the evidence in favor of a link between childhood malignancies and postnatal X-ray exposure has depended on case/control comparisons of arguable validity. We have therefore attempted to assess the evidence by means of comparisons within the case and the control series, using the following argument. In a "normal" group of children, such as our own controls, the percentage who have ever been X-rayed should steadily increase with age, for each year adds to the number of children who are X-rayed for the first time. For the sake of simplicity we shall assume that the percentage of "first" X-ray exposures is normally the same in each of the first ten years of life. In order to test this assumption we have calculated for the control children the "expected" percentages of children ever X-rayed in each of the five age groups shown in Table 17. In the first two columns of Table 18 these expected figures are shown in italics together with the actual percentages and numbers. It will be seen that the correspondence between the two sets of figures is not exact but lies well within the limits of chance fluctuation (P>0.1). It follows that the original assumption is a reasonable one. Now, if the postnatal X-ray exposure had *not* influenced the risk of the children dying later of malignant diseases, the correspondence between the actual and expected figures for the case series should be much the same as in the control series. But the discrepancies are much greater in the case series than in the control. Subdivision of the cases into leukemias and other cancers

shows that in the second age group of the leukemia series (which includes children who developed leukemia between their second and fourth birthdays) the proportion of "X-rayed children" is actually higher than the proportion in the third age group, although for these children the period during which they had an opportunity to be X-rayed was half as long again. For children with other cancers the largest discrepancy is in the first age group, where the actual number of children X-rayed (14) is nearly twice the expected number (7.43).

In earlier parts of this paper (and again in Section IV) we discuss evidence which indicates that the decisive factor in some of the cases, particularly in the leukemia series, dates back to a period well before birth. If this is so then there must be, in the newborn population, a number of children in what may be loosely called a "premalignant state." The present analysis of postnatal X-ray exposures suggests that if such children are X-rayed during infancy overt signs of the disease may appear relatively quickly.

This inference can be drawn from the tables already given, but is perhaps better illustrated by the distribution of cases and controls according to the interval between the first postnatal X-ray exposure and the final date. For children X-rayed in the first three years of life this was:

Interval, first exposure to the final date	Cases	Controls
Up to 11 months	12	11
12 to 47 months	62	26
Longer intervals	33	37

Table 18. Distribution (by age at onset date) of children with postnatal X-ray exposure compared with the distribution expected on the basis of a regular increase with age of the percentage of children ever X-rayed since birth.

Age of children at onset date (years)	Controls		All cases		Leukemia		Other cancers	
	Actual / Expected		Actual / Expected		Actual / Expected		Actual / Expected	
	%	No.	%	No.	%	No.	%	No.
0, 1	4.9 / 3.5	17 / 12.28	5.8 / 3.7	20 / 12.76	4.4 / 3.8	6 / 5.25	6.7 / 3.6	14 / 7.43
2, 3	7.2 / 10.6	27 / 40.03	15.4 / 11.0	58 / 41.61	17.9 / 11.4	35 / 22.37	12.7 / 10.7	23 / 19.30
4, 5	19.7 / 17.7	57 / 51.15	15.2 / 18.4	44 / 53.16	16.1 / 19.0	23 / 27.20	14.4 / 17.8	21 / 25.95
6, 7	25.9 / 24.8	49 / 46.83	18.0 / 25.8	34 / 48.67	18.3 / 26.6	17 / 24.77	17.7 / 24.9	17 / 23.89
8, 9	32.2 / 31.9	28 / 27.71	33.3 / 33.1	29 / 28.80	31.1 / 34.2	14 / 15.41	35.7 / 32.0	15 / 13.44
Total	13.8 / 13.8	178 / 178.00	14.4 / 14.4	185 / 185.00	15.4 / 15.4	95 / 95.00	13.4 / 13.4	90 / 90.01
$\chi^2_{(4)}$ Value of P	7.622 >0.10		19.414 <0.001		12.478 <0.02		11.015 <0.05	

This interpretation would also explain the deficiency on the case side of X-rayed children who developed the fatal disease between their fourth and eighth birthdays (see Table 17). For, if irradiation in infancy hastens overt signs of the disease, then there must be some "vulnerable" children who survive a comparatively long time partly because they have not been X-rayed. If this is so, we would expect the percentage of X-rayed children in the older half of the case series to be below the level for healthy children.

Pedoscopes

We must now reconsider the records for shoe-shop X-ray exposures. The same rays are emitted from pedoscope machines as from diagnostic X-ray sets. If, therefore, the medical X-ray examinations have had an effect, one would expect the pedoscope records to show the same signs. A possible reason for there being no such excess has already been mentioned—namely, inclusion on the control side of children whose first pedoscopic examination was later than the onset date. Another reason should now be apparent. The data on medical X-ray examina-

tions suggest a risk only when the first exposure takes place before the third birthday—that is to say, during a period when very few children will have had shoe-shop X-ray exposures. The relevant data cannot be analyzed by age at first exposure, but if the cases with pedoscope exposures are examined in relation to the age at death some suggestive figures emerge. Only seven children dying before the age of 2 had been X-rayed in a shoe-shop, but six of them had leukemia. The other pedoscope histories included 37 children who developed leukemia between 2 and 4 years of age (18 percent of such cases), but only 17 (or 10 percent) of the children who developed other cancers between these ages. Thus there is no inconsistency between the figures for medical and shoe-shop X-ray exposures.

Comment

To sum up: there are two reasons for thinking that X-ray films taken shortly after birth influence the distribution of childhood deaths from malignant disease. In the first place, there is a significant case excess for X-ray exposures during infancy. Secondly, children who died of leukemia at the age of 2 and 3 years were concentrated within the group of cases exposed to X rays in infancy. The effect of postnatal X-ray exposure appears to be more marked in respect of leukemia than other cancers and to be much weaker than the effect of prenatal X-ray exposure. It may in fact be restricted to speeding the date of death in children who are already predisposed to leukemia.

The lack of any association between the parts of the body exposed to X rays and subsequent developments may be related to the fact that in infancy the reticulo-endothelial system is so widespread that it is likely to be involved in any exposure.

SECTION V. CHILDREN'S ILLNESSES AND THEIR TREATMENT

In this section we consider: (1) congenital defects, (2) acquired diseases during the preonset period, and (3) two classes of drugs—sulphonamides and antibiotics. Again we discriminate between accurately dated illnesses and ones which might have happened after the onset date.

Congenital Defects

These were mentioned in 75 of the case and 46 of the control records, but only two conditions, mongolism and naevi, were more common among the cases.

Mongols. There were 17 mongols in the leukemia series, one among the other malignant disease, and none in the control group, though one child placed first on a control selection list was said to be a mongol and to have been in an institution since infancy, and was for this reason not chosen (see Section I). Until two years ago only four cases of leukemia associated with mongolism had been reported. Since then Krivit and Good (*12*), Merrit and Harris (*13*), Carter (*14*), and Paterson (*9*), have between them reported 13 cases. With the present series this makes a total of 34 reported cases. Since the incidence of mongolism in the present leukemia series (2.6 percent) is nearly 20 times as high as the incidence of mongolism in 14 000 consecutive births (*15*), the association is evidently not a fortuitous one. We have already shown that excessive maternal age at the time of the child's birth (which undoubtedly pre-

disposes to mongolism) also predisposes to leukemia (see Section I). It is therefore more likely that the two diseases are influenced by a common factor than that the antecedent condition, mongolism, predisposes to the later condition, leukemia. If this is so, then for some of the cases of leukemia the decisive event must date back at least to the onset of the mongolism; that is to say, at the latest to the second month of gestation. A number of facts relating to the mongols in the survey are shown in Table 19. The mongol who developed a glioma had been X-rayed 71 days before birth, but none of the mongols who died of leukemia had been irradiated *in utero*. Four mothers had had previous abortions, but there were no threatened abortions in the relevant pregnancy and no previous stillbirths. One mother was married to a second cousin.

Nevi. These were reported 34 times on the case side and 21 times on the control side. As previously stated, eight of the cases and three of the controls were treated with X rays. The overall difference between cases and controls is not statistically significant, and might be due to underreporting on the control side of a condition which is only cosmetically important. For girls there were 18 cases and 14 controls, and for boys 16 cases and 7 controls.

The other congenital defects took various forms and were evenly distributed between the two series, with 25 records on the case side and 25 on the control side.

Other Diseases of Childhood

It was clearly important to exclude all illnesses which happened after the onset date. This raised two problems: what to do with an illness which appeared to coincide with the onset of the fatal disease; and what to do with an inaccurately dated event which might or might not have preceded this date. An illustration of the first problem is provided by a case record which stated: "Following measles the child was always ailing. The measles was complicated by pneumonia then. . . ." In this case we should have placed the onset date immediately after the measles and excluded all subsequent events, even the so-called pneumonia.

The second problem arose when an illness was not more precisely dated than the year in which it happened or the age, in years, of the

Table 19. Features of the 18 mongols included in the survey.

Cause of death	Cell type (Leukemias)	Sex	Birth rank	Age at death		Age of mother[a]
Cerebral glioma	—	M	4	3 years	5 months	40
leukemia	Myeloid	M	7	2 years	11 months	44
"	"	M	2	1 year	2 months	44
"	Lymphatic	F	8	1 year	6 months	43
"	"	F	4	5 years	0 months	42
"	Myeloid	M	5	2 years	1 month	40
"	N/R	F	2	2 years	8 months	39
"	Lymphatic	M	3	1 year	11 months	38
"	"	M	2	4 years	9 months	36
"	Monocytic	M	2	5 years	11 months	34
"	Lymphatic	F	1	2 years	0 months	34
"	Myeloid	F	4	2 years	6 months	34
"	Lymphatic	F	1	2 years	0 months	32
"	"	F	2	1 year	5 months	32
"	Aleukemic	F	3	8 years	4 months	29
"	Lymphatic	M	1	6 years	5 months	26
"	Monocytic	M	1	4 years	6 months	26
"	Lymphatic	M	1·	6 years	11 months	19

[a] Age at birth of survey child.

child at the time. In such cases we have assumed that the event occurred midway between the limiting dates. It follows that an illness dated, say, "1953" would have been counted in the pre-onset period if the onset date was July 1 or later, but not otherwise. Similarly an illness occurring "at 4 years of age" would be counted in the pre-onset period if the onset date was 4 years and 6 months or over, but not otherwise.

It follows that, though some illness must have been wrongly placed, the errors in placing are likely to have canceled out, leaving an approximately correct total in the two series; where there was possible confusion between a previous illness and an early but unrecognized manifestation of the fatal disease, the illness has not been included in the following analyses.

In Table 20 the illnesses allocated to the pre-onset period have been classified as *recent* if within two years of the onset date, and *remote* if two or more years before this date. Events which could not be placed in one or other of these subgroups have been relegated to a separate column and are not included in the total of dated illnesses. The Table deals with illnesses, not injuries, and is restricted to relatively acute episodes which could be more or less precisely dated. A number of chronic diseases, injuries, operations, and ill-defined conditions not included in the Table are mentioned in the text.

The first part of Table 20 deals with the six

infectious diseases which comprise nearly 80 percent of all dated illnesses and of all illnesses in the *recent* period. The exclusion of cases of uncertain date has still left an excess on the control side, but this is slight and confined to three diseases—measles, chickenpox, and whooping-cough. As this comparison might have been affected by the deficit of first-born children in the control group, a rough standardization for birth rank was made. This had very little effect, particularly on the comparison between illnesses which happened within two years of the onset date, where the difference between cases and controls was mainly concentrated. Hence the popular idea that an infectious illness occasionally initiates a malignant process (or provokes a premalignant state) receives no support from the present survey. To argue the other way and say that the survey findings suggest an antagonism between exanthema and malignant diseases would also be wrong. Only in the *recent* period and for one disease (chickenpox) was there a significant excess of controls, and for this disease there was a deficiency of control records in the *remote* period, which reduces the overall excess to a nonsignificant level.

The second part of Table 20 shows that acute pulmonary infections were relatively uncommon, but for every three cases with such infections there were only two controls. In the *recent* period there were nearly twice as many records of acute bronchitis or pneumonia on the case side, and in the leukemia series (not distinguished in the Table) the case/control contrast was greater than in the other malignant series. Compared with all controls, the excess in the leukemia series was highly significant (P<0.001) and indicates in this series an "extra" 24 cases of acute bronchitis or pneumonia in the two years before the onset date. If this is accepted as evidence of a causal relationship, then about 4 percent of leukemia cases might be ascribed to a recent acute pulmonary infection. The corresponding figure (less than 2 percent) for other cancers was of borderline significance. Since there is no excess on the case side of acute pulmonary infections in the *remote* period, the recent infections are more likely to have accelerated overt signs of malignant diseases in vulnerable children than to have initiated the malignant process.

These estimates all relate to single acute episodes. A much smaller number of children were said to have recurrent attacks of bronchitis (often associated with teething), and these were also in the ratio of approximately three cases to two controls. Such reports are necessarily suspect and difficult to date, so the excess is less certainly a genuine finding. Nevertheless for three infections of the respiratory tract, which were suspect in the same way, there was an excess on the control side: these were "frequent colds" (242/295), "recurrent sore throat" (27/39), and "sinusitis" (10/21).

Clear-cut acute attacks of tonsillitis and otitis media are shown in the third part of Table 20. The slight excess of tonsillitis on the case side is confined to the *recent* period, and the figures for otitis media are roughly equal on the two sides. Not mentioned in the Table are 35 case children and 29 controls who had their tonsils removed within two years of the onset date, also 10 cases and 19 controls with chronically discharging ears.

The fourth part of Table 20 includes a number of illnesses which were either too rare or too

Table 20. Childhood illnesses in 1299 pairs of survey (M) and control (C) children.

	Illness within 2 years of onset date		Illness more than 2 Years before onset date		Total of dated illnesses		Additional illnesses of uncertain date	
	M	C	M	C	M	C	M	C
Measles	208	235	236	219	444	454	60	70
Chickenpox	131	173	125	102	256	275	46	55
Whooping cough	105	136	154	158	259	294	48	36
Mumps	57	61	45	38	102	99	10	22
Rubella	47	46	34	34	81	80	12	23
Scarlet fever	20	24	19	15	39	39	4	6
Total	568	675	613	566	1181	1241	180	212
Bronchitis	38	24	19	19	57	43	6	3
Bronchopneumonia	39	17	37	32	76	49	2	1
Total	77	41	56	51	133	92	8	4
Acute tonsillitis	30	22	14	12	44	34	1	4
Acute otitis media	20	25	15	9	35	34	0	2
Total	50	47	29	21	79	68	1	6
Other infections	88	54	65	47	153	101	12	9
Other illnesses	29	12	29	12	58	24	1	3
Total	117	66	94	59	211	125	13	12
Grand total	812	829	792	697	1604	1526	202	234

M = Survey children (all malignant diseases). C = Controls.

vaguely described to be considered separately. In both periods there was a marked excess on the case side, but since the risk of "inflated reporting" by bereaved mothers is probably at a maximum with minor or ill-defined conditions (which form the bulk of this section), we prefer to draw no conclusions from these figures. Trivial conditions not included in the Table are "feeding difficulties" (254 cases, 198 controls), allergic conditions (28 cases, 25 controls), worm infections (89 cases, 82 controls), and frequent colds (already mentioned). The even distribution of cases and controls for three of these four conditions does not suggest underreporting on the control side; it is therefore possible that the figures in the fourth section of Table 20 and the figures for recurrent attacks of bronchitis indicate a genuine excess on the case side.

Finally, some reference must be made to injuries and operations. A vast number of minor injuries, including bruises, were recorded, but only two types were regarded as important enough to merit analysis, and then only if they happened within two years of the onset date. In this period there were 44 fractures (26 cases, 18 controls) and 28 burns or scalds (16 cases, 12 controls). The case excess lay entirely within the leukemia series, and for the two items combined these children produced 28 records, compared with 14 for the children with other cancers. For recent operations, other than tonsillectomy, the figures were 16 cases and 17 controls.

In summary: Neither in their lifetime as a whole, nor in the two years immediately preceding the fatal illness, did the children with leukemia and other cancers have an excessive number of the common infectious diseases of childhood. If anything they experienced less chickenpox and fewer throat and ear infections than usual. On the other hand, the children with leukemia had a noticeable heavy incidence of acute pulmonary diseases and severe injuries during the two years before they showed signs of the fatal disease.

Sulphonamides and Antibiotics

There were three reasons why the interviewing doctors were specifically asked to record treatments with sulphonamides and antibiotics. In the first place, being new drugs, they might have contributed to the recent increase in leukemia mortality. Secondly, intensive treatment with sulphonamides occasionally causes aplastic anemia. Finally, it was thought that the mother would know, if not what exactly was given to the child, at least whether sulpha drugs or penicillin had been prescribed, and how these drugs had been administered.

In the following analyses we have omitted all local applications (drops, powders, and ointments) and made no distinction between oral and parenteral administrations. The conventions which were used to decide whether the drugs were actually given in the pre-onset period were the same as for the illnesses but, as Table 21 shows, there was a higher proportion of undated drugs than illnesses. This is due to the fact that in some of the records it was impossible to say which of the dated illnesses had been treated in this way. The Table reveals an even distribution of adequately dated treatments

Table 21. Treatment of children's illnesses with sulphonamides and antibiotics.

Treatments	Leukemia (619 pairs)		Other cancers (680 pairs)		Total (1299 pairs)		Case/control ratios
	Cases	Controls	Cases	Controls	Cases	Controls	
Sulphonamides:							
Adequately dated	94	96	84	61	178	157	1.13
Not adequately dated	30	18	26	34	56	52	1.08
Total	124	114	110	95	234	209	1.12
Antibiotics:							
Adequately dated	109	83	95	77	204	160	1.28
Not adequately dated	36	36	29	41	65	77	0.84
Total	145	119	124	118	269	237	1.14

with sulphonamides, but the corresponding figures for antibiotics show a small case excess. Since the high incidence of pulmonary infections on the case side was likely to have influenced these figures, Table 22 has been prepared in which the children who had such an illness in the two years before the onset date are shown separately. The effect of doing this is to reduce the case/control ratio for antibiotics from 1.28 (all treatments) to 1.18 (treatments other than those probably but not certainly related to a recent pulmonary infection). At this level it is within the conventional limits of chance fluctuation (P = approximately 1 in 15). The relatively high case/control ratio for both types of drugs in this Table probably reflects the fact (not yet mentioned) that in the case series these infections were usually more severe, as well as more numerous, than in the control series, and for this reason were more likely to receive antibiotics or sulphonamides.

A record was also kept of treatments with ultraviolet light. These were reported for 50 cases and 40 controls. No conclusions can be drawn from these small numbers.

We conclude that there is no evidence for a direct relationship between childhood malignancies and the drugs considered here. There may, however, be an indirect relationship between antibiotics and leukemia. In recent years antibiotics have revolutionized the prognosis for acute pulmonary infections and have undoubtedly kept alive children who would otherwise have died. If these infections occasionally provoke a latent leukemic process, then, by increasing the number of children who survive, antibiotics may indirectly increase the prevalence of leukemia.

SECTION VI. FEEDING HABITS AND HOME BACKGROUND OF THE SURVEY CHILD

Concern is often expressed about the widespread use of new chemicals, particularly food preservatives and detergents, on the grounds that these may be carcinogenic. In the present survey no attempt was made to collect information about exposure to specific chemicals, but the mothers were asked a number of questions about their own habits and what they allowed their children to eat and drink.

Feeding Habits

The survey doctors were told to ask whether the children had been given certain foods and drinks every day, less than daily but at least once a week, less often, or never. They were also asked to state when these foodstuffs were first given; and what the mother thought the child had consumed in the way of colored sweets. The completed records showed that a few control mothers had reported foods which were so unlikely to have been given during the pre-onset period—for example, fish and chips before the age of one—that the analysis has been restricted to case/control pairs for whom the age at the onset date was not less than an arbitrarily chosen "qualifying age" for each foodstuff (see Table 23).

The figures shown in this Table relate to children who had ever been given a food regardless of the reported frequency. In aggregate the case/control differences for the eight foodstuffs considered appear to be statistically significant (P<0.05), but only two foods—tinned vegetables and colored drinks—showed a significant difference, and both were reported more often

Table 22. Sulphonamide and antibiotic treatments, distinguishing children who had an acute pulmonary infection within two years of the onset date.

| | All cases | | All controls | | Ratio[a] |
	No.	%	No.	%	
Sulphonamide:					
Children who had acute pulmonary infection within two years of onset date	22/77	28.57	10/41	24.39	1.17
Remainder	156/1222	12.77	147/1258	11.69	1.09
Antibiotics:					
Children who had acute pulmonary infection within two years of onset date	36/77	46.75	13/41	31.71	1.48
Remainder	168/1222	13.75	147/1258	11.69	1.18

[a] Case/Control incidence ratio.

Table 23. Feeding habits; percentage of cases and controls who had ever taken certain foodstuffs.

Item	Qualifying age	% of children who had ever taken this item		$\chi^2_{(1)}$	P approx.
		Cases	Controls		
Dried milk	3 days	69.6	67.1	1.718	0.19
Fruit juice	1 month	90.6	90.7	0.002	0.96
Tinned sieved vegetables	4 months	61.1	58.2	1.976	0.16
Other tinned vegetables		55.1	60.6	6.797	0.009
Highly colored cakes		33.5	33.7	<0.001	>0.98
Highly colored fruit drinks	12 months	47.4	52.6	5.729	0.017
Colored sweets[a]		32.6	33.0	0.018	0.90
Shop-fried fish and chips		43.2	43.9	0.066	0.79
Total				16.306	0.05>P>0.02

[a] For this item "over" = more than ¼ lb. (113 g.) per week.

on the control than on the case side. For these two items the qualifying age may have been set too low, thus permitting some upward bias on the control side. If such bias exists, the case/control ratios for other items may have been underestimated, but the reported percentages are so nearly level that it is unlikely that any important differences have been missed.

The foodstuffs listed on Table 23 were also considered from the point of view of "dosage." Three of them showed a case excess in the highest consumption category:

Colored Cakes. Daily consumption of these was reported for 45 cases and 16 controls, but when this and the next-highest "dose" were combined the figures became 125 cases (11.3 percent) and 111 controls (10.0 percent).

Colored Sweets. At an estimated level of 12 oz. (340 g.) or more sweets per week there appeared to be an excess of cases (7.0 percent) over controls (4.4 percent), but this was balanced by an excess on the control side of children who usually ate between 3 and 12 oz. (85 and 340 g.) per week. As already shown, there was no deficiency of cases in the lowest consumption group.

Shop-Fried Foods. There was no difference in the proportion of cases and controls who had never had these foods, but consumption of fish and chips as often as once a week was reported by 191 cases and 140 controls. Once again the balance was made up by an excess of control children among those who occasionally had fish and chips.

In short, for none of the eight foodstuffs considered was there either a significant excess in the percentage of case children who had ever consumed them, or a consistent association between the amount consumed and subsequent events.

Other Factors

Contraception. An attempt was made to discover whether there had been any attempt at family planning and if so what methods had been used. The proportion of completed records for contraception (89 percent) was lower than for most items, but the numbers of case and control mothers who gave satisfactory answers were similar (1158 and 1143). Chemical contraceptives were used by 124 case mothers (10.7 percent of those giving full information) and 107 control mothers (9.4 percent). The small difference arose principally in the leukemia series, but these mothers did not differ significantly either from their own control pairs (P = approximately 0.21) or from the mothers of other cases (P = approximately 0.37).

Detergents. The percentage of case mothers who stated that they used synthetic detergents was 61.3 percent—very similar to, but slightly below, the figure of 63.6 percent for mothers of controls.

Smoking. Under this heading interviewers were asked to place the mother and father in one of the following categories: heavy, moderate, or light smokers, and nonsmokers (the instructions gave quantitative definitions for these four categories). The figures quoted here relate only to "smokers" (at least one cigarette or pipe a day) and "nonsmokers." The percentages of fathers and mothers in both series recorded as smokers were slightly higher than those recently reported for men and women of comparable age by Research Services Ltd. (*16*). For fathers of cases the proportion was 82.9 percent and for fathers of controls 80.9 percent, and for mothers 47.8 percent and 43.8 percent, respectively. These percentages indicate a significant ($P \approx 0.04$) excess among mothers of cases, but the difference is a small one (case/control ratio of 1.09), and we have not attempted to relate it to age, income, or number of children, as would be necessary before concluding that the mothers' smoking habits had affected their children. One factor which might well produce a genuine but irrelevant difference between mothers of cases and controls was, of course, the bereavement itself.

SECTION VII. FAMILY HISTORIES

Sibs. The records gave a complete tally of all the mothers' pregnancies up to the date of the interview, including those which ended with an abortion or stillbirth. As Table 24 shows, there was no case/control difference in respect of stillbirths, but the case excess for abortions is at least suggestive, particularly as it is concentrated (like the case excess for threatened abortions during the "relevant" pregnancy) in the leukemia series. The numbers of deaths among the liveborn sibs of the cases and controls were 132 and 129, respectively. This implies a very similar total mortality, since the numbers of liveborn sibs in the two series were almost equal (2119 and 2155) and the average number of years at risk was only slightly greater on the control side. Although most individual causes of death were equally common in the two series,

deaths from malignant disease among the case sibs numbered eight as against only two for the controls. On the basis of the relatively high national mortality rates in 1953–5, and without allowing for reduction of the population at risk by other deaths, the expected number of deaths from malignant disease among the sibs of the cases is 2.15. It follows that the total of eight malignant deaths on the case side is significantly higher than expectation ($P = 0.001$) (see Table 25). Even five cancer deaths—that is, after the exclusion of three cases which were not certainly cancers—namely, the "acute anemia," the "brain tumor," and the "growth in abdomen"—represent a significant case excess ($P < 0.05$).

Parents. One reason for not obtaining the first name on a control selection list was death of the mother; therefore, little meaning attaches to the excess of dead parents in the case series (20) as compared with the controls (5). Among nine dead parents in the leukemia series two had died of leukemia and one of lymphosarcoma. Among 11 dead parents in the other cancer series four had died of some form of malignant disease. One of the five deaths among parents of control children was attributed to leukemia and two to other malignant diseases.

Grandparents. A total of 4508 deaths of grandparents were reported. Judged by the proportions of deaths for which the cause was unknown or attributed to "senility," mothers gave better information about their own than about their husbands' parents, but there was no difference between the standard of information supplied by case and control mothers. Overall mortality was almost identical in the two series, the number of surviving grandparents being 2936 in the case and 2948 on the control side. Among 53 specified causes of death the largest proportional discrepancies between cases and

Table 24. **Miscarriages and stillbirths (up to the date of the survey child's death).**

	Leukemia		Other Cancers		Total	
	Cases	Con- trols	Cases	Con- trols	Cases	Con- trols
Mothers reporting abortions	129	93	119	118	248	211
Total no. of abortions	173	122	153	156	326	278
Mothers reporting stillbirths	26	23	27	23	53	46
Total no. of still births	26	28	32	25	58	53

Table 25. Siblings of cases with death attributed to malignant disease.

		Index case			Sibling	
Serial no.	Sex	Diagnosis	Age at death (years)	Sex	Diagnosis	Age at death (years)
122	F	Lymphosarcoma	6	M	"Acute anemia"	1
289	F	Acute lymphatic leukemia	1	F	Leukemia	1
290	F	Acute recticular leukemia	0	F	Leukemia	0
347	M	Acute lymphatic leukemia	5 {	M	Generalized lymphosarcoma	3
				M	Retroperitoneal sarcoma	2
476	F	" " "	5	M	"Brain tumor"	4
1293	F	Acute stem-cell leukemia	1	F	"Growth in abdomen"	2
1656	M	Neuroblastoma	1	M	Lymphatic leukemia	5

controls were war injuries (60/95) and renal conditions (32/54), the excess in each case being on the control side. For malignant diseases as a whole there was a proportionally smaller but significant excess on the case side, the totals being 387 for cases and 316 for controls. This excess ran uniformly through the records (Table 26). The proportion of case children with an affected grandparent varied very little between the main diagnoses in the case series. There was no detectable variation in the sex ratio of cases as between groups with an affected grandparent on the paternal or maternal side, nor when these relatives were subdivided into father's father, father's mother, etc. One tabulation which did appear to show some variation was that of the reported site of the cancer in the grandparents. For example, lung cancers in grandparents showed *no* excess of cases over controls (52/55), but a relatively high case/control ratio was observed for breast and genital cancers (cases 58, controls 37).

Uncles and Aunts. The total number of uncles and aunts was much the same for cases and controls (9578 for cases, 9425 for controls). Only deaths attributed to malignant disease were coded for these relatives, the numbers being: uncles and aunts of cases, 77; of controls, 55. The case/control ratio of 1.20 is almost identical with that for grandparents. In the case series there was no significant variation between the diagnostic subgroups, but the cancers in the uncles and aunts seemed to parallel two features noted in the grandparents. Thus cancers of the respiratory system showed no case excess (8/13), while breast and genital cancers showed a relatively large case excess (18/8).

Remoter Relatives. Rather more case mothers volunteered statements about cancer in relatives beyond the second degree than control mothers, and this revealed one interesting cancer pedigree. This concerned a boy who died at the age of six from "cancer of the liver and bowel" and had five relatives on the father's side who had also died of bowel cancer—the father himself, the grandfather, the greatgrandfather, and two aunts.

Consanguinity. The number of cousin marriages in the case series was not large either in relation to the controls or in relation to the frequency in the general hospital population (*17*). Of the 10 consanguineous matings reported in the case series, only 5 (0.4 percent) were between first cousins. To these should be added one case (not fully followed up and not included in the 1299 pairs) in which a father-daughter mating resulted in the birth of a girl who died at the age of 5 months from Letterer-Siwe's disease.

Table 26. Reports of malignant disease in grandparents of cases and controls.

	Cases	Controls	Ratio
Grandparents of leukemia series	172	140	1.23
Grandparents of other malignant series	215	176	1.22
All paternal grandparents	186	152	1.22
All maternal	201	164	1.23

Discussion

All scientific investigations are faced with the problem of eliminating unknown bias from test and control observations. Where, as in the present case, the findings are based on human data and involve comparisons between facts which have been obtained by different observers from inexpert witnesses the main sources of such bias are: (1) unequal recording of events by different observers; (2) unequal reporting of events by the individuals chosen to represent case and control groups; and (3) faulty selection of cases and/or controls.

The first source of error has been controlled by insisting on the same doctor seeing each member of a given case/control pair. By so doing, errors due to lack of skill in interviewing and recording should be equally represented on the case and control sides. The same device might be expected to control the second source of error; but here we were on less certain ground, and have therefore applied other tests of reliability. Thus for several items specified in the questionaries the proportions of completed records in the two samples have been calculated and found to be alike. To illustrate this point we have summarized the findings for six items in which a low response rate might, with some justification, have been expected (Table 27). By these criteria it would seem that the doctors were equally pertinacious when questioning the cases and controls, and the mothers were equally helpful when replying to the doctors' questions.

Other safeguards include repeated demonstration that significant differences between cases and controls are not compatible with any *general* tendency on the part of control mothers to be unduly forgetful or uncooperative. For instance, the case excess for two maternal diseases which might have affected fetal development—virus infections and threatened abortions in the relevant pregnancy—were not accompanied by a case excess for other maternal illnesses, either during this period or previously. Again, the case excess for pulmonary diseases in childhood must be viewed against a background of almost equal numbers of all childhood diseases in the two groups, and the case excess for X-ray exposure in infancy against almost equal numbers for postnatal X-ray exposure as a whole.

The third source of bias—namely, faulty selection of cases and controls—has been dealt with in the following ways. The cases were drawn from the total number of cases for a three-year period, and those actually included in the survey represent such a high proportion of this total that, however atypical the *lost cases* may be, the consequences would remain numerically unimportant. The controls were drawn from the general population of surviving children, thus avoiding some of the confusion which might have resulted from using more accessible children—for example, other hospital patients, children attending welfare clinics, or siblings of cases. The controls actually included in the survey have been shown to differ in two important respects (first-born children and twins) from the national population. But because the numbers in these classes can be calculated from official vital statistics, it has been possible to show that the deficiencies in the control group had a negligible effect on the main finding—namely, a large excess for direct fetal irradiation in the case series. We have also shown that this finding was not affected either by systematic checking of the mother's statements against hospital records, or by the publication of a preliminary report half-way through the survey. Finally, we already know

Tale 27. **Response of case and control mothers to certain questions.**

Items	Response rate (i.e., percentage of complete answers)	
	Cases	Controls
Family income	87	88
Contraception	88	89
Dated illnesses (children)	89	87
" (antibiotics and sulpha drugs) (children)	76	71
" post-natal X-ray exposure	85	78
Specific cause of death (grandparents)	82	81

that at least one independent observer has tested this main finding and used different methods to obtain virtually the same result.

We are therefore confident that the finding in respect of direct fetal irradiation is not an artifact. Nor have we any reason to doubt that there are genuine case/control differences in other respects—namely, maternal age at the time of conception, postnatal pulmonary infections, and X-ray exposure in infancy. All these factors appear to have a "causal" association with childhood malignancies, but we do not suggest that any one of them is either a necessary or a sufficient cause of the malignant changes. The special risks associated with these events may perhaps be compared with the well-known risk of being a male child. Thus boys are known to run a higher risk than girls of developing cancers, but no one ever cites the Y-chromosome as a "cause" of cancer. Nor do we claim that any of the associations are quantitatively important. The number of childhood malignancies which they might account for is small even in relation to the recent increase of these deaths reported during the last two decades—about 60 percent for children under five years (see *18*).

Summary and Conclusions

The prenatal and postnatal experiences of a large group of children who recently died of malignant diseases have been compared, point by point, with the experiences of a similar group of live children.

The frequency of three prenatal events—namely, direct fetal irradiation, virus infections, and threatened abortion—was significantly higher among the dead children than among the live children.

One other prenatal influence—namely, excessive maternal age—appears to increase the risk of leukemia in childhood and to be related to the fact that this disease and mongolism tend to occur together.

The frequency of three postnatal events—namely, X-ray exposures in infancy, acute pulmonary infections and severe injuries—was significantly higher for children who subsequently died of leukemia than for other children. In the "pre-antibiotic era" some of these children might have died before showing signs of the leukemia.

The health of the mothers and the home background of the children were not significantly different in the two groups, but there were minor points of difference in the family histories of cancer and leukemia.

Our final conclusions are that fetal irradiation does not account for the recent increase in childhood malignancies, but the finding of a case excess for this event does underline the need to use minimum doses for essential medical X-ray examinations and treatments.

A survey on the scale achieved could never have been contemplated without the active cooperation of doctors and health visitors too numerous to mention by name. Principal medical officers of health of local authority areas assumed responsibility for the field work of the investigation and completed the whole of their arduous and self-imposed task in the short space of 18 months. The interviews were done either by principal or by assistant medical officers of health, and health visitors did invaluable work in tracing cases and controls. We record with gratitude the high standard of the work in all regions.

We are also indebted to the Lady Tata Memorial Trust, which defrayed all costs other than those borne by the Health Departments and Oxford University; to the General Register Office, which provided essential data; to the Medical Research Council Working Party on Leukemia, who gave us constant encouragement and advice; and to the mothers of the dead children, who had the courage to reopen a painful topic and so often expressed the hope that by doing so they might be helping other children.

Finally, we thank two members of our own staff: Miss Dawn Giles, who, while holding the Mary Goodger Research Scholarship, helped with the organization of the survey and the coding of records, and W. E. C. Brooksbank, who was responsible for the machine sorting of the data.

References

(1) Hewitt, D. *Br J Prev Soc Med* 9:81, 1955.
(2) Registrar-General. Annual Statistical Review of England and Wales, 1953–5. Part 1 Tables, Medical. London, H.M.S.O., 1954–6.
(3) Stewart, A., J. Webb, D. Giles, and D. Hewitt. *Lancet* 2:447, 1956.
(4) Logan, W.P.D. and E.M. Brooke. *The Survey of Sickness, 1943–1952.* General Register Office Studies on Medical and Population Subjects, No. 12. London, H.M.S.O., 1957.

(5)   Registrar-General. Annual Statistical Review of England and Wales, 1943–55. Part II Table, Civil. London, H.M.S.O., 1945–56.

(6)   Manning, M.D. and B.E. Carroll. *J Natl Cancer Inst* 19:1087, 1957.

(7)   Court-Brown, W.M. and R. Doll. *Spec Rep Med Res Counc (Lond).* No. 295. London, H.M.S.O., 1957.

(8)   Faber, M. Radiation-induced leukemia in Denmark. In *Advances in Radiobiology.* London, Oliver and Boyd, 1957.

(9)   Paterson, J.C.S. Personal communication, 1958.

(10)   World Health Organization. *Manual of the International Statistical Classification of Diseases, Injuries, and Causes of Death.* 6th revision, 1948. London, H.M.S.O., 1949.

(11)   Simpson, C.L. and L.H. Hempelmann. *Cancer* 10:42, 1957.

(12)   Krivit, W. and R.A. Good. *Am J Dis Child* 91:218, 1956.

(13)   Merrit, D.H. and J.S. Harris. *Am J Dis Child* 92:41, 1956.

(14)   Carter, C.O. *Br Med J* 2:993, 1956.

(15)   Malpas, P. *J Obstet Gynecol Br Emp* 44:434, 1937.

(16)   Todd, G.F. (Ed.). *Statistics of Smoking.* Research paper No. 1. London, Tobacco Manufacturers Standing Committee, 1957.

(17)   Bell, J. *Ann Eugen (Lond)* 10:370, 1940.

(18)   McKenzie, A., R.A.M. Case, and J.T. Pearson. *Cancer Statistics for England and Wales, 1901–1955.* General Register Office Studies on Medical and Population Subjects. No. 13. London. H.M.S.O., 1957.

(19)   Registrar-General. Decennial Supplement, England and Wales, 1951. Occupational Mortality, Part 1. London, H.M.S.O., 1954.

STATISTICAL ASPECTS OF THE ANALYSIS OF DATA FROM RETROSPECTIVE STUDIES OF DISEASE

Nathan Mantel and William Haenszel[1]

SUMMARY

The role and limitations of retrospective investigations of factors possibly associated with the occurrence of a disease are discussed and their relationship to forward-type studies emphasized. Examples of situations in which misleading associations could arise through the use of inappropriate control groups are presented. The possibility of misleading associations may be minimized by controlling or matching on factors which could produce such associations; the statistical analysis will then be modified. Statistical methodology is presented for analyzing retrospective study data, including chi-square measures of statistical significance of the observed association between the disease and the factor under study, and measures for interpreting the association in terms of an increased relative risk of disease. An extension of the chi-square test to the situation where data are subclassified by factors controlled in the analysis is given. A summary relative risk formula, R, is presented and discussed in connection with the problem of weighting the individual subcategory relative risks according to their importance or their precision. Alternative relative-risk formulas, R_1, R_2, R_3, and R_4, which require the calculation of subcategory-adjusted proportions of the study factor among diseased persons and controls for the computation of relative risks, are discussed. While these latter formulas may be useful in many instances, they may be biased or inconsistent and are not, in fact, averages of the relative risks observed in the separate subcategories. Only the relative-risk formula, R, of those presented, can be viewed as such an average. The relationship of the matched-sample method to the subclassification approach is indicated. The statistical methodology presented is illustrated with examples from a study of women with epidermoid and undifferentiated pulmonary carcinoma.

INTRODUCTION

A retrospective study of disease occurrence may be defined as one in which the determination of association of a disease with some factor is based on an unusually high or low frequency of that factor among diseased persons. This contrasts with a forward study in which one looks instead for an unusually high or low occurrence of the disease among individuals possessing the factor in question. Each approach has its advantages. Among the desirable attributes of the retrospective study is the ability to yield results from presently collectible data, whereas the forward study usually requires future observation of individuals over an extended period (this is not always true; if the status of individuals can be determined as of some past date, the data for a forward study may already be at hand). The retrospective approach is also adapted to the limited resources of an individual investigator and places a premium on the formulation of hypotheses for testing, rather than on facilities for data collection. For especially rare diseases a retrospective study may be the only feasible approach, since the forward study may prove too expensive to consider and the study size required to obtain a respectable number of cases completely unmanageable.

Source: *Journal of the National Cancer Institute* 22(4):719-747, 1959.
[1] Biometry Branch, National Cancer Institute, Bethesda, Maryland; National Institutes of Health, Public Health Service, U.S. Department of Health, Education, and Welfare.

In the absence of important biases in the study setting, the retrospective method could be regarded, according to sound statistical theory, as the study method of choice. This follows from the much reduced sample sizes required by this approach and may be illustrated by the following extreme example. If a disease attack rate of 10 per 100 000 among 50 percent of the population free of some factor were increased tenfold among the other half of the population subject to the factor, a retrospective study of 100 cases and 100 controls would, with high probability, reveal this significantly increased risk. On the other hand, a forward study covering 2000 persons, half with and half without the factor, would almost certainly fail to detect a significant difference. For comparable ability to find the type of increased risk just indicated, a forward study would need to cover about 500 times as many individuals as the corresponding retrospective study. The disparity in the required number of persons to be studied could, of course, be reduced by lengthening the follow-up period for forward studies to increase the experience in terms of person-years observed. The larger sample size required for the forward study reflects principally the infrequent occurrence of the disease entity under investigation. In the example illustrated, uncovering 100 cases of disease in a forward study would require either 100 000 individuals with the factor or 1 million without. For diseases with a higher probability of occurrence the disparity in required size between retrospective and forward studies would be progressively reduced.

The retrospective study might be looked upon as a natural extension of the practice of physicians since the time of Hippocrates, to take case histories as an aid to diagnosis. Its guise has varied with respect to the means of measuring the prevalence of the suspect factor among diseased persons and the criteria for determining unusual departures from normal experience. When an association is so marked, as in Percival Pott's observations on the representation of chimney sweeps among cases of scrotal cancer, no further quantitative data are required to perceive its significance.

The retrospective approach has often been employed in studies of communicable diseases, one illustration being Snow's observations (1) on a common water supply for cholera cases in an area served by several sources (there would have been no element of unusualness had there been but one water supply). When a disease is epidemic in a circumscribed locality, the disease-free population in the same area offers a natural contrast. The method may be used successfully for endemic diseases as well. Holmes, in reaching his conclusions on the communicable nature of puerperal fever (2), noted particularly that a large number of women with puerperal fever had been attended by the same physicians. In this context it should be emphasized that communicable disease investigations have often combined retrospective and forward study methods. For example, Snow supplemented his retrospective observations on water supply by a contrast of cholera rates among subscribers of the Southwark and Vaûxhall water company with the experience of persons served by the Lambeth water company within the same area.

When a disease occurs sporadically, or its occurrence is not confined to a well-defined group (such as women at childbirth), a choice of controls is not immediately evident. For cancer and other diseases characterized by high fatality rates, a study restricted to decedents might use persons dying from other causes as controls. Rigoni Stern adopted this technique in deducing the relationship of cancer of the breast and of the uterus to pregnancy history (3). Some contemporary studies have also used deaths from other causes as controls (4, 5).

The present-day controlled retrospective studies of cancer date from the Lane-Claypon paper on breast cancer published in 1926 (6). This report is significant in setting forth procedures for selecting matched hospital controls and relating them to a consideration of study objectives. Retrospective techniques have since been applied in several investigations of cancer, including the following partial list of current references for a few primary sites: bladder (7-10), breast (11-13), cervix (13-16), larynx (17, 18), leukemia (19), lung (18, 20-27), and stomach (13, 28-30).

Statisticians have been somewhat reluctant to discuss the analysis of data gathered by retrospective techniques, possibly because their training emphasizes the importance of defining a universe and specifying rules for counting events or drawing samples possessing certain properties. To them, proceeding from "effect to cause," with its consequent lack of specificity of a study population at risk, seems an unnatural approach. Certainly, the retrospective study raises some questions concerning the representative nature of the cases and controls in a given situation which cannot be completely satisfied by internal examination of any single set of data.

Only a few published papers have treated the statistical aspects of retrospective studies. Cornfield discussed the problem in terms of estimated measures of relative and absolute risks arising from contrasts of persons with and without specified characteristics (*31*). His paper was concerned with the simple situation of a homogeneous population of cases and controls, presumably alike in all characteristics except the one under investigation, which could be represented by a single contingency table. In a later contribution he handled the problem of controlling for other variables by adjusting the distribution of controls to the observed distribution of cases (*16*). Dorn briefly mentions retrospective studies with emphasis on such topics as sources of data, choice of controls, and validity of inferences (*32*).

This paper presents a method for computing relative risks for retrospective study contrasts, which controls for the effects of other variables by use of the basic statistical principle of subclassification of data. The related problem of significance testing is also considered. Since details of statistical treatment are conditioned by study objectives, data collection methods, choice of a control series, and the use of matched or unmatched controls, these topics are also discussed briefly.

OBJECTIVES

Restrospective studies are relatively inexpensive and can play a valuable role as scouting forays to uncover leads on hitherto unknown effects, which can then be explored further by other techniques. The effects may be novel and not suggested by existing data, as in the pioneer work on the association of smoking and lung cancer or the association of blood type and gastric cancer, or they may represent refinements of current knowledge. The latter category might include collection of lifetime residence and/or work histories to elaborate differences in incidence and mortality which appear when some diseases are classified by last place of residence or last occupation of the newly diagnosed case or decedent.

With diseases of low incidence the controlled retrospective study may be the only feasible approach. Here emphasis should be placed on assembling results from several studies. Before accepting a finding and offering an interpretation, scientific caution calls for ascertaining whether it can be reproduced by others and in other administrative settings having their own peculiar biases.

A primary goal is to reach the same conclusions in a retrospective study as would have been obtained from a forward study, if one had been done. Even when observations for a forward study have been collected, a supplementary retrospective approach to the same body of material may prove useful in collecting more data on points not covered in the original study design or in amplifying suggestive associations appearing in the initial forward-study results.

The findings of a retrospective study are necessarily in the form of statements about associations between diseases and factors, rather than about cause and effect relationships. This is due to the inability of the retrospective study to distinguish among the possible forms of association—cause and effect, association due to common causes, etc. Similar difficulties of interpretation arise in forward studies as well. A forward study, to avoid these difficulties, would need to be performed with the preciseness of a laboratory experiment. For example, such a study of associations with cigarette smoking would require that an investigator randomly assign his subjects in advance to the various smoking categories, rather than simply note the categories to which they belong. The inherent practical difficulties of such an enterprise are evident.

In addition to the failings shared with the forward study, the retrospective study is further exposed to misleading associations arising from the circumstances under which test and control subjects are obtained. The retrospective study picks up factors associated with becoming a diseased or a disease-free *subject*, rather than simply factors associated with presence or absence of the disease. The difficulties in this regard may be most pronounced when the study group represents a cross section of patients alive at any time (prevalence), including some who have been ill for a long period. Inclusion of the latter may lead to identification of items associated with the course of the illness, unrelated to increased or decreased risk of developing the disease. The theoretical point has been raised that factors conducive to longer survival of patients may be found in "prevalence" samples and interpreted erroneously as being associated with excess liability to the disease (*33*). Loopholes of this type are minimized when investigations are restricted to samples of newly diagnosed patients (incidence).

A partial remedy for these uncertainties lies in employing a conservative approach to interpretation of the associations observed. Recognizing the ease with which associations may be influenced by extraneous factors, the investigator may require not only that the measure of relative risk be significantly different from unity but also that it be importantly different. He may, for instance, require that the data indicate an increased relative risk for a characteristic of at least 50 percent, on the assumption that an excess of this magnitude would not arise from extraneous factors alone. However, the use of such conservative procedures emphasizes a corresponding need to pinpoint the disease entity under study. A strong relationship between a factor and a disease entity might fail to be revealed, if the entity was included in a larger, less well-defined, disease category. After the event from data now at hand, we know that a study of the association of cigarette smoking with epidermoid and undifferentiated pulmonary carcinoma is more revealing than an inquiry covering all histologic types of lung cancer.

MULTIPLE COMPARISON PROBLEM

The present-day retrospective study is usually concerned with investigating a variety of associations with a disease, little effort being involved in acquiring, within limits, added information from respondents. The results may be analyzed in a number of ways: the various factors may be investigated separately, without regard to the other factors; they may be investigated in conjunction with each other, a particular conjunction being considered a factor in its own right; or, more commonly, a factor may be tested with control for the presence or absence of other factors. Thus, if the roles of cigarette smoking and coffee drinking in a given disease are under study, the possible comparisons include the relative risk of disease for

individuals who both smoke and drink as opposed to all other persons, or as opposed to those who neither smoke, nor drink coffee. In addition, the relative risk associated with smoking might be obtained separately for drinkers and nondrinkers of coffee, with a weighted average of these two relative risks constituting still another item. Conversely, risks associated with coffee drinking, with adjustments for cigarette smoking, could be computed.

The potential comparisons arising from a comprehensive retrospective study can be large. Almost any reasonable level of statistical significance used to test a single contrast, when applied to a long series of contrasts, will, with a high degree of probability, result in some contrasts testing significant, even in the absence of any real associations. The usual prescription for coping with this multiple comparison problem—requiring individual comparisons to test significant at an extreme probability level to reduce the number of associations incorrectly asserted to be true—would result only in making real associations difficult to detect.

However, the multiple comparison problem exists only when inferences are to be drawn from a single set of data. If the purpose of the retrospective study is to uncover leads for fuller investigation, it becomes clear there is no real multiple significance testing problem—a single retrospective does not yield conclusions, only leads. Also, the problem does not exist when several retrospective and other type studies are at hand, since the inferences will be based on a collation of evidence, the degree of agreement and reproducibility among studies, and their consistency with other types of available evidence, and not on the findings of a single study.

Nevertheless, it would be wise to employ testing procedures which do not lead to a superabundance of potential clues from any one study. This may be achieved by employing nominal significance levels in testing factors of primary interest incorporated into the design of an investigation and applying more stringent significance tests to comparisons of secondary interest or to comparisons suggested by the data. For the usual problem of multiple significance testing, this would be equivalent to allocating a large part of the desired risk of erroneous acceptance of an association as real to a small group of comparisons where fruitful results were anticipated, and parceling out the remainder of the available risk to the large bulk of comparisons of a more secondary nature. This minimizes the risk of diluting, through inclusion of many secondary comparisons, the chances for detecting an important primary effect.

REPRESENTATIVE NATURE OF DATA

The fundamental assumption underlying the analysis of retrospective data is that the assembled cases and controls are representative of the universe defined for investigation. This obligates the investigator not only to examine the data which are the end product but also to go behind the scenes and evaluate the forces which have channeled the material to his attention, including such items as local practices of referral to specialists and hospitals and the patient's condition and the effect of these items on the probability of diagnosis or hospital admission. We reemphasize that this requires the exercise of judgment on the potential magnitude of biases and as to whether they could result in factors seeming to be related to a disease, in the absence of a real association of the factor with presence or absence of the disease. The danger of bias may be greatest in working with material from a single diagnostic source or institution.

Among the more important practical considerations affecting retrospective studies is that they are ordinarily designed to follow the line of least resistance in obtaining case and control histories. This means that cases and controls will often be hospital patients rather than persons in the general population outside hospitals. As a result, any factor which increases the probability that a diseased individual will be hospitalized for the disease may mistakenly be found to be associated with the disease. For example, Berkson (34) and White (35) have pointed out that positive association between two diseases, not present in the general population, may be produced when hospital admissions alone are studied, because persons with a combination of complaints are more likely to require hospital treatment. In theory, bias might also be produced in reverse manner, if the suspect factor diminished the probability of hospitalization for other diagnoses used as controls. The difficulties are not unique for hospital patients. Similar loopholes in interpretation

may be advanced for any special groups used as sources of cases and controls.

However, a mere catalogue of biases arising from the possibly unrepresentative nature of a sample of cases and controls should not *ipso facto* invalidate any study findings. This is a substantive issue to be resolved on its merits for a specific investigation. Collateral evidence may provide information on the potential magnitude of bias and the size of spurious associations which could result. In some situations the difference between cases and controls may be so great that postulation of an unreasonably large bias would be required. Whether he consciously recognizes it or not, the investigator must always balance the risks confronting him and decide whether it is more important to detect an effect, when present, or to reject findings, when they may not reflect the true situation. If opportunities for further testing exist, one should not be too hasty in rejecting an association as an artifact arising from the method of data collection, and in foreclosing exploration of a potentially fruitful lead.

Because of the important role retrospective studies play in studies of human genetics, mention may be made of a bias frequently encountered in studies dealing with the familial distribution of diseases. A frequently used procedure takes a group of diagnosed cases for a disease in question and a group of controls and compares the prevalence of this disease among relatives of the probands and controls. The bias arises from the unrepresentative nature of the probands with respect to familial distribution and is known in other fields as "the problem of the index case" or "the effect of method of ascertainment." It has long been recognized that the characteristics for a random sample of families will differ from those for families to whom the investigator's attention has been directed because the family rosters include individuals selected for study on the basis of a specified attribute. For example, data on family size (number of children) obtained from siblings, rather than parents, are biased, since two or three potential index cases are present in the population for two- and three-child families as opposed to one for one-child families and none for childless couples. The analogy for disease occurrence is apparent. Families with two or three cases of the disease under study may have double or triple the probability of being represented by individuals in source material and having a representative selected as a proband than families with only one case. An appropriate analysis for this situation in studies of family size and birth order has been discussed by Greenwood and Yule (*36*), which takes account of the probability of family representation in proband data. Haenszel (*37*) has applied their correction to gastric-cancer data reported by Videbaek and Mosbech (*38*) and found the correction to reduce the originally reported fourfold excess of gastric cancer among relatives of probands, as compared to relatives of controls, to one of about 60 percent.

One remedy for the weakness of the retrospective approach to problems involving association of diseases and familial distribution would be to place greater reliance on forward observations of defined cohorts for data on these topics.

CONTROLS

While easier accessibility to and lesser expense of hospital controls are important considerations, they should not deter one from collecting control data for a sample representing a more general population, if the latter are demonstrably superior. Some of the uncertainties about the superiority of hospital or general population controls arise from the need to maintain comparability in responses. The dependence of retrospective studies on comparability of responses from cases and controls cannot be overemphasized. When more accurate answers can be obtained from controls in a medical-care environment, the gain in comparability of responses for these controls could outweigh the other advantages to be derived from the more representative nature of general population controls. The difficulties may be illustrated by the experience with smoking histories. Hospital controls invariably yield a higher proportion of smokers for each sex than controls of comparable age drawn from the general population (*27*). Does this mean more complete smoking histories are collected in hospitals or does it imply that smokers have higher hospital admission rates? If the first alternative is correct, hospital controls are the appropriate choice for measuring the association of smoking history with a given disease. The second alternative calls for general population controls and

in this situation the use of hospital controls yields underestimates of the degree of association.

Dual hospital and general population controls would have some merit. If control data from the two sources were in agreement, this would rule out some alternative interpretations of the findings. In the event of disagreement, its extent could be measured and alternate calculations made on the degree of association between an event and a suspect antecedent characteristic. Where the two sets of controls lead to substantially different results, a cautious and conservative interpretation is indicated.

Some topics, such as those bearing on sex practices and use of alcohol, may be amenable to study only within a clinical setting, and the collection of general population data on these items may prove impractical. The limitations of general population controls in this regard may have been overstressed, and empirical trials to test what information can be collected in household surveys should be encouraged instead of dismissing the possibility with no investigation whatsoever. Whelpton and Freedman, for example, have reported some success in collecting histories of contraceptive practices in interviews of a random sample of housewives (*39*).

When hospital controls are chosen, some precautions may be built into the study. Within limitations on the nature of controls imposed by a study hypothesis, controls drawn from a wide variety of diseases or admission diagnoses should be preferred. This permits examination of the distribution of the study characteristics among subgroups to check on internal consistency or variation among controls. This affords protection against two sources of error: *a*) attributing an association to the disease under investigation, when the effect is really linked to the diagnosis from which controls were drawn, and *b*) failure to detect an effect because both the study and control diseases are associated with the suspect factor. The latter is far from impossible. Both tuberculosis and bronchitis have exhibited association with smoking history and the use of one disease or the other as a control could easily lead to missing the association with smoking history. Similarly, patients with coronary artery disease would not constitute suitable controls for a study of the relationship of smoking and bladder cancer and *vice versa*, since the investigator would probably conclude that smoking was not related to either disease, when in truth it appears related to both. When there is definite evidence that two diseases are associated, for example, pernicious anemia and stomach cancer, the use of one as a control for the other is contraindicated, unless the study is specially designed to elucidate some aspects of the relationship.

It is always advantageous to include several items in a questionnaire for which general population data are available. This could be considered a partial substitute for dual hospital and general population controls. Disparity among cases, hospital controls, and general population controls on several general characteristics unrelated to the study hypothesis may be regarded as warning signals of the unrepresentative nature of the hospital cases and controls.

Where possible, interviews should be conducted without knowledge of the identity of cases and controls to guard against interviewer bias, although administrative reasons will often prevent attainment of "blind" interviews. In cooperative studies employing several interviewers, the magnitude of interviewer bias may be diminished, since it is unlikely that all interviewers will share the same bias in concert. In special circumstances, such as those prevailing at Roswell Park Memorial Institute, admissions may be interviewed before diagnosis, and hence before the identity of cases and controls is established. This feature requires a comprehensive, general purpose interview routinely administered to all admissions, which may restrict its use to publicly supported institutions diagnosing and treating neoplastic diseases or other specialized disease entities. Several epidemiological contributions for specific cancer sites have been based on the unique control data available from Roswell Park Memorial Institute (*9, 11, 12, 30, 40-43*), which are particularly valuable for collation with studies depending on more conventional sources of controls to evaluate interviewer bias and related issues.

Some patients interviewed as diagnosed cases will subsequently have their diagnoses changed. This may be turned to advantage. If scrutiny of the data for the erroneously diagnosed group reveals they had histories resembling those for the control rather than the case series, as Doll and Hill found in their study of smoking and lung cancer (*21*), this would constitute evidence against interviewer bias.

In investigations of a cancer site the association of a factor may often be restricted to a specific histologic type or a well-defined portion of an organ. The finding that epidermoid and undifferentiated pulmonary carcinoma is more strongly related to smoking history than adenocarcinoma of the lung is now well established. The range of explanations for the observed deficit of epidermoid carcinoma of the cervix in Jewish women as compared to other white women is greatly circumscribed by the presence of about equal numbers of adenocarcinoma of the corpus in both groups. When these finer diagnostic details or their significance are unknown to the interviewer, another check on interviewer bias is provided. Furthermore, the confirmation in repeated studies of an association limited to a specific histologic type or a detailed site will lend credence to an etiological interpretation of the association. Repeated confirmation is an essential element. Otherwise, a very specific association may be a reflection of the multiple comparison problem; if enough contrasts are created by fractionation of a single set of data, some apparently significant result is likely to appear. For this reason it would be desirable to reproduce such provocative results as Wynder's finding that use of alcohol was more strongly associated with cancer of the extrinsic larynx than of the intrinsic larynx (*18*), and Billington's report that prepyloric and cardiac neoplasms of the stomach were associated with blood group A and those located in the fundus with blood group O (*44*).

Discussion of matched controls in relation to the analysis and the computation of relative risks is deferred to a later section. One consideration on matched controls arising in the planning and development of a study should be mentioned here. Obviously, if the risk of disease changes with age an apparent association of the disease with other age-related factors may result. Other apparent associations with race, sex, nativity, etc., may arise in a similar manner. In devising rules for selecting controls, those factors known or strongly suspected to be related to disease occurrence should be taken into account if unbiased and more precise tests of the significance of the factors under investigation are desired. A sensible rule is to match those factors, such as age and sex, the effect of which may be conceded in advance and for which strong evidence is available from other sources, such as mortality data and morbidity surveys. When a factor is matched, however, it is eliminated as an independent study variable; it can be used only as a control on other factors. This suggests caution in the amount of matching attempted. If the effect of a factor is in doubt, the preferable strategy will be not to match but to control it in the statistical analysis. While the logical absurdity of attempting to measure an effect for a factor controlled by matching must be obvious, it is surprising how often investigators must be restrained from attempting this.

When a minimum of matching is involved, the importance of establishing, precisely and in advance, the method by which controls are selected for study increases. The rule should be rigid and unambiguous to avoid creating effects by subconscious selection and manipulation of controls. The problem is similar to that encountered in therapeutic trials where a protocol spelling out all the contingencies and actions to be taken in advance is, along with random assignment of cases and controls, the major bulwark against bias.

To reduce interview time and expense there are advantages in procedures for selecting controls which permit a case and the corresponding controls to be interviewed in a single session, particularly if travel to several institutions is involved. In practice, this favors selecting controls from a hospital patient census rather than from hospital admission lists. The difficulty with hospital admissions is that there is no guarantee that the controls will be available in the hospital at the time the diagnosed case is interviewed. This point seems more important than the fact that patients with diagnoses requiring long-term stays are overrepresented in a current hospital census (*45*). If the latter is an important issue, it may be handled in analysis through subclassification of controls by diagnosis.

Normally there will be little difficulty in reconciling these considerations into a harmonious set of rules. The items to be matched often lend themselves to a procedure for specifying controls. In a recent study on female lung cancer we found that the definition of two controls as the next older and the next younger women in the same hospital service, present on the day the case was interviewed, met the requirements just outlined (*27*). The controls were uniquely defined, the records establishing their identity were readily available on the service floor, inter-

views could be completed in one day, and a provision for balancing ages of cases and controls was incorporated. Simultaneous interviews of cases and controls may be more than an administrative convenience. If the prevalence of the associated factor is rapidly shifting over time, failure to control time of interview could obscure or exaggerate an association.

SOME STATISTICAL TOOLS

To progress further, questions on the representative nature of the case and control series must have been resolved affirmatively. With this condition in mind, let us suppose that a controlled retrospective study has been conducted and that the number of diseased cases, N_1, consists of A individuals with the factor being investigated and B free of the factor, while the number of controls, N_2, consists of C individuals with, and D individuals without, the factor. Let $M_1 = A + C, M_2 = B + D, T = N_1 + N_2 = M_1 + M_2 = A + B + C + D$. What statistical evidence is there for the presence of an association and what is an appropriate measure of the strength of the association?

A commonly employed statistical test of association is the chi-square test on the difference between the cases and controls in the proportion of individuals having the factor under test. A corrected chi square may be calculated routinely as

$$(|AD - BC| - \tfrac{1}{2}T)^2 T / N_1 M_1 N_2 M_2$$

and tested as a chi square with 1 degree of freedom in the usual manner.

A suggested measure of the strength of the association of the disease with the factor is the apparent risk of the disease for those with the factor, relative to the risk for those without the factor. Consider that a population falls into the four possible categories and in the proportions indicated by the following table:

	With factor	Free of factor	Total
With disease	P_1	P_2	$P_1 + P_2$
Free of disease	P_3	P_4	$P_3 + P_4$
Total	$P_1 + P_2$	$P_3 + P_4$	1

The proportion of persons with the factor having the disease is $P_1/(P_1 + P_3)$, while the corresponding proportion for those free of the factor is $P_2/(P_2 + P_4)$. Relatively then, the risk of the disease for those with the factor is $P_1(P_2 + P_4)/P_2(P_1 + P_3)$. On a sampling basis this quantity may be estimated either by drawing a sample of the general population and estimating P_1, P_2, P_3, and P_4 therefrom or estimating $P_1/(P_1 + P_3)$ and $P_2/(P_2 + P_4)$ separately from samples of persons with, and persons free of, the factor.

It may be noted, however, that if the relative risk as defined equals unity, then the quantity P_1P_4/P_2P_3 will also equal unity. Further, for diseases of low incidence where the values for P_1 and P_2 are small in comparison with P_3 and P_4 it follows, as has been pointed out by Cornfield (*31*), that P_1P_4/P_2P_3 is also a close approximation to the relative risk. This latter approximate relative risk can properly be estimated from the two sample approaches described or from samples drawn on a retrospective basis; that is, separate samples of persons with, and persons free of, the disease. The sample proportions of persons with, and free of, the factor in the retrospective approach provide estimates of $P_1/(P_1 + P_2)$ and of $P_2/(P_1 + P_2)$ from the sample having the disease and of $P_3/(P_3 + P_4)$ and of $P_4/(P_3 + P_4)$ from the disease-free sample. The estimate of P_1P_4/P_2P_3 is obtained by appropriate multiplication and division of these four quantities.

Whichever of the three methods of sampling is employed, the estimate of the approximate relative risk, P_1P_4/P_2P_3, reduces simply to *AD/BC*, where A, B, C, and D are defined in the manner stated in the first paragraph of this section. Also, the chi-square test of association given, which is essentially a test of whether or not the relative risk is unity, is equally applicable to all three sampling methods.

In the foregoing the two basic statistical tools of the epidemiologist for retrospective studies, the chi-square significance test and the measure of a relative risk, have been described for a relatively simple situation, one in which to all intents there is a single homogeneous population. The more complex situations confronting the epidemiologist in actual practice and the corresponding modifications in the statistical procedures will be presented.

Two other statistical problems may be noted here. One is the determination of how large a retrospective study to conduct. This depends on how sure we wish to be that the study will yield clear evidence that the relative risk is not unity, when it in fact differs from unity to some important degree. Application of this statistical technique requires reinterpreting a relative risk greater than unity into the corresponding difference between the diseased and the disease-free groups in the proportion of persons with the factor. For example, suppose an attack rate of 20 percent, given a normal rate of 10 percent, is worth uncovering. Suppose further that the factor associated with the increased disease rate affects 20 percent of the population. The population would then be distributed as follows:

	With factor	Free of factor	Total
With disease	$P_1 = 4\%$	$P_2 = 8\%$	12%
Free of disease	$P_3 = 16\%$	$P_4 = 72\%$	88%
Total	20%	80%	100%

The required retrospective study should be large enough to differentiate between a 33.3 percent $[P_1/(P_1 + P_2)]$ relative frequency of the factor among diseased individuals and an 18.2 percent $[P_3/(P_3 + P_4)]$ relative frequency among disease-free individuals. The usual procedures for determining required sample sizes to differentiate between two binomial proportions are applicable in this situation.

While rigorous extension of this procedure to the more complex situations to be considered is not too simple, it can readily be adapted to secure approximations of the necessary study size. One might, for example, start by estimating the overall required sample size following the procedure just indicated for differentiating between two sample proportions, assuming that cases and controls are homogeneous with respect to factors other than the one under investigation. Suppose on an overall basis it is determined that the study should include $N_1 = 200$ disease cases and $N_2 = 200$ controls, but that the study data will be subclassified for purposes of analysis. Ignoring mathematical complications resulting from variations in binomial parameter values within individual subclassifications, we may interpret the above values of N_1 and N_2 as roughly meaning that the total information required for the study is $N_1N_2/(N_1 + N_2) = 100$. The objective should then be to assign values to N_{1i} and N_{2i} to obtain a total score of 100 for the cumulated information over all the subclassifications, $\Sigma N_{1i}N_{2i}/(N_{1i} + N_{2i})$, where N_{1i} and N_{2i} are the number of cases and controls in the *ith* subclassification.

This formulation of required total information brings out some aspects of retrospective study planning which are considered later in this paper. For instance, if any N_{1i} or N_{2i} is zero, no information is available from that particular category. Much of the benefit of a large N_{1i} (or N_{2i}) in any particular category is lost if the corresponding N_{2i} (or N_{1i}) is small. It is normally desirable to have N_{1i} and N_{2i} values commensurate with each other; for fixed totals, ΣN_{1i} and ΣN_{2i}, the total information in an investigation will be at a maximum if the degree of crossmatching is equal in all subclassifications with a constant case-control ratio of $\Sigma N_{1i}/\Sigma N_{2i}$. Maintaining a fixed case-control ratio among categories need not preclude assigning more cases and controls to specific categories. Larger numbers may be desired for categories of crucial interest to the study or for categories which represent greater segments of the population.

The information formula also reveals the limits for adjusting the relative numbers of diseased and control cases. It shows that if the number of controls (N_2) becomes indefinitely large, the required N_1 value can at most be reduced only by a factor of 2. Furthermore, this reduction in required diseased cases may be inappropriate if one wishes to obtain clear results for the separate subcategories.

The study size requirements suggested by the information formula may be seriously in error if the binomial parameters show excessive variation among subcategories. Ordinary precautions, however, should serve to keep the formula useful. In some situations it may be desirable to modify the information formula indicated above to reflect the contribution due to variation in the binomial parameters involved.

The second statistical procedure involves setting reasonable limits on the relative risk when it is in fact different from unity. For the homogeneous case considered, formulas for such limits have been published in (*46*). The chi-square test as stated is essentially a test of whether or not the confidence limits include unity. Extension of this procedure to more complex cases is fairly involved and depends primarily on the measure of relative risk adopted. In the absence of a clear justification for any single measure of overall relative risk, the burden of extremely involved computation of confidence limits in such cases would not seem warranted. Instead, we feel that emphasis should be directed to obtaining an overall measure of risk, coupled with an overall test of statistical significance.

STATISTICAL PROCEDURES FOR FACTOR CONTROL

A major problem in any epidemiological study is the avoidance of spurious associations. It has been remarked that where the risk of disease changes with age, apparent association of the disease with other age-related factors can result. However, there are appropriate statistical procedures for controlling those factors known or suspected to be related to disease occurrence. They serve not only to remove bias from the investigation but, in addition, can add to its precision.

Two simple procedures for obtaining factor control may first be mentioned. One is simply to restrict the investigation to individuals homogeneous on the factors to be controlled. For this situation the statistical procedures already outlined would be appropriate. The potential number of individuals available for such a study would, of course, be sharply restricted.

There is also the matching case method. A sample of N diseased individuals is drawn and the characteristics of each individual noted with respect to the control factors. Subsequently, a sample of N well individuals is drawn, with each individual matched on the control factors to one of the diseased individuals. The statistical procedures to be presented can be shown to cover the matched-sample approach as a special case, and a discussion of the analysis of such data will be given in that context. Some difficulties of the matched-sample study may be mentioned here. One is that when matching is made on a large number of factors, not even the fiction of a random sampling of control individuals can be maintained. Instead, one must be grateful for each matching control available. Another difficulty is that the method cannot be applied to factors under control, since diseased and control individuals are identical with respect to these factors. Conversely, factors under study in matched samples cannot themselves be controlled statistically. They can be analyzed separately or in particular conjunctions but cannot be employed as control factors.

An alternative to case matching is to draw independent samples of cases and controls, and adjust for other factors in the analysis. This approach requires simply the classification of individuals according to the various control and study factors desired, and an analysis for each separate subclassification as well as an appropriate summary analysis. Its success will depend on a reasonable degree of cross-matching between observations on diseased and control persons. In a small study various devices for reducing the number of subclassifications and for increasing the chances of cross-matching may be necessary, including a limit on the number of factors on which individuals are classified in any one analysis and the use of broad categories for any particular classification. Thus, a 10-year interval for age classification might permit a reasonable degree of cross-matching, whereas a 1-month interval would not.

The need for some degree of deliberate matching, even when the classification approach is employed, can be seen. If the disease under consideration occurs at advanced ages, little cross-matching would result if controls were selected from the general population. The remedy lies in deliberately selecting controls from the same age groups anticipated for persons with the disease, perhaps even matching one or more controls on age for each diseased person. This principle can be extended to matching on several control factors, *solely for the purpose of increasing the extent of cross-matching in the analysis*.

One of the subtle effects which can occur in a retrospective study, even with careful planning, may be pointed out. It can be shown, for instance, that within a given age interval the average age of individuals with cancer of certain sites will be greater than the average age of individuals from the general population in the same age interval. This can arise when incidence increases rapidly with age and may pose a serious problem with broad age intervals. This effect can be offset by close matching of cases and controls on age in drawing samples, even though they are classified by a broad age category in the analysis.

When a random sample of diseased and disease-free individuals is classified according to various control factors the distribution of the factor under study within the *ith* classification may be represented as follows:

	With factor	Free of factor	Total
With disease	A_i	B_i	N_{1i}
Free of disease	C_i	D_i	N_{2i}
Total	M_{1i}	M_{2i}	T_i

Within this subgroup the approximate relative risk associated with the disease may be written as $A_i D_i / B_i C_i$. One may compare the observed number of diseased persons having the factor, A_i, with its expectation under the hypothesis of a relative risk of unity, $E(A_i) = N_{1i} M_{1i} / T_i$. The discrepancy between A_i and $E(A_i)$ (which is also the discrepancy for any other cell within a 2×2 table) can be tested relative to its variance which, subject to the fixed marginal totals—N_{1i}, N_{2i}, M_{1i}, and M_{2i}—is given by $V(A_i) = N_{1i} N_{2i} M_{1i} M_{2i} / T_i^2 (T_i - 1)$. The corrected chi square with 1 degree of freedom $(| A_i - E(A_i) | - \frac{1}{2})^2 / V(A_i)$ reduces in this case to $(| A_i D_i - B_i C_i | - \frac{1}{2} T_i)^2 (T_i - 1) / N_{1i} N_{2i} M_{1i} M_{2i}$. This formula for the variance of A_i is obtained as the variance of the binomial variable $N_1 PQ (P = M_1/T, Q = M_2/T)$, multiplied by a finite population correction factor $(T - N_1)/(T - 1) = N_2/(T - 1)$. The earlier chi-square formula, which is ordinarily used, essentially employs a finite population correction factor of N_2/T.

There is thus a difference between the two chi-square formulas of a factor of $(T - 1)/T$ which, though trivial for any single significance test with respectably large T, can become important in the overall significance test. It is with the latter formula, just presented, that chi square is computed as the ratio of the square of a deviation from its expected value to its variance.

The adjustment for control factors is at this point resolved for the resulting separate subclassifications. The problem of overall measures of relative risk and statistical significance still remains. A reasonable overall significance test which has power for alternative hypotheses, where there is a consistent association in the same direction over the various subclassifications between the disease and a study factor, is provided by relating the summation of the discrepancy between observation and expectation to its variance. The corrected chi square with 1 degree of freedom then becomes $(|\Sigma A_i - \Sigma E(A_i)| - \frac{1}{2})^2 / \Sigma V(A_i)$ where $E(A_i)$ and $V(A_i)$ are defined as above.

The specification of a summary estimate of

the relative risk associated with a factor is not so readily resolved as that for an overall significance test, and involves consideration of alternate approaches to a weighted average of the approximate relative risks for each subclassification $(A_i D_i / B_i C_i)$. If one could assume that the increased relative risk associated with a factor was constant over all subclassifications, the estimation problem would reduce to weighting the several subclassification estimates according to their respective precisions. The complex maximum likelihood iterative procedure necessary for obtaining such a weighted estimate would seem to be unjustified, since the assumption of a constant relative risk can be discarded as usually untenable.

Another possible criterion for obtaining a summary estimate of relative risk would involve weighting the risks for subclassification by "importance." A twofold increase of a large risk is more important than a twofold increase of a small risk. An increased risk for a large group is more important than one for a small group. An increased risk for young individuals may be more important than for older individuals with a shorter life expectation. Difficulties arise in attempts to weight relative risk by measures of importance. For one, the necessary information on importance, in terms of the size of the populations affected or in terms of the absolute level of rates prevailing in the subgroups, is generally not contained within the scope of the investigation. A problem in definition of the precise terms of the weighted comparison also appears. Does one want to adjust the risks of disease among persons with the factor to the distribution of the population without the factor, or *vice versa*, or adjust the risks for the populations with and without the factor to a combined standard population? These procedures, and the different phrasing of the comparisons which they entail, could yield different answers. If only a small proportion of the population with the factor was in a subcategory with a high relative risk, while most of the factor-free population fell into this subcategory, and in other categories the relative risk associated with the factor was less than unity, the factor would appear to exert a protective influence under one set of weights but a harmful effect under the other.

Published instances of summary relative risks do not fall clearly into either of the two categories—weighting by precision or weighting by importance. They do follow an approach usually employed in age-adjusting mortality data. Since the relative risk for a single 2×2 table can be obtained from the incidence of the factor among diseased and well individuals, the problem would appear translatable into terms of obtaining overall, category-adjusted incidence figures. Direct or indirect methods of adjustment can be used, employing as a standard of reference the frequency distribution or rates corresponding to the sample of diseased persons, of controls, or the diseased persons and controls combined.

While such adjustment procedures provide weighting by importance in their customary application to mortality rates, this is not so in the relative risk situation. This may be illustrated in the following extreme example. Suppose that in each of two subcategories the approximate relative risk for a contrast between the presence and absence of a factor is about 5, which arises in the first subcategory from contrasting percentages of 1 and 5, and in the second subcategory from contrasting percentages of 95 and 99. If these percentages were based on equal numbers of individuals, all methods of category adjusting would yield contrasting adjusted summary percentages of 46 and 52, and a resultant relative risk of slightly less than 1.3. Some other approach for obtaining category-adjusted relative risks would seem desirable. However, to the extent that such extreme situations are not encountered in actual practice, results based on these more conventional adjustment procedures will not be grossly in error.

A suggested compromise formula for overall relative risk is given by $R = \Sigma(A_i D_i / T_i) / \Sigma(B_i C_i / T_i)$. As a weighted average of relative risks this formula would, in the illustration given, yield the overall relative risk of 5 found in each of the two subcategories. The weights are of the order $N_{1i} N_{2i} / (N_{1i} + N_{2i})$ and as such can be considered to weight approximately according to the precision of the relative risks for each subcategory. The weights can· also be regarded as providing a reasonable weighting by importance.

An interesting property of this summary relative risk formula is that it equals unity only when $\Sigma A_i = \Sigma E(A_i)$ and hence the corresponding chi square is zero. From the fact that $A_i - E(A_i) = (A_i D_i - B_i C_i)/T_i$, it follows that when $\Sigma A_i = \Sigma E(A_i)$, $\Sigma A_i D_i / T_i$ will equal $\Sigma B_i C_i / T_i$, chi square will be zero, and R will be unity. The chi-square significance test can thus be construed as a significance test of the departure of R from unity.

Of some other procedures for measuring overall relative risks, the one following also has the interesting property of being equal to unity when $\Sigma(A_i) = \Sigma E(A_i)$ and therefore subject to the chi-square test:

$$R_1 = \frac{\Sigma A_i \Sigma D_i}{\Sigma B_i \Sigma C_i} \bigg/ \frac{\Sigma E(A_i)\Sigma E(D_i)}{\Sigma E(B_i)\Sigma E(C_i)}$$

$$\text{where } E(A_i) = N_{1i}M_{1i}/T_i, \ E(B_i)$$

$$= N_{1i}M_{2i}/T_i, \ E(C_i) = N_{2i}M_{1i}/T_i,$$

$$\text{and } E(D_i) = N_{2i}M_{2i}/T_i.$$

In this formula the numerator represents the crude value for the relative risk, which would result from pooling the data into one table and ignoring all subclassification on other factors. The denominator represents the crude value for relative risk, which would have resulted from pooling in the situation where all relative risks within each subclassification were exactly unity. Readers familiar with the "indirect" method of computing standardized mortality ratios will recognize an analogy between the "indirect" method and the above procedure.

The estimator R_1 can be seen to have a bias toward unity. One reason is covered by the illustration which indicated that adjusted percentages (or frequencies) do not yield an appropriate adjusted relative risk. In addition, when either cases or controls have little representation in a subcategory, there will be lack of cross-matching and little information about relative risk, and the observed cell frequencies and their expectations will be numerically close. Such results will, in the process of summation used by the estimator, tend to force its value toward unity. This weakness will not be too important if the degree of cross-matching is roughly equal in the various subclassifications—an optimum goal one would normally attempt to achieve. The bias will become more pronounced as the number of control factors increases and as the prospects for good cross-matching become poorer.

We used the estimator R_1 in a recent paper (27), knowing its potential weaknesses. This was done to present results more nearly comparable with those reported by other investigators using

similarly biased estimators. One set of results from this paper on lung cancer among women illustrates the conservative behavior of estimator R_1 compared with R, as additional factors are controlled. The relative risk (R_1) for epidermoid and undifferentiated pulmonary carcinoma associated with smoking more than one pack of cigarettes daily as compared to non-smokers decreased from 7.1 (controlled for age) to 5.6 (controlled for age and coffee consumption). The corresponding figures, with R as a measure of relative risk, were 9.7 and 9.9.

Computational procedures for R and R_1 are presented in Table 1, drawing on material comparing smoking histories of women diagnosed as cases of epidermoid and undifferentiated pulmonary carcinoma with those of female controls. For simplicity in presentation only two smoking levels are considered—nonsmokers and smokers of more than one pack of cigarettes daily. An extension of the significance testing procedures to the case of study factors at more than two levels is discussed later. The control factors are age and occupation. The basic data are given in the first 9 columns. Columns 10 and 11 carry the derivative calculations required for R. Columns 12 and 13 are used in the computation for R_1 and for the variance estimate in column 14—the latter being needed for the chi-square test. Only columns 1 to 10, 12, and 14 would be necessary to compute chi square, R and R_1. Column 13 is not essential for the computation of $E(D)$ but simplifies computation of $V(A)$, while providing a check on $E(A)$. Column 11 serves as a check on 10 and 12. A system of checks and computations is outlined at the bottom of Table 1. Not all the computations shown would ordinarily be necessary for an analysis.

The corrected chi-square value of 30.66 (1 degree of freedom) would indicate a highly significant association between epidermoid and undifferentiated pulmonary carcinoma and cigarette smoking in women, after adjusting for possible effects connected with age or occupation. The value of R implies that the risk of these cancers is 10.7 times as great for women currently smoking in excess of one pack a day than for women who never used cigarettes. The value of R_1, 7.05, is almost identical with the crude relative risk, 7.10, which results from pooling the data with no attention to the control factors. The difference from the published R_1

Table 1. Illustrative computations for chi square and for summary measures of relative risk (R, R_1, R_2, R_3, and R_4) relating to the association of epidermoid and undifferentiated pulmonary carcinoma in women with smoking history.

Group	Epidermoid-undifferentiated pulmonary carcinoma			Controls			Cases and controls			Derivative computations								
	1+ pack cigarettes daily	Nonsmokers	Total	1+ pack cigarettes daily	Nonsmokers	Total	1+ pack cigarettes daily	Nonsmokers	Total	$\frac{AD}{T}$	$\frac{BC}{T}$	$E(A)$	$E(D)$	$V(A)$	$\frac{N_1C}{N_2}$	$\frac{N_1D}{N_2}$	$\frac{N_2A}{N_1}$	$\frac{N_2B}{N_1}$
	A	B	N_1	C	D	N_2	M_1	M_2	T	$\frac{(1)(5)}{(9)}$	$\frac{(2)(4)}{(9)}$	$\frac{(3)(7)}{(9)}$	$\frac{(6)(8)}{(9)}$	$\frac{(12)(13)}{(9)-1.0}$	$\frac{(3)(4)}{(6)}$	$\frac{(3)(5)}{(6)}$	$\frac{(1)(6)}{(3)}$	$\frac{(2)(6)}{(3)}$
	(1)	(2)	(3)	(4)	(5)	(6)	(7)	(8)	(9)	(10)	(11)	(12)	(13)	(14)	(15)	(16)	(17)	(18)
House-wives under age 45	0	2	2	0	7	7	0	9	9	0	0	0	7.000	0	0	2.000	0	7.000
45–54	2	5	7	1	24	25	3	29	32	1.500	0.156	0.656	22.656	0.480	0.280	6.720	7.143	17.857
55–64	3	6	9	0	49	49	3	55	58	2.534	0	0.466	46.466	0.380	0	9.000	16.333	32.667
65 and over	0	11	11	0	42	42	0	53	53	0	0	0	42.000	0	0	11.000	0	42.000
White-collar workers under age 45	3	0	3	2	6	8	5	6	11	1.636	0	1.364	4.364	0.595	0.750	2.250	8.000	0
45–54	2	2	4	2	18	20	4	20	24	1.500	0.167	0.667	16.667	0.483	0.400	3.600	10.000	10.000
55–64	2	4	6	2	23	25	4	27	31	1.484	0.258	0.774	21.774	0.562	0.480	5.520	8.333	16.667
65 and over	0	6	6	1	11	12	1	17	18	0	0.333	0.333	11.333	0.222	0.500	5.500	0	12.000
Other occupations under age 45	1	0	1	3	10	13	4	10	14	0.714		0.286	9.286	0.204	0.231	.769	13.000	0
45–54	4	1	5	1	12	13	5	13	18	2.667	0.056	1.389	9.389	0.767	0.385	4.615	10.400	2.600
55–64	0	6	6	1	19	20	1	25	26	0	0.231	0.231	19.231	0.178	0.300	5.700	0	20.000
65 and over	1	3	4	0	15	15	1	18	19	0.790		0.211	14.211	0.166	0	4.000	3.750	11.250
Total	18	46	64	13	236	249	31	282	313	12.825	1.201	6.375	224.375	4.036	3.325	60.675	76.960	172.040

Checks: Total discrepancy, Y, $= \Sigma A - \Sigma E(A) = \Sigma(1) - \Sigma(12) = 11.625$
$= \Sigma D - \Sigma E(D) = \Sigma(5) - \Sigma(13) = 11.625$
$= \Sigma(AD/T) - \Sigma(BC/T) = \Sigma(10) - \Sigma(11) = 11.625$

$\Sigma(15) + \Sigma(16) = 64.000$; $\Sigma(3) = 64$
$\Sigma(17) + \Sigma(18) = 249.000$; $\Sigma(6) = 249$

Derivative computations: $\Sigma E(B) = \Sigma(2) + Y = 57.625$
$\Sigma E(C) = \Sigma(4) + Y = 24.625$
$\Sigma(AT/N_1) = \Sigma(1) + \Sigma(17) = 94.960$
$\Sigma(BT/N_1) = \Sigma(2) + \Sigma(18) = 218.040$
$\Sigma(CT/N_2) = \Sigma(4) + \Sigma(15) = 16.325$
$\Sigma(DT/N_2) = \Sigma(5) + \Sigma(16) = 296.675$

Chi-square: $X^2 = (|\text{discrepancy}| - 0.5)^2/\Sigma V(A) = (|Y| - 0.5)^2/\Sigma(14) = 30.66$
Relative risk: $R = \Sigma (AD/T)/\Sigma(BC/T) = \Sigma(10)/\Sigma(11) = 10.68$

R_1 $\begin{cases} \text{crude relative risk, } r = \Sigma A\Sigma D/\Sigma B\Sigma C = \Sigma(1)\Sigma(5)/\Sigma(2)\Sigma(4) = 7.10 \\ \text{adjustment factor, } f = \Sigma E(A)\Sigma E(D)/\Sigma E(B)\Sigma E(C) = \Sigma(12)\Sigma(13)/\Sigma E(B)\Sigma E(C) = 1.0081 \end{cases}$

$R_1 = r/f = 7.05$

$R_2 = \Sigma A\Sigma(N_1D/N_2)/\Sigma B\Sigma(N_1C/N_2) = \Sigma(1)\Sigma(16)/\Sigma(2)\Sigma(15) = 7.14$
$R_3 = \Sigma(N_2A/N_1)\Sigma D/\Sigma(N_2B/N_1)\Sigma C = \Sigma(5)\Sigma(17)/\Sigma(4)\Sigma(18) = 8.12$
$R_4 = \Sigma(AT/N_1)\Sigma(DT/N_2)/\Sigma(BT/N_1)\Sigma(CT/N_2) = 7.91$

Note: Figures shown are rounded from those actually calculated and consequently are not fully consistent. Column totals and figures shown do not necessarily agree.

value of 6.3 in (27) arises from the exclusion in the illustrative example, of data for women currently smoking one pack a day or less and for occasional or discontinued smokers.

The computation of three other summary estimates of relative risk is also outlined in Table 1. The additional derivative computations required for this purpose appear in columns 15 to 18. All three estimates are based on a direct method of category adjustment, that is, the use of a standard distribution to which both the case and control distributions are adjusted. If the distribution of diseased cases is taken as the standard distribution to which the controls are adjusted, the estimator becomes

$$R_2 = \frac{\Sigma A_i \Sigma \left(D_i \times \dfrac{N_{1i}}{N_{2i}} \right)}{\Sigma B_i \Sigma \left(C_i \times \dfrac{N_{1i}}{N_{2i}} \right)}.$$

Estimator R_2 was used by Wynder *et al.* in a study of the association of cervical cancer in women with circumcision status of sex partners (16). The merit of employing the cervical cancer case-distribution as the standard presumably rests on the fact that this distribution at least would be well defined by the study.

If the distribution of control cases is taken as standard the estimator becomes

$$R_3 = \frac{\Sigma \left(A_i \times \dfrac{N_{2i}}{N_{1i}} \right) \Sigma D_i}{\Sigma \left(B_i \times \dfrac{N_{2i}}{N_{1i}} \right) \Sigma C_i}.$$

If the combined distribution is taken as standard the estimator becomes

$$R_4 = \frac{\Sigma \left(A_i \times \dfrac{T_i}{N_{1i}} \right) \Sigma \left(D_i \times \dfrac{T_i}{N_{2i}} \right)}{\Sigma \left(B_i \times \dfrac{T_i}{N_{1i}} \right) \Sigma \left(C_i \times \dfrac{T_i}{N_{2i}} \right)}.$$

If any N_{1i} or N_{2i} should equal zero, the estimator R_4 would not be defined. R_2 is not defined for any zero-valued N_{2i}, and R_3 is not defined for any zero-valued N_{1i}. In these instances it would be necessary to exclude the zero-frequency categories to define the estimators. The estimator R_1 retains these categories to define the estimators. The estimator R_1 retains these categories at the expense of greater bias toward unity. The estimator R gives such categories zero weight, since they contain no information about relative risk. The chi-square significance test gives no weight to these categories.

While R_4 is clearly a direct adjusted estimate of relative risk employing the combined distribution as standard, R_2 and R_3 may be viewed alternatively as either direct or indirect adjusted estimates. The same estimates will result if a direct adjustment is made using the distribution of cases as standard, or an indirect adjustment is made using the factor incidence rates for controls as the standard rates.

It may be noted that in the example used, the values for R_2, R_3, and R_4 (7.14, 8.12, and 7.91, respectively) were roughly comparable to R_1, and all were smaller than R. The example was selected because all the N_{1i} and N_{2i} values were non-zero, so that the values of R_2, R_3, and R_4 were all defined.

The overall relative risk estimates are averages and as averages may conceal substantial variation in the magnitudes of the relative risk among subgroups. Ordinarily, the individual subcategory data should be examined, paying special attention to relative risks based on reasonably large sample sizes. This will provide protection against the potential deficiencies of any particular summary relative risk formula employed. The overall chi-square significance test in any case will remain appropriate for detecting any strong general tendency for the risk of disease to be associated with the presence or absence of the test factor.

THE MATCHED-SAMPLE STUDY

The matched-sample study previously described can be considered a special case of the classification procedure with the number of classifications equal to the number of pairs of individuals. The status of pairs of well and diseased individuals classified with respect to the presence or absence of the suspect factor in each individual will be represented as F, G, H, or J in the following fourfold table. The meanings attached to the marginal totals A, B, C, and D are the same as those in the first schematic representation.

Well individuals	Diseased individuals		
	With factor	Free of factor	Total
With factor	F	G	C
Free of factor	H	J	D
Total	A	B	N

In the absence of association between the disease and the factor, we expect the same number of individuals with the factor to appear among both diseased and well individuals; that is, we expect $A(=F + H)$ to equal $C(=F + G)$. This can occur only when $G = H$ and the statistical test is simply whether or not G differs significantly from 50 percent of $G + H$. G is tested as a binomial variable with parameter ½, $G + H$ being the number of cases. G thus has expectation ½$(G + H)$, variance ¼$(G + H)$ and the corrected chi square with 1 degree of freedom can readily be shown to reduce to $(| G - H | - 1)^2/(G + H)$.

Treating the data as consisting of N classifications each with $N_{1i} = N_{2i} = 1$, $T_i = 2$ and applying the previously described procedures will lead to the same value of chi square. For F of the N classifications, $A_i = 1, M_{1i} = 2, M_{2i} = 0, E(A_i) = 1, V(A_i) = 0$; for G classifications $A_i = 0, M_{1i} = M_{2i} = 1, E(A_i) = ½, V(A_i) = ¼$; for H classifications $A_i = 1, M_{1i} = M_{2i} = 1, E(A_i) = ½, V(A_i) = ¼$; and for J classifications, $A_i = 0, M_{1i} = 0, M_{2i} = 2, E(A_i) = 0, V(A_i) = 0$. Thus, $\Sigma A_i = F + H, \Sigma E(A_i) = F + ½(G + H), \Sigma V(A_i) = ¼(G + H)$, and the resultant corrected chi square can again be seen to be $(| G - H | - 1)^2/(G + H)$.

It is of interest to observe that the summary chi-square formula is appropriate in the matched-sample case, even though the frequencies for each of the separate subclassifications are small. Its appropriateness, despite the small frequencies, stems from the fact that it is a test on a summation of random variables, A_i, and thus tends to approach normality rapidly, making the chi-square test valid, even though the individual A_i's are not normally distributed. This property of the chi-square formula applies in the general classification as well as the matched-sample situation. Only substantial lack of cross-matching in the general case would tend to make the chi-square test invalid. It is also essential, of course, that there be some

appreciable variation in the presence or absence of the factor under study.

It should be noted that in the matched-sample study with $T_i = 2$ for each of the N pairs of individuals, the variances of the A_i's would have been understated by a factor of 2, had $T - 1$ been replaced by T in the variance formulas. The usual formula for chi square does essentially make this replacement, but it is usually of little consequence if T is of any reasonable magnitude. The formulas for relative risk in the matched-sample study reduce simply to the following: $R = H/G; R_1 = R_2 = R_3 = R_4 = AD/BC$.

STUDY FACTORS AT MORE THAN TWO LEVELS

The preceding discussion on the analysis of retrospective data has been in terms of the test factor under study taking only two values. This framework has sufficed for discussion of the underlying statistical ideas and issues. In practice, the study factor will frequently take on more than two, perhaps many, potential values. When the number of study factor values is large, grouping can reduce them to manageable proportions.

The need to consider only a limited number of classes for the study factor stems from the fact that, when an association is anticipated, most of the significant information about the association will come from the results for the more extreme values of the study factor. While it is efficient to concentrate attention on the test factor classes expected to show the greatest differences in association with the disease, it is also profitable to consider intermediate values for the test factor to seek evidence for a consistent pattern of association. For example, in Table 1, a highly significant difference between nonsmokers and women currently smoking more than one pack of cigarettes daily was illustrated. Inclusion of data for smokers of one pack or less a day showing results intermediate between the other classes would have added little, if anything, to the statistical significance of the results, and might actually lower it, if one made an overall test of the differences among the three smoking classes. However, the observation that the intermediate smoking class does, in fact, show an intermediate relative risk contributes to an orderly pattern and increases our confidence in the conclusions suggested by the data for the remaining two classes.

For any two particular test-factor levels, the relative risk for one over the other may be calculated using only the data pertaining to those two levels or by using the results for all test levels. In the formulas previously given for R, R_1, R_2, R_3, and R_4, the difference between the two calculating procedures is simply one of setting the values of N_{1i}, N_{2i}, and $T_i = N_{1i} + N_{2i}$ in terms of number of cases and controls occurring at the two study-factor levels only, or defining them in terms of total number of cases and controls in the entire study. When total cases and controls are used in defining N_{1i}, N_{2i}, and T_i, it can be shown that for R_1, R_2, R_3, and R_4 the various relative risks will be internally consistent with each other. If the relative risk for the first level is twice that for the second level, which in turn is twice that for the third level, then the relative risk for the first level will be four times that of the third. These exact relationships do not hold for R as an estimator of relative risk, and a somewhat sophisticated extension of the formula for R would be required to secure this property.

The problem of obtaining a summary chi square when the study factor is at more than two levels is complicated by the fact that the deviations from expectation at the various study-factor levels are intercorrelated. When there are but two levels, the two deviations will have perfect negative correlation, and attention need be directed to only one of the deviations. Irrespective of the number of levels, at any one level the deviation from expectation among diseased persons will be equal, but opposite in sign, to the deviation from expectation among controls, so that attention can be confined to the deviations for diseased persons.

The problem can be stated as one of reducing a set of correlated deviations into a summary chi square. Table 2 applies this process for obtaining a summary chi square to the study of the association of epidermoid and undifferentiated pulmonary carcinoma in women and maximum cigarette-smoking rate, classified into three levels, after adjustment for age and occupation.

The general expressions for the expectations and variances of the number of cases at a particular test-factor level are given in the lower right section of Table 2. Also shown is the expression for the covariance between the number of cases at two different test-factor levels. Since the total of all the deviations is zero, one would in general need the variances of, and covariances between, the number of cases at all but one of the levels. The number of covariance terms will rise sharply as the number of test levels are increased. At 3 test levels, there are 2 variance terms and 1 covariance term, while at 10 test levels, there would be 9 variances and 36 covariance terms of interest.

For the general case the burden of computation could be heavy. After all the necessary computation for the deviations, their variances and covariances, there would still remain the problem of converting these, presumably by matrix methods, into a summary chi square. Since the retrospective problem will normally involve only a limited number of test-factor levels, precise procedures will be given only for the three-level situation, and approximate procedures outlined for the general case.

The exact computation procedure for the three-level case is detailed in Table 2. Lines (1), (2), and (4) show the total observed and expected frequencies and variances of the number of cases (and controls) at each of the three smoking-rate levels, after adjusting for age and occupation. These are the summary totals over each subclassification obtained by application of the formulas appearing in Table 2.

Lines (5) and (6) give the chi squares corresponding to the total deviation from expectation at each of the smoking-rate levels. The chi squares in line (5) are corrected for continuity. They relate to the difference of the particular level to which they apply, from the two other levels combined. Following the usual practice of making no continuity corrections when chi squares with more than 1 degree of freedom are under consideration, line (6) shows the uncorrected chi squares.

The computing procedure of Table 2 takes advantage of the fact that, since the sum of the deviations from expectation is zero, the variance of the third deviation must equal the sum of the other two variances plus twice the covariance for the first two deviations. The covariance of the first two deviations is readily obtained as illustrated and is used in calculating the summary chi square. The summary chi square is obtained as the sum of squares of two orthogonal deviates, with each square adjusted

Table 2. Illustrative computation of summary chi square, when there are three levels for study factor. The data relate to the association of epidermoid and undifferentiated pulmonary carcinoma in women with smoking history;

	1+ pack cigarettes daily			1 pack or less of cigarettes daily			Occasional or nonsmokers			Total		
	Epidermoid-undifferentiated pulmonary carcinoma	Controls	Total (ΣM_1)	Epidermoid-undifferentiated pulmonary carcinoma	Controls	Total (ΣM_2)	Epidermoid-undifferentiated pulmonary carcinoma	Controls	Total (ΣM_3)	Epidermoid-undifferentiated pulmonary carcinoma (ΣN_1)	Controls (ΣN_2)	Total (ΣT)
(1) Total observed frequencies	19	17	36	32	71	103	51	251	302	102	339	441
(2) Total expected frequencies, adjusted for age and occupation	9.09	26.91	36	23.76	79.24	103	69.15	232.85	302	102	339	441
(3) Total deviation from expectation (1)–(2)	$+9.91 = Y_1$			$+8.24 = Y_2$			$-18.15 = Y_3$					
(4) Variance of total observed frequencies, subject to fixed marginal totals in each age and occupation group	$5.9163 = V_1$			$12.2900 = V_2$			$14.0723 = V_3$					
(5) Individual corrected chi squares $(|Y| - 0.5)^2/V$	$14.97 = X^2_{1c}$			$4.88 = X^2_{2c}$			$22.15 = X^2_{3c}$					
(6) Individual uncorrected chi squares Y^2/V	$16.60 = X^2_1$			$16.60 = X^2_2$			$16.60 = X^2_3$					
(7) Covariance (Y_1, Y_2) $(V_2 - V_1 - V_2)/2$				-2.0670								
(8) Adjusted Y_2 $Y_2 - (7) Y_1/V$				11.70								
(9) Adjusted V_2 $V_2 - (7)^2/V_1$				11.5678								
(10) Adjusted X^2_2 $(8)^2/(9)$				$11.83 = X^2_2$ (ad.)								
(11) Summary chi square (2 degrees of freedom) $X^2_1 + X^2_2$ (ad.)						$16.60 + 11.83 = 28.43$						

For the general situation the total expected case frequency at the jth level of a test factor is

$$\Sigma N_{1i}M_{ji}/T_i$$

The variance of the total case frequency is

$$V_i = \sum_i \frac{N_{1i}N_{2i}M_{ji}(T_i - M_{ji})}{T_i^2(T_i - 1)}$$

The covariance of the total case frequencies at test levels j and k is

$$-\sum_i \frac{N_{1i}N_{2i}M_{ji}M_{ki}}{T_i^2(T_i - 1)}$$

The index of summation, i, represents the various subclassifications into which the results are divided

For 3 test levels only, since $Y_3 = -(Y_1 + Y_2)$, it follows that $V_3 = V_1 + V_2 + 2$ Covariance (Y_1, Y_2)

for its own variance. The first deviate squared is simply the uncorrected chi square at the first level in line (6)—the variance of the deviate remaining as initially calculated. The second deviate is the deviation at the second level adjusted for its correlation with the first deviation [adjusted $Y_2 = Y_2 - b_{21}Y_1$; b_{21} = covariance (Y_1, Y_2)/variance Y_1)]. The variance of the adjusted second deviate is the initial value reduced by that portion of the variation accounted for by the first deviation [Var. (adjusted Y_2) = variance Y_2—covariance² (Y_1, Y_2)/variance Y_1)].

In the present instance the summary chi square with 2 degrees of freedom is 28.43 [line (11)]. This presumably is close to the chi square with 1 degree of freedom which would have been obtained had only the two most extreme smoking classes been compared. If one examines the individual uncorrected chi squares [line (6)], their total is found to be 45.55, the maximum individual figure being 23.42. *It will necessarily be true that the summary chi-square value will lie between the largest of the three chi squares and their total. At almost any reasonable probability level these limits would be sufficient to establish statistical significance without further calculation.* In our companion paper (27) this rule sufficed in almost all instances to separate the significant from the nonsignificant results.

COMMENTS ON EXTENSIONS TO MORE THAN THREE FACTORS

Two procedures can be suggested for getting approximate summary chi squares, when there are a large number of levels for the test factors, without the burden of computation that the exact method would entail. Both methods calculate the approximate summary chi square as a sum of squares of approximately orthogonal standardized deviates.

In the first method one computes an uncorrected chi square with 1 degree of freedom for the difference of the first level from all the remaining levels combined (the same first step as in the illustration for the three-level case). Discarding the data from the first level, a second chi square is computed for the difference between the second test-factor level and the remaining levels combined. This is done successively up to and including the last two remaining levels. The approximate summary chi square is then the sum of the separate chi

squares with the number of degrees of freedom being one less than the number of test levels.

Exactly orthogonal standardized deviates would be obtained if, in the summary analysis, as each successive total deviation from expectation were evaluated, it was adjusted for its multiple regression on the preceding deviations, and then standardized by the adjusted variance. This, of course, would no longer be a simplified approximate procedure. However, it can be shown that for a single classification, in the multiple regression of any deviation from expectation on any subset of deviations, the regression coefficients will all be equal; the multiple regression on the set of deviations will be the same as the simple regression on their sum. The equality of regression coefficients, while holding true exactly for deviations in the separate subclassifications, will hold only approximately for the total deviations from expectation (it would hold exactly if equal numbers of individuals were observed from level to level at each subclassification). Nevertheless, this result suggests that approximately orthogonal deviates would be obtained if, in evaluating each successive total deviation, it were adjusted for the cumulative total of deviations already evaluated. Computing procedures to accomplish this can readily be devised.

Both approximate chi-square procedures just outlined, which may have merit when more than three groups are being compared simultaneously, should, in theory, yield linear combinations of independent chi squares. While testing the chi-square values obtained as though they were exact is not likely to be too inappropriate, it may be more correct to obtain a modified number of degrees of freedom, along the lines suggested by Satterthwaite (47) for problems involving such linear combinations. What the modified number of degrees of freedom would be has not been investigated by us, and it may prove as easy to apply the exact chi-square procedure, indicated later, as to determine the appropriate degrees of freedom for the approximate chi square.

It is of interest that a somewhat similar task of obtaining an appropriate summary chi square appears in the birth-order problems described by Halperin (48). There, it was necessary to compare a set of total observations (across family sizes) with a set of total expectations, one for each birth order. Halperin described a matrix-inversion procedure for reducing the set of correlated deviations into a summary chi square. In that problem it can be shown that all the regression coefficients are equal in the multiple regression of the deviation at a particular birth order on the set of deviations at all succeeding birth orders. The second approximate method described previously for the present problem could thus be used exactly for the birth-order problem, permitting simplified computation of chi square. The procedure indicated by Halperin has the advantage of generality and could be applied to the current and related problems, if one obtained all the necessary variances and covariances and inverted the resulting matrix.

References

(1) Snow, J. On the mode of communication of cholera. In *Snow on Cholera*. New York, The Commonwealth Fund, 1936, pp. 1-139.

(2) Holmes, O.W. The contagiousness of puerperal fever. In *Medical Classics*. Baltimore, Williams & Wilkins Co., 1936, vol. 1, pp. 211-243.

(3) Stern, R. Nota sulle ricerche del dottore Tanchon intorno la frequenza del cancro. *Annali Universali di Medicina* 110:484-503, 1844.

(4) Stocks, P. and J.M. Campbell. Lung cancer death rates among non-smokers and pipe and cigarette smokers. *Brit M J* 2:923-929, 1955.

(5) Wynder, E.L. and J. Cornfield. Cancer of the lung in physicians. *New Engl J Med* 248:441-444, 1953.

(6) Lane-Claypon, J.E. A further report on cancer of the breast, with special reference to its associated antecedent conditions. *Rept Publ Health & M Subj* no. 32, pp. 1-189, 1926.

(7) Clemmesen, J., K. Lockwood, and A. Nielsen. Smoking habits of patients with papilloma of urinary bladder. *Danish M Bull* 5:123-128, 1958.

(8) Denoix, P.R. and D. Schwartz. Tobacco and cancer of the bladder. (Bulletin de L'Association Francaise pour l'étude du Cancer.) *Cancer* 43:387-393, 1956.

(9) Lilienfeld, A.M., M.L. Levin, and G.E. Moore. The association of smoking with cancer of the urinary bladder in humans. *AMA Arch Int Med*, 1956.

(10) Mustacchi, P. and M.B. Shimkin. Cancer of the bladder and infestation with *Schistosoma hematobium*. *J Nat Cancer Inst* 20:825-842, 1958.

(11) Lilienfeld, A.M. The relationship of cancer of the female breast to artificial menopause and marital status. *Cancer* 9:927-934, 1956.

(12) Lilienfeld, A.M. and M.L. Levin. Some factors involved in the incidence of breast cancer. In *Proc Third National Cancer Conference*, Philadelphia, J.B. Lippincott Co., 1957, pp. 105-112.

(13) Segi, M., I. Fukushima, S. Fujisaku, M. Kurihara, S. Saito, K. Asano, and M. Kamoi. An epidemiological study on cancer in Japan. *Gann Supp* 48, 1957.

(14) Dunham, L.J., L.B. Thomas, J.H. Edgcomb, and H.L. Stewart. Some environmental factors and the development of uterine cancers in Israel and New York City. To be published in *Acta Unio internat contra cancrum*.

(15) Stocks, P. Cancer of the uterine cervix and social conditions. *Brit J Cancer* 9:487-494, 1955.

(16) Wynder, E.L., J. Cornfield, P.D. Schroff, and K.R. Doraiswami. A study of environmental factors in carcinoma of the cervix. *Am J Obst & Gynec* 68:1016-1052, 1954.

(17) Mills, C.A. and M.M. Porter. Tobacco smoking habits and cancer of the mouth and respiratory system. *Cancer Res* 10:539-542, 1950.

(18) Wynder, E.L., I.J. Bross, and E. Day. A study of environmental factors in cancer of the larynx. *Cancer* 9:86-110, 1956.

(19) Manning, M.D. and B.E. Carroll. Some epidemiological aspects of leukemia in children. *J Nat Cancer Inst* 19:1087-1094, 1957.

(20) Breslow, L., L. Hoaglin, G. Rasmussen, and H.K. Abrams. Occupations and cigarette smoking as factors in lung cancer. *Am J Pub Health* 44:171-181, 1954.

(21) Doll, R. and A.B. Hill. A study of the aetiology of carcinoma of the lung. *Brit M J* 2:1271-1286, 1952.

(22) Levin, M.L. Etiology of lung cancer; present status. *New York J Med* 54:769-777, 1954.

(23) Sadowsky, D.A., A.G. Gilliam, and J. Cornfield. The statistical association between smoking and carcinoma of the lung. *J Nat Cancer Inst* 13:1237-1258, 1953.

(24) Watson, W.L. and A.J. Conte. Lung cancer and smoking. *Am J Surg* 89:447-456, 1955.

(25) Wynder, E.L. and E.A. Graham. Tobacco smoking as possible etiologic factor in bronchiogenic carcinoma. *JAMA* 143:329-336, 1950.

(26) Wynder, E.L., I.J. Bross, J. Cornfield, and W.E. O'Donnell. Lung cancer in women. *New Engl J Med* 255:1111-1121, 1956.

(27) Haenszel, W., M.B. Shimkin, and N. Mantel. A retrospective study of lung cancer in women. *J Nat Cancer Inst* 21:825-842, 1958.

(28) Aird, I., H.H. Bentall, and J.A.F. Roberts. A relationship between cancer of stomach and the ABO blood groups. *Brit M J* 1:799-801, 1953.

(29) Buckwalter, J.A., C.B. Wohlwend, D.C. Colter, R.T. Tidrick, and L.A. Knowler. The association of the ABO blood groups to gastric carcinoma. *Surg Gynec & Obst* 104:176-179, 1957.

(30) Kraus, A.S., M.L. Levin, and P.R. Gerhardt. A study of occupational associations with gastric cancer. *Am J Pub Health* 47:961-970, 1957.

(31) Cornfield, J. A method of estimating comparative rates from clinical data. Applications to cancer of the lung, breast, and cervix. *J Nat Cancer Inst* 11:1269-1275, 1951.

(32) Dorn, H.F. Some applications of biometry in the collection and evaluation of medical data. *J Chron Dis* 1:638-664, 1955.

(33) Neyman, J. Statistics—servants of all sciences. *Science* 122:3166, 1955.

(34) Berkson, J. Limitations of the application of fourfold table analysis to hospital data. *Biometrics Bull* 2:47-53, 1946.

(35) White, C. Sampling in medical research. *Brit M J* 2:1284-1288, 1953.

(36) Greenwood, M. and G.U. Yule. On the determination of size of family and of the distribution of characters in order of birth from samples taken through members of the siblings. *Roy Stat Soc J* 77:179-197, 1914.

(37) Haenszel, W. Variation in incidence of and mortality from stomach cancer with particular reference to the United States. *J Nat Cancer Inst* 21:213-262, 1958.

(38) Videbaek, A. and J. Mosbech. The aetiology of gastric carcinoma elucidated by a study of 302 pedigrees. *Acta med scandinav* 149:137-159, 1954.

(39) Whelpton, P.K. and R. Freedman. A study of the growth of American families. *Am J Sociol* 61:595-601, 1956.

(40) Levin, M.L., H. Goldstein, and P.R. Gerhardt. Cancer and tobacco smoking. *JAMA* 143:336-338, 1950.

(41) Levin, M.L., A.S. Kraus, I.D. Goldberg, and P.R. Gerhardt. Problems in the study of occupation and smoking in relation to lung cancer. *Cancer* 8:932-936, 1955.

(42) Lilienfeld, A.M. Possible existence of predisposing factors in the etiology of selected cancers of nonsexual sites in females. A preliminary inquiry. *Cancer* 9:111-122, 1956.

(43) Winkelstein, W., Jr., M.A. Stenchever, and A.M. Lilienfeld. Occurrence of pregnancy, abortion and artificial menopause among women with coronary artery disease: a preliminary study. *J Chron Dis* 7:273-286, 1958.

(44) Billington, B.P. Gastric cancer—relationships between ABO blood-groups, site, and epidemiology. *Lancet* 2:859-862, 1956.

(45) Schwartz, D. and G. Anguera. Une cause de biais dans certaines enquêtes médicales: le temps de séjour des malades a l'hôpital. Communication à l'Institut International de Statistique, 30ème Session. Stockholm, 1957.

(46) Cornfield, J. A statistical problem arising from retrospective studies. *Proc Third Berkeley Symposium on Mathematical Statistics and Probability* 4:135-148, 1956.

(47) Satterthwaite, F.E. Synthesis of variance. *Psychometrika* 6:309-316, 1941.

(48) Halperin, M. The use of X^2 in testing effect of birth order. *Ann Eugenics* 18:99-106, 1953.

A CONTROLLED STUDY OF FATAL AUTOMOBILE ACCIDENTS IN NEW YORK CITY[1]

James R. McCarroll,[2] and William Haddon, Jr.[3]

An estimated 1.4 *million* persons have been killed in motor vehicle accidents in the United States alone in the past sixty years (1901-1960) (*1*). Despite this, only two adequately controlled investigations of the factors associated with the occurrence of such *fatal* accidents have been inititated and completed anywhere to date. The first of these, concerned with fatal, adult pedestrian accidents in Manhattan, demonstrated the feasibility of tightly controlled accident research under complex urban conditions. It found large differences between the characteristics of fatally injured pedestrians and those of noninvolved but similarly exposed individuals (*2*). The second study, reported here, represents an extension to the driver-fatal accident of the design and technics developed and employed in the first.

In both of these controlled studies the objective was to compare those fatally injured with noninvolved persons similarly exposed. This was accomplished by matching the exposure of the case and control groups by obtaining the latter in an arbitrary manner at the same sites, on the same days of week, at the same times of day. By thus matching for exposure, artifacts were avoided which had been introduced into other types of accident investigations because of case-control variations in exposure.

CASE SERIES

The case series consisted of forty-three (93 percent) of the forty-six drivers of noncommercial automobiles fatally injured in New York City, exclusive of Staten Island, in the periods of June 1, 1959-October 24, 1959 and June 1, 1960-October 24, 1960. The forty-six deaths represent all those known to the Office of the Chief Medical Examiner of New York, and to the Accident Investigation Squad (A.I.S.), New York City Police Department. Twenty-four of these, twenty-three of which were included in the forty-three in the series, occurred in 1959. Only one driver was killed in each of the forty-six accidents.

Postmortem inspections or examinations were performed in all cases. Analyses for alcohol, based either on brain, or on heart or great vessel blood, were performed by the Office of the Chief Medical Examiner using the method of Gonzales *et al.* (*3*) routinely employed by the Medical Examiner's Office in cases of violent death. Data with respect to the deceased and the circumstances of each accident were obtained from both the Office of the Chief Medical Examiner and from the A.I.S. It is pertinent that the characteristics of case-series members from the two years were not statistically significantly different, and that the numbers of such accidents have shown but little variation from year to year.

CONTROL GROUP

Each accident site was visited on a subsequent date, but on the same day of week and at the same time of day at which the accident had occurred. Site-visit dates were chosen days or weeks in advance without reference to probable weather, and all site visits were made in 1960, within a few weeks of the calendar week of occurrence.

Each site-visit team consisted of one or both of the authors, medical students, and one to eight police. Routinely, on arrival, an *n* between 1 and 20 was chosen. Then each *n*th noncommercial, passenger motor vehicle proceeding in the same direction as that driven by the case-series driver was stopped by the police until a

Source: *Journal of Chronic Diseases* 15:811-826, 1962.
[1] The investigation was supported, in part, by research grants (RG-5937) and (2G-558) from the United States Public Health Service, and by the New York State Departments of Health and Motor Vehicles.
[2] Director, Division of Epidemiologic Research, Department of Public Health, Cornell University Medical College, New York.
[3] Director, Epidemiology Residency Program, New York State Department of Health, Albany; formerly, Director, Driver Research Center, New York State Department of Health—State Department of Motor Vehicles.

total of six had been stopped and successfully interviewed. At many locations with low traffic density an *n* of one was chosen and the *first* six vehicles were stopped. At high-density sites a larger *n* was employed.

Each *n*th driver on being stopped was requested, in a manner similar to that employed previously with pedestrians (*2*), to cooperate anonymously. Despite some initial apprehension and occasional hostility, and in one case an initial plea of diplomatic immunity, only one of 259 drivers stopped (0.4 percent) refused complete interview and breath specimen. The remaining 258 (six from each of the forty-three site visits) constituted the control group. The breath specimens were collected in special Saran bags (*4*), processed as previously described (*2*), and analyzed in a "Breathalyzer"(*2*, *5*).

RESULTS

Figure 1 shows the distribution of cases in the four boroughs Manhattan, Queens, Brooklyn, and Bronx. The Borough of Richmond (Staten Island) was omitted.

Prior to the analysis of the data, each accident in which a member of the case series was fatally injured was placed in one of six categories based upon the type of accident in which he was involved:

I. Only one vehicle involved, its driver fatally injured.
II. More than one vehicle involved, but only one in motion, its driver fatally injured.
III. More than one vehicle involved and in motion, driver in responsible vehicle fatally injured.
IV. More than one vehicle involved, but only one in motion, driver of nonmoving vehicle fatally injured.
V. More than one vehicle involved and in motion, driver in nonresponsible vehicle fatally injured.
VI. More than one vehicle involved and in motion, not known whether fatally injured driver's vehicle was responsible or not.

The category assignment was based on the A.I.S. report without reference either to the blood alcohol concentration of the case series member or to other postmortem finding. Multi-

Figure 1. Locations of forty-three accidents in which drivers of passenger cars were fatally injured in New York City exclusive of Staten Island.

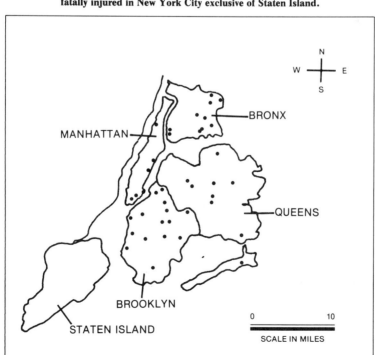

vehicle accidents in which the only evidence as to responsibility was the disclaimer of a surviving driver were placed, because of the frequent unreliability of such statements, in category VI. As appropriate in the tabulations which follow, the thirty responsible drivers in accident categories I, II, and III have been grouped together for analysis, as have the thirteen questionably responsible drivers in accident categories IV, V, and VI (see Table I and Discussion). Cases in the first, responsible, group (I-III) comprised 70 percent (30/43) of the case series. On the basis of the category of each accident, the control subjects from the same site have been similarly categorized and grouped.

Table 1. Categories of accidents from which case-series members were derived.

Accident category[a]	Number of accidents in category[b]
I	19
II	7
III	4[c]
IV	1
V	1[d]
VI	11

[a] See text.
[b] Only one driver was fatally injured in each accident contributing to the case series.
[c] One of these resulted in the death of the driver of a fleeing stolen car who went through a red light and hit another car broadside. A second accident in this category resulted when the vehicle driven by a case-series member crossed into the opposite lane on a Brooklyn to Manhattan bridge and hit an oncoming car head on. The third accident in this category involved a driver seen to be slumped over his wheel before hitting two pedestrians and another car. As the car approached the pedestrians, its estimated speed was only 10-15 miles per hour. The fourth accident resulted when the case-series driver, a transit bus driver by occupation, was seen by two independent witnesses to slump over his wheel and lose control of the car he was driving. It is not known whether or not the drivers in the last two of these accidents were literally "fatally injured," but for lack of further evidence these accidents have been classified as listed. (See also footnotes, Table 5.)
[d] This accident resulted when a car crossed a center island and hit an oncoming car, the driver of which was killed. (See also footnotes, Table 5.)

There were significantly ($P = 0.005$) more accidents (27/43) on weekends (Friday, Saturday, and Sunday) than in the remainder of the week. There was also a significant association ($P = 0.05$) between time of day and accident occurrence, with more accidents from 6 p.m.-5 a.m. than from 6 a.m.-5 p.m. There was no statistically significant association ($P = 0.75$)

between time of day of occurrence and accident category, comparing the time of day distribution (6 a.m.-5 p.m. and 6 a.m.-5 a.m.) of accidents in the responsible (I-III) group with that of those in the questionably responsible (IV-VI) group. In addition, there was no statistically significant association ($P = 0.38$) between road condition (wet or dry) and accident occurrence (see Table 2 and Discussion).

Table 2. Road condition at time of accidents and at subsequent site visits.[a]

	Accident	Site visit[b]	Total
Number wet	9	6	15
Number dry	34	37	71
Total	43	43	86

$$P = 0.38$$

[a] Includes all sites at which the road was wet from any cause, for example, from concurrent or recent rain or from the use of street-washing equipment.
[b] See text.

The case subjects were suggestively *older* in both responsible (I-III) and questionably responsible (IV-VI) groups. However, the differences were not statistically significant ($P > 0.05$) (Table 3). As a result, no age adjustment has been made in the case-control comparisons which follow. In this respect, the analyses presented here differ from those of the pedestrian accident report (2), since in that instance a highly significant, seventeen year case-control age difference made age-adjusted case-control comparisons mandatory.

Table 3. Median age of fatally injured and control group drivers.

Accident category[a]	Cases	Controls
I, II, III	37.0	34.5
IV, V, VI	47.5	35.0
Total I-VI	39.0	35.0

$$P > 0.05 \text{ (Kolmogorov-Smirnov Test}$$

[a] See Table 1 and text.

The ages of the vehicles, taken as the calendar year-model year difference, in the case and control groups were not significantly different ($P > 0.05$) in any of the groups studied (I-III, IV-VI, and I-VI), allowance being made in the case of the twenty-three 1959 accidents for the fact that their controls were obtained one year later (*q.v.*). Also, there was no statistically significant association between car age and time of day in either the accident-responsible case (*P* > 0.9) or control (*P* > 0.2) groups. Further, there was no significant association (*P* > 0.05) between car age in case and control groups and drivers' blood alcohol concentrations. The difference in the case group, however, was suggestive. The median age of the cars of the accident-involved drivers (I-VI) with blood alcohol concentrations (see below) of 100 mg % and higher was 4.5 years in comparison with 3.3 years in the case of case-series drivers with concentrations below 100 mg %. In the control group, the age differences, although not significant (*P* > 0.05), were reversed, 3.0 years (≥ 100 mg %) and 3.8 years (< 100 mg %).

Males were driving all but 11 percent (29 female drivers/258 total) of the *non*involved cars sampled at the times and places of the accidents (Table 4). They were nonetheless significantly overrepresented in the all-male case group (I-III, *P* = 0.04; I-VI, *P* < 0.01). As far as race and place of birth were concerned, no significant case-control differences were found.

The *case*-series' alcohol concentrations by time of day and accident category are given in Table 5 with pertinent additional data, where available. High alcohol concentrations (≥ 100 mg %) were found significantly more often in both the accident responsible group (I-III, *P* < 0.03), and in the total group of accident-involved drivers (I-VI, *P* < 0.01) in the eve-

ning, nighttime, and early morning hours (6 p.m.–5 a.m.) than during the day. In all of the comparisons involving alcohol, only the thirty-seven cases in which postaccident survival was less than six hours have been used—together with their 222 site-matched controls. This was done to avoid the artifacts which would have arisen from including cases in which prolonged postaccident survival had permitted substantial metabolic lowering of the alcohol concentrations present at the times of the accidents. This necessary precaution is seldom taken in the analysis of motor vehicle accident data (*2, 6*).

Alcohol was not detected in the case of the majority (76 percent) of the 258 drivers in the entire *control* group (Table 6). However, 13 percent (34/258) had concentrations in the 20–99 mg % range in which driving deterioration begins and 3 percent (9/258) had concentrations in the high, 100–249 mg %, range.

The percentage of *case*-series members in the accident-responsible group (I-III) with blood alcohol concentrations in the very high 250 mg % and over range was 46 percent (12/26), whereas *no* member of the six-times-as-large control group was in this range (Table 6). Using partial χ², the case-control difference among drivers with concentrations ≥ 100 mg % was highly significant (*P* < 0.001). In the entire group of accident-involved drivers (I-VI), which contained in categories IV-VI a number of drivers not responsible for their accidents and deaths, 41 percent (15/37) of those dying within six hours were in the 250 mg % and over range, in comparison with 0 percent (0/222) in

Table 4. Sex of driver.

Accident category[a]		Male	Female	Total	*P*[b]
I, II, III	Cases	30	0	30	
	Controls	160	20	180	0.04
IV, V, VI	Cases	13	0	13	
	Controls	69	9	78	0.23
I-VI	Cases	43	0	43	0.01
	Controls	229	29	258	
Total		272	29	301	

[a] See Table 1 and text.
[b] In each grouping the probability is the exact probability of obtaining 0 females.

Table 5. Alcohol concentration of fatally injured drivers dying within 6 hours of their accidents, by time of day and accident category.

Accident category[a]	a.m.				p.m.			
	12-2	3-5	6-8	9-11	12-2	3-5	6-8	9-11
III	+3[b]	+3	0	+3	0	0[e]	+3	+3
	+3	+3		No test	0	0	+1[g]	+3
	+3	+2				No test[f]	+1[h]	+3
	+3	0[d]						+1
	+3							
	+2							
	0[c]							
V, VI	+3	+3		0	0	0	0	0[i]
		+3		No rep				0
		0						

[a] See Table 1 and text.

[b] Within each 3 hour period, equivalent alcohol concentrations have been grouped together. The semiquantitative notation used here and the equivalent concentrations are those given by Gonzales et al. (2). See text. 0 = no alcohol detected; $tr > 0$, < 20 mg percent; $+1 = \geq 20$, < 100 mg percent; $+2 = \geq 100$, < 250 mg percent; $+3 = \geq 250$, < 400 mg percent.

[c] Twenty-six-year-old driver of fleeing stolen car hit ramp divider. Driver thrown to pavement. The postmortem examination report records no nontraumatic pathology.

[d] Sixteen-year-old driver of fleeing stolen car fatally injured when he went through a red light and hit a second car broadside. The postmortem examination report records no nontraumatic pathology.

[e] Nineteen-year-old driver of following car in drag race hit puddle and went out of control. The postmortem examination revealed no nontraumatic pathology.

[f] Fifty-seven-year-old driver was seized with chest pains and collapsed. Examination revealed no external signs of trauma.

[g] Fifty-nine-year-old driver was seen to be collapsed over wheel prior to collision with two pedestrians and another vehicle. Postmortem examination revealed occlusive coronary arteriosclerosis, myocardial fibrosis, and cardiac hypertrophy. Cause of collapse not known.

[h] Fifty-two-year-old driver, by occupation a transit bus operator, was seen to slump prior to accident. Postmortem examination revealed no pertinent nontraumatic pathology. Cause of collapse not known.

[i] Fifty-nine-year-old driver found at postmortem examination to have a ruptured cerebral aneurysm. As is commonly the case where medical factors are considered possible, the accident report attributed the accident to a "heart attack" (23).

Table 6. Blood alcohol concentration of fatally injured drivers dying within 6 hours compared with those of noninvolved drivers at the same accident sites.[a]

Accident category[b]		Blood alcohol concentration in mg (%)[c]	00	< 20	20–99	100–249	250–399	Lab. loss no test no report	Total
I, II, III	Cases[d]	(#)	7	0	3	2	12	2	26
		(%)	27	0	12	7	46	8	100
	Controls	(#)	115	4	27	8	0	2	156
		(%)	74	3	17	5	0	1	100
IV, V, VI	Cases[d]	(#)	7	0	0	0	3	1	11
		(%)	64	0	0	0	27	9	100
	Controls	(#)	50	5	7	1	0	3	66
		(%)	76	8	11	2	0	5	102
Total	Cases	(#)	14	0	3	2	15	3	37
		(%)	38	0	8	5	41	8	100
	Controls	(#)	165(195)	9(14)	34(34)	9(9)	0(0)	5(6)	222(258)
		(%)	74(76)	4(5)	15(13)	4(3)	0(0)	2(2)	99(99)

[a] Cases in which postaccident survival was 6 hours or more have been omitted to avoid the artifacts introduced by postaccident, antemortem metabolic lowering of the alcohol concentrations present at the times of the accidents. However, for completeness with respect to the noninvolved drivers, the figures in parenthesis give the data for the drivers sampled at *all* accident sites, regardless of the duration of survival of the corresponding, fatally injured drivers.

[b] See text.

[c] 10 mg. = 0.01 % by wt. = 0.1 per mille.

[d] See footnotes, Table 5.

the corresponding control group, a highly significant difference. The case-control difference in the numbers of drivers in the accident-responsible group (I-III) with no detectable alcohol (negative) was not significantly different ($P = 0.66$) from that of drivers with relatively low concentrations (> 0, < 100 mg %).

Within the married group there was a significant difference in blood alcohol concentration ($P < 0.001$) between the accident-responsible case and control subjects (Table 7). The married *case*-series members more often had higher concentrations (≥ 100 mg %) than the married control-group members. Within the nonmar-

ried group (composed of the never married, widowed, separated, and divorced) a similar difference was found ($P < 0.001$). Marital status (married, nonmarried) was also significantly associated with alcohol concentration ($P < 0.01$). The nonmarried in the entire case-control group more often had high blood alcohol concentrations (≥ 100 mg %). Also, unmarried persons, without reference to their alcohol concentrations, were significantly ($P = 0.02$) over-represented in the entire forty-three member case group in comparison with the 258 member control group. Forty-nine percent of the cases were married, in comparison with 67 percent of the controls.

No statistically significant difference ($P = 0.20$) was found between accident-responsible drivers and their site-matched control drivers with respect to socioeconomic status, as classified using the U.S. Census Classification of Occupations. Also, no significant associations were found with respect to socioeconomic status in relation to alcohol concentration in the accident-responsible case ($P = 0.17$) and control ($P = 0.60$) groups. Finally (Table 8), case drivers were significantly more often closer to their residences than were the noninvolved, control-group drivers.

Table 7. Marital status and alcohol concentration of fatally injured, accident responsible drivers, dying within 6 hours of their accidents, and of their site-matched controls.

Marital status[a]		Alcohol concentration		
		0-99 mg %	≥ 100 mg %	Total
Married[b]	Cases	5	4	9
	Controls	103	5	108
Non-married[c]	Cases	5	10	15
	Controls	43	3	46
Total[d]		156	22	178

[a] Two I-III group case-series members and two controls not tested have been omitted.
[b] The case-control difference in alcohol level within the married group is highly significant ($P < 0.001$, partial χ^2).
[c] The case-control difference in alcohol level within the nonmarried group is highly significant ($P < 0.001$, partial χ^2).
[d] In the entire case-control group there was also a very significant ($P < 0.01$, partial χ^2)-association between marital status and alcohol concentration.

DISCUSSION

A seldom-recognized problem in accident-causation research results from the inclusion in case groups of individuals not responsible for

Table 8. Place of residence of fatally injured and control group drivers.

	Cases		Controls	
	Number	Percent	Number	Percent
Residence and accident site in same borough	35(25)[a]	81(83)[a]	166(108)[a]	64(60)[a]
Residence in different borough of New York	6(4)	14(13)	44(35)	17(19)
Residence elsewhere in New York state	2(1)	5(3)	29(20)	11(11)
Other U. S.	0(0)	0(0)	19(17)	7(9)
Total	43(30)	100(99)	258(180)	99(99)

[a] The parentheses give the data from accidents in Categories, I, II, III, and from their site-matched controls.
$P = 0.04$ (χ^2) for the entire (I-VI) case-control residence difference.
$P = 0.03$ (χ^2) for the accident-responsible (I-III) case-control residence difference.
$P = 0.03$ (partial χ^2) for entire (I-V) case-control residence difference comparing residence in New York City with residence elsewhere.
$P = 0.02$ (partial χ^2) for accident responsible (I-III) case-control residence difference comparing residence in New York City with residence elsewhere.

their accidents. To a corresponding extent, case series tend to include members whose characteristics are similar to those of the noninvolved populations at risk (2). This decreases the magnitude of case-control differences relative to those which would be observed if it were possible to compare uncontaminated groups of the accident-responsible with the remainder of the population at risk. Hence, it is desirable, when possible, to subdivide case series according to probable responsibility. This has been done effectively, for example, in a previous study in which the distribution of a group of drivers' alcohol concentrations was compared with the distribution of their probable responsibilities, independently rated (7). An additional reason for subdivisions into more homogeneous groups stems from the fact that given factors may vary in importance from one such group to the next, as demonstrated by Barmack and Payne (8-10).

The drivers (together with their vehicles) in accidents in categories I, II and III may reasonably be considered, on the basis of the available evidence, to have been responsible in most or all cases for their accidents. For this reason the case-series members from these accidents have been grouped together in the analyses of the data, and referred to as "accident-responsible." A second group comprised of the remaining case-series members, those from accidents in categories IV, V and VI, have been referred to as "questionably responsible." It is recalled that the "accident-responsible" group (I-III) constituted 70 percent (30/43) of the case series. Further, since the accidents in the questionably responsible group (IV-VI) involved some nonresponsible drivers, the fraction of all the accident-responsible drivers in the *entire* case series derived from the I-III group was undoubtedly considerably higher than 70 percent.

The inclusion in the questionably responsible group (IV-VI) of some nonresponsible drivers would be expected to have shifted the characteristics of drivers from this group to a position intermediate between those of the accident-responsible group and those of the corresponding controls. Insofar as the relatively small numbers in the questionably responsible group permitted analyses, this was consistently found to be the case, as can be seen in several of the tables.

The very significant preponderance of Friday, Saturday, and Sunday accidents is consistent with the distributions almost invariably observed elsewhere. The significant preponderance of evening, nighttime, and very early morning accidents has also been often previously observed. It is worth noting, however, that the periods with the highest numbers of accidents, 12-2 and 3-5 a.m., have relatively light traffic. In contrast, the smallest number of accidents (one) in any three-hour period occurred in the three hours ending at 9 a.m., a period during which the city's traffic greatly increases. These data are very similar to those obtained in the Manhattan pedestrian accident study, and suggest, as stated previously, that gross exposure *per se* is not the major determinant of such accidents, and that the factors of importance are more active at other times of the day (2). This also must lead to the questioning of the appropriateness of using the *unqualified* total of miles driven as the demoninator of accident rates calculated for research and other purposes.

The predominance of evening, nighttime, and early morning accidents again underscores the importance of emphasizing the same period in the organization of emergency medical care, "a point of general relevance in the motor-vehicle accident picture"(2). For example, only six of the forty-three member case series survived six hours or more and thirty-four were either dead on arrival at the medical facilities to which they were taken, or were dead within one hour of their accidents. Further, among the twenty-nine injured between 6 p.m. and 9 a.m., only three were alive at 9 a.m. Consequently, prompt medical care during these off-hours is essential. However, since death was immediate in many cases, only the better packaging of the vehicle occupants could have contributed, once their accidents had been initiated, to the possible survival of many of those killed.

The lack of a significant association between road condition and accident occurrence (Table 2) was also seen in the pedestrian-accident study. However, as noted in that context, the design employed does not correct for possible weather-associated shifts in density (2).

It is generally accepted that young drivers have higher fatal, injury-producing, and property-damage accident rates *per license holder* than do those in following decades (11). This has been widely interpreted to indicate that such drivers drive more dangerously. However, such intergroup differences in rate per license holder can result: (1) exclusively from differences in the quantity *and* quality of exposure; (2) from differences in the risks assumed, exposure remaining constant; or (3) from a combination of both. Although the potential importance of such differences in the quality and quantity of exposure has been emphasized by some authorities, for example, by McFarland and Moore (*12*), it has often been overlooked in the discussion of highway accidents and in the design of accident countermeasures.

If younger drivers tend to drive more dangerously under the same conditions of exposure, the age of drivers in accidents should tend to be lower than that of the non-involved similarly exposed. In the investigation reported here, the fatally injured drivers were found to be *older* as a group, though not significantly so, than non-involved drivers similarly exposed (Table 3). This finding is consistent with the possibility that the age-associated differences in accident rates per license holder, referred to above, result primarily from age-associated differences in the quality and quantity of exposure, rather than from differences in risk per unit of exposure, for example, per mile driven, otherwise unqualified. The series reported here, however, is of only moderate size, consisting of forty-three cases and their 258 controls, and as such the data relative to this point should be regarded, pending confirmation, as suggestive rather than conclusive.

This investigation was not designed to determine directly the role of the vehicle itself either from the standpoint of accident causation, or from the standpoint of crash-injury production. The lack of significant case-control differences in car age, however, does not lend support to the possibility that factors associated with vehicle aging contributed prominently to the causation of the fatal accidents studied. This does not, however, rule out either vehicle factors of types which are less commonly contributory than the factors elicited or those which are not significantly associated with vehicle age. Since accidents which result from both use-associated mechanical failures and faulty design and manufacture are known to occur (*13*), the determination of the role of such factors in causation should be elicited by adequately controlled and designed studies in which such vehicle variables are directly studied. This was not the objective

of the work reported here.

The most commonly observed characteristic of the drivers killed, other than maleness, was an extremely high alcohol concentration (Table 5). This was particularly the case during late evening and early morning hours. For example, of the fifteen killed in the 9 p.m.–5 a.m. period, twelve had been drinking heavily (2, 3 +), one moderately (1 +) and only two, both drivers of stolen cars, not at all. In the accident-responsible case group (I-III), 14/26 (54 percent) of all of the drivers had alcohol concentrations ≥ 100 mg % and 12/26 (46 percent) had concentrations ≥ 250 mg %! To put these concentrations in perspective, a 155-lb man, for example, drinking within 1 hour or less and within 2 hours of eating an average meal, would have to consume a minimum of approximately 5 oz. of 80 proof (U.S.) spirits to reach a blood alcohol concentration of 50 mg %, 7.5 oz to reach 100 mg %, and 15.5 oz to reach 250 mg % (*14*).

It is noteworthy that, despite the fact that the site vists were predominantly in the evening and nighttime, 76 percent (195/258) of the drivers in the entire control group had not been drinking to a measurable extent. Nonetheless, a substantial minority, in addition to the drivers in the accidents, had been drinking, since 13 percent had concentrations of 20-99 mg %, and 3 percent had 100-249 mg %. The conjunction of drinking and driving at the times and places of accidents must be regarded, as a result, as by no means rare. It is not the purpose of this report to discuss the considerable evidence that driving performance deteriorates with increasing alcohol concentration. However, it has been repeatedly demonstrated that the driving performance of some individuals begins to deteriorate at concentrations of less than 50 mg %, and that, in the words of an expert committee, "... as the blood alcohol concentration increases, a progressively higher proportion of such individuals are so affected until at a blood alcohol concentration of ... (100 mg %) ... all individuals are definitely impaired" (*15*). Similarly, the report of a special committee of the British Medical Association stated, "The committee considers that a concentration of 50 mg of alcohol in 100 ml of blood while driving a motor vehicle is the highest that can be accepted as entirely consistent with the safety of other road users. While there may be circumstances in which individual driving ability will not depreciate significantly by the time this level is reached, the committee is impressed by the rapidity with which deterioration occurs at blood levels in excess of 100 mg/100 ml. This is true even in the case of hardened drinkers and experienced drivers. The committee cannot conceive of any circumstances in which it could be considered safe for a person to drive a motor vehicle on the public roads with an amount of alcohol in the blood greater than 150 mg/100 ml" (*16*). Such statements are derived from a large, well-documented, and internally consistent body of evidence derived from laboratory, field-trial, and epidemiological investigations (*7, 14, 17-21*). This evidence is reviewed elsewhere (*22*).

Several of the accidents in which alcohol was either present in low concentration or absent involved other circumstances which may reasonably be presumed to have been responsible for the deaths involved (Table 5). Aside from the issue as to whether or not an accident *preceded* by the death or incapacitation of the driver on another basis than drunkenness should be counted as a fatal motor vehicle accident, in the accident-responsible group (I-III) the accidents involving very high alcohol concentrations (≥ 250 mg %) (*12*), fleeing stolen cars (*2*), drag races (*1*), and presumably medical factors (*3*), totaled 69 percent (18/26) of the accident-responsible group herein defined. Drunkenness of the marked degree present in the twelve cases (≥ 250 mg %) referred to was not found in a single member of the control group (Table 6). Further, none of these other events were observed in connection with the control group or its collection. Consequently, the factors just listed, as a group, distinguished between cases and controls in 69 percent (18/26) of the cases in the accident-responsible group. As a group, these same factors, particularly drunkenness, were also represented in the composite, questionably responsible group (IV-VI) but not in the corresponding control group (Tables 5, 6).

There is considerable evidence that a similar situation with respect to the importance of drunkenness in driver-fatal accidents exists in other areas. However, apparently only one previous study of driver-fatal accidents has used an adequately defined and collected case series (*6*), and the methods usually used, discussed elsewhere (*6, 22*), tend to result in substantial underestimates of the actual frequency and extent

of alcohol involvement. In the one adequate study, descriptive of the alcohol concentration distribution of drivers fatally injured in single vehicle accidents in Westchester County, adjacent to New York City, 70 percent had concentrations of 50 mg % or higher; 57 percent, 100 mg % or higher; and 49 percent, 150 mg % or higher. These data are similar to those now reported for the accident-responsible group, and should, together with the data from the noninvolved drivers similarly exposed, leave little further doubt as to the genesis of a remarkably substantial portion of the heterogenous, fatal accident problem. There is also considerable evidence of the importance of alcohol in *non*fatal motor vehicle accidents of various types (*7-10, 21*), but much further work remains to be done.

The presumably medical episodes noted in Table 5 are consistent with previous knowledge (*23*), but the fraction of the case series involved should not, because of the statistically small numbers involved, be taken as indicative of the prominence of such factors in the fatal-accident picture. Further, as pointed out elsewhere (*23*), although such accidents do occur, this knowledge should *not*, per se, be used as the basis of or justification for programs of medical license restriction. It is easily shown that the great rarity of such events in the huge driving population at risk and the practical difficulties inherent in medical screening programs of the types often proposed make such programs both theoretically and practically unreasonable on the basis of present knowledge (*23, 24*). It is also of interest in connection with the proposals which have been made to restrict older drivers, that none of the drivers in this group were sixty years of age or older.

Within both the married and unmarried groups the case-series members had significantly higher alcohol concentrations (Table 7). This is consistent with the data in Table 6 and with other evidence (*q.v.*) documenting the marked increase in risk associated with high alcohol concentration. The significant negative correlation between marital status and alcohol level and the significant overrepresentation of the nonmarried in the case group are of greater interest, and should be the subject of further research. It is very possible that these case-control differences would have been augmented if it had been possible to measure the stability of the marital and other social adjustments of those in the case and control groups. Considerable support for the importance of such social variables has come from the work of others. For example, Tillmann and Hobbs (25) found, in a controlled investigation of taxi drivers with high and low accident rates, that those with high rates had less stable marital adjustments. Also, Tillmann, and McFarland et al. (11) found that among commercial operators those with high rates had significantly more frequent contacts with credit bureaus and with various social agencies. The importance of social and psychological variables in accidents among airmen has also been well documented by Barmack and Payne (8, 10). In addition to their relationship to such other reports, the present findings should also be considered in relation to the "considerable body of literature dealing with alcoholism and marriage," recently reviewed by Bailey (26).

It is not possible on the basis of present evidence to determine the extent to which the alcoholic, as opposed to the nonalcoholic, drinker is contributing to the substantial fraction of fatal and, apparently, also non-fatal accidents in which alcohol is involved. However, the fact that a very substantial proportion of the driver-responsible accidents in which alcohol was a factor involved exceptionally high alcohol concentrations (e.g., 46 percent ≥ 250 mg %) suggests that something more than merely social drinking was involved in the same cases. Consequently, as noted in connection with the discussion of the same problem among pedestrians, many of the strategies implicit in present control measures may be inappropriate to the problem since the alcoholic would not be expected to be appreciably influenced by the approaches used (2, 22, 27).

There is great need for research with respect to the relationship both of drinkers who are not alcoholics, and those who are, to the motor-vehicle accident problem, since it is increasingly likely that the largely ignored problem of alcoholism in the modern community is accounting for substantial fractions of the totals of motor vehicle accidents and deaths. There is also a great need for research with respect to the circumstances under which the drinking which precedes alcohol-involved accidents takes place, and an excellent beginning in this respect has been made by Barmack and Payne (8).

Despite the fact that alcohol-concentration distributions, similarly heavily weighted with exceptionally high values, have been reported previously, for example, from Westchester (6) and Baltimore (28), the impression is growing in the literature that the concentrations found among accident-responsible individuals are *usually* in the much lower range frequently reached by ordinary social drinkers. It is well documented that many accident-responsible drivers and pedestrians do have much lower concentrations, and that such individuals are significantly overrepresented in case series. Nevertheless, the assumption that persons with such low concentrations greatly predominate among accident-responsible drivers in most alcohol-involved accidents is not warranted by the present evidence, at least in so far as fatal accidents are concerned.

The question of whether men or women are safer drivers has long been argued, and lower accident rates per license holder among women are usually cited in favor of women drivers, without information as to whether or not women drive as much, or under the same conditions as men. It is noted that there were no women in the case series. Also, considering the time of day of many of the accidents in the series, it not surprising that few women appeared in the control group (Table 4). Nonetheless, men were significantly overrepresented in the case series. Differences of this type may quite possibly be due to differences in the cultural, social, and personal circumstances under which the members of the two sexes drive, as suggsted, for example, by McFarland and Moore (12). For example, it may be that very high alcohol concentrations are more common among men than among women similarly exposed and that this underlies one portion of the disparity observed. The question, however, is complex and will require much further research.

The significantly greater proximity of the case subjects than of the control subjects to their homes is of interest (Table 8) first, because it duplicates the same finding in the case of fatally injured pedestrians (2), and, second, because it confirms for an urban area the same finding obtained with respect to accidents in a group of rural areas (29). Although the reasons for this greater proximity cannot be determined without further reearch, it might be expected that

drivers drinking very excessively might be
closer to home than other drivers in the same
areas. The data in Table 8 are of further interest because they show that, like the pedestrian-
accident problem, the problem of the driver-
fatal accident in New York is predominantly of
very local origin. Unlike the non-accident-in-
volved drivers similarly exposed, eighty-three
percent (25/30) of the drivers in the accident-
responsible group were fatally injured in the
same borough as their homes, and only one of
the thirty accident-responsible drivers was from
outside the city.

SUMMARY

Drivers of noncommercial automobiles fatally
injured in accidents in New York City were compared with noninvolved drivers passing the accident sites at the same times of day and on the
same days of the week. The greatest difference
between the two groups was in the prior use of
alcohol. Among drivers rated as probably responsible for their accidents, 73 percent had
been drinking to some extent whereas only 26
percent of the similarly exposed, but noninvolved drivers had been drinking. Forty-six percent of the accident-responsible group had
blood alcohol concentrations in the very high,
250 mg % and over, range. In contrast, not a
single one of the drivers in the large control
group had a concentration in this range.

Also represented in the fatally injured group,
but not in the control group, were drivers of
fleeing stolen cars, one driver killed in a drag
race, and a small group of drivers, all in the
fifth decade of life, whose accidents resulted
from the prior, medical incapacitation. It is
pointed out that all of the drivers in these latter
categories were sober, and that the occurrence
of accidents in the medical group should not
per se be used in justification of programs of
medical license restrictions on the basis of present evidence.

Those fatally injured were significantly closer
to home than were the similarly exposed, but
noninvolved, drivers and almost none of those
fatally injured lived outside the city.

The case group was composed entirely of
males. Although few women were driving at the
times and places of the predominantly nighttime and early morning accidents, males were
nonetheless significantly overrepresented in the

case group. The fatally injured were also significantly less often married, and in the entire case-
control group those not married had significantly higher alcohol concentrations than those
married.

The fatally injured drivers were not significantly different in age or socioeconomic status
from the similarly exposed but noninvolved
controls, and no association between accident
involvement and vehicle age was found.

Finally, it is suggested that alcoholism rather
than merely social drinking was involved in the
case of the drivers with very high alcohol concentrations.

ACKNOWLEDGMENTS

This work would not have been possible without the superb cooperation of Dr. Milton Helpern, Chief Medical Examiner, City of New York,
and of the officers and men of the New York
City Police Department. The authors particularly wish to thank former Police Commissioner
Stephen P. Kennedy; Assistant Chief Inspector
John J. King, Commanding Officer, Safety Division; Captain Milton Zarchin, Commanding Officer, Accident Investigation Squad; Lieutenant
James Donnelly, Commanding Officer, Accident Records Bureau; and Lieutenant Hugh A.
Cleary and Sgt. Joseph Cea of the Accident
Investigation Squad.

In addition, Blaine A. Braniff, Robert B.
McFadden and Richard M. Sallick of Cornell
Medical College, and Robert E. Carroll, Albany
Medical College, carried a large share of the
burden imposed by the often inconvenient site
visits, and this, together with the high level of
professional competence with which they
worked, are greatly appreciated. The authors
also wish to thank Dr. Alan M. Gittelsohn, Director, Office of Biostatistics, New York State
Department of Health, and Mrs. Wilhemina
Calhoun for their very considerable assistance
in the evaluation of the data, and the staffs of
the Division of Epidemiologic Research and the
Epidemiology Residency Program for their continued support.

References

(1) National Safety Council. *Accident Facts.* (1961
Edition.) Chicago, 1961.
(2) Haddon, W., Jr., P. Valien, J.R. McCarroll, and
C.J. Umberger. A controlled investigation of the char-

acteristics of adult pedestrians fatally injured by motor vehicles in Manhattan. *J Chron Dis* 14:655, 1961.

(3) Gonzales, T.A., M. Vance, M. Helpern, and C.J. Umberger. *Legal Medicine Pathology and Toxicology* (2d Edition). Appleton-Century-Crofts, New York, 1954, p. 1095.

(4) Salem, H., G.H.W. Lucas, and D.M. Lucas. Saran plastic bags as containers for breath samples. *Canad Med Ass J* 82:682, 1960.

(5) Friedmann, T.E., and K.M. Dubowski. Chemical testing procedures for the determination of ethyl alcohol. *JAMA* 170, 47, 1959. Also published by: American Medical Association's Committee on Medicolegal Problems. *Chemical Tests for Intoxication Manual*. Chicago, 1959.

(6) Haddon, W., Jr., and V.A. Bradess. Alcohol in the single vehicle fatal accident: Experience of Westchester County, New York. *JAMA* 169:1587, 1959; reprinted in *Traff Saf Res Rev* 3, 1959.

(7) Smith, H.W. and R.E. Popham. Blood alcohol levels in relation to driving. *Canad Med Ass J* 65:325, 1951.

(8) Barmack, J.E. and D.E. Payne. Injury-producing private motor vehicle accidents among airmen: Psychological models of accident-generating processes. *J Psychol* 52:3, 1961.

(9) Barmack, J.E. and D.E. Payne. Injury-producing private motor vehicle accidents among airmen: I. The role of drinking. *Highw Res Bd Bull* 285, 1961.

(10) Barmack, J.E. and D.E. Payne. Injury-producing private motor vehicle accidents among airmen: II. Background correlates of the lost-time accident. *Highw Res Bd Bull* 285, 1961.

(11) McFarland, R.A., R.C. Moore, and A.B. Warren. *Human variables in motor vehicle accidents: A review of the literature*. Harvard School of Public Health, 1955.

(12) McFarland, R.A. and R.C. Moore. *Youth and the automobile*. Presented at the White House Conference on Children and Youth, 1960; reprinted by the Association for the Aid of Crippled Children.

(13) *Comstock vs. General Motors et al.*, 358 Mich. 163, 99 N.W. 2d 627, 1959.

(14) Coldwell, B.B. (Editor). *Report on impaired driving tests*. Crime Detection Laboratory, Royal Canadian Mounted Police, Queen's Printer, Ottawa, 1957.

(15) *Proceedings of the symposium on alcohol and road traffic, 1958*. Indiana University, 1959.

(16) Alcohol and road accidents: Report of Special British Medical Association Committee. *Brit Med J* 1:269, 1960.

(17) Loomis, T.A. and T.C. West. The influence of alcohol on automobile driving ability: An experimental study for evaluation of certain medicolegal aspects, *Quart J Stud Alcohol* 19:30, 1958.

(18) Drew, G.C., W.P. Colquhoun, and H.A. Long. Effect of small doses of alcohol on a skill resembling driving. *Brit Med J* 2,5103,1958; reprinted in *Traff Saf Res Rev* 1:4, 1959.

(19) Bjerver, K. and L. Goldberg. Effect of alcohol ingestion on driving ability: Results of practical road tests and laboratory experiments. *Quart J Stud Alcohol* 11:1, 1950.

(20) Cohen, J., E.J. Dearnaley, and C.E.M. Hansel. The risk taken in driving under the influence of alcohol. *Brit Med J* 15:1438, 1958.

(21) Lucas, G.H.W., W. Kalow, J.D. McColl, B.A. Griffith, and H.W. Smith. Quantitative studies of the relationship between alcohol levels and motor vehicle accidents. *Proceedings of the Second International Conference on Alcohol and Road Traffic, Toronto*, 139, 1953.

(22) Haddon, W., Jr. Alcohol and highway accidents. Presented at the American Medical Association Symposium on the medical aspects of automobile injuries and deaths. One Hundred and Tenth Annual Meeting, New York City, June 27, 1961.

(23) Haddon, W., Jr. In *The Heart in Industry*. L.J. Warshaw, Editor. New York, P.B. Hoeber, 1960, pp. 406-407.

(24) Haddon, W., Jr. Drivers' licenses. *AMA News (Letters)* 4, 1961.

(25) Tillmann, W.A. and G.E. Hobbs. The accident-prone automobile driver: A study of the psychiatric and social background. *Amer J Psychiat* 106:321, 1949.

(26) Bailey, M.B. Alcoholism and marriage, a review of research and professional literature. *Quart J Stud Alcohol* 22, 81, 1961.

(27) Schmidt, W.S. and R.G. Smart. Alcoholics, drinking, and traffic accidents. *Quart J Stud Alcohol* 20:631, 1959.

(28) Freimuth, H.C., R.W. Spencer, and R.S. Fisher. Alcohol and highway fatalities. *J. Forens Sci Soc* 3, 65, 1958; reprinted in *Traff Saf Res Rev* 4, 23, 1960

(29) Anonymous. *The federal role in highway safety*. U.S. Government Printing Office, 1959.

AGE AT FIRST BIRTH AND BREAST CANCER RISK[1]

B. MacMahon,[2] P. Cole,[3] T. M. Lin,[4] C. R. Lowe,[5] A. P. Mirra,[6] B. Ravnihar,[7] E. J. Salber,[8] V. G. Valaoras,[9] and S. Yuasa[10]

An international collaborative study of breast cancer and reproductive experience has been carried out in seven areas of the world. In all areas studied, a striking relation between age at first birth and breast cancer risk was observed. It is estimated that women having their first child when aged under 18 years have only about one-third the breast cancer risk of those whose first birth is delayed until the age of 35 years or more. Births after the first, even if they occur at an early age, have no, or very little, protective effect. The reduced risk of breast cancer in women having their first child at an early age explains the previously observed inverse relationship between total parity and breast cancer risk, since women having their first birth early tend to become ultimately of high parity. The association with age at first birth requires different kinds of etiological hypotheses from those that have been invoked in the past to explain the association between breast cancer risk and reproductive experience.

One of the most consistently observed epidemiological characteristics of breast cancer is the inverse association between the number of children a woman has borne and her risk of developing the disease. This association has been observed in all geographic areas and ethnic groups in which it has been studied. The association has been interpreted as indicating that some concomitant of pregnancy protects against the later development of breast cancer, the amount of protection being related to the number of pregnancies.

Analyses of data from a recent international collaborative study have shown that breast cancer risk is strongly correlated with age at first pregnancy (1, 2, 3, 4, and Lin, Chen, and MacMahon; Ravnihar, MacMahon, and Lindtner; Mirra and Cole, unpublished data). These analyses were based on the women's ages at their first pregnancy, even if that pregnancy aborted. Differences between cases and controls with respect to frequency of abortion were observed in only a few centers and were in the direction which suggested increased risk associated with abortion—contrary to the reduction in risk associated with full-term births. Therefore, it seemed worthwhile to conduct analyses restricting attention to the age at which the first full-term birth occurred. The details are presented in this paper. The analysis has also been extended to take a more detailed account of possible interrelationships with other variables and to examine the effect of age at confinements, other than the first.

METHODS

The case-control study which is the source of these data, has been described previously (5). It was conducted in seven areas of the world; the

Source: *Bulletin of the World Health Organization* 43:209-221, 1970.

[1] This study was supported by Grant E-385 A from the American Cancer Society; Grant 402-C-200 from the Boris Kidric Fund of Yugoslavia; a grant from the Medical Research Council of Great Britain; a grant from the Ministry of Health and Welfare, Japan; Grant 5 POI CA 06373 from the U.S. National Cancer Institute; a grant from the National Council for Science of China (Taiwan); and Grants R/00057, R/00062, R/00072 and C2/18/24 from the World Health Organization.

[2] Professor, Department of Epidemiology, Harvard School of Public Health, Boston, Mass., U.S.A.

[3] Assistant Professor, Department of Epidemiology, Harvard School of Public Health, Boston, Mass., U.S.A.

[4] Associate Professor, Department of Epidemiology, College of Medicine, National Taiwan University, Taipei, Taiwan.

[5] Mansel Talbot Professor, Department of Social and Occupational Medicine, Welsh National School of Medicine, University of Wales, Cardiff, Wales.

[6] Director, Central Cancer Registry, São Paulo, Brazil.

[7] Professor, Institute of Oncology, Medical Faculty, University of Ljubljana, Yugoslavia.

[8] Senior Research Associate, Department of Epidemiology, Harvard School of Public Health, Boston, Mass., U.S.A.

[9] Professor, Department of Hygiene and Epidemiology, University of Athens, Athens, Greece.

[10] Medical Officer, Department of Epidemiology, Institute of Public Health, Tokyo, Japan.

populations included exhibited a wide range of incidence rates for breast cancer—from a high of 55 per 100 000 persons per year in Boston, U.S.A., to about 10 per 100 000 persons in Tokyo, Japan, and Taipei, Taiwan. As far as possible, the cases included all female residents of the study areas who were hospitalized for a first diagnosis of breast cancer during the study period. The controls were patients hospitalized in the same hospitals for conditions other than breast cancer. The three eligible patients in the beds closest to that of the index case were interviewed for each breast cancer patient interviewed. Eligibility required being a resident of the study population, never having had cancer of the breast, and being over 35 years of age (unless the breast cancer patient was under 35 years of age, in which event an age-match within two years of the breast cancer patient's age was required). The interview form and the study protocol were the same for all centers. Coding, data-processing, and analyses for all study areas were carried out in a single co-ordinating center.

In all, more than 4000 breast cancer cases and nearly 13 000 control patients were interviewed. In five of the centers, the breast cancer cases included 80 percent or more of the cases known to have occurred during the study period. In two centers total ascertainment was not possible but the interviewed cases are believed to have represented about 50 percent of all incident cases in one (Tokyo) and about 70 percent in the other (São Paulo, Brazil).

For the purpose of the present analyses, her age at the time of birth of each of her full-term children was computed for each woman from her own and her children's dates of birth. Abortions—defined as pregnancies with fetal death prior to the fifth month—were excluded, but children stillborn at five or more months' gestation were included. "Parity" is also defined in terms of births at or after the fifth month of pregnancy, whether liveborn or stillborn. Single and ever-married women are included. In five of the seven centers (all but Slovenia and São Paulo), single women were not questioned about their reproductive histories and have been assumed to be nulliparous. A few interviews (56 cases, 128 controls) were rated as "unreliable" by interviewers; these have been excluded. Also excluded are 11 cases and 31 controls for whom age at first birth is unknown. The numbers of women on whom the present analyses are based are given in Table 1.

FINDINGS

Age at first birth

Table 2 shows the relationship between total parity and breast cancer risk. In this table, the risk for women of any specified parity relative to that of nonparous women is calculated from the usual formula ad/bc, where a is the number of cases of that parity, b the number of controls in the same parity, and c and d the number of nonparous cases and controls, respectively. The trends are not regular but, except in Slovenia where the trend is weak and in Tokyo where it is strong, estimated risks for women of parity five or more are between 40 percent and 60 percent

Table 1. Number of breast cancer cases and controls interviewed in the various study centers.

Center	Numbers included in present analyses						Numbers excluded[a]	
	Cases			Controls				
	Non-parous	Parous	Total	Non-parous	Parous	Total	Case	Control
Boston, U.S.A.	203	374	577	467	1262	1729	29	78
Glamorgan, Wales	161	446	607	321	1492	1813	12	37
Athens, Greece	216	579	795	554	1910	2464	4	6
Slovenia, Yugoslavia	153	601	754	419	1862	2281	18	27
São Paulo, Brazil	112	420	532	229	1298	1527	5	28
Taipei, Taiwan	34	177	211	55	589	644	3	4
Tokyo, Japan	224	623	847	409	1832	2241	2	9
All centers	1103	3220	4323	2454	10 245	12 699	73	189

[a] Women whose interview was rated "unreliable" by the interviewer and those for whom parity or age at first birth was not recorded are excluded.

of those of the nulliparous. This is the usual relationship between parity and breast cancer risk, as observed many times by previous workers.

Table 3 shows the association of breast cancer risk with age at first birth. In all seven centers,

Table 2. Estimates of relative risk[a] of breast cancer, by parity.

Center	0	1	2	3	4	≥5
			Parity			
Boston	100	76	81	64	59	54
Glamorgan	100	68	60	63	61	42
Athens	100	76	93	77	68	58
Slovenia	100	93	89	84	83	90
São Paulo	100	78	87	60	62	57
Taipei	100	74	48	41	47	48
Tokyo	100	82	84	60	59	34

[a] Risk relative to an arbitrary risk of 100 for the nonparous (see text).

risk increases with increase in the age at which a woman bore her first child. In five of the centers the trend is strong and regular, with women who had their first birth when under 20 years of age having only about one-third the risk of those whose first birth occurred at the age of 35 years or older. In Slovenia, the trend appears not to be as strong as in the other centers. In this center, for women with first births after the age of 20 years, the trend is consistent with that in other centers, but the relative risk for women with births under the age of 20 years is inconsistently high. In Taipei, the trend is irregular, perhaps as a consequence of the small numbers in this center, but the impression of low breast cancer risk for women having their first birth at an early age is present. It is interesting that the trend is reasonably consistent between centers in spite of the considerable differences in the distribution of women by age at first birth. For example, nearly 30 percent of the women in

Table 3. Percentage distribution of cases and controls, and estimates of relative risk of breast cancer, by age at first birth.

Group	Center	Nulli-parous	<20	20-24	25-29	30-34	≥35	Total
			Parous, age at first birth being:					
Cases	Boston	35.2	3.1	19.6	23.4	12.5	6.2	100.0
	Glamorgan	26.5	3.8	27.2	24.5	11.7	6.3	100.0
	Athens	27.2	8.2	22.5	22.5	14.0	5.7	100.1
	Slovenia	20.3	5.0	27.4	28.4	12.6	6.2	99.9
	São Paulo	21.5	20.5	39.1	13.2	3.4	2.3	100.0
	Taipei	16.1	16.6	41.7	14.7	8.1	2.8	100.0
	Tokyo	26.5	2.8	29.4	27.9	9.1	4.4	100.1
	All centers	25.5	7.4	27.9	23.4	10.7	5.1	100.0
Controls	Boston	27.0	7.5	27.2	23.5	10.7	4.1	100.0
	Glamorgan	17.7	6.7	37.0	24.6	10.6	3.4	100.0
	Athens	22.5	13.2	26.1	23.6	10.9	3.7	100.0
	Slovenia	18.4	5.7	33.7	27.3	10.2	4.8	100.1
	São Paulo	15.0	29.3	42.1	9.8	2.9	0.9	100.0
	Taipei	8.5	16.2	48.5	20.7	4.8	1.4	100.1
	Tokyo	18.2	7.5	41.4	24.5	6.2	2.2	100.0
	All centers	19.3	11.2	34.9	22.7	8.6	3.2	99.9
Relative risk[a]	Boston	100	32	55	76	90	117	
	Glamorgan	100	38	49	67	73	124	—
	Athens	100	51	71	79	106	127	—
	Slovenia	100	81	74	94	112	118	—
	São Paulo	100	49	65	94	84	175	—
	Taipei	100	54	45	37	89	106	—
	Tokyo	100	26	49	78	100	138	—
	All centers	100	50	60	78	94	122	—
Married only[b]	All centers	100	48	59	76	91	119	—

[a] Estimated risk relative to a risk of 100 for the nonparous.
[b] Relative risk based on married women only.

São Paulo, but only 7 percent of those in Glamorgan, Wales, had a birth before the age of 20 years, but the relative risks for women in this group are similar in the two centers. It is also of interest that the reduction in relative risk appears not to be dependent on the overall level of breast cancer rates in a particular area.

The risks for women who had their first birth between the ages of 30 and 34 years approach those of nonparous women, and, in all centers, women whose first birth was delayed until the age of 35 years or over actually had higher risks than nulliparous women.

In view of the general similarity of these trends, it seemed reasonable to pool the data for all centers. Table 3 gives an estimate, from the pooled data, that the breast cancer risk for women having their first birth under the age of 20 years is about half that for nulliparous women and 40 percent of that for women whose first birth is delayed until the age of 35 years or over.

To evaluate the effect of the assumption made in five centers, that single women were non-parous, the bottom row of Table 3 shows the pooled relative risks based on married women only. The values are almost identical with those based on all women, and the remaining analyses are therefore based on all women regardless of marital status.

Pooling of the data from all centers enables estimates of relative risk for individual years of age at first birth to to be made. These values, for ages of 14 years to 41 years, inclusive, are plotted in the accompanying figure. The figure suggests that, at least up to about 30 years of age, breast cancer risk increases linearly with increasing age at first birth. For women having

first births when under 20 years of age, the risk continues to decrease as age at first birth decreases; women with first births when under 18 years of age have only about one-third of the breast cancer risk of those with first births when over 35 years. The number of women having first births in the individual ages after 30 years is small, even when the data for all centers are combined, and the estimates of relative risk have fairly large variances. It is not clear, therefore, whether the linear trend continues for first births after the age of 30 years.

Relationship to total parity

We must of course examine the possibility that the association of breast cancer risk with age at first birth reflects merely the low parity of the breast cancer patients—women of low parity tending to begin their reproductive lives late. The fact that, in all centers except Taipei, the relative risks associated with first birth under the age of 20 years (Table 3) are lower than those for women of parity five or more (Table 2) suggests that age at first birth is the more relevant variable. However, the question can be approached more directly.

Table 4 shows the observed numbers of cases with first births under the age of 20 years, together with expected values based on the control series adjusted for pertinent variables, including parity. The use of parity-specific rates in the control series does shift the expected values towards the observed values in all centers. However, the shifts are small and, except in Slovenia and Taipei where the differences were small even before correction for parity, substantial differences remain after this adjustment.

Table 4. Observed number of breast cancer cases with first births when under 20 years of age and expected values computed from the control series.

Center	Observed	Expected,[a] with adjustment for:			
		No. variables	Parity	Age at interview	Duration of schooling
Boston	18	38.2	34.7	37.7	37.5
Glamorgan	22	36.5	33.5	35.9	35.4
Athens	65	98.2	94.0	99.7	93.2
Slovenia	38	41.6	41.4	41.8	41.6
São Paulo	117	144.6	135.8	144.2	140.5
Taipei	35	31.3	32.6	33.6	28.1
Tokyo	24	57.1	47.8	52.5	52.5

[a] The expected values are based on the distribution of the control series, specific for the stated variables.

Figure 1. Relative risk[a] of breast cancer according to age at first birth; data for all centers combined.

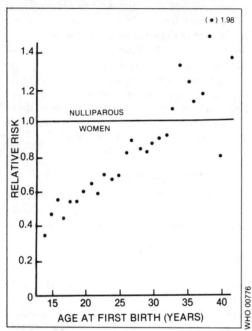

[a]Relative to a risk of 1.0 for nulliparous women.

That the association of breast cancer risk with age at first birth is not merely a reflection of the low parity of breast cancer patients can also be demonstrated by restricting attention to women who have borne only one child. Relative risks for such women, according to age at which their only birth occurred, are shown in Table 5. Except in Slovenia and Taipei, which again show irregular patterns, there is in each center a sharp increase in risk as age at confinement increases.

Births after the first

Since the increased risk associated with delayed first birth is not explained by the low parity of breast cancer patients, we must consider the possibility that the late first births of such women explain the previously noted association of risk with low parity. Table 6 shows observed and expected numbers of cases having births after the first. In this table expected values are based on the distribution of the controls specific for each individual year of age at first birth. If births after the first were associated with decreased breast cancer risk, the number of cases who had no births after the first would be higher than the expected value; it is actually slightly lower. There is a deficit of cases with four or more births after the first (observed 600, expected 668.1), but the risk for this category is reduced only to 93 relative to 100 for the women having no subsequent births. Moreover, the deficit of cases with four or more subsequent births is substantial only in Tokyo. It seems, therefore, that births after the first have relatively little influence on breast cancer risk, and the relationship between breast cancer risk and parity results primarily from the fact that age at first birth and ultimate total parity are highly correlated.

We must still inquire whether births after the first may exert a protective influence if they

Table 5. Estimates of relative risk of breast cancer by age at delivery, for women of parity one only.

Center	Relative risks,[a] age at delivery being:						No. of:	
	<20	20-24	25-29	30-34	≥35	Any age	Cases	Controls
Boston	19	72	60	107	118	76	77	233
Glamorgan	(50)[b]	29	100	55	106	68	117	345
Athens	44	64	65	120	81	76	129	433
Slovenia	123	81	83	126	88	93	136	399
São Paulo	66	70	102	74[b]	(175)[b]	78	63	165
Taipei	(92)[b]	(61)[b]	(121)[b]	(50)[b]	(81)[b]	74	22	48
Tokyo	52	61	67	119	152	82	135	302
All centers	58	62	77	98	104	78	679	1925

[a] Relative risks are expressed relative to a risk of 100 for nonparous women. Estimates are based on direct comparison of cases and controls, without adjustment.
[b] Values for cells containing less than 20 controls are shown in parentheses.

Table 6. Observed and expected numbers of breast cancer cases having specified numbers of births after the first, adjusted for age at the first birth.

Center	No. of cases having one or more births	None		1		2		3		4-8		≥9	
		Obs.	Exp.[a]	Obs.	Exp.[a]	Obs.	Exp.[a]	Obs.	Exp.[a]	Obs.	Exp.[a]	Obs.	Exp.[a]
Boston	374	77	78.6	122	109.2	75	77.4	42	46.2	58	59.4	0	3.3
Glamorgan	446	117	122.5	138	137.6	91	85.4	51	42.7	45	53.8	4	4.1
Athens	579	129	148.4	210	178.1	109	105.5	64	69.1	62	74.2	5	3.7
Slovenia	601	136	137.8	163	161.5	110	114.6	75	77.8	106	100.9	11	8.4
São Paulo	420	63	58.4	100	79.7	59	68.9	47	50.8	118	122.9	33	39.4
Taipei	177	22	19.4	26	24.7	29	34.0	29	29.3	62	62.6	9	7.1
Tokyo	623	135	128.6	186	150.4	120	121.6	95	94.2	86	123.3	1	5.0
All centers	3220	679	693.7	945	841.2	593	607.4	403	410.1	537	597.1	63	71.0
Relative risk[b]	—	100		116		101		102		93		92	

[a] Expected values are based on rates in the control series specific for individual years of age at first birth.
[b] Relative to a risk of 100 for women having no births after the first; data for all centers combined.

occur at a young age. Table 7 shows observed and expected distributions of women who had at least one birth when under the age of 25 years according to the number of births they had under that age. The expected values are computed, taking account of the specific year of age at the first birth. Using the pooled data from all centers, there is a suggestion that the risk for women having more than one birth when under the age of 25 years is somewhat lower than for those having only one. However, the reduction is relatively small. Thus, among women who had a second birth when under the age of 25 years, the mean age at the second birth (all centers combined) was 22.1 years. The figure indicates that a first birth at this age would be associated with a reduction in risk of about 40 percent. The data in Table 7 indicate that the additional reduction of risk associated with more than one birth when under the age of 25 years is about 13 percent.

In all centers combined, there were 319 cases in which a first birth occurred under the age of 20 years. Of these, 78 had more than one birth

Table 7. Observed and expected numbers of breast cancer cases with specified numbers of births prior to the age of 25 years.

Center	No. of Cases	1		2		≥3	
		Obs.	Exp.[a]	Obs.	Exp.[a]	Obs.	Exp.[a]
Boston	131	89	76.0	31	38.3	11	16.7
Glamorgan	187	122	113.3	46	51.6	19	22.1
Athens	243	137	125.3	67	76.6	39	41.1
Slovenia	245	158	143.9	64	68.7	23	32.4
São Paulo	321	109	97.9	117	115.7	95	107.4
Taipei	123	46	52.1	47	39.3	30	31.6
Tokyo	272	172	173.9	80	76.7	20	21.5
All centers	1522	833	782.4	452	466.9	237	272.8
Relative risk[b]	—	68		61		55	

[a] The table is based on women with at least one birth before the age of 25 years. Expected values are based on rates in the control series specific for individual years of age at first birth.
[b] Relative to a risk of 100 for women with no births before the age of 25 years.

Table 8. Observed and expected numbers of breast cancer cases having births other than the first at the age of 35 years or older.

Center	Women whose first birth occurred at 35 years of age or older			Women whose first birth occurred under 35 years of age		
	No. of women	No. having one or more other births		No. of women	No. having one or more births at 35 years of age or older	
		Obs.	Exp.[a]		Obs.	Exp.[a]
Boston	36	18	17.9	338	118	124.6
Glamorgan	38	12	8.6	408	131	125.3
Athens	45	25	11.7	534	127	116.0
Slovenia	47	28	21.9	554	221	183.7
São Paulo	12	6	4.9	408	94	93.6
Taipei	6	4	3.3	171	54	50.5
Tokyo	37	12	12.5	586	141	175.8
All centers	221	105	80.8	2999	886	869.5
Relative risk[b]	—	157		—	103	

[a] Expected values are based on rates in the control series specific for individual years of age at first birth.

[b] Relative to a risk of 100 for women in the same age-at-first-birth category who had no subsequent births when aged 35 years or more.

when under this age. The expected number having more than one birth when under the age of 20 years (68.5), computed with adjustment for age at which the first birth occurred, is actually lower than the observed. If births other than the first at an early age conferred additional protection, the expected value would of course be higher than the observed. In summary, it seems that if births after the first have any additional protective influence it is substantially less than that of a first birth at the same age.

Table 3 indicates that women with first births when over 35 years of age have higher risks than nonparous women. In Table 8, therefore, relative risks associated with births other than the first occurring over the age of 35 years are examined. The data are shown separately for women whose first birth occurred at 35 years of age or over and for women whose first birth occurred before the age of 35 years. In each case, expected values are based on the control series with adjustment for age at first birth. In women whose first birth was delayed until the age of 35 years, additional births do seem to be associated with an increase in risk. However, no such increase in risk is seen for women having

births when over the age of 35 years if their first birth occurred prior to that age.

Socioeconomic status

Socioeconomic status, being related to both age at first birth and breast cancer risk, must also be examined as a possible confounding variable. In our data, the duration of a patient's schooling was found to be the measure of socioeconomic status most closely related to breast cancer risk. As shown in Table 4, adjustment for this variable does reduce the expected values for patients with births under the age of 20 years but, again, the reductions are relatively small and substantial differences between expected and observed values persist after the adjustment.

We have also examined the possibility that the association of breast cancer risk with age at first birth may explain the previously observed association of the disease with socioeconomic status. However, in those centers where differences exist between cases and controls with respect to socioeconomic status—in particular Athens, São Paulo, and Tokyo—the extent of the differences is not substantially changed by adjusting for age at first birth.

Age at diagnosis of cancer

In at least some of the areas included in this study, changes have occurred over time in the usual age at first confinement in the female population. We must therefore consider the possible effect of age differences between cases and controls at the time of interview—in effect, the age at diagnosis of breast cancer. The computation of expected values using age-specific rates (Table 4) leaves the expected values virtually unchanged, and age at interview can be ignored as a variable likely to confound the association of breast cancer risk with age at first birth.

It is also of interest to know whether the association of breast cancer risk with age at first birth differs between cases diagnosed at different ages. Table 9 shows the risks for women with first births when under the age of 25 years relative to those for women with first births when aged 30 years or over, according to age at diagnosis of cancer. Two estimates are given of the values for the pooled data. One of these, A, is based on the simple sums of the numbers of cases and controls in the specific age group in all centers. This estimate has the disadvantage that the different centers contribute in different proportions to the several age-at-diagnosis groups and also exhibit different strengths of the association between breast cancer risk and

age at first birth. For example, the association with age at first birth appears to be particularly strong in Tokyo (Table 3) and the age distribution of the cases in Tokyo is lower than that in the other centers. A second estimate for the pooled data, B, is therefore derived by obtaining a weighted mean of the values shown for individual centers, the weights being the numbers of controls in the various centers. The weights are the same in all age-at-diagnosis groups.

Within individual centers, trends in Table 9 are irregular—presumably because of the small numbers in many of the cells. Both sets of estimates from the pooled data suggest less reduction in the relative risk among cases first diagnosed after 65 years of age than in younger age groups. However, this difference is relatively small and a protective effect of a first pregnancy under the age of 25 years is seen in all age categories.

Age at marriage

Since the risk of breast cancer in married, nulliparous women is similar to that in single women (5), there seems no reason to suspect that the association observed with age at first birth is an indirect expression of an association between breast cancer risk and age at marriage. However, this question can be explored directly by examining the age at marriage of nulliparous women. Such an examination is shown in Table 10.

Table 9. Estimates[a] of risk of breast cancer for women with first births before the age of 25 years, relative to risks for women with first births at 30 years or older, by age at diagnosis of cancer.

Center	Age at diagnosis				
	<45	45-54	55-64	65-74	≥75
Boston	56	28	68	81	62
Glamorgan	54	61	51	63	72
Athens	63	54	37	92	77
Slovenia	65	66	75	57	113
São Paulo	42	64	82	—	—
Taipei	70	29	—	—	—
Tokyo	38	60	33	37	—
All centers					
A[b]	54	55	59	62	70
B[c]	55	55	56	66	81

[a] Estimates are not shown for cells containing less than five expected cases.
[b] Estimates derived from actual sums of the data in each age group from all centers.
[c] Weighted means of the values shown for individual centers. Weights are the number of controls included, as shown in Table 1.

Table 10. Observed and expected numbers of breast cancer cases, by marital status and age at first marriage; nonparous cases only.

Center	Observed or expected	Never married	Ever-married, age at first marriage being:					
			<20	20-24	25-29	30-34	≥35	Total
Boston	Obs.	114	8	16	25	8	28	199
	Exp.[a]	108.0	7.3	21.7	19.4	12.1	30.5	199.0
Glamorgan	Obs.	61	3	25	32	12	27	160.0 [b]
	Exp.[a]	61.2	3.8	28.5	28.4	12.3	25.9	160.1
Athens	Obs.	80	16	27	29	25	34	211
	Exp.[a]	74.5	27.5	32.1	31.3	20.4	25.2	211.0
Slovenia	Obs.	92	1	13	17	16	17	156
	Exp.[a]	89.9	1.9	11.7	17.9	12.0	22.6	156.0
São Paulo	Obs.	67	18	17	3	3	8	116
	Exp.[a]	55.2	26.0	20.1	7.8	3.1	3.9	116.1
Taipei	Obs.	1	10	14	4	2	2	33
	Exp.[a]	8.2	8.6	11.8	0.9	0.6	2.9	33.0
Tokyo	Obs.	65	20	66	40	17	15	223
	Exp.[a]	58.3	18.6	75.7	46.4	13.6	10.5	223.1
All centers	Obs.	480	76	178	150	83	131	1098
	Exp.[a]	455.3	93.7	201.6	152.1	74.1	121.5	1098.3
Relative risk,[c] all centers		105	81	88	99	112	108	—
Relative risk,[c] all centers except Athens and São Paulo		102	104	90	104	109	96	—

[a] Expected values are derived from the control group of the same center, adjusted for age at interview (5-year groups).
[b] Excludes 1 case with unknown age at marriage.
[c] Relative to a risk of 100 in all nonparous women.

Again, numbers are too small for examination of trends in individual centers. The pooled data for all centers do suggest lower risks for nulliparous women married under the age of 25 years than for those married later. However, relative to the trend in risks associated with age at first birth (Table 3), that with age at marriage is weak. In addition, the deficit of cases observed among nulliparous women first married under the age of 20 years is confined to two centers. If these are excluded (bottom line of Table 10), the trend disappears. We have no explanation for the appearance of this feature in these two centers. In view of the relatively small change in risk associated with it and its limitation to two of the seven centers, we conclude that early marriage is not associated with reduction in risk of cancer of the breast, unless it is associated with early confinement.

DISCUSSION

This is by no means the first study in which a difference between breast cancer cases and controls in age at first birth has been observed. In many previous comparisons of breast cancer cases and unaffected women, the cases have been found to be, on average, older at marriage, at first pregnancy, or at both (6, 7, 8, 9, 10, 11, 12). However, previous workers seem not to have considered the differences to be sufficiently important to warrant detailed exploration. An apparent lack of interest in the relationship may have resulted from failure to realize the magnitude of the differences in relative risk that underlie it. This lack of recognition of the strength of the relationship can be attributed primarily to analyses utilizing summary statistics such as means and ridits. In countries where most epidemiological studies of this disease have been undertaken, the proportion of women who have their first birth at an early age is relatively small, and summary statistics fail to reveal the high risks experienced by small segments of the population. For example, in the present data from Boston, the mean age at first birth was 27.1 years in the cases and 25.5 years in the controls. While this difference is statistically highly significant, it would hardly lead one to suspect the almost fourfold range of relative risks shown in Table 3.

Most previous workers have given more attention to the relationship of breast cancer with total parity than to that with age at first birth. Stocks (*13*), among past workers, appears to have come closest to elucidating the nature of the relationship between reproductive experience and breast cancer risk. In a series of 421 breast cancer cases and 718 age-matched controls, he noted a deficit of cases first married before the age of 25 years. He also noted that, when differences in age at marriage were allowed for, breast cancer cases first married under the age of 25 years had a relative deficit of confinements whereas those first married over the age of 25 years did not. Stocks did not consider age at first birth directly and so did not note that the deficit of confinements among cases married when under 25 years occurred solely with respect to the first confinement. The strength of the relationship was not as clear as it would have been if the group first married under the age of 20 years had been separated from those first married between the ages of 20 and 25 years. Nevertheless, Stocks (*13*) was able to conclude that a dearth of confinements during the first 10 years or so of reproductive life increases the risk of breast cancer but that, if marriage is delayed, the number of confinements is unimportant. Kaplan and Acheson (*14*) confirmed the first part of this conclusion, noting a deficit of births within 10 years of menarche among breast cancer cases which was statistically highly significant even though based on only 86 cases and 87 controls.

Our findings suggest that:

(1) The protective effect of early reproductive experience is related to age at confinement, rather than to age at marriage.

(2) The effect is a function particularly of age at first confinement, although it is possible that subsequent deliveries, if they also occur at an early age, may have some additional protective effect.

(3) The relationship is much stronger than previously suspected, women first confined under 18 years of age having only 40 percent of the breast cancer rates of nulliparous women, and even lower relative risks in some areas.

(4) Age at first confinement is a much more important factor than the total number of births; indeed, the latter probably has no association with breast cancer risk except through its association with age at first birth.

Several aspects of these findings make it necessary to revise existing hypotheses about the protective mechanisms of pregnancy. The striking reduction of risk associated with a single pregnancy of only 9 months' duration implies that the reduction is not explained by decreased exposure to causative agents during the pregnancy alone. The pregnancy must be associated with changes that bring about reduction either in exposure or in response to exposure over a prolonged period of time.

That it is the *first* confinement with which reduction in risk is associated suggests that the first pregnancy induces irreversible changes that either render the breast tissue itself less susceptible to induction of cancer or reduce the carcinogenic stimulus to the breast. The fact that early first pregnancy is associated with reduction in breast cancer risk even among women aged 75 years and older indicates the long duration of the changes that must be induced.

The effect of the first pregnancy being more marked the earlier it occurs might be explained by one or more of several mechanisms. First, a pregnancy at a young age, because of special characteristics of such pregnancies, may be particularly protective. Second, exposure to carcinogens may be particularly high in younger women—pregnancy in the young would then exert its protective effect during a period which would otherwise be associated with high risk of tumor induction. Third, the first pregnancy may act as, or possibly is itself made possible by, a threshold type of biological phenomenon which brings to an end a period of high risk of tumor induction; the earlier the pregnancy, the shorter would then be the period of risk and the lower the probability of induction.

It has recently been suggested—in part on the basis of the known protective effect of early pregnancy—that the specific estrogen fractions produced by a woman in the decade or so after puberty are important determinants of her lifetime breast cancer risk (*15, 16*). The data presented here would be compatible with this hypothesis if an early first pregnancy is associated with a favorable alteration in the estrogen profile, or if the first pregnancy induced changes in the breast tissue rendering it less susceptible to estrogen carcinogenesis. Data that would allow evaluation of either of these possibilities are lacking. Whether or not this specific hypothesis is correct, it is clear that there must be some potential carcinogenic experience to which postpubertal girls are exposed and which can be markedly influenced by pregnancy.

In addition to indicating a protective influence of early pregnancy, our data suggest that late first pregnancies may actually increase risk. Women who had their first delivery after the age of 35 years had risks approximately 20 percent higher than those who were nulliparous. If a woman had had a first birth at an earlier age, later births after the age of 35 years did not appear to be associated with increased risk. However, if the first birth was delayed until the age of 35 years, subsequent births appeared to be associated with an additional increase in risk (Table 8). This phenomenon most likely has a mechanism quite different from that underlying the protective effect of early pregnancy. Of possible relevance are observations of the effect of pregnancy on chemically induced mammary tumors in the rat. A single pregnancy prior to the feeding of a carcinogen results in a decreased frequency of mammary tumors; further pregnancies do not greatly influence the number of tumors (*17*). The situation appears therefore to be quite analogous to the effect of early pregnancy in women. However, pregnancy occurring *after* chemical induction of breast tumors in rats is associated with acceleration of tumor growth and increase in the number of active centers per rat (*18*). If, in humans, breast cancer is induced at some point during the reproductive years, the later a woman has her first pregnancy, the more likely it is that an antecedent neoplastic change has occurred. In view of the rapid proliferation of breast tissue during pregnancy, it is understandable that pregnancy could be associated with stimulation and proliferation of any cancerous cells present in the breast tissue at the time of the pregnancy.

Thus, early first pregnancies may tend to occur prior to induction and confer protection, while late first pregnancies may be likely to occur after induction and produce a deleterious effect.

ACKNOWLEDGMENTS

This study was made possible by the cooperation of our colleagues who gave access to their records and permission to interview their patients. More detailed recognition than can be given here of our indebtedness to these individuals and to our staff who conducted the interviews has been given in the reports from the individual centers.

We are grateful to Mrs. Hazel Coven, Mrs. Joyce Berlin, and Mrs. Linda Desmond who have been responsible for the coding, data processing, and computer programming, respectively, and to Dr. Dimitrios Trichopoulos for assistance in the statistical analysis.

For encouragement and counsel at all stages of the investigation, we are indebted to staff of the World Health Organization.

References

(*1*) Lowe, C.R. and B. MacMahon. *Lancet* 1:153-156, 1970.

(*2*) Salber, E.J., D. Trichopoulos, and B. MacMahon. *J Nat Cancer Inst* 43:1013-1024, 1969.

(*3*) Valaoras, V.G., B. MacMahon, D. Trichopoulos, and A. Polychronopoulou. *Int J Cancer* 4:350-363, 1969.

(*4*) Yuasa, S. and B. MacMahon. *Bull WHO* 42:195-204, 1970.

(*5*) MacMahon, B., T.M. Lin, C.R. Lowe, A.P. Mirra, B. Ravnihar, E.J. Salber, D. Trichopoulos, V.G. Valaoras, and S. Yuasa. *Bull WHO* 42:185-194, 1970.

(*6*) Lane-Claypon, J.R. A further report on cancer of the breast with special reference to its associated antecedent conditions. Report on Public Health and Medical Subjects, No. 32. H.M. Stationery Office, London, 1926.

(*7*) Wainwright, J.M. *Amer J Cancer* 15:2610-2645, 1931.

(*8*) Gilliam, A.G. *J Nat Cancer Inst* 12:287-304, 1951.

(*9*) Stocks, P. *Schweiz Z Path* 18:706-717, 1955.

(*10*) Segi, M., I. Fukushima, S. Fujisaku, M. Kurihara, S. Saito, K. Asano, and M. Kamoi. *Gann* 48, Suppl.:1-63, 1957.

(*11*) Wynder, E.L., I.J. Bross, and T. Hirayama. *Cancer* 13:559-601, 1960.

(*12*) Levin, M.L., P.R. Sheehe, S. Graham, and O. Glidewell. *Amer J Publ Hlth 54:580-587, 1964.*

(13) Stocks, P. *Practitioner* 179:233-240, 1957.

(14) Kaplan, S.D., and R.M. Acheson. *J Chron Dis* 19:1221-1230, 1966.

(15) Cole, P. and B. MacMahon. *Lancet* 1:604-606, 1969.

(16) MacMahon, B., and P. Cole. *Cancer* 24:1146-1150, 1969.

(17) Moon, R.C. *Int J Cancer* 4:312-317, 1969.

(18) Dao, T.L., and J. Sunderland. *J Nat Cancer Inst* 23:567-585, 1959.

INCREASED RISK OF ENDOMETRIAL CARCINOMA AMONG USERS OF CONJUGATED ESTROGENS

Harry K. Ziel[1] and William D. Finkle[1]

ABSTRACT

The possibility that the use of conjugated estrogens increases the risk of endometrial carcinoma was investigated in patients and a twofold age-matched control series from the same population. Conjugated estrogens (principally sodium estrone sulfate) use was recorded for 57 percent of 94 patients with endometrial carcinoma, and for 15 percent of controls. The corresponding point estimate of the (instantaneous) risk ratio was 7.6 with a one-sided 95 percent lower confidence limit of 4.7. The risk-ratio estimate increased with duration of exposure: from 5.6 for 1 to 4.9 years' exposure to 13.9 for seven or more years. The estimated proportion of cases related to conjugated estrogens, the etiologic fraction, was 50 percent with a one-sided 95 percent lower confidence limit of 41 percent. These data suggest that conjugated estrogens have an etiologic role in endometrial carcinoma.

Between 1962 and 1973, dollar sales of estrogen quadrupled in the United States (1, 2). Conjugated estrogens (Premarin, Ayerst Laboratories) containing principally sodium estrone sulfate constituted the vast majority of the quantity supplied. A recent series of articles by Siiteri and his colleagues (3-5) has suggested that the estrone form of estrogen might be associated with the development of endometrial cancer. Siiteri's theory is consistent with previous data from animal experiments indicating carcinogenicity of estrogen. (6-9). In addition, MacMahon (10) cites clinical and epidemiologic evidence that exogenous estrogen increases the risk of the development of endometrial cancer.

The present work addresses the relation of estrogen to endometrial cancer using the case-control approach. Members of the Kaiser Foundation Health Plan with endometrial cancer who were reported to the tumor registry of the Kaiser Permanente Medical Center, Los Angeles, were compared with control subjects selected from the same Health Plan population and matched for age, duration of Health Plan membership, and area of residence.

Source: *New England Journal of Medicine* 293(23): 1167-1170, 1975.

[1] From the Department of Obstetrics and Gynecology, Kaiser Permanente Medical Center, Los Angeles and the Department of Medical Economics, Kaiser Foundation Health Plan, Southern California Region.

SUBJECTS AND METHODS

Patients

Between July 1, 1970, and December 31, 1974, the diagnosis of endometrial cancer was made in 94 patients at the Kaiser Permanente Medical Center, Los Angeles, and reported to its tumor registry. The criterion for the definition of endometrial cancer was a pathological diagnosis of endometrial adenocarcinoma or adenoacanthoma; mixed Müllerian sarcoma and choriocarcinoma were excluded.

Control Subjects

Control subjects were selected in the following way. The membership files of the Southern California Kaiser Foundation Health Plan population were reviewed, and all members in the vicinity of the Los Angeles facility whose record designations ended in arbitrarily selected numbers were identified and listed. From the list, two control subjects were selected for each patient and matched for birth date within one year, area of residence by postal zip code, duration of Health Plan membership (each control subject had been a member at least as long as the associated patient), and potential for the development of endometrial cancer by the control subject's having an intact uterus. The patient and the two control subjects thus constituted a matched triple.

Record Review

The data source for the 94 matched triples was the clinic record. To avoid information bias that could result from the more probing clinical history-taking after identification of the cancer, the following procedure was employed for each matched triple. A medical-records clerk requested all three records from the record room and reviewed those of the control subjects to determine whether they had an intact uterus. Subjects without an intact uterus were replaced by selection of others from the original list. The clerk determined the date of diagnosis for each patient, and then the date one year before that diagnosis (the reference date). The clerk concealed all information in the record after the reference date. For control subjects, information recorded during the same period was similarly concealed. The record was then given to an abstractor, who filled out the abstract form without knowing whether the record was that of a patient or a control.

RESULTS

For any given triple, there were six possible combinations of conjugated-estrogen use: all three were users; the patient and one of the control subjects were users; and so forth. The

observed frequencies for each of the six possible combinations for each of the 94 triples are shown in Table 1. These data were used to estimate the risk ratio associated with the use of conjugated estrogens and the etiologic fraction (the proportion of cases due to conjugated estrogens). The (maximum-likelihood) point estimate of the relative risk ($\hat{RR}$) is 7.6 *(11)*.[2] The significance test statistic (χ^2_1) is 49 (P << 10^{-8}) *(12)*. The approximate 95 percent one-sided lower confidence limit of the risk ratio (RR) is 4.7 *(13)*. The point estimate of the etiologic fraction ($\hat{EF}$) is 50 percent *(14)*. For this parameter, Miettinen's proposed (test-based) computation *(15)* of the 95 percent one-sided lower confidence limit (EF) yields 41 percent.[3]

Data on the relation of risk ratio to duration of exposure are given in Table 2. Even with only 1.0 to 4.9 years of use, the point estimate is 5.6, with a corresponding 95 percent one-sided confidence limit of 2.7. For uses of less than one

---

[2] The computations for the point estimate and significance test were performed according to Miettinen, *(11)* and *(12)* respectively. The 95 percent confidence interval *(13)* was computed according to: $(\underline{RR},\overline{RR}) = \hat{RR}^{1\pm Z_{1-\alpha}/x} = 7.6^{1\pm1.96/6.98} = (4.3, 13.4)$.

[3] The point estimate of EF was calculated by $\hat{EF} = [(\hat{RR}-1)/RR]$ (exposure rate of the cases) *(14)*. The 95 percent confidence interval was calculated by: $(\underline{EF}, \overline{EF}) = 1 - (1 - \hat{EF})^{1\pm Z_{1-\alpha}/x} = 1 - (1 - 0.50)^{\chi1\pm1.96/6.98} = (0.39, 0.59)$.

Table 1. History of conjugated-estrogen use among 94 patients with endometrial cancer and 188 matched[a] control subjects.

Patients' use of conjugated estrogens	Controls' use of conjugated estrogens			
	both	one	neither	totals
Used	1	16	37	54
Did not use	0	11	29	40
Totals	1	27	66	94

Exposure rates:	Used conjugated estrogens		Did not use conjugated estrogens		Totals
	No.	%	No.	%	
Patients	54	(57)	40	(43)	94
Controls	29	(15)	159	(85)	188

[a] The matching criteria were age, area of residence, duration of Health Plan membership, and potential for development of uterine cancer.

Table 2. Duration of conjugated-estrogen use[a] by patients with endometrial cancer and by control subjects, with risk-ratio analysis: point estimate ($\overline{RR}$), 95 percent one-sided lower confidence bound ($\underline{RR}$), and chi-square test statistic (χ_1^2).

Group	Duration of exposure (yr)						
	Unknown	≥7	5.0-6.9	1.0-4.9	<1	Non-exposed	Totals
Patients (No.)	14	14	9	14	3	40	94
Controls (No.)	6	4	5	10	4	159	188
RR		9.3	13.9	7.2	5.6	$(1.0)^b$	
(RR)		4.2	6.0	2.8	2.7		
χ_1^2		22	26	12	15		
P		$<10^{-5}$	$<10^{-5}$	$<.01$	$<.01$		

[a] Duration of use for both patients and controls was defined by difference in year between date of most recent prescription for conjugated estrogens and date of first such prescription given in record. If a first prescription date was given, but subsequent prescription dates were absent, a statement in the record, such as "conjugated estrogens for five years" was acceptable as a statement of duration. If a first prescription date was given, but subsequent dates were absent and no summary of conjugated estrogens use was in the record, the duration of use was defined as unknown.
[b] By definition.

year's duration, the data are too scanty to be informative.[4]

DISCUSSION

The apparent association between conjugated estrogen use and the development of endometrial cancer requires consideration of several explanations other than causality.

Information bias, particularly bias in ascertaining the use of conjugated estrogens, is an unlikely explanation. The history of such use was ascertained from pre-existing records, which covered at least as many years of care for the controls as for the patients. The original notations on the record, and the subsequent notations used to determine duration of use of conjugated estrogens, were made at least one year before detection of the cancer, Moreover, the method of record abstraction was expressly designed to eliminate bias in the process of extracting data.

As for selection bias, the ascertainment of subjects (patients and controls) does not appear to have depended directly upon use of conju-

gated estrogens. The vast majority of cases are reported to the cancer registry, regardless of whether the patient used conjugated estrogens, and the controls were selected from a defined population by a procedure that precluded selection on the basis of a history of such use.

Among various potential confounding factors, age, duration of Health Plan membership, and area of residence are controlled by (matching and) stratification. Among other known correlates of risk of development of endometrial cancer *(10)*, parity, excessive weight, and age at menopause deserve consideration.

In the present data, the risk of endometrial cancer of nulliparas was estimated to be 1.5 times that of parous women, and their rate of conjugated-estrogen use was also somewhat higher. However, the estimate of the confounding risk ratio *(16)* from subjects with parity recorded (90 percent of patients and 84 percent of controls) was as low as 1.18. This small ratio, together with an overall crude risk ratio of 6.7, implies a confounding effect of only $(1.18 - 1)/[6.71/1.18) - 1] = 4$ percent.

To estimate the confounding risk ratio and confounding effect for subjects with height and weight recorded, Quetelet's index (Wt/Ht^2) was employed. The risk of endometrial cancer for the patients in the upper third of the weight index was estimated to be twice that for patients in the lower two thirds, and their use of conjugated estrogens was also slightly higher. Data could be obtained from 89 percent of the pa-

[4] Data were also recorded on the use of conjugated estrogens by control subjects who had been excluded from the study because of hysterectomy or radiation therapy to the uterus. If the restrictive criterion of an intact uterus in the control subjects had not been applied, the estimated relative risk and etiologic fraction would have been 4.9 and 46 percent respectively.

tients and 80 percent of the controls; the confounding risk ratio, crude risk ratio, and confounding effect were estimated as 1.1., 5.7, and 2 percent respectively.

The analogous calculations for confounding by the risk factor "age at menopause" were as follows. The risk ratio for endometrial cancer for subjects with an age at menopause of 51 years or more versus those with an age at menopause below 51 was estimated to be 1.3, and the rate of conjugated-estrogen use was slightly lower in the former age group. On the basis of data obtained from 90 percent of the case records and 70 percent of the control records, the confounding risk ratio, crude risk ratio, and confounding effect were estimated as 1.08, 5.6, and 2 percent, respectively.

From these considerations, it is apparent that the observed association between conjugated-estrogen use and the development of endometrial cancer cannot be explained to any appreciable extent by confounding due to age, parity, excessive weight, or age at menopause. It is possible, of course, that there could be a major confounding effect by other, unknown factors that lead to the development of endometrial cancer.

As an overall check on the validity of the method, data were also collected on the use of diazepam (Valium), reserpine, and thyroid drugs by both patients and controls. The point estimates of the risk ratio were 0.7, 0.5, and 0.9, respectively. All these estimates are small in comparison with the estimated risk ratio of 7.6 that was found for conjugated estrogens. In addition, data were collected on the indications given in the record for prescribing conjugated estrogens. Where an indication was recorded (for 54 percent of patients and 72 percent of controls), it was "hot flashes" for 72 percent of patients and 71 percent of controls, indicating that the reasons for prescribing this drug were similar for patients and controls. Chance is an extremely unlikely explanation, considering the magnitude of the P value.

Causal explanation of the association involves the difficulty of explaining why an association of this magnitude has remained undetected until now. Estrogens have been used extensively only during the last decade or two (1, 2), and if the results of this study are generalizable to all post-menopausal women, there should have been an appreciable increase in the occurrence of endometrial cancer. Specifically, the present data imply that the etiologic fraction for conjugated estrogens has a point estimate as high as 50 percent, with a 95 percent one-sided lower confidence limit of 41 percent. A 50 percent etiologic fraction would correspond to a 100 percent increase in the incidence of this cancer. Whether an increase of this order of magnitude has occurred in regions of high estrogen use, such as the one in which this study was conducted, is difficult to assess, but no such increase is believed to have occurred. Analysis of the Second and Third National Cancer Surveys suggests that the incidence of endometrial cancer did not increase appreciably in the United States between 1947 and 1971 (17). The same conclusion holds for England, Wales, and Canada (18).

These surveys, however, are affected by a major bias. The incidence rates are in reference to the total female population, whereas the rates should be expressed in reference to women at risk (18). For the 1950s, the frequency of hysterectomy must be surmised from incidental sources, which suggest that 10 to 15 percent of postmenopausal women had undergone hysterectomy (19-22). MacMahon and Worcester (23) and Hammond (24) provide evidence of increased prevalence of hysterectomy in this age group during the early 1960s. Recent national survey data show much higher frequencies and continued increase in the rate of hysterectomy. By 1968, the prevalence of hysterectomy among American women at the age of 60 years was 31 percent (25); in the period from 1968-1973, the incidence rate in women 15 years of age or older rose from 6.8 per 1000 woman-years (26) to 8.6 per 1000 woman-years (27). It is apparent, therefore, that the incidence rate of the development of endometrial cancer for women at risk (those with an intact uterus) has increased dramatically during the past decade or so.

Another difficulty in employing the 1969 and 1971 Third Survey to assess the impact of use of conjugated estrogens on the incidence of endometrial cancer is that the survey may have been performed too early for this purpose. The Kaiser Permanente Medical Center's tumor-registry data are not particularly helpful in settling the question of increase in the incidence of endometrial cancer, owing to uncertainty about the completeness of reporting over time, particularly before 1971. However, the data do indicate a significant increase (uncorrected for hysterectomy) in 1972 to 1974.

Causal interpretation of the association between conjugated-estrogen use and the development of endometrial cancer has some biologic credibility. Carcinogencity of estrogens has been demonstrated in laboratory animals at various sites *(6-9)*, including the endometrium *(9)*. In addition, the cases of endometrial cancer observed in surgically castrated women or in girls with ovarian dysgenesis exceed the expected number *(28-33)*, and these women receive replacement estrogen therapy. Moreover, endometrial cancer has been found to be associated with high estrogen-producing granulosatheca ovarian tumors *(34-36)*.

Recently, Siiteri et al. *(3-5)* have suggested a theory of hormone conversion that implies a higher level of estrone in women in whom endometrial cancer develops than in those in whom it does not. They found rates of conversion of androstenedione to estrone two to three times as high in women with endometrial cancer or hyperplasia (a precursor of endometrial carcinoma) *(37,38)* as in women without such cancer. Confirming Siiteri's findings, Schindler and his associates *(36)* discovered that adipose tissues of patients with endometrial cancer converted androstenedione to estrone nearly four times as fast as those of subjects without cancer.

The evidence for a connection between the use of conjugated estrogens and the development of endometrial cancer seems rather persuasive. Caution is urged, however, in view of the absence of data both from similar epidemiologic studies in other populations and from follow-up studies. Such information is necessary before policy conclusions can be drawn. Further studies are necessary to evaluate the possible relation between the use of other estrogens and endometrial cancer.

We are indebted to our primary consultant, Dr. Olli Miettinen; to Drs. Robert Brook, Brian Henderson, Robert Hoover, Thomas Mack, Malcolm Pike, and Noel Weiss, and Mrs. Kathleen N. Williams for criticism of the paper; and to the abstractors for the study, David Harrison, Susan Lieberman, Mary Rambo, and Sandra Tyson.

References

(1) Shipments of Pharmaceutical Preparations, Except Biologicals, 1962, U.S. Bureau of the Census Current Industrial Reports, Series M28G[62]-1. Washington, D.C., Government Printing Office, 1963.

(2) Pharmaceutical Preparations, Except Biologicals, 1973, U.S. Bureau of the Census Current Industrial Reports, Series Ma-28G[73]-1. Washington D.C., Government Printing Office, 1975.

(3) Siiteri, P.K., B.E. Schwartz, I. Moriyama, et al. Estrogen binding in the rat and human. *Adv Exp Med Biol* 36:97-112, 1973.

(4) Siiteri, P.K. and P.C. MacDonald. The role of extraglandular estrogen in human endocrinology. *Handbook of Physiology.* Section 7, Endocrinology, Vol. 2, Part 1. Edited by R.O. Greep and E.B. Astwood. Washington, D.C., American Physiological Society, 1973, pp. 615-629.

(5) Siiteri, P.K., B.E. Schwartz, and P.C. MacDonald. Estrogen receptors and the estrone hypothesis in relation to endometrial and breast cancer. *Gyneco Oncol* 2:228-238, 1974.

(6) Cook, J.W. and E.C. Dodds. Sex hormones and cancer-producing compounds. *Nature* 131:205-206, 1933.

(7) Perry, I.H. and L.L. Gintzon. The development of tumors in female mice treated with 1:2:5:6-dibenzanthracene and theelin. *Am J Cancer* 29:680-704, 1937.

(8) Gardner, W.U. Tumors in experimental animals receiving steroid hormones. *Surgery* 16:8-32, 1944.

(9) Meissner, W.A., S.C. Sommers, and G. Sherman. Endometrial hyperplasia, endometrial carcinoma, and endometriosis produced experimentally by estrogen. *Cancer* 10:500-509, 1957.

(10) MacMahon, B. Risk factors for endometrial cancer. *Gynecol Oncol* 2:122-129, 1974.

(11) Miettinen, O.S. Estimation of relative risk from individually matched series. *Biometrics* 26:75-86, 1970.

(12) ———. Individual matching with multiple controls in the case of all-or-none responses. *Biometrics* 25:339-355, 1969.

(13) ———. Simple interval-estimation of risk ratios. *Am J Epidemiol* 100:515-516, 1974.

(14) ———. Proportion of disease caused or prevented by a given exposure, trait, or intervention. *Am J Epidemiol* 99:325-332, 1974.

(15) ———. Estimability and estimation in case-referent studies. *Am J Epidemiol* (in press).

(16) ———. Components of the crude risk ratio. *Am J Epidemiol* 96:168-172, 1972.

(17) Cramer, D.W., S.J. Cutler, and B. Christine. Trends in the incidence of endometrial cancer in the United States. *Gynecol Oncol* 2:130-143, 1974.

(18) Kinlen, L.J. and R. Doll. Trends in mortality from cancer of the uterus in Canada and in England and Wales. *Br J Prev Soc Med* 27:146-149, 1973.

(19) McMahon, B. and M. Feinleib. Breast cancer in relation to nursing and menopausal history. *J Natl Cancer Inst* 24:733-753, 1960.

(20) Lilienfeld, A.M. The relationship of cancer of the female breast to artificial menopause and marital status. *Cancer* 9:927-934, 1956.

(21) Herrel, W.E. The relative incidence of oophorectomy in women with and without carcinoma of the breast. *Am J Cancer* 29:659-665, 1937.

(22) Lane-Claypon, J.E. A Further Report on Cancer of the Breast, with Special Reference to Its Associated Antecedent Condition. Ministry of Health, Reports on Public Health and Medical Subjects, No. 32. London, His Majesty's Stationery Office, 1926.

(23) MacMahon, B. and J. Worcester. Age at menopause, United States 1960-1962, Vital and Health Statistics: Data from the National Health Survey, Series II, No. 19. Rockville, Maryland, U.S. National Center for Health Statistics, Health Services and Mental Health Administration, 1966.

(24) Hammond, E.C. The early diagnosis of uterine cancer. The Early Diagnosis of Cancer of the Cervix: A symposium held at the University of Hull, 20 March 1970, as part of the 11th annual general meeting of the British Association for Cancer Research. Edited by J.M. Riggott. Hull, England, University of Hull, 1971.

(25) Bunker, J.P. and Brown, B.W., Jr. The physician-patient as an informed consumer of surgical services. *N Engl J Med* 290:1051-1055, 1974.

(26) Mead, S. Surgical operations in short-stay hospitals. United States, 1968. Department of Health Education and Welfare Publication No. HSM 73-1796. Rockville, Maryland, U.S. National Center for Health Statistics, Health Services and Mental Health Administration, January 1973.

(27) Hospital discharge survey data, Monthly Vital Statistics Report. Department of Health, Education and Welfare Publication No. [HRA] 75-1120, Vol. 24, Suppl. 3, Rockville, Maryland, U.S. National Center for Health Statistics, Health Services and Mental Health Administration, May 30, 1975.

(28) Cutler, B.S., A.P. Forbes, F.M. Ingersoll, et al. Endometrial carcinoma after stilbestrol therapy in gonadol dysgenesis. *N. Engl J Med* 287:628-631, 1972.

(29) Dowsett, J.W. Corpus carcinoma developing in a patient with Turner's syndrome with endometrial adenocarcinoma and stilbestrol therapy. *Am J Obstet Gynecol* 86:622-625, 1963.

(30) Wilkinson, E.J., E.G. Friedrich, R.F. Mattingly, et al. Turner's syndrome with endometrial adenocarcinoma and stilbestrol therapy. *Obstet Gynecol* 42:193-200, 1973.

(31) Dewhurst, C.J., E.B De Koos, and R.M. Haines. Replacement hormone therapy in gonadal dysgenesis. *Br J Obstet Gynaecol* 82:412-416, 1975.

(32) Roberts, G. and A. L. Wells. Oestrogen-induced endometrial carcinoma in a patient with gonadal dysgenesis. *Br J Obstet Gynaecol* 82:412-416, 1975.

(33) McCarroll, A.M., D.A.D. Montgomery, J. Mc.D.G. Harley, et al. Endometrial carcinoma after cyclical oestrogen-progestogen therapy for Turner's syndrome. *Br J Obstet Gynecol* 82:421-423, 1975.

(34) Greene, J.W., Jr. Feminizing mesenchymomas (granulosa-cell and theca cell tumors) with associated endometrial carcinoma: review of the literature, and a study of the ovarian tumor registry. *Am J Obstet Gynecol* 74:31-41, 1957.

(35) Ingram, J.M., Jr. and E. Novak. Endometrial carcinoma associated with feminizing ovarian tumors. *Am J Obstet Gynecol* 61:774-789, 1951.

(36) Mansell, H. and A.T. Hertig. Granulosa-theca cell tumors and endometrial carcinoma: a study of their relationship and survey of 80 cases. *Obstet Gynecol* 6:385-394, 1955.

(37) Hertig, A.T. and S.C. Sommers. Genesis of endometrial carcinoma. I. Study of prior biopsies. *Cancer* 2:946-956, 1949.

(38) Taylor, H.C.J.R. Endometrial hyperplasia and carcinoma of the body of the uterus. *Am J Obstet Gynecol* 23:309-332, 1932.

(39) Schindler, A.E., A. Ebert, and E. Friedrich. Conversion of androstenedione to estrone by human fat tissue. *J Clin Endocrinol Metab* 35:627-630, 1972.

A STUDY OF THE RELATION OF FAMILY INCOME AND OTHER ECONOMIC FACTORS TO PELLAGRA INCIDENCE IN SEVEN COTTON-MILL VILLAGES OF SOUTH CAROLINA IN 1916

Joseph Goldberger, G. A. Wheeler, and Edgar Sydenstricker

In the spring of 1916 we began a study of the relation of various factors to pellagra incidence in certain representative textile-mill communities of South Carolina. On a varying scale the study was continued through 1917 and 1918. The results of the first year's (1916) study with respect to diet (1, 2), to age, sex, occupation, disabling sickness (3, 4), and to sanitation (5) have already been reported. At the present time we wish to record the results of the part of the study dealing with the relation of conditions of an economic nature to the incidence of the disease.

REVIEW OF LITERATURE

A close association of pellagra with poverty has been repeatedly remarked upon since the time of the first recognition of the disease. In the earliest account, Casal (6, p. 93), discussing the diet of those persons attacked by the disease, remarks that "they eat meat very rarely since most pellagrins are poor field laborers, and this circumstance does not permit them to eat meat daily nor even from time to time." Continuing, he says: "Their only beverage is water. Their clothes, beds, habitations, etc., are strictly in keeping with their extreme poverty." Further along, discussing the treatment of the disease, Casal states that "milk, thanks to the butter it contains, is certainly capable of supplying the nutritive lack of the other foods; they use it but rarely without having first removed the butter, since these poor people sell the butter in order that they may be able to buy other necessaries, thus using in their own diet what remains in the milk after having thus treated it."

Much more definite and direct is Strambio (7) who states that "thus much is certain, that pellagra is most at home where poverty and misery reign and increases as they increase."

Source: *Public Health Reports* 35 (46) 2673-2714, 1920.

Very interesting and significant is Marzari's observation (cited by Russell, 8, p. 167). "I have several times observed," he states, "that if a villager falls into poverty, as happens so often as a result of a storm, drought, or other calamity, pellagra does not fail to crown his misfortune and put an end to his miserable existence."

Holland (9), in introducing his discussion of the cause and symptoms of pellagra in a paper read in 1817, based on observations of his own and on information secured from Italian physicians in the course of a journey to Italy, remarks: "The pellagra is a malady confined almost exclusively to the lower classes of the people, and chiefly to the peasants and those occupied in the labors of agriculture." He repeats this two or three times in other connections. In his discussion of the etiology of the disease (p. 322) we find the following highly suggestive statements: "Though I have spoken of Lombardy as one of the most fertile portions of Europe, yet to those who consider the little certain relation between mere productiveness of soil and the prosperity or comforts of the population dwelling upon it, it will not appear very extraordinary that the peasants of this district should be subject to various physical privations unknown to the people of countries which are much less favored by nature. The fact unquestionably is, whatever be our speculations as to the cause, that the peasants of Lombardy do for the most part live in much wretchedness, both as regards the quantity and quality of their diet and the other various comforts of life. It further seems probable, if not certain, that this evil has been progressively augmenting within the last 50 years; partly, perhaps, an effect of the wars which have so often devastated the country by marches and military contributions; partly a consequence of the frequent changes of political state; together with the insecurity, the variable system of government, and the heavy taxes and imposts attending such changes. To these causes may be added a decaying state of commerce and a faulty system of arrangement between landlords and the cultivators of the soil, all tending to depress agriculture and to reduce the peasantry at large to a state of much misery and privation." Continuing this discussion, Holland remarks further (p. 333): "Animal food rarely forms a part of their diet, and although living on a soil which produces wine their poverty almost precludes the use of it, even when sickness and debility render it most needful. The same condition of poverty is evident in their clothing, in their habitations, and in the want of all the minor necessaries and comforts of life. The immediate effect of these privations is obvious in the aspect of squalid wretchedness and emaciation which forms so striking a spectacle at the present time throughout the greater part of Lombardy. I say particularly *at the present time* (italics in original), because whatever may have been the progress of misery among the peasants of this country during the last half century it appears to have increased in a tenfold ratio during the last two years, the effect of bad harvests added to the preceding wars and political changes which have distressed this part of Italy."

Hameau (*10*), in the first recorded observations of pellagra in France, reported that "this disease attacks individuals of both sexes and all ages, but I have not yet seen it in any but the poor and uncleanly who subsist on coarse food."

Lalesque (*11*), in his account of pellagra of the Landes, cites a number of instances illustrating the conditions of misery under which pellagra occurred, finally exclaiming (p. 421): "These are the individuals attacked by pellagra, for it attaches itself to poverty as the shadow to the body."

In a discussion of pellagra in Gorz-Gradisca, Berger (*12*), very significantly observes: "The appearance during the last decennium of diseases of the vine, the reduction in value of the product of the soil because of foreign competition, crop failures, increase in taxes, increasing living costs, all operated to undermine economic conditions, particularly of the poorer country folk, and thus prepared favorable conditions for the spread of the disease."

Discussing the therapy and prophylaxis of pellagra in Bessarabia, V. Rosen (*13*) bewails the attendant difficulties "in that, on the one hand, the alimentation with cornmeal porridge is a deeply rooted national custom, and, on the other, that the disease attacks the poorest class of the population; 'N'am vaca, n'am lapte a casa' ('I have no cow and no milk in the house') is uniformly the reply of the patient to questions in relation to this subject," and Sofer (*14*, p. 219), discussing the economic status of pellagrins (in Austria), remarks that "89.9 percent haven't even a cow."

The extremely unfavorable economic conditions of those subject to pellagra (in Austria-Hungary, at least) is further strikingly suggested by the character of some of the recommendations for its control. Thus Von Probizer (*15*, p. 141) urged, as a necessary measure, "pecuniary aid by the Government in view of the deplorable condition of the peasantry in the affected localities."

V. Babes (*16*), writing on pellagra in Roumania, remarks (p. 1187) that "practically all pellagrins are very poor"; and goes into some detail in describing the unfavorable economic condition of the Roumanian peasant, which leaves him in debt to the landowner and the tax collector.

In modern Spain we have Calmarza (*17*) remarking (p. 66) that although he had seen cases in well-to-do individuals, the disease only exceptionally occurred in those of this class. He adds (p. 67) also that in his experience, unlike the reported observations of others (Roussel, *18*, p. 431), pellagra is quite common in beggars. In discussing the etiological role of widowhood, this keen observer expresses the opinion (p. 68) that this plays a part only in proportion as it tends to bring about a depression in economic well-being and a consequent insufficient alimentation. Huertas (*19*) describes the disease as occurring among the most miserable class of the population of Madrid, who live on the food picked from the city's garbage.

In Egypt Sandwith (*20*) found the disease highly prevalent among the poorer peasants of Lower Egypt. "In one village," he reports, "where the inhabitants are especially well to do because they get regular pay throughout the year from the Domains administration, there were only 15 percent of pellagrous men, while among the men of the village which has the reputation of being the poorest, the percentage rose as high as 62."

Gaumer (*21*), discussing pellagra in Yucatan,

states that the disease did not become epidemic in that state until 1884, two years after a destructive invasion by locusts or grasshoppers. "Among the better classes the disease seldom made its appearance. . . . It was the middle and lower classes who, from reduced circumstances, were obliged to purchase the cheapest corn in the market that suffered most from the ravages of the disease.

"From 1891 to 1901 Yucatan produced sufficient corn for home consumption, and new cases of pellagra were no longer to be found. . . .

"From 1901 to 1907 the corn crops were almost total failures and corn was again imported in greater quantities than ever before. . . .

"Pellagra again became epidemic, but was not then confined to the middle and lower classes, as in the former invasion. The wealthy hemp owners, on account of the exorbitant prices paid for hemp, found it was more profitable to import than to raise corn for home consumption, thus compelling even well-to-do people to consume the imported article," which was believed to have been spoiled in transport from the United States. "Pellagra then spread alike among the rich and poor, until by the close of 1907 about 10 percent of the inhabitants were victims of the disease. . . ."

In Barbados, B. W. I., the disease, according to Manning (22), is "confined to the laboring classes and is most prevalent among those who are badly off or poverty stricken. It is very seldom found among the whites, but cases do occur among those in straitened circumstances." In the pioneer reports on pellagra in the United States such references as are made to the relation of economic status to the disease are of a very general character and appear for the most part to be echoes of European opinion. So far as we are aware, credit for the first study of this relationship is due to Siler and Garrison (23). This study was made in South Carolina in 1912 and relates to pellagrins alone. In recording their data relating to the economic conditions under which the patients lived, Siler and Garrison adopted five classes, namely, squalor, poverty, necessities, comfort, and affluence. Of the 277 cases so classified, the economic conditions were reported as poor (squalor, poverty, necessities) in 83 percent, within the average (comfort) in 15 percent, and well above the average (affluence) in 2 percent.

Jobling and Petersen (24) in their second year's study of the epidemiology of pellagra in Nashville, Tenn., "endeavored to make a most accurate study of the economic condition of pellagrous patients. In order to do this," they state that their examiners "ascertained the average rentals for the entire city, the weekly income of the pellagrin when a wage earner, and the total income of the pellagrous family." From these data the amount of money available for each pellagrin per week was computed by dividing the total income by the number of individuals, children being accorded the same value as adults.

They found that 70 percent of their white adult male pellagrins were wage earners, more than 60 percent of whom earned $10 or more per week. Of the white adult females, 22 percent were wage earners, and of these, 56 percent earned less than $10 per week. Of the colored wage earners, 66 percent of the males earned less than $10 per week, while a similar percent of the females earned under $8 per week.

When the amount of money available for each pellagrin per week was estimated, Jobling and Petersen found that of the whites 56.5 percent and of the colored 24 percent had an available income of $2.50 or more per week.

These workers also made an estimate of the economic status of the pellagrous class on the basis of rentals, which they considered a "fairly reliable basis" for this purpose. They found that of the whites 11 percent and of the colored 16 percent owned their own homes or were buying them on the installment plan. "The rentals paid by the balance were practically all under $15 per month, only 3 percent of the cases occurring in families paying more than this amount. Of the colored families few pay more than $8 per month."

It will be observed that the study of Jobling and Petersen, like that of Siler and Garrison, concerns itself exclusively with the pellagrin. Neither study affords any basis for a comparison with the economic distribution of the general population so that neither these nor, so far as we are aware, any previous observations give us any means of measuring in a definite objective manner the degree of association between economic status and pellagra incidence. This deficiency we have endeavored to repair by the study that we shall now proceed to detail.

PLAN AND METHODS OF PRESENT STUDY

Locality

The study was made in seven representative cotton-mill villages situated in the northwestern part of South Carolina.

Population

The villages were of about average size; none had over 800 or less than 500 inhabitants. Each constituted a distinct, more or less isolated community in close proximity to a cotton-cloth manufacturing plant and was composed practically exclusively of the mill employees and their families. The few Negro families present and living somewhat apart were not considered, so that our study deals with an exclusively white population, which, with hardly a single exception, was of Anglo-Saxon stock born in this country of American-born parents. Besides the Negroes, there were also excluded from this study the mill executives, store managers, clerks, and their households, so that we had left for study an exceptionally homogeneous group with respect to racial stock, occupation, and general standard of living, including dietary custom. An enumeration of the population was made in May and June in connection with the collection of our dietary and economic data, and totaled about 4160 people, included in about 750 households.

Pellagra Incidence

The procedure adopted for determining the incidence of pellagra in this population has been described at length in a previous paper of this series (2).

Briefly, in order to ascertain the incidence of the disease as completely as possible, the expedient of a systematic biweekly house-to-house search for cases was employed and practically exclusively depended on.

Only cases with a clearly defined, bilaterally symmetrical dermatitis were recorded as pellagra; cases with poorly defined eruptions, or those with more or less suggestive manifestations but without clearly marked eruption, were recorded at most as "suspects" and are excluded from present consideration.

Just as in our study of pellagra incidence in relation to diet, so here, in relating pellagra incidence to economic conditions, no distinc-

tion is made between first and recurrent attacks, but all active cases as above defined are considered. So-called inactive or quiescent cases, that is, individuals who had had the disease in a previous year but during 1916 presented no definite eruption or evidence sufficient to be classed as "suspects," are considered as nonpellagrous.

As a considerable proportion of the population of any village is of transient character (see in this connection, 3) and as much of the pellagra occurs in this class (tabulation deleted, ED.), some assumption was necessary on the basis of which cases might be assigned to households and villages. Accordingly the rule was adopted that a case was to be charged to a household or village only if the affected individual had been a member of that household or had resided in the village not less than 30 days immediately preceding the beginning of the attack (as above defined).

Season

It would seem reasonable to expect, if diet, economic status, or other factor has any influence in relation to the seasonal rise in incidence of the disease, that this influence is most effective during a period immediately anterior to the sharp rise and peak of incidence. Such statistics of pellagra morbidity as were available to us at the beginning of our study indicated that the rise of the seasonal curve of pellagra incidence in the southern states began in the late spring and reached its peak in June. It was assumed, therefore, that the factors favoring the production of pellagra were most effective during the season beginning some time in the late winter or early spring and continuing up to or possibly somewhat into June. The period actually selected by us as representative of this season extended from April 16 to June 15, 1916. Information relating to family income, household food supply, and the composition of the households, etc., for sample sections of this period was secured by trained enumerators who canvassed the village in successive 15-day periods under the immediate direction and supervision of one of us (E. S.).

Dietary Data

The methods adopted for securing data relating to diet have been described fully in a previous communication (2). It will suffice in the present connection to recall that these data relate to the food supply of the household, not to that of the individual, and so do not indicate the differences that may have existed in the diets of the individual members. It being impracticable to secure our dietary data simultaneously in all villages, the record of household food supply secured in the several villages was for successive 15-day periods between April 16 and June 15. It was assumed that an accurate record for a 15-day period would be a sufficiently representative sample of the supply of the season immediately anterior to the peak of seasonal incidence of the disease, that is, of what may be considered as the pellagra-producing season.

Data Relating to Economic Conditions

Since nearly 90 percent of the individuals composing the population studied were found to be dependent upon the income of family groups composed of more than one person, family income was adopted as the basis for classifying the population according to economic status.

Family Income

The data relating to family income were secured by inquiries of the housewife or of some other responsible member or members of each family, supplemented by data from the mill payrolls. For the latter we are greatly indebted to the willing cooperation of the administrative officials of the mills.

The information obtained from the families covered (a) the rate of daily earnings of each member earning wages during the half month preceding the week of the canvass and the various rates of daily earnings of all members who had been employed during the 12 preceding months; (b) the days not at work for all members who had worked for wages during the 12 preceding months; (c) the income from all other sources during the preceding half month as well as during the preceding 12 months, this information being secured in detail for each source of income. On the basis of this information it was possible to approximate the total income of each family for the half month preceding the visit of the enumerator, and, roughly, for any part or all of the preceding year.

Finding that approximately 90 percent of the total income of the families studied came from the earnings of wage-earning members, the family statements of earnings during this half-month period were compared with the records on the mill payrolls, and, in the great majority of instances, were found to agree closely with them; but in order to reduce the error arising from even slightly inaccurate statements as to wages, the payroll records instead of the family statements have been used to supply the earnings data. For that small proportion of family income made up of wages earned in employment outside of the mills and of the amounts derived from other miscellaneous sources, the family statement was necessarily accepted.

On the basis of the results of some preliminary tabulations it was decided that the family income during the half month preceding the week of the enumerator's canvass would be a fairly accurate indication of family income during the season selected as most significant in relation to the occurrence of pellagra. The basis for classifying families with respect to income was, therefore, the total cash income of each during a 15-day period between April 16 and June 15, 1916. A half-month sample period was used, partly because it corresponded to the sample period for which dietary data were secured and partly because a majority of the mills in the villages paid at semimonthly intervals. The payroll data from other mills were adjusted to a half-month basis.

In the course of the canvass of the homes of the mill workers' families other data affecting the economic status of the families were also collected. These related principally to length of experience in mill work, occupational status of wage earners, and the amount and incidence of disabling sickness (4) among wage-earning and other members of households.

Availability of Food Supply

With the view of studying the relation of food availability to pellagra incidence, information was collected under the immediate direction of one of us (E. S.), relating to conditions that might affect the supply of a given food or foods. In collecting and recording this information a uniform method was followed as closely as possible except where specific points suggested the advisability of special inquiry. The principal sources of information and the nature of the information sought were as follows:

(1) Statements were obtained from households as to the immediate source of every article of food entering into their half-month's supplies. Thus it was ascertained, for example, whether the fresh milk used by the household was produced at home, purchased from another mill worker's household in the village, or from some specific farmer, dairy, or store, or donated by a relative, neighbor, or other person. In the event that a household had a source of supply not common generally to households in the village, inquiries were directed with a view of ascertaining the length of time the household had had such a supply, particularly, with respect to the period after January 1, 1916.

(2) From farmers, hucksters, or "peddlers" selling from house to house, statements were secured relating to the quantities sold, prices, frequency of selling, and character of produce sold since January 1, 1916.

(3) From managers and clerks in the stores, markets, and other retail establishments at which mill workers' households largely dealt, data were secured relating to (a) prices during the 15-day period and price changes during 1916; (b) sources of each food sold, whether direct from nearby farms or through middlemen from local agricultural territory or from other sections of the United States; (c) names of brands and quantities of the foods sold; (d) practices with respect to credit to mill workers' households, especially as affected by the amount of earnings by the mill workers.

Economic Classification

Method of Classification According to Economic Status

As has already been mentioned, the great majority of the individuals composing the population studied were members of families who subsisted on the income of families composed of several persons; the small proportion not subsisting on such family income were boarders living under substantially the same conditions as the families with which they boarded. It would seem permissible, therefore, to classify these economically with the members of the family with which they boarded, although it is fully recognized that in so doing a certain,

though, for the present purpose, unimportant, error is involved.

In classifying this population according to economic status on the basis of family income the conventional method of using total family income for a given period was found to be so inaccurate in many instances as to be misleading. The average total annual cash income of all of the families for which income data were secured was about $700, and relatively few had annual incomes of over $1000. Thus the range of total income was relatively small and the families were, from this point of view, fairly homogeneous. They differed, however, very markedly in size and with respect to the age and sex of their members. Manifestly it was improper to classify, for example, a family whose half-month's income was $40, and was composed of only a man and his wife, with one whose half-month's income was also $40, but was composed of a man, his wife, and several dependent children. Since family income, for the purpose of this study, was used as an index of the economic status of individuals who composed the family group, it was necessary to take into consideration the number of such individuals in comparing one family with another. A per capita statement of income, however, while more accurate than the statement of total income, was subject to the inaccuracy arising from differences in the age and sex of members of the families to be compared. It appeared advisable, therefore, to employ a common denominator to which the individuals of both sexes and of all ages could be reduced in order to obtain a more accurately representative method of expressing the relative size of the families to be compared.

In the absence of a better common denominator for this purpose, the Atwater (25) scale of food requirements was employed, and the size of each family was computed according to this scale and expressed in terms of "adult male units." The scale used appears below. The assumption in the use of this scale was that the expenditures for total maintenance for individuals varied according to sex and age in the same proportion as did their food requirements. The assumption is by no means as accurate as could be desired; in its favor, however, it may be said that since family expenditures in the great majority of cases equaled total family income, and since food expenditures were nearly half (among poorer families consider-

Age	Equivalent adult male unit	
	Male	Female
Adult (over 16)	1.0	0.8
15 to 16	0.9	0.8
13 to 14	0.8	0.7
12	0.7	0.6
10 to 11	0.6	0.6
6 to 9	0.5	0.5
2 to 5	0.4	0.4
Under 2	0.3	0.3

ably more than half) of total expenditures, a scale based on food requirements alone is obviously very much more accurate than one omitting any consideration whatsoever of the number, sex, and age of the individuals composing the families to be compared with respect to income.[1] For the present purpose, therefore, the total income of each family as defined above, has been divided by the number of "adult male units" subsisting on the family income, and the resulting figure has been termed the "family income per adult male unit."

Results of Classification

The 747 families for which income data were sufficiently accurate and complete for consideration have been classified by this method and grouped into four convenient classes, each containing a fair proportion of the total number. Table 1 presents this classification and also the resulting distribution of individuals and their equivalent "adult male units."

---

[1] In order to establish a more accurate basis for computing the size of families in comparing their incomes, a detailed study of expenditures for individuals in a number of representative families in cotton-mill villages was undertaken during 1917. While the tabulations of these data were not completed in time for use in the study of the data collected in 1916, it appears that the Atwater scale is roughly indicative of the variations, according to sex and age, in the consumption of all articles for which there are individual expenditures. It should be noted that before using the Atwater scale in the preliminary computations of family income, several published estimates of the cost of maintenance for individuals of various ages were examined. These estimates were based, in several instances, upon the results of investigation of actual expenditures of individual members of families. Using the estimated expenditures for an adult male as 100, the estimates for individuals of other ages of either sex were expressed relatively and compared with the Atwater scale. It appeared that, in most instances, the scales were fairly similar. [Tabulation of data deleted. ED.]

Table 1. Number of families and members of families and their equivalents in adult male units in seven cotton-mill villages of South Carolina, classified according to family income during a fifteen-day period between April 15 and June 16, 1916.

Half-month family income per adult male unit	Families	Persons[a]	Equivalent adult male units[b]
	Number		
Less than $6.00	217	1289	866.2
$6.00–$7.99	183	972	675.9
$8.00–$9.99	139	704	529.2
$10.00 and over	208	800	607.1
All incomes	747	3765	2678.2
	Percent	Percent	Percent
All incomes	100.0	100.0	100.0
Less than $6.00	29.1	34.2	32.4
$6.00–$7.99	24.5	25.8	25.2
$8.00–$9.99	18.6	18.7	19.8
$10.00 and over	27.9	21.3	22.6

[a] Exclusive of persons paying board and including only those dependent upon family income.
[b] According to the Atwater scale for food requirements.

The differences in income are also indicated in Table 2, which permits of a comparison of the results of classification on the basis of the average income during the half-month period per family, per person, and per "adult male unit." It will be noted that the same *general* differences in *average* incomes for the four groups are indicated by any of the three methods of classification. For reasons already stated, however, the "adult male unit" method is believed to be more accurately representative of actual conditions than either of the others and, therefore, to be preferred for the classification of individual families; it is the method hereinafter employed.

Before entering upon a consideration of the relation of family income to pellagra incidence it will be desirable to make brief reference to the factors affecting family income. An analysis of our data with a view of determining, so far as practicable, what these were, showed the principal ones to be as follows: (*a*) Supplemental income, chiefly from boarders; (*b*) the number of dependent persons, principally children, in proportion to the number of wage-earning persons in the family; and (*c*) the earning capacity

Table 2. Average half-month family income, computed in terms of "per family," "per person," and "per adult male unit,"[a] for various income classes of the population in seven cotton-mill villages in South Carolina.

Half-month family income per adult male unit	All family income during a half month	Average income during a half month		
		Per family	Per person	Per adult male unit[b]
Less than $6.00	$3990.45	$18.38	$3.09	$4.61
$6.00–$7.99	4780.85	26.12	4.92	7.07
$8.00–$9.99	4642.29	33.40	6.55	8.77
$10.00 and over	7777.99	37.39	9.72	12.81
All incomes	21 191.58	28.36	5.63	7.92

[a] According to the Atwater scale for food requirements.
[b] Exclusive of persons paying board and including only those dependent upon family income.

of the wage earners, including chiefly the factors of natural ability, length of training, and state of health. In the classification of this population according to "family income per adult male unit," those persons in the higher income classes appeared distinctly to have the advantage in each of these respects over those in the lower income classes.

PELLAGRA INCIDENCE ACCORDING TO ECONOMIC STATUS

Having considered the methods employed for securing the basic data relating to the occurrence of the disease and for securing those relating to the classification of the population with respect to economic status, we may now proceed to determine the relationship existing between the economic status of the family and the degree of incidence of the disease.

We have, in all, 747 households for which our data are sufficiently complete and accurate to permit of classification according to income. There were recorded among the members of these households 97 definite cases of pellagra. In Table 3 we have distributed these households in accordance with the family income per "adult male unit" during the sample half-month period and have indicated therein also the number and percent of the households in each of the resulting five income classes that were affected with pellagra to the extent of (a) one or more cases, (b) two or more cases, and (c) three or more cases.

It will be observed that the proportion of families affected with pellagra declines with a marked degree of regularity as income increases. This inverse correlation is even more clearly shown when weight is given to households with more than one case of the disease,[2] as is done in Table 4, in which the incidence of pellagra is expressed as a rate per 1000 persons in each income class.

The occurrence of multiple-case families, especially from the point of view of difference in income, invites special comment. The 97 cases of pellagra occurred in 61 families. In each of 24 of these families, two or more cases occurred, while in each of 8, three or more cases developed. Taking into consideration the size of the families and assuming that all individuals were equally susceptible to the disease,[3] a computation of the probability of the occurrence of multiple-case families according to purely chance distribution indicated that in the 747 families we should expect about 90 families with one case each, about 8 families with two or more cases, while the probability of households each with three or more cases would be less than 2 in 10 000. The actual occurrence of 24 families with two cases each and of 8 families with three or more cases would thus seem to be far in

[2] Upon the basis of the average half-month income per adult male unit for each of the income classes and the corresponding pellagra rate per 1000 persons, the Pearsonian coefficient of correlation is -0.91 ± 0.05. While the small number of classes considered must, of course, be taken into account, the expression indicates high degree of correlation (-1.0 being perfect inverse correlation).

[3] So far as sex and age are concerned, all families (with but few exceptions) contained fairly comparable proportions of "susceptible" individuals.

Table 3. Number and percent of households of different income classes affected with pellagra in seven cotton-mill villages of South Carolina in 1916.

Half-month family income per adult male unit	All households	Pellagrous households in which were:		
		One or more cases of pellagra	Two or more cases of pellagra	Three or more cases of pellagra
		Number		
Less than $6.00	217	28	17	7
$6.00–$7.99	183	21	3	1
$8.00–$9.99	139	8	4	0
$10.00–$13.99	144	3	0	0
$14.00 and over	64	1	0	0
All incomes	747	61	24	8
		Percent		
Less than $6.00	100.00	12.9	7.8	3.2
$6.00–$7.99	100.00	11.5	1.6	.5
$8.00–$9.99	100.00	5.8	2.9	0.0
$10.00–$13.99	100.00	2.1	0.0	0.0
$14.00 and over	100.00	1.5	0.0	0.0
All incomes	100.00	8.2	3.2	1.1

excess of the result of chance.[4] The fact that multiple-case families occurred only in the lower-income classes and that families with three or more cases occurred practically only in the lowest-income class plainly shows that the tendency toward concentration of cases in certain families increases as income diminishes. Pellagra incidence in the population studied therefore not only varied inversely according to family income, but with decreasing income it seemed to show an increasing tendency to affect members of the same family.

Discussion

The very marked inverse correlation between low income and pellagra incidence naturally calls for explanation. Under the conditions of the study the following possibilities in this regard suggested themselves for consideration: (a) Bad hygiene and sanitation; (b) Difference in sex and age composition of the population in the several income classes; and (c) Difference in diet.

(a) Bad Hygiene and Sanitation

[These factors] are in general closely associated with poverty so that the incidence of a disease, the dissemination of which is favored by such conditions, may be expected to be unusually high in the lower economic strata. Consequently it is natural to suspect that a disease found to be highly prevalent in an environment of poverty is dependent on the almost inevitably attendant unhygienic and unsanitary conditions for its propagation, and to assume that it is of microbial origin. The possibility of an essential infective etiological factor in this disease has therefore been given careful consideration, and in a previous paper (5) we reported the results of our study of the relation of certain factors of a sanitary character to the incidence of pellagra in these villages. No consistent correlation was found.[5] This, coupled with the results of the other of our own studies (see 5, pages 36-41) and of the studies of other investigators (26,

---

[4] Acknowledgment is made to Associate Statistician F. M. Phillips, United States Public Health Service, for assistance in this computation.

[5] The data collected during 1916 were not in a form to permit the study of the relation of crowding in the home to pellagra incidence. We may state, however, that a preliminary analysis of a considerable mass of data bearing on this point, collected during 1917, shows very little, if any, correlation between them when the effect of income is minimized.

Table 4. Number of definite cases of pellagra and rate per 1000[a] among persons of different income classes in seven cotton-mill villages of South Carolina in 1916.

Half-month family income per adult male unit	Total			Males			Females		
	Number of persons	Number of cases	Rate[a] per 1000	Number of persons	Number of cases	Rate per 1000	Number of persons	Number of cases	Rate per 1000
Less than $6.00	1312	56	42.7	650	20	30.8	662	36	54.4
$6.00–$7.99	1037	27	26.0	521	6	11.5	516	21	40.7
$8.00–$9.99	784	10	12.8	376	4	10.7	408	6	14.7
$10.00–$13.99	736	3	4.1	363	0	0.0	373	3	8.0
$14.00 and over	291	1	3.4	161	1	6.2	130	0	0.0
All incomes	4160	97	23.3	2071	31	14.9	2089	66	31.6

Comparison of crude pellagra rates and of rates after adjustment for age
to a standard population for each income class
(Standard population-total population, all incomes)

Family income per adult male unit	Case rate per 1000	
	Crude	Adjusted
Less than $6.00	42.7	41.0
$6.00–$7.99	26.0	24.8
$8.00–$9.99	12.8	14.2
$10.00–$13.99	4.1	5.2
$14.00 and over	3.4	2.5

[a] Since a marked variation in the pellagra rate according to age and sex was found for the population studied (*3*), and since, ordinarily, differences in the distribution of persons according to age occur in different economic groups, computation of rates adjusted to a standard population was made. The influence of differences in the sex distribution in any age group was insignificant, and practically the same incidence rates were obtained after making adjustments to a standard age distribution, as is shown in the above table.

27), and with the fact of the complete absence of any unequivocal evidence in support of an essential infective etiological factor in this disease, not only renders discussion of hygienic and sanitary factors in the present connection unnecessary but, we believe, permits of their dismissal from further serious consideration.

(b) Differences in Sex and Age Composition of the Population in the Several Income Classes

We have shown in a previous communication (*3*) that the incidence of the disease in the population of these villages differs markedly in the sexes and at certain age periods; it is conceivable, therefore, that differences in the sex and the age distribution in the different income classes might give rise to the phenomenon under discussion. That this is not the case, however, is evident (1) when it is recalled that we are dealing with a population composed of family units and (2) when we compare the indications afforded by Tables 4 and 5, showing, respec-

tively, the sex and the age distribution of the population of each economic class, and note the agreement in the indications afforded by the crude rates and by the rates after adjustment to a standard population (footnote to Table 4).

(c) Differences in Diet

The results of budgetary investigations have repeatedly demonstrated the association of marked variations in diet with variation in family income. (In this connection, see *28*) It seemed doubly pertinent, therefore, to inquire what, if any, variations in diet were associated with variations in income among the families of our cotton-mill villages. Accordingly, we prepared Table 6, showing the average food supply of the households of the several income classes. To facilitate comparison between the averages thus presented, indices have been computed, the figures for the households with the highest income being used as the base. It will be noted

Table 5. Number and percent of persons in each income class, classified according to age, in seven cotton-mill villages of South Carolina in 1916.
(The classes being divided from each other at those ages at which the pellagra incidence rate for the whole population varies most sharply.[a])

Half-month family income per adult male unit	All ages	Under 5 years	5–9	10–19	20–29	30–44	45–54	55 years and over
			Number					
Less than $6.00	1312	260	251	317	162	217	49	56
$6.00–$7.99	1037	162	166	270	172	166	60	41
$8.00–$9.99	784	104	108	229	149	114	48	32
$10.00–$13.99	736	95	69	173	215	102	46	36
$14.00 and over	291	27	15	71	91	63	9	15
All incomes	4160	648	609	1060	789	662	212	180
			Percent					
Less than $6.00	100	19.8	19.1	24.2	12.4	16.5	3.7	4.3
$6.00–$7.99	100	15.7	16.0	26.0	16.6	16.0	5.8	3.9
$8.00–$9.99	100	13.3	13.8	29.2	19.0	14.5	6.1	4.1
$10.00–$13.99	100	12.9	9.4	23.5	29.2	13.9	6.2	4.9
$14.00 and over	100	9.3	5.2	24.4	31.3	21.6	3.1	5.2
All incomes	100	15.6	14.6	25.5	19.0	15.9	5.1	4.3

[a] See (2).

that, from the point of view of income, the following general tendencies are suggested:

1. The smaller the income the smaller were the supplies purchased of all meats (except salt pork), green vegetables, fresh fruits, eggs, butter, cheese, preserved milk, lard, sugar (including syrup), and canned foods.
2. The smaller the income the larger were the supplies purchased of salt pork and cornmeal.
3. In the households of the various income classes the quantities of the purchased supplies[6] of dried peas and beans, potatoes, dried fruits, wheat flour and bread, fresh milk, and rice appeared without any consistent trend.

Thus it appears that there were associated with differences in family income quite definite differences in household food supplies. In

order to determine the outstanding differences more clearly, the households with intermediate incomes were disregarded and comparison was made of the food supplies in households presenting the greatest contrast from an economic standpoint (i.e., those households representing the respective extremes of family income), with the result that not only did the differences already noted stand out more clearly, but, in addition, it appeared that the supplies of wheat flour and bread and of fresh milk were appreciably smaller in the poorest households.

In that part of our study dealing with the relation of household food supply to pellagra incidence (2) a very definite significant relationship between the character of the diet and the incidence of the disease was demonstrated, and since, as we have seen above, a marked inverse correlation exists between the amount of family income and the degree of incidence of the disease, it follows that the character of the diet of the population under consideration may be expected to vary with the amount of family income, in the sense at least that the lower the income the more the character of the diet will tend to approach that associated with pellagra.

[6] Practically all food supplies, with the exception of fresh milk, were purchased (i.e., not home-produced) during the season (the late spring) of the year under consideration. Households securing supplies of milk from home-owned cows have not been included in Table 6, since supplies of food from this source constitute a factor affecting the diet of the population apart from the factor of family income. They are considered in another connection.

Table 6. Average supply (per adult male unit) during a fifteen-day period between April 15 and June 16, 1916, of various purchased articles of food[a] in households of different income classes and in the group of households in each of which two or more cases of pellagra occurred prior to August 1, 1916.

Grams per adult male unit per day

Half-month family income per adult male unit	Salt pork	Corn meal and grits	Dried peas and beans	Potatoes	Dried fruits	Wheat flour, bread	Fresh milk (bought)	Sugar syrup	Butter	Rice	Canned vegetables	Preserved milk	Lard and lard substitutes	Canned meats	Cheese	Eggs	Green vegetables[b]	Fresh fruits	Canned corn	Canned fruits	Jellies and jams	Fresh meats	Canned peas and beans	Cured lean meats
$14.00 and more	39	126	31	71	10	447	319	59	30	8	58	4	63	20	3	59	105	41	9	27	11	47	9	53
$10.00–$13.99	49	152	31	107	9	434	302	61	35	6	36	4	54	12	3	57	63	33	10	26	10	32	6	28
$8.00–$9.99	54	151	35	97	9	410	342	67	14	5	37	3	49	16	3	44	60	31	8	24	8	30	4	24
$6.00–$7.99	56	174	33	88	9	460	317	55	19	4	46	1	49	14	2	38	61	30	6	14	9	21	5	20
Less than $6.00	54	169	31	73	10	399	282	50	19	5	35	2	37	12	2	33	49	19	4	12	5	19	2	12
Pellagrous households	65	150	34	60	10	361	127	48	11	6	20	2	35	16	c	31	61	10	6	16	6	16	2	8

Relative numbers. Base: Supply per adult male unit per day in households with highest incomes

Half-month family income per adult male unit	Salt pork	Corn meal and grits	Dried peas and beans	Potatoes	Dried fruits	Wheat flour, bread	Fresh milk (bought)	Sugar syrup	Butter	Rice	Canned vegetables	Preserved milk	Lard and lard substitutes	Canned meats	Cheese	Eggs	Green vegetables[b]	Fresh fruits	Canned corn	Canned fruits	Jellies and jams	Fresh meats	Canned peas and beans	Cured lean meats
$14.00 and more	100	100	100	100	100	100	100	100	100	100	100	100	100	100	100	100	100	100	100	100	100	100	100	100
$10.00–$13.99	126	121	100	151	90	97	95	103	117	75	62	100	86	60	67	97	60	81	111	96	91	68	67	53
$8.00–$9.99	138	120	113	137	90	92	107	114	47	63	64	75	78	80	100	75	57	76	89	89	73	64	44	45
$6.00–$7.99	144	138	107	124	90	103	99	93	63	50	79	25	78	70	67	64	58	73	67	52	82	45	56	38
Less than $6.00	138	134	100	103	100	89	88	85	63	63	60	50	59	60	67	56	47	46	44	44	45	40	22	23
Pellagrous households	167	119	110	85	100	81	40	81	37	75	34	50	55	80	..	53	58	24	67	59	55	34	22	15

a For explanation of terms, see (3), appendix.
b Includes string beans.
c Less than 0.5 of a gram.

595

This is confirmed by the quite definite differences in food supply above actually shown to be associated with differences in family income, and further by the fact that when comparison is made, such as Table 6 permits, it is found that in a general, but quite definite, way the food supply of the households of the lowest-income class tends to be similar to that of the group of pellagrous households in each of which at least two cases of pellagra occurred prior to August 1, 1916; that is, similar to that of the group whose food supply more closely approximates a representative sample of a pellagra-producing diet than does any other afforded by our study. [Graphic comparison deleted. ED.]

Differences in Incidence Among Households

From the foregoing considerations the conclusion would seem to be suggested that the inverse correlation between pellagra incidence and family income depended in large measure, if not entirely, on the unfavorable effect of a low income on the character of the diet. In this connection, however, it must be noted and consideration must be given to the fact that a large proportion of households with low incomes were not affected with the disease.

(Similarly, a large proportion of the members of pellagrous households were apparently unaffected by the disease. As has already been stated, the present study deals with the household, not with the individual, excepting only as to pellagra incidence. We have, therefore, no special data on which an explanation of the exemption of the unaffected members of a household might be based. Nevertheless, in the light of (a) certain general observations and (b) of analogies to such food deficiency diseases as scurvy and beriberi, together with (c) the knowledge gained as the result of the newer work of many students in the field of diet and nutrition, the following suggestions may properly be submitted for consideration in this connection:

1. *Differences in Diet Consumed Among Individuals of the Household.* Although all members of a household presumably have the same diet available, as the result of individual likes and dislikes, observable at almost any table, slight differences in diet actually consumed are common and marked differences, amounting in some instances to outstanding individual eccen-

tricities, are not rare. Furthermore, differences in diet actually consumed may arise from, or be accentuated by, food eaten between meals and by supplemental foods of one kind or another in respect to which individuals of the same household may differ considerably. Clearly, then, a knowledge of the exact composition of the diet of a household or other dietary group does not necessarily justify the assumption of a knowledge of the composition of the diet consumed by an individual member of such household or group. Failure to appreciate this, it may be noted, has been a frequent cause of serious error and consequent confusion in connection with studies of food-deficiency diseases.

2. *Differences in Individual Susceptibility or Resistance.* Assuming identity of diet actually consumed, differences in incidence among individuals of the same household or other dietary group may result from individual variation in resistance or susceptibility, which may conceivably be related to (a) an inherent individual characteristic, (b) the age or sex of the individual, (c) the existence of some exhausting underlying disease or condition (hookworm, dysentery, duodenal fistula), or (d) to unlike physical strain or exertion.

3. *Combinations of Factors 1 and 2.* Thus, in the village of *In*, where the highest of the incidence rates observed by us in 1916 occurred and where the rate among persons constituting the households with incomes under the average was 90 per 1000, over 65 percent of these poorer households appeared not to be affected, and, in varying degree, this was true of each of the seven villages studied. That the exemption of these families from pellagra was not due to a lack of subjects of "susceptible" sex is evident from what has already been said on this point; and that it could not be attributed to lack of human material of "susceptible" age appears very clearly when the distribution of the population according to age is compared for the pellagrous and for the poorer nonpellagrous households in a representative village, as is done in Table 7. Manifestly, therefore, the amount of family income—that is, money income (in the sense here used), such as wages, cash payments from boarders, cash receipts from sales of supplies, and other sources—was not the sole factor determining the character of the household diet.

Table 7. Age distribution of population constituting the nonpellagrous households with low family income[a] and the pellagrous households of the mill village of In.

Households	All ages	Under 5	5-9	10-14	20-29	30-44	45-54	55 and over
				Age groups				
			Number of persons					
Nonpellagrous	265	52	53	61	33	45	14	7
Pellagrous	168	31	32	49	19	31	5	1
All households	433	83	85	110	52	76	19	8
			Percent					
Nonpellagrous	100.0	19.6	20.0	23.0	12.5	17.0	5.3	2.6
Pellagrous	100.0	18.5	19.0	29.2	11.3	18.5	3.0	.6
All households	100.0	19.2	19.6	25.4	12.0	17.5	4.4	1.8

[a] That is, under $8 per adult male unit during a half-month period in the late spring of 1916.

This is quite in accord with common experience, which teaches that there are many factors that, singly or in varying combinations, may have an important influence on the character of the diet and that may vary among and thus may distinguish different households of the same income. In illustration of this, reference may be made to the group of factors that tend to determine the amount and proportion of family income available for the purchase of food, an example of which is the occurrence of sickness or injury, making an unusual draft on the family income. Related to such factors are the general spirit of the household with respect to thrift (which, when unwisely directed, may be harmful) and the intelligence and ability of the housewife in utilizing the available family income.

More tangible than these, and perhaps of more immediate practical importance in its effect on the household diet, is the difference among households with respect to the availability of food supplies. We found that, among households with similar incomes and of the same village and thus with access to the same markets, there were some more favorably situated in having sources of food supplies that others either did not possess or possessed in a lesser degree. Such sources frequently were gardens, home-owned cows, swine, poultry, and the like.

Differences in Incidence Among Villages

Besides differences among households with similar incomes and of the same village, quite marked differences in pellagra incidence were also observed, as has already been pointed out, among the villages themselves. We have sought to determine the explanation of this by considering in order the various possibilities that suggested themselves.

(*a*) The general environment (except as to condition of sanitation and food supply), the origin and type of the population, the character of work, and the general habits of living among these populations being, as we have already stated, strikingly similar, do not call for consideration in the present connection.

(*b*) Differences in sanitary conditions among villages were noted and their relation to differences in the incidence of the disease was studied without, however, discovering any consistent correlation among them. Reasons have been given why hygienic and sanitary factors might be dismissed from consideration in the attempt to explain the inverse correlation between family income and the incidence of pellagra (see p. 592). Further discussion of these factors in the present connection would therefore seem to be unnecessary.

(*c*) The marked association between low family income and pellagra incidence suggested the possibility that the difference in incidence among villages might be associated with a difference in the proportion of families of low incomes included in the populations of the several villages. But if the differences in the proportion of the population which had low incomes in the various villages be compared with the differences in pellagra incidence, as is done in Table 8, no consistent correlation is disclosed. Clearly the differences in pellagra incidence among these villages cannot be accounted for by differences in the economic status of the populations concerned.

(*d*) As family income is simply an index of the power to buy, and as this power is obviously

Table 8. Comparison of the relation of rate of pellagra incidence to proportion of population of low family income in seven mill villages of South Carolina in 1916.

Village	Percent of population whose half-month family income per adult male unit was less than:		Pellagra rate per 1000 population (all incomes in 1916)
	$6.00	$8.00	
All villages	31.5	56.5	23.4
At	37.0	64.3	20.7
In	40.9	66.6	64.6
Ny	26.2	45.7	0.0
Rc	13.2	23.7	24.9
Sn	38.3	58.1	10.9
Sa	28.3	57.4	25.7
Wy	31.0	64.0	18.7

Pearsonian coefficient of correlation: $r = 0.33 \pm 0.23$.

limited by the cost of the thing desired (in this instance food), the thought naturally suggests itself that differences in prices in the different villages might be of importance in the present connection. That this was a negligible factor, however, is shown by the fact that we found no significant differences in food prices in the different villages.

(*e*) That individuals of "susceptible" ages may have been present in relatively insignificant numbers in the villages among whose poorer households few if any were affected by the disease, and that this may account for the differences, is an explanation that may be dismissed from consideration when the age distribution of the population is compared according to village, as may be seen by reference to Table 9.

(*f*) We thus come to a consideration, finally, of differences among villages with respect to availability of food supplies on the local markets or from home production. More or less marked differences in this respect were found to exist. In relating these to differences in pellagra incidence it should be borne in mind that the availability to a consumer of a supply of a given

Table 9. Comparison of the age distribution of the population constituting the households with low family incomes[a] of seven cotton-mill villages of South Carolina.

Villages	All ages	Classified by age periods (years)						
		Under 5 years	5-9	10-19	20-29	30-44	45-54	55 and over
				Number of persons				
At	367	65	65	82	63	59	18	15
In	433	83	85	110	52	76	19	8
Ny	331	60	56	87	45	57	15	11
Rc	206	37	42	50	34	32	5	6
Sn	338	65	46	69	61	52	14	31
Sa	268	51	51	68	40	34	14	10
Wy	407	62	72	120	39	73	24	17
All villages	2350	423	417	586	334	383	109	98
				Percent				
At	100.0	17.5	17.5	22.3	17.2	16.1	4.9	4.1
In	100.0	19.2	19.6	25.4	12.0	17.5	4.4	1.8
Ny	100.0	18.1	16.9	26.3	13.6	17.2	4.5	3.3
Rc	100.0	18.0	20.4	24.3	16.5	15.5	2.4	2.9
Sn	100.0	19.2	13.6	20.4	18.0	15.4	4.1	9.2
Sa	100.0	19.0	19.0	25.4	14.9	12.7	5.2	3.7
Wy	100.0	15.2	17.4	29.5	9.6	17.9	5.9	4.2
All villages	100.0	18.0	17.7	24.9	14.2	16.3	4.6	4.2

[a] That is, under $8 per adult male unit during a half month in the late spring of 1916.

article or group of articles of food is often involved in a number of interrelated conditions, the influence of any one of which may be difficult to measure. Therefore, in analyzing community conditions affecting the supply of any article or articles of food, only the outstanding and clearcut differences between localities can be considered. Furthermore, since even considerable differences in pellagra incidence among localities of small population are not necessarily a reflection of community conditions, it seemed desirable to select for the study of the relationship under consideration villages presenting the most marked contrast in the incidence of the disease, thereby avoiding the possibly confusing effects of irregularities likely to arise in attempts to relate community conditions of food availability to pellagra rates for which community conditions were possibly responsible only in part or not at all. There was, moreover, the compelling practical consideration to thus restrict ourselves in the fact that the amount of labor involved in a detailed study of conditions in each of our villages was beyond the physical capacity of the available personnel to perform. Accordingly we selected for study *Ny* village, with no pellagra, and *In* village, with a rate of not less than 64.6 per 1000 during 1916. The facts, as we were able to determine them relating to the availability of supplies of various foods in these two villages, are briefly summarized in the following:

(1) *Retail grocery establishments.* In both villages the mill workers' households purchased their supplies of all foods from the company stores and from grocery stores in adjacent communities, with the exception of fresh meats, fresh milk, and varying proportions of their supplies of eggs, butter, green vegetables, and fresh fruits. Exclusive of the articles named, the availability of supplies of all foods appeared to be the same in both villages for the reasons that (*a*) in both villages there existed company stores which carried in stock practically the same kinds of foods and were operated along similar lines from the point of view of credit allowances to mill workers, and (*b*) within a mile of either village were general grocery stores carrying in stock the same kinds and varieties of foods as those sold at the company stores. The company stores at *Ny*, however, did not sell fresh vegetables, potatoes, and fresh fruits, there being an

agreement with the lessee of the village market to the effect that the latter should have the exclusive store privilege of selling these articles. A much more regular and abundant supply of fresh vegetables and fruits was available at the *Ny* market than at the *In* company store.

It is of interest to note that the *In* households, whose incomes were less than the average income for the two villages, relied to a greater extent upon the company store than the *Ny* households with similar incomes. This is indicated by the purchase and food supply records during the 15-day period from May 16 to May 30, 1916, which show that 60 percent of the *In* households purchased all of their groceries (exclusive of home produce and produce from nearby farms) from the company store as compared with only 13 percent of the *Ny* households.

(2) *Fresh-meat markets.* In *Ny* there was a fresh-meat market which had been open seven days in the week the year round for several years. This market, as already noted, also sold fresh fruit and vegetables. The nearest other market was one mile away, and this market operated a wagon which regularly had taken orders and delivered fresh meat in the village at the doors of the mill workers' households during the spring and the preceding fall and winter. At the town of Seneca, four miles away, there were two other fresh-meat markets which were occasionally patronized by *Ny* mill workers. In *In* village there was no fresh-meat market, and there had not been any since the last of February, 1916. In October, 1915, a privately operated market was opened in the basement of the company store building. This market was kept open every week day until about January 1, 1916, but, from all accounts, it was poorly managed. For this reason and for the reason that locally produced fresh meats became scarce after January 1, the market was open only one or two days a week during January and February and its credit trade was severely curtailed, being now limited to those households which had been prompt in settlements. In the latter part of February the market ceased to be operated. In the town of Inman, a mile or more from the mill village, there was a market selling fresh meat for cash only, which had a few regular customers among the mill workers. No other market was accessible except in the city of Spartanburg, 13 miles away.

With the exception of a small amount of poultry purchased at home or purchased from nearby farmers, the sole sources of fresh meats in the two villages during the late spring of 1916 were these fresh-meat markets. The difference in availability of a fresh meat supply in the two villages is clearly reflected in the records of actual purchases during the 15-day period May 16–30, 1916, illustrated in Table 10, thereby suggesting a marked contrast in fresh-meat consumption between the two villages for households of similar incomes.

(3) *Produce from adjacent farm territory.* The two villages presented a striking contrast with respect to the availability of food supplies from adjacent farm territory.

In the mill village of *In* there were no regular sellers of farm produce during the spring of 1916; farmers visited the village only occasionally and then practically solely in order to dispose of such goods as they had been unable to sell in the nearby town of Inman. The absence of hucksters was so marked that repeated and detailed inquiries were made of mill workers' households and of other persons living in or in close touch with the village, and the village was several times canvassed in order to secure as complete and accurate information as possible in relation thereto. *Ny*, on the other hand, appeared to be a center for marketing produce from nearby farms. In addition to a number of farmers who marketed their produce in that village occasionally, not less than 22 farmers who habitually sold in the village at retail were found and interviewed in a single canvass of the adjacent territory. These regular hucksters came to the village once a week or oftener prac-

tically the year round. Of the 22 who were interviewed, 15 sold fresh milk and butter, 10 sold eggs, 7 sold poultry, 5 sold fresh pork, 2 sold fresh beef, and practically all of them sold potatoes and vegetables. Those selling milk and butter delivered regularly throughout the year and marketed other produce in different seasons. Thus, eggs were sold principally in the spring, poultry in the summer, autumn, and winter, fresh beef and pork in the autumn and winter, and green vegetables in the spring, summer, and autumn. On the basis of statements made by those selling produce regularly, not less than 41 000 quarts of fresh milk (about 790 quarts weekly), 12 000 pounds of butter (about 230 pounds weekly), 1800 dozen eggs, and 4200 pounds of live poultry, fresh beef, and fresh pork were sold during the 12 months ending May 30, 1916. These totals do not include quantities sold by other farmers or by stores and markets.

This contrast in available sources of farm produce is indicated also by the statements of actual purchases by the households in the respective villages, secured in the course of the dietary canvass. These statements have been summarized for households of similar incomes in Table 11. A striking difference is shown in the extent to which the households in *Ny* and *In* relied upon nearby farms for supplies of certain foods.

The difference between *Ny* and *In* in availability of food supplies from adjacent farm territory was so pronounced that further inquiries were made into some of the underlying conditions in order to discover, if possible, what other economic factors were responsible for bringing

Table 10. Comparison of availability of fresh meat as shown by the number of purchases and the average daily supply of this food during the period May 16–30, 1916, in households, with family incomes less than the average, of two mill villages of South Carolina.

Number of purchases during 15-day period	Village of Ny (average daily supply per adult male unit, 31.2 grams)		Village of In (average daily supply per adult male unit, 7.0 grams)	
	Number of households purchasing	Percent of total households	Number of households purchasing	Percent of total households
None	17	31.0	46	65.8
1	6	10.9	18	25.7
2	7	12.7	4	5.7
3	7	12.7	1	1.4
4	6	10.9	1	1.4
5	6	10.9	0	0.0
More than 5	6	10.9	0	0.0

Table 11. Comparison of availability of certain foods in two cotton-mill villages of South Carolina, as indicated by the proportion of the households with family incomes under the average of the contrasted villages purchasing the specified articles from nearby farms during the period May 16–30, 1916.

Article purchased	Ny			In		
	Average quantity per household purchasing	Households purchasing		Average quantity per household purchasing	Households purchasing	
		Number	Percent of total households		Number	Percent of total households
Fresh milk	22.5 qts.	24	51.0	29.3 qts.	3	4.5
Butter	3.4 lbs.	23	49.0	4.0 lbs.	1	1.5
Eggs	2.9 doz.	19	40.5	6.0 doz.	1	1.5
Fresh vegetables		31	66.0		1	1.5
Fresh fruit		8	17.0		0	0.0
Poultry	4.0 lbs.	1	2.1	3.0 lbs.	1	1.5
Any of the above articles		40	83.3		6	9.0
None		8	16.7		61	91.0

this about. From these inquiries it appeared that at least two conditions were important in causing the difference in availability of the supply of the foods in question: namely (*a*) differences in the kind of agriculture in the territory adjacent to the villages, and (*b*) differences in marketing conditions. The two are closely related, but for the sake of clearness it will be advantageous to discuss them separately.

(*a*) Contrast in the kinds of agriculture near the two villages. A census of the farm products in the agricultural territory adjacent to the two villages was not undertaken, but from observation in the course of several trips and canvasses in the sections in question it was quite clear that a marked contrast existed in the kinds of agriculture pursued. The territory around *In* was planted principally in cotton, and relatively little diversification in crops existed. Truck farming on any considerable scale was not engaged in. Few beef cattle were raised and milch cows apparently were usually not more than sufficient to supply the household needs of the farmers. Many farmers had no cows or pigs or even poultry. The agriculture in the *In* section seemed rather typical of the cotton areas in South Carolina. Cotton was the predominant crop; all other products were incidental, none of them constituting the principal output of any farm, so far as was observed. The territory around *Ny*, on the other hand, was exceptional for South Carolina in that a considerable amount of diversified farming was carried on, although not fully comparable in this respect

with the farming sections in states where one-crop agriculture has not been the rule. Cotton was a relatively less important crop, and beef cattle, swine, poultry, and milch cows seemed much more abundant than in the *In* section. Apparently greater emphasis was given to gardens, and the amount of truck produce was noticeably larger. The physical character of the section apparently was one cause of this difference in products. The land around *In* is almost level, lies well below the foothills of the Blue Ridge Mountains, and is well suited for the growing of cotton. The land around *Ny* is quite rolling and even hilly, being, in fact, in the foothills of the mountains and thus not so well suited to cotton growing. Land not suitable for the cultivation of cotton and, hence, available and used for corn and truck products was consequently far more abundant near *Ny* than near *In*.

(*b*) Contrast in market conditions. Conditions affecting the market for farm produce from the two sections were quite different in some important respects. The village of *Ny* is itself more isolated than the village of *In* and is not near any important community. The nearest railway station is a mile away and is surrounded by only about a dozen houses, including three small stores. Seneca, the nearest town of any size (population 1313 in 1910), is some 4 miles from *Ny*, and Greenville, the nearest city (population 15 741 in 1910), is about 40 miles distant. Seneca exports comparatively little produce and hence its market is limited to local needs which are not sufficient to absorb all the miscellaneous farm products of the vicinity. *Ny* is thus a competitor for such produce as the adjacent farm territory affords. The village itself has been in existence without much change in size for about 25 years, and we found that some of the sellers of farm produce had been visiting it regularly for over 10 years. On the other hand, *In* mill village is almost on the outskirts of the town of Inman (population 474 in 1910), which is on the railroad connecting Spartanburg, S. C., with Asheville, N. C. The demands of the Inman market for farm products are far from being confined to securing sufficient supplies for the needs of its townspeople, since several resident buyers purchase the surplus produce of the adjacent territory and ship it to Spartanburg. Since Spartanburg (population 17 517 in 1910) is but 13 miles distant along a good highway, buyers from that city cover the territory around *In* village fairly thoroughly, and farmers having produce to market often take it to the city when they go there to avail themselves of Spartanburg's superior shopping advantages. The position of *In* village appears, therefore, to be distinctly disadvantageous with respect to farm produce since it must compete for this not only with the town of Inman but, more important, also with the city of Spartanburg. So far as could be ascertained in 1916, no regular trade with nearby farms

had been established, and, as has been pointed out, such casual trade as existed was only that afforded by occasional visits of hucksters who, after making the rounds in the town of Inman, had unsold remnants of produce.

(4) *Home-provided foods.* Specific inquiries were made of all mill workers' households regarding their possession of cows, poultry, and gardens and, as far as practicable, regarding their importance particularly during the spring of 1916. Different proportions of the households in the two villages were found to have such sources of food supplies.

(a) Milch cows. There was but little difference in the proportion of households in either village owning productive cows during the spring of 1916, the percentage being 17.2 for *Ny* and 23.3 for *In* among households having less than the average income. Such difference as existed in this respect was in favor of *In*. But it should be noted in this connection that 33.3 percent of the *In* households had no fresh-milk supply at all during the 15-day period for which household supply records were kept, as against only 8 percent of the *Ny* households (see Table 12). This difference in distribution was caused by the larger proportion of *Ny* households that purchased milk from hucksters, since, as shown in Table 11, 51 percent of *Ny* households purchased fresh milk from hucksters as against 4.5 percent of *In* households.

Table 12. Percentages of cotton mill operatives' households having supplies of various articles of food in different quantities per adult male unit per day, compared for the mill villages of Ny and In, South Carolina.
(All households considered have incomes of less than the average for the two villages.)

			Percent of households whose average daily supply per adult male unit was:			
Article of food	Village	Average daily supply per adult male unit (grams)	None	Some, but less than one-third of the average of all households	One-third or more, but less than the average of all households	The average or more than the average of all households
Fresh meats	Ny	34	31.2	6.2	16.7	45.8
	In	7	67.2	10.4	13.4	9.0
Cured lean meats	Ny	24	37.5	4.2	27.1	31.2
	In	20	46.3	6.0	14.9	32.8
Canned meats	Ny	19	22.9	10.4	37.5	29.2
	In	17	35.8	3.0	31.3	29.9
Eggs	Ny	34	31.2	4.2	31.2	33.3
	In	50	7.5	6.0	26.9	59.7
Fresh milk	Ny	426	8.3	10.4	45.8	35.4
	In	457	33.3	0.0	30.2	36.5
Preserved milk	Ny	1	87.5	2.1	2.1	8.3
	In	3	73.6	1.5	1.5	22.4

Table 12. (Continued.)

| Article of food | Village | Average daily supply per adult male unit (grams) | Percent of households whose average daily supply per adult male unit was: | | | |
			None	Some, but less than one-third of the average of all households	One-third or more, but less than the average of all households	The average or more than the average of all households
Butter	Ny	26	16.7	10.4	33.3	39.6
	In	30	14.9	16.4	21.4	46.3
Cheese	Ny	3	87.5	2.1	0.0	10.4
	In	b	97.0	0.0	0.0	3.0
Dried peas and beans	Ny	32	25.0	14.6	29.8	39.6
	In	25	32.8	7.5	29.9	29.9
Canned peas and beans	Ny	2	83.3	0.0	0.0	16.7
	In	4	85.1	0.0	0.0	14.9
Wheat flour	Ny	358	6.2	0.0	43.7	29.2
	In	358	18.5	3.1	32.3	46.2
Wheat bread, cakes, and crackers	Ny	13	18.7	12.5	33.3	35.4
	In	18	25.4	6.0	22.4	46.3
Cornmeal	Ny	139	29.8	4.3	29.8	36.2
	In	180	20.9	0.0	17.9	61.2
Grits	Ny	4	87.5	0.0	0.0	12.5
	In	2	95.6	0.0	0.0	4.5
Rice	Ny	4	75.0	0.0	0.0	25.0
	In	5	70.2	0.0	0.0	29.9
Salt pork	Ny	54	4.3	4.3	57.2	34.0
	In	53	10.4	0.0	41.8	47.8
Lard and lard substitutes	Ny	41	6.2	4.2	52.1	37.5
	In	40	10.4	3.0	37.3	49.3
Green string beans	Ny	11	68.7	0.0	0.0	31.2
	In	1	100.0	0.0	0.0	0.0
Canned string beans	Ny	1	97.9	0.0	0.0	2.1
	In	4	89.5	0.0	0.0	10.5
Green vegetables (bought)	Ny	88	14.6	12.5	39.6	33.3
	In	46	22.7	16.7	37.9	22.7
Other canned vegetables	Ny	36	29.2	2.1	22.9	45.8
	In	36	26.9	7.5	28.4	37.3
Fresh fruits	Ny	40	25.0	10.4	20.8	43.7
	In	20	43.9	9.1	28.8	18.2
Dried fruits	Ny	12	53.2	0.0	17.0	29.8
	In	8	70.2	1.5	6.0	22.4
Canned fruits	Ny	10	66.7	0.0	2.1	31.2
	In	20	56.7	0.0	1.5	41.8
Irish potatoes	Ny	34	45.8	4.2	20.8	29.2
	In	60	53.7	3.0	3.0	40.3
Fresh sweet potatoes	Ny	0	0.0	0.0	0.0	0.0
	In	0	0.0	0.0	0.0	0.0
Canned sweet potatoes	Ny	5	81.2	0.0	0.0	18.7
	In	3	88.1	0.0	0.0	11.9
Sugar	Ny	46	10.4	4.2	45.8	39.6
	In	39	9.0	9.0	43.3	38.8
Syrup	Ny	17	68.7	0.0	2.1	29.2
	In	17	64.2	0.0	0.0	35.8
Jellies and Jams	Ny	3	70.2	0.0	4.3	25.5
	In	9	40.3	2.5	0.0	58.2

[a] Tabulation of approximate average daily supply of various foods in these same households deleted. ED.
[b] Less than 0.5 gram.

(b) Swine. Slaughtering of hogs is done in autumn and winter. This is a general practice and prevailed in *Ny* as well as in *In*. Home-produced pork did not figure in the spring food supply of mill workers' households in either village, except in the form of cured and salt meat. Of the *Ny* households, 17 percent slaughtered home-raised hogs as compared with 33.3 percent of *In* households. All of these households slaughtered their hogs before February 1, 1916, the majority in either village slaughtering before Christmas, 1915. Of the *Ny* households, 11 percent cured home-slaughtered meat, as compared with 29 percent of *In* households; but very little of this meat was on hand for use in the late spring. Inquiries of households slaughtering swine revealed the fact that in less than 5 percent of such households were there any supplies of home-cured pork on hand on May 16, 1916, these being principally salt pork. The home-produced pork, therefore, did not appear to enter in significant degree into the spring food supply of the households in either village.

(c) Poultry. Inquiries of households having less than the average income showed that 40 percent of the *Ny* households and 25 percent of the *In* households either did own poultry during the winter and spring months ending May 30, 1916, or were owning poultry at the time of the canvass (from June 1 to June 10, 1916). The average number of poultry consumed per household during the preceding year was 22 in *Ny* and 8 in *In*. The percent of *Ny* households reporting consumption of home-owned poultry during the spring of 1916 was 19, as against 3 percent for *In*. Thirty-two percent of *Ny* households reported a fairly regular supply of eggs from home-owned hens as against 21 percent of *In* households. It appears that the advantage in the supplies of home-produced poultry and eggs during the preceding winter and spring lay distinctly with *Ny* households.

(d) Gardens. Home gardens were much more generally found in the village of *In* than in *Ny*. Nearly 92 percent of the *In* households had gardens planted on June 1, 1916, as against less than 23 per cent of *Ny* households. The opportunity afforded by suitable garden space was decidedly better in *In* than in *Ny;* practically every home in *In* had a good-sized garden plot, whereas many of the *Ny* households had no suitable space at all.

It was quite evident, however, that home gardens contributed but very slightly, if at all, to the food supply of households in either village during the spring of 1916. With the exception of an occasional ("rare" is perhaps a more accurate term) "mess" or dish of greens, a very little lettuce, and a few young onions, the gardens had yielded no supplies during 1916 up to about June 1. Not until after June 15 did garden produce become abundant, a condition that was somewhat contrary to the expectation of the authors, who had anticipated finding considerably earlier garden production in this section. The principal reason for this tardiness appears to be the fact that gardens in mill villages are usually planted later than gardens elsewhere in this section. Difficulty in getting the ground prepared early enough, owing in part to the fact that the long hours of work in the mill leave no available daylight for gardening until well along in the spring, lack of initiative in making other preparations, and possibly other causes, apparently almost preclude good early spring gardens in most of the mill villages studied, including *Ny* and *In*, although climatic conditions ordinarily are such that gardens can be made to yield supplies of early varieties of vegetables during May and even in April. Aside from a half dozen households reporting that they had had radishes, lettuce, or English peas, only about one-third of the *In* households reported that they had had greens or young onions even occasionally and in small quantities before this date. In *Ny* the proportion was even less.

Summing up the principal differences in availability of food supplies during the spring of 1916 as between *Ny* and *In*, it may be said that (1) supplies of fresh milk, butter, green vegetables, and fresh fruit were available to a greater degree (better distributed among the households) in *Ny* than in *In*, because, in the farm territory adjacent to *Ny*, there was a larger production of these articles of food and because *Ny* occupied a more advantageous location as a market for such products, and (2) that a supply of fresh meat was available to a greater degree in *Ny* than in *In* because of the existence of a fresh-meat market in *Ny* all the year round. In practically all other respects the availability of food supplies appeared to be generally similar in the two villages.

The conditions outlined above are reflected

in a comparison of the total food supplies during the 15-day period May 16–30, 1916, of households in *Ny* and *In*. In this comparison (Table 12) in order to eliminate as far as practicable the influence of differences in economic status, only those households with less than the average of incomes[7] have been considered.

In Table 12 is shown the average quantity of each article of food for all the households considered, as well as the percentages of the households in each village which had various quantities of each article of food, such quantities being expressed in terms of the average for all households in order to shorten the statistical presentation.

This comparison indicates that during the 15-day period, May 16–30, 1916, (1) supplies of fresh meat, fresh milk, green vegetables, and fresh fruit were more abundant (i.e., better distributed) in *Ny* than in *In* households; (2) supplies of cured and canned meats, salt pork, butter, flour, lard, and lard substitutes, and dried peas and beans in *Ny* households were quite similar to those in *In* households; and (3) supplies of eggs, corn meal, Irish potatoes, and most canned goods were more abundant in *In* than in *Ny* households. Other differences in the supplies of articles of food occurring either rarely or in small quantities are indicated.

From the foregoing considerations it clearly appears that the character of the household food supply in the two villages was considerably influenced by the availability of certain foods, notably fresh meats, fresh milk, green vegetables, and fresh fruits, all of which were relatively less abundant or less equally distributed in *In* than in *Ny*. It is clear also that these differences in the food supply of *Ny* and *In* households are quite similar to the differences which, as already reported, we found to exist in the food supply of nonpellagrous and of pellagrous households (*1, 2*).

We have here, therefore, a striking and significant correspondence between the differences in the availability of certain foods (and thus, it is permissible to assume, in the character of the diet) in the two villages, on the one hand, and the difference with respect to the incidence of pellagra among their households on the other.

Since between these two villages no other differences to which significance could properly be attached were disclosed by our study, the conclusion would seem to be warranted that the difference in the availability of food supplies above summarized was the outstanding determining factor in relation to the marked difference in the incidence of the disease.

Thus, of all the factors we have studied in relation to differences in pellagra incidence among our villages, the factor of food availability is the only one in connection with which significant evidence of such relationship was found. The conclusion would, therefore, seem to be warranted that in this factor we have the explanation for the differences among the villages studied in the incidence of the disease, so far as this incidence was a reflection of community conditions.[8]

DISCUSSION

From the data presented in the foregoing pages it is evident that a variety of factors of an economic nature, through their effect on the character of the household diet, had an important influence on the incidence of pellagra in the communities studied. Among these factors family income and food availability stand out most conspicuously.

As has been seen, the data presented reveal a very marked inverse correlation between family income and the incidence of the disease. When it is recalled that the range of income enjoyed by our families was small (see Table 2), that the amount of income of even the highest of our

---

[7] The average half-month family income per adult male unit for all households in *Ny* and *In* was $7.99. Hence, all households with such incomes under $8 were considered.

[8] If such factor as food availability operated to affect the rate of pellagra incidence in our villages, then it may be reasonably expected that in the locality with exceptionally unfavorable conditions of food availability, family income would be less efficient as a protective factor than in other similar localities with better conditions of food availability. With a view to testing this we compared the pellagra incidence rate for each of our income classes of *In* village in which we believed food availability conditions were least favorable with that of a group of five villages in which conditions in respect to food availability are believed to have been better. It was seen that (1) the incidence rate in those income groups in which a significant number of cases occurred was decidedly higher in *In* village; and (2) that the curve of incidence showed a highly suggestive tendency to extend to a higher plane of income in *In* village than in the group of five villages. The indications thus afforded would, therefore, appear to be consistent with and to bear out the assumption which was tested. [Tabulation deleted. ED.]

income classes was actually quite low (but few had annual incomes of over $1000), the reduction of incidence to the point of practical disappearance of the disease in this income class is all the more striking and significant. It would seem quite impressively to indicate that the occasional occurrence of the disease in well-to-do individuals must be regarded as a relatively quite exceptional occurrence, and that the explanation of such occurrence must be sought in circumstances of a special or exceptional character.

Cases in the well-to-do, instances of which have been observed repeatedly since the time of Strambio (7), are of more than ordinary interest because of the perplexity and confusion to which they tend to give rise with respect to the etiology of the disease. Favorable economic status of the individual tends to create the presumption that diet can have little or no etiological significance, since there can be no question of the ability of such individual to provide himself with a liberal diet. Natural as this presumption may be under the circumstances, it nevertheless involves danger of serious error. This results from the implied assumptions that because of financial ability, not only was a satisfactory diet available, but that such was also consumed. Even granting what is not necessarily the case, that financial ability to provide may be assumed to be invariably synonymous with the actual provision of a good diet[9] and that a liberal diet was actually available to the individual, it by no means follows that such diet was in fact consumed. For such assumption would totally ignore the existence of individual likes and dislikes, more or less marked examples of which may be observed at almost any family table.

A great variety of causes may operate to bring about individual peculiarities of taste with respect to food. They may have their origin in the seemingly inherent human prejudice against the new and untried food or dish; they may date from some disagreeable experience associated with a particular food; they may arise as the result of ill-advised, self-imposed, or professionally directed dietary restrictions in the treatment of digestive disturbances, kidney disease, etc.; they may originate as a fad; and in the insane they may arise because of some delusion such as the fear of poisoning, etc.

The individual peculiarities of taste which may thus arise have a significance in relation to pellagra that has been but little appreciated until recently (29, 30). In much the greater proportion of a moderate number of cases in well-to-do individuals with a good diet presumably available, coming under our observation, a significant eccentricity in diet could readily be determined (unpublished observations). Vedder (81—pages 157–160) and Roberts (32) have reported observations of a similar character. It is of interest to note also that analogous facts have been recorded in connection with beriberi (33—pages 154, 156, 171, 180, 184). Therefore, in seeking to explain cases of pellagra in individuals believed to have a good diet available, this factor must be given due consideration.

With conditions (including labor supply) in the cotton-milling industry substantially stable, family income may, in general, be expected to fluctuate but little from year to year. With conditions unsettled, family income may either fall or rise very considerably; a depression, accompanied by increasing unemployment and, possibly, reductions in wage rates will be reflected in a reduced family income, while industrial prosperity, with a diminution of unemployment and, possibly, increased wage rates, will be reflected in larger family income. In the former event we may have a diminution in family income to the point of inability to provide the family with a proper diet, with a consequent danger of the development of pellagra and thus with a more or less marked rise in the incidence rate of the disease. In the latter event we have the opposite effects, with a tendency to a reduction in or practical disappearance of the disease. In this we have, we believe, an illustration of the manner of operation of one of the most powerful factors in relation to the endemic and epidemic prevalence of the disease. Through its effect on diet, economic status is also an important element in, if not the entire explanation of, the oft repeated observation of the occurrence of a marked increase in the incidence or the development of an epidemic of the disease fol-

---

[9] In this connection the following from Roussel (1866, pp. 430–431) is of interest: "Almost all the individual histories, found in the literature of pellagra in the well-to-do, are remarkable because of this constant fact . . . namely, that because of some misfortune or by reason of some unwholesome trait (mauvaises habitudes), such as avarice, these well-to-do or wealthy pellagrins subsisted exactly as did the poor pellagrins about them."

lowing on crop failure[10] (*34*—page 327) or other cause of "hard times," as was actually observed in the United States in 1915, following depression consequent on the outbreak of the World War in 1914, and as there is some reason to fear may again be observed in the spring of 1921 if the present depression, especially in the price of cotton and cotton-textile manufacturing, continues.

At this juncture it may be well to point out that family income should always be considered in connection with living (food) costs if confusion and error are to be avoided. It is the purchasing power of family income that is significant and not necessarily its absolute amount.

Although economic status (as typified by family income) is, ordinarily, perhaps the most important factor (particularly in industrial communities) in relation to fluctuation in incidence of pellagra in different years,[11] marked changes in food availability conceivably play a similar role (particularly in agricultural communities). The reported occurrence, in some localities, of a sharp increase in the prevalence of the disease following an epizootic among swine or cattle (*35*) or after the loss of these through floods, we believe, is to be explained, in part, at least, in this manner.

The very great importance of food availability in relation to pellagra prevalence seems heretofore not to have been very clearly recognized. Under some circumstances, as we have shown, this factor may operate notably to affect the character of the diet and thus the incidence of the disease. Our data dealt with differences in availability between localities of relatively small area, but it is readily conceivable that analogous differences may exist between areas of great extent such as there is reason to believe actually is the case between the northern and southern parts of the United States. This difference is probably an important factor (together with the well-known difference in dietary habit, *28*) in the notable inequality in the incidence of the disease in these two sections of the country.

The results of the present study clearly suggest fundamental lines along which efforts looking to the eradication of the disease should be directed, namely, (1) economic, by improvement of economic status (income), and (2) food availability, by improvement in availability of food supplies.

Measures for improving the economic status of those people most subject to the disease, are in the main, outside of the sanitarian's sphere and but little subject to his influence. While much the same may be said to apply to the conditions of food availability, this field is more easily accessible, both directly and indirectly, to his activities and influence. Thus, for instance, by avoiding ill-considered regulations governing milk production he can, negatively at least, favor an adequate supply of this invaluable food. Furthermore, he can and should aid in improving the conditions of food availability by lending his powerful influence in support of and, by cooperating with, the agencies at work in this field, in their efforts to stimulate milk production (particularly through cow ownership) and to induce the farmer to adopt a suitable system of crop diversification.

And in this connection it may perhaps be remarked that certain preliminary observations have created in our minds a rather strong suspicion that the single-crop systems practiced in at least some parts of our southern states, by reason of apparently unfavorable conditions of food supply and of other conditions of an economic character bound up therein, will be found indirectly responsible for much of the pellagra morbidity and mortality with which local agricultural labor is annually afflicted.

Although considerable study will be required to determine definitely the factors responsible for the high incidence of the disease in the rural areas in question, it would, nevertheless, seem to be the better part of wisdom to make an earnest effort to improve conditions in the ways suggested above.

SUMMARY AND CONCLUSIONS

1. In the present paper are reported the results of the part of the pellagra study of cotton-mill villages, during 1916, dealing with the relation of conditions of an economic nature to the incidence of pellagra. It is the first reported study in which the degree of the long-recog-

---

[10] It should not be forgotten that overproduction, by glutting the market, may affect family income (of the farmer) as disastrously as may crop failure.

[11] We hope to consider the relation of economic status to the course of the disease from year to year in a separate paper.

nized association between poverty and pellagra incidence is measured in a definite, purely objective manner.

2. The study was made among the white mill operatives' households in seven typical cotton-mill villages of South Carolina. Pellagra incidence was determined by a systematic, biweekly, house-to-house canvass and search for cases, only active cases being considered. Information relating to household food supply, family income, etc., was secured by enumerators for a sample section of the period April 16 to June 15, assumed to be representative of the season during which the factors favoring the production of pellagra were assumed to be most effective.

3. Family income was made the basis of classification according to economic status, the Atwater scale for food requirements being used for computing the size of families in comparing their incomes.

4. In general, pellagra incidence was found to vary inversely according to family income. As the income fell, the incidence of the disease rose and showed an increasing tendency to affect members of the same family; as the income rose, incidence fell, being reduced almost to the point of practical disappearance in the highest of our income classes, although the income enjoyed by this class was comparatively quite low.

5. The inverse correlation between pellagra incidence and family income depended on the unfavorable effect of low income on the character of the diet; but family income was not the sole factor determining the character of the household diet.

6. Differences in incidence among households of the same income class are attributable to the operation of such factors as tend to determine the amount and proportion of family income available for the purchase of food, the intelligence and ability of the housewife in utilizing the available family income, and to the differences among households with respect to availability of food supplies from such sources as home-owned cows, poultry, gardens, etc.

7. Differences in incidence among villages whose constituent households are economically similar, are attributable to differences among them in availability of food supplies resulting from differences (a) in the character of the local markets, (b) in the produce from adjacent farm territory, and (c) in marketing conditions.

8. The most potent factors influencing pellagra incidence in the villages studied were: (a) low family income, and (b) unfavorable conditions regarding the availability of food supplies, suggesting that under the conditions obtaining in some of these villages in the spring of 1916 many families were without sufficient income to enable them to procure an adequate diet, and that improvement in food availability (particularly of milk and fresh meat) is urgently needed in such localities.

References

(1) Goldberger, J., G.A. Wheeler, and E. Sydenstricker. A study of the diet of nonpellagrous and of pellagrous households, etc. *JAMA*, 71:944-949, 1918.

(2) Goldberger, J. A study of the relation of diet to pellagra incidence in seven textile-mill communities of South Carolina in 1916. *Public Health Rep* 35:648-713, 1920.

(3) Goldberger, J. Pellagra incidence in relation to sex, age, season, occupation, and 'disabling sickness' in seven cotton-mill villages of South Carolina during 1916. *Public Health Rep* 35:1650-1664, 1920.

(4) Sydenstricker E., G.A. Wheeler, and J. Goldberger. Disabling sickness among the population of seven cotton-mill villages of South Carolina in relation to family income. *Public Health Rep* 33:2038-2051, 1918.

(5) Goldberger, J. A study of the relation of factors of a sanitary character to pellagra incidence in seven cotton-mill villages of South Carolina in 1916. *Public Health Rep* 35:1701-1714, 1920.

(6) Casal, G. Obra postuma del Dr. Casal publicada en 1762. *Corresp Med* (Madrid) 5:78, 1870.

(7) Strambio, G. *Abhandlungen ueber das Pellagra*. Leipzig, 1796.

(8) Roussel, T. *La Pellagre*. Paris, 1845.

(9) Holland, H. On the pellagra, a disease prevailing in Lombardy. *Med Chir Trans (London)* 8:313-346, 1820.

(10) Hameau. Note sur une maladie peu connue observée dans les environs de la teste (Gironde). *Jour de Med Prat (etc.) de la Soc Roy de Med de Bordeaux* 1:310-314, 1829.

(11) Lalesque, fils. *Actes de l'Acad Roy d Sc (etc.) de Bordeaux*. p. 421, 1846.

(12) Berger, L. Pellagra. *Wiener Klinik Wien* 16:161-179, 1890.

(13) Rosen, H.V. Ueber die pellagra in Russland, Petersburg. *Med Wchnschrft n. F.* 11:21-23, 1894.

(14) Sofer, T. Die pellagra in Oesterreich und ihre Bekampfung als Volkskrankheit. *Therap Monatshefte* 23:216, 219, 1909.

(15) Probizer, von. Die Pellagra. *Die Heilkunde (Wien)* 4:139-142, 1899.

(16) Babes, V. Ueber Pellagra in Rumanien. *Wien Med Presse* 44:1184-1239, 1903.

(17) Calmarza, J.B. *Memoria Sobre La Pelagra*. Madrid, 1870.

(*18*) Roussel, T. *Traité de la Pellagre,* . . . Paris, 1866.

(*19*) Huertas, F. La pelagra en España. *Arch Latin de Med y de Biol (Madrid)* 1:9-15, 1903.

(*20*) Sandwith, F.M. How to prevent the spread of pellagra in Egypt. *Lancet* 1:723, 1903.

(*21*) Gaumer, G.F. Pellagra in Yucatan. *Trans Nat'l Conf on Pellagra* (Columbia, S.C., 1910), pp. 101-107.

(*22*) Manning, C.J. Report on Certain Cases of Psilosis Pigmentosa Which Have Recently Occurred at the Lunatic Asylum. Barbados, 1907.

(*23*) Siler, J. and P. E. Garrison. An intensive study of the epidemiology of pellagra. *Am J Med Sci* 146:July and August, 1913.

(*24*) Jobling, J.W. and W. Petersen. The epidemiology of pellagra in Nashville, Tennessee, II. *J Infec Dis* 21:109-131, 1917.

(*25*) Atwater, W. O. Principles of Nutrition and Nutritive Value of Food. *Farmers' Bull (US Dept of Agric* 142:33, 1915.

(*26*) White, R.G. *Report on an Outbreak of Pellagra Among Armenian Refugees at Port Said, 1916-1917,* Cairo, Egypt, 1919.

(*27*) Boyd, F. D. and P. S. Lelean. *Report of a Committee of Enquiry Regarding the Prevalence of Pellagra Among Turkish Prisoners of War* Alexandria, Egypt, 1919. Also *J Roy Army Med Corps* 33:426 et al., 1919.

(*28*) Sydenstricker, E. The prevalence of pellagra—Its possible relation to the rise in the cost of food. *Public Health Rep* October 22, 1915.

(*29*) Goldberger, J. The cause and prevention of pellagra. *Public Health Rep* 29:2354-2357, 1914.

(*30*) Goldberger, J. Pellagra—Causation and a method of prevention *JAMA* 66:471-476, 1916.

(*31*) Vedder, E. B. Dietary deficiency as the etiological factor in pellagra. *Arch Int Med* 18:137-172, 1916.

(*32*) Roberts, S.R. Types and treatment of pellagra *JAMA* 75:21-25, 1920.

(*33*) Vedder, E. B. *Beriberi.* New York, 1913.

(*34*) Weiss, E. Die pellagra in Sudtirol und die staatliche bekampfungsaktion. *Das Osterreichische Sanitätswesen (Wien)* 26:309-331, 1914.

(*35*) Niederman, J., E. Konrad, and E. Farkas. A report on pellagra in Transylvania (abstract). *Lancet* 2:164, 1898.

MORTALITY FROM LUNG CANCER IN ASBESTOS WORKERS

Richard Doll[1]

Sixty-one cases of lung cancer have been recorded in persons with asbestosis (1, 2) since Lynch and Smith (3) reported the first case. In view of the infrequency of asbestosis, this large number of cases suggests—but does not prove—that lung cancer is an occupational hazard of asbestos workers. The strongest evidence that it may be a hazard has been produced by Merewether and by Gloyne. Merewether (4) found that lung cancer was reported at necropsy in 13.2 percent of cases of asbestosis (31 out of 235) but in only 1.3 percent of cases of silicosis (91 out of 6884) and Gloyne (5), on personal examination, found lung cancer in 14 percent of necropsies on subjects with asbestosis (17 out of 121) against 6.9 percent in silicotics (55 out of 796). Neither author gave full details of the sex composition of the groups examined, but since women form a higher proportion of asbestos workers than of persons employed in occupations liable to give rise to silicosis (coal-miners, stonemasons, pottery workers, foundrymen, metal grinders) and since lung cancer is less common among women, the differences in the proportions of cancer cases cannot be accounted for by differences in sex distribution. In fact the proportions which are more properly comparable with the findings in silicotic subjects are the proportions of lung cancer found among men with asbestosis, 17.2 percent in Merewether's series and 19.6 percent in Gloyne's.

Animal experiments are inconclusive. A positive result was reported by Nordmann and Sorge (6) who found that of 10 mice which had been exposed to asbestos dust and survived for 240 days, two developed lung carcinoma. Smith (7), however, considers that one of the "carcinomas" was, in fact, an example of squamous metaplasia and that the other, an adenocarcinoma, may have developed spontaneously from the common mouse adenoma. A negative result has been reported by Vorwald and Karr

(8). The majority of workers (cited in 2) consider that a causal relationship between asbestosis and lung cancer is either proved or is highly probable and the reality of the relationship was agreed at the recent International Symposium on the Endemiology of Lung Cancer (9). A minority, however, remains sceptical (10, 11), and, according to Hueper (2), Lanza and Vorwald, so that it was thought desirable to undertake a fresh investigation.

NECROPSY DATA

Since 1935, records have been collected of all the coroners' necropsies on persons known to have been employed at a large asbestos works.[2] Pathological diagnoses in 105 consecutive cases are summarized in Table 1. Details of the cases

Table 1. Causes of death diagnosed at necropsy among persons employed at an asbestos works (1933-52).

Cause of death	Asbestosis present	Asbestosis absent	All cases
"Heart failure"	34	11	45
Pulmonary tuberculosis	12	9	21
Lung cancer	15	3	18
Other diseases of the respiratory system	10	4	14
Other diseases	4	3	7
All causes	75	30	105

in which lung cancer was found are shown in Table 2. During the first half of the period eight deaths occurred in which lung cancer was found in association with asbestosis, while in the second half of the period there were seven such cases and a further three in which lung cancer was found without asbestosis. The number of asbestos workers employed at the works increased steadily from 1914, and a great increase in the number of lung cancer deaths was also

Source: *British Journal of Industrial Medicine* 12:81-86, 1955.
[1] From the Statistical Research Unit, Medical Research Council, London.

[2] Necropsies on asbestos workers are ordered by the coroner when, in his opinion, there may be a question of asbestosis being a contributory cause of death.

Table 2. Occupational history and necropsy data of asbestos workers with primary lung cancer.

Year of death	Sex and age	Occupation	Period of exposure	Years of exposure	Years of exposure before Jan. 1, 1933	Years from first exposure to death	Years from last exposure to death	Asbestosis	Histological type of primary lung cancer
1935	M.62	Weaver	1919-32	13	13	16	3	Present	"Carcinoma"
1935	M.54	Weaver	1909-32	23	23	26	3	"	Epithelial carcinoma
1936	M.65	Fiberizer	1913-36	23	19	23	Less than 1	"	Endothelioma of pleura
1938	M.47	Weaver	{ 1910-12, 1920-37 }	19	14	28	1	"	"Carcinoma"
1939	M.49	Disintegrater	{ 1910-14, 1919-39 }	24	17	29	Less than 1	"	"Carcinoma"
1940	M.52	Disintegrater	{ 1911-15, 1919-21, 1923-39 }	22	15	29	Less than 1	"	"Carcinoma"
1941	M.52	Weaver	{ 1913-19, 1924-38 }	20	14	28	3	"	Oat-celled carcinoma
1942	M.59	Bag carrier	1913-41	28	19	29	1	"	Oat-celled carcinoma
1948	M.59	Weaver	{ 1912-14, 1918-48 }	32	16	36	Less than 1	"	Anaplastic carcinoma
1948	M.53	Weaver	1922-35	13	10	26	13	"	"Carcinoma"
1948	M.48	Spinner	1922-48	26	10	26	Less than 1	"	"Carcinoma"
1948	M.65	Maintenance man	1919-48	29	13	29	Less than 1	"a	Oat-celled carcinoma
1950	F.51	Spinner	1915-42	27	17	35	8	"	"Carcinoma"
1951	M.74	Fiberizer	1917-43	26	15	34	8	"	Adenocarcinoma
1951	M.60	Weaver	{ 1919-25, 1929-50 }	27	9	32	1	"	"Carcinoma"
1944	M.36	Weaver	1942-44	2	0	2	Less than 1	Absent	Oat-celled carcinoma
1951	M.43	Fiberizer	1939-48	9	0	12	3	"	Anaplastic carcinoma
1952	M.51	Weaver	{ 1941 (3/12), 1945-52 }	7	0	11	Less than 1	"	"Carcinoma"

a Also pulmonary tuberculosis.

recorded among the whole population of England and Wales over the same period. It might, therefore, have been anticipated that a larger number of cases in which the two conditions were associated would have been found in the last 10 years. National regulations for the control of asbestos dust were, however, introduced in 1931 (*12*) and the precautions taken to prevent dust dissemination in the works had become effective by the end of the following year. All the subjects in whom the two diseases were found together had been employed for at least nine years under the old conditions, and although 11 of the 15 men and women died within 30 years of their first exposure, the association of the two conditions has not yet been found in any person taken into employment during the last 31 years (1923-1953). It is, therefore, possible that the reason more cases were not found in the second half of the period is that reduced exposure to dust has already begun to lessen the incidence and severity of asbestosis.

METHOD OF ESTIMATION OF RISK

Although the necropsy data shown in Tables 1 and 2 suggest (1) that some groups of asbestos workers have suffered an increased risk of lung cancer, and (2) that the risk may now have decreased, it is not possible to be certain of either of these propositions without a more detailed knowledge of the whole mortality experience of the workers. The first proposition has, therefore, been tested by comparing the mortality experienced by that section of the male employees of the works referred to above, who had worked for at least 20 years in "scheduled areas,"[3] with the mortality recorded for all men in England and Wales; and the second proposition by comparing the incidence of lung cancer among men employed for different periods under the pre-1933 conditions. The investigation was limited to the small group of men who had been employed for at least 20 years, since the labor involved in searching out the individual records of men employed for shorter periods would be disproportionately great and, so far as was known from Table 2, would be comparatively unrewarding.

[3] By "scheduled areas" is meant those areas where processes were carried on which were scheduled under the Asbestos Industry Regulations of 1931 as being dusty.

The date of birth, date of completing 20 years' work in the "scheduled areas", and, where applicable, date of ceasing employment and date and cause of death were obtained, for each man, from the records of the firm's Personnel Officer. Full details were, in most instances, already available for the men who had ceased employment as well as for the greater number who continued to be employed, since some of those who had left were registered as having asbestosis and the attention of the firm had been drawn to the death of others, in view of the possibility of the cause of death being industrial in origin. All the remaining men were successfully traced and the relevant details obtained. This was not difficult since, by limiting the study to men who had been employed in one place for 20 years, few were found to have changed their job or to have moved out of the region.

From the data the numbers of men alive in each five-year age group were counted separately for each of the years from 1922 (the first in which a man was recorded as having had 20 years' service) to 1953. A man who had completed the 20 years before the beginning of a year and who was alive at the end of it was counted, for that year, as one unit; a man who completed the period before the beginning of a year but who died during it, and a man who completed the period during a year and who survived to the end of it, were each counted, for that year, as half a unit; the one man who died the same year as he completed his 20-year period was counted as a quarter of a unit.

The causes of death were recorded as they were given on the death certificate or, when available, as they were finally determined by necropsy. The causes were classified in five categories (see Table 4), and the numbers in each category were then compared with those which might have been expected to occur by multiplying the numbers of men alive in each five-year age group by the corresponding mortality rates for men in England and Wales over the same period. Because of the small numbers, however, the populations were not considered separately for each year, but were added together to form five groups living in the periods 1922-1933, 1934-1938, 1939-1943, 1944-1948, and 1949-1953, and the mortality rates used for each group were those for the years 1931, 1936, 1941, 1946, and 1951. The rates for 1931 were used for the period 1922-1933, rather than those for the mid-years, since disproportionately few men were under observation during the early part of the period. As an example of the method, the mortality rate for all neoplasms other than lung cancer among men in England and Wales aged 55 to 59 in 1951 was 2.778 per 1000. The numbers of years lived in this age group in the five years 1949-1953 were respectively 15 years, 15 years, 17½ years, 19 years, and 19 years. The number of deaths expected in the period was, therefore, estimated to be (15 + 15 + 17½ + 19 + 19) × 2.778/1000 = 0.238. The total number of deaths expected from each category of diseases was obtained by adding the numbers thus calculated for each age group for each of the five periods.

The great majority of the men lived and, when they died, died in the town in which the works was situated, so that it would have been preferable to have based the calculation of the expected deaths on the death rates observed in that town rather than on the rates for all England and Wales. These, however, were not known in sufficient detail. Little error in the expected number of deaths from lung cancer is likely to have been introduced on this account since, according to Stocks (*13*), the age-adjusted death rate for lung cancer among men in the town concerned was 96 percent of the rate for England and Wales. Stock's figure was calculated only for the period 1946-1949, but the proportion is unlikely to have varied greatly over the longer period of the investigation. The expected number of deaths from all causes is, however, likely to be somewhat underestimated since the age-adjusted death rate from all causes for the town is about 25 percent higher than the England and Wales rate (*i.e.* the excess was 22 percent in 1950, 28 percent in 1951, and 22 percent in 1952).

RESULTS

The number of men studied was 113; the numbers of man-years lived in each of the five periods in each age group are shown in Table 3. The total number of deaths from all causes and the number of deaths observed in each of the five disease categories, together with the expected number of deaths, are shown in Table 4. From Table 4 it appears that the men who had been exposed to asbestos dust suffered an increased mortality from lung cancer, other respiratory diseases, and cardiovascular diseases, in association with asbestosis, but that their mortality from other diseases was close to that expected.

Four explanations of the findings are possible: (1) that all the men who had died of lung cancer were recorded because of interest in the condition, but that some of the records of other men dying of other diseases or still alive were omitted, with consequent underestimation of the expected number of deaths; (2) that lung cancer was incorrectly and excessively diagnosed among the asbestos workers; (3) that lung cancer was insufficiently diagnosed among the general population of England and Wales; or (4) that the asbestos workers studied suffered an excess mortality from lung cancer.

Table 3. Number of man-years lived by men with 20 or more years of work in a "scheduled area."

Age (years)	Period					All periods
	1922-33	1934-38	1939-43	1944-48	1949-53	
30-	0	0.5	1.5	0	0	2
35-	4.5	2	11	17.5	9	44
40-	9.5	16	33.5	48	55	162
45-	9.5	19.5	50	78.5	84	241.5
50-	6.5	25.5	39.5	85	96.5	253
55-	12	6	30	52	85.5	185.5
60-	15	3	5.25	25.5	36	84.75
65-	1	13.5	3	10	21.5	49
70-	0	2	9	3	3.5	17.5
75-79	0	0	1	1.5	0.5	3
All ages	58	88	183.75	321	391.5	1042.25

Table 4. Causes of death among male asbestos workers compared with mortality experience of all men in England and Wales.

Cause of death	No. of deaths		Test of significance of difference between observed and expected (value of P)
	No. observed	Expected on England and Wales rates	
Lung cancer:[a]			
with mention of asbestosis	11	—	} <0.000001
without mention of asbestosis	0	0.8	
Other respiratory diseases (including pulmonary tuberculosis) and cardiovascular diseases:			
with mention of asbestosis	14	—	} <0.001
without mention of asbestosis	6	7.6	
Neoplasms other than lung cancer	4	2.3	} <0.1
All other diseases[b]	4	4.7	
All causes	39	15.4	<0.000001

[a] Including one case with pulmonary tuberculosis.

[b] Including two cases (benign stricture of esophagus and septicemia) in which asbestosis was present but was not thought to have been a contributory cause of death.

It certainly cannot be claimed that the records of the Personnel Office were necessarily complete, but they were believed to be complete and no deficiency on this score would account for the total excess of deaths unless it were so gross that more than half the defined population had been omitted. Moreover, the number of deaths due to conditions unrelated to asbestosis was close to the estimated number and this is unlikely to have happened unless the population had been estimated approximately correctly and the deaths from all causes fully reported.

All the 11 deaths attributed to lung cancer were confirmed by necropsy and histological examination so that the excess number cannot be attributed to incorrect diagnosis among the group of asbestos workers. Some of the excess may well be due to an underestimation of the expected deaths since part of the increase in mortality attributed to lung cancer over the past 30 years is certainly due to improvements in diagnosis and in therapy (*14*). Even, however, if it were postulated that the whole of the recorded increase between 1931 and 1951 was spurious and that the real mortality from the disease throughout was that ascribed to it in

1951, the expected number of deaths is increased to only 1.1 and the observed excess is still grossly significant. For the actual number of lung cancer cases to be so little in excess of the expected as to be reasonably attributable to chance, it would be necessary for the expected cases to be 6.2, that is 5.6 times the number estimated on 1951 rates. In other words, it would be necessary to postulate that in 1951 (and throughout the previous 20 years) there was 5.6 times as much cancer of the lung as was recognized in 1931, which would mean that the condition would have to have been present and capable of detection in over 20 percent of all men at death. Moreover, even if this were so, it would still not account for the fact that all the cases of lung cancer were found in association with asbestosis.

It is, therefore, concluded that the fourth explanation is the most reasonable one and that the asbestos workers who had worked for 20 or more years in the "scheduled areas" suffered a notably higher risk from lung cancer than the rest of the population.

To test if the risk has altered since the 1931 regulations were introduced, it is not only necessary to make allowance for duration of employment before the end of 1932, but also to allow for the men's ages and for the total durations of their employment in the "scheduled areas", since the men employed in the earlier periods can also have been employed longer and lived to be older. On the other hand, there is no need to consider the changing incidence of lung cancer in the total population of England and Wales since the non-industrial risk has been shown to be small in comparison with the industrial one. The data required for comparing the risks among men employed for under 10 years, for 10 to 14 years, and for 15 years and over in the pre-1933 conditions are shown in Table 5. The ages shown are the ages at death of the men who have died and the ages in mid-1953 for the men who are still alive. The expected numbers of men in each pre-1933 employment group found to have asbestosis or asbestosis and lung cancer are estimated by multiplying the numbers in each age, total employment, and pre-1933 employment subgroup by the proportions of men with asbestosis or with asbestosis and lung cancer in the same age and total employment group for all lengths of pre-1933 employment combined. For example, three out of the nine men aged 50 to 54 years who had been employed for 20 to 24 years in the areas in which they might be exposed to asbestos dust were found to have asbestosis and lung cancer. Since three men had worked for under 10 years in the pre-1933 conditions, three had worked for 10 to 14 years, and three had worked for 15 or more years, the expected number of cases in each of the pre-1933 employment groups would have been the same, i.e., $3 \times 3/9$, or 1. In fact, the numbers of cases found were 0, 1, and 2. The total numbers expected in each pre-1933 employment group are obtained by adding the numbers calculated for each of the age and total employment groups within it. The results are as follows:

The differences between the numbers of men observed and the numbers expected in each employment group, had the incidence of the conditions remained steady throughout, are statistically significant (total asbestosis, $\chi^2 = 7.52$, n = 2, p = 0.025; asbesotsis and lung cancer, $\chi^2 = 8.74$, n = 2, P = 0.01).[4] They are highly so if the trend, that is, the biologically important reduction in the proportion between observed and expected numbers as the length of pre-1933 employment is reduced, is also taken into consideration. It is clear, therefore, that the incidences both of asbestosis and of lung cancer associated with asbestosis have become progressively less as the number of years during which men were exposed to the pre-1933 conditions has decreased.

The extent of the risk of lung cancer over the whole period among the men studied appears to have been of the order of 10 times that experienced by other men. This agrees well with the data reported by Merewether (4), but it is somewhat greater than that suggested by Gloyne's data (5). The great reduction in the amount of dust produced in asbestos works during the period has been accompanied by a reduction in the incidence of lung cancer among the workmen so that the risk before 1933 is likely to have been considerably greater—perhaps 20 times the general risk. Whether the specific industrial risk of lung cancer has yet been completely eliminated cannot be determined with certainty; the number of men at risk, who have been exposed to the new conditions only and who have been employed for a sufficient length of time, is at present too small for confidence to be placed in their experience. It is clear however, that the risk has for some time been greatly reduced. The extent of the reduction is particularly striking when it is recalled that between 1933 and 1953 the incidence of the disease among men in the country at large has increased sixfold.

		Length of employment before January 1, 1933		
		Under 10 yrs.	10–14 yrs.	15 yrs. +
Total number of men with asbestosis	observed	13	14	16
	expected	21.9	10.3	10.8
Number of men with asbestosis and lung cancer	observed	1	3	7
	expected	5.5	2.4	3.1

[4] The expected numbers of lung cancer are small and the probability that the differences could arise by chance has consequently been somewhat, but not seriously, underestimated. If all men with more than 10 years pre-1933 employment are grouped together and Yales' correction made for small numbers, $\chi^2 = 5.82$, n = 1, P = 0.02.

Table 5. Numbers of men employed for different periods before 1933 and numbers known to have asbestosis and lung cancer in association with asbestosis divided by total duration of employment in a scheduled area and by age.

Total length of employment in "scheduled area" (years)	Age at June 30, 1953, or at death (years)	Length of employment before January 1, 1933									All Lengths of employment before January 1, 1933		
		0-9 Years			10-14 Years			15+ Years					
		No. of men	No. of men with asbestosis	No. of men with cancer of lung	No. of men	No. of men with asbestosis	No. of men with cancer of lung	No. of men	No. of men with asbestosis	No. of men with cancer of lung	No. of Men	No. of men with asbestosis	No. of men with cancer of lung
20-24	35-	1	—	—	1	1	—	0	—	—	2	1	—
	40-	4	—	—	1	1	—	0	—	—	5	1	1
	45-	7	1	—	0	0	1	1	1	2	8	2	3
	50-	3	2	—	3	3	—	3	3	0	9	8	0
	55-	5	3	—	2	1	—	0	—	—	7	4	—
	60-	3	1	—	1	1	—	1	1	1	5	3	1
	65-	2	0	—	0	—	—	1	1	—	3	1	—
	70-	0	0	—	0	—	—	1	1	—	1	1	—
	75-9	1	1	—	0	—	—	0	—	—	1	1	1
25-29	40-	3	0	—	0	—	—	0	—	—	3	0	—
	45-	10	2	—	2	1	—	0	—	—	12	3	1
	50-	6	2	1	0	—	—	0	—	—	6	2	1
	55-	6	1	—	8	4	0	1	1	0	15	6	0
	60-	3	0	—	1	1	0	3	3	—	7	4	0
	65-	1	0	—	1	1	—	0	—	—	2	1	—
	70-	0	—	—	0	—	—	1	0	1	1	0	1
	75-	0	—	—	0	—	—	1	1	0	1	1	0
	80-4	0	—	—	0	—	—	1	0	1	1	0	1
30-34	45-	2	—	—	0	—	—	0	—	—	2	0	—
	50-	2	—	—	5	—	—	2	2	—	9	0	—
	55-	1	—	—	1	—	—	3	2	1	5	2	1
	60-	0	—	—	0	—	—	3	1	—	3	1	—
	65-	0	—	—	0	—	—	0	—	—	0	—	—
	70-4	0	—	—	0	—	—	1	1	—	1	1	—
35+	55-	0	—	—	0	—	—	1	0	—	1	0	—
	60-	0	—	—	0	—	—	1	0	—	1	0	—
	65-9	0	—	—	0	—	—	2	0	—	2	0	—

Table 5. (Continued.)

Total length of employment in "scheduled area" (years)	Age at June 30, 1953, or at death (years)	Length of employment before January 1, 1933									All Lengths of employment before January 1, 1933		
		0-9 Years			10-14 Years			15+ Years					
		No. of men	No. of men with asbestosis	No. of men with cancer of lung	No. of men	No. of men with asbestosis	No. of men with cancer of lung	No. of men	No. of men with asbestosis	No. of men with cancer of lung	No. of men	No. of men with asbestosis	No. of men with cancer of lung
	35-	1	—	—	1	1	—	0	—	—	2	1	—
	40-	7	—	—	1	1	—	0	—	—	8	1	—
	45-	19	3	—	2	1	1	1	1	1	22	5	2
All lengths of employment in a "scheduled area" (20 yrs.)	50-	11	4	1	8	3	1	5	3	2	24	10	4
	55-	12	4	—	11	5	0	5	3	1	28	12	1
	60-	7	1	—	2	2	0	7	5	1	16	8	1
	65-	3	0	—	1	1	1	3	1	—	7	2	2
	70-	0	0	—	0	—	—	3	2	0	3	2	0
	75-	1	1	—	0	—	—	1	1	1	2	2	1
	80-84	0	—	—	0	—	—	1	0	—	1	0	1
	All ages	61	13	1	26	14	3	26	16	7	113	43	11

617

SUMMARY

The cause of death, as determined at necropsy, is reported for 105 persons who had been employed at one asbestos works. Lung cancer was found in 18 instances, 15 times in association with asbestosis. All the subjects in whom both conditions were found had started employment in the industry before 1923 and had worked in the industry at least nine years before the regulations for the control of dust had become effective.

One hundred and thirteen men who had worked for at least 20 years in places where they were liable to be exposed to asbestos dust were followed up and the mortality among them compared with that which would have been expected on the basis of the mortality experience of the whole male population. Thirty-nine deaths occurred in the group whereas 15.4 were expected. The excess was entirely due to excess deaths from lung cancer (11 against 0.8 expected) and from other respiratory and cardiovascular diseases (22 against 7.6 expected). All the cases of lung cancer were confirmed histologically and all were associated with the presence of asbestosis.

From the data it can be concluded that lung cancer was a specific industrial hazard of certain asbestos workers and that the average risk among men employed for 20 or more years has been of the order of 10 times that experienced by the general population. The risk has become progressively less as the duration of employment under the old dusty conditions has decreased.

I would like to offer my thanks to the management of the firm concerned for permission to carry out this work and to the Medical Officer and members of the staff of the works where the men were employed, who carried out the greater part of the work on which this report is based.

References

(*1*) Boemke, F. *Med Mschr* 7:77, 1953.

(*2*) Hueper, W. C. *Proceedings of the Seventh Saranac Symposium.* To be published.

(*3*) Lynch, K.M. and W.A. Smith. *Am J Cancer* 24:56, 1935.

(*4*) Merewether, E.R.A. *Annual Report of the Chief Inspector of Factories for the Year 1947.* London, H.M.S.O., 1949.

(*5*) Gloyne, S.R. *Lancet* 1:810, 1951.

(*6*) Nordmann, M. and A. Sorge. *Z Krebsforsch* 51:168, 1941.

(*7*) Smith, W.E. *Arch Industr Hyg* 5:209, 1952.

(*8*) Vorwald, A.J. and J.W. Karr *Am J Path* 14:49, 1938.

(*9*) Council of the International Organizations of Medical Sciences. *Acta Un Int Cancer* 9:443, 1953.

(*10*) Cartier, P. *Arch Industr Hyg* 5:262, 1952 (contribution to discussion).

(*11*) Warren, S. *Occup Med* 5:249, 1948.

(*12*) Asbestos Industry Regulations. Statutory Rules and Orders, 1931, No. 1140. London, H.M.S.O., 1931.

(*13*) Stocks, P. *Br J Cancer* 6:99, 1952.

(*14*) Doll, R. *Br Med J* 2:521, 1953.

AN APPROACH TO LONGITUDINAL STUDIES IN A COMMUNITY: THE FRAMINGHAM STUDY[1]

Thomas R. Dawber, William B. Kannel, Lorna P. Lyell

Those concerned with community health have a legitimate interest in all matters related to promoting the health of the community. These interests may vary depending on the purposes for which the health agency was organized, its location, the skills and resources available to it, and many other factors. In general, the major objective of community health activities is to prevent, or improve the medical care of, existing disease.

In the past, research engaged in by health agencies has usually been initiated because of some real or suspected problem affecting the health of their community. Because of inability to answer certain crucial questions pertaining to the problem, an investigation is undertaken to attempt to provide the desired information. Studies might be undertaken to assist in administrative planning concerning the number of beds required for some major emergency or to meet changing patterns of disease incidence, or of ways to convert existing facilities for such purposes, e.g., conversion of tuberculosis sanatoria to chronic disease hospitals. Research may be required to discover ways of improving medical care for particular diseases by determining methods required to bring persons with given diseases under medical care early in the course of the illness, in order to minimize disability. This type of research has usually been done with specific uses in mind and can be considered under the category of applied research.

In addition to research aimed directly at solving immediate local problems, it is now increasingly common for health agencies to ask how the facilities and resources available to them can best be used for purposes of research to increase general knowledge without necessarily being motivated by the immediate needs of the particular health agency. Studies may be carried out to evaluate the manner in which a particular problem has already been solved or to indicate the desirable approach to a particular health problem.

Community health agencies are especially fitted for the conduct of edemiologic studies which require access to large populations and resources for handling large numbers of subjects. For this reason, a large proportion of community health research projects are of this type. Because of the classic contributions of the epidemiologic method in determining the causes and methods of prevention of infectious and nutritional diseases, this method has been applied in an attempt to unravel the problems surrounding chronic diseases of unknown etiology. Although notable progress is being made, it remains to be demonstrated whether this approach will prove as valuable in solving the problems surrounding chronic disease.

It is difficult to delineate the boundaries of epidemiologic research and to indicate in what way this method differs from other research methods. Epidemiology may be considered the study of the circumstances under which a disease arises and flourishes in its natural surroundings. It constitutes an approach to the unraveling of nature's secrets pertaining to the development of a disease through the identification of factors which are directly or indirectly associated with the disease. It involves the study of the distribution and determinants of disease prevalence and incidence. This requires analysis and interpretation of distribution patterns of disease in terms of possible causal factors. However, in the final analysis, the epidemiologic study suggests guilt by association. Proof of causal association between a factor and a disease is seldom provided by an epidemiologic study. More often, important clues to pathogenesis of disease are uncovered which require more fundamental laboratory or clinical research to demonstrate a cause and effect relationship.

Source: *Annals New York Academy of Sciences* 107:539–556, 1963.
[1] Heart Disease Epidemiology Study, Framingham, Mass. and the National Heart Institute, National Institutes of Health, Public Health Service, U.S. Department of Health, Education, and Welfare, Washington, D.C.

Clinical, laboratory, and animal experimental studies, as well as epidemiologic studies, attempt to associate certain factors with the development or existence of disease. Experimental studies can control the environment and more precisely define the conditions of the experiment. Epidemiologic studies most often must observe interrelationships as they occur spontaneously, and attempt to evaluate the interplay of the various factors acting on the subject, in relation to development of disease, without controlling the conditions of the "natural" experiment. Only one type of epidemiologic study can approach the experimental study, i.e., the field trial, in which the environment is modified in a specified way and the outcome noted in relation to some hypothesis. Experimental studies deal with individual persons or animals, epidemiologic studies tend to deal with populations or subgroups of populations.

It is because of the need for the study of general populations in epidemiologic studies that community health agencies are particularly fitted for this type of investigation. Other health facilities are primarily concerned with persons already ill, and, although such populations may be used for certain types of retrospective studies, they cannot be used to determine the relative risk of developing a disease at a time when preventive measures could be instituted with a reasonable hope of influencing development or progression of the disease.

Determining whether associations which exist between certain specified characteristics in a population, and either the existence of or subsequent development of disease are "causal" or only secondary, is often difficult. Causal associations are more probable if the suspected characteristics can be shown to precede the development of disease by some appropriate period, if the association is quite strong, and if the association is consistent with or suggests some reasonable pathogenetic mechanism for the disease in question.

It is unusual for an epidemiologic study to provide positive proof of the "cause" of a disease, although the epidemiologic study which attempts to determine if some modification of environmental characteristics of a population produces predicted modifications of the disease pattern in the population, comes closest to accomplishing this goal. More often epidemiologic studies point the way to fruitful areas for definitive research into the causal factors of a disease. Such studies can point the way to its prevention long before the cause or cure for the disease is discovered.

Epidemiologic studies may be retrospective or prospective. In general, the former is of value in suggesting hypotheses for study by longitudinal prospective studies. The study of diseased persons, and their comparison to those found free of disease, may bring to light significant differences in the two groups. The causal relation of these differences to disease development is by no means as strongly suggestive as it is when the suspected factors are known to be present prior to the onset of the disease. A long-term prospective study of a disease has the advantage of studying the population long before clinical disease is evident, relating host and environmental factors found relatively early in life to the development of disease later in life. It is far more likely that favorable change in these factors many years before the disease may be expected to demonstrate itself will be of benefit in the prevention of chronic diseases.

The requirements for a longitudinal prospective epidemiologic study include: (1) An appropriate population sample of the proper size, which can be kept under surveillance for a long period of time without excessive loss to follow-up; (2) an estimate of the expected incidence of disease development in the population; (3) hypotheses to be tested; (4) planned observations and measurements determined to a large extent by the hypothesis to be tested; (5) some idea of the size of the risk anticipated to be associated with the characteristic under study; (6) an examination procedure capable of detecting the disease in question reliably; and (7) a capable staff willing to participate in the study for a long period in order to assure uniformity.

Although the successful completion of longitudinal epidemiologic studies in the community in general depends on the same basic ingredients that go to make up any good scientific study, there are certain features of this type of study which make consideration of the methodology involved worthwhile for those who may be concerned with such studies.

THE FRAMINGHAM STUDY

For the past 13 years the National Heart Institute of the Public Health Service, acting through the Massachusetts Department of Public Health and the Framingham Health Department, has been conducting a long-term study of coronary heart disease in the town of Framingham, Massachusetts. A number of reports of the progress of this study have been made *(1–4)*. The authors have been engaged in the conduct of this study from its inception, and their experience gained in this undertaking serves as the basis for a discussion of the methodology of longitudinal community studies of which the Framingham Study will serve as a prototype.

The Framingham Study was set up as a community-wide study of the general adult population of a town. It is a prospective study concerned with the incidence of coronary heart disease and with the study of those factors, both host and environmental, which may contribute to its development.

It is safe to say that up to the present time this study has been considered reasonably successful. It is customary to attribute success to such factors as careful planning and hard work. Such ingredients are admittedly necessary. It is not customary to point out that "success" in epidemiologic studies usually depends on finding significant associations between some factors and disease development, i.e., having the good fortune to select those factors for study which turn out to be related to the disease. If all of the factors studied had turned out not to be associated with coronary heart disease, this study would have been considered a failure, and it would probably have been abandoned. Nevertheless, such a study might have been almost as valuable, and the methodology just as worthwhile, even if it only showed that large numbers of factors did not appear to be related to disease development, particularly if the factors studied were widely accepted as being causally related.

The methodology of the Framingham Study should not, therefore, be evaluated in terms of the "success" or "failure" of this project to turn up positive findings, but rather on whether it was, in fact, able to study a population adequately for a reasonable length of time in order to determine whether or not the factors studied could be demonstrated to be associated with coronary heart disease development.

OBJECTIVES OF THE STUDY

The first aspect of any study to warrant attention is that of its objectives. As previously indi-

cated, research is generated by the existence of a problem. The problem may be peculiar to a particular community, in which case its solution will be solely of benefit to that community, or it may be one in which the local interest is only part of a general concern. A number of questions will need to be answered in order to solve the particular problem. The objectives of the study developed will be to answer some or all of the specified questions for which the investigator is unable to find an answer from available information.

The investigator then formulates a study designed to answer the questions asked. The more clear-cut and specific the questions, the better the study can be designed to provide clear-cut answers. The more vague or general the questions, the less clear-cut and useful will the answers be.

Because of the difficulties of securing and following a large general population there is a tendency to increase the scope of the study to include a great many observations well beyond the limits of the original concept. The investigator is under pressure to include a few questions on an additional aspect of the disease or about another disease which, it would appear, could also be studied without much additional effort. There is also a tendency to shift from the study of certain specific aspects of a disease problem to the study of the whole problem of the disease in the community. In so doing, the ability to accomplish the basic objectives may be jeopardized.

The problem with which the organizers of the Framingham Study were concerned was that of the increasing importance of coronary heart disease as a cause of mortality and morbidity. While the decreasing incidence of infectious and other diseases of adult life were partly responsible for the apparent increase in coronary heart disease, there were also signs pointing toward a real, as well as a relative, increase in this disease. Some information, e.g., sex differences in incidence and probable incidence differences in grossly different populations, was already available. As a major step toward the possible control of coronary heart disease, further information concerning the epidemiology of the disease was needed.

In order to describe what specific pieces of information were required, a committee of cardiologists and others concerned with the problem was assembled, and asked to provide a number of working hypotheses based on their knowledge of the disease. As a result of their help and that of many others who were asked for similar advice, it was possible to arrive at a number of specific hypotheses which were subject to study. A number of specific questions were thus formulated which could be answered by the appropriate research. These questions involved the relationship of age, sex, family history, occupation, educational level, national origin, serum lipid levels, and physical activity (among others) to the development of coronary heart disease.

The hypotheses, in the main, were developed as a result of observations of the characteristics of persons with already developed disease in comparison to "controls."

Armed with these specific hypotheses it was possible to design a study which might be expected to provide the data necessary to test these hypotheses. It was concluded that a long-term prospective study of a population free of coronary heart disease was required to meet these expectations.

Since the magnitude of the risk of development of disease associated with the characteristics under study was to be estimated, and susceptible individuals identified, a prospective study was mandatory. A prospective study would also avoid the biases of retrospective studies which are restricted to information from persons already diseased.

SELECTION OF A POPULATION FOR STUDY

Selection of the most appropriate population for study is of prime importance. A cooperative population willing to participate over a long period of observation is required. The community must be of the proper size to provide enough individuals for study. It should also be compact so that the study population can be observed conveniently. The location selected must contain enough socio-economic, ethnic, or other particular subgroups of the population, with the characteristics required for study. Presumably the greatest variability in such factors is to be found in a general population rather than in any subgroup thereof. For this reason it seemed wise to undertake the Framingham investigation in a general population, even though it would manifestly have been easier to

obtain access to one or more special groups e.g., industrial populations, prison populations, etc. If it is desired to limit the objectives of the study to certain restricted hypotheses, the selection of certain specific subgroups of the population may be desirable. Access to such subgroups may be easier, the variability between them greater, the population size needed for study smaller, and continued cooperation of such a study group may be more readily obtained.

It is desirable that the population be stable so that loss to follow-up can be kept at a minimum. For this reason the geographic area should have a stable economy. Diversification of employment opportunities should be such that closing of a principal industry will not cause a large proportion of the population to move elsewhere seeking employment. It is also desirable that the geographic location be near a medical center since it is then possible to obtain the necessary consultation, skills, laboratory facilities, and statistical assistance required. It is also desirable that the medical profession in the community be sympathetic, competent, and cooperative.

The location should contain a good general hospital, and preferably only one, since this makes surveillance of the population admissions to the hospital much easier. It is desirable that the population use the local hospital almost exclusively. A town of limited size is preferable to a large metropolis since it is then possible to obtain closer surveillance of the population through neighbors, friends, the local medical profession, and the local hospital. It is also helpful if the town keeps accurate annual lists of its residents. A competent, cooperative medical examiner is most desirable as an aid to assessing deaths which occur outside the hospital or under unexpected circumstances. A well-organized health department will assist in obtaining death certificate information and other vital statistics, and can help in the organization of the community for participation.

SIZE OF POPULATION

The determination of the appropriate size of a population for study is often difficult. It requires the estimation of the number of persons expected to develop the disease under study in a given length of time. Estimates of the absolute incidence of disease are usually not difficult to make. The size of the population for study, based on absolute estimates of disease incidence, may be inadequate for the demonstration of significant differences in relative disease incidence in making comparisons between subgroups of the population. If the factors to be investigated are strongly related to the disease, this estimate of the population size will probably be adequate. If, however, the factor bears only a weak relationship to the disease, a much larger population, and/or a longer period of observation will be needed. It cannot be hoped to study a population large enough to provide answers as to the effects of factors, regardless of the potency of their effect, or their distribution in the population. The major determining factor must be the expected incidence of the disease and the assumption that at least some of the factors operating are strongly enough associated so that within-group comparisons will show significant differences. Since it is usually not possible to estimate reliably the potency of the characteristic under investigation in relation to development of disease before the study is undertaken, it is necessary, arbitrarily, to assign some potency to the characteristic in estimating the size of the population sample required to demonstrate statistically significant differences. In making this decision, one is motivated by how large a difference would be biologically meaningful or important.

AGE OF POPULATION

Intimately related to the problem of size of the population is that of the age distribution if the disease is age related, as was clearly the case with coronary heart disease. In diseases which require years before the development of overt manifestations, a serious problem is encountered. In the desire to observe the development of new cases of disease in a relatively short time, the tendency is to select populations in age groups with high incidence. Such a procedure, although defensible in diseases with short incubation periods, may be very misleading in the study of diseases requiring years to develop, and in which the "disease" measured is merely the endpoint in a prolonged process. It is necessary to distinguish between the factors relating to the underlying process of a disease and the factors relating to the overt clinical manifestations of the disease.

The practical person also is concerned about the fact that if the population selected is so young that it is still highly mobile, the difficulty in follow-up may be insurmountable. In diseases which develop later in life, the period of follow-up may be so prolonged that the loss to follow-up becomes prohibitively high if a young population has been selected for study.

With the above considerations in mind, the problem in selecting a population for the epidemiologic study of coronary heart disease may be more readily understood. It was known that little clinical evidence of coronary heart disease is manifest before the age of 30, even in males. It was also recognized that below age 30, not only would the yield of new "cases" be extremely low but the mobility of the population would be such that great difficulty would be experienced in following the population. It was also apparent that the clinical syndromes found in coronary heart disease were due to coronary atherosclerosis which may well have begun to develop many years before age 30 and that the study of the older population might, in fact, be primarily a study of the precipitating factors.

Taking all these factors into consideration, the decision was reached to select a population age 30–59. It was estimated that from a population of 5000 persons in this age range, approximately 1500 new "cases" would develop over a 20-year period. It was believed that such a population would be sufficient to demonstrate any significant relationships between important population characteristics and the development of coronary heart disease. It will be readily apparent that in a disease as highly age related as coronary heart disease, the wide age range of this population could create problems. Such has been the case. If subgroups based on age ranges which can be considered homogeneous are selected, the numbers may be too small for study. If a given characteristic is also age related, e.g., cholesterol level in women, this poses still further problems.

OBTAINING POPULATION SUPPORT

Having decided on the size, age, and sex distribution, and type of population desired, the next task was that of finding the population. Inquiry had been made through several state health departments as to the possible communities where such a study could be carried out. As a result of such inquiries, several localities were recommended. On the basis of size of the community, medical facilities available, and acceptability of the proposed project to the medical community and civic leaders, the town of Framingham was selected. Of all the factors, it seems that the most important one that influenced the decision to utilize Framingham for this study was that of community acceptability. This factor is clearly the *sine qua non* of community studies, and probably the only one that cannot be overcome in some way.

The town of Framingham at the time of its selection was a self-contained community, 20 miles west of Boston, with a population of some 28 000 persons of whom about 10 000 were adults in the age range 30–59. It had been estimated that if it were possible to obtain the support of 6500 persons in this age range, it would be possible to obtain 5000 people free of coronary heart disease and suitable for a prospective study.

METHOD OF SAMPLING

In the selection of population samples for study, a great deal of emphasis has been placed on the need for random sampling. Whether a random sample, a volunteer group, or a special subgroup is used should be determined by the study objectives. Each of these sampling methods has merit.

If the objective is to determine the absolute prevalence or incidence of a disease, or to compare any findings from the study with other population groups, then random sampling would seem to be essential. If the objectives relate to comparisons of subgroups within the population, e.g., incidence of disease in persons with high serum cholesterol *versus* those with low serum cholesterol, the need for random sampling becomes less important. Except for the fact that volunteers might have less variability in their characteristics than randomly selected persons, either population would seem to be suitable for a study of within-group comparisons.

While it is true that the greatest variability of population characteristics would be found in a randomly selected general population, some of this variability may be lost unless close to a hundred percent response is obtained. In fact, un-

less the cooperation of the population is essentially complete, it is difficult, if not impossible, to consider it a random sample and representative of a larger population. If the characteristics to be studied influence the cooperation of the population and in effect determine the response rate, it is conceivable that a systematic bias may be introduced, thus making random sampling highly desirable for such studies. If, however, the personal traits under consideration are apparently unrelated to population response, the use of volunteers would seem to be adequate. If the objective in random sampling is to insure that the sample be representative of the entire community, steps must also be taken to ascertain the degree to which the population sample represents larger population segments such as the county, the state, the country, etc.

At the inception of the Framingham Study it was believed that the selection of a sample should be made by random sampling methods, to provide a study population representative of the town. If a truly random sample could have been obtained, it would then have been possible to have made observations on the absolute prevalence and incidence of coronary heart disease which could then be compared with estimates of prevalence and incidence in other locations. Since the major effort of the Framingham Study involved within-group comparisons, it would appear that a great deal of unnecessary effort may have been expended in attempting to get a random sample of the Framingham population.

The possibility that studies of other population groups may obtain data on coronary heart disease in a similar manner may yet justify the effort expended in trying to get a "representative sample." To date, however, this effort seems to have been unwarranted.

A two-thirds random sample of the adult population age 30–59 of the town of Framingham was selected, and an attempt made to bring in those selected for examination and continued follow-up.

A systematic sampling scheme was used, arranging persons by precincts of residence and by size of family grouping; and two out of every three family groupings were selected.

This method was chosen over a geographic sampling, presumably on the basis that the sample obtained would be more representative of the entire town. The major difficulty encountered by the use of such a random sample was the inability to explain the relatively complicated method of selection to the townspeople by mass communication methods. Such a difficulty would not have been encountered if a simpler method had been used, sampling by precincts, widening of the sample to include the whole town, or the selection of a town of approximately the size to contain the study population required. When attempts were made to encourage participation, the confusion resulting from lack of ability to explain the basis for selecting the participants was so great that mass communication methods had to be abandoned.

ORGANIZING THE COMMUNITY

To obtain community participation, a committee of civic leaders willing to support the study was assembled through the efforts of a health educator assigned to the local Health Department. This committee, in turn, suggested the names of other persons active in civic endeavors throughout the town. A large number of small committees were thus organized and made aware of the Study objectives. From the list of selected subjects, these committee members chose individuals well-known to them. Many of the committee members, all of whom had been offered a clinic examination and were familiar with the examination procedures, were able to answer any questions and so reassure prospective participants. They attempted to obtain the support of the selected participants to the point of agreeing to come to the clinic which had been set up for examination purposes. Committee members reported back to the clinic staff the results of their efforts to secure participation. A telephone call or personal visit was then made to arrange an appointment for a clinic visit.

As a result of this approach in which the only contact with the subjects was made by non-professional volunteers, it was possible to bring in for initial examination 4469 persons out of the 6507 originally selected (Table 1).

In other than general population samples, Civil Service employees, physicians, etc., higher response rates may be expected *(5,6)*. Similarly, in prevalence studies, much higher response rates can be achieved than is possible in incidence studies which will require continued participation over many years.

Table 1. Derivation of Framingham study group.

	Total	Men	Women
Random sample	6507	3074	3433
Respondents	4469	2024	2445
Volunteers	740	312	428
Respondents free of CHD	4393	1975	2418
Volunteers free of CHD	734	307	427
Total free of CHD: Framingham study group	5127	2282	2845

The question remains whether this approach was the most effective one, or whether some other method of soliciting support would have fared better. This question cannot be answered. In one precinct an attempt was made by the clinic personnel to contact all persons in that precinct who had refused to participate when approached by the volunteers. Of the 80 persons re-approached, three came in for examination but failed to return for any further visits. It was concluded, on the basis of this unsuccessful attempt, that any further approach to the non-respondent group was not warranted.

In addition to obtaining initial population cooperation, the problem of continued cooperation must be examined. It is this aspect of a longitudinal prospective study which is probably most important, and one on which the success of the undertaking may depend.

Each of the subjects was advised at the initial interview that it was intended to reexamine him at two-year intervals, and that he would be approached directly at the appropriate time. The names of a relative, a friend, and the family physician were all recorded so that the subject could be traced in case he moved during the interval. An abstract of the initial examination was sent to the family physician and the subject was advised by letter as to whether the physician should be consulted or not. The objective of this procedure was to provide some tangible benefit to the subject other than the knowledge of his contribution to medical science. At the same time, care was taken not to become involved in the medical management of the subject and to avoid interfering in any way with the relationship between the subject and his physician. This helped to maintain rapport, not only with the subjects themselves, but with the medical community as well.

The need to obtain the support of the local medical community seems self-evident. It is difficult to assess the impact of the physicians' support in obtaining population cooperation, but it is a definite impression from experience in Framingham that, without strong support of the local physicians, it would be impossible to conduct such a study with any degree of success.

Not only was the role of the private physician of great value in obtaining the initial cooperation of the population, but also in promoting their continued support. It is the Framingham experience that many subjects continued to participate in the study only because of the encouragement of their private physicians.

The continued interest of the community physicians in the Study project has been sustained by deliberate attempts to refrain from interfering in any patient-doctor relationship, by making available to the physicians, medical records of past clinic examination, by participating in the educational program of the local hospital and medical society, and by frequent progress reports of the results of the study.

The prestige of a successful research venture serves to stimulate continued interest on the part of both the medical community and the study participants. It is necessary not only to keep the medical community informed of any significant findings and to indicate their impor-

tance and implications, but also to keep the lay community informed as well.

At the time of the subsequent examination the subject was again contacted by telephone or in person, and offered an appointment for re-examination. The same approach has been used at each subsequent examination, and no one initially seen has been dropped from follow-up. Figure 1 shows the extent of follow-up over ten biennial examinations.

In assessing the success of follow-up, it is necessary to take into consideration all information available in addition to the direct interview and examination of those still living and able to visit the clinic. Deaths require death certificates, medical examiner's reports, and hospitalization and physicians' reports and, when documented, constitute a satisfactory follow-up. Records of hospitalization or physicians' reports may be just as valuable as, or supplementary to, a personal interview and examination. Evaluation of other less definite information, e.g., work records, reports from relatives, etc., is more difficult and hardly can be considered adequate medical follow-up.

It would seem that the follow-up of this population has been adequate for the purposes intended and that, in terms of coronary heart disease, essentially no disease has developed of which the study is unaware.

As indicated in Figure 1, in addition to bien-

Figure 1. Ten year Framingham follow-up.

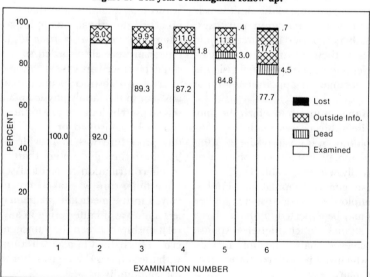

nial clinic examinations, follow-up also has consisted of surveillance of the study population with respect to hospital admissions, records of interim illnesses obtained from subjects, physicians, relatives and friends, medical examiner reports, and death certificates.

On the basis of all information available for each subject, conclusions have been reached as to the state of health with particular reference to cardiovascular disease.

The need to consider changes in concepts of disease, in laboratory procedure, and in observers is peculiar to longitudinal studies. It is necessary, therefore, to consider modifying criteria and laboratory methodology when better information concerning these develops. In so doing, it is necessary to consider the effect of such changes on the continuity of information. Changes in the subjects must be distinguished from changes in method. Unless previous observations are proved invalid by more recent knowledge, it is not desirable to make frequent or drastic changes in study techniques.

Since the inception of the Framingham Study, enzyme studies for the detection of myocardial infarction have been introduced. These have been incorporated in the diagnostic criteria to supplement electrocardiographic information.

CRITERIA FOR DISEASE

Methodology for the development of a clinic, the examination of the subjects, and the determination of population characteristics for cardiovascular epidemiology has been described in detail elsewhere *(7,8)*.

Determination of criteria for the various diagnostic categories and for the population characteristics were based on procedures which could be carried out in a large volunteer population. The important consideration in establishing criteria for diagnostic categories of coronary heart disease was the desire to keep the diseased group as free as possible of subjects who might, in fact, be free of disease. It was apparent that a relatively small percentage of the nondiseased persons placed in the diseased category might so dilute this subgroup that the importance of some of the characteristics as factors in the development of coronary heart disease might be lost.

The components of the criteria must consist of procedures actually carried out on the study population.

Similarly, observation and recording of population characteristics must be made so as to produce clear-cut groups. Where possible, the measurements should be objective and recorded on a quantitative basis using the actual measurements, e.g., the number of cigarettes smoked per day rather than a classification as "heavy" or "light" smoker. Qualitative characteristics should be classified into simple groups with little overlap. Observations should be made reliably, in a standard specified manner. Care must be taken to assure that reliable data are being systematically obtained.

Insofar as possible, the diagnostic criteria should be as objective as possible. For purposes of the Framingham Study it was possible to distinguish several clinical categories of coronary heart disease.

1. Myocardial infarction—based on changes in the electrocardiogram considered diagnostic of this clinical entity.
2. Angina pectoris—a subjective syndrome of chest discomfort.
3. Coronary insufficiency—prolonged chest discomfort, often with transient electrocardiographic changes, but with no evidence of heart muscle necrosis.
4. Sudden death in a matter of minutes in persons apparently well.
5. Death apparently due to coronary heart disease occurring in persons in whom a specific clinical diagnosis could not be made.

It was recognized that each of the above syndromes representing coronary heart disease was not equally reliable as an indicator of coronary heart disease. It was also recognized that the demonstration of differences in the pathological state of the coronary arteries between persons presenting these syndromes and others of the same age and sex with no symptoms were essentially of degree rather than kind. It was therefore not possible to make a diagnosis of coronary artery atherosclerosis, but only of the overt clinical manifestations of coronary heart disease. Care has been taken, therefore, to point out that it is the epidemiology of coronary heart disease, not coronary atherosclerosis, which is being studied.

Although an attempt was made to make the diagnoses as objective as possible, it is recognized that even such objective measurements as an electrocardiogram require interpretation. Interpretation of the same electrocardiogram may differ from physician to physician, and over a period of time in the hands of the same physician. This difficulty was partly corrected by periodic review of records by all the medical staff. Exchange of electrocardiograms with other groups working in the field also has helped to standardize electrocardiographic reading.

The use of computers in this field would be of great value if their ability to detect specific patterns uniformly and reliably could be established.

Diagnoses based on subjective assessment, e.g., angina pectoris and coronary insufficiency, present additional problems. By insisting that two independent observers both agree on the diagnosis before the subject be placed in a definite disease category, and that those in whom there was any disagreement be considered in a doubtful category, these diagnoses were made more firm. Use of standard forms requiring that all of the features of the syndrome be covered and recorded also helped.

Review of all deaths, including all pertinent information, allowed classification of cardiovascular deaths with reasonable accuracy.

ANALYSIS OF DATA

The nature of the analytical problems in longitudinal prospective studies, such as Framingham, are such that machine processing of data is imperative. Since the incidence of disease has been relatively low and a large population has been required, the difficulty in handling longitudinal data collected on such a large population under continuous surveillance for so many years has made the use of machines mandatory. Huge quantities of data on personal characteristics and environmental influences collected continuously throughout a long period of observation must be tabulated and cross-classified. While this is a counting and sorting operation, the large numbers of observations make use of machines necessary not only for tabulation, but also for storage and retrieving of information.

Up to the present time, analysis of data has been based on an assumed uniform period of observation of all persons initially examined.

Characteristics of subjects in the study population, determined at the initial examination, have been used to define subgroups. On the basis of these subgroups with specified characteristics, and identification of those individuals within each group who have developed disease under observation within the specified period of follow-up, it has been possible, with the use of simple tabulations, to show significant relationships between certain factors under study and the development of coronary heart disease. The magnitude of the risk associated with each of these characteristics, singly and in combination, has been assessed. In this way, highly susceptible individuals in the population have been identified (Figures 2 and 3).

Figure 2. Risk of developing "heart attack" in ten years according to initial serum cholesterol level, men 30-59 at entry; Framingham heart study.

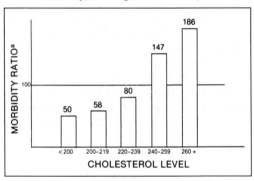

$$^a\text{Morbidity ratio} = \frac{\text{Observed cases}}{\text{Expected cases}} \times 100$$

Figure 3. Risk of developing "heart attack" in ten years according to antecedent abnormalities.[a] Men 30-59 years and women 40-59 years at entry; Framingham heart study.

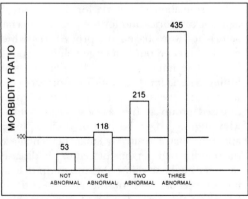

[a]High blood pressure 160/90; ECG: LVH, NSA, IVB; Cholesterol 250 or over

Serum cholesterol level, blood pressure, electrocardiographic abnormalities not considered diagnostic of coronary heart disease, weight, cigarette smoking habits, and vital capacity are factors which, by simple analysis, have been demonstrated to be significantly associated with the development of coronary heart disease. Assessment of the independent contribution of each of these often interrelated factors to the development of coronary heart disease has required detailed, rather cumbersome, analysis which would have been almost impossible if done by hand.

Because of the many observations on such a large population, even relatively simple operations of counting, sorting, classifying, and cross-classifying of information would have been tedious and prohibitively time-consuming if done by hand. Calculations of means, standard deviations, and correlation coefficients, while perfectly feasible with the use of a desk type calculating machine, are extremely time-consuming when done on such a large number of observations.

As the data from the repeated biennial examinations have accumulated, the number of ways in which these data can be examined seems infinite. To date, analysis has been based on observations made at the initial examination in relation to the subsequent development of disease. Since these initial characteristics may have been lost, acquired, or otherwise changed through the years on repeated observation, it will be desirable to know whether some parameter of these continuous observations, e.g., trends, means, variability, etc., will improve the ability to predict disease or give further insight into the mechanism of disease production. Accumulation of the additional persons in the population at risk, by making use of all the longitudinal observations, allows more detailed analysis of the relationship of a characteristic under observation to development of disease. Data analysis, accounting for changes in characteristics or personal attributes with the passage of time in relation to development of disease, requires use of computers so that variable periods of follow-up from the onset, loss, or change of some characteristic to development of disease can be taken into account.

From the beginning of the Framingham Study, plans were made to analyze data by means of machine tabulators and computers.

As indicated, the size of the population and the multiple observations being made were the major factors which made such a decision necessary. As a means toward implementing this procedure, forms were designed with the necessity of coding the data for machine application constantly in mind. Forms were modified to assist the coding procedure and, whenever possible, the procedure of original recording of the data and coding were combined. In this way, X-ray readings were recorded in such a way that the original entries of X-ray data were made on a code sheet. Since physicians may not be sufficiently motivated to become expert coding clerks, it is important to keep such coding procedures quite simple and almost self-evident.

Difficulty in realizing the potentialities of machine tabulation can be responsible for problems in handling data. Grouping of data and combining of factors under study, rather than coding of the actual measurements, has been the most prominent error made. It is difficult to decide before the distribution of the particular characteristic is determined, what groupings should be made. Comparisons of results of one study with another may be impossible if different groupings are used.

With the broadening of responsibility of community health activities to include noncontagious disease, health agencies are becoming increasingly involved in research towards control of chronic disease of unknown etiology. Epidemiologic studies constitute the most suitable type of research for community health agencies to undertake because of their access to, and ability to cope with, large population groups. Because of the inadequacies of prevalence or "cross-sectional" studies, incidence or prospective longitudinal studies are being undertaken with increasing frequency in an attempt to find solutions to pressing local and national health problems. Through a knowledge of the epidemiology of chronic disease, methods of control and prevention may be developed and susceptible individuals in the population identified. Experience in methodology for the conduct of such studies is accumulating, and dissemination of this information seems highly desirable.

While the successful execution of a longitudinal study is a difficult task and "ideal" studies in a free-living population are, for practical purposes, usually impossible, less than "perfect" studies may nevertheless be valuable as a basis for implementing community health activities. In the course of investigating a population, an increased public awareness of health problems occurs which, in itself, is valuable from a health education standpoint.

SUMMARY

1. The expanding role of community health agencies, particularly in epidemiologic research, is discussed.

2. The nature of epidemiologic research and the requirements for its conduct are considered.

3. A brief description of the Framingham Study is presented.

4. The importance of selecting precise, limited objectives, based on hypotheses for study, is stressed.

5. Factors important in the selection of a population for study, and in eliciting its cooperation, have been described.

6. Factors influencing the extent and adequacy of follow-up have been assessed.

7. Principles governing the development of criteria for use in longitudinal studies are reviewed.

8. Problems involved in processing and analysis of data are examined.

References

(1) Dawber, T.R., G.F. Meadors, and F.E. Moore, Jr. Epidemiologic approaches to heart disease: the Framingham study. *Am J Pub Health* 41: 279–286, 1951.

(2) Dawber, T.R., F.E. Moore, and G.V. Mann. Coronary heart disease in the Framingham study. *Am J Pub Health* 47: 4–24, 1957.

(3) Dawber, T.R., W.B. Kannel, N. Revotskie, J. Stokes III, A. Kagan, and T. Gordon. Some factors associated with the development of coronary heart disease: six years' follow-up experience in the Framingham study. *Am J Pub Health* 49: 1349–1356, 1959.

(4) Kannel, W.B., T.R. Dawber, A. Kagan, N. Revotskie, and J. Stokes III. Factors of risk in the development of coronary heart disease—six-year follow-up experience: the Framingham study. *Ann Internal Med* 55: 33–50, 1961.

(5) Doyle, J.T., A.E. Heslin, H.E. Hilleboe, P.F. Formel, and R. F. Korns. A prospective study of degenerative cardiovascular disease in Albany: report of three years' experience—I. Ischemic heart disease. *Am J Pub Health* 47: 25–32, 1957.

(6) Drake, R.M., R.W. Buechley, and L. Breslow. An epidemiological investigation of coronary heart disease in the California health survey population. *Am J Pub Health* 47: 43–57, 1957.

(7) Report of the Conference on Longitudinal Cardiovascular Studies at the Hotel Beaconsfield, Brookline, Massachusetts, June 17–18, 1957.

(8) Epidemiology of cardiovascular diseases methodology—hypertension and atherosclerosis. Report of Conference, Princeton, N.J., April 24–26, 1959. Supp. to *Am J Pub Health* 50: 1–124, 1960.

MORTALITY IN RELATION TO SMOKING: TEN YEARS' OBSERVATIONS OF BRITISH DOCTORS

Richard Doll[1] and Austin Bradford Hill[2]

In previous papers we have described how at the end of October 1951 we sent a short and simple questionary to the 59 600 men and women whose names were on the current British *Medical Register* and who were then resident in the United Kingdom. In addition to giving name, address, and age, they were asked to say whether *(a)* they were, at that time, smokers of tobacco, *(b)* they had previously smoked but had given up, or *(c)* they had never smoked regularly which we defined as having never smoked as much as one cigarette a day, or its equivalent in pipe tobacco or cigars, for as long as one year). The smokers and ex-smokers were asked the age at which they had started smoking, the amount that they smoked, and the method by which they smoked either at the time of reply or when they last gave up, and, when appropriate, the age at which they had stopped.

We deliberately limited our inquiries to these very few questions, partly to encourage a large number of answers and partly because we believed that these were questions that could be answered with reasonable accuracy. For such reasons we did not ask for a life-history of smoking habits nor did we, at that time, inquire into the habit of inhaling.

DATA

To this request we had 40 637 replies sufficiently complete to be used—34 445 from men and 6192 from women. From a 1 in 10 random sample of the register that we subsequently drew and analyzed we estimate that these figures represent answers from 69 percent of the men and 60 percent of the women alive at the time of the inquiry.[3] (These numbers differ slightly from those we published in 1956; from answers to our second questionary (see below) we learned that we had allotted the wrong sex to a few subjects and had included a few forms that had come from relatives who were not doctors.)

Selective Sample

We may feel sure that the doctors who chose to answer were not representative of the total. The seriously ill would have been unable to respond, and thus, as we showed in our previous paper, the mortality of the group who replied would be, at least for a time, abnormally low. In fact, using the 1 in 10 sample as a basis, we calculated that the standardized death rate of those who replied to us had been only 63 percent of the death rate for all doctors in the second year of the inquiry, and 85 percent in the third year. In the fourth to tenth years the proportion varied about an average of 93 percent, and there was no evidence of any regular change with the further passage of years. Evidently the effect of selection did not entirely wear off, but after the third year it had become slight.

One factor in this favorable mortality is the presence among those who replied of a relatively large number of nonsmokers and a relatively small number of heavier cigarette smokers. This feature, which we previously suspected, can now be shown from a small inquiry we undertook in 1961. We then drew two small samples of *(a)* those who *had* replied to us in 1951 and *(b)* those who had *not*. Eliminating those who had died between 1951 and 1961 we had 267 previous "answerers" and 213 previous "nonanswerers." We asked them their smoking habits in 1961, and 261 (98 percent) of the

Source: *British Medical Journal* 1:1399-1410 and 1460-1467, June, 1964.

[1] Director of the Medical Research Council's Statistical Research Unit, University College Hospital Medical School, London.

[2] Emeritus Professor of Medical Statistics in the University of London.

[3] This sample was not quite representative of the total to whom we wrote, since we drew it some months later and by then some of the original population would have been removed from the *Register* by death and other causes; no other names had, however, been added and the error is small.

answerers and 179 (84 percent) of the non-answerers responded. Comparison of these two groups shows 21 percent (answerers) and 6 percent (nonanswerers) as nonsmokers and 15 percent (answerers) and 28 percent (nonanswerers) as moderate or heavy cigarette smokers (15 or more daily). While these differences are large and must contribute measurably to the continuing favorable mortality of the group that replied in 1951, they are unlikely to account for it wholly. As a further factor we suspect (but obviously cannot prove) that there may be some more general association between mortality and the tendency not to reply to such an inquiry—whether the tendency be due to a deliberate refusal (which is rare) or a mere neglect of these things (which is frequent) In this respect it is perhaps not too fanciful to note that one non-replier died of smallpox and another of diabetic coma.

Second Questionary

According to the doctors' replies in 1951 we allocated them to the appropriate nonsmoking or smoking groups (subdivided by manner and amount, continuing or stopped). Our previous calculations of their subsequent death rates were based upon the number of persons in each of those groups at that time. We knew nothing about any subsequent change of smoking habits, either in the dead or in the living, and the further we moved from 1 November 1951 the more likely it was that changes in habits had occurred. In particular, it was probable that a large number of doctors had given up cigarette smoking. We therefore decided to approach again all the survivors of those who had previously replied, and, taking advantage of this opportunity, we added questions on: (1) the past use of cigarettes by pipe and cigar smokers, and (2) inhaling (a factor that had since become prominent in argument). Allowing for repeated inquiries, we sought answers from men between 1 November 1957 and 31 October 1958, and from women between 1 November 1960 and 31 October 1961.

Between the issue of our first and second questionaries 2579 of the men and 320 of the women had died; seven men had been struck off the *Register*, and these we omitted. Of the remaining 31 859 men and 5872 women, all but 2 percent replied to our second approach. Of the 651 men and 122 women who did not do so, 182 (28 percent) and 24 (20 percent) died within the year of inquiry or were reported to be too ill; 433 (67 percent) and 90 (74 percent) could not be traced or would make no reply; and a very small number (36 men and 8 women) refused to answer.

Fortunately, these 2 percent are not wholly lost to us as they would be in a first approach. We can retain them under their 1951 habits, and, in view of their small number, do so without appreciable error.

Deaths

Through the courtesy of the Registrars-General in the United Kingdom, a form with particulars of the cause of death has been provided to us for every death since November 1951 identified as referring to a medically qualified person. We have also obtained lists of deaths notified to the General Medical Council and of those recorded by the British Medical Association, and we have sought information from the records of the fighting Services and from other sources at home and abroad. A few deaths came to light from our second questionary. As a result of these several approaches we believe that very few deaths can have been missed. In fact, combining their total numbers appropriately with our 10 percent sample of non-repliers gives us a mortality rate for all British doctors which is 93 percent of the corresponding mortality of all males in England and Wales. This figure compares well with the standardized mortality ratio of 89 percent that the Registrar-General gives for doctors aged 20-64 and 65-74 years in his Occupational Mortality Supplement for 1949-1953.

In total, in the ten years to which this paper relates (1 November 1951 to 31 October 1961) there have been 4597 deaths of men and 366 deaths of women. (Preliminary data for the eleventh year give another 472 deaths of men and 48 deaths of women, and these will also be used for analyses where the numbers would otherwise be too few.) Except for deaths attributed to cancer of the lung, we have accepted without further inquiry the certified cause of death, and (unless otherwise mentioned) have classified these deaths according to the specified underlying causes. In only one case have we failed to obtain any evidence of the cause of death.

Cancer of the lung was given as the underlying cause in 216 men and 7 women and as a contributory cause in 6 men. For each of these deaths we sought confirmation of the diagnosis from the doctor who certified the death, and, when necessary, from the consultant to whom the patient had been referred. We thus obtained information on the nature of the evidence in all but one case. As a result we have accepted 212 deaths from carcinoma of the lung in men (5 being contributory causes) and 6 in women, and we have rejected 10 in men and 1 in a woman.[4] The 10 deaths of men we have reclassified, on the information given, to cancer of the stomach, cancer of the bladder, cancer of the rectum, cancer of the trachea, peripheral neuritis, atheroma of the aortic valves, collapse of lung, heart failure, and (in two cases) cancer primary site unknown; while these last two may have been primary carcinomas of the lung, the evidence was lacking. With the woman, the histological report was sarcoma of the lung (the specimen had been lost and could not be reviewed). All these reclassifications were made on the advice of a colleague (Dr. J. R. Bignall), who had no knowledge of the smoking history of the patient.

Use of Questionaries

It is important to remember that we can use the information given by our second questionary only prospectively from 1 November 1958. For example, we may find that a doctor cut down from the 30 cigarettes a day he reported at 1 November 1951 to 10 a day soon after and remained at that level. We can use that information to see what happens to him (and similar persons) *after 1 November 1958;* but we cannot change his group from the earlier date when he changed his habits, since we have no such information for doctors who died between 1951 and 1958. We cannot adjust the denominators of the death rates when we are unable to adjust the numerators. In particular we can study the effects of inhaling only in the events that reveal themselves after 1 November 1958. On the other hand, the increase in the number of doctors who reported giving up smoking is imme-

diately valuable in that if we know that a doctor stopped smoking in 1952 we can at 1 November 1958 begin to measure the effects of having stopped for six years.

As a result of these features we can analyze the data in three ways: (A) we can relate the deaths of the whole ten years to the smoking habits as recorded in the 1951 questionary; (B) we can relate the deaths reported during the first seven years to the smoking habits recorded on the first questionary (1951) and the deaths of the last three years, 1958 to 1961, to the smoking habits recorded on the second questionary (1957 to 1958); and (C) we can relate the deaths of the last three years, 1958 to 1961, to the information recorded *only* on the second questionary.

In considering whether to adopt the simplicity of method A or the slightly more complex method B we have studied the changes reported in smoking habits (Tables 1, 2, and 3). Table 1 shows the changes in the *method* of smoking; the main features are: (1) 75 percent of the population had not changed; (2) only 3 percent of nonsmokers had started smoking but 12 percent of ex-smokers had restarted; (3) 19 percent of smokers had given up, and the proportion is much the same for the various methods of smoking.

In examining changes in the *amount* of smoking (Table 2) we may regard a smoker's change of one to four cigarettes a day (or the equivalent in pipe tobacco) as being a negligible movement, probably well within the error of reporting. On this basis 69 percent of the men had not changed their habits, 23 percent had reduced their smoking (including those who gave up entirely), and 8 percent had increased it (including those who started or recommenced).

Of *pure cigarette smokers* in 1951 (men who were smoking only cigarettes and were not known to have smoked pipes or cigars regularly in the past), 64 percent were still smoking approximately the same—that is, remained in the same or an adjacent category—2 percent had increased their smoking, 29 percent had decreased including those who had given up), and 5 percent had changed to pipes and/or cigars (Table 3).

We have, secondly, to consider that we have seven years of deaths to place against the 1951 habits and only three years of deaths against the revised 1958 habits. When this and the magni-

---

[4] A further 16 deaths of men and 1 of a woman were attributed to cancer of the lung in the 11th year of the study: in each case further information was obtained and the diagnosis was accepted.

Table 1. Method of smoking in 1951 and 1958, men.

Habits in 1951	Habits in 1958					
			Current smokers			
	Non-smokers	Ex-smokers	Pipe or cigar	Cigarette and other	Cigarette only	Total
Nonsmokers	5272	—	54	13	100	5439
Ex-smokers	—	4247	207	65	293	4812
Current smokers:						
Pipe or cigar	—	707	2575	213	118	3613[a]
Cigarette and other	—	520	629	2083	570	3802
Cigarette only	—	2840	641	787	9274	13 542
Total	5272	8314	4106[b]	3161	10 355	31 208

[a] Including 153 cigar.
[b] Including 608 cigar.

Table 2. Amount of smoking in 1951 and 1958, men, all forms of smoking.

Habits in 1951	Habits in 1958										
		Some tobacco (g/day)									
		Reduced by					Increased by				
	No tobacco	15 or more	10-14	5-9	1-4	No change	1-4	5-9	10-14	15 or more	Total
Nonsmokers	5272						67	47	24	29	5439
Ex-smokers	4247						135	144	122	164	4812
Smokers of (g/day):											
1-4	591				139	473	242	68	21	35	1569
5-9	808			115	487	938	322	154	53	32	2909
10-14	854		60	436	569	1439	376	289	98	38	4159
15-19	629	27	190	427	394	1504	289	244	67	31	3802
20-24	677	131	290	453	300	1991	160	216	128	39	4385
25+	508	392	336	373	162	1832	153	183	116	78	4133
Total	13 586	550	876	1804	2051	8177	1744	1345	629	446	31 208

Table 3. Pure cigarette smokers in 1951 and their smoking habits in 1958, men.

Habits in 1951 (No. smoked per day)	Habits in 1958									
	Stopped smoking	Changed to pipes and/or cigars	Continued smoking cigarettes, no. per day							Total
			1-4	5-9	10-14	15-19	20-24	25+	Total	
1-4	328	31	301	65	18	11	8	3	406	765
5-9	481	72	171	495	101	25	19	5	816	1369
10-14	550	120	125	280	920	188	88	23	1624	2294
15-19	438	101	59	156	240	1056	191	79	1781	2320
20-24	557	163	54	87	268	213	1753	316	2691	3411
25+	397	130	31	43	90	149	222	2027	2562	3089
Total	2751	617	741	1126	1637	1642	2281	2453	9880	13 248[a]

[a] This total is less than the total of men smoking only cigarettes shown in Table 1 since it excludes 294 men who were known to have smoked pipes or cigars regularly at some previous time.

tude of the changes in habits are both taken into account it is not surprising to find that the principal results of the inquiry are practically the same irrespective of whether we use method A or method B. We have therefore used the simpler method A throughout except (1) for the analysis of the effects of giving up smoking when method B is the method of choice, and (2) for the analysis of the effects of inhaling when method C must be employed.

Calculation of Rates

For each of the subgroups defined by smoking habits, sex, and age we have calculated the number of person-years of exposure between 1951 and 1961 (as described in our 1956 paper). On this basis we have calculated sex and age specific death rates from the different causes of death. By applying these specific rates to the 1956 male population of England and Wales (as given by the Registrar-General) we have calculated standardized death rates at all ages.

MORTALITY AMONG MALE DOCTORS

Principal Comparisons

By such means we can compare the mortality from all causes and from separate causes among: (1) smokers and lifelong nonsmokers, (2) cigarette smokers and pipe smokers, (3) smokers who had given up before 1 November 1951 and those who were continuing to smoke at that date, and (4) those who smoked different daily numbers of cigarettes or different quantities of pipe tobacco. The results for male doctors are presented in Tables 4 to 24. Study of the mortality among men who had stopped smoking for different lengths of time and among men with different inhaling habits is made later (see p. 648). Analysis of the mortality among women is also deferred (see p. 653), since the deaths (366) are too few to allow similar detailed comparisons.

All Causes

The total mortality rate was 19 percent higher among smokers (14.32)[5] and 28 percent

[5] All the mortality rates referred to are rates per 1000 persons per year and are standardized for age unless stated otherwise.

higher among cigarette smokers (15.38) than among nonsmokers (12.06). In contrast, the mortality among men who had smoked only pipes or cigars and were not known to have smoked cigarettes (12.23) was only 1 percent greater than among the nonsmokers. As would be anticipated from these data the mortality among men who were known to have smoked cigarettes as well as pipes or cigars—referred to subsequently as mixed smokers—was intermediate between the figures for the two separate types (13.34). Very few doctors in Britain have smoked only cigars, and the rate for men in this category in 1951 (10.78) is based on the experience of only 127 men and may therefore not be very accurate (95 percent confidence limits 6.57 and 14.99).

Among cigarette smokers the rate was substantially higher among those who were still smoking at 1 November 1951 (16.32) than among those who had given up (12.68), and among the continuing smokers there was a progressive increase in mortality from those smoking 1-14 a day (14.44) to those smoking 15-24 a day (15.47) and to those smoking 25 or more cigarettes a day (19.67). Among the last group the mortality was 63 percent greater than that of the lifelong nonsmokers and 55 percent greater than that of men who had smoked cigarettes but, at 1 November 1959, had given up. (The rates quoted above can be found in the bottom lines of Tables 23 and 24.)

The numbers of deaths in most of these categories are so large that tests of statistical significance are hardly necessary. As would be expected, there are highly significant differences (P<0.001) between nonsmokers and all smokers, nonsmokers and all cigarette smokers, cigarette smokers and pipe and/or cigar smokers, ex- and continuing cigarette smokers, and light and heavy cigarette smokers. In contrast the differences between nonsmokers and pipe or cigar smokers and between nonsmokers and ex-cigarette smokers are not significant (P>0.05).

While the simplest interpretation of these differences is that cigarette smoking is an important factor contributing to death, it is not the only possible explanation. We must consider whether smoking habits may be determined by the presence of disease or whether they are not associated with some other factor, environmental or constitutional, to which the cause of death is more directly related. For example, a man who suspects that he has developed a fatal disease is unlikely to quit smoking; therefore men who have recently given it up may form a relatively healthy group. Again, men who drink heavily tend also to be heavy smokers, and any mortality attributable to alcoholism will accordingly tend to raise the mortality of heavy smokers above that of non-smokers.

These figures for total mortality should not, therefore, be intrepreted until the mortality of each of its principal disease components has been separately studied.

Cancer of the Lung

Mortality from cancer of the lung is examined in Tables 4 to 11, where we have included the five deaths for which cancer of the lung was mentioned on the death certificate as contributory with the 207 in which it was given as the underlying cause.[6] Many of the rates, however, are based on small numbers, and although they may contribute usefully to the general picture they cannot be relied on individually. In spite of this there is a steadily rising death rate with increasing consumption of cigarettes at every age above 45 years (Table 4). For all ages a more detailed analysis in Figure 1 indicates a linear relationship, the death rate rising step by step from the 0.07 per 1000 in nonsmokers to 3.15 per 1000 per annum in men smoking 35 or more cigarettes daily.

In examining the effect of the *method* of smoking (Table 5), we are dependent upon the

---

[6] Ten certified deaths were excluded because additional evidence suggested that the diagnosis was incorrect (see p. 633).

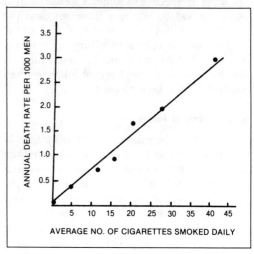

Figure 1. Death rate from lung cancer, standardized for age, among men smoking different daily numbers of cigarettes at the start of the inquiry (men smoking pipes or cigars as well as cigarettes excluded).

smoking habits reported at the time of our first questionary, and we did not, in that inquiry, ask whether pipe smokers had ever previously smoked cigarettes. We have learned subsequently, from the response to the second questionary, that 40 percent of the pipe smokers had regularly smoked cigarettes at some time previously, so that the excess death rate of pipe and/or cigar smokers over that of nonsmokers (0.43 against 0.07) may be partly due to this previous consumption of cigarettes. We cannot yet test this directly by examining the mortality of the 60 percent of pipe smokers who never smoked cigarettes regularly, since their number is small and we have not observed them for long

Table 4. Age and number of cigarettes smoked: death rates per 1000 per annum from cancer of the lung (numbers of deaths in parentheses).

Age	Nonsmokers	Cigarettes per day[a]		
		1-14	15-24	25+
35-44	0.05 (1)	0.07 (1)	0.00	0.11 (1)
45-54	0.00	0.31 (3)	0.62 (9)	0.75 (8)
55-64	0.00	0.48 (3)	2.31 (20)	3.88 (26)
65-74	0.00	2.69 (9)	5.16 (17)	6.48 (14)
75 and over	1.11 (2)	2.68 (6)	7.27 (8)	16.33 (8)
All ages	0.07 (3)	0.57 (22)	1.39 (54)	2.27 (57)

[a] Number reported at 1 November 1951 for men continuing to smoke cigarettes only at that time.

Table 5. Method of smoking: standardized death rates from cancer of the lung.

Method of smoking	Death rate per 1000 (No. of deaths)	
Cigarette (current and ex)[a]	0.96	(143)
Mixed (current and ex)[a]	0.53	(42)
Pipe and/or cigar (current and ex)[a]	0.43	(24)
Pipe and/or cigar (current):[a]		
1-14 g. daily	0.42	(12)
15-24 g. daily	0.45	(6)
25+ g. daily	0.96	(3)

[a] At 1 November 1951.

enough to obtain a reliable estimate of their death rate. However, although the numbers of deaths are very few the rates in Table 5 do show an increase in lung cancer mortality with increasing amounts of pipe tobacco consumed. On these data, together with the total rate, we could hardly exonerate the pipe from all risk.

We are still less inclined to do so after examining the data in Table 6, which show the death rates of men who were continuing to smoke at 1 November 1951 and of those who had stopped. For each type of smoking (cigarettes alone,

mixed, pipe and/or cigar alone) the rate of continuing smokers is higher than that of those who had stopped, and the rate in ex-cigarette smokers (0.24) is notably less than that in current pipe smokers (0.47).

The difference between the ex-smokers and the continuing smokers is most marked for those who smoked cigarettes, where the rate for those who had given up is only 19 percent of the rate for those who continued. This difference, moreover, may well underestimate the true difference, since in this analysis we take no account of the changes in habits in the years following 1951. (See p. 648, where allowance has been made for some of the changes in habits which took place and where comparison is made between men who have given up smoking for different lengths of time.)

In Table 7 we consider the nature of the evidence available to the doctors who certified cancer of the lung as the cause of death (excluding the one case for which this information was refused to us). In more than half of the deaths (56 percent) there was histological, cytological, or necropsy evidence together with X-ray or bronchoscopic confirmation of the site of the primary growth. In another 38 percent an X-

Table 6. Continuity of smoking: standardized death rates from cancer of the lung.

Continuity of smoking	Death rate per 1000 (No. of deaths)		
	Cigarette smokers	Mixed smokers	Pipe and/or cigar smokers
Continuing at 1/11/51	1.25 (133)	0.59 (36)	0.47 (21)
Stopped before 1/11/51	0.24 (10)	0.48 (6)	0.23 (3)

Table 7. Standard of diagnosis: standardized death rates from cancer of the lung.

Standard of diagnosis[a] (No. of deaths)	Death rate per 1000						
	Non-smokers	All smokers	Cigarette smokers[b]				
			Continuing	Given up	1-14 daily	15-24 daily	25+ daily
Grade 1 (118)	0.01	0.41	0.68	0.17	0.37	0.76	1.02
" 2 (81)	0.03	0.28	0.52	0.05	0.15	0.60	1.21
" 3 (12)	0.03	0.04	0.04	0.03	0.02	0.03	0.05
All grades (211)	0.07	0.73	1.24	0.24	0.54	1.39	2.27

[a] Grade 1 = Necropsy evidence *or* histological *or* cytological together with evidence of primary from x-ray picture or bronchoscopy. Grade 2 = Clinical evidence together with evidence of primary from x-ray picture or bronchoscopy. Grade 3 = Evidence from history and physical examination alone.

One case for which information was refused has been excluded (a man aged 74 smoking 14 cigarettes a day).

[b] At 1 November 1951.

ray picture or bronchoscopy supported the clin- ical evidence. In both these groups the various associations of mortality with smoking are quite distinct. On the other hand, it is of interest that for the 12 cases in which the diagnosis rested on history and physical examination there is no clear evidence of association. In other words, these figures show that doctors are not diagnos- ing cancer of the lung in their colleagues with- out adequate evidence, and that in the few less definite cases they are not making such a diag- nosis merely because the sick person was a heavy cigarette smoker.

Similarly Table 8 shows no marked associa- tions with smoking in the 13 cases of adenocar- cinoma, whereas they are distinct with both the squamous and the oat and anaplastic growths. Taking the death rate of the continuing ciga- rette smokers in each histological group as stan- dard (100), we have ratios for those smoking 1 to 14, 15 to 24, and 25 or more daily, of 68, 104, and 139 percent in the squamous group, and 44, 91, and 169 percent with the oat celled and anaplastic group.

The rise in lung cancer mortality with in- creasing number of cigarettes smoked occurred in all types of area, and the rates in Table 9 provide no reason to suppose that the associa- tion was any closer in big towns than in small towns or in the countryside. It is, however, pos- sible that the rural mortality is affected by the retirement there of men who had passed their active lives in towns. We therefore consider in Table 10 doctors under 65 years of age. The number of deaths in the different areas is then small, but they do suggest that there is a lower lung cancer mortality in the rural, and possibly the small town, areas which is not due to differ- ences in amounts smoked.

Table 11 shows the mortality in the principal smoking categories for two periods of time—1 November 1951 to 31 October 1956 and 1 No- vember 1956 to 31 October 1961. The first of these quinquennia followed immediately after the questionaries were sent out. Although the majority were returned within a few weeks, there were some which were not returned for several months, so that the first year of observa- tion was biased by the inclusion of some months of observation for which there could not be any corresponding mortality. A much more impor- tant type of bias is the differential selection of healthy men among the repliers, and we have shown that the total mortality rate was lower during the early years of follow-up than in any subsequent period. Clearly, therefore, we would expect the mortality from lung cancer to be higher in the second quinquennium and that

Table 8. Histological type: standardized death rates from cancer of the lung.

Histological type (No. of deaths)	Death rate per 1000						
	Non-smokers	All smokers	Cigarette smokers				
			Contin-uing	Given up	1-14 daily	15-24 daily	25 + daily
Squamous (55)	0.00	0.19	0.32	0.09	0.22	0.33	0.45
Oat and ana-plastic (40)	0.01	0.14	0.22	0.05	0.10	0.20	0.38
Adenocarcinoma (13)	0.00	0.05	0.07	0.03	0.03	0.12	0.07

Table 9. Place of residence: standardized death rates from cancer of the lung.

Place of residence	Death rate per 1000				No. of deaths
	Non-smokers	Cigarettes per day[a]			
		1-14	15-24	25 +	
Conurbation	0.03	0.48	1.31	1.90	49
Large towns	0.00	0.32	1.88	4.43	34
Small "	0.11	0.87	1.06	2.20	32
Rural areas	0.12	0.52	1.15	1.17	18

[a] For men continuing to smoke cigarettes only at 1 November 1951.

Table 10. Place of residence: standardized death rates[a] at ages 25-64 years.

Place of residence	Death rate per 1000		
	Non-smokers	Cigarette smokers[b]	No. of deaths
Conurbation	0.04	0.62	31
Large towns	0.00	0.65	17
Small "	0.00	0.52	16
Rural area	0.00	0.40	8

[a] Standardized for age and amount smoked.
[b] Men continuing to smoke cigarettes only at 1 November 1951.

Table 11. Period after start of inquiry: standardized death rates from cancer of the lung.

Period (No. of deaths)	Death rate per 1000							
	All men	Non-smokers	All cigar-ette smokers	Cigarette smokers		Current cigarette smokers		
				Current	Ex-	1-14/d	15-24/d	25 + /d
1951-6 (102)	0.69	0.05	0.98	1.22	0.41	0.64	1.20	2.25
1956-1 (110)	0.64	0.08	0.95	1.28	0.09	0.50	1.53	2.32

the effect of any selective bias would show itself most markedly during the first. In fact, the association with smoking was similar in both periods—though somewhat closer in the second period than in the first. Few, if any, of the doctors who died of lung cancer in the second period could have suspected that they had the disease in November 1951, and it is thus impossible to attribute this association to a selective bias in answering the questionary.

It is notable also that the mortality of ex-smokers decreased in the second quinquennium, when—on average—they had given up smoking for a longer time, and that it also decreased among the doctors as a whole. This last decrease was not large (from 0.69 to 0.64 per 1000 men per year), but it took place in spite of an increase in the mortality from all causes (from 13.46 to 14.56) and despite a steady increase during these years in the mortality from lung cancer in the male population of the whole country.

Other Cancers

Data for cancers other than cancer of the lung are shown in Tables 12 to 15. The number of deaths attributed to each type is small—in some cases very small—but we have given the results separately to enable them to be compared with other series.

Table 12 shows the mortality from cancer of (1) the mouth, pharynx, or nose; (2) the larynx or trachea; and (3) the esophagus. In each case the rates are higher in smokers than in non-smokers (columns 4 and 5), but they are not specifically higher in cigarette smokers than in other smokers (columns 6, 7, and 8). In Table 13, therefore, the rates are examined only for all smokers classed together, equating 1 g. of pipe or cigar tobacco with 1 cigarette. The most marked feature is a substantially increased death rate for each type of cancer in the heavily smoking men (25 g. or more a day), and it is evidently to this group that the excess mortality of smokers over nonsmokers is largely due. Only cancer of the esophagus shows a progressive increase in mortality with an increase in the amount smoked, and only this type of cancer shows any important difference in the death rates between men who have stopped smoking and those who have continued. It must be remembered, however, that the numbers of deaths attributed to cancer of the mouth, pharynx, or nose (19) and to cancer of the larynx or trachea (16) are very small. If all these cancers of the upper respiratory and digestive tracts are grouped together the combined results show

Table 12. Standardized death rates from cancers of the upper respiratory and digestive tracts.

		Death rate per 1000					
Site (1)	No. of deaths[a] (2)	All men (3)	Non-smokers (4)	All smokers[b] (5)	Cigarette smokers[b] (6)	Mixed smokers (7)	Pipe or cigar smokers[b] (8)
Mouth, pharynx, or nose	19 (2)	0.06	0.00	0.06	0.05	0.10	0.04
Larynx or trachea ..	16 (5)	0.05	0.00	0.06	0.05	0.03	0.10
Esophagus	29 (1)	0.09	0.04	0.10	0.06	0.19	0.08
Total	64 (8)	0.20	0.04	0.22	0.16	0.32	0.22

[a] The numbers in parentheses are of deaths (included in the total figure) in which cancer of the specified site was certified as being associated with the death but not its direct or underlying cause.
[b] Currently smoking or past smokers in 1951.

Table 13. Standardized death rates from cancer of the upper respiratory and digestive tracts in relation to the amount smoked.

	Death rate per 1000				
	Amount of tobacco smoked daily (g.)[a]				
Site	1-14	15-24	25 +	All amounts	Given up smoking
Mouth, pharynx, or nose	0.04	0.01	0.21	0.07	0.06
Larynx or trachea	0.02	0.02	0.15	0.06	0.05
Esophagus	0.08	0.14	0.20	0.12	0.02
Total	0.13	0.17	0.56	0.24	0.13

[a]Continuing smokers at 1 November 1951.

significant differences between smokers and nonsmokers (P = 0.02) and between heavy smokers and light smokers (P<0.001), but not between continuing smokers and men who have stopped (P>0.1).

Tables 14 and 15 show no clear evidence of an association for any of the other forms of cancer, either with method of smoking or with amount. As would be expected with eight groups, the individual figures show considerable variation, but in no case is this more than can reasonably be attributed to chance. Moreover, the total mortality from all these cancers is closely similar among nonsmokers (1.87), cigarette smokers (1.72) and pipe or cigar smokers (1.77).

Other Respiratory Diseases

Mortality from respiratory diseases other than cancer of the lung is given in Tables 16 and 17. For chronic bronchitis there is a close—and statistically highly significant—association with smoking. While this was most marked when chronic bronchitis was described as the underlying cause of death, it was also clearly present when chronic bronchitis served as a contributory cause in cardiovascular mortality. For pulmonary tuberculosis the evidence is much less clear. The mortality was higher in cigarette smokers than in nonsmokers, in continuing cigarette smokers compared with those who had stopped, and in heavy cigarette smokers compared with light. The deaths were, however, few, and none of these differences was statistically significant. Moreover, the few additional deaths for which pulmonary tuberculosis was described as a contributory cause tend to diminish the relationship rather than reinforce it. In other words, the data suggest that *death* from pulmonary tuberculosis may be associated with smoking, while the disease itself is not.

Table 14. Standardized death rates from cancer of other sites.

Site	No. of deaths	All men	Non-smokers	All smokers	Cigarette smokers	Mixed smokers	Pipe or cigar smokers
Bladder	38[a]	0.11	0.17	0.11	0.13	0.12	0.07
Stomach	84	0.26	0.27	0.25	0.30	0.14	0.30
Bowel	97	0.30	0.31	0.30	0.26	0.32	0.39
Rectum	35	0.11	0.05	0.11	0.12	0.12	0.08
Prostate	69	0.21	0.33	0.20	0.18	0.16	0.26
Other sites	194	0.61	0.64	0.61	0.68	0.52	0.51
Primary site unknown	27	0.08	0.09	0.08	0.05	0.09	0.15
Total	542	1.67	1.87	1.65	1.72	1.45	1.77

[a] Two deaths from other causes in which cancer of the bladder was mentioned as contributory are included in this category, but are excluded from the total cancer deaths.

Table 15. Standardized death rates from cancer of other sites in relation to the amount smoked.

| | Death rate per 1000 | | | | |
| | Amount of tobacco smoked daily (g.)[a] | | | | |
Site	1-14	15-24	25+	All amounts	Given up smoking
Bladder	0.10	0.11	0.13	0.12	0.08
Stomach	0.28	0.28	0.26	0.28	0.18
Bowel	0.37	0.22	0.44	0.32	0.23
Rectum	0.10	0.06	0.22	0.11	0.12
Prostate	0.16	0.19	0.12	0.17	0.28
Other sites	0.57	0.59	0.83	0.63	0.54
Primary site unknown	0.10	0.07	0.06	0.09	0.05
Total	1.67	1.52	2.03[b]	1.71	1.49

[a] Continuing smokers at 1 November 1951.
[b] See footnote to Table 14.

Table 16. Standardized death rates from respiratory diseases.

Cause of death	No. of deaths	All men	Non-smokers	All smokers	Cigarette smokers	Mixed smokers	Pipe or cigar smokers
Chronic bronchitis	111	0.34	0.05	0.37	0.51	0.33	0.15
Chronic bronchitis as associated cause[a]	55	0.17	0.03	0.18	0.20	0.21	0.12
Pulmonary tuberculosis	42	0.13	0.06	0.14	0.15	0.11	0.11
Pulmonary tuberculosis as associated cause	14	0.04	0.05	0.04	0.05	0.02	0.04
Other respiratory diseases	181	0.54	0.63	0.53	0.55	0.49	0.47

[a] In association with cardiovascular disease.

Table 17. Standardized death rates from respiratory diseases in relation to the number of cigarettes smoked.

Cause of death	Death rate per 1000				
	No. of cigarettes smoked daily			All amounts	Given up smoking cigarettes
	1-14	15-24	25+		
Chronic bronchitis	0.34	0.64	1.06	0.58	0.38
Chronic bronchitis as associated cause[a]	0.15	0.20	0.30	0.21	0.16
Pulmonary tuberculosis	0.10	0.16	0.26	0.17	0.12
Pulmonary tuberculosis as associated cause	0.05	0.09	0.02	0.06	0.11
Other respiratory diseases	0.41	0.68	0.40	0.51	0.61

[a]In association with cardiovascular disease.

All other respiratory diseases (including 116 deaths due to pneumonia, 21 deaths due to influenza and other acute infections and 44 deaths due to other causes) show no association with smoking. In our previous report (2) we suggested that some of the excess mortality attributed to chronic bronchitis among heavy cigarette smokers might be due to a tendency to diagnose chronic bronchitis rather than some other respiratory disease in patients with a chronic cough. With the present greater numbers the evidence for a negative association between other respiratory diseases and smoking has disappeared and it is clear that such a bias (if it exists at all) could not account for the results with chronic bronchitis.

Cardiovascular Disease

In Tables 18 and 19 we set out the data relating to mortality from cardiovascular diseases—due to nephritis. With the deaths attributed to cardiovascular accidents or to coronary disease we have .separately considered those in which reference was made on the death certificate to the presence of hypertension, for these deaths might be related to the causes of hypertension more closely than to any other factor.

For the 138 deaths in which hypertension was given as the primary cause there is no association with smoking habits—neither with method (Table 18) nor with the amount of cigarette smoking (Table 19). This is equally true for the 143 cerebrovascular accidents and for the 89 coronary disease deaths in which hypertension was also mentioned. Adding the three hyper-

tensive groups together gives, with one exception, remarkably similar rates in all the smoking categories, varying only between 1.26 per 1000 in nonsmokers and 1.10 per 1000 in men who had given up smoking (the final lines of Tables 18 and 19). The exception lies in the rather low death rate of 0.81 per 1000 in pipe and/or cigar smokers, a figure which is based upon only 53 deaths, and has 95 percent confidence limits of 0.69 and 0.93.

We can also conclude from these tables that there is no association with smoking habits in the 135 deaths from "other heart diseases" (rheumatic heart 35, other valvular disease 22, other diseases 78) nor in the 135 from "other cardiovascular diseases" (general arteriosclerosis 64, dissecting and atherosclerotic aneurysm of the aorta 47, and other vascular diseases 24). With the larger group of cerebrovascular accidents without reference to hypertension, there also seems to be no association. Though the death rate of all smokers at 1.41 per 1000 is a trifle above that of the nonsmokers (1.24), this small excess is not related specifically to one method of smoking (Table 18), and there is no clear gradient with number of cigarettes smoked nor fall in the death rate on giving up smoking (Table 19).

With the 337 deaths attributed to myocardial degeneration and the 43 deaths attributed to nephritis there is some suggestion of an association, but the evidence is slight. With myocardial degeneration there is a substantial—and statistically significant (P<0.01)—difference between smokers (1.02) and non-smokers (0.59), but there is no difference between the different methods of smoking (Table 18) and no gradient with the number of cigarettes smoked. With nephritis the maximum mortality falls on the heaviest smoking category and mortality declines with giving up smoking, but the differ- ences are small; none of them is statistically significant.

In short, we would conclude from these data that the only cardiovascular cause of mortality to show any association with smoking habits is

Table 18. Standardized death rates from cardiovascular diseases.

Cause of death		No. of deaths	Death rate per 1000					
			All men	Non-smokers	All smokers	Cigarette smokers	Mixed smokers	Pipe or cigar smokers
Cerebro-	(a)[a]	462	1.39	1.24	1.41	1.48	1.27	1.44
vascular	(b)[b]	143	0.45	0.51	0.44	0.50	0.44	0.23
accidents	All	605	1.84	1.76	1.85	1.98	1.71	1.67
	(a)[a]	1287	3.99	3.31	4.08	4.39	3.87	3.18
Coronary	(b)[b]	89	0.28	0.30	0.28	0.26	0.37	0.21
disease	All	1376	4.26	3.61	4.36	4.65	4.25	3.39
Myocardial degen- eration		337	0.97	0.59	1.02	1.01	0.98	1.00
Hypertension		138	0.42	0.45	0.42	0.45	0.36	0.37
Other heart diseases		135	0.41	0.41	0.41	0.42	0.43	0.33
Other cardiovascu- lar diseases		135	0.41	0.41	0.41	0.46	0.38	0.35
Nephritis		43	0.13	0.09	0.14	0.14	0.13	0.12
Total		2769	8.44	7.32	8.61	9.11	8.24	7.23
Total hypertensive		370	1.15	1.26	1.14	1.22	1.17	0.81

[a] Without reference to hypertension on the death certificate.
[b] Hypertension referred to on the death certificate.

Table 19. Standardized death rates from cardiovascular diseases in relation to the number of cigarettes smoked.

Cause of death		Death rate per 1000				Given up smoking cigarettes
		No. of cigarettes smoked daily				
		1-14	15-24	25 +	All amounts	
Cerebro-	(a)[a]	1.46	1.43	1.69	1.49	1.42
vascular	(b)[b]	0.46	0.48	0.54	0.51	0.51
accidents	All	1.93	1.91	2.23	2.00	1.93
	(a)[a]	4.35	4.28	4.97	4.57	3.73
Coronary	(b)[b]	0.29	0.29	0.18	0.28	0.19
disease	All	4.65	4.57	5.16	4.86	3.92
Myocardial degeneration		1.10	0.94	0.97	1.07	0.87
Hypertension		0.44	0.45	0.45	0.46	0.40
Other heart diseases		0.32	0.59	0.21	0.41	0.41
Other cardiovascular diseases		0.41	0.45	0.62	0.54	0.25
Nephritis		0.16	0.14	0.29	0.17	0.08
Total		9.01	9.05	9.93	9.51	7.86
Total hypertensive		1.20	1.22	1.17	1.25	1.10

[a] (a) Without reference to hypertension on the death certificate.
[b] (b) Hypertension referred to on the death certificate.

Table 20. Death rate from coronary thrombosis by age[a]

Age in years	No. of deaths	Death rate per 1000				
		Non-smokers	Current cigarette smokers smoking daily			All cigarette smokers, ex and current
			1-14	15-24	25+	
35-44	38	0.11	0.41	0.49	1.50	0.61
45-54	149	1.12	1.66	3.40	2.73	2.40
55-64	319	4.90	6.81	7.03	8.81	7.20
65-74	389	10.83	16.44	13.04	17.59	14.69
75-84	314	21.20	21.22	15.04	17.30	19.18
85+	78	32.35	33.06	58.54	—[b]	35.93
All ages	1287	3.31	4.36	4.28	4.97	4.39

[a] Includes all deaths attributed to coronary thrombosis, except those for which hypertension was mentioned as a contributory cause (89).

[b] Very small total number of man-years at risk (27½)—no deaths due to coronary thrombosis.

coronary disease, unrelated to hypertension, and that even here the differences in rates are not very marked. The death rate of all smokers (4.08) is 23 percent higher than that of non-smokers (3.31), and this excess appears to be limited to the cigarette smokers (4.39, or 33 percent above the nonsmokers, Table 18). There is certainly no clear gradient with number of cigarettes smoked, but the highest mortality is found among the heaviest smokers and there appears to be a fall in mortality on giving up smoking (Table 19). We examine these finding more closely in Table 20, which shows the age-specific death rates from coronary disease. These figures show that a rising gradient of mortality from nonsmokers to heavy cigarette smokers is clearly present at ages under 65, doubtful at ages 65-74, and absent at age 75 years and over.

We have not sought clinical information about the large number of deaths in this cardiovascular group and consequently have not felt justified in trying to separate a group of deaths which might be ascribed to "cor pulmonale." We noted earlier that 55 cardiovascular deaths included a reference to chronic bronchitis on the death certificate (coronary thrombosis 24, myocardial degeneration 15, hypertension 2, other heart disease 4, and cerebrovascular accidents 10), and it was shown in Tables 16 and 17 that these deaths were closely associated with smoking. It is possible that in a few of them the primary cause was really chronic bronchitis—particularly perhaps among those attributed to

myocardial degeneration or "other heart disease"—and that these constitute another cardiovascular group which is also associated with smoking. On the evidence available, however, this group would not appear to be large enough to have materially affected the results. Possibly most such deaths among doctors are attributed directly to chronic bronchitis.

Other Diseases

Finally, in Tables 21 and 22 we set out the mortality observed in all other diseases. Some associations with smoking are seen in peptic ulcer, in cirrhosis of the liver and alcoholism, and in "other digestive diseases," but none in genitourinary diseases other than nephritis, deaths due to violence, indefinite causes, and a miscellaneous group of other causes to which many diseases each contribute a handful of cases.

The 54 deaths ascribed to peptic ulcer include 15 in which peptic ulcer was referred to only as a contributory cause and two deaths attributed to hematemesis (a man of 64 smoking 30 cigarettes a day and a man of 82 smoking 16 g. a day in a pipe who have been included here rather than with the group of indefinite causes as peptic ulcer is most likely to have been the correct diagnosis). For these deaths the association with smoking is not close—for example, the mortality is higher among men smoking 15 to 24 cigarettes a day (0.31) than among heavier smokers (0.22)—but the difference between the

Table 21. Standardized death rates from other diseases.

Cause of death	No. of deaths	Death rate per 1000					
		All men	Non-smokers	All smokers	Cigarette smokers	Mixed smokers	Pipe or cigar smokers
Peptic ulcer	54[a]	0.17	0.03	0.18	0.21	0.16	0.12
Cirrhosis of liver and alcoholism	33	0.10	0.00	0.11	0.12	0.11	0.05
Other digestive diseases	87	0.26	0.07	0.28	0.32	0.20	0.25
Genito-urinary diseases[b]	82	0.24	0.33	0.24	0.27	0.21	0.22
Indefinite causes	50	0.15	0.17	0.14	0.13	0.12	0.20
Violence	248	0.77	0.94	0.75	0.79	0.68	0.64
All remaining causes of death	150	0.46	0.50	0.47	0.49	0.48	0.45

[a] Including 15 deaths in which peptic ulcer was certified as being associated with the death but not its direct or underlying cause.

[b] Excluding nephritis.

mortality rates for smokers (0.18) and non-smokers (0.03) is sufficiently great to be unlikely to be due to chance (P = 0.05).

With alcoholism (6 deaths) and cirrhosis of the liver (27 deaths) the association is strong. No deaths from these causes occurred among nonsmokers, and, like cancers of the mouth, pharynx, and larynx, the mortality fell almost wholly on the heaviest smokers.

The evidence relating to other digestive diseases is inconclusive. This is a heterogeneous group, the major components of which were 11 deaths from appendicitis, 12 from hernia, 18 from obstruction, 9 from diverticulitis, and 17 from gallstones or cholecystitis. Several of these

conditions are normally treated by surgery, and it would be reasonable to assume that their mortality rate was related to smoking, because of the resulting chest complications, rather than the incidence of the conditions themselves. The numbers of deaths, however, are too few to justify separate examination of the various diseases. The difference in mortality between smokers and nonsmokers for the group as a whole is statistically significant (P = 0.03), but there is very little trend with the amount smoked and no difference between continuing smokers and ex-smokers. Until further evidence is obtained, we have tentatively classified the group as unrelated to smoking.

Table 22. Standardized death rates from other diseases in relation to the number of cigarettes smoked.

Cause of death	Death rate per 1000				Given up smoking cigarettes
	No. of cigarettes smoked daily				
	1-14	15-24	25 +	All amounts	
Peptic ulcer[a]	0.07	0.31	0.22	0.21	0.16
Cirrhosis of liver and alcoholism	0.05	0.08	0.43	0.15	0.03
Other digestive diseases	0.26	0.33	0.36	0.32	0.32
Genito-urinary diseases[a]	0.28	0.29	0.29	0.29	0.21
Indefinite causes	0.21	0.12	0.12	0.16	0.08
Violence	0.85	0.57	1.15	0.83	0.65
All remaining causes of death	0.53	0.34	0.53	0.45	0.55

[a] See footnotes to Table 21.

Related and Unrelated Causes

From this examination of the mortality rates by cause we believe that we can now reasonably and usefully divide them into two groups: (*a*) those that have revealed associations with smoking, and (*b*) those that have not. Thus we reach the death rates summarized in Tables 23 and 24. (In these tables we have ignored the contributory causes of death and have included each death once only under that condition given on the death certificate as the underlying cause.)

Causes of death that we have regarded as related to smoking account, it will be seen, for 39 percent of all deaths (1775 of 4597). In this group the mortality among smokers (5.74) is 63 percent more than in nonsmokers (3.53) and that among cigarette smokers (6.39) 81 percent more; and the mortality in continuing cigarette smokers (7.01) is 50 percent more than in ex-

Table 23. Standardized death rates from causes related to smoking and from causes unrelated to smoking.

Cause of death	No. of deaths	Death rate per 1000					
		All men	Non-smokers	All smokers	Cigarette smokers	Mixed smokers	Pipe or cigar smokers
Related causes:							
Cancer of lung	207	0.65	0.07	0.71	0.93	0.52	0.43
Other upper respiratory and digestive cancers	56	0.17	0.04	0.20	0.15	0.28	0.16
Chronic bronchitis	111	0.34	0.05	0.37	0.51	0.33	0.15
Coronary disease without hypertension	1287	3.99	3.31	4.08	4.39	3.87	3.18
Peptic ulcer (including hematemesis)	39	0.12	0.00	0.13	0.13	0.12	0.10
Cirrhosis of liver and alcoholism	33	0.10	0.00	0.11	0.12	0.11	0.05
Pulmonary tuberculosis	42	0.13	0.06	0.14	0.15	0.11	0.11
Total	1775	5.49	3.53	5.74	6.39	5.33	4.17
Unrelated causes:							
Other cancers	542	1.67	1.87	1.65	1.72	1.45	1.77
Other respiratory disease	181	0.54	0.63	0.53	0.55	0.49	0.47
Cerebrovascular accidents without hypertension	462	1.39	1.24	1.41	1.48	1.27	1.44
Myocardial degeneration	337	0.97	0.59	1.02	1.01	0.98	1.00
All hypertension	370	1.15	1.26	1.14	1.22	1.17	0.81
Other heart disease	135	0.41	0.41	0.41	0.42	0.43	0.33
Nephritis	43	0.13	0.09	0.14	0.14	0.13	0.12
Other cardiovascular disease	135	0.41	0.41	0.41	0.46	0.38	0.35
Other digestive disease	87	0.26	0.07	0.28	0.32	0.20	0.25
Violence	248	0.77	0.94	0.75	0.79	0.68	0.64
Remainder	282	0.85	1.00	0.85	0.89	0.81	0.87
Total	2822	8.55	8.53	8.58	8.99	8.00	8.06
All causes	4597	14.05	12.06	14.32	15.38	13.34	12.23

Table 24. Standardized death rates from causes related to smoking and from causes unrelated to smoking in relation to the number of cigarettes smoked.

Cause of death	Death rate per 1000				
	No. of cigarettes smoked daily				Given up smoking cigarettes
	1-14	15-24	25 or more	All amounts	
Related causes:					
Cancer of lung	0.57	1.29	2.23	1.20	0.24
Other upper respiratory and digestive cancers	0.04	0.18	0.43	0.20	0.05
Chronic bronchitis	0.34	0.64	1.06	0.58	0.38
Coronary disease without hypertension	4.35	4.28	4.97	4.57	3.73
Peptic ulcer (including hematemesis)	0.02	0.18	0.19	0.13	0.12
Cirrhosis of liver and alcoholism	0.05	0.08	0.43	0.15	0.03
Pulmonary tuberculosis	0.10	0.16	0.26	0.17	0.12
Total	5.48	6.81	9.56	7.01	4.67
Unrelated causes:					
Other cancers	1.77	1.56	2.31	1.82	1.47
Other respiratory disease	0.41	0.69	0.40	0.51	0.61
Cerebrovascular accidents without hypertension	1.46	1.43	1.69	1.49	1.42
Myocardial degeneration	1.10	0.94	0.97	1.07	0.87
All hypertension	1.20	1.22	1.17	1.25	1.10
Other heart disease	0.32	0.59	0.21	0.41	0.41
Nephritis	0.16	0.14	0.29	0.17	0.08
Other cardiovascular disease	0.41	0.45	0.62	0.54	0.25
Other digestive disease	0.26	0.33	0.36	0.32	0.32
Violence	0.85	0.57	1.15	0.83	0.65
Remainder	1.02	0.75	0.94	0.90	0.84
Total	8.96	8.66	10.11	9.31	8.02
All causes	14.44	15.47	19.67	16.32	12.68

cigarette smokers (4.67). The mortality in men who smoke 25 or more cigarettes a day (9.56) is 74 percent more than in those who smoke under 15 a day (5.48) and 171 percent more than in nonsmokers (3.53). In contrast, the mortality in pipe or cigar smokers (4.17) is only 18 percent more than in nonsmokers.

In contrast, the remaining 2822 deaths (61 percent of the total) provide mortality rates that are closely similar in all the smoking categories. Among smokers as a whole the mortality from these causes (8.58) is 1 percent more than in nonsmokers (8.53) and the mortality among cigarette smokers (8.99) is raised by only 5 percent. There is a somewhat greater difference— 16 percent—between men who continued to smoke cigarettes (9.31) and those who stopped (8.02), but, as will appear later, this may be an artifact due to the self-selection of men who stop smoking (see p. 649). The mortality in pipe and/or cigar smokers (8.06) is 6 percent less than that in nonsmokers (8.53), but neither this difference (0.3<P<0.4) nor that between non-smokers and cigarette smokers (P = 0.09) is statistically significant.

MORTALITY OF MEN WHO HAVE GIVEN UP SMOKING

Cigarette Smokers

For detailed study of the mortality of the men who have given up smoking (ex-smokers) we have used the information given on both questionaries (see Method of Analysis, B) and have calculated man-years at risk at different ages for men who had given up for less than 5, 5-9, 10-19, and 20 years and over. For example, a man who stated on both questionaries that he gave up smoking in 1950 at 37 years of age is calculated to have been at risk for three-and-a-half years in the group that had stopped smoking for under five years (one-and-a-half years in the age group 35-39 years and two years in the age group 40-44 years), for five years in the group that had stopped smoking for five to nine years (three years in the age group 40-44 years and two years in the age group 45-49 years), and for one-and-a-half years in the group that had stopped for 10-14 years (in the age group 45-49 years). A man who was smoking in 1951 but who stated on the second questionary that he gave up in 1955 at age 52 years is recorded as an ex-smoker of three-and-a-half years' duration at the end of 1958, contributing one-and-a-half years at risk to the group that had given up for under five years and one-and-a-half years to the

group that had given up for five to nine years (all in the age group 55 to 59 years).

Thus we have studied the mortality among ex-smokers from (*a*) cancer of the lung; (*b*) chronic bronchitis; (*c*) coronary disease without mention of hypertension; (*d*) other cancers of the upper respiratory and upper digestive tract together with pulmonary tuberculosis, peptic ulcer, and cirrhosis of the liver and alcoholism—that is, all other causes of death related to smoking grouped together because of the small numbers of deaths attributed to each; and (*e*) all causes unrelated to smoking (see Table 25). In Table 25 allowance has been made for the amount smoked by calculating separately for each age group the deaths from each disease that would be expected among men smoking 1-14, 15-24, or 25 or more cigarettes daily, if death from the disease was unrelated to stopping smoking. The numbers of expected deaths were summed for each age and amount of smoking category and the standardized death rates calculated indirectly by multiplying the rate for all cigarette smokers (current and ex) by the ratio between the observed and expected numbers of deaths.

The results show three distinct patterns of behavior. For cancer of the lung (Figure 2) and the group of other diseases related to smoking, the mortality rates decline immediately and become progressively smaller as the length of time increases since smoking has been given up. Thus after 20 years the rates are only 15 and 34 percent, respectively, of the level for continuing smokers, although they are still two to three

Table 25. Mortality among cigarette smokers at different times after stopping smoking (numbers of deaths in parentheses).

Cause of death	Continuing cigarette smokers[a]	Death rate per 1000				
		Cigarette smokers stopped for (years)				Nonsmokers[a]
		<5	5-9	10-19	20 or more	
Lung cancer	1.28 (124)[b]	0.67 (5)	0.49 (7)[c]	0.18 (3)	0.19 (2)	0.07 (3)
Chronic bronchitis	0.58 (48)	0.71 (5)	0.81 (11)	0.06 (1)	0.30 (4)	0.05 (2)
Coronary disease without hypertension	4.72 (464)	3.52 (28)	4.17 (61)	3.87 (59)	3.74 (40)	3.34 (113)
Other related causes	0.65 (69)[c]	0.50 (4)	0.40 (6)	0.33 (5)	0.22 (2)	0.10 (3)
Unrelated causes	9.43 (865)	6.26 (49)	8.49 (120)	9.27 (136)	8.80 (105)	8.52 (315)
All causes	16.62 (1566)	11.62 (91)	14.25 (204)	13.60 (204)	13.38 (153)	12.09 (436)

[a] Calculate by method B (see text) and therefore not in all cases exactly the same as the rates in previous Tables.
[b] Including three deaths, also included under their primary cause, in which the specified disease was a contributory cause.
[c] Including one death, also included under its primary cause, in which the specified disease was a contributory cause.

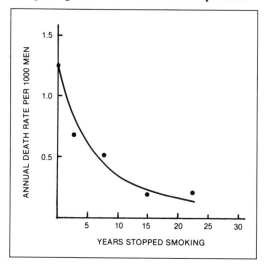

Figure 2. Death rate from lung cancer, standardized for age and amount smoked, among men continuing to smoke cigarettes and men who had given up smoking for different periods (men who had regularly smoked pipes or cigars as well as cigarettes excluded). The corresponding rate for nonsmokers was 0.07 per 1000.

times the rates of nonsmokers. On the other hand, for chronic bronchitis the mortality at first increases and then, after 10 years from giving up, falls well below the rate for men who continued to smoke. Lastly, for coronary disease without hypertension and for the unrelated causes of death the pattern is complex. In both groups the mortality falls quite sharply in men who have recently stopped, but it then rises again to fall finally to a figure which, 20 or more years after stopping smoking, is only slightly above that for the nonsmokers.

Clearly these different patterns cannot be due to a single cause, and we must postulate the interaction of several, probably competing, factors. For cancer of the lung and the group of other related diseases the results can be simply explained if cigarette smoking (or some factor commonly associated with it) is a direct etiological agent. With chronic bronchitis, however, clinical experience suggests that the rates will be influenced by the tendency of patients to give up smoking because of the increasing severity of their symptoms. Thus the group of men who have given up smoking will include a disproportionate number of severe cases of chronic bronchitis, and, as a corollary, the mortality from this

disease will remain higher in the ex-smokers compared with the smokers until, in the long run, the change in habits can exert a beneficial effect on the disease in the survivors.

For the unrelated diseases selective factors might operate in just the reverse way. A doctor who realizes that he may have a carcinoma of the large bowel or who has recently recovered from a stroke will hardly have the normal incentives to renounce smoking. There is little point in giving up if one is in danger of death and the act of smoking cannot influence it. It would not be surprising, therefore, if the doctors who chose to stop smoking were, so far as such diseases are concerned, the relatively healthy. From Table 25 it appears that this may well have happened and that the selective effect described has not fully worn off until smoking has been stopped for at least ten years. For coronary disease we believe the situation may lie between that for the related and that for the unrelated diseases: in other words, the mortality from the disease may be reduced by stopping smoking (directly or indirectly through some etiological agent associated with smoking) but that effect will be complicated by a tendency for doctors not to modify their smoking habits after the disease is first suspected.

In short, the doctors who stop smoking are not a randomly selected cross-section, as one would ideally wish, but will include those whose actions have been influenced by the presence (or absence) of symptomatic disease. Assessment of the effects of stopping smoking must take this situation into account. The influence of such selective mechanisms will, clearly, be most marked during the first years after stopping smoking and are likely to wear off in time. We have therefore compared in Table 26 the mortality of men who have given up for more than five years with that of all other men who have either continued to smoke cigarettes or have given up for less than five years. In other words, those who recently selected themselves are put back in the smoking population, which is then compared with those who selected themselves as long as five years ago (and in many of them very much longer). For cancer of the lung, chronic bronchitis, and the group of other related causes the contrast between continuing and ex-smokers is increased. For coronary disease it is slightly lessened. For the unrelated diseases it is so appreciably diminished that there is only a 3 percent difference between the rates.

We conclude that the fall in mortality with the stopping of smoking is a real effect so far as the "related" diseases are concerned, while for the "unrelated" diseases it is an artifact due to selection. With the related diseases the fall in cancer of the lung stands out remarkably.

With such a fall in mortality—and the much smaller falls with other diseases—it might well be asked how far these changes are directly due to the stopping of smoking and how far to the "stoppers" being different in their previous smoking habits from the general run of smokers—for example, being late starters, noninhalers, or smokers of lesser amounts. The answer is that such features are unlikely to account for the results. Differences in amount of smoking have already been allowed for in Tables 25 and 26 by the use of rates standardized for amount. Table 27 shows that the average age at which these men started to smoke grows a little less as the number of cigarettes smoked daily increases, but there are not appreciable nor progressive differences between men who continue to smoke cigarettes and those who have stopped.

Ex-smokers do include a higher proportion of noninhalers (Table 28). This difference, however, is found mainly among light smokers and therefore cannot have an important effect, since this particular group contributes only a small proportion of the excess mortality from the related diseases. We have too few data to measure the effect more quantitatively.

That factors of this nature are unlikely to be influential is also indicated by the results of the two halves of our study. The data, shown in Table 29, are classified according to the smoking habits recorded in the first questionary (and

Table 26. Mortality among cigarette smokers: effect of grouping men who had stopped smoking for less than five years with continuing smokers.

	Death rate per 1000			Death rate per 1000		
Cause of death	All ex-smokers (A)	Continuing smokers (B)	A as percentage of (B)	Ex-smokers of 5 years or more (C)	All other smokers (D)	C as percentage of (D)
Lung cancer	0.35[b]	1.28[a]	27	0.29[b]	1.24[a]	23
Chronic bronchitis	0.42	0.58	72	0.37	0.59	63
Coronary disease without hypertension	3.88	4.72	82	3.95	4.63	85
Other related causes	0.36	0.65[b]	55	0.33	0.64[b]	52
Unrelated causes	8.44	9.44	89	8.86	9.18	97
All causes	13.42	16.62	81	13.77	16.23	85

[a] See footnote[a] to Table 25.
[b] See footnote[b] to Table 25.

Table 27. Average age at starting to smoke among cigarette smokers divided by continuity and amount smoked (standardized for age at inquiry).

	Average age at starting when daily number of cigarettes last smoked was:		
Group	1-14	15-24	25 or more
Smoking at 1/11/51	20.3	19.7	19.1
Stopped less than 10 years	20.7	19.9	19.8
" 10 years or more	19.6	19.3	19.3

[a] The ages are somewhat higher than would be anticipated from present experience: they refer, however, to a section of the population composed of university graduates, some of whom completed their education before the first world war. The average is heavily weighted by the few doctors who began to smoke after 25 years of age; in each group the commonest age at starting was one to two years less than the average.

Table 28. Percentage of inhalers among cigarette smokers, divided by continuity and amount smoked (standardized for age at inquiry).

Group	Percentage of inhalers when daily number of cigarettes last smoked was:		
	1-14	15-24	25 or more
Smoking at 1/11/51	68	80	81
Stopped less than 10 years	59	77	80
" 10 years or more	34	72	73

Table 29. Mortality from various causes in first and second quinquennia of observation: continuing and ex-cigarette smokers

Cause of death	Death rate per 1000			
	Continuing smokers		Ex-smokers	
	1st 5 years	2nd 5 years	1st 5 years	2nd 5 years
Lung cancer[a]	1.22	1.28	0.41	0.09
Chronic bronchitis	0.55	0.61	0.45	0.32
Coronary disease without hypertension	4.50	4.64	3.19	4.17
Other related causes	0.67	0.64	0.36	0.30
Unrelated causes	9.14	9.37	7.51	8.63
All causes	16.02	16.48	11.93	13.51

[a] Including four deaths among continuing cigarette smokers in which lung cancer was certified as a contributory cause (method A).

include the results for lung cancer already given in Table 11). For the three groups of diseases that are closely related to cigarette smoking the mortality among men who had stopped smoking was lower than that among men who continued to smoke and fell further with the passage of time. It is difficult to see how these results could have been produced if the fact of stopping smoking had not at the same time reduced the extent of exposure to some specific etiological agent.

It is shown in Table 23 that pipe and cigar smokers had a mortality from all causes (12.2) negligibly higher than that of nonsmokers (12.1). Although, at the same time, there was evidence that pipe or cigar smoking contributes to the development of cancers of the upper respiratory and digestive tracts and to chronic bronchitis, the effect on the total mortality was clearly small. It is not surprising, therefore, to find no reduction in total mortality when pipe or cigar smoking has been stopped. On the contrary, the death rate in ex-pipe or cigar smokers (13.8) is slightly higher than that among men who have continued to smoke (11.9). The information obtained from both questionaries shows that this excess mortality is entirely limited to men who have given up for under five years (35.8) and that men who have stopped for five years or more have a death rate that is even less than among nonsmokers (9.8 compared with 12.1; P = 0.02).

The numbers of deaths among ex-pipe or cigar smokers are too few to allow us to make any useful calculations for different causes of death. It may be noted, however, that for the first five years after stopping smoking there is an increased mortality from diseases that are unrelated to smoking as well as from related diseases. The most likely explanation for this increased mortality would seem to be that it was an artifact due to the effect of illness on smoking. If this is so, it follows that among doctors the effect varies with the method of smoking—pipe or cigar smokers tending to stop and cigarette smokers tending to continue (Table 25).

MORTALITY IN RELATION TO INHALING

Information about inhaling was obtained on our second (1957) questionary, and the deaths observed in the subsequent three years have been used to calculate mortality rates for men who said they inhaled and for those who said they did not. To these deaths we have added, to obtain more data, those that occurred in the eleventh year of the study. A few of these eleventh-year deaths—that is, occurring before 1 November 1962—may not yet have been reported, and the death rates may therefore very slightly underestimate the true figures; they may also be diminished by our failure to obtain replies from all the doctors in 1957, and some of them are known not to have replied because they were ill. The proportion not replying was, however, very small (2 percent), and this selective failure to reply cannot have appreciably affected the contrast between the rates.

In several previous studies it has been shown that inhaling varies with age, with the method of smoking, and with the amount smoked. Sim-

ilar trends were observed in this study and also for length of time stopped smoking (Tables 28 and 30). It is necessary, therefore, to allow for all these factors when comparing the incidence of deaths from different causes among inhalers and noninhalers. The rates shown in Table 31 are therefore limited to pure cigarette smokers, and they have been standardized for amount smoked (using the three categories 1-14, 15-24, and 25 or more a day) as well as for age. Further, to avoid complications due to giving up smoking, the calculations have been confined to men who were still smoking only cigarettes at the time of the second inquiry.

The results show that while the mortality from all causes was slightly higher in inhalers (17.73) than in noninhalers (15.83) the difference varies very considerably with cause of death. The largest relative excess was observed

Table 30. Inhaling habits by age, method of smoking, and amount smoked; (Male doctors aged 25 years and over).

Age (years)	Percentage of inhalers among						
	Continuing cigarette smokers smoking daily			All continuing cigarette smokers	Ex-cigarette smokers	Continuing smokers, cigarette and other	Continuing pipe and/or cigar[a] smokers
	1-14	15-24	25 or more				
25-34	85	93	95	90	82	74	12
35-44	78	89	89	85	76	60	10
45-54	65	78	81	75	62	47	7
55-64	54	70	73	66	57	36	5
65-74	49	66	59	58	49	30	4
75 or more	38	47	46	41	41	26	4
All ages	67	81	81	76	63	47	7

[a] Figures for the few cigar smokers are almost identical with those for pipe smokers.

Table 31. Mortality among continuing cigarette smokers according to inhaling habits, compared with non-smokers (numbers of deaths in parentheses).

Cause of death	Death rate per 1000 men per year		
	Continuing cigarette smokers		Nonsmokers
	Inhalers	Noninhalers	
Lung cancer	1.88 (33)[a]	1.10 (11)	0.03 (1)
Chronic bronchitis	0.72 (12)	0.51 (7)	0.07 (1)
Coronary disease without hypertension	5.22 (113)	5.09 (60)	3.29 (50)
Other related causes	0.70 (17)	0.48 (4)	0.12 (2)
Unrelated causes	9.27 (171)	8.65 (99)	7.32 (112)
All causes	17.73 (345)	15.83 (181)	10.82 (166)

[a] Including one death, also included under its primary cause, in which lung cancer was certified as a contributory cause.

with lung cancer (71 percent, P=0.10) and the next largest with chronic bronchitis (41 percent) and the group of other related causes[7] (46 percent). Only small and statistically insignificant differences were observed in coronary disease without hypertension (3 percent excess in inhalers) and in the large group of unrelated causes (7 percent excess in inhalers). With each cause the rate for noninhalers was higher than that for nonsmokers, but the excess is least for the unrelated diseases (only 18 percent).

With only 44 deaths from lung cancer, comparison of the rates among men who have smoked different numbers of cigarettes must be highly unreliable. Nevertheless, the figures shown in Table 32 may give an indication of the likely pattern—that is, that the importance of inhaling is most marked among light smokers (none of whom died of lung cancer if they did not inhale) and is least marked among heavy smokers. Among the light and moderate smokers the excess mortality of inhalers is significant (P=0.01). Among the heavy smokers the rate was actually higher among noninhalers, but the difference could here have arisen by chance (0.4<P<0.5).

Table 32. Mortality from lung cancer according to number of cigarettes smoked and inhaling habits (numbers of deaths in parentheses).

Number of cigarettes smoked daily	Death rate per 1000 continuing cigarette smokers per year	
	Inhalers	Noninhalers
1-14	1.59 (11)	0.00
15-24	1.95 (13)	0.86 (4)
25 or more	2.16 (9)[a]	2.98 (7)

[a] See footnote to Table 31.

MORTALITY AMONG WOMEN

The women doctors available for study number less than a fifth of the male doctors (18 percent) and fewer of them are in the age groups of high mortality rate (40 percent were under 35 years of age against 29 percent of men, and 5 percent were 65 years or over

[7] Other upper respiratory and upper digestive diseases, pulmonary tuberculosis, peptic ulcer, and cirrhosis of the liver and alcoholism.

against 12 percent). The observed deaths are therefore far fewer, and very little information can be obtained about the causes of death. To increase the numbers we have therefore included 48 deaths which occurred in the eleventh year of the study, and this brings the total number of deaths of women to 414.

Table 33 shows the mortality in each of the six groups of diseases which were shown to be related to smoking in men and for the remaining unrelated causes of death. The results agree with those for men in showing no relation with smoking in these "unrelated" causes—and with women they account for four-fifths of all deaths. The mortality among cigarette smokers (6.60) is identical with that among nonsmokers (6.60). The 11 deaths attributed to cancer of the lung, cancer of the rest of the respiratory and upper digestive tracts, and chronic bronchitis were, as in men, concentrated among smokers; but cirrhosis of the liver and alcoholism (4 deaths) and coronary disease in the absence of hypertension (56 deaths) showed no such relation. (Only one death was attributed to pulmonary tuberculosis and none to peptic ulcer.) For coronary disease the mortality of male doctors who smoked cigarettes was only 10 percent greater than that of nonsmokers, and the 56 deaths of women are really too few to be confident that the experience of the two sexes is different. It may, moreover, be noted that at ages under 65 years—at which the relation among men was most marked—the mortality rate of women was higher among cigarette smokers (0.35) than among nonsmokers (0.26).

Examination of the few data for lung cancer shows that the mortality rate is highest among women who smoked 15 or more cigarettes a day (the rate was lower among the 244 women in the heaviest category of smokers—that is, those smoking 25 or more a day—but is based upon only one death). All the rates are lower (sometimes substantially) than those of men, and even with these minute numbers it seems that some factor other than the amount smoked is necessary to account for the difference.

Other features of the smoking history may indeed play a part, particularly: (1) the age at starting to smoke, and (2) the proportion of inhalers. Women doctors who were continuing to smoke cigarettes in 1951 began to smoke on average when aged 24.7 years—4.5 years older than the corresponding male doctors (see Table

Table 33. Standardized death rates from various causes among women doctors in relation to smoking habits.

Cause of death	No. deaths	All women	Non-smokers	Smokers	Ex-smokers	Continuing smokers	1-14	15-24	25 or more
								Death rate per 1000 women per year	
							No. of cigarettes daily (continuing smokers)		
Lung cancer	7	0.08	0.03	0.13	0.08	0.15	—	0.41	0.22
Other respiratory and upper digestive cancer	2	0.04	—	0.07	—	0.11	—	0.27	0.22
Chronic bronchitis	2	0.04	—	0.08	—	0.11	0.05	0.27	—
Pulmonary tuberculosis	1	0.03	0.04	—	—	—	—	—	—
Cirrhosis of liver and alcoholism	4	0.06	0.04	0.07	0.16	0.03	—	0.10	—
Coronary disease without hypertension	56	1.14	1.25	0.99	1.26	0.84	0.41	1.25	2.62
Other causes (unrelated)	342	6.72	6.60	6.60	5.94	6.93	6.30	8.60	5.70
All causes	414	8.10	7.95	7.94	7.44	8.17	6.76	10.89	8.76

[a] Only one woman said she smoked a pipe as well as cigarettes and no women smoked only pipes or cigars. For the purpose of this analysis the small additional amount of pipe tobacco has been ignored.

27). Among doctors aged 55 years and over in 1951—that is, those who have contributed most of the cases of lung cancer—the difference was greater; women of these ages began to smoke at an average age of 28.3 years compared with 20.2 years for men.

Differences in inhaling habits are shown in Tables 30 and 34. At each level of smoking and at each age the inhalers were fewer among women than among men—and the difference was most marked at 55 years and over, when the risk of cancer was highest. At these ages and at each level of smoking the proportion of inhalers was approximately twice as great in men as in women.

We have not sufficient data to take these differences into account, but it appears (from Table 32) that the difference in inhaling will lower the female mortality rate in relation to the male, and it is reasonable to suppose that the later average age at starting to smoke would have a similar effect. These differences, too, may affect not only the relative lung cancer mortality rate in the two sexes, but also, to a

Table 34. Inhaling habits by age and amount smoked; women doctors aged 25 years and over.

Age (years)	1-14	15-24	25 or more
	Percentage of inhalers among continuing smokers		
	Number of cigarettes smoked daily		
25-34	73	91	78[a]
35-44	63	71	43
45-54		59	54
55-64	26	34	47
65-74	17	26	25[a]
75 or more	17	18	
All ages	44	55	58
Women aged 55 years or more[b]	22	29	36
Men aged 55 years or more[b]	50	65	64

[a] Age groups combined because number of women in one age group was less than 10.
[b] Standardized for age.

greater or less extent, the rates for all the other "related diseases."

GENERAL DISCUSSION

In the preceding sections we have set out our observations. We turn now to their interpretation. We have to consider, as is true in nearly every problem of human epidemiology, observed *associations*—in the present instance between smoking habits and features of mortality. We have to decide from these associations, together with all other available evidence in man and animal, whether association implies *causation*.

In so doing we can consider our rates of mortality in at least two ways: (1) we can calculate the *absolute* difference between them, and (2) we can calculate the *ratio* of one to the other. For example, we have found death rates per 1000 per annum from cancer of the lung of 0.07 in nonsmokers, 0.93 in cigarette smokers, and 2.23 in cigarette smokers of 25 or more cigarettes a day (Tables 23 and 24). With these figures we can say that the excess mortality in cigarette smokers over nonsmokers has been 0.86 deaths per 1000 and in heavy cigarette smokers over nonsmokers 2.16 deaths per 1000—that is, the absolute differences. Alternatively we can say that the death rate of cigarette smokers from cancer of the lung has been thirteen times the rate of nonsmokers, and that the death rate of heavy cigarette smokers has been over thirty times the rate of nonsmokers—that is, the ratios.

Both these ways of looking at the data are legitimate, both have their uses. If we wish to know how many extra deaths will result from smoking (presuming for the moment causation) then clearly we must calculate the absolute differences. We may, of course, find that quite a small proportional rise in mortality from a common cause of death, such as coronary thrombosis, has a greater effect upon total mortality than a pronounced rise for a less common cause, such as cancer of the lung. But, despite Berkson's (3) opinion, it certainly does not follow that this best measure of the effect upon total mortality is also the best measure in relation to etiology. Here the contrasts given by the ratios may be far more informative and convincing. Indeed, in many epidemiological investiga-

tions of the past the clue to etiology lay in the pronounced ratio of the attack rates in consumers versus nonconsumers of, for example, water or of foodstuff, and not in the absolute difference between their attack rates. That there were proportionately in the consumers 20 victims, say, to every one in the nonconsumers stands out starkly. In general we shall follow that example. On this basis we have no associations to inquire into in the numerous causes of death, which comprise 60 percent of the total mortality. But, in contrast, in the remaining 40 percent there are seven causes (or groups of causes) which present a prima-facie case of cause and effect. Each of these we must examine separately.

Cancer of the Lung

With cancer of the lung our figures wholly confirm and, with larger numbers of deaths, strengthen those we have previously published. They also agree closely with those obtained by Hammond and Horn (4) and by Dorn (5) and with other studies summarized in the Report of the Advisory Committee to the Surgeon General of the U.S. Public Health Service (6). With the larger numbers we now present, the approximately linear relation that emerges between mortality and number of cigarettes smoked daily is particularly striking (Figure 1). There is no evidence here of any threshold that must be passed before a response in mortality takes place. On the other hand, there is evidence of so close a relation that it becomes increasingly difficult to envisage any other feature of the environment correlated with cigarette smoking as being the real and underlying cause. Equally striking and informative is the fall in mortality that rapidly follows the cessation of smoking. Unexpected as this may be at first sight, it is entirely consistent with the findings of Auerbach, Stout, Hammond, and Garfinkel (7) on the pathological abnormalities to be seen in the bronchial epithelium of smokers and ex-smokers. Cells with "atypical nuclei comparable to the cells in lung cancer" were observed in 93 percent of their sections of the bronchi from 72 current cigarette smokers and in only 6 percent of the sections from 72 matched ex-cigarette smokers. Further, a peculiar type of cell with a disintegrating nucleus was seen in the ex-smokers and only in the ex-smokers, 43 of whom had these "unique cells."

This feature of an increasing fall in mortality with the passage of time since smoking was given up cannot, we believe, be explained in terms of genetics. If, on Fisher's (8) hypothesis, the smokers who selectively choose to give up smoking are those who would in any event suffer a relatively low mortality from cancer of the lung, then this relatively low mortality should be an unchanging feature of the group. That would be their genetic fate at all points of time. Table 29, however, gives a very different picture. While the death rate of the continuing smokers from cancer of the lung is unchanged, we see in ex-smokers a rate of 0.41 per 1000 during our first five years of observation which falls to 0.09 in the second five-year period. These results are amplified in Table 25; among continuing cigarette smokers the rate is 1.28 per 1000 whereas among ex-smokers it is 0.67 within the first five years of giving up, 0.49 during the fifth to ninth year, 0.18 during the 10th to 19th year, and 0.19 after 20 years or more. In terms of environment we can explain this sequence simply. We see the effects of exposure to an environmental factor diminishing the further one goes in time.

There is another feature of these data which refutes the argument that the excess of cancer of the lung in smokers compared with non-smokers is merely a feature of their differing genetic constitutions. During the 10 years of this inquiry the death rate from cancer of the lung of all men aged 25 and over in England and Wales has risen by 22 percent (from 1.04 per 1000 in 1952-6 to 1.27 per 1000 in 1957-61). On the other hand, looking at our population of male doctors *as a whole* we find that their mortality from cancer of the lung has fallen (Table 11). Thus during the first five years, 1951-6, the death rate was 0.69 per 1000 per annum, and during the second five years, 1956-61, it was 0.64, a fall of 7 percent—and this figure must understate the real change, since in the first year or two of the inquiry we know that the mortality we recorded was unduly favorable[8] (see p. 631). Since we are considering

the whole population no selective factors can explain this change, and we believe it to be a reflection of the concurrent change in the doctors' smoking habits. Of the 31 208 men in 1951 roughly 17 500 were smoking cigarettes (alone or mixed); in 1958 the number had fallen to 13 500 (Table 1). Of those smoking cigarettes only in 1951, 29 percent had decreased their amount in 1958 (including those who had given up entirely), 5 percent had switched to pipe and/or cigars, and only 2 percent had increased their smoking (Table 3).

Our data on inhaling are another new feature of this inquiry. In this respect we may recall that our retrospective investigations of patients and paired controls showed very little difference between them (9). In total (men and women) 64.6 percent of the patients with lung cancer and 66.6 percent of the patients with other diseases said that they inhaled, and similar results were found for men and women separately. Looking back, one feature that must have contributed to this equality was our inclusion of patients in the control group who were suffering from diseases that today we find are also affected by inhaling—for example, bronchitis. Still subject to this same defect, a later analysis by number of cigarettes smoked gave the results shown in Table 35.[9] With light and medium smokers we again find but little difference, while with the heavy smokers there is a drop in the proportion with cancer of the lung who said that they inhaled, and this is much less apparent in the controls.

In the similar large-scale inquiry carried out in Paris by Schwartz, Flamant, Lellouch, and Denoix (11) the results were different. They show a very large excess of inhalers in the cancer of the lung group in the light smokers. On the other hand, the excess diminishes with increased smoking, and, as in our own figures, is reversed at the highest level of smoking. Spicer (12), in an extensive study carried out in conjunction with the British Tuberculosis Association, also found the same trend.

With our present prospective inquiry the numbers of deaths are so far small, but they also seem to indicate a hazard in inhaling at the

---

[8] This feature must also contribute to the difference between the doctors and the general population in the first five years of the inquiry. Other factors will include a substantially higher proportion of non-smokers among the doctors who replied to us and possibly other differences in smoking habits.

[9] These figures differ from those published by R. A. Fisher, (10), who, when we provided him with these data, used only those from the first half of our inquiry.

Table 35. Retrospective inquiries into the frequency of inhaling.

No. of cigarettes per day	Doll and Hill % inhalers		Schwartz *et al.* 1961 % inhalers	
	Cancer of lung patients	Control patients	Cancer of lung patients	Control patients
1-4	50	48	50	29
5-9				
10-14	81	79		
15-19			59	46
20-24	72	82		
25-29			61	46
30+	62	71		
			60	72

lower levels of smoking and its disappearance at high levels. For this latter phenomenon we have no explanation. But there are, of course, many facets to smoking of which we are ignorant. Do, for instance, very heavy smokers who inhale smoke less of the cigarette? Does the heavy smoker inhale the smoke so deeply that it is deposited in the alveoli instead of in the bronchi (13)? And so on.

Such questions arise acutely, we have shown, in the comparison of the mortality of men with that of women. With a higher age of starting to smoke and far less inhaling in women, allowance made merely for the amount smoked is clearly insufficient. Whether, therefore, cigarette smoking alone is adequate to account for the large sex difference in mortality remains open to question; certainly it cannot be asserted that it is not.

One feature that is striking is the very low mortality in both sexes in nonsmokers. With quite large numbers of doctors at risk we have seen in ten years only three deaths from cancer of the lung in men and one in women.[10] Most

doctors in the United Kingdom must practice in urban areas, and in the absence of smoking they have not derived cancer of the lung from the air pollution of the type and level to which they have been exposed in the last 50 to 60 years. This, of course, does not deny the possibility of some urban factor acting synergistically with smoking. What it does show is that in the absence of any smoking the rate would be only 11 percent of that actually prevailing. We cannot necessarily pass from doctors to the general population with its different smoking habits and some occupational hazards. The estimated death rate of our nonsmoking doctors is, however, similar to the rates derived from other populations in other studies, including our own large retrospective inquiry (9, 14). It seems probable, therefore, that without smoking the lung cancer mortality in England and Wales could also be at a similar low level.

We have already shown that a reduction of the present death rate would be likely to follow quite rapidly on a reduction in cigarette smoking.

How smoking exerts its effects remains open to doubt. Experimentally, applied to the skin of laboratory animals, the tar from tobacco smoke is carcinogenic (15), though not, it generally appears, very strongly so; however, it has also a substantial promoting action (16). If either of these observations is relevant, the latter may be the more important, since the rapid fall in the deaths from lung cancer on stopping smoking is similar to the reduction in skin cancers in animals when the application of a promoting agent is stopped (17, 18). The suggestion that the effect may merely be to hasten the appearance of cancer, in a "cancer prone" individual, and to localize it in a particular site (19) is not sup-

---

[10] It is very doubtful if one of them was in fact due to primary lung cancer. A man aged 79 presented with diarrhea and loss of weight and was diagnosed by a consultant physician on the strength of a single chest x-ray examination as having a bronchogenic carcinoma. The x-ray films were submitted to us and we sought the opinions of two radiologists. Both reported independently that there were multiple rounded opacities in both lungs and that the lesions were most probably secondary to a primary cancer elsewhere. Of the other three diagnoses, one (in a man also aged 79) was made on the basis of a three-months history of weakness, dyspnea, cough, and blood-stained sputum; edema appeared in the right leg after three weeks and death occurred two months later. A barium-meal examination was negative; a chest x-ray examination was refused. The two other diagnoses (in a man aged 37 and a woman aged 63) were confirmed histologically; in both cases the tumor was an oatcelled carcinoma.

ported by the evidence. If such an effect exists there should be less cancer in other sites among smokers than among nonsmokers. In fact, there is no evidence of this until after 75 years of age (Table 36). Moreover, other evidence from both family and industrial studies (20-22) weighs heavily against the existence of any general "cancer proneness" in man.

Cancers of the Upper Respiratory and Digestive Tracts

This group includes several different types of cancer which vary in their incidence in different populations independently, it appears, of one another. They are likely, therefore, to have different causes. Yet there is much evidence to suggest that most of them are to some extent related to tobacco consumption in one form or another. This relation has been demonstrated repeatedly in retrospective studies of patients and is borne out in all the prospective studies reviewed by the Surgeon General's Advisory Committee. However, unlike lung cancer, the association is less characteristic of cigarette smoking, and, indeed, in several studies the relationship is equally close, or closer, with the smoking of pipes or cigars. In the present study we have too few deaths to examine each of the sites separately, but, taking the group as a

whole, our results agree with those of other studies and indicate that these cancers are about five times as common in smokers as in nonsmokers.

Whether this observation should be interpreted to mean that such cancers are caused by smoking is, however, open to doubt. That they may be would seem to follow from the fact that tobacco smoke must pass through the mouth and larynx before it reaches the bronchi, and that in the bronchi it is carcinogenic. Two pieces of evidence, however, weigh against it. First, the mortality from some of these cancers has fallen in recent years, whereas the consumption of tobacco and the mortality from lung cancer have both risen. For example, between 1942 and 1962, while the number of deaths attributed to lung cancer in England and Wales rose by 325 percent, the number attributed to esophageal cancer rose by only 8 percent and the numbers attributed to laryngeal cancer and to cancer of the oral cavity and pharynx *fell* by 22 percent and 36 percent, respectively. Such wide differences cannot be explained by different trends in the fatality rate, nor, we think, by a differential change in the standards of diagnosis. To some extent they may be due to a change in the way tobacco has been smoked (from pipes to cigarettes). We do not know enough about the mechanism and time rela-

Table 36. Death rate from related and unrelated cancers by smoking habits and age (numbers of deaths in parentheses).

Age (years)	Death rate per 1000			
	Cancer of lung and upper respiratory and digestive tracts		Other cancers	
	Nonsmokers	Smokers	Nonsmokers	Smokers
25-29	—	—	0.19 (1)	0.49 (5)
30-34	—	—	0.20 (2)	0.23 (6)
35-39	0.10 (1)	0.03 (1)	0.57 (6)	0.27 (10)
40-44	—	0.08 (3)	0.24 (2)	0.39 (15)
45-49	—	0.18 (6)	0.82 (5)	0.56 (19)
50-54	—	0.69 (21)	0.66 (3)	1.18 (36)
55-59	—	1.32 (36)	1.16 (4)	1.11 (30)
60-64	—	2.52 (51)	1.76 (4)	2.82 (57)
65-69	—	2.95 (44)	6.02 (9)	3.89 (58)
70-74	0.92 (1)	2.94 (34)	2.75 (3)	6.41 (74)
75-79	2.34 (2)	4.06 (33)	12.87 (11)	8.00 (65)
80-84	—	4.52 (22)	16.46 (10)	12.92 (63)
85 and over	—	3.35 (8)	32.35 (11)	13.82 (33)
25 and over[a]	0.11 (4)	0.91 (259)	1.87 (71)	1.65 (471)

[a] Standardized rates.

tions of cancer induction to estimate any possible effect of this change, but it is difficult to believe that it is the whole explanation.

Secondly, all these cancers have been reported as closely related to alcohol consumption, and this alone must result in some association with smoking, since heavy drinkers tend also to be heavy smokers (see p. 662). In this respect it is perhaps notable that our results show that the excess mortality among smokers as a whole is largely due to a greatly increased mortality among the heavy smokers, a situation similar to that observed for the 33 deaths attributed to cirrhosis of the liver or alcoholism. We sought no data on alcohol consumption in our study, and thus it is impossible to assess the effect of the two factors separately. However, according to Schwartz, Denoix, and Anguera (23) and to Wynder and Bross and their colleagues (24-26) who have made detailed retrospective studies of patients with all of these cancers, alcohol and tobacco both exert independent effects. According to Wynder and Bross the effect of alcohol is unlike that of smoking, in that it is not proportional to the amount drunk, but is principally concentrated on heavy drinkers. If that be so, it might account for much of the discrepancy in the trends in the death rates from the different cancers.

On present evidence the most reasonable conclusion is that tobacco and alcohol both play some part in their production, but the two factors are correlated and it is not possible to estimate their separate effects quantitatively.

Chronic Bronchitis

The association of chronic bronchitis and emphysema with smoking that we observe in doctors has been a conspicuous feature of other prospective as well as retrospective studies and also of carefully conducted surveys of various populations. Thus, bringing together the results of seven prospective studies (including our own), the Surgeon General's Advisory Committee calculates that cigarette smokers died of chronic bronchitis and emphysema six times more frequently than nonsmokers (546 observed deaths to only 89 expected). In all but one of these studies the excess is marked.

As an example of a retrospective study we may cite the comparison made by Oswald, Harold, and Martin (27) of 300 chronic bron-

chitics with 300 controls of similar age, sex, and social status. Of the latter, 21 percent reported themselves as nonsmokers compared with only 9 percent of the former. These findings have been strongly supported by surveys of specific and general population groups in which smokers compared with nonsmokers have been found to have more frequent respiratory symptoms, more frequent chest illnesses, and, on average, a diminished respiratory efficiency—for example, Higgins (28), Olsen and Gilson (29), Fletcher and Tinker (30), Anderson and Ferris (31); for a full review see the reports of the Royal College of Physicians (32) and the Surgeon General's Advisory Committee.

There is undoubtedly also good evidence in this country associating chronic bronchitis with air pollution independently of smoking—for example, Reid and Fairbairn (33). Clearly the two characteristics may act independently or, perhaps more probably, synergistically. However that may be, the strong evidence on smoking has led Fletcher and Tinker (30) to suggest that it is not unreasonable to conclude that cigarette smoking is one of the more important etiological factors in chronic bronchitis in Great Britain. The death rates we have found in this present inquiry in doctors are certainly in keeping with this concept of the disease. Thus we have the very marked gradient in mortality with increasing amount smoked (Table 17), we have its concentration on cigarette smokers (Table 16), we have a higher death rate in inhalers (Table 32), and we have, after the initial period of self-selection, a decline in mortality after the giving up of smoking (Tables 25, 26, and 30). We may note also that the relationship, as would be anticipated, is less marked for those deaths in which chronic bronchitis was mentioned as only a contributory and not the underlying cause.

Finally, the thesis is supported by both histological and experimental evidence. Auerbach and his colleagues (7, 34, 35), for example, found frequent epithelial changes in the bronchial tree and alveoli of cigarette smokers, and Hilding (36) and Ballenger (37), among many others, found that cigarette smoke had an inhibitory effect on human and on animal respiratory cilia. Taking all this evidence into account, we conclude that there is here, as with cancer of the lung, a direct causal relationship between smoking and mortality.

That being so, and seeing that chronic bronchitis is a common disease in this country, we must naturally anticipate the clinical finding that chronic bronchitis and cancer of the lung will quite frequently occur together in the same person. It is, of course, possible that the chronic bronchitis itself plays a part in producing cancer of the lung (*38*), and figures published in a retrospective inquiry by Campbell and Lee (*39*) somewhat support that view. For the prospective inquiry, however, what we need is to observe the incidence of cancer of the lung in *nonsmokers* suffering from chronic bronchitis; and with its rarity in the absence of smoking the problem is to obtain enough of them.

Pulmonary Tuberculosis

The relationship between smoking and mortality from pulmonary tuberculosis is quite distinct, though it is based, we should observe, upon only 42 deaths. The further 14 deaths in which the presence of the disease was mentioned as a contributory and not as the primary cause of death reveal no such association. It is therefore possible that smoking may hinder recovery from the infection or, as Lowe (*40*) has concluded from his retrospective survey, it may conceivably re-aggravate a quiescent lesion. We see nothing unlikely in that. On the other hand, Kissen (*41*) suggests that anxiety is one reason for a poor prognosis in tuberculosis and also one reason for smoking. Without, therefore, more—and more precise—data on a disease so influenced by social factors, we hesitate to conclude that a direct causal relationship of mortality with smoking does exist.

Coronary Thrombosis

Deaths attributed to coronary disease amount, in our data, to 30 percent of the total deaths (1376 out of 4597). The great majority are described as due to coronary thrombosis or myocardial infarction, but there is a small proportion described less specifically as due, for example, to "coronary-atheroma," "coronary ischemia," or "angina pectoris with myocardial degeneration." With so many deaths it was not practicable to check the diagnoses as we did with cancer of the lung, and it is probable that many of them, particularly at ages over 75 years, were not, in fact, associated with an acute episode of thrombosis.

In 89 instances (6 percent of the total) hypertension was also mentioned on the certificate, and these cases, examined separately, showed no relationship with smoking (Tables 18 and 19).

For the remaining 1287 deaths the results are very similar to those we previously reported with less than half the number of cases (*2*), and, although the differences in mortality between cigarette smokers and nonsmokers (33 percent) and between heavy and light cigarette smokers (14 percent) are not great, the numbers are so large that there can be no doubt that the relationship with cigarette smoking is not due to chance (P = 0.001 and P = 0.04, respectively). The results are, moreover, similar to those obtained in the six other large prospective studies reviewed by the Surgeon General's Advisory Committee, all of which show that the observed mortality from coronary disease among cigarette smokers is from 1.7 to 2.0 times the mortality expected from the experience of the nonsmokers. Similar results have also been obtained in Albany and Framingham by Doyle, Dawber, Kannel, Heslin, and Kahn (*42*), who followed 4120 initially healthy men and found that the incidence of myocardial infarction was 2.4 times higher in cigarette smokers than in nonsmokers and 1.3 times higher in men smoking more than 20 cigarettes a day than in men smoking less. In all these studies as well as in our data the relationship is specific for cigarette smokers, and no excess mortality has been observed among pipe or cigar smokers.

According to Hammond and Horn (*4*) and to Buechley, Drake, and Breslow (*43*), the relationship is more marked at younger ages than at old. In our data this feature is distinct (Table 20) and the 38 deaths that occurred at the early age of 35-44 years show a relationship with smoking that is only a little less close than that for chronic bronchitis. At these ages the mortality among nonsmokers is extremely low (0.11 per 1000 per year), so that although the rate of 0.61 among cigarette smokers is only 0.50 per 1000 higher the ratio of the rates is 5.5 to 1. Over the next four decades the mortality of nonsmokers increases to 10.83 and of smokers to 14.69; in other words, though the ratio of the rates has become quite small, the excess mortality of 3.86 is seven times the excess at ages 35-44 years. At the oldest ages (75 years and over) the difference between smokers and nonsmokers disappears, but here the accuracy of many of the certified causes of death must be in serious doubt.

As with the other related diseases the mortality is lower among cigarette smokers who have stopped than among those who have continued, and, although the difference appears to be substantial, it has been shown that much of it may be an artifact, due merely to the selective failure of doctors to give up smoking when they are already ill (see p. 649). When, to correct for this selection, the data for the first five years after stopping are omitted the results are less impressive. There is still evidence of a reduction in mortality, but the maximum effect is reached only slowly. Five to nine years after stopping the excess mortality has been reduced to 60 percent of that among continuing smokers, 10 to 19 years after to 38 percent, and 20 or more years after to 29 percent (Table 25). Hammond and Horn (4) also found a reduction in mortality with the passage of time after smoking had been stopped, and Doyle *et al.* (42), studying men who were initially free from heart disease, found the subsequent incidence of myocardial infarction to be the same in both ex-smokers and non-smokers. The number of cases in their study was, however, small.

If the reduction in mortality is due to stopping smoking it would seem from these data that the effect takes place only slowly and over a long period of years. Many people, however, eat more when they stop smoking, and it is possible that the effect may be complicated by the effect of changing weight.

Our data on inhaling are still few, being based on only four years' observations, and the results are correspondingly unreliable. So far as they go they suggest that the mortality is higher among inhalers than among noninhalers, but the difference is small and it is not statistically significant (Table 31). Schwartz, Anguera, and Lenègre (44), on the other hand, carried out a retrospective study on nearly 1000 patients with coronary atherosclerosis and found a highly significant excess of inhalers over a matched control series. Their data suggested that there was practically no difference in risk between noninhalers and nonsmokers and that the risk for heavy cigarette smokers could be almost entirely attributed to the fact that heavy smokers also tended to inhale.

The evidence from all these studies, there-fore, is compatible with the belief that cigarette smoking is one of the causes of coronary thrombosis, and, in particular, one of the more important causes under 55 years of age. That it has an effect on the cardiovascular system is undisputed—the effect being probably due to the action of nicotine on the sympathetic ganglia or on the chromaffin cells, liberating noradrenaline and adrenaline. Even one or two cigarettes can increase the heart rate by 15-25 beats a minute, raise the blood-pressure by 10-20 mm. Hg, and increase both the stroke volume and the cardiac output. The skin blood-flow is reduced, but the coronary flow is either increased or, with regular smoking, held stationary. Why these effects should be harmful is less clear. Smoking does not precipitate pain in the great majority of patients with angina pectoris, and true cases of tobacco angina (45, 46) are so rare that it is difficult to believe that they provide a model for the substantial mortality that is apparently related to smoking.

It is, however, possibly more relevant that smoking may also have an effect on the level of serum lipids and on the control of intravascular coagulation. Many investigators have found that the serum cholesterol is, on average, higher in cigarette smokers than in nonsmokers;[11] only two studies have been negative—one limited to young men who could not have smoked for more than a few years (48) and the other to men over 65 years of age (49). No change in serum cholesterol is, however, found immediately after smoking, the immediate effects being a decrease in serum triglycerides and an increase in free fatty acids (47, 50). No effect has been noted on blood coagulation, but Mustard and Murphy (51) found that smoking had an effect on the blood platelets, decreasing their duration of survival *in vivo*.

Alternatively, cigarette smoking and coronary thrombosis may be related to one another only indirectly through some other factor. It may be, for example, that men with a raised serum cholesterol or of a particular physical constitution (52) or who tend to take little physical exercise also tend to take up cigarette smoking, and that these factors contribute to the production of the disease. Such a hypothesis is not, at first sight, unattractive, since the ratio of the mortality rate

---

[11] References are given by the Surgeon-General's Advisory Committee and by Konttinen and Rajasalmi (47).

of smokers to nonsmokers is relatively small. But it becomes difficult to accept when all the evidence is taken into account—namely, the much closer relationship at young ages, the increase in mortality with increased amount smoked, the difference between cigarette and pipe smoking and between inhaling and not inhaling, the reduction in mortality with increasing time after smoking has been stopped, and the many physiological effects of smoking on the cardiovascular system. In short, that cigarette smoking is a cause of coronary thrombosis is not, we think, proved; but it is the most reasonable interpretation of the available facts.

Peptic Ulcer

Even including 15 deaths in which peptic ulcer was certified as being contributory though not the underlying cause, the total number (54) is too small to allow us to examine gastric and duodenal ulcers separately. Classed together as peptic ulcer, the results agree with those of 12 other studies in which the relationship between smoking and peptic ulcer has been specially examined (five retrospective, six prospective, and one cross-sectional survey, Surgeon General's Advisory Committee). In all the retrospective studies the proportion of nonsmokers was higher in the control group than in the ulcer group, and in all the prospective studies the mortality was higher in smokers than in nonsmokers. In all studies in which gastric and duodenal ulcers have been separated the relationship has been stronger with gastric ulcer than with duodenal, and, when the type of smoking has been examined, the relationship has been closer with cigarette smoking than with the smoking of pipes or cigars.

An unusual feature of the prospective studies has been that the mortality has been maximum in the moderate or light smokers rather than in the heavy cigarette smokers. This is shown in the present data (Table 22), and a comparable result was obtained in the one large-scale retrospective study in which this aspect was examined in detail (53).

It is difficult to believe that these findings mean that smoking is a direct cause of gastric ulcer, since gastric ulcers have been decreasing in incidence over the long period of time in which cigarette smoking has been increasing. Duodenal ulcers, admittedly, have increased in incidence, but with them the relationship with smoking is less close. The worldwide distribution of gastric and duodenal ulcers is also quite unlike the distribution of cigarette smoking. If, therefore, smoking is a direct cause it is only one among many and not the most important. The excess mortality could, of course, be obtained if smoking affected the fatality of the disease without affecting the incidence—if, for example, it increased the risk of respiratory complications following operation. This, however, could not account for the excess morbidity. An alternative explanation would be that smoking habits are affected by the disease or result from the same factors as give rise to the disease. Thus many physicians believe that psychic factors play a part in producing ulcers, and there is evidence to suggest that they are also related to cigarette smoking (54-56). It is reasonable also to attribute the concentration of deaths among moderate smokers to a reduction, in the amount smoked.

On the other hand, not all physicians are impressed by the importance of psychic factors in producing peptic ulcers, and few would suggest that they were more important in gastric than in duodenal ulcers. There is, moreover, one piece of evidence to suggest that smoking has a direct effect on the healing of gastric ulcers. Doll *et al.* (53) carried out a controlled clinical trial on 80 patients and found that the ulcer healed, on average, by 78 percent of its initial size in those who were advised to stop smoking and by only 57 percent in those who were not so advised and all of whom continued to smoke.

From this we conclude that smoking plays some part in preventing the healing of a chronic gastric ulcer and that it may thereby have an effect on the mortality rate, both by maintaining the activity of the ulcer and by adversely affecting the fatality rate in the presence of complications. Some of the association, however, may well be secondary and of no etiological significance, particularly, perhaps, with duodenal ulcer.

Cirrhosis of the Liver and Alcoholism

These two conditions show a close association with smoking, most marked with cigarettes and particularly with the smoking of more than 25 a day. We know of no evidence from retrospective studies, but the six other prospective studies in Canada and the U.S.A. all agree in showing an increased mortality in smokers compared with nonsmokers (range 1.3 to 1 to 4.0 to 1, Surgeon General's Advisory Committee). It is conceivable that very heavy smoking may exert a toxic effect on the liver—particularly, perhaps, if the liver is already damaged by other agents—but it seems more likely that the association with cirrhosis is secondary to an association with alcoholism. Several studies have shown that heavy drinkers tend also to be heavy cigarette smokers (24, 57), but without precise figures and an estimate of the proportion of cases that are due to alcoholism in Britain it is impossible to test the hypothesis.

Other "Unrelated" Diseases

With the large group of other and "unrelated" diseases the death rates of all the smoking subgroups lie, with one exception, in the narrow range of 8 to 9 per 1000 (nonsmokers 8.53, cigarette smokers 8.99, mixed smokers 8.00, pipe and/or cigar smokers 8.06, ex-cigarette smokers 8.02, 1-14 cigarettes daily 8.96, 15-24 cigarettes daily 8.66, 25 + cigarettes daily 10.11; Tables 23 and 24). This close similarity makes it unlikely that we have overlooked any major relationship between smoking and mortality. The only departure from the prevailing pattern is the rather high death rate of 10.11 per 1000 in the heaviest cigarette smokers, an excess of 19 percent over the rate for nonsmokers. This excess comes from only 7 of the 11 causes of death shown in Tables 23 and 24, and could, we believe, be partly due not to smoking *per se* but to other features of life, both environmental and constitutional, which are correlated with it—for example, the psychological and possibly physical characteristics of heavy smokers and their habits of eating and drinking, etc. It is also likely that some of the excess is due to errors in the certification of the cause of death. Unless 100 percent accuracy was achieved in death certification—and we know that it is never so—the "unrelated" causes must inevitably include some deaths that should in fact have been classified as related. The "unrelated" causes will thereby share some of the excess mortality of heavy cigarette smokers that is characteristic of the related causes. In short, we conclude that smoking bears no direct or causal relationship to some 60 percent of the total death rate.

That is not to say that our related causes necessarily include all the diseases in which smoking is of direct etiological importance. We have no evidence on nonfatal diseases such as tobacco amblyopia, and very little for many rare diseases or diseases with a low fatality rate. There is, for example, strong evidence to inculpate smoking as a cause of thromboangiitis obliterans (Buerger's disease), but in our data no deaths were attributed to it.

Paucity of cases may also be the explanation of our failure to find any association of smoking with cancer of the bladder. Four retrospective studies have shown an increased mortality for this site among cigarette smokers—of the order of two to three times the rate in nonsmokers—and a still higher rate of mortality in heavy cigarette smokers (44, 58-60). Moreover, similar results have been obtained in all the other six prospective studies (Surgeon General's Advisory Committee). Our data are based on only 38 cases—six of which occurred in nonsmokers—and with this small number of deaths it would not be surprising if by chance we had failed to demonstrate a weak association with cigarette smoking. But it does not appear that there can be a strong relationship. (Since the conclusion of the ten-year period of observation a further 14 deaths with bladder cancer have been reported—six among cigarette smokers, eight among other smokers, and none in nonsmokers.)

In the studies of Hammond and Horn (4) and Dorn (5) several other broad groups of diseases have also been reported to show an excess mortality with smoking. The excesses have mostly been quite small, and, with the exception of a heterogeneous group of "other circulatory diseases" (Surgeon General's Advisory Committee), none have consistently shown a mortality among cigarette smokers as much as double that among nonsmokers. Such differences, we believe, could easily be due to the same causes as we have suggested above may account for the excess mortality from "unrelated" diseases in doctors who are heavy cigarette smokers. We may also note that the very large populations studied by Hammond and Horn (4) and by Dorn (5) have necessarily been heterogeneous in many respects. Their results may thereby be influenced to some extent by the social distribution of smoking. Doctors, on the other hand, are a more homogeneous group of one social class and one profession. Environmental factors that may be associated with smoking in the population at large will play a less important part. Further, the cause of death may be more accurately assessed among doctors, so that spurious associations due to errors in certification will be less likely to arise.

Finally, we have found no evidence of any cause of death, the rate of which is lessened by smoking. There were, of course, several diseases in which the mortality was lower among smokers than among nonsmokers, but in no case was this difference statistically significant and none showed a progressive decrease with increase in the amount smoked. This was slightly surprising, as morbidity studies have provided consistent evidence that the average blood pressure is lower among cigarette smokers than among nonsmokers (61-65). Yet, in our data, the mortality from hypertension was remarkably similar in all the categories of smokers and nonsmokers. In the corresponding American studies (Surgeon General's Advisory Committee) the mortality was either unaltered or was slightly higher among smokers. Evidently, therefore, if smoking reduces the casual blood pressure it does not affect the pressure sufficiently to have any measurable effect upon the death rate.

Mortality Attributable to Smoking

It was shown in Tables 23 and 24 that the annual death rate of cigarette smokers, including both those continuing and those giving up,

was 29 percent greater than that of nonsmokers; in men who were continuing to smoke cigarettes at the start of the inquiry it was 35 percent greater. These figures, we pointed out, do not necessarily mean that cigarette smoking increases the death rate by such amounts, since other explanations are possible. However, after our separate and detailed examination of the principal causes of death we have concluded that cigarette smoking is likely to be responsible for at least the greater part of the excess.

The results of our assessment are summarized in Table 37, where we divide the excess death rate in smokers of different ages into three categories. (1) The first category comprises the excess deaths from the "unrelated" diseases and from cirrhosis of the liver and alcoholism. Conceivably some small part of this excess may be due to cigarette smoking, insofar as it is due to errors in the diagnosis of the cause of death; the greater part, however, is likely to be either an artifact (due to the selective failure of doctors to stop smoking when they develop a serious illness; Table 25 and p. 649), or a secondary effect of the association of cigarette smoking with some other factor which itself predisposes to disease and death—for example, heavy drinking or excessive anxiety. (2) The second category includes deaths from cancers of the upper respiratory and upper digestive tracts, from peptic ulcer, and from pulmonary tuberculosis. Some of these deaths are, we suggest, directly attributable to smoking, but it is impossible to say how many, since the effect of smoking is complicated by other factors, en-

Table 37. Excess death rate among cigarette smokers.

Age (years)	Non-smokers	Causes not attributable to smoking	Causes partly attributable to smoking	Causes attributable to smoking	Cigarette smokers all causes
		Death rate per 1000 — Excess among cigarette smokers			
25-44	1.12	0.48	0.04	0.39	2.04
45-54	4.12	1.02	0.22	2.25	7.62
55-64	12.08	2.37	0.92	5.33	20.70
65-74	30.56	6.72	0.82	10.87	48.96
75+	114.29	-11.64	2.09	6.64	111.37
All ages standardized	12.06	0.93	0.40	2.93	16.32
Percentage of nonsmokers	100	8	3	24	135

vironmental and constitutional, with which it is associated. (3) The third and largest category includes deaths from lung cancer, chronic bronchitis, and coronary thrombosis. The first two, we conclude, are the direct result of the habit. With coronary thrombosis we feel less certainty, but at ages under 65 years we believe it only reasonable to regard smoking as the dominant factor. That being so, Table 37 shows that during the ages of 45-54 and 55-64 years approximately 50 percent is added to the death rate by smoking. One of the most striking characteristics of British mortality in the last half-century has been the relatively poor improvement in the death rate of men of ages 45-64 years. In cigarette smoking may, it seems, lie one prominent cause.

We have not made similar calculations for pipe or cigar smokers, since their total death rate is only 1 percent more than that of nonsmokers in our inquiry and is only slightly raised in the four other prospective studies which provide these data. Thus the combined figures for all five studies show an excess death rate of only 6 percent (Surgeon General's Advisory Committee). Our examination of the separate causes of death, in the light of the findings for cigarette smokers, suggests, however, that pipe smoking is probably responsible for some cases of cancer of the lung and of the upper respiratory and digestive tracts and of chronic bronchitis. For these three causes of death we report an excess mortality in pipe and cigar smokers of 0.58 per 1000 per annum, which is more than the total excess from all causes (0.17). The deficiency of deaths among pipe and cigar smokers compared with nonsmokers for all other causes of death (0.41) may well be due to chance (P = 0.4), but it is possible that pipe smokers also differ from nonsmokers in other ways that tend to reduce their mortality. We cannot be sure, therefore, that a change in the method of smoking from cigarettes to pipes or cigars would necessarily result in as large a reduction in the death rate as would appear from the present figures—particularly if the ex-cigarette smokers were to continue to inhale (Table 30).

Summary

The mortality of nearly 41 000 medically qualified men and women in the United Kingdom has been observed for 12 years.

During the first 10 years 4597 of the men and 366 of the women died. These deaths have been analyzed in relation to the smoking habits reported by doctors in reply to a questionary dispatched to them in 1951 (both sexes) and again in 1957 (men) and 1960 (women).

An association with smoking is found, in differing degrees, in men for seven causes of death—namely, cancer of the lung, cancers of the upper respiratory and digestive tracts, chronic bronchitis, pulmonary tuberculosis, coronary disease without hypertension, peptic ulcer, and cirrhosis of the liver and alcoholism. No association is found with the remaining 61 percent of the death rate, and this includes such major causes as other forms of cancer, cerebrovascular accidents, hypertension, myocardial degeneration, suicide, and accident.

In women the few deaths at present available show an association only between smoking and cancer of the lung.

The most pronounced association is shown by cancer of the lung for which the annual death rate rises linearly from 0.07 per 1000 in men who are nonsmokers to 3.15 per 1000 in men smoking 35 or more cigarettes daily. This linear rise from nonsmokers to light smokers to medium smokers to heavy smokers indicates no smoking threshold which must be reached before the death rate from cancer of the lung shows a response.

In men who have given up cigarette smoking the death rate from cancer of the lung falls substantially. It continues to fall step by step the longer smoking has been given up. This trend can be explained in terms of a diminishing risk from the previously operative environmental agent, but not in terms of genetic selection of those who choose to give up.

Between 1952 and 1961 the death rate from cancer of the lung in all men aged 25 years and over in England and Wales *increased* by 22 percent. In the doctors here studied it has slightly *declined* (7 percent) between 1951-1956 and 1956-1961, and this fall can be attributed to the concurrent change in their smoking habits. Many have given up smoking and many have reduced their consumption.

The very low death rate from cancer of the lung in nonsmokers of both sexes in a population that must live largely in urban areas does not suggest that air pollution *per se* has been an important factor in the production of the disease. Whether smoking acts synergistically with air pollution upon the respiratory tract is not known.

Mortality from cancer of the lung is certainly not closely associated with pipe smoking, but it does not appear that pipe smoking is entirely without risk.

The death rate from cancer of the lung is higher for light and medium smokers who inhale than for those who do not inhale. With heavy smokers this extra hazard is not apparent.

With cancers of the upper respiratory and digestive tracts the association with smoking is not specific to cigarette smoking, and the excess mortality of smokers in these present observations of British doctors is mainly due to a greatly increased death rate of the heavy smokers. Taking all evidence into account the most reasonable conclusion would appear to be that tobacco and alcohol consumption both play some part in their production.

Though there is good evidence that in this country air pollution plays some part in the etiology or aggravation of chronic bronchitis, the association of the disease with smoking has been a conspicuous feature of nearly every form of inquiry. As with cancer of the lung, there is no reason to doubt that there is a direct and important causal relationship between smoking and mortality.

The relationship between smoking and mortality from pulmonary tuberculosis is distinct, but with a disease so influenced by social factors more precise data are needed to justify a direct cause and effect hypothesis.

In the group of diseases and conditions leading to cardiovascular mortality the only cause associated with smoking habits is coronary disease without hypertension, of which the excess mortality is limited to cigarette smokers (a death rate 33 percent greater than the death rate of non-smokers); this association is marked at ages under 55 but it disappears at ages over 75 (where errors in diagnosis may be relatively frequent).

A reduction in coronary disease follows the giving up of smoking but appears to do so somewhat slowly.

The evidence from this and other studies supports the belief that cigarette smoking is one of the causes of coronary thrombosis under the age of 75.

Though the association between smoking and mortality from peptic ulcer is significant it is not very close, and some part of it may well be secondary to other factors, either constitutional or environmental. There is, however, evidence that continued smoking may prevent or delay the healing of a chronic gastric ulcer and thereby it may increase the mortality rate.

Mortality from alcoholism and cirrhosis of the liver is specially high in heavy smokers. Heavy drinkers tend to be also heavy cigarette smokers, and this may well be the explanation of the increased death rate.

With the large group of diseases unrelated in these data to smoking—and comprising 61 percent of the total mortality—the death rates of the several and different smoking categories (with the one exception of continuing heavy cigarette smokers) all lie in an exceedingly narrow range. There appears to be no cause of mortality which is lessened by smoking.

If the excess deaths in smokers under the age of 65 years from (a) cancer of the lung, (b) chronic bronchitis and emphysema, and (c) coronary thrombosis without hypertension be taken as attributable to their cigarette smoking, then the total mortality from all causes at ages 45-64 years is increased thereby by approximately 50 percent.

One of the striking characteristics of British mortality in the last half-century has been the lack of improvement in the death rate of men in middle life. In cigarette smoking may lie one prominent cause.

This work was made possible by the cooperation of the thousands of doctors who completed our two questionaries, and we are most grateful to them for their assistance. We are also indebted to the many doctors who gave us details of the evidence on which their diagnoses were based; to Dr. J. R. Bignall, who advised on the diagnosis in particularly difficult cases; to the British Medical Association, who helped in tracing individual doctors; to the Registrars-General of the United Kingdom and the Registrars of the General Medical Council and its branch councils in Ireland and Scotland, who provided information about doctors' deaths; and to the combined tabulating installation of Her Majesty's Stationery Office, who undertook the mechanical analysis of much of the data. We are grateful also to Miss Margaret Devine, who programmed the more complex data for analysis by the London University Computer Unit's Mercury; to Mrs. Janet Pixner, who carried out the greater part of the calculations; and to Mrs. Jean Gilliland, who was responsible for the onerous work of maintaining and coding the mass of individual records.

References

(1) Doll, R. and A. B. Hill. *Br Med J* 1:1451, 1954.
(2) ———— *Br Med J* 2:1071, 1956.
(3) Berkson, *J Proc Mayo Clin* 34:206, 1956.
(4) Hammond, E. C. and D. Horm. *JAMA* 166:1159, 1294, 1958.
(5) Dorn, H. F. *Public Health Rep* 74:581, 1959.
(6) Report of the Advisory Committee to the Surgeon General of the US Public Health Service. *Smoking and Health.* Public Health Service Publication No. 1103. Washington, D.C., U.S. Government Printing Office, 1964.
(7) Auerbach, O., A. P. Stout, E. C. Hammond, and L. Garfinkel. *New Engl J Med* 267:119, 1962.
(8) Fisher, R. A. *Br Med J* 2:43, 297, 1957.
(9) Doll, R. and A. B. Hill. *Br Med J* 2:1271, 1952.
(10) Fisher, R. A. *Smoking: The Cancer Controversy. Some Attempts to Assess the Evidence.* Edinburgh, Oliver and Boyd, 1959.
(11) Schwartz, D., R. Flamant, J. Lellouch, and P. F. Denoix. *J Natl Cancer Inst* 26:1085, 1961.
(12) Spicer, C. C. To be published, 1964.
(13) Davies, C. N. *Br Med J* 2:410, 1957.
(14) Doll, R. *Br J Cancer* 7:303, 1953.
(15) Wynder, E. L., E. A. Graham, and A. B. Croninger. *Cancer Res* 15:445, 1955.
(16) Roe, F. J. C., M. H. Salaman, and J. Cohen. *Br J Cancer* 13:623, 1959.
(17) Pike, M. C. and F. J. C. Roe. *Br J Cancer* 17:605, 1963.
(18) Roe, F. J. C. and J. Clack. *Br J Cancer* 17:596, 1963.
(19) Goodhart, C. B. *Practitioner* 182:578, 1959.
(20) Case, R. A. M. *Br Med J* 2:987, 1954.
(21) Murphy, D. P. and H. Abbey. *Cancer in Families.* Cambridge, Massachusetts, Harvard University Press, 1959.
(22) Hauge, M. and B. Harvald. *Acta Genet (Basel)* 11:372, 1961.
(23) Schwartz, D., P. F. Denoix, and G. Anguerra. *Bull Ass Fr Cancer* 44:336, 1957.
(24) Wynder, E. L.' I. J. Bross, and E. Day. *Cancer* 9:86, 1956.
(25) Wynder, E. L., I. J. Bross, and R. M. Feldman. *Cancer* 10:1300, 1957.
(26) Wynder, E. L. and I. J. Bross. *Cancer* 14:389, 1961.
(27) Oswald, N. C., J. T. Harold, and W. J. Martin. *Lancet* 2:639, 1953.
(28) Higgins, I. T. T. *Br Med J* 2:1198, 1957.
(29) Olsen, H. C. and J. C. Gilson. *Br Med J* 1:450, 1960.

(30) Fletcher, C. M. and C. M. Tinker. *Br Med J* 1:1491, 1961.
(31) Anderson, D. O. and B. G. Ferris, Jr. *New Engl J Med* 267:787, 1962.
(32) Royal College of Physicians. *Smoking and Health.* London, Pitman, 1962.
(33) Reid, D. D. and A. S. Fairbairn. *Lancet* 1:1147, 1958.
(34) Auerbach, O., A. P. Stout, E. C. Hammond, and L. Garfinkel. *New Engl J Med* 265:253, 1961.
(35) ——————. *New Engl J Med* 269: 1045, 1963.
(36) Hilding, A. C. *New Engl J Med* 254:1155, 1956.
(37) Ballenger, J. J. *New Engl J Med* 263:832, 1960.
(38) Case, R. and A. J. Lea. *Br J Prev Soc Med* 9:62, 1955.
(39) Campbell, A. H. and E. J. Lee. *Br J Dis Chest* 57:113, 1963.
(40) Lowe, C. R. *Br Med J* 2:1081, 1956.
(41) Kissen, D. M. *Health Bull (Edinb)* 18:38, 1960.
(42) Doyle, J. T., T. R. Dawber, W. B. Kannel, A. S. Heslin, and H. A. Kahn. *New Engl J Med* 266:796, 1962.
(43) Buechley, R. W., R. M. Drake, and L. Breslow. *Circulation* 18:1085, 1985.
(44) Schwartz, D., G. Anguera, and J. Lenègre. *Rev Fr Etud Clin Biol* 6:645, 1961.
(45) Pickering, G. W. and P. H. Sanderson. *Clin Sci* 5:275, 1945.
(46) Oram, S. and E. Sowton. *Quart J Med* 32:115, 1963.
(47) Konttinen, A. and M. Rajasalmi. *Br Med J* 1:850, 1963.
(48) Konttinen, A. *Br Med J* 1:1115, 1962.
(49) Acheson, R. M. and W. J. E. Jessop. *Br Med J* 2:1108, 1961.
(50) Kershbaum, A., S. Bellet, E. R. Dickstein, and L. J. Fainberg. *Circ Res* 9:631, 1961.
(51) Mustard, J. F. and E. A. Murphy. *Br Med J* 1:846, 1963.
(52) Seltzer, C. C. *JAMA* 183:639, 1963.
(53) Doll, R., F. A. Jones, and F. Pygott. *Lancet* 1:657, 1958.
(54) Lilienfeld, A. M. *J Natl Cancer Inst* 22:259, 1959.
(55) Eysenck, H. J., M. Tarrant, M. Woolf, and L. England. *Br Med J* 1:1456, 1960.
(56) Kissen, D. M. *Med Offr* 104:365, 1960.
(57) Heath, C. W. *Arch Intern Med* 101:377, 1958.
(58) Lilienfeld, A. M., M. L. Levin, and G. E. Morore. *Arch Intern Med* 98:129, 1956.
(59) Lockwood, K. *Acta Pathol Microbiol Scand* 51 (suppl. 145):1, 1961.
(60) Wynder, E. L., J. Onderdonk, and N. Mantel. *Cancer* 16:1388, 1963.
(61) Brown, R. G., T. McKeown, and A. G. W. Whitfield. *Br J Prev Soc Med* 11:162, 1957.
(62) Karvonen, M., E. Orma, A. Keys, F. Fidanza, and J. Brozek. *Lancet* 1:492, 1959.
(63) Edwards, F., T. McKeown, and A. G. W. Whitfield. *Clin Sci* 18:289, 1959.
(64) Miall, W. E. *Proc WHO Czech Cardiol Soc Symp on Pathogenesis of Essential Hypertension, Prague,* 1960.
(65) Thomas, C. B. *Ann Intern Med* 53:697, 1960.

FINAL REPORT OF A PROSPECTIVE STUDY OF CHILDREN WHOSE MOTHERS HAD RUBELLA IN EARLY PREGNANCY

Mary D. Sheridan[1]

A controlled prospective inquiry regarding the effects of rubella and other virus infections in pregnancy, beginning early in 1950 and ending in December 1952, and sponsored by the Ministry of Health, was fully reported by Manson, Logan, and Loy (1). The total number of pregnancies complicated by rubella available for analysis was 578. The controls numbered 5717. Follow-up of the infants showed that when rubella occurred during the first 16 weeks of pregnancy the incidence of congenital abnormalities in the children was significantly raised. When the infection occurred after the 16th week the incidence of abnormalities in the children of the rubella mothers was no higher than in the controls.

The number of pregnancies complicated by rubella in the first 16 weeks was 279. Of these, 11 ended in abortion and 11 in stillbirth, and 16 children died before 2 years of age, leaving 241 in the original group. A number of medical officers of health continued to send in records of children born in 1953 whose mothers had been notified for rubella before the end of 1952. Since these cases fulfilled the criteria laid down by Logan (2), a further 18 infants whose mothers had rubella in the first 16 weeks of pregnancy were added to the original group. This gave a final total of 259 children available for assessment at 2 years, by which age it had been anticipated that all major abnormalities would have been diagnosed. This examination is designated No. 1 in Table 1.

In order to check the possibility of hitherto unidentified defects, however, full pediatric and otological examination of 57 "early rubella" children and 57 controls living in the London and Middlesex areas was undertaken in 1956-7 by Jackson and Fisch (3), the children concerned being then between the ages of 3 and 6 years. The results of their inquiry indicated that the proportion of children suffering from significant hearing loss had been underestimated at the original examination. It was therefore considered advisable to extend the inquiry to "early rubella" children living in the rest of the country. Reports for 237 children were received and the results were included in the report of Manson et al. (1). This examination is designated No. 2 in Table 1.

Finally, in order to discover how they developed in later childhood a third inquiry was carried out in 1962, when the children were between the ages of 8 and 11 years. The present paper reports the results of this examination, which is designated No. 3 in Table 1, in relation to findings of the previous examinations.

THE REPORT FORM

The medical officers of health were requested to provide the following particulars: (1) Any abnormality of the eyes: visual acuity right and left, distant and near, without and with spectacles if worn. (2) Any abnormality of the ears: hearing right and left for quiet conversational voice without lip-reading at 3 and 10 ft. (0.9 and 3 m.). Also a full pure-tone audiogram. (3) Condition of the heart as reported by a cardiologist or pediatrician. (4) Intelligence quotient, naming testing scale used. (5) Assessment of the child's emotional development and social behavior. (6) Any other pathological condition present. (7) Type of school attended.

A total of 227 completed reports were received. Of the remaining 32, one child had emigrated, the parents of five children refused to participate, and 26 were untraced.

Owing to the wide geographical distribution of cases and the large number of medical examiners concerned, it was inevitable that the reports received were not equally informative, but the general standard of recording was high. Assessment of an abnormality as major or minor on the evidence available sometimes re-

Source: *British Medical Journal* 2:536-539, 1964.
[1] Ministry of Health.

Table 1.ᵃ

Week	No. of children	No. with abnormalities	No. of abnormalities per child	Nature of abnormalities and when first noted
1	11	Major 1	5	Cataracts 1; deafness 2; C. heart 1; subnormality 1; motor handicap 3
		Minor 1	2	Malformed right ear 1, with unilateral deafness 3; undescended testicles 3
2	6	Major 0	—	—
		Minor 1	1	Defective vision 3
3	8	Major 1	1	Congenital heart 1
		Minor 2	1 1	Mild deafness right and left 2. Heart murmur 3
4	16	Major 2	2 1	Cataract left and right squint 1. Severe deafness 2
		Minor 4	2 1 1 1	Mild deafness right and left and heart murmur 3. Deafness right and left 3. Heart murmur 3. Heart murmur 3
5	14	Major 4	3 2 2 1	Cataracts 1; C. heart 3; maladjusted 3. Squint 3; deafness 2. Deafness 2; C. heart 2. Deafness 1
		Minor 1	2	Deafness right and left 3; heart murmur 3
6	5	Major 1	3	D. vision 3; deafness 2; heart murmur 3
		Minor 3	2 2 1	Squint 3; heart murmur 3. Deafness right and left 3; heart murmur 3. Squint 3
7	11	Major 3	4 1 1	Squint with d. vision 1; deafness 3; C. heart 1; undescended testicle 3. C. heart 1. Deafness 1
		Minor 2	1 1	Minor C. heart 1. Heart murmur 3
8	22	Major 5	3 3 2 2 1	Cataract R. 1; deafness 2; C. heart 1. D. vision 3; deafness 1; spasticity 1. Deafness 1; C. heart 1. Pyloric stenosis 1; asthma 1. Deafness 2
		Minor 3	2 2 1	D. vision 3; deafness right and left 3. Deafness 3; squint 3. Unilateral deafness 3
9	14	Major 4	4 4 2 1	Cataract right and left 1; deafness 1; C. heart 1; spastic 1. Cataract left 1; deafness right and left 3; C. heart 1; E.S.N. 3. Cataract left 1; C. heart 1. Duodenal stenosis 1
		Minor —	—	—
10	16	Major 4	1 1 1 1	Deafness 1. Deafness 1. Deafness 1. Pyloric stenosis 1
		Minor 2	1 1	Heart murmur 3. Deafness right and left 3
11	17	Major 1	3	Deafness 3; heart murmur 3; asthma 3
		Minor 0		
12	20	Major 5	3 2 2 1 1	Deafness 2; C. heart 3; aphasia 2. Squint with d. vision 3; deafness 1. Deafness 1; migraine 2. Deafness 2. C. heart 3
		Minor 7	1 1 1 1 1 1 1	Unilateral amblyopia L. 3. Unilateral deafness 2. Unilateral deafness 2. Unilateral deafness 3. Deafness 3. Heart murmur 3. Heart murmur 3
13	16	Major —	—	
		Minor 1	1	Unilateral deafness 3
14	15	Major 0	—	
		Minor 3	2 1 1	Unilateral deafness 3; undescended testicles 3. D. vision 3. Deafness 3
15	24	Major 2	4 2	D. vision 3; deafness 1; E.S.N. 1; undescended testicles 3. Unilateral amblyopia 3; asthma 3
		Minor 6	2 1 1 1 1 1	Deafness 3; heart murmur 3. Unilateral amblyopia 3. Deafness 2. Deafness 2. Heart murmur 3. Heart murmur 3
16	12	Major —	—	
		Minor 1	1	Heart murmur 3
Totals	227	Major 33	Major 15%	
		Minor 37	Minor 16%	

ᵃ The figures 1, 2 and 3 in the last column refer to the number of the examination (see text).

quired much thought, and final classification is necessarily the result of my personal judgment. For this reason, and because there were no controls, it proved difficult to submit the very varied information collected to any sophisticated statistical analysis. It has therefore been decided to present it in tabulated form.

The final outcome of this prospective study has confirmed the findings of previous, mainly retrospective, inquiries regarding the special vulnerability to rubella infection of the eyes, ears, and heart of the developing fetus during the first 16 weeks of pregnancy. It does not, however, bear out the very pessimistic evaluations of attendant risks which have sometimes been offered on the basis of retrospective studies. *Major* abnormalities were present in 33 (15 percent) children, 20 of whom had more than one abnormality. *Minor* abnormalities were noted in 37 (16 percent) children, of whom 9 had another abnormality. In both groups, particularly the latter, it is probable that some of the children included were suffering from conditions unrelated to the rubella infection, al-

though in compiling the tables only those children whose abnormalities were considered from the information available to be certainly or possibly due to rubella have been included. Hence 11 children showing single abnormalities which were either known or thought unlikely to be connected with the maternal rubella infection have been omitted from the tables—that is, two cases of myopia developing in middle childhood, two cases of hearing loss associated with active otitis media, six cases of uncomplicated educational subnormality, and one case of paralytic poliomyelitis.

Table 1 summarizes according to the pregnancy week of rubella infection the number of children at risk, the number showing abnormalities, and the number and nature of the abnormalities occurring in each affected child.

Major Abnormalities.—The number and associations according to week of infection are shown in Table 2.

Minor Abnormalities.—The associations and number of cases are shown in Table 3.

Table 2.

No. of abnormalities	Nature	Week
5	Bilateral cataract, deafness, congenital heart, spasticity, mental defect	1
	Squint, deafness, congenital heart, undescended testicle	7
	Bilateral cataract, deafness, congenital heart, spasticity	9
4	Unilateral cataract, deafness, congenital heart, E.S.N.	9
	Defective vision, deafness, E.S.N., undescended testicles	15
	Bilateral cataract, congenital heart, emotional maladjustment	5
	Defective vision, deafness, heart murmur	6
3	Unilateral cataract, deafness, congenital heart	8
	Defective vision, deafness, spasticity	8
	Deafness, heart murmur, asthma	11
	Deafness, congenital heart, aphasia	12
	Unilateral cataract, paralytic squint	4
	Pyloric stenosis, asthma	8
	Deafness, congenital heart (2 cases)	5, 8
2	Squint, deafness (2 cases)	5, 12
	Unilateral cataract, heart murmur	9
	Deafness, migraine	12
	Unilateral amblyopia, asthma	15
	Deafness (8 cases)	4, 5, 7, 8, 10, 10, 10, 12
Single	Congenital heart (3 cases)	3, 7, 12
	Duodenal stenosis	9
	Pyloric stenosis	10

Table 3.

No. of abnormalities	Nature	No. of cases
2	Malformation of right ear with unilateral deafness, undescended testicles	1
	Bilateral deafness, heart murmur	4
	Squint, heart murmur	1
	Squint, bilateral deafness	1
	Defective vision, bilateral deafness	1
	Unilateral deafness, undescended testicle	1
Single	Squint	1
	Unilateral amblyopia	2
	Defective vision	2
	Bilateral deafness	7
	Unilateral deafness	5
	Congenital heart	1
	Heart murmur	10

EYE DEFECTS

Cataract was noted in seven cases and never as a single abnormality: six of these children had congenital lesions of the heart and five of them were also deaf; the remaining child had a paralytic squint. The cataract was bilateral in three cases and unilateral in four. All seven were associated with infection in the first to ninth week. Visual acuity was recorded for all but 4 of the 227 children: two of these were blind and two were noted as having been successfully operated upon—one for cataract and the other for squint. Squint was noted in seven cases, five of them for the first time at the third examination. Defective vision was noted in eight cases for the first time at the third examination, and unilateral amblyopia was noted three times—one in association with another disability. Some of these visual defects may have been due to causes other than maternal rubella. In the absence of any note to the contrary, it is not possible to differentiate. Nevertheless, the need for continual reassessment before and after school entrance is clearly indicated.

EAR DEFECTS

The inquiry has shown up very clearly the importance of rubella in early pregnancy as a cause of congenital deafness. The cases were associated with infection from the first to the fifteenth week. Pure-tone audiograms as well as the results of clinical voice tests—that is, quiet conversational voice without lip-reading at 3 and 10 ft. (0.9 and 3 m.) right and left were available for 179 (79 percent) children and the results of clinical tests alone were available for 46. The remaining two were attending schools for the deaf, and were incapable of responding to either test. In assessing the audiograms for summary in the tables it was necessary to adopt some standard of classification. It was finally decided that hearing loss over 20 decibels must be shown for at least two adjacent frequencies and the degree of deafness was evaluated as follows: Mild deafness = loss of 20-45 db., moderate deafness = loss of 45-70 db., and severe deafness = loss of 70 + db. On these standards, 43 (19 percent) children had a significant hearing loss: 23 (10 percent) had severe or moderate bilateral deafness necessitating some form of special education; 14 had mild bilateral loss; and 6 had unilateral deafness which was moderate or severe. These last 20 (9 percent) children were able to attend ordinary school, some of them wearing hearing-aids, and others receiving speech therapy or other forms of special help.

No fewer than 17 cases with significant degrees of deafness were noted for the first time at the third examination, and in 10 of these the hearing loss was bilateral. Five of the ten showed a serious loss, three of these five children had additional abnormalities, which had been duly recorded at previous examinations. The need for thorough periodic investigation of the hearing in all children at risk, whether or not there is another presenting abnormality, is obvious. It is, of course, possible that some of these late discoveries were children whose deafness was not due to rubella, but there was no suggestion of other causation in the reports.

Of the 43 children with significant hearing loss 36 audiograms were available. Of the other seven, two were in schools for the deaf, four were in ordinary schools wearing hearing-aids, and one was the multi-handicapped child in hospital. Of the 36 available audiograms, 26 showed a flat loss over the whole speech range and 10 showed curves sloping from left to right—that is, high-tone deafness—thus confirming the original observations of Fisch (4) regarding the audiometric patterns commonly associated with rubella deafness.

HEART DEFECTS

The amount of information available regarding cardiac abnormalities was particularly satisfactory. The report of a cardiologist or consultant pediatrician was available for all except about a dozen children whose attendance at hospital or special clinic had been too difficult to arrange. In these cases the school medical officer had examined the child. Fourteen cases were definitely diagnosed as congenital lesions, the weeks of infection being from 1 to 12. In 10 cases the cardiac lesion was associated with another abnormality; in four it was the sole abnormality noted. Eighteen heart murmurs described as "innocent" or "of no significance" were recorded (16 of them for the first time at the third examination), but it is noteworthy that nine of these (seven of the 16) were associated with another abnormality.

OTHER CONDITIONS

Asthma was noted three times and migraine once, all in association with another abnormality. Four cases of undescended testicles were noted, also in association with another abnormality. Spasticity of the limbs was noted in three cases, and all three children had other handicaps. Two cases of pyloric stenosis and one of duodenal stenosis, which were reported at previous examinations as having been successfully operated upon during infancy, were noted to be doing well.

SOCIAL ADJUSTMENT

It has been suggested that rubella children often show emotional instability and difficult behavior, but although the information was specifically requested there was little supportive evidence in the reports. Twelve children were variously noted as "shy," "immature," "lacking in concentration," or "liable to outbursts of temper," but only one, a blind child, was reported as "psychologically difficult."

INTELLIGENCE

Intelligence quotients were available for 191 (84 percent) children and teachers' assessments for the remaining 36. The testing scales were Terman-Merrill (174), WISC (14), and other standard scales (3). In the circumstances it was thought permissible to combine these to plot a curve of distribution, which is shown in [Figure 1]. It proved to be strikingly normal.

The mean I.Q. was 106.8, with a range of 63 to 160. The teachers' estimates for the remaining 36 were as follows: 27 average, 1 above average, 6 below average, 1 borderline, and 1 mentally handicapped. The number of children concerned, range of I.Q., and teachers' assessment according to the week of maternal rubella are given in Table 4. It is worthy to note that of the 37 children with I.Q.s under 85, or designated "below average," 13 had a significant hearing loss, which raised the question to what extent their lowered performance on tests was due to their sensory disability. Although it is convenient for statistical purposes to record the results of intelligence tests in terms of a numerical I.Q., it needs to be kept in mind that the results of testing (British) handicapped children with intelligence scales standardized on a normal (North American) child population can only be justified clinically by using some such form of words as "the I.Q. is not less than. . . ." It can safely be said that this inquiry has produced no evidence that mental subnormality is a common sequel of early maternal rubella.

EDUCATION

The educational placement of the 227 children is shown in Table 5. Thus 206 (92 percent) of the children were attending ordinary schools. Of these seven (3 percent) are noted as having special provision such as hearing-aids, speech therapy, remedial teaching, etc. Twenty children were attending special schools or classes, including the child whose handicap was the result of paralytic poliomyelitis. The majority of those in special schools were severely deaf. The child receiving home tuition was blind and maladjusted. He had also been operated upon for a congenital heart lesion, a residual murmur being present. The child who was in a hospital for the mentally subnormal had multiple handicaps.

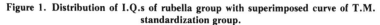

Figure 1. Distribution of I.Q.s of rubella group with superimposed curve of T.M. standardization group.

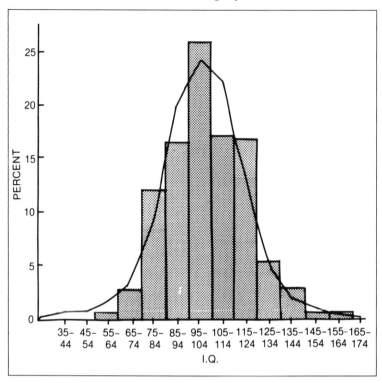

Table 4. Intelligence. Distribution according to time of rubella infection.

| Week | No. of cases | I.Q. | | | Additional assessments |
		Given	Mean	Range	
1	11	9	102	88–141	1 below average, 1 severely subnormal
2	6	4	116	83–131	2 average
3	8	8	110	96–139	
4	16	11	103	80–128	5 average
5	14	13	101	71–150	1 average
6	5	5	112	80–130	
7	11	10	103	80–142	1 average
8	22	19	108	84–134	2 average, 1 borderline
9	14	13	95	63–110	1 average
10	16	11	107	82–160	4 average, 1 below average
11	17	17	107	83–140	
12	20	15	107	70–143	2 average, 3 below average
13	16	14	110	80–133	1 above average, 1 average
14	15	14	103	83–134	1 average
15	24	18	109	70–145	5 average, 1 below average
16	12	10	116	93–143	2 average

[a] I.Q. mean for 191 cases = 106.8.

Table 5.

Ordinary school	199
Ordinary school with special help	7
Special schools or classes, etc.:	
For deaf or partially deaf	15
For partially sighted	1
For speech defectives	1
For E.S.N.	1
Home tuition	1
Hospital for mentally subnormal	1
[P.H. school—paralytic polio (not rubella)	1

BIRTH WEIGHTS

Birth rates were available for 226 of the 227 children. The missing record referred to a (fifth week) child with multiple major abnormalities. The figures (Table 6) show a suggestive trend.

MISSING CASES

In order to complete this record the previous reports of the missing 32 children were scrutinized. Four of them had abnormalities associated with maternal rubella in the first, eighth and eleventh weeks of pregnancy as follows:

Week 1: Severe unilateral deafness noted at second examination.

Week 8: Congenital heart noted at first examination; and at the second examination reported as having had a successful operation at 2½ years.

Week 8: Unilateral deafness noted at second examination.

Week 11: Squint, severe deafness, talipes, and mental subnormality noted at first examination; no record of any second examination.

SEASONAL DISTRIBUTION

It has often been suggested that a larger proportion of handicapped children are born in the months of winter and early spring than in the summer. The months of birth of the 259 early rubella children, with and without abnormalities, are given in Table 7.

Although the larger number of "early rubella" children were born in the months October to February inclusive, reflecting the usual springtime incidence of rubella epidemics, there was no significant difference in the proportion of handicapped and non-handicapped children born at any season of the year.

Table 7. Months of birth for whole series of 259 early rubella children with and without defects.

Month	Normal	Abnormal	Total
January	21	15	36
February	18	3	21
March	6	4	10
April	5	1	6
May	1	1	2
June	2	1	3
July	4	2	6
August	6	5	11
September	21	6	27
October	34	6	40
November	35	18	53
December	32	12	44
Total	185	74	259

Table 6. Birth weight of 226 children.

Children	Mean			Range			
	lb.	oz.	g.	lb. oz.	lb. oz.		g.
Normal (157)	7	2	3230	4 10 –	10 2		2100–4590
With minor abnormalities (37)	6	10	3005	3 13 –	10 6		1730–4705
With major abnormalities (32[a])	6	4½	2850	3 13 –	8 8		1730–3855
With multiple major abnormalities (19)	5	14	2665	4 6 –	8 4		1985–3740

[a] These 32 cases include the 19 with multiple major abnormalities.

SUMMARY

A controlled prospective inquiry regarding mothers who had rubella during the first 16 weeks of pregnancy was begun during 1950-2.

Three follow-up medical examinations of the children resulting from these pregnancies were carried out, the first at 2 years (259 children), the second between 3 and 6 years (237 children), and the third between 8 and 11 years (227 children).

The results of the first two examinations were published by Manson, Logan, and Loy (*1*).

This paper reports the final outcome of the inquiry, with special reference to the findings of the three examinations.

Major abnormalities, mainly of the eye, ear, and heart, occurred in 15 percent of the children, 8 percent having more than one abnormality. Minor abnormalities were present in a further 16 percent, 4 percent having more than one abnormality. These are outside estimates, as it is possible that some of the abnormalities discovered were due to causes other than maternal rubella.

The distribution of intelligence among the children was normal.

The need for long-term follow-up and periodic full reassessment of children known to be at risk from maternal rubella during the first 16 weeks of pregnancy was clearly demonstrated.

This inquiry would not have been possible without the generous help of medical officers of health throughout Britain. Dr. M.A. Heasman, of the Ministry of Health's Medical Statistics Section, kindly prepared the graph for the [Figure].

References

(*1*) Manson, M.M., W.P.D. Logan, and R.M. Loy. *Reports on Public Health and Medical Subjects*, No. 101. London, H.M.S.O., 1960.

(*2*) Logan, W.P.D. *Br Med J* 2:641, 1951.

(*3*) Jackson, A.D.M. and L. Fisch. *Lancet* 2:1241, 1958.

(*4*) Fisch, L. *J Laryng* 69:479, 1955.

RADIATION-RELATED LEUKEMIA IN HIROSHIMA AND NAGASAKI, 1946-1964[1]
I. DISTRIBUTION, INCIDENCE, AND APPEARANCE TIME

O. Joseph Bizzozero, Jr.,[2] Kenneth G. Johnson,[3] and Antonio Ciocco,[4] with the collaboration of Takashi Hoshino, Takashi Itoga, Shigeki Toyoda, and Sho Kawasaki

The role of human exposure to radiation in the genesis of leukemia has been recognized since 1925. In recent times many authors have reported cases of leukemia occurring in irradiated persons (1-14). Several reports of the Atomic Bomb Casualty Commission have verified the development of leukemia at an excessive rate in the survivors of the atomic bombings (15-25). The literature on the relation of ionizing radiation to leukemia has been summarized in the past by others (26-28) and most recently by Miller (29).

The previous findings of the Commission have demonstrated an excess of leukemia developing in those more proximal to the hypocenter at the time of the bombings. This effect was first noted in 1948 and has persisted, with a peak rate observed in 1951. The greatest increase for any specific type was in the incidence of chronic granulocytic leukemia.

This report summarizes the experiences of the Commission in the detection of leukemia during 1946-1964, with particular reference to the rates of occurrence and the time of appearance.

Source: *The New England Journal of Medicine* 274(20): 1095-1101, 1966.

[1] From the Atomic Bomb Casualty Commission, a cooperative research agency of the United States National Academy of Sciences-National Research Council and the Japanese National Institute of Health of the Ministry of Health and Welfare, with funds provided by the United States Atomic Energy Commission, the Japanese National Institute of Health, and the United States Public Health Service. . . .

[2] Surgeon, United States Public Health Service Division of Radiological Health assigned to the Atomic Bomb Casualty Commission.

[3] Chief of Medicine, Atomic Bomb Casualty Commission: associate professor of clinical medicine, Yale University School of Medicine.

[4] Professor of biostatistics and chairman of the Department of Biostatistics, University of Pittsburgh School of Medicine; formerly, chief of statistics, Atomic Bomb Casualty Commission.

MATERIALS AND METHODS

Since its establishment in 1946 the Commission has maintained a continuous surveillance of cases of leukemia occurring in Hiroshima and Nagasaki. In addition, parallel efforts are made to obtain adequate data for evaluating cases of leukemia occurring in survivors of the bombings living outside these cities. Each case of leukemia is carefully investigated and reviewed at frequent intervals by the current investigative and consultant staff. The type of leukemia is decided after review of all available data and material; the certainty of diagnosis, expressed as definite, probable, or possible, is based on established criteria. This program of case finding and review is described elsewhere (30). *Definite leukemia* is defined as follows: cases with good clinical information and a history of well studied and convincing morphologic documentation of the disease by earlier investigators of the Commission even though the material currently is not at hand; cases with good clinical and hematologic material that provide convincing evidence for the diagnosis of leukemia; and cases with morphologic confirmation and a clinical history not inconsistent with leukemia, even though the clinical information is scanty.

The definition of *probable leukemia* is as follows: cases with convincing clinical information for the diagnosis of leukemia but with little or no morphologic material; cases with inadequate clinical information but with good morphologic material consistent with leukemia; cases clinically consistent with the diagnosis and with adequate documentation of morphologic material studied by earlier physicians of the Commission, and cases with adequate clinical and morphologic material in which it is only remotely possible that some other clinical syndrome caused the hematologic abnormality.

The following characteristics are included in the definition of *possible leukemia*: cases with

Table 1. Accuracy of diagnosis in 1098 cases of leukemia, 1946-64.

Diagnosis	Hiroshima no. of cases	Nagasaki no. of cases	Total no. of cases	Percentage
Definite and probable	562	397	959	87.3
Possible	63	66	129	11.7
Information incomplete	4	6	19	1.0

only death-certificate information; cases with inadequate clinical information and no morphologic examination by the Commission; and cases with scanty clinical information and insufficient morphologic evidence for a diagnosis.

During January 1946 through December 1964, 1098 cases of leukemia were recorded at the Commission; 959 (87.3 percent) were definite and probable cases, of which 562 occurred in Hiroshima and 397 in Nagasaki. Possible cases of leukemia and cases with incomplete information numbered 139, or 12.7 percent. Tables 1 and 2 show the distribution of the definite and probable cases according to city, exposure status, and chronicity.

Of the 959 definite and probable cases, 738 occurred in persons born before the atomic bombs were dropped in August 1945, and 221 in persons born after the bombings. The distribution according to year of onset for the 738 persons alive at the time of the bombings is shown in Figure 1.

All data available on these 738 cases have been reviewed to recheck criteria of type of leukemia, date of onset, certainty of diagnosis, exposure status, age, and sex. Pertinent clinical and laboratory data were recorded. We conferred with staff and consultant hematologists regarding problems, and the solution followed

the detection-program procedures of the Commission (*30*).

Month and year of onset of leukemia were determined after a study of all collected data. Acute leukemia produces dramatic changes in the person's health status, permitting more satisfactory dating of its onset than that of chronic leukemia. In any case the date represents the best estimate by a group of hematologists.

The subject's distance in meters from the bomb's hypocenter has proved to be a useful equivalent of radiation dosage in previous studies by the Commission (*22, 24*) and is used here as an index of exposure.

Since 1950 every effort has been made to collect all cases of leukemia in both cities. Previously, emphasis had been on the verification of cases in subjects exposed up to 10 000 meters from the hypocenter. It is possible that some cases of leukemia for the period 1946-1949 were missed in those beyond 10 000 meters or in those who moved into the cities after August 1945.

This report, then, deals principally with 326 cases of leukemia occurring in survivors located up to 10 000 meters from the hypocenter. Two exposure groupings are used, one up to 1500 meters (160 cases), and the second 1501 to 10 000 meters from the hypocenter (166 cases).

Table 2. Exposure category in 959 cases of definite and probable leukemia, 1946-64.

Type of leukemia	City	Distance from hypocenter			Patients born after Aug. 1945
		0-1500 meters	1501-10 000 meters	>10 000 meters	
		no. of cases	*no. of cases*	*no. of cases*	*no. of cases*
Acute	Hiroshima	74	66	171	122
	Nagasaki	30	62	154	89
Chronic	Hiroshima	46	25	52	6
	Nagasaki	10	13	35	4
Total		160	166	412	221

Figure 1. Total cases of leukemia (acute and chronic, definite and probable), Hiroshima and Nagasaki, 1946-1964.

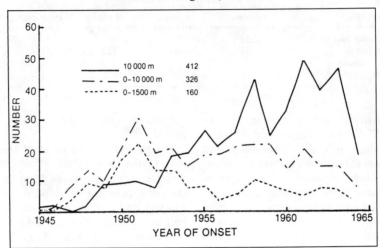

RESULTS

Leukemia in the Group Exposed up to 1500 Meters from the Hypocenter

During 1946-1964, leukemia developed in 160 persons who were up to 1500 meters from the hypocenter (Figure 2). The distribution curve according to year of onset for this exposure group suggests bimodality, with peaking in 1951 and 1958. The separation of these cases according to chronicity demonstrates that the distribution of acute cases appears bimodal (1951, 1958), whereas the distribution curve for chronic leukemia has a broad single peak (1950-1953). The ratio of acute to chronic leukemia in the group up to 1500 meters from the hypocenter was 2.1 in 1951 and 4.1 in 1958. Regrouping these cases before 1956 and after discloses that 64 percent (103) of all cases, 53.8 percent (47) of the chronic cases occurred during 1946-1955. During 1956-1964, 36 percent (57) of all cases, 46.2 percent (48) of acute cases, and 17.5 percent (9) of chronic cases developed.

Figure 2. Definite and probable cases of leukemia among persons within 1500 meters of the hypocenter, Hiroshima and Nagasaki.

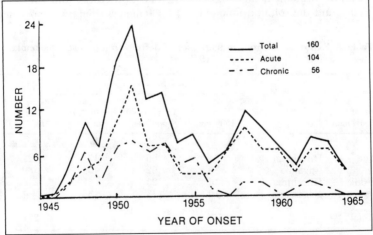

Figure 3. Definite and probable cases of leukemia among persons 1500 to 10 000 meters from the hypocenter, Hiroshima and Nagasaki.

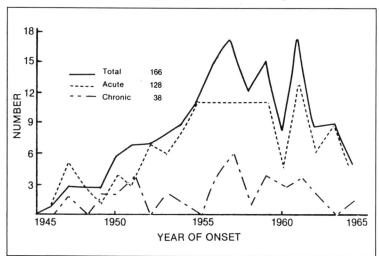

Leukemia in the Group 1501 to 10 000 Meters from the Hypocenter

Leukemia occurred in 166 persons in this group. A distribution curve according to time and chronicity is shown in Figure 3. The increased number of cases occurring between 1956 and 1964 is consistent with the increased spontaneous incidence for all Japan. The distribution in this relatively nonexposed group differs in that most cases and especially those of chronic leukemia in the group up to 1500 meters from the hypocenter occurred during the earlier period, 1946-1954.

In this group during 1946-1955, 36.4 percent (60) of all cases occurred, 36.7 percent (47) of the acute and 35.1 percent (13) of the chronic type. During the second period (1956-1964) 63.5 percent (106) of all cases occurred, 63.3 percent (81) of the acute and 64.9 percent (25) of the chronic type.

The case distribution curves in Figure 4, with special reference to the intervals 1946-1955 and 1956-1964, show that the differences between

Figure 4. Distribution of cases of leukemia according to distance from the hypocenter.

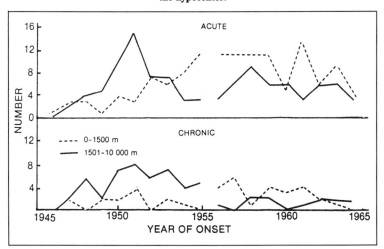

exposure groups were characterized in the early period by greater numbers and a higher proportion of chronic cases in the group up to 1500 meters from the hypocenter. The second period, 1956-1964, is of interest in that the ratio of acute to chronic leukemia in the group up to 1500 meters from the hypocenter is similar to that of the group 1501 to 10 000 meters away. The latter half of each set of curves is similar after 1956.

Leukemia According to Morphologic Type

The distribution of type-specific leukemia (Table 3) shows a larger proportion of acute lymphocytic leukemia in the group up to 1500 meters and a curious increase of monocytic and myelomonocytic leukemia in the group 1501 to 10 000 meters from the hypocenter (the virtual absence of chronic lymphocytic leukemia reflects its extremely low rate in Japan—*31-35*). The distribution in the former is characterized further by 31.8 percent (55 of 160 cases) of chronic granulocytic leukemia as compared with only 20.4 percent (34 of 166 cases) in the latter.

In the group up to 1500 meters from the hypocenter the early peak in 1951 was a mixture of acute and chronic leukemias, but the second peak in 1958 was mainly acute leukemia.

Occurrence of Leukemia in a Defined Population

The Life Span Study (*36*) sample of the Commission (referred to by Heyssel et al.—*24*—as

"Master Sample") consists of approximately 100 000 survivors and nonexposed subjects who were resident in the two cities on October 1, 1950. This population is under continuous surveillance for ascertaining deaths through daily checking of deaths in both cities, receiving all death certificates and periodically checking the *Koseki* (family registry) of each member. Thus, population denominators are available classified according to age at the time of the bombings and exposure status (distance in meters from the hypocenter) for this sample. Among the subjects in this sample who were located up to 10 000 meters from the hypocenter 88 cases of leukemia occurred between 1946 and 1964, with death between 1950 and 1964; of these, 61 were in the group up to 1500 meters and 27 were in the group 1501 to 10 000 meters from the hypocenter. Observations are summarized in Table 4 and Figure 5.

The distribution according to time and types of leukemia is also presented and parallels the observations already made in the analysis of the larger number of cases for the combined populations of the cities.

Estimated Rates of Leukemia in the Exposed Populations

The chief value in studying a defined population is that rates for diseases causing death can be more accurately estimated. Any effort to calculate rates for leukemia for both cities immediately founders on the formidable problem of establishing a population denominator for *all*

Table 3. Total definite and probable cases of leukemia according to type.

Type of leukemia		Distance from hypocenter			
		0-1500 meters		1501-10 000 meters	
		no. of cases	%	*no. of cases*	%
Acute:	Granulocytic	32	30.7	44	34.4
	Lymphocytic	35	33.7	22	17.2
	Monocytic	6	5.8	14	10.9
	Myelomonocytic	6	5.8	17	13.3
	Stem cell	10	9.6	8	6.2
	Unknown	9	8.7	18	14.1
	Other	6	5.8	5	3.9
	Total	104		128	
Chronic:	Granulocytic	55	98.2	34	89.5
	Lymphocytic	0	—	4	10.5
	Other	1	1.8	0	—
	Total	56		38	

Table 4. Leukemia occurring in the Life Span Study sample, 88 cases, according to type.

Type of leukemia		Distance from hypocenter			
		0-1500 meters		1501-10 000 meters	
		no. of cases	*%*	*no. of cases*	*%*
Acute:	Granulocytic	13	34.2	4	22.2
	Lymphocytic	12	31.6	5	27.8
	Monocytic	4	10.5	1	5.5
	Myelomonocytic	3	7.9	4	22.2
	Stem cell	4	10.5	2	11.2
	Unknown	1	2.6	1	5.5
	Other	1	2.6	1	5.5
	Total	38		18	
Chronic:	Granulocytic	22	95.7	9	100.0
	Lymphocytic	0		0	
	Other	1	4.3	0	
	Total	23		9	

persons at risk according to exposure status. Thus, what one sacrifices in dealing with a relatively small number of cases in a defined, continuously surveyed population is regained by the avoidance of a poorly measurable but important factor.

The incidence of leukemia per 100 000 persons for both exposure groups is presented in Table 5. The excessive rate in the group up to 1500 meters from the hypocenter has been observed since 1950, was greatest during 1950-1954 but persists to the present at a relatively high rate. The rates for the other group

are within the spontaneous case rates observed for all Japan (*37*), which have been sharply increasing since 1950. It is wise to consider as an underestimate the yearly rates presented between 1946 and 1949 because the patients involved must have been alive in 1950 to be included in the Life Span Study. The possibility exists that if the Life Span Study sample had been established earlier (that is, in 1945), the rate would have been higher during 1946-1949.

The rate of chronic leukemia in the members of the group up to 1500 meters from the hypocenter who were less than 15 years of age at the

Figure 5. Distribution of leukemia in the Life Span Study sample.

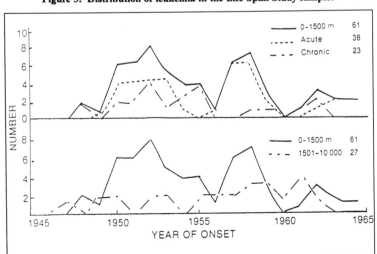

Table 5. Average annual rate of leukemia per 100 000 population in the Life Span Study sample.

Type	Year of onset							
	1946-49		1950-54		1955-1959		1960-1964	
	no. of cases	*rate/ 100 000*	*no. of cases*	*rate/ 100 000*	*no. of cases*	*rate/ 100 000*	*no. of cases*	*rate/ 100 000*
Exposure, 0-1500 meters from hypocenter								
Acute	1	2.07	17	28.21	15	26.24	5	9.24
Chronic	2	4.15	12	19.91	6	10.50	3	9.54
Total	3	6.22	29	48.12	21	36.74	8	14.78
Exposure, 1501-10 000 meters from hypocenter								
Acute	0		4	1.32	10	3.46	4	1.46
Chronic	3	1.24	2	0.66	2	0.69	2	0.73
Total	3	1.24	6	1.98	12	4.15	6	2.20

time of the bombings (Figure 6) invites particular attention since it is clearly excessive and contrasts with a null incidence in the other exposure group (Figure 6). The contrast between groups is not altered appreciably if the group up to 1500 meters is extended to less than 30 years at the time of the bombings. No type-specific leukemia tables are available for Japan, but reference to either a published report by MacMahon and Clark (*38*) of the spontaneous incidence of leukemia during 1943-1952 in the white population of Brooklyn or the general experience of Japanese hematologists confirms the unique nature of this excessive rate of chronic leukemia in persons less than 40 years of age.

Figure 6. Average annual rate, per 100 000 population, of cases of acute and chronic leukemia.

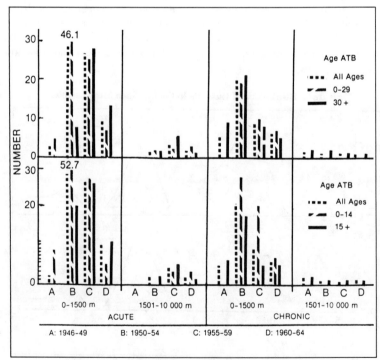

Appearance Time

This term is used to express in years the interval between the age at the time of the bombings and the age at onset—that is, between exposure to radiation and the onset of leukemia (Table 6).

Acute Leukemia. All persons in whom acute leukemia developed who were exposed up to 1500 meters from the hypocenter and who were less than 30 years of age at the time of the bombings had a significantly shorter appearance time (8.6 years for those under 15 and 9.4 for those 15 to 29 years of age) than persons with the same type of leukemia in the sample age group, but exposed between 1501 and 10 000 meters (11.6 years under 15 and 11.6 years 15 to 29 years of age). These differences are statistically significant (p less than 0.025) but are not seen in persons who were 30 years of age and over at the time of the bombings (13 years for those exposed up to 1500 meters and 11.6 years for those 1501 to 10 000 meters from the hypocenter).

Chronic Leukemia. All persons exposed up to 1500 meters in whom chronic leukemia developed experienced a shorter appearance time in all age groups than those with chronic leukemia exposed at greater distances. The probability values for both these groups are statistically significant (p less than 0.005).

The length of appearance time in the group exposed 1501 to 10 000 meters from the hypocenter for both types of leukemia and for all age groups (mean, 11.4 years) is remarkably consistent.

Analysis according to 100-meter bands in the range of 500 to 1500 meters and according to sex has not provided a differential definition of the length of appearance time. A future analysis based on actual estimates of rad dosage related to distance will be attempted when the 1965 revision of radiation dose estimates is available.

DISCUSSION

This report, based as it is on the collected observations of leukemia in the cities of Hiroshima and Nagasaki during the years 1946-1964, affirms the unquestioned role of radiation in leukemogenesis. Heyssel's report (*24*) for the period 1946-1957 has been extended. In this seven-year interval the group exposed within 1500 meters continued to experience an excessive rate of leukemia although the rate has declined since 1959. In general, we have confirmed the findings of this previous study by the Atomic Bomb Casualty Commission. The longer experience and the larger number of cases have permitted a more meaningful computation of incidence, with the Life Span Study serving as a fixed denominator.

The total period of observation (1946-1964) suggests that the radiation effect was more specifically recognizable in the early period (Figures 2 and 3) by the lower ratio of acute to chronic, the presence of chronic leukemia in the young and higher rates of all leukemia in the group exposed within 1500 meters of the hypocenter.

Table 6. Leukemia appearance time according to age at time of bombings and type of leukemia.

Age at time of bombing	Distance from hypocenter							p Value
	0-1500 meters				1501-10 000 meters			
yr.	yr.	no.	variance		yr.	no.	variance	
Acute leukemia:								
0-14	8.6	38	19.9		11.6	36	23.7	<0.005
15-29	9.4	40	22.1		11.6	29	17.1	<0.025
30+	13.0	26	14.3		11.6	63	16.4	N.S.
Chronic leukemia:								
0-29	8.1	30	17.3		11.7	16	18.3	<0.005
50+	7.2	26	10.5		10.3	22	17.8	<0.005

During the second period (1956-1964) the radiation effect appeared to decline. Leukemia by chronicity was similar in both exposure groups. The sole expression of radiation appeared in the higher rate for the group within exposure up to 1500 meters. But the analysis of this second period is complicated by a steep increase in the rate of spontaneous leukemia for all Japan (*37*). This unexplained increase, probably environmental but not radiation in origin, should be affecting the rates in both exposure groups.

The shorter appearance time of leukemia in the group exposed within 1500 meters of the hypocenter is a reflection of the events of the early period. The almost fixed appearance time of the cases in the other group calls attention once again to the possible effects of the demographic phenomenon of a rising leukemia rate.

At no point has the effect of radiation succeeded in the induction of chronic lymphocytic leukemia in our population, in which spontaneous occurrence of this type of leukemia is virtually absent (*31-35*).

It is indicative of progress in the understanding of leukemia and human radiation effects that the unitarian concept of a radiation event producing in time an effect related to dose alone without consideration of other factors is no longer tenable.

Our interpretation of the composite picture of human radiation effects does not allow a simple dependence on the linearity of the dose-response curve. The order of magnitude of freedom or escape from a radiation-related disease, such as leukemia, in persons of the same age and sex groups, similarly exposed, cannot be dismissed without further thought. In this report we have called attention to the age at the time of the bombings as a covariable of distance in the appearance time of leukemia. Our experience of an excess of thyroid neoplasia in females exposed within 1500 meters of the hypocenter would add yet another variable, a discriminatory sex effect (*39*).

A further consideration in the understanding of radiation effect is the recorded cases in human beings of chromosomal damage persisting for months after diagnostic X-ray studies (*40*) and for years after radiotherapy (*41*). Parenthetically, the demonstration of chromosomal aberrations in leukemia (*42*) is an interesting parallel. Thus, one cannot assume that

single exposures to radiation have a limited temporal effect in vivo.

Reports of the association of leukemia with mongolism (*43-46*) and of the genetic or environmental effects of familial and geographic clustering (*29*), as well as mounting support for a viral etiology of leukemia (*29, 47*), strengthen the hypothesis that many factors are involved in the genesis of leukemia.

We interpret the effect of radiation in a human experience such as Hiroshima and Nagasaki, with particular reference to leukemia, as a burden imposed on a human being who had a genetic predisposition to viral and environmental factors, arranged so as to constitute a proclivity for leukemia.

The observations that we have made on appearance time demonstrate that in persons in the youngest age group at the time of the bombings *acute* leukemia developed sooner if they were more proximally exposed, but the proximally exposed in all age groups acquired *chronic* leukemia sooner than those persons distally exposed. Furthermore, the high rate of chronic leukemia in the youngest age group is strikingly different from the usual distribution of spontaneous leukemia and suggests a radiation effect independent of age.

One interpretation of the uniformly decreased appearance time in chronic leukemia is that the effect of radiation is bidirectional, *accelerating* in the older group a common form of leukemia, but *inducing* in the youngest age group a relatively uncommon form of leukemia at a remarkably high rate. In this sense chronic granulocytic leukemia is a more specific type of radiation-induced leukemia.

Assuming genetic homogeneity and the linearity of a radiation effect in acute leukemia, the shift of the appearance time in persons with exposure within 1500 meters but over 30 years of age at the time of the bombings may be ascribed to the combination of increased age and a randomization of environmental factors.

However, the assumption of genetic homogeneity in most human situations is probably invalid. In experimental circumstances the success of producing leukemia varies in genetically different strains of the same species. Upton (*48*) has reported studies on the effects of different genetic strains and age, as well as method of administration of radiation, in the successful induction of leukemia in mice. The human counterpart of this observation of a possible genetic effect has been provided by MacMahon and Levy (*49*) in their demonstration of an excessive rate of leukemia in the twins of patients with leukemia.

The rates of leukemia in the Life Span Study for the two exposure categories and for the periods 1946-1949, 1950-1954, 1955-1959 and 1960-1964, indicating an absolute increase in incidence for those persons exposed within 1500 meters of the hypocenter and the demonstration of a shorter appearance time and, subsequently, earlier development of leukemia for this group, can be construed to mean that radiation accelerated the development of leukemia. The declining rates over time suggest either that the subgroup of persons with the genetic and environmental mosaicism that prefigured the development of leukemia has been consumed, or that a radiation-produced loss of specificity at a cellular level promoting an undirected cellular proliferation has been repaired.

SUMMARY

The observation of the occurrence of leukemia in Hiroshima and Nagasaki for the period 1946-1964 are presented.

During this period leukemia developed excessively in persons exposed within 1500 meters from the hypocenter.

A decreased appearance time, defined as the interval between exposure to radiation and the clinical or symptomatic onset of leukemia, was noted in patients exposed within 1500 meters. Attention is invited to the role of age as a covariable to distance in the appearance time of acute leukemia developing in such persons.

In this group chronic granulocytic leukemia developed in persons up to 29 years of age at the time of the bombings in the period 1946-1955 at a disproportionate rate as compared to the distally exposed and the pattern of spontaneous leukemia for this age group.

We are indebted to our predecessors at the Atomic Bomb Casualty Commission, whose careful labor made this study possible, and especially to the present consultants, Dr. S.C. Finch, of Yale University, Professor M. Tomonaga, of Nagasaki University, and Professor G. Wakisaka, of Kyoto University, and the present staff statisticians, Drs. R.C. Milton and P.G. Archer and Mr. K. Omae, as well as to Mr. G. Day for preparation of the tables and figures.

References

(*1*) Court-Brown, W.M. and J.D. Abbatt. Incidence of leukaemia in ankylosing spondylitis treated with x-rays: Preliminary report. *Lancet* 1:1283-1285, 1955.

(*2*) Court-Brown, W.M. and R. Doll. Leukaemia and aplastic anaemia in patients irradiated for ankylosing spondylitis. *Med Res Coun Spec Rep Series* Number 295. 135 pp. London, Her Majesty's Stationery Office, 1957.

(*3*) Murray, R., P. Heckel, and L.H. Hempelmann. Leukemia in children exposed to ionizing radiation. *New Engl J Med* 261:585-589, 1959.

(*4*) Simpson, C.L., L.H. Hempelmann, and L.M. Fuller. Neoplasia in children treated with x-rays in infancy for thymic enlargement. *Radiology* 64:840-845, 1955.

(*5*) MacMahon, B. Prenatal x-ray exposure and childhood cancer. *J Nat Cancer Inst* 28:1173-1191, 1962.

(*6*) Stewart, A., J. Webb, and D. Hewitt. Survey of childhood malignancies. *Br Med J* 1:1495-1508, 1958.

(*7*) Stewart, A., W. Pennybacker, and R. Barber. Adult leukaemias and diagnostic x-rays. *Br Med J* 2:882-890, 1962.

(*8*) March, H.C. Leukemia in radiologists, ten years later: With review of pertinent evidence for radiation leukemia. *Am J Med Sci* 242:137-149, 1961.

(*9*) Peller, S. and P. Pick. Leukemia and other malignancies in physicians. *Am J Med Sci* 224:154-159, 1952.

(*10*) Ulrich, H. Incidence of leukemia in radiologists. *New Engl J Med* 234:45, 1946.

(*11*) Gunz, F.W. and H.R. Atkinson. Medical radiations and leukaemia: Retrospective survey. *Br Med J* 1:389-393, 1964.

(*12*) Moloney, W.C. Leukemia and exposure of x-ray: Report of 6 cases. *Blood* 14:1137-1142, 1959.

(*13*) Pochin, E.E. Leukaemia following radioiodine treatment of thyrotoxicosis. *Br Med J* 2:1545-1550, 1960.

(*14*) Modan, B. and A.M. Lilienfeld. Polycytemia vera and leukemia—role of radiation treatment: Study of 1222 patients. *Medicine* 44:305-344, 1965.

(*15*) Valentine, W.N. Present status of study of incidence of leukemia among individuals surviving exposure to atomic bomb: Hiroshima and Nagasaki. Progress Report, Atomic Bomb Commission, Hiroshima, Japan, 1951, p. 34.

(*16*) Folley, J.H., W. Borges, and T. Yamawaki. Incidence of leukemia in survivors of atomic bomb in Hiroshima and Nagasaki, Japan. *Am J Med* 13:311-321, 1952.

(*17*) Lange, R.D., W.C. Moloney, and T. Yamawaki. Leukemia in atomic bomb survivors. I. General observations. *Blood* 9:574-585, 1954.

(*18*) Moloney, W.C. and M.A. Kastenbaum. Leukemogenic effects of ionizing radiation on atomic bomb survivors in Hiroshima City. *Science* 121:308, 1955.

(*19*) Moloney, W.C. Leukemia in survivors of atomic bombing. *New Engl J Med* 253:88-90, 1955.

(*20*) Wald, N. Leukemia in Hiroshima City atomic bomb survivors. *Science* 127:699, 1958.

(*21*) Watanabe, S., M. Wago, and T. Ito. Trend in incidence and mortality rate of leukemia among persons who had been exposed to atomic radiation at Hiroshima in 1945. *Acta Haemat Japonica* 21 (Supp. 2):301-308, 1958.

(*22*) Atomic Bomb Casualty Commission. Tomonaga, M., et al. Leukemia in Nagasaki Atomic Bomb Survivors. Technical Report 11-15, Hiroshima, Japan, 1959, pp. 1-72.

(*23*) Heyssel, R.M., et al. Leukemia in Hiroshima atomic bomb survivors. *Blood* 15:313-331, 1960.

(*24*) Brill, A.B., M. Tomonaga, and R.M. Heyssel. Leukemia in man following exposure to ionizing radiation: Summary of findings in Hiroshima and Nagasaki, and comparison with other human experience. *Ann Int Med* 56:590-609, 1962.

(*25*) Moloney, W.C. and R.D. Lange. Leukemia in atomic bomb survivors. II. Observations on early phases of leukemia. *Blood* 9:663-685, 1954.

(*26*) Cronkite, E.P. Etiologic role of radiation in development of leukemia. *Blood* 18:370-376, 1961.

(*27*) Cronkite, E.P., W.C. Moloney, and V.P. Bond. Radiation leukemogenesis: Analysis of problem. *Am J Med* 28:673-682, 1960.

(*28*) Hempelmann, L.H. Epidemiological studies of leukemia in persons exposed to ionizing radiation. *Cancer Research* 20:18-27, 1960.

(*29*) Miller, R.W. Radiation, chromosomes and viruses in etiology of leukemia: Evidence from epidemiological research. *New Engl J Med* 271:30-36, 1964.

(*30*) Atomic Bomb Casualty Commission. Finch, S.C., et al. Detection of Leukemia and Related Disorders, Hiroshima and Nagasaki. Technical Report 5-65, Hiroshima, Japan, 1965, pp. 1-22.

(*31*) Wakisaka, G. Clinical and statistical study of leukemia in Japan, especially in Kinki District. *Acta Haemat Japonica* (Supp.) 21:240-257, 1958.

(*32*) Ota, K. Clinical and statistical study of leukemia in Tokai District. *Acta Haemat* (Supp.) 21:279-285, 1958.

(*33*) Nakajima, A. Statistical and clinical studies on leukemia (Kanto Area)—especially around Tokyo Prefecture. *Acta Haemat Japonica* (Supp.) 21:269-278, 1958.

(*34*) Wakisaka, G. et al. Two cases of chronic lymphocytic leukemia. *Acta Haemat Japonica* 25:109-117, 1962.

(*35*) Wakisaka, G. et al. Present status of leukemia in Japan with special reference to epidemiology and studies of effect of chemotherapy. *Acta Haemat Japonica* 31:214-224, 1964.

(*36*) Atomic Bomb Casualty Commission. Ishida, M. and G.W. Beebe. Research Plan for Joint NIH-ABCC Study of Life Span of A-Bomb Survivors. Technical Report 04-59, Hiroshima, Japan, 1959, pp. 1-89

(*37*) Segi, M., M. Kurihara, and T. Matsuyama. *Cancer Mortality in Japan (1899-1962)*. Sendai, Tohoku University School of Medicine, Department of Public Health, 1965, pp. 14, 23, and 45.

(*38*) MacMahon, B. and D.W. Clark. Incidence of common forms of human leukemia. *Blood* 11:871-881, 1956.

(*39*) Atomic Bomb Casualty Commission. Johnson, K.G. and A. Ciocco. Human Radiation Effects: Report from the Atomic Bomb Casualty Commission. Technical Report 10-65, Hiroshima, Japan, 1965, pp. 1-20.

(*40*) Bloom, A.D. and J.H. Tjio. In vivo effects of diagnostic x-irradiation on human chromosomes. *New Engl J Med* 270:1341-1344, 1964.

(*41*) Court-Brown, W.M., K.E. Buckton, and A.S. McLean. Quantitative studies of chromosome aberrations in man following acute and chronic exposure to X rays and gamma rays. *Lancet* 1:1239-1241, 1965.

(*42*) Gunz, F.S. and P.H. Fitzgerald. Chromosomes and leukemia. *Blood* 23:394-400, 1964.

(*43*) Merrit, D.H. and J.S. Harris. Mongolism and acute leukemia: Report of 4 cases. *J Dis Child* 92:41-44, 1956.

(*44*) Krivit, W. and R.A. Good. Simultaneous occurrence of leukemia and mongolism: Report of four cases. *J Dis Child* 91:218-222, 1956.

(*45*) Krivit, W. and R.A. Good. Simultaneous occurrence of mongolism and leukemia: Report of nationwide survey. *J Dis Child* 94:289-293, 1957.

(*46*) Wald, N., W.H. Borges, C.C. Li, J.H. Turner, and M.C. Harnois. Leukaemia associated with mongolism. *Lancet* 1:1228, 1961.

(*47*) Heath, C.W., Jr. and W.C. Moloney. Familial leukemia: Five cases of acute leukemia in three generations. *New Engl J Med* 272:882-887, 1965.

(*48*) Upton, A.C. Studies on mechanism of leukemogenesis by ionizing radiation. *In* Ciba Foundation Symposium on Carcinogenesis: Mechanisms of Action. Edited by G.E.W. Wolstenholme and M. O'Connor. Boston, Little, Brown, 1959, pp. 249-268.

(*49*) MacMahon, B. and M.A. Levy. Prenatal origin of childhood leukemia: Evidence from twins. *New Engl J Med* 270:1082-1085, 1964.

INCIDENCE AND PREDICTION OF ISCHEMIC HEART DISEASE IN LONDON BUSMEN

J. N. Morris,[1] Aubrey Kagan,[2] D. C. Pattison,[2] M. J. Gardner,[2] P. A. B. Raffle[3]

Between 1956 and 1960 A. K. examined a sample of 687 drivers and male conductors working on London Transport's central buses. The examination included many factors known, or suspected, to be related to the incidence of ischemic heart disease, and about five years later D. C. P. reexamined the men. Ninety-three percent have now been seen (or have died) and useful medical information is available on most of the remainder. During this follow-up we found that ischemic heart disease had developed in 47 of the men. We describe here the incidence of the disease in terms of the observations made at the initial examination and attempt to see how individuals at high and low risk might be predicted.

METHODS

We examined the men in first-aid, or similar rooms, in garages when they came off duty and under conditions as uniform as possible. The examination included a familial, personal, and clinical history, blood-pressure readings, urinalysis, standard 12-lead electrocardiography at rest, measurements of physique and skin fold thickness, and blood-lipid estimations. The 7 percent of the men who have not been directly accounted for were not atypical for any of the variables investigated. All examination findings are confidential between the unit, the men, and, as required, their general practitioners; by agreement of all parties no information on any individual has been disclosed to the London Transport Board.

Criteria of Ischemic Heart Disease

We have classified the disease into four clinical categories and give the number of cases which developed during follow-up.

I: "sudden" death from ischemic heart disease. Death within 24 hours of the first clinical attack. There were seven cases during the five years; in six the diagnosis was confirmed at necropsy.

II: myocardial infarction not "suddenly" fatal. Twenty-seven other men had suffered a typical first infarction as judged by standard clinical and electrocardiographic criteria; three of them died within a few days. In 25 cases diagnosis was confirmed by a consultant in the National Health Service.

III: angina. Questioning elucidated that seven men not included in category II had developed angina of effort during the five years.

IV: Q.QS changes. Six of the men developed these major abnormalities on the electrocardiogram (corresponding to the Minnesota code I_{1-2}, Blackburn et al., *1*); they had no other evidence of ischemic heart disease. Changes were agreed by three observers.

At the initial examination, 20 men were found to have ischemic heart disease of categories II/IV; they have not been considered further in this incidence study. We are dealing therefore with a sample of 667 busmen—who when first examined had no evidence of infarction or angina nor a pathological Q wave—47 of whom developed ischemic heart disease during five years of observation.

RESULTS

Incidence of Ischemic Heart Disease

Age

Six of the 128 men who were in their forties when first examined newly developed the disease (an incidence rate during the period of

Source: *The Lancet.* September 10, 1966, pp. 553-559.

[1] Director, Medical Research Council's Social Medicine Research Unit, The London Hospital, London E.1.

[2] Member, Medical Research Council's Social Medicine Research Unit, The London Hospital, London E.1.

[3] Deputy Chief Medical Officer, London Transport Board, London, S.W.1.

Table 1. Incidence of ischemic heart disease in sample of London busmen during five years, by age at initial examination.[a]

Age (yr.)	No. of new cases in 5 years	No. of men examined	Incidence rate per 100 men in 5 years	No. of man-years of observation	Incidence rate per 100 man-years of observation
30-39	1	32	(3.1)	175	(0.6)
40-49	6	128	4.7	689	0.9
50-59	24	300	8.0	1461	1.6
60-64	13	170	7.6	917	1.4
65-69	3	37	(8.1)	207	(1.4)
Total	47	667	7.0	3449	1.4

[a] Figures in parentheses are incidence rates calculated from very small numbers of cases. All men were born in the British Isles.

observation of 4.7 per 100 men); and so on for other ages (Table 1). The average period of observation was just over five years and most men were seen at four to six years. Thus Table 1 also gives the incidence rates per 100 man-years of observation. These rates are just under a fifth of the former rates and since this was true throughout the analysis they will not be quoted further. (In the tables, we give incidence rates per 100 men during the period of observation described as "five years," though it averaged just over five years.)

Occupation

Table 2 gives incidence rates of ischemic heart disease for conductors and drivers separately. As expected (2, 3), the conductors of these double-decker buses have a lower inci-

dence. This, again as expected, is particularly evident in early middle age but the number of men under 50 is very small.

At the time of their initial examination most of the men had been in the same job for over 20 years; only 4 of the 47 men who developed ischemic heart disease had been driving or conducting for less than 10 years, a fraction typical of the whole sample.

On average, drivers earned only a few shillings per week more than conductors and standards of living are thus about the same.

Blood Pressure

The incidence is strongly associated with the casual systolic blood pressure (S.B.P.). This was taken very soon after the man entered the examination room and while he was sitting. We

Table 2. Incidence of ischemic heart disease in conductors and drivers during five years, by age at initial examination.

Age (yr.)	Conductors			Drivers		
	No. of new cases in 5 years	No. of men examined	Incidence rate per 100 men in 5 years	No. of new cases in 5 years	No. of men examined	Incidence rate per 100 men in 5 years
30-39	0	7	—	1	25	(4.0)
40-49	1	62	(1.6)	5	66	7.6
50-59	6	117	5.1	18	183	9.8
60-69	5	68	7.4	11	139	7.9
Total	12	254	4.7	35	413	8.5[a]

[a] When standardized on the age structure of the conductors this was 8.6 per 100 men in 5 years.

Allowing for consistency by age, $p<0.05$, for occupational difference.

The rates per 100 man-years of observation were 0.9 in the conductors and 1.7 in the drivers, the drivers' rate again being standardized for age.

used the same standard manual mercury sphygmomanometer (cuff 14 cm.) throughout, and read the levels to the nearest even number.

We divided the drivers into four groups, by using the quartile points of the distribution of casual systolic B.P. for each 10-year age group to produce as nearly equal "quarters" as possible. Thus (Table 3) the drivers in the top quarters had levels over 153 mm Hg at ages 40–49; over 171 at 50–59; and over 175 at 60–69; these drivers may be considered to have "high" blood pressure. We divided the conductors in the same way. Next, we identified the new cases of ischemic heart disease within the quarters; the results are shown in Table 3. There are 23 in the "high" quarters (last column of the Table) and 6 in the "low" quarters. The incidence among the hypertensive men (those in the "high" quarters), is several times that in the "low" quarters. Grouping the men into quarters is a useful, if arbitrary, way of handling the data, but the number of new cases did not permit a finer breakdown.

Figure 1a gives the incidence in terms of casual systolic B.P. for all the men, regardless of age or occupation.

Again there were 23 in the "high" quarter and 6 in the "low"; the net result of the distribution of new cases is the same as in Table 3. This is so, with only minor differences, throughout the analysis and further results are simplified as in Figure 1a.

Systolic and diastolic B.P. in middle age are highly correlated, but the casual diastolic reading by itself is not quite so effective a predictor,

the number of new cases from high to low quarters being: 19, 16, 5, and 7. B.P. was also taken at rest and after mild exercise; simple combinations of these various pressures, for example by adding the three systolic or diastolic readings together, have not been more powerful in identifying future ischemic heart disease than the casual systolic (or diastolic) reading alone.

Very few of the men in the high quarters of S.B.P. distributions initially had any symptoms referable (even with hindsight) to the cardiovascular system and, of course, none showed evidence of ischemic heart disease. No systematic search was made for "secondary" hypertension other than analysis for proteinuria.

Blood Pressure and Occupation

There are two connections between S.B.P., occupation, and ischemic heart disease. Drivers aged over 50 have higher S.B.P. than conductors—higher average pressures and more men with "high" pressures (Table 3). This is a factor, therefore, in the higher incidence of the disease among drivers. Secondly, there is an indication that at the same level of S.B.P. drivers have a higher incidence than conductors (Table 4).

Incidence in Relation to Initial Blood-lipid Levels

We took a sample of blood from each man and the Courtauld Institute made various estimations for us. The plasma was analyzed by the micromethod 10 of Cohn et al. (5) into fractions containing the α and β lipoproteins. Cholesterol in these fractions and in the origi-

Table 3. Incidence of ischemic heart disease in conductors and drivers during five years, by age and casual systolic blood-pressure level at initial examination.

Quarter	No. of new cases among conductors aged:				No. of new cases among drivers aged:				All busmen	
	40–49	50–59	60–69	40–69	40–49	50–59	60–69	40–69	No.	No. of cases
High	1	2	2	5	1	10	7	18	168	23
Second	0	2	0	2	1	3	2	6	165	8
Third	0	2	1	3	1	3	2	6	164	10[a]
Low	0	0	2	2	2	2	0	4	167	6
Total	1	6	5	12	5	18	11	34	664[b]	47

The quartile points (mm. Hg) for each column were, from high to low: (1) 153, 137, 125; (2) 161, 143, 131; (3) 165, 153, 143; (4) 153, 135, 125; (5) 171, 153, 137; and (6) 175, 159, 145.

[a] 1 case was aged 39, a driver, systolic B.P. 128 mm. Hg.

[b] The casual pressure of 3 men was not recorded.

Figure 1. Incidence of ischemic heart disease in sample of London busmen during 5 years by findings at initial examination: (a) By casual systolic B.P. (664 men); P < 0.001. (b) By total plasma cholesterol (607 men); P < 0.001. (c) By stature (663 men); P < 0.1. (d) By skin-fold thickness at right suprailiac crest (658 men); P < 0.2. Probability levels in figures 1, 3, and 4 have been calculated using a test for trend in proportions (4).

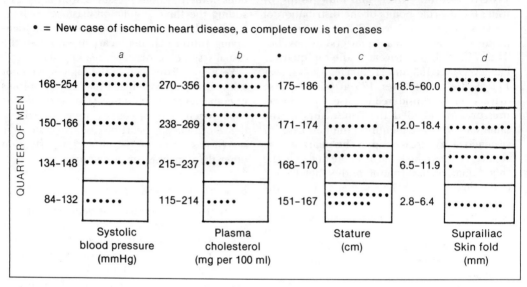

Table 4. Incidence of ischemic heart disease in conductors and drivers during five years, by casual systolic blood pressure level at initial examination.

Quarters of casual systolic B.P. (mm. Hg)	Age-standardized[a] incidence rate per 100 men in 5 years		
	Conductors	Drivers	Total busmen
168–254	8.5	15	13[b]
150–166			4.7
134–148	3.9	5.6	5.7 ⎫ 4.9[b]
84–132			4.1

664 men.

[a] Standardization by indirect method.

[b] "Morbidity ratios" are 190 ± 40 and 69 ± 14.

There was 1 case among the 7 conductors whose systolic B.P. was 200 mm. Hg and over, and 2 among the 16 such drivers.

nal plasma was determined by the Liebermann-Burchard reaction as described by Dodds and Mills (6). Total plasma-cholesterol in 607 men—measured regardless of season of year, time of day, or time of last meal—is a good predictor (Figure 1b), with 19 new cases in the high quarter and 5 in the low. β-lipoprotein cholesterol seems to be the effective fraction—19, 11, 6, and 3 new cases occurring in the quarters from high to low—but the number of estima-

tions was less again (544 men). With α-lipoprotein cholesterol the figures are 6 cases in the high quarter, then 10, 14, and 9 in the other quarters. The very low density lipoproteins, $S_f 20$–400, that carry much of the plasma-triglyceride (7) were also estimated. They showed an inconsistent trend with incidence of ischemic heart disease; we will report when more cases have accumulated.

Drivers have substantially higher blood-lipid levels than do conductors of the same age, and this is another factor in the higher incidence of ischemic heart disease in the drivers.

These connections between age, occupation, S.B.P., and blood-lipid levels and the subsequent incidence of ischemic heart disease are the main findings; we report briefly on five others, none of them statistically significant.

Parental Mortality. The circumstances of the examination were not suitable for taking a detailed family history of health but we did try to get information on age of parents at death (8). The 5 years' incidence of ischemic heart disease is 9.1 per 100 among busmen one or both of whose parents died at 40–64 (they are later described as "positive" in this respect), and 5.9 per 100 in men whose parents lived to age 65.

Stature. The incidence of ischemic heart disease is greatest among the shortest men (Figure 1c), and the same is true measuring "sitting-height." Gertler and White (*9*) have noted this association. There is no excess of high s.b.p. among the 160 shortest men, but the 40 hypertensive (as defined) in this group have a particularly high incidence—with 10 new cases, compared to 7 in the other 120 men of similar height. The short hypertensive men who developed the disease were not particularly obese, nor did they have especially high blood-cholesterol levels.

Obesity. We measured skin fold thickness at three sites (the triceps, subscapular, and suprailiac) on the right side of the body, using a Harpenden calliper (*10*). There is a trend for increasing incidence of ischemic heart disease with increasing fatness; this is most striking for the skin fold thickness at the suprailiac crest (Figure 1d).

Cigarette Smoking. Unfortunately, the number of men who had never smoked cigarettes was small (45 of the 667 in the sample). But cigarette smokers at the time of the initial examination do show a greater incidence of ischemic heart disease than all current nonsmokers—7.9 and 4.7 per 100 men, respectively.

Electrocardiographic Abnormalities at Initial Examination. The electrocardiogram was taken at rest using a portable direct writer (Phillips). We consider three types of change to be important while not acceptable as ischemic heart disease. Abnormalities (Minnesota code) were noted in 68 cases as follows: 59 cases with st depression and/or t-wave flattening or inversion (IV$_{1-3}$, V$_{1-3}$); 6 cases with left ventricular preponderance with st/t wave changes as above (III$_1$); and 3 cases with left bundle-branch block (VII$_1$). Three observers agreed on these findings.

When first seen, then, 68 of the men presented such abnormality without evidence of ischemic heart disease. Eight of them (12 percent) subsequently developed the disease compared with 6.5 percent of the 599 men who did not show such changes.

In the 599 men, we include 37 with miscellaneous electrocardiographic changes of left ventricular hypertrophy, right bundle-branch block, sinus arrhythmia, etc. As a group these men show about the same incidence of ischemic heart disease during the 5 years as the rest of the 599 men; numbers are too small for calculations to be done for individual abnormalities.

Other Factors. Many other factors were examined and found to have no or negligible relationship, taken singly or in various combinations, to the development of ischemic heart disease. These include body-weight, relative weight, ponderal index, arm circumference, waist, biacromial diameter, chest expansion, hemoglobin level, civil state, number of siblings and children, social class of father, and alcohol consumption. We will not mention these further.

Multiple Factors and Individual Risk

Levels of s.b.p. and plasma-cholesterol thus stand out as predictors of the incidence of ischemic heart disease. The correlation between s.b.p. and plasma-cholesterol is low ($r = +0.28$ for 604 men) and many men with "high" levels of one have "low" levels of the other. Together (Figure 2) "high" levels of s.b.p. or cholesterol contain about three-quarters of the new cases of ischemic heart disease. For this population, therefore, we may postulate that the 40 percent of the men with either level "high" (or both) contain the epidemic disease. These 34 new cases occurred among 240 men; their *individual risk* of having ischemic heart disease within the five years is thus 1 in 7 (and almost exactly the same on life-table calculation for the varying periods of follow-up). We attempted next to improve prediction of individual risk by considering actual values of s.b.p. and cholesterol and not merely the quarter of the distribution in which they occurred; and by including at the same time the other seven factors reported. Several investigations have shown these to be relevant; in the present study they behave as postulated. All the factors are interrelated, moreover, so this aspect must also be examined. Many of the interrelationships—e.g., the strong connection between obesity, blood-lipids and b.p.—are interesting but will not be considered further here. Our concern is with net effects on the incidence of ischemic heart disease.

Discriminant Analysis

We adopted the method of linear discriminant function analysis (*11, 12*). Multivariate analysis of a large set of data is more practicable now that there is direct access to electronic computers and some library programs are available. In discriminant analysis, a single "score," based on the observed values of factors, is given to

Figure 2. Incidence of ischemic heart disease in London busmen during 5 years of casual systolic B.P. and plasma cholesterol at initial examination (604 men; P < 0.0001).

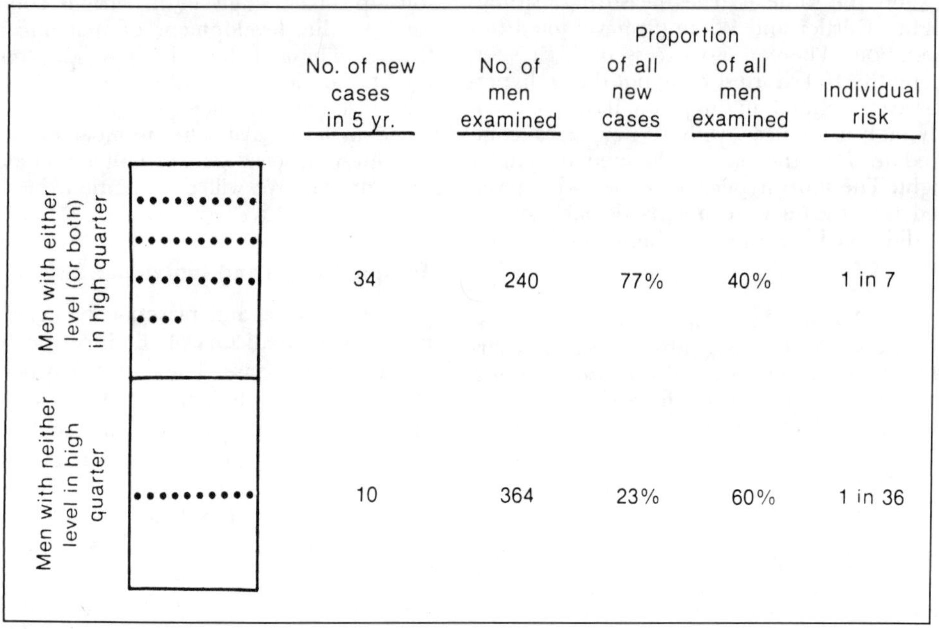

	No. of new cases in 5 yr.	No. of men examined	Proportion of all new cases	of all men examined	Individual risk
Men with either level (or both) in high quarter	34	240	77%	40%	1 in 7
Men with neither level in high quarter	10	364	23%	60%	1 in 36

each man. In this instance, the score is a measure in terms of the factors studied of an individual's risk of developing ischemic heart disease, and is calculated as a weighted addition of their values. The weights are determined to produce as small a range of scores as possible within each of the two groups (with or without the disease) and as little overlap as possible between the groups. The efficiency of the discriminant score for selecting men at greater or lesser risk will be evident to the degree that the new cases have higher values than the remainder; its efficiency diminishes the more the scores for the two groups overlap. The more efficient the score in this sense, the better will it be as a predictor of the small group of men (*a*), who are at a particularly high risk (*b*), and among whom the majority of the future cases in the population will occur (*c*). At present in the U.K., about 20 percent of men, we may estimate, develop clinical ischemic heart disease during middle age; in these terms the group is small. (*a*), (*b*), and (*c*) are related, each is a function of the other two (the argument is briefly set out in an appendix to this article).

Theoretical requirements of the mathematical model underlying the technique of discriminant analysis are not strictly met in the present exercise. Thus, the distribution of s.b.p. is not normal but skewed; logarithmic transformation while overcoming this makes little difference to the power of the discriminant. Moreover, "qualitative" factors, for example whether a man was driver or conductor at the initial examination, had to be included and "quantified." But we went ahead on the grounds that the first essential of any tool is that it should be useful and, of the multivariate techniques now available, the discriminant seems the best for the particular question we are asking.

We cannot include all our men in this analysis because data on some of them are incomplete. The nine factors already considered are completely specified for 593 men, 43 of whom developed ischemic heart disease. These factors are:

(X_1) Age (in years) at first examination.
(X_2) History of parental mortality in middle age (negative 0, positive 1).
(X_3) Stature (cm.).
(X_4) Skin fold thickness at suprailiac crest (mm.).
(X_5) Occupation (conductor 0, driver 1).

(X_6) Current cigarette smoking (nonsmoker 0, smoker 1).

(X_7) Casual systolic b.p. (mm. Hg).

(X_8) Total plasma-cholesterol (mg per 100 ml).

(X_9) Non-ischemic electrocardiographic abnormality of the three types described (absent 0, present 1).

It is helpful at this point to think of the natural history of a chronic disease like ischemic heart disease in "stages" (*3*). Thus it is possible to postulate:

(1) the *causes* in inheritance, experience, and mode of life;
(2) the *precursor* pathology, as causes begin to show effects in disturbed function and structure, without as yet any evidence of the disease; then comes the
(3) *early incidence* as disease, possibly reversible, appears; and so on to established and advanced disease, etc.

Several postulated *causes* of ischemic heart disease are included in our study, and two evident *precursors*—high levels of b.p. and plasma-cholesterol—the minor electrocardiographic abnormalities may be regarded as *early disease*.

So we organized these factors to give some picture of *causes* (X_1-X_6), *precursors* (X_7 and X_8), and *early disease* (X_9).

We consider the *causes* first. By obtaining a weighted score (as described) from factors X_1-X_6, we sought to combine their individual predictive powers in an effective way; at the same time the method indicates the extent to which the factors are contributing independently—this is essential in view of known interrelationships, for example of age, obesity, and occupation. We calculated a score for each of the 593 men, divided them into "quarters" of about 150 and identified the number of new cases occurring in each. Figure 3a shows that these *causes* by themselves go some way to building a predictive device: the individual risk of a man with a high score is several times greater than that of a man with a low score. Occupation is the most powerful of these *causes;* stature and obesity contribute little to the prediction in the presence of the other factors.

Next we produced a score, using only the measurements of s.b.p. and plasma-cholesterol. The equation shows the weights attaching to the two factors and how the score is obtained:

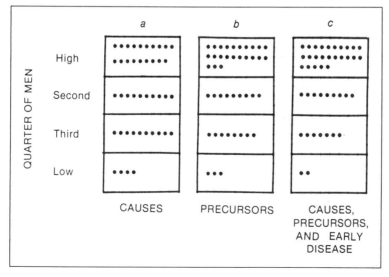

Figure 3. Incidence of ischemic heart disease in London busmen during 5 years by findings at initial examination. Quarters of men identified by linear discriminant function analysis including stated factors (see text). (a) *Causes* (X_1-X_6); P < 0.01. (b) *Precursors* (X_7-X_8); P < 0.0001. (c) *Causes*, *precursors*, and *early disease* (X_1-X_9); P < 0.00001. 593 men.

Score = 0.139 × systolic B.P. (mm Hg) + 0.055 × cholesterol (mg per 100 ml) − 34.1.[4]

The standard errors of the weights are 0.045 for s.b.p., and 0.025 for plasma-cholesterol; each factor is therefore contributing significantly ($p < 0.01$ and $p < 0.05$, respectively) to the discriminant function. Men with higher levels of each of these *precursors* have a greater risk, men with lower levels a lesser risk of developing ischemic heart disease. The quartile points of the distribution of the combined score are − 3.3, − 0.3, and + 3.1, the lowest score is − 13.9 (a man with systolic B.P. of 100 mm Hg and plasma-cholesterol of 115 mg per 100 ml) and the highest + 16.8 (240 mm Hg, 319 mg per 100 ml). The distribution of new cases of ischemic heart disease is shown in Figure 3b: over half the cases occurred in the quarter of men with highest scores.

Figure 3c combines these *causes, precursors,* and *early disease.* Individual prediction is now a little more effective again: 25 new cases were among the men with high scores; about 1 in 6 of

them developed ischemic heart disease. Dividing the men into five groups (instead of four) for all these factors, yields 21, 10, 6, 6, and 0 new cases in each. If we extend this process to six groups of about a hundred men, there are 18 new cases in the group with highest scores, then 9, 7, 5, 4, and 0 in the remainder. *Early disease* (X_9) contributes very little.

One point is clear: the levels of s.b.p. and plasma-cholesterol predominate, and adding the other factors achieves little net improvement in prediction. Comparing Figures 3b and 3c, it seems that these *causes* (occupation, obesity, and the rest), operate largely through these *precursors.* Moreover, comparing Figures 3a and 3b, and in light of their many known and demonstrated connections, it seems that much of the predictive power of these *precursors* is due to these *causes.*

Finally, for the moment, we contrast in "profile" the sizable groups of men placed (Figure 3c) in opposite quarters of risk by scores based on all the factors. In terms of these factors, and of the occurrence of new cases of ischemic heart disease, the men in the "low" and "high" quarters are very different (Table 5). In detail, for instance, 37 of the 46 busmen having a casual systolic B.P. reading less than 120 mm Hg are in the "low" group as are 63 of the 88 men with cholesterol levels under 200 mg per 100 ml.

---

[4] The effect of the constant (− 34.1) in the equation is that the average score for all the men is 0. Transforming both factors to the same scale (i.e., adjusting to the same mean and variance) to compare their independent contributions, produces weights of 3.36 and 2.37, respectively, both having a standard error of 1.10. These weights are not significantly different.

Table 5. Profile of "low" and "high" quarters of the sample of London busmen for risk of developing ischemic heart disease during five years.

		Quarter of men	
	Finding at initial examination	At "low" risk (n = 150)	At "high" risk (n = 147)
X_1	Mean age (yr.)	52	58
X_2 {	Parental mortality (−)	71%	37%
	Parental mortality (+)	29%	63%
X_3	Mean stature (cm.)	173	170
X_4	Mean suprailiac skin fold (mm.)	11	17
X_5 {	Conductors	59%	17%
	Drivers	41%	83%
X_6 {	Non-cigarette smokers	37%	15%
	Smokers	63%	85%
X_7	Mean casual systolic B.P. (mm. Hg)	131	176
X_8	Mean plasma-cholesterol (mg. per 100 ml.)	205	272
X_9	Non-ischemic electrocardiograph abnormalities: Absent	96%	77%
	Present	4%	23%
	No. of new cases	2	25
	Incidence rate per 100 men in 5 years	(1.3)	17
	Individual risk	1 in 75	1 in 6

There are many older drivers, smokers, men who are fat and have a bad family history in the "high" group; and there are many thin conductors with a good family history and an unblemished electrocardiograph in the "low" group. Individually, there are interesting placements of men with high S.B.P. or plasma-cholesterol in the "low" group (none of these men have developed ischemic heart disease) through the compensating advantages in other factors. In this way we can move towards a picture of the individual who is susceptible to ischemic heart disease and, equally interesting though not elaborated here, the individual least likely to develop the disease.

DISCUSSION

We comment briefly that these results though limited in themselves are strongly in line with much American work (*6, 13-20*). Our findings illustrate two advantages of prospective studies of incidence. Thus, 10 of the 47 new cases were rapidly fatal, and liable to be missed in a cross-sectional survey at any one time. Moreover, 6 of the 47 new events had silent Q-wave abnormality only, compared to 9 of the 20 cases found at the initial examination. The method of sampling (*21*) excluded men absent from work because of their first clinical attack of ischemic heart disease; these could have added only another 1-3 cases, probably with acute infarction, to the original 20. In this population, therefore, the clinical pictures of incidence and prevalence are very different. Secondly, the predictive value of any factor, such as B.P., for the development of ischemic heart disease can only be demonstrated prospectively. It is also interesting that hypertension is particularly related to the incidence of rapidly fatal infarction. Of 10 men who died within a few days, 8 were hypertensive for their age, but there were only 7 hypertensive men among the 24 with less severe infarction. Adequate study of the association of risk factors with type of disease will need more cases; comparison of these findings with the American likewise must wait.

Figure 3 demonstrates some of the possibilities of "explaining" the occurrence of epidemic ischemic heart disease in middle-aged men: but greater explanation can be expected all along the front. Thus, Figure 3a surely understates the position on *causes*. The number of men is small, especially those aged under 50, but apart from this, the data do little justice to the cigarette smoking (*22*) or the genetic (*23*) contributions to the etiology; and the "personality" factor is virtually ignored (if the findings of Rosenman et al., *24*, are confirmed, this last may prove to be a major gap). The observations take a step further the hypothesis that physical activity of occupation is a protection against ischemic heart disease. The levels of S.B.P. and blood-lipids seem to be importantly involved: middle-aged conductors have lower levels of both. But, even in this instance, it may be questioned whether this is the best test of the hypothesis, whether bus conductors are typical of "active" workers—they seem to have almost as high an incidence of ischemic heart disease as physicians (*25*). Such studies need to be repeated on general population samples, including physically active occupations without the particular nervous strains of bus-conducting. We ignored nutrition, but in the present study it seems to play no part in determining casual blood-lipid levels (*26*), nor is there much evidence for its effect on B.P. The diet of drivers and conductors is very similar, although conductors eat more calories per lb body-weight (*27*).

At the stage of measurement of *precursors*, also, better methods can be expected. β-lipoprotein cholesterol may yet prove a more powerful predictor than total cholesterol. Casual S.B.P., which is proving so predictive, is at present measured crudely; perhaps this can be remedied (*28*), though it could be that its usefulness lies in the way it is measured at present. Adjusting B.P. for arm-circumference and body-weight (*29*) makes very little difference to our findings. Factors not included may also be useful predictors—e.g., blood-sugar (*18*). Of 15 busmen with glycosuria at the initial examination, 1 has developed ischemic heart disease, but no loading tests were done. Similarly, the attempt to detect *early disease* should include a challenge (*30, 31*).

More powerful prediction thus will probably come, as also may easier methods (although the tests used at present could readily be done in a few minutes by any doctor, or his auxiliary, with the backing of a modern laboratory). At the most elementary stage of all—the diagnosis of the disease—there is much scope for improvement. We used a clinical rather than epidemiological approach *(32).* And at the other end, better mathematical models will surely come; the linear discriminant function (designed for addition of normally distributed variables exerting direct effects) by no means simulates what is already known of the natural history of ischemic heart disease. The results of the present exercise are interesting enough, but the inadequacy of the model is evident in the very modest improvement of prediction achieved by Figure 3 over the simple sums in Figure 2.

In conclusion we raise some larger issues. There is a new optimism that the modern epidemic of ischemic heart disease of middle age can be controlled. In the first place, investigators are adjusting themselves to the idea of "multiple causes"—their existence, identity, how they connect, and that conceivably there is no essential cause except perhaps for some threshold of nutrition which must be reached. Public health campaigns relating to these causes—e.g., education on the dangers of cigarette smoking or on the need for sedentary workers to take regular exercise—could be effective. But the dominant hope today is that action at the stage of precursor pathology (hypertension and hypercholesterolemia in particular) may still achieve true primary prevention. Individuals shown to be susceptible will be identified and prophylactic measures directed at them. Prevention will be translated into the clinical field.

In these terms, three-quarters of the total incidence (Figure 2) is already a worthwhile prediction: this is the main community problem. Reduction of disease in this high-risk group to that of the remainder would reduce the overall incidence among the busmen by about half. And an individual risk over five years of one in seven (about five times that of the remainder) is already serious enough to warrant attempts at individual prevention. Moreover, the prediction is for the next five years only. Trends of vascular disease with age suggest that the incidence in a further five-year period will be the same at least: the high individual risk may eventually become one in three, or even more, for the whole span of middle age. In the long run, the number of "false-positives" treated on such a simple method of identifying susceptibles might not be unreasonably large. Cerebrovascular disease has also to be considered. Even in middle age numbers are appreciable,

and its incidence is strongly connected with levels of s.b.p. if not of blood-lipids. Figure 4 shows the five-year incidence of recognized new major vascular disease in these busmen relative to initial systolic B.P. Since clinical ischemic disease is so common—affecting perhaps 20 percent of middle-aged men—it has to be recognized that individual approaches to its prevention are likely to have only a limited place. The approach to all who are clearly susceptible would involve more than 20 percent of middle-aged men and so, with foreseeable methods of prevention, would be impracticable. It seems likely that the eventual approach will be to combine mass campaigns with personal treatment for special individuals—e.g., those who can be identified as early candidates for the disease, or the most severe disease, for example.

So the grand question is whether reduction of symptomless hypertension and hypercholesterolemia from early middle age will re-

Figure 4. Incidence of cardiovascular disease in London busmen during 5 years by casual systolic B.P. level at initial examination. (664 men; P < 0.00001.) Age-standardized incidence rates per 100 men in 5 years in the four quarters are 22.3, 7.6, 9.2, and 5.2 from "high" to "low." Two men developed two conditions, but are counted only once.

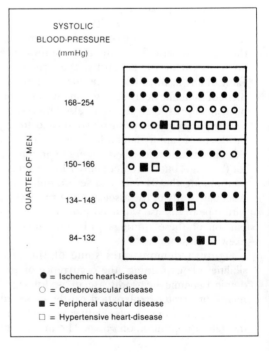

duce the subsequent incidence of ischemic heart disease. There are signs of acceptable means of lowering high blood-cholesterol, and a trial is under way to discover whether there is any advantage for an otherwise healthy population in doing so. To assess the prophylactic value of long-term lowering of mild and moderate hypertension by large-scale experiment is now an urgent task for preventive medicine, though it is doubtful if any of the available agents are suitable. The tantalizing situation today in ischemic heart disease is that the main causes probably are known, and the main mechanisms also. But how to prove it, and benefit from the knowledge? Preventive studies on an adequate scale if only they can be organized—and they give rise to quite new issues for medicine and the public—could give the answer. In a situation where animal experiment is progressing so slowly, and where multiple interrelated factors render human observation so difficult to interpret, no other method is in sight for getting an answer. Such studies in the free-living population could have tremendous theoretical importance in determining whether the evident precursors are in fact important mechanisms of the disease, in distinguishing causes from mere association, and in assessing the roles of inheritance, experience, and mode of life in the modern epidemic of ischemic heart disease.

SUMMARY

A sample of 667 middle-aged London busmen who showed no evidence of ischemic heart disease when first examined were followed up for five years. During this period 47 of them developed the disease—an incidence rate of seven percent. The incidence is higher in later than in early middle age, in men with a bad family history of parental death, in drivers than conductors, in cigarette smokers, in the more obese, and in the shortest men.

Levels of casual systolic blood-pressure (s.b.p.) and of plasma-cholesterol are, however, the predominant predictive factors. Three-quarters of the new cases were among the men who were in the top quarter of the distribution of either s.b.p. or plasma-cholesterol. The risk, during five years, for such an individual of developing the disease was about one in seven—several times the risk for the remainder.

The *causes* studied strongly affect the levels of s.b.p. and plasma-cholesterol and seem to be effective mainly through the levels of these. Most of the new disease can in fact be explained by these two factors and little improvement in prediction was obtained by including the rest.

Since it is clear that men with low b.p. and plasma-cholesterol are less likely to have ischemic heart disease than men with high values, the important question today is whether long-term reduction of hypertension and hypercholesterolemia will in turn reduce the incidence of the disease.

Large-scale preventive trials are needed to give the answer and, generally, new types of population studies will have to be done to test the reality and relative contributions of the multiple causes and mechanisms of ischemic heart disease which are now postulated.

APPENDIX

However a vulnerable or "high-risk" group is defined, and taking:

N = number of individuals in the total population (or sample).
R = number of individuals in the high-risk group (as defined).
n = number of new cases occurring in the population during any defined follow-up period.
r = number of these new cases in the high-risk group, then—

Incidence of disease during follow-up period in population is n/N and also:

(a) proportion of the population included in the high-risk group is R/N;
(b) incidence of new cases of disease during follow-up period in high-risk group is r/R; and
(c) proportion of the new cases of disease included in high-risk group is r/n.

These ratios are related as shown in the following equation:

Incidence in high-risk group $(r/R) =$

$$\frac{\text{Proportion of all new cases included } (r/n)}{\text{Proportion of population included } (R/N)}$$

$\times$ Incidence in population (n/N)

Also, the individual risk for a man in the high-risk group of developing the disease is 1 in R/r.

At any point of time during the follow-up period the incidence of new disease in the total population will be known. Thus the incidence (or, derived from it, the individual risk) in a defined high-risk group will be larger when the proportion of new cases of the disease which are included is greater, and when the high-risk group as a proportion of the total population is smaller (see equation).

The proportion of new cases of disease included in the high-risk group is a measure of the "sensitivity" of the method by which the vulnerable group is defined—i.e., these new cases are true-positives in the sense that the disease subsequently develops. The remaining men in the high-risk group can be regarded, meanwhile, as "short-term" false-positives, since some of them during further follow-up may develop ischemic heart disease.

We are deeply grateful to the following: the busmen; the London Transport Board; the officials of the Transport and General Workers Union; the chief depot inspectors at the garages; the departmental staffs of the operating manager (central buses); the staff administration officer and the chief medical officer of the London Transport Board; to Dr. G. L. Mills of the Courtauld Institute of Biochemistry, for the lipid analyses; to Dr. Marvin Bierenbaum, Dr. Wallace Brigden, Dr. William Evans, and Dr. H. G. Lloyd-Thomas for reading electrocardiograms; to Mr. W. Abbott and the staff of the London Hospital Computer Unit; to hospital physicians and pathologists, general practitioners, and Executive Councils in the National Health Service; to the General Register Office and the Ministry of Pensions and National Insurance; and to our colleagues in the Social Medicine Research Unit, in particular Miss J. Sullivan, secretary.

References

(1) Blackburn, H., A. Keys, E. Simonson, P. Rautaharju, and S. Punsar. *Circulation* 21:1160, 1960.

(2) Morris, J. N., J. A. Heady, P. A. B. Raffle, C. G. Roberts, and J. W. Parks. *Lancet* ii:1053, 1111, 1953.

(3) Morris, J. N. *Uses of Epidemiology.* Edinburgh, 1964.

(4) Armitage, P. *Biometrics* 11:375, 1955.

(5) Cohn, E. J., F. R. N. Gurd, D. M. Surgenor, B. A. Barnes, R. K. Brown, G. Derouaux, J. M. Gillespie, F. W. Kahnt, W. E. Lever, C. H. Lin, D. Mittleman, R. F. Mouton, K. Schmid, and E. Uroma. *J Am Chem Soc* 72:465, 1950.

(6) Dodds, C. and G. L. Mills. *Lancet* i:1160, 1959.

(7) Gofman, J. W., W. Young, and R. Tandy. *Ischaemic Heart Disease, Artherosclerosis, and Longevity.* Livermore, California, 1966.

(8) Morrison, S. L. and J. N. Morris. *Lancet* ii:829, 1960.

(9) Gertler, M. M. and P. D. White. *Coronary Heart Disease in Young Adults.* Cambridge, Massachusetts, 1954.

(10) Edwards, D. A. W., W. H. Hammond, M. J. R. Healy, J. M. Tanner, and R. H. Whitehouse. *Br J Nutr* 9:133, 1955.

(11) Fisher, R. A. *Ann Eugen* 7:179, 1936.

(12) Cornfield, J. *Fedn Proc Fedn Am Soc Exp Biol* 21:58, 1962.

(13) Keys, A., H. L. Taylor, H. Blackburn, J. Brozek, J. T. Anderson, and E. Simonson. *Circulation* 28:381, 1963.

(14) Paul, O., M. H. Lepper, W. H. Phelan, G. W. Dupertuis, A. MacMillan, H. McKean, and H. Park. *Circulation* 28:20, 1963.

(15) Chapman, J. M. and F. J. Massey. *J Chron Dis* 17:933, 1964.

(16) Gertler, M. M., L. D. Cady, and H. H. Whiter. *Am J Med Sci* 248:377, 1964.

(17) Doyle, J. T. *Mod Concepts Cardiovasc Dis* 35:81, 1966.

(18) Epstein, F. H. *Proc R Soc Med* (in press), 1966.

(19) Kannel, W. B., T. R. Dawber, and P. M. McNamara. *J Iowa Med Soc* 56:26, 1966.

(20) Stamler, J., D. M. Berkson, H. A. Lindberg, Y. Hall, W. Miller, L. Mojonnier, M. Levinson, D. B. Cohen, and Q. D. Young. *Med Clin North Am* 50:229, 1966.

(21) Heady, J. A., J. N. Morris, A. Kagan, and P. A. B. Raffle. *Br J Prev Soc Med* 15:143, 1961.

(22) Doyle, J. T., T. R. Dawber, W. B. Kannel, S. H. Kinch, and H. A. Kahn. *JAMA* 190:886, 1964.

(23) Epstein, F. H. *Am Heart J* 67:445, 1964.

(24) Rosenman, R. H., M. Friedman, R. Straus, M. Wurm, D. Jenkins, H. B. Messinger, R. Kositcheck, W. Hahn, and N. T. Werthessen. *JAMA* 195:86, 1966.

(25) Morris, J. N. *Proc R Soc B* 159:65, 1963.

(26) Morris, J. N., J. W. Marr, J. A. Heady, G. L. Mills, and T.R.E. Pilkington. *Br Med J* i:571, 1963.

(27) Marr, J. W. Unpublished, 1966.

(28) Holland, W. W. In *Epidemiology: Reports on Research and Teaching 1962* (edited by J. Pemberton) Oxford, 1963, p. 271.

(29) *Lancet* i:414, 1966.

(30) Rumball, A. and E. D. Acheson. *Br Med J* i:423, 1963.

(31) Bruce, R. A. and S. R. Yarnall. *J Chron Dis* 19:473, 1966.

(32) Reid, D. D., W. W. Holland, S. Humerfelt, and G. Rose. *Lancet* i:614, 1966.

AN OVERVIEW OF THE RISK FACTORS FOR CARDIOVASCULAR DISEASE

William B. Kannel

A number of factors have been identified and firmly established as risks for cardiovascular disease (CVD). Support for the risk factor concept derives from epidemiological studies that have compared CVD mortality rates among countries and occupational, racial, and religious groups. The most important evidence comes from prospective investigations of the development of CVD within populations in relation to antecedent suspected risk factors. Over the past three decades a number of longitudinal prospective epidemiological studies were undertaken that involved tens of thousands of participants in various population samples (1-3). These prospective studies were all natural experiments, not controlled trials. Hence, unequivocal causal relationships of risk factors to the incidence of CVD cannot be claimed on this evidence alone. It remains for other methods to provide additional evidence. Since etiology is only inferred, the host and environmental factors epidemiologically linked to the incidence of CVD have been designated as risk factors or disease predictors.

For such data to be considered etiologically relevant, a number of criteria should be met. Epidemiologically demonstrated associations are more likely to be causal if they precede the disease and are strong and dose related, consistent, predictive of disease in other populations, independent of other risk factors, pathogenetically plausible, and supported by animal experiments and clinical investigation. The major identified risk factors meet most of these criteria. Although epidemiology deals chiefly with the way disease evolves in population samples, the findings have great relevance to the understanding of the development of disease in individuals. In view of my personal involvement with the Framingham Study, most of this chapter will deal with that body of data. . . .

Most of the evidence relating risk factors to atherosclerotic CVD deals with its major and most lethal manifestation, coronary heart disease (CHD). Although the same risk factors do, in general, apply to other clinical atherosclerotic events, such as atherothrombotic brain infarction, occlusive peripheral arterial disease, and cardiac failure, some important differences exist. Table 1 gives the comparative relative strengths of the relationships between the various risk factors and the major cardiovascular events in terms of their regression, in coefficients standardized to place them on equal footing for the different units of measurement. The higher the coefficient, the stronger is the relationship between the risk factor and the cardiovascular event. As an example of the different roles of various risk factors, note that hypertension is the most powerful contributor to stroke and cardiac failure, but that it contributes less to occlusive peripheral arterial disease. Diabetes and cigarette smoking are more powerful contributors to the development of this disease. Serum total cholesterol is feebly related to stroke and cardiac failure. Because of the importance of CHD as the most common and highly lethal manifestation of atherosclerosis, this chapter on cardiovascular risk factors will focus mainly on this cardiovascular event.

CLASSIFICATION OF RISK FACTORS

The concept of risk factors evolved from prospective epidemiological studies in the 1950's relating personal characteristics of participants to subsequent incidence of CHD. Risk factors are based only on associations demonstrated in epidemiological studies; hence they may be directly causative, secondary manifestations of more basic underlying metabolic abnormalities or early symptoms of the disease. Also, risk can be expressed in terms of absolute risk, relative risk ratios, or attributable risks. A high relative

Source: *Excerpted from Prevention of Coronary Heart Disease: Practical Management of the Risk Factors.* Edited by Norman M. Kaplan and Jeremiah Stamler. Philadelphia, W.B. Saunders Company, 1983.

Table 1. Coefficients for regression[a] of specified cardiovascular events on cardiovascular risk factors, for men and women, ages 45 to 74, in the Framingham Study, over 20-year follow-up.

Risk factors	Cardiovascular disease		Cardiac failure		Intermittent claudication		Brain infarction		Coronary disease	
	Men	Women	Men	Women	Men	Women	Men	Women	Men	Women
Cigarettes	.198	.029[b]	.087[b]	.195	.372	.217[b]	.190[b]	.042[b]	.168	−.023[b]
ECG-LVH	.222	.219	.394	.316	.158	.287	—	—	.212	.174
Serum cholesterol	.236	.255	.161[b]	.133[b]	.271	.244	.154[b]	.104[b]	.255	.314
Diabetes	.160	.192	.196	.325	.316	.358	.244	—	.117	.201
Hypertension	.414	.509	.616	.504	.362	.529	.682	.717	.338	.483
Heart rate	.144	.058[b]	.293	.201	.170[a]	−.060[b]	.305	.105[b]	.125	.053[b]
Relative weight	.156	.219	.227	.387	−.192	.193[b]	.130[b]	.359	.206	.223
Vital capacity	−.179	−.330	−.392	−.667	−.264	−.469	−.214[b]	−.264	−.116	−.292
Proteinuria	.090	.062[b]	—	—	.027[a]	—	—	—	.094	.120

[a] These numbers represent the strength of the relationships between the risk factor and the cardiovascular event. The higher the number, the stronger is the relationship.
[b] Not statistically significant at $P = <0.05$.
— = Insufficient data.

risk, comparing people with and without the risk attribute, can mean little if the absolute risk (i.e., average annual incidence of disease) is low or if the prevalence of the risk factor is so rare that the amount of disease that is attributed to the risk factor (i.e., population attributable risk) is also low.

The major identified cardiovascular risk factors can be logically categorized as: (1) atherogenic personal attributes, (2) living habits or less discretionary environmental factors that promote these host factors, (3) signs of preclinical disease, and (4) host susceptibility to all these various influences. Most of the risk factors can be assessed in unprepared persons and require no more than ordinary office procedures and simple laboratory tests. By placing the risk factor information into a composite cardiovascular risk profile, their joint effects can be estimated. In this way risk can be estimated over a wide range, and a segment of the asymptomatic population can be identified who are prime candidates for CVD and who require personalized management by prevention-minded physicians. The risk factor concept is not merely mindless numerology alien to the practice of medicine. There is a probabilistic basis to most of what we do in the practice of medicine in relation to diagnosis or prognostication. In dealing with individual patients, we must always apply knowledge from a large case series in order to determine the best course of action for the case at hand. We must assume that the patient is likely to have the average experience of

the group to which he belongs. This is exactly what we do when we apply population data in a probabilistic way to assess risk for individuals, whether they be detected in a mass screening program or the physician's office.

Because of the pervasiveness of predisposing factors, the entire population could benefit from public health measures to alter the ecology to one more favorable to cardiovascular health and from hygienic advice that would allow people to protect themselves and their families from the faulty life style that endangers them.

Atherogenic Traits

The atherogenic risk attributes include the blood lipids, blood pressure (BP), and clinical diabetes. These factors jointly play a large role in determining the pace of atherogenesis (Figure 1). Each has been repeatedly shown to be independently related to the rate of development of clinical CHD and to the extent of occlusive coronary atherosclerosis as shown on angiography. Gout or hyperuricemia may be an additional factor.

Blood Lipids

The evidence incriminating the serum total cholesterol in the evolution of CHD is extensive and unequivocal (3, 4). Atherosclerosis has been produced in animals by hypercholesterolemia-inducing diets; the lesions have been shown to contain the lipid, derived from plasma; CHD cases have been shown to have higher choles-

Figure 1. The risk of coronary heart disease according to the number of risk factors[a] at initial exam in men aged 30 to 49 over 20-year follow-up, in the Framingham Study.

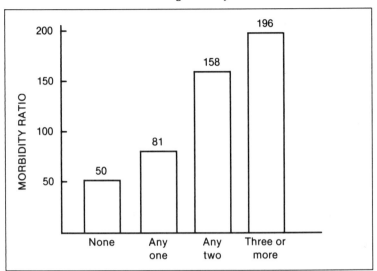

[a]*Risk Factors:*

Hypertension
Cholesterol ≥ 250
Diabetes
Cigarettes ≥ Pkg Day
ECG-ABN

terol values; persons with genetic hypercholesterolemia develop premature coronary disease; and epidemiological studies have shown that CHD mortality mirrors the serum cholesterol values of populations around the world. Finally, prospective epidemiological studies have also shown that CHD evolves in direct relation to cholesterol values.

In both sexes the risk of CHD in people under age 50 is independently related to their serum total cholesterol. Within the range of values usually encountered in countries with a high CHD incidence (185 to 335 mg/dl), there is a fivefold range of risk with no discernible critical value (Table 2). A total serum cholesterol of 260 mg/dl is associated with twice the standard risk. Populations with a good life expectancy and a low CHD incidence have average cholesterol values in the 160 to 180 mg/dl range, and this would appear to be optimal.

At any given total cholesterol, the risk of CVD has been found to vary depending on the individual's age and sex, and the level of other cardiovascular risk factors (see Table 2). The risk at any given cholesterol level is lower in women than in men and depends on the lipoprotein-cholesterol fractions.

The atherogenicity of the serum total cholesterol is dependent on its relative proportions in the high-density and low-density lipoproteins (HDL and LDL). The fraction of the serum total cholesterol that is carried in the LDL has been shown to be the atherogenic component. It is this fraction that is chiefly responsible for the association between the total cholesterol and CHD incidence. In contrast, the HDL cholesterol fraction is *inversely* related to CHD risk and appears to reflect processes of removal of cholesterol from the tissues.

Determination of these cholesterol-lipoprotein fractions is particularly useful when individuals are beyond age 55, when the serum total cholesterol no longer identifies high-risk CHD candidates. Fractionation into the lipoprotein components restores the ability of the serum total cholesterol to predict CHD. Prospective data from the Framingham Study indicate that the LDL and HDL cholesterol are each inde-

Table 2. Eight-year probability (per 100) of developing CVD in a 40-year-old man.

	Does not smoke cigarettes								Smokes cigarettes						
SBP:[a]	105	120	135	150	165	180	LVH-ECG negative	SBP:	105	120	135	150	165	180	195
Chol[b]								Chol							
185	1	2	2	2	3	4	Glucose intolerance	185	2	3	3	4	5	6	8
210	2	2	2	3	4	5	absent	210	3	3	4	5	7	8	10
235	2	3	3	4	5	6		235	4	4	6	7	9	11	13
260	3	3	4	5	7	8		260	5	6	7	9	11	14	17
285	4	4	6	7	9	11		285	6	8	9	12	14	17	21
310	5	6	7	9	11	14		310	8	10	12	15	18	22	26
335	6	8	9	12	14	17		335	10	13	15	19	23	27	32
185	2	3	3	4	5	7	Glucose intolerance	185	4	5	6	7	9	11	13
210	3	4	4	6	7	9	present	210	5	6	7	9	11	14	17
235	4	5	6	7	9	11		235	6	8	10	12	15	18	21
260	5	6	8	9	12	14		260	8	10	12	15	18	22	27
285	6	8	10	12	15	18		285	11	13	16	19	23	28	33
310	8	10	13	15	19	22		310	13	16	20	24	29	34	39
335	11	13	16	19	23	28		335	17	21	25	30	35	40	46

[a] SBP = systolic blood pressure.
[b] Chol = serum cholesterol.

pendently related to CHD incidence, with the protective influence of HDL possibly even stronger than the atherogenic influence of LDL, particularly in individuals beyond age 50. The joint effect of the two lipids is substantial and augmented by BP (Figure 2).

To facilitate incorporation of the HDL cholesterol into a lipid risk profile, a ratio of LDL/HDL cholesterol or, even more practicable, a total/HDL cholesterol is recommended (Figure 3). Because of the generally high correlation between LDL and total cholesterol, the latter can serve as a surrogate for the former. Since as little as a 10 mg/dl difference in HDL cholesterol is associated with as much as a 50 percent difference in risk of CHD, accuracy in the assay is essential.

Striking correlations have been found between the average intake of fat and the mean levels of cholesterol in population samples around the world. Metabolic ward studies in humans indicate a predictable joint influence of dietary saturated fat and cholesterol on the serum cholesterol (and LDL) (5-7). The whole spectrum of atherosclerotic lesions seen in humans has been produced in a variety of experimental animals, including nonhuman primates, by feeding them diets enriched with cholesterol and fat so as to induce hypercholesterolemia. It has also been shown that atherosclerosis can regress upon elimination of the offending nutrients (8).

Thus, international dietary comparisons, human metabolic investigations, and animal experiments clearly incriminate dietary cholesterol and saturated fat as major contributors to the high serum cholesterol and LDL-cholesterol values characteristic of populations with a high CHD incidence (9, 10). This association is augmented by excessive calorie intake. The nutrients affecting HDL cholesterol are still poorly

Figure 2. The risk of coronary heart disease according to levels of HLD-cholesterol in men aged 55 over 24-year follow-up.

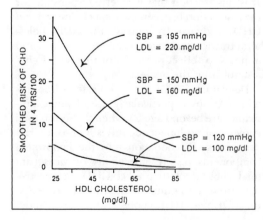

Figure 3. The 4-year risk of coronary heart disease according to the ratio of cholesterol lipoprotein fractions, in the Framingham Study, exam II.

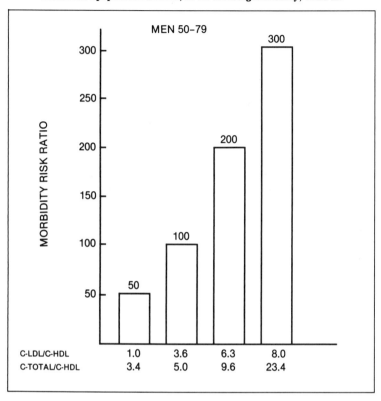

understood and are under intensive investigation, although it is known that excessive calories definitely lower this lipoprotein. A high intake of complex carbohydrates is definitely associated with a low CHD mortality, particularly when they are eaten in place of saturated fats. Calorie balance has been clearly shown to improve the LDL/HDL cholesterol ratio. Conclusive demonstration of the relationship of diet to CHD or hyperlipidemia within typical American population samples is difficult because of the generally high consumption of the incriminated nutrients and inadequate methods of quantifying both the intakes and energy expenditures of individuals (11-13).

Serum triglyceride values and the very low-density lipoproteins (VLDL), which transport the triglycerides, are also positively associated with CHD risk, but most prospective studies indicate that this excess risk is dependent on coexisting low HDL values, high LDL cholesterol, obesity, and impaired glucose tolerance.

Persons with elevated triglycerides should be investigated for increased LDL cholesterol, depressed HDL cholesterol, hyperglycemia, obesity, and alcohol abuse, and appropriate countermeasures should be implemented.

Blood Pressure

Hypertension, whether labile or fixed, borderline or definite, casual or basal, systolic or diastolic, at any age and in either sex, is a common and powerful contributor to atherosclerotic CVD. As an individual factor, the casual office BP is as accurate a predictor of CHD as the level of blood sugar, the level of cholesterol, or the amount of cigarette smoking. The contribution of BP to CHD incidence is powerful even taking other risk factors into account (Figure 4). The blood pressure impact is also, however, markedly influenced by the other risk factors.

Elevated BP, whether systolic or diastolic, is predictive of CHD (*14*). Morbidity and mortality increase progressively with the degree of BP elevation of either component, with no discernible critical value. At any level of pressure, the absolute risk is greater for men; however, the risk gradients and population attributable risks are just as great for women (*14, 15*). At a given average BP, the degree of lability of the pressure has no influence on risk (*15*).

It is unwise to use the lowest pressure recorded to judge the risk if the average of three office pressures is high. Lability of BP increases with the level of BP, so that pressures usually judged to be "fixed hypertension" are actually more labile than those commonly characterized "labile hypertension."

Although BP generally rises with age in most cultures in the modern world, there is no indication that elevated pressure is any less of a risk factor in the elderly than in the young. Neither absolute, relative, nor attributable risks are any lower in the elderly (*14*). Moreover, it is imprudent to dismiss isolated systolic hypertension as an innocuous accompaniment of aging; it is definitely associated with an increased risk of CHD (*14*).

Diabetes

Prospective epidemiological studies have confirmed the clinical observation that diabetes predisposes individuals to CVD (*16, 17*). Although some have reported that asymptomatic

Figure 4. The 8-year probability per 1000 men aged 40 of cardiovascular disease, according to systolic blood pressures from 105 to 195 mmHg at specified levels of other risk factors, in the Framingham Study. (Source: Monograph No. 28)

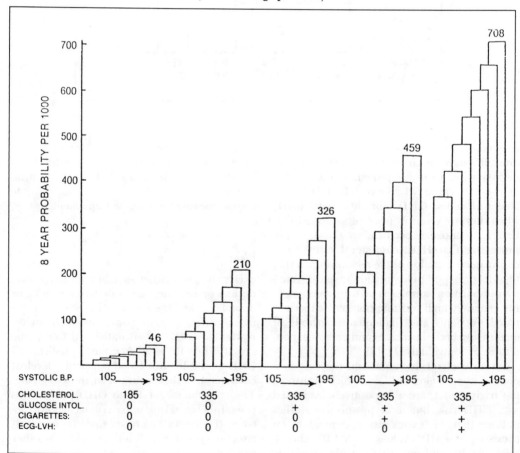

hyperglycemia is not hazardous, some studies have indicated that hyperglycemia, an abnormal glucose tolerance test, or even a high casual blood sugar, is associated with an increased risk of CVD (*18*). In western industrial society, asymptomatic hyperglycemia may well be an independent risk factor for atherosclerotic disease.

In the Framingham cohort, diabetes was found to double cardiovascular mortality (*17, 18*). Its relative impact is substantially greater in women than in men, tends to diminish with advancing age, and varies widely depending on the level of coexisting risk factors (Figure 5).

The cardiovascular risk is not entirely a result of associated higher levels of other risk factors; nor is their evidence that the other risk factors exert a greater impact on the diabetic (*17*). Insulin-dependent and noninsulin-dependent diabetic adults appear to be at increased risk of developing CHD (*19*). In early-onset diabetes, microvascular manifestations are prominent, and mortality from renal disease appears to be the disease's greatest hazard (*20*). In adult-onset diabetes, the *relative* impact is greatest for occlusive peripheral arterial disease, but CHD is still the most common sequela in absolute incidence. Diabetes also appears to damage the

Figure 5. The risk of cardiovascular disease with glucose intolerance according to the level of other risk factors in men aged 40, over 18-year follow-up, in the Framingham Study. (Source: Monograph No. 28.)

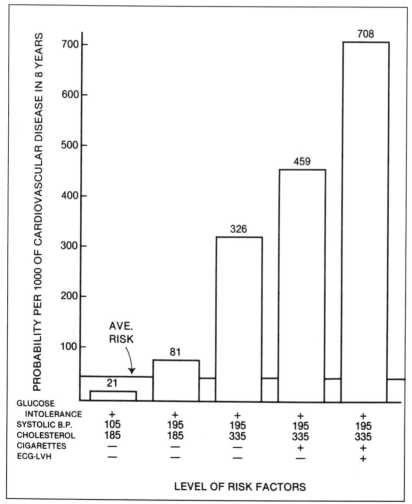

myocardium directly, predisposing the individual to cardiac failure (*21*). Diabetes appears to be less dangerous in some parts of the world, which suggests that cofactors, such as exercise, obesity, cigarette smoking, diet, and form of treatment, may be of great importance.

Gout

Gout or hyperuricemia appears to be indirectly atherogenic, an effect most likely mediated through associated hypertension, hyperlipidemia, and obesity (*22, 23*). There is little net contribution of gout or hyperuricemia to development of CHD in men when the associated atherogenic traits are taken into account. Nonetheless, gouty arthritis has been found to be associated with a doubled risk of CHD (*22*), and there seems to be an association between asymptomatic hyperuricemia and the development of CHD. The relation of hyperuricemia induced by diuretics to the development of CHD is not established.

Living Habits

The life style that predisposes individuals to CVD is characterized by a diet too rich in calories, saturated fat, cholesterol, and salt and by physical indolence, unrestrained weight gain, cigarette smoking, and alcohol abuse.

Cigarette Smoking

Prospective epidemiological studies covering 12 million person-years of experience document the association between cigarette smoking and myocardial infarction (MI) and CHD mortality (*23*). As compared with nonsmokers, male cigarette smokers have 60 percent more overall mortality; pipe and cigar smoking is less hazardous (*23*). Cigarette smoking doubles the risk for CVD in general (see Table 2).

There is convincing evidence supporting the strong relationship of cigarette smoking to CHD. The effect of cigarette smoking is dose related as well as powerful, according to all prospective studies with sufficient data (*23*). The data are reasonably consistent and from a variety of sources, and the effect of cigarette smoking has been demonstrated, taking into account all the associated cardiovascular risk factors (see Table 2). Finally, those who quit smoking have been found to have only half the risk of CHD of those who continue to smoke (*24*). As opposed

to the pulmonary consequences, the excess CHD risk in ex-smokers seems to decline substantially within a year (*24*).

Although cigarette smoking is less consistently related to overall CHD incidence in women, both sexes appear to exhibit the same increased inconsistency to MI. This vulnerability derives from the inexplicable weak relationship of cigarette smoking to angina pectoris, the most common manifestation of CHD in women (*16*). This lack of a consistent relationship of cigarette smoking to angina pectoris is curious, since smoking has been shown to decrease exercise tolerance in people with angina pectoris (*25*).

The demonstrated effects of nicotine and carbon monoxide on the heart, the coronary arteries, and the blood provide a reasonable pathogenic mechanism. Nicotine has been shown to transiently increase heart rate and BP, to increase myocardial oxygen needs, and to lower the fibrillation threshold. Carbon monoxide build-up has been shown to diminish oxygen transport and utilization. Smoking also adversely affects platelet adhesiveness and injures the arterial endothelium and depresses HDL cholesterol (*25*). Thus, cigarette smoking may well have both an acute noncumulative, reversible effect, precipitating occlusive and electrical events in those with a compromised circulation, and a long-term atherogenic effect.

Although cigarette smoking contributes independently to the development of coronary attacks, as regards absolute risk, this influence is particularly pernicious in those predisposed by other risk factors (Figure 6). Risk of MI and sudden death are promoted by cigarette smoking, and this liability is evidently eliminated by quitting cigarette smoking (*24*).

Obesity

Obese persons in the Framingham Study developed twice as much cardiac failure and brain infarction and a more modest excess of CHD (*18*). The impact of obesity upon CHD was greater for men than for women and was most impressive for angina and coronary attacks (Figure 7). The incidence of sudden death was related to relative weight, and the fraction of CHD deaths that were sudden also increased progressively with the degree of overweight, suggesting a specific relationship.

Although it is generally agreed that obesity is associated with CHD (*18*), its independent contribution to the disease has been questioned (*26*). Several studies have found that the association with CHD is accounted for by the other cardiovascular risk factors that tend to accompany obesity (*16, 24*). Overweight has been found to be strongly associated with adverse lipid profiles, hypertension, and glucose intolerance (*27*). Change in weight is mirrored by corresponding changes in these cardiovascular risk factors (*27*).

Although the contribution of obesity to CHD incidence may be largely mediated through effects on the major cardiovascular risk factors, obesity must nevertheless be considered an important modifiable risk factor for the disease. There is also some evidence from the Framingham Study that there is a net contribution of obesity to CHD incidence in men, even taking these risk factors into account; this evidence is corroborated by studies of Hawaiian Japanese and cohorts of young subjects (*28*).

Physical Activity

Epidemiological evidence strongly suggests that endurance exercise protects against CHD (*29*). Overall mortality, cardiovascular mortality, and CHD mortality, in particular, all have been found to be inversely related to the level of physical activity in the Framingham cohort (*30*). The protection seems to be confined to men and is modest compared with the effects of major cardiovascular risk factors, but it persists even when the risk factors are taken into account. The protection in men can be demonstrated into advanced age (Table 3).

The amount of exercise required to achieve the benefits of physical activity has not been

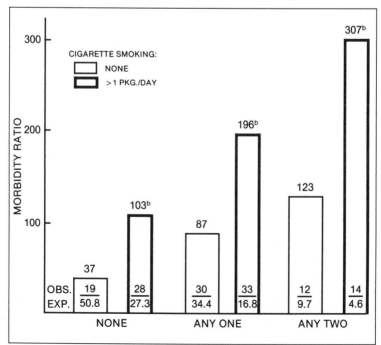

Figure 6. The risk of coronary heart disease (12 years) according to cigarette smoking habit and presence of "predisposing factors"[a] in men aged 30 to 59 at entry in the Framingham Study. OBS refers to the number of coronary heart disease events observed, EXP to the number of events expected for this portion of the population. The OBS divided by the EXP provides the morbidity ratio.

[a]Predisposing factors: cholesterol ≤ 250; hypertension; diabetes.
[b]Significantly different from "nonsmoker" P < .05.

Figure 7. The risk of manifestations of coronary heart disease according to the obesity status of men and women aged 45 to 74 years, over 20-year follow-up, in the Framingham Study.

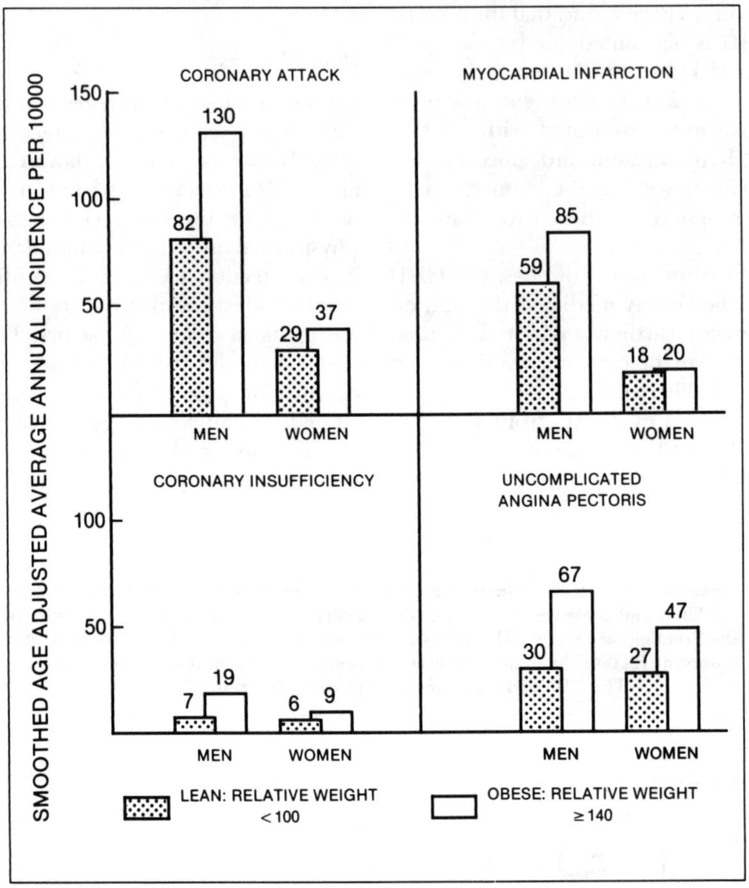

quantified. Epidemiological data based on general population samples indicate that moderate amounts of exercise will suffice. Yet exercise

Table 3. Fourteen-year incidence of cardiovascular mortality according to physical activity, for men aged 35 to 64.

Physical activity index[a]	Rate (%) in 14 years			All ages adjusted
	35-44	45-64	55-64	
24-29	3.5	12.6	22.5	12.1
30-33	4.0	10.5	19.1	10.6
34-37	1.8	10.2	12.0	7.7
38-83	1.4	9.6	9.1	6.5
t-Value	−1.74	−0.55	−2.85	−2.86

[a] The higher the index, the greater the degree of physical activity.

physiologists advocate strenuous and prolonged exercise to achieve a "training effect." There is also uncertainty as to whether the physiological effects are directly on the heart or on peripheral circulation and whether the improved risk is largely a product of attendant alteration of the other risk factors. It is also not known whether exercise alone can produce substantial improvements in the various cardiovascular risk factors. Yet to be determined is whether exercise alone can produce substantial improvements in the various cardiovascular risk factors independent of weight change or changes in diet, both of which often accompany exercise programs. Judging from the experience in Finland, where there is a high CHD mortality despite a high occupational level of physical exertion, physical activity is evidently not powerful enough to overcome the effects of other atherogenic influences.

Psychosocial Influences

Societally conditioned psychosocial factors influence various important aspects of life style, such as eating, drinking, smoking, and inactivity, and hence must be important in the evolution of atherosclerotic CVD. The exact role of various emotional and social factors in the evolution of CHD remains speculative, perhaps because definition and quantification of these factors remain imprecise. Reviews of the role of psychosocial factors have indicated some inconsistent associations with CHD. It is suspected that sustained overstimulation of the central nervous system may lead to CHD, and depression, sleep disturbance, prolonged anxiety, and Type A behavior have also been incriminated. Less consistently associated factors are work overload, life dissatisfactions, social mobility, and status incongruity. Social deprivation involving low income and low education have been implicated, though social status, when considered in isolation, appears to bear no consistent relationship to CHD incidence (*31*).

An overdeveloped sense of time-urgency, preoccupation with deadlines, competitive drive, and work-oriented behavior, all characterized as Type A, have been found to be related to the development of CHD (*32*). The Western Collaborative Study Group found that Type A men had a doubled risk of CHD compared with those characterized as antithesis, Type B (*32*). The Framingham Study confirmed this finding in men and demonstrated similar excess risks for Type A women (*33*). Two prospective studies have shown that the Type A behavior precedes CHD, that its effect is independent of associated risk factors, and that risk is proportional to the degree of Type A behavior exhibited (*32, 33*). However, both the Multiple Risk Factor Intervention Trial and the Aspirin Myocardial Infarction Study recently reported no relationship between type and risk of CHD death (*34*).

Among women in the Framingham Study a number of psychosocial factors have been found to be related to CHD (Table 4). Working women in the Framingham Study were more likely than housewives to report Type A behavior, marital disagreements, job mobility, daily stress, or marital dissatisfaction. Although employment itself is not associated with CHD in women, the working environment (a nonsupportive boss, decreased job mobility), personality (suppressed hostility), and economic stress appear to be determinants of vulnerability to CHD.

Diet

Beyond the effects of dietary saturated fat and cholesterol, higher consumption of sucrose and glucose and reduced amounts of fiber in processed foods have been incriminated in the development of CHD, diabetes, obesity, and hyperlipidemia (*35*). Animal experiments, however, have not corroborated any association between dietary sucrose, or carbohydrates in general, and the development of atherosclerosis. Feeding animals carbohydrates has been shown to produce only a transient elevation of plasma triglycerides (*3, 9*). In fact, most populations with a low CHD incidence derive from 65 to 80 percent of their energy from grains and potatoes. Although not clearly linked to CHD incidence, fiber does appear to influence ab-

Table 4. Somatic strain scores among CHD cases and non-cases in the Framingham Study, for women ages 45 to 64.

	Any clinical manifestation of CHD		Uncomplicated angina pectoris	
	Cases	Non-cases	Cases	Non-cases
Tension state	0.58	0.38[a]	0.67	0.38[a]
Daily stress	0.37	0.30	0.46	0.30[b]
Anxiety symptoms	0.53	0.20[a]	0.59	0.21[a]
Anger symptoms	0.49	0.30[a]	0.54	0.31[a]

[a] $P = <0.01$.
[b] $P = <0.05$.

sorption of lipids and carbohydrates (*35*). Recent evidence now connects cholesterol, polyunsaturated and saturated fats in the diet, and serum cholesterol to coronary mortality prospectively in men (*13*). Positive calorie balance produces an unfavorable LDL/HDL cholesterol ratio, impaired glucose tolerance, hyperuricemia, and hypertension, promoting accelerated atherogenesis.

Sodium

A high sodium content in the diet can produce hypertension in genetically predisposed animals (*36*). Some cross-population epidemiological studies have suggested a strong association between sodium intake and the prevalence of hypertension (*36*). Restriction of sodium intake has been shown to be helpful in patients being treated for hypertension (*36*). The connection between salt intake and hypertension is hard to establish in humans because of the difficulty in assessing their salt intake and in accounting for such confounding influences as weight, potassium intake, and alcohol usage. There is also no good index of individual susceptibility to the effect of sodium aside from a family history of hypertension. Perhaps measurement of intracellular sodium concentration and fluxes may prove helpful in this regard, but the evidence currently available is too sparse to be definitive.

Common Beverages

Caffeine-containing beverages, because they can produce transient changes in hemodynamics, have been suspect as contributors to CHD. Data from a number of prospective studies that took cigarette use into account have failed, however, to corroborate retrospective studies implicating coffee (*37*).

Alcohol is a toxic substance that may contribute to cancer, hypertension, hypertriglyceridemia, and psychosocial problems. In excessive amounts it can damage the myocardium and make it more irritable. In moderate amounts, however, there is little evidence that alcohol increases the risk of coronary attacks, and some evidence suggests a preventive effect, reflected in an inverse relationship to CHD incidence (Figures 1-8). Other investigators, however, have found either a positive association or none at all (*38*). Alcohol appears to raise HDL cholesterol, but the benefits of a high HDL so induced remain to be shown.

Less Discretionary Environmental Factors

Climate, air pollution, trace metals, and water softness have been implicated in CHD, but the evidence supporting their roles remains tenuous. An inverse relationship has been noted between hardness of drinking water and regional cardiovascular mortality (*39*). Efforts to

Figure 8. The risk of coronary heart disease and angina according to alcohol intake in men aged 50 to 62 over 18-year follow-up, in the Framingham Study.

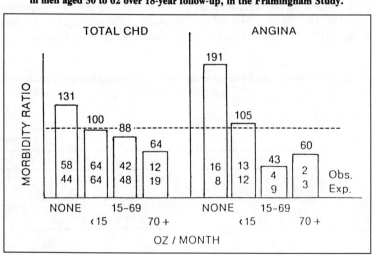

identify specific chemical components of the water that might be responsible for the protective effect have not been too productive. Protection against CHD has been linked to magnesium, selenium, and zinc; harm has been attributed to cadmium, manganese, and lead. Unfortunately there is no firm basis for recommending alteration of the hardness or chemical composition of drinking water because of the inconsistency of the findings and the fact that other sources of some of these trace metals are not adequately considered. Exposure to industrial toxins, such as carbon disulfide and aliphatic nitrates, has also been incriminated.

Coronary heart disease mortality appears to vary widely among different countries and even within countries. In the United States high mortality rates are noted along the southeastern Atlantic coast, in the deep South from Georgia to Alabama, and in the industrial Northeast and Midwest. The lowest CHD mortality rates are found in the mountain states and in the Great Plains. Adequate explanations for the large variations in mortality have not been found. Climatic variation, such as extremes of temperature and snowfall, has been implicated (40).

Minor and Other Risk Factors

Because the currently identified risk factors do not appear to completely explain the differences in CHD mortality observed between areas of high and low CHD incidence, there is a suspicion that other unknown major risk factors may well exist. This suspicion may well be justified, but not on the grounds that the major risk factors do not explain the variance in incidence of CVD. There is some doubt as to whether it is reasonable to expect that 100 percent of the variance in CVD should be explained by even a complete set of variables. In any event, before concluding that unknown major risk factors exist, it is required that all of the relevant ones be included. Thus far, none of the multivariate analyses attempting to test whether the variance in incidence is completely explained has dealt with all the relevant variables. Also, measurements of various life styles generally do not encompass a lifetime experience.

A variety of other risk factors have been incriminated but fail to meet as many of the aforementioned criteria to qualify as major risk factors and, therefore, are less likely to be causal. High normal hemoglobin values have been

found to be associated with an increased risk of CHD (18). Vital capacity was noted to be inversely and independently related to CHD and cardiac failure in the Framingham Study (18). Blood group investigations indicate that type O persons may be at slightly reduced risk compared to those with type A blood. Patients with rheumatoid arthritis are alleged to have a low incidence of CHD. Although this could be an autoimmune phenomenon, such as has been suspected in thyroiditis, it may well be a consequence of aspirin therapy, affecting platelet function.

Oral Contraceptives

The use of oral contraceptives has been associated both retrospectively and prospectively with an increased risk of CHD (41). Adverse effects are more likely in women who are cigarette smokers, are over age 35, have hypertension, hypercholesterolemia, or diabetes, and are long-term users of oral contraceptives. The hazards associated with oral contraceptive use include the adverse effects of the major cardiovascular risk factors, alteration in blood clotting and platelet factors, histochemical vascular alterations, and thromboembolic events. In a few susceptible women, oral contraceptives may provoke severe hypertension, marked hyperlipidemia, and overt diabetes. Even in those not so predisposed, oral contraceptives tend to shift the distribution of these cardiovascular risk factors upward, which could have serious consequences once the women are beyond child-bearing age. The adverse effects are more common in the oral contraceptives containing larger amounts of estrogen. Although progestin-containing pills have less overall impact on cardiovascular risk factors, they tend to lower HDL cholesterol, which estrogen raises.

Host Susceptibility

It was formerly believed that the atherosclerotic diseases were largely an inevitable consequence of aging and genetic make-up. But the progressive rise in CHD mortality in the 1940s and 1950s and its decline since 1968 have been too rapid to be explained by genetic factors. Also the rates of CHD mortality vary widely among populations with similar genetic make-ups (1, 2). Migrants from low to high incidence geographical areas tend to acquire the increased vulnerability of their adopted environment (*1, 2*).

Genetic factors do have a role in the development of CHD. People who have or develop CHD are concentrated in fewer families than chance allows. Such clustering cannot be attributed entirely to the demonstrated component of lipid and BP abnormalities.

Indicators of innate susceptiblity include a family history of premature CVD, diabetes, hypertension, hypercholesterolemia, or gout. In the Framingham Study, the incidence of MI in older brothers was significantly related to the MI experience of the younger brothers even when the data were controlled for a shared tendency towards hypertension or hypercholesterolemia and for the cigarette habit (Table 5).

Though these data indicate that the family tendency to CHD is not entirely a function of a higher level of shared predisposing risk factors, it is conceivable that genetically predisposed individuals tolerate a given burden of risk factors less well than those not so predisposed.

The demonstration of familial aggregation of CHD risk does not necessarily differentiate between genetic and environmental influences on disease or predisposing factors. Families also share environment.

Age and Sex

Mortality from each of the atherosclerotic diseases is strikingly related to age in each sex and in all races. Although uncommon in young white women, CHD is already a major cause of death for men aged 35 to 44 years. By ages 55 to 64, 40 percent of all deaths among men are due to this single cause.

The male predominance in CHD mortality applies for both whites and nonwhites but is more striking in whites and is greater at younger than older ages. Rates for white and nonwhite men are similar. Female rates lag behind those of men by 10 years for whites and by about 7 years for nonwhites. Despite the male predominance, CHD is still a very common disease in women and their leading cause of death.

The male predominance cannot be explained on the basis of a lower level of risk factors, since at any level of risk factors, singly or combined, women exhibit an advantage over men. Diabetes is the only common risk factor that can eradicate this advantage.

An escalation of CHD incidence and a dramatic increase in the severity of the disease are noted in women after menopause (Table 6). In the Framingham Study, women in their 40's and 50's who underwent menopause were found to have more than double the incidence of CHD of women the same age who remained premenopausal. Although menopause is associated with a change in some of the major risk factors, these do not account for the prompt escalation of risk noted. In those with a surgical menopause there was an excess risk whether the ovaries were removed or not (Table 6). Postmenopausal women on hormones had a doubled risk. These data suggest that estrogen is not responsible for the relative immunity of premenopausal women to CHD. Estrogens do not reduce the risk of developing CHD in older women and increase CHD risk when given to young women or to men.

Table 5. Predictive value of CHD in older brothers on CHD risk in younger brothers in association with other variables, in the Framingham Study.[a]

Risk factor variables	Total CHD	CVD other than CHD	Myocardial infarction	CHD mortality
CHD in brother	.156	.351[b]	.471[c]	.512[c]
Age	.185	−.056	−.100	.412
Systolic blood pressure	.325[b]	.555[c]	.452[c]	.720[c]
Serum total cholesterol	.157	.422[c]	.349[b]	.415
Metropolitan relative weight	.383[b]	−.102	−.017	−.212
Smoking (yes/no)	.165	.008	.154	.245

[a] These are standardized multivariate logistic coefficients and represent the strength of the relationships between risk factors and the occurrence of various aspects of coronary heart disease.

[b] † P = <0.05.

[c] ‡ P = <0.01.

Table 6. Age-adjusted[a] CHD incidence rates for women having surgical menopause in the Framingham Study, over a 24-year follow-up.

	Person years	CHD	
		No.	Rate/1000
Premenopausal	8384	6	0.95
Postmenopausal	6848	26	2.95
Ovaries removed			
0	1396	7	3.24
1 or 2	4544	17	2.87
Unspecified	908	2	1.42

[a] Indirect method.

A recent study with a larger number of cases has indicated that women who have had a hysterectomy without bilateral oophorectomy have a greater risk of MI than premenopausal women (*42*). In this study, however, women who had a hysterectomy at younger ages did not have a greater increase in risk. Reports on their influences in older women are inconsistent; some indicate that estrogen has a protective effect against CHD, others do not.

Endogenous estrogens may reduce a woman's risk of ischemic heart disease (*43*) if it is true that bilateral oophorectomy is associated with a greater increase in risk of MI than that associated with hysterectomy without bilateral oophorectomy. More data are evidently needed on this issue.

Preclinical Signs

Atherosclerotic CVD is an insidious process, so that coronary attacks or strokes often strike without warning. Coronary events generally occur in subjects who, despite lack of symptoms, have severe occlusive disease in two or three major coronary artery branches. Not only can advanced coronary disease exist without symptoms, but it may progress to an actual MI without typical symptoms. In fact, about one in four MIs is either asymptomatic or so atypical that it goes unrecognized. Less specific indications of ischemic myocardial involvement may also occur in persons with a hazardous coronary risk profile. Thus there may be electrocardiographic evidence of left ventricular hypertrophy (LVH), blocked intraventricular conduction, or nonspecific S-T segment and T wave repolarization abnormalities. When these occur without other explanation in persons with an unfavorable risk profile, it is reasonable to assume that the patient has a compromised coronary circulation. Such persons have been shown to have an increased risk of coronary events (*18*).

In coronary candidates with a normal resting ECG, a compromised coronary circulation may be revealed by exercise testing to elicit acute coronary insufficiency, impaired ventricular performance, or transient subendocardial ischemia. Positive reactors have been shown to be at greatly increased risk of symptomatic coronary disease. Other noninvasive procedures, including nuclear imaging techniques and echocardiography, may also be useful in detecting a compromised coronary circulation and impaired myocardial function.

MULTIVARIATE RISK PROFILES

Optimal risk predictions require a quantitative synthesis of the various independently contributing risk factors into a composite estimate. For this purpose multivariate risk functions are employed to quantify the combined effect of those interrelated risk factors (*44*). This concept takes into account the multifactorial elements of cardiovascular risk and the continuous gradient of response.

Categorical assessment of risk by assignment of arbitrary values to designate the point at which a continuous variable such as blood pressure or blood lipid is to be considered a risk factor has pragmatic utility, the risk of CVD rising with the number of risk factors (see Figure 1). This procedure is not efficient, however, because it tends to overlook those at high risk because of multiple modest abnormalities. This is an important consideration because it is from this segment of the population that the bulk of individuals with CVD emerges. With use of multivariate risk formulations incorporating the major identified risk factors, it is possible to assess risk quantitatively over an extremely wide range (see Table 2). With this procedure it is possible to identify a fifth of the asymptomatic population from which 40 percent of the CHD, 58 percent of the occlusive peripheral arterial disease, 80 percent of brain infarction, and 73 percent of the cardiac failure will evolve. For office use in assessing risk, handbooks have been devised based on these multiple logistic risk formulations. The handbooks provide estimates of risk for various combinations of risk factors at specified ages for each sex (see Table 2).

These risk formulations have been shown to predict disease accurately given the risk factor make-up in American population samples. The multivariate risk formulations can predict in the elderly about as well as in the younger population samples. However, since most risk factors are more potent on a relative scale early in life rather than later, and early lesions are apt to be more reversible, it would seem more important to identify and treat young people who are susceptible.

It is likely that the risk formulations can be further improved by the incorporation of additional risk factor information. The Type A or B pattern of behavior can be incorporated into the quantitative risk model. It is estimated that Type A behavior pattern would increase the probabilities as indicated from the conventional risk profile by 20 percent and decrease them by 20 percent for Type B. New data on the influence of the cholesterol-lipoprotein fractions can also be used, and it is likely that the total cholesterol/HDL-cholesterol ratio will replace the cholesterol' in the standard risk formulation (see Figure 3). Some other risk factor information, on the other hand, adds little to the multivariate risk formulation. For example, the addition of diastolic pressure does not enhance the risk estimation if systolic pressure is already contained in the equation. Obesity or relative weight does not further enhance the multivariate model presumably because obesity increases risk largely by promoting the other atherogenic risk factors.

PREVENTION

Prospects for Secondary Prevention

Although primary prevention is paramount, secondary prevention is also an urgent necessity because almost half of male coronary deaths arise from those with prior overt disease (45). The risk of an early death or reinfarction following a first MI is serious, particularly in the first six months to one year, especially in women and for those with evidence of extensive myocardial damage. Following an initial MI, about 20 percent of men and 40 percent of women can be expected to succumb within the first year (46).

High-risk subgroups can be identified among convalescent patients with MIs who, within the first year, have as high as a 50 percent risk of death. A positive submaximal ECG exercise test or ambulatory ECG monitoring indicating ischemic changes, arrythmias, or inappropriate heart rate or BP responses just prior to discharge will predict angina, excess mortality, and sudden death. Evaluation of left ventricular function with radionuclide and angiographic studies to determine the extent of coronary artery disease can furnish prognostic information in high-risk subjects. An enlarged heart on X-ray or ECG-LVH triples the risk of death following an MI. Any hint of cardiac failure in the convalescent stage is of ominous import.

After this period of high early mortality, the average mortality is about 5 percent per annum, which is still three to four times that of the general population (46). Even apparently mild unrecognized or silent MIs carry the same serious prognosis. Although coronary recurrences and mortality decline progressively with time after an infarction, the long-term outlook for those surviving the initial high-risk interval remains precarious.

Following the period of high early mortality, when the severity of the attack and the extent of coronary artery disease are the chief determinants of mortality, conventional risk factors may have utility for identifying high-risk candidates for recurrences and death. The coronary event may, however, alter the cardiovascular risk attributes, confounding the interpretation of their relationship to prognosis. For example, a *fall* in BP, cholesterol, or relative weight carries an adverse prognosis. By taking this change in risk factor level into account, the rate of recurrences and mortality is better shown to be related to conventional risk factors.

A variety of cardiovascular risk factors have been found to be related to mortality and reinfarction following the occurrence of coronary events. These factors include hypertension, cigarette smoking, physical inactivity, diabetes, and ECG abnormalities following onset of angina. By combining these risk variables it is possible to identify a tenth of the postmyocardial infarction population from which 31 percent of the deaths will arise. The Type A score has been found to be a good predictor of recurrent MI, even taking other risk factors into account.

The utility of correcting many of the risk factors following the onset of CHD remains to be demonstrated but seems rational and without great hazard. Comprehensive multifactorial management along with careful surveillance and prompt management of complications has been found to lower the rate of new coronary events (47). Smokers should be advised to quit, since stopping smoking has been found to reduce mortality to half that of those who continue to smoke (47). Hypertension should be controlled and weight reduction should increase exercise tolerance, reduce postinfarction angina, and help control risk factors, although evidence of benefit from these measures is still lacking. Supervised exercise and lipid control may be helpful in reducing the rate of new coronary events, but evidence of efficacy is still limited.

Primary Preventive Implications

Because of the nature and magnitude of the problem of CHD, it is not reasonable to rely upon modern innovations in the diagnosis or treatment of CHD, no matter how sophisticated these may have become. Only a primary preventive approach has the potential to make a substantial impact.

Each year about 640 000 Americans succumb to CHD and one fourth of these deaths occur in people under the age of 65. Almost 70 percent of these deaths occur outside the hospital, and more than half of these are sudden, unexpected deaths. Even among those who manage to survive, the chances of their dying over the ensuing five years are five times that of the general population, and 90 percent of these deaths will occur from recurrent cardiovascular catastrophes.

Beyond this appalling mortality, disability and illness are also considerable. One in every five American men can expect to develop CHD before age 60 (1). Infarctions spawn angina and limit the physical activity of half of those surviving. The fact that vulnerable persons can be easily selected from the general population and the fact that correctable risk factors have been identified seem cause for optimism about prevention of CVD.

Recent trends in CHD mortality indicate that prevention already has been effective. After rising for decades and leveling off in the late 1950s and early 1960s, CHD and CVD mortality rates in the United States have exhibited a steady year by year decline since at least 1968. At the same time that the United States mortality rates were falling more than 30 percent, the rates in other countries have been either continuing to rise or declining less dramatically. Although one can only speculate as to the reason for the decline, it is interesting to note that it accompanied reductions in the major cardiovascular risk factors and in the consumption of foods high in fat and cholesterol.

Although the final link in the chain of evidence incriminating CHD risk factor remains to be forged for many of the suspected contributors, a number of recommendations are warranted. In subjects with an ominous cardiovascular risk profile, serious attention to modifiable risk factors is amply justified. The primary approach should be hygienic. Because of the high prevalence of predisposing factors and the generally high risk, public health measures for the general population are also required.

Blood Lipids

In the management of most lipid problems, the focus should be on diet, weight control, and exercise. Since dietary cholesterol and saturated fat have both been shown to raise LDL cholesterol, intake of these nutrients should be reduced. Excessive calories raise both LDL and VLDL and lower HDL, making weight control important. HDL can also be raised by exercising, quitting cigarette smoking, increasing fish intake, and moderating use of alcohol. Although some measures taken to reduce LDL occasionally lower HDL as well, the LDL/HDL ratio is usually improved, suggesting a lessened atherogenic effect. Women taking oral contraceptives usually develop a rise in triglycerides which may influence their HDL, depending on the estrogen-progestin composition of the pill. Oral contraceptives of predominantly progestin composition may reduce HDL. In high-risk coronary candidates unresponsive to hygienic measures, an improvement in the LDL/HDL ratio may be achieved by lipid-lowering drugs. Of these, clofibrate and nicotinic acid also raise HDL. Trials involving clofibrate have not been encouraging. Diet, cholestyramine, and nicotinic acid have been shown to reduce cholesterol by 30 to 40 percent when used in combination.

The atherogenic effects of blood lipids require decades to produce clinical disease, and hence, clinical benefits cannot be expected from corrective measures in a short period of time. The improvement in the lipid profile should be discernible in a month. Although cellular fatty deposits may shrink in weeks, extracellular fatty deposits require one or more years to change significantly. Even the mass of fibrous lesions can be reduced but only after four or more years of vigorous treatment.

Obesity

The control of obesity, particularly on a fat-modified diet, is one of the chief hygienic measures available to control the major cardiovascular risk factors, including hypertension, lipid abnormalities, and hyperglycemia. It is easier to avoid than to correct long-standing obesity. A greater sense of urgency is needed concerning correction of modest weight gain, since this often leads insidiously to intractable obesity.

Diabetes

The efficacy of treating diabetes to prevent cardiovascular sequelae is in doubt. The University Group Diabetes Program investigated the effects of several oral hypoglycemic agents and two insulin regimens in patients with adult-onset diabetes and found no significant benefits over placebo treatment. No current regimen confined to the control of hyperglycemia alone appears able to moderate the atherosclerotic sequelae. It would appear more rational to redefine control to include normalization of all the multiple metabolic aberrations common to the diabetic state, including the blood lipids,

overweight, and hypertension and to restrict cigarette smoking.

Physical Activity

It does not seem wise to rely upon physical exercise programs alone to protect against fatal coronary attacks. Physical exercise is best prescribed as one component of a comprehensive program for avoiding CHD. Activities requiring movement over a distance seem most valuable. Sustained regular exercise of moderate intensity (50 to 75 percent of capacity) for 15 to 30 minutes at least every other day is required to maintain a training effect. There is some evidence, however, that lesser levels of exercise may also be beneficial. A vigorous walking program may be more prudent for middle-aged, flabby, deconditioned Americans. This will also tend to minimize the considerable orthopedic side effects of vigorous exercise such as jogging. Swimming and bike riding also have the merit of not being weight bearing.

Hypertension

Because even moderate degrees of hypertension have been shown to double the risk of a coronary event and the Hypertension Detection and Follow-up Program has demonstrated the efficacy of treating this mild hypertension, it is especially important to treat this group. It can be shown, however, that the bulk of the cardiovascular sequelae over the first decade in this mild hypertension is concentrated in a small percentage who have other accompanying cardiovascular risk factors and hence a poor cardiovascular risk profile. It would seem best to reserve drug treatment for these and use hygienic treatment with weight reduction and salt and alcohol restriction for the rest. The regimen must be followed, since hypertension tends to progress and drug treatment may be required at a later stage.

Cigarette Smoking

Despite mandatory warnings on each package that cigarette smoking is hazardous to health and public health campaigns, teenagers take up the habit too often and are only lately beginning to heed warnings. Physicians as a group have shown a greater decline in smoking than the general population and can serve as a good role model. However, more vigorous and conscientious efforts in dispensing this advice and checking on compliance are needed. Physicians should always raise the question of smoking in connection with the findings of CVD and even in general health exams. They should more often solicit help from the family in getting the patient to quit.

Because of the tenaciousness of the cigarette habit and powerful vested interests in protecting the tobacco industry, an attempt to develop a "safer" cigarette has been undertaken. The tar and nicotine content has been reduced, largely through the introduction of filter cigarettes. Preliminary evidence from the Framingham Study indicates that this has been of little benefit in reducing the hazard of CVD. Men under 55 in the Framingham Study were classified as to whether they smoked filter cigarettes or nonfilter cigarettes. The 58 percent who smoked filter cigarettes tended to have slightly less prior smoking exposure, but despite this, they did not have lower CHD incidence than nonfilter smokers (*48*). Filter cigarette smokers tend to smoke more vigorously, getting as much nicotine and carbon monoxide as nonfilter cigarette smokers.

CONCLUSION

Effective risk factor control will require mobilization of community resources to assist in the endeavor. Such measures should be multifactorial and should be begun as early in life as possible, when the faulty habits are conditioned and lesions are still only in the formative stages. The entire family should be involved in the risk factor modification of the high-risk candidate. Physicians must develop the preventive skills needed to encourage the behavior modification required. Although the rewards may lie decades in the future, the physicians must recognize that such an endeavor will have a greater impact on his patients' ultimate well-being than almost anything else he might do for them.

References

(*1*) Intersociety Commission for Heart Disease Resources: Primary prevention of the atherosclerotic diseases. *Circulation* 42:A-55, 1970.

(*2*) Keys, A. Coronary heart disease—the global picture. *Atherosclerosis* 22:149-192, 1975.

(*3*) Stamler, J. Lifestyles, major risk factors, proof and public policy. *Circulation* 58:3-19, 1978.

(*4*) Kannel, W.B., W.P. Castelli, and T. Gordon. Cholesterol in the prediction of atherosclerotic disease. New perspectives based on the Framingham Study. *Ann Intern Med* 90:85-91, 1979.

(*5*) Hegsted, D.M., R.B. McGandy, M.L. Nyers, and F.J. Stare. Quantitative effects of dietary fat on serum cholesterol in man. *Am J Clin Nutr* 17:281-295, 1965.

(*6*) Keys, A., J.T. Anderson, and F. Grande. Serum cholesterol response to changes in the diet. IV. Particular saturated fatty acids in the diet. *Metabolism* 14:776-787, 1965.

(*7*) Mattson, F.H., B.A. Erickson, and A.M. Kligman. Effect of dietary cholesterol on serum cholesterol in man. *Am J Clin Nutr* 25:589-594, 1972.

(*8*) Vesselinovitch, D., R.W. Wissler, R. Highes, and J. Borensztajn. Reversal of advanced atherosclerosis in rhesus monkeys. I. Light-microscope studies. *Atherosclerosis* 23:155-176, 1976.

(*9*) Glueck, C.J. Dietary fat and atherosclerosis. *Am J Clin Nutr* 32:2703-2711, 1979.

(*10*) McGill, H.C., Jr. The relationship of dietary cholesterol to serum cholesterol concentration and to atherosclerosis in man. *Am J Clin Nutr* 32:2664-2702, 1979.

(*11*) Beaton, G.H., J. Midner, P. Corey, et al. Sources of variance in 24 hour dietary recall data: implications for nutrition study design and interpretation. *Am J Clin Nutr* 32:2546-2559, 1979.

(*12*) Liu, K., J. Stamler, A. Dyer, and P. McKeever. Statistical methods to assess and minimize the role of intra-individual variability in obscuring the relationship between dietary lipids and serum cholesterol. *J Chron Dis* 31:399-418, 1978.

(*13*) Shekelle, R.B., A.M. Shryock, O. Paul, et al. Diet, serum cholesterol and death from coronary heart disease. The Western Electric Study. *N Engl J Med* 304:65-70, 1981.

(*14*) Kannel, W.B., T.R. Dawber, and D.L. McGee. Perspectives on systolic hypertension. The Framingham Study. *Circulation* 61:1179-1182, 1980.

(*15*) Kannel, W.B., P. Sorlie, and T. Gordon. Labile hypertension: a faulty concept? The Framingham Study. *Circulation* 61:1183-1187, 1980.

(*16*) *Report of the National Commission on Diabetes.* Washington, DC, DHEW Publ. No. (NIH) 76-1022, 1975.

(*17*) Kannel, W.B. and D.L. McGee. Diabetes and cardiovascular risk factors: the Framingham Study. *Circulation* 59:8-13, 1979.

(*18*) Kannel, W.B., and T. Gordon. The Framingham Study: an epidemiological investigation of cardiovascular disease. Section 30. Some characteristics related to the incidence of cardiovascular disease and death: the Framingham Study. 18 year follow-up. US Dept. of Health, Education, and Welfare. Public Health Service. National Institutes of Health. DHEW Publ No. (NIH) 74-599, 1974.

(*19*) Garcia, M.J., P.M. McNamara, T. Gordon, and W.B. Kannel. Morbidity and mortality of diabetes in the Framingham population. 16 year follow-up. *Diabetes* 23:105-111, 1976.

(*20*) Knowles, H.C., Jr. Magnitude of the renal failure problem in diabetic patients. *Kidney International* Vol. 6, No. 4, Suppl. I. New York, Springer Verlag, 1974.

(21) Kannel, W.B., M. Hjortland, and W.P. Castelli. Role of diabetes in congestive heart failure. The Framingham Study. *Am J Cardiol* 34:29-34, 1974.

(22) Persky, V.W., A.R. Dyer, E. Idris-Soven, et al. Uric acid: a risk factor for coronary heart disease? *Circulation* 59:969-977, 1979.

(23) US Public Health Service. The Health Consequences of Smoking. Washington DC, Government Printing Office, 1971.

(24) Gordon, T., W.B. Kannel, D.L. McGee, and T.R. Dawber. Death and coronary attacks in men after giving up cigarette smoking. A report from the Framingham Study. *Lancet* 2:1345-1348, 1974.

(25) Aronow, W.S. Effect of cigarette smoking and of carbon monoxide on coronary heart disease. *Chest* 70:514-518, 1976.

(26) Keys, A. Overweight and the risk of heart attack and sudden death. In: *Bray, Georgia: Obesity in perspective*. Vol. 2. Part 2. Washington DC, DHEW Publ. No. (NIH) 75-708, 1976, p. 215.

(27) Ashley, F.W. and W.B. Kannel. Relation of weight change to changes in atherogenic traits. The Framingham Study. *J Chronic Dis* 27:103-114, 1974.

(28) Kagan, A., T. Gordon, G.G. Rhoads, and J.C. Schiffman. Some factors related to CHD incidence in Honolulu Japanese men: the Honolulu Heart Study. *Int J Epidemiol* 4:271-279, 1975.

(29) Wyndham, C.H. The role of physical activity in the prevention of ischaemic heart disease. *S Afr Med J* 36:7-13, 1979.

(30) Kannel, W.B., T. Gordon, P. Sorlie, and P.M. McNamara. Physical activity and coronary vulnerability: the Framingham Study. *Cardiology Digest* 6:28-40, 1971.

(31) Jenkins, C.D. Recent evidence supporting psychologic and social risk factors for coronary disease. *N Engl J Med* 294:1033-1088, 1976.

(32) Friedman, H. and R.H. Rosenman. *Type A Behavior and Your Heart*. New York, Alfred A. Knopf, 1974.

(33) Haynes, S.G., M. Feinleib, and W.B. Kannel. The relationship of psychosocial factors to coronary heart disease in the Framingham Study. III. Eight-year incidence of CHD. *Am J Epidemiol* 3:37-58, 1980.

(34) Shekelle, R.B., S. Hulley, J. Neaton, et al. Type A behavior and risk of coronary death in MRFIT. *Proceedings of the Council on Epidemiology, American Heart Association. San Diego, California, March 3, 1983*.

(35) Kritchevsky, D. Dietary fiber and other dietary factors in hypercholesteremia. *Am J Clin Nutr* 30:979-984, 1977.

(36) Page, L.B. Epidemiologic evidence on etiology of human hypertension and its possible prevention. *Am Heart J* 91:527-534, 1976.

(37) Dawber, T.R., W.B. Kannel, and T. Gordon. Coffee and cardiovascular disease. Observations from the Framingham Study. *N Engl J Med* 291:871-874, 1974.

(38) Stason, W.B., R.K. Neff, O.S. Miettinen, and H. Jick. Alcohol consumption and nonfatal myocardial infarction. *Am J Epidemiol* 104:603-608, 1976.

(39) Crawford, M.D., D.G. Clayton, F. Stanley, and A.G. Shaper. An epidemiological study of sudden death in hard and soft water areas. *J Chronic Dis* 30:69-80, 1977.

(40) Rogot, E. and S.J. Padgett. Association of coronary and stroke mortality with temperature and snowfall in selected areas of the United States 1962-1966. *Am J Epidemiol* 103:565-575, 1976.

(41) Pfeffer, R.I., G.H. Whipple, T.T. Kurosaki, and J.M. Chapman. Coronary risk and estrogen use in postmenopausal women. *Am J Epidemiol* 107:479-497, 1978.

(42) Rosenberg, L., C. Hennekens, B. Rosner, et al. Early menopause and risk of myocardial infarction. *Am J Obstet Gynecol* 139:47-57, 1981.

(43) McGill, H.C., Jr. and M.P. Stern. Sex and atherosclerosis. *Atheroscler Rev* 4:157-242, 1979.

(44) *Coronary Risk Handbook. Estimating Risk of Coronary Heart Disease in Daily Practice.* New York, American Heart Association, 1973.

(45) Gordon, T. and W.B. Kannel. Premature mortality from coronary heart disease. The Framingham Study. *JAMA* 215:1617-1625, 1971.

(46) Kannel, W.B., P.D. Sorlie, and P.M. McNamara. Prognosis after myocardial infarction: the Framingham Study. *Am J Cardiol* 44:53-59, 1979.

(47) Vedin, A., C. Wilhelmsson, G. Tibblin, and L. Wilhelmsen. The post-infarction clinic in Göteborg, Sweden. A controlled trial of therapeutic organization. *Acta Med Scand* 200:453-456, 1976.

(48) Castelli, W.P., R.J. Garrison, T.R. Dawber, et al. The filter cigarette and coronary heart disease: the Framingham Study. *Lancet* 4:109-113, 1981.

PSYCHIATRIC DISORDERS IN FOSTER HOME REARED CHILDREN OF SCHIZOPHRENIC MOTHERS[1]

Leonard L. Heston[2]

INTRODUCTION

The place of genetic factors in the etiology of schizophrenia remains disputed. Several surveys have demonstrated a significantly higher incidence of the disorder in relatives of schizophrenic persons as compared to the general population. Furthermore, the closer the relationship, the higher the incidence of schizophrenia. The studies of Kallmann (1) and Slater (2) are especially significant and the research in this area has been thoroughly reviewed by Alanen (3).

Although the evidence for a primarily genetic etiology of schizophrenia is impressive, an alternative explanation—that schizophrenia is produced by a distorted family environment—has not been excluded. A close relative who is schizophrenic can be presumed to produce a distorted interpersonal environment and the closer the relationship the greater the distortion.

This study tests the genetic contribution to schizophrenia by separating the effects of an environment made "schizophrenogenic" by the ambivalence and thinking disorder of a schizophrenic parent from the effects of genes from such a parent. This is done by comparing a group of adults born to schizophrenic mothers where mother and child were permanently separated after the first two postpartum weeks with a group of control subjects.

SELECTION OF SUBJECTS

The Experimental subjects were born between 1915 and 1945 to schizophrenic mothers confined to an Oregon State psychiatric hospital. Most of the subjects were born in the psychiatric hospital; however, hospital authorities encouraged confinement in a neighboring general hospital whenever possible, in which case the children were delivered during brief furloughs. All apparently normal children born of such mothers during the above time span were included in the study if the mother's hospital record (1) specified a diagnosis of schizophrenia, dementia precox, or psychosis; (2) contained sufficient descriptions of a thinking disorder or bizarre regressed behavior to substantiate the diagnosis; (3) recorded a negative serologic test for syphilis and contained no evidence of coincident disease with known psychiatric manifestations; and (4) contained presumptive evidence that mother and child had been separated from birth. Such evidence typically consisted of a statement that the mother had yielded the child for adoption, a note that the father was divorcing the mother, the continued hospitalization of the mother for several years, or the death of the mother. In practice these requirements meant that the mothers as a group were biased in the direction of severe, chronic disease. No attempt was made to assess the psychiatric status of the father; however, none were known to be hospital patients. The 74 children ascertained as above were retained in the study if subsequent record searches or interviews confirmed that the child had had no contact with its natural mother and never lived with maternal relatives. (The latter restriction was intended to preclude significant exposure to the environment which might have produced the mother's schizophrenia.)

All of the children were discharged from the State hospital within three days of birth (in accordance with a strictly applied hospital policy) to the care of family members or to foundling homes. The records of the child care institutions made it possible to follow many subjects through their early life, including, for some, adoption. The early life of those subjects discharged to relatives was less completely known,

Source: *British Journal of Psychiatry* 112:819-825, 1966.

[1] This research was supported by the Medical Research Foundation of Oregon.

[2] Resident in Psychiatry, University of Oregon Medical School; Guest Worker, Psychiatric Genetics Research Unit, Maudsley Hospital, London.

although considerable information was developed by methods to be described.

Sixteen subjects were dropped because of information found in foundling home records; six children, four males and two females, died in early infancy. Ten others were discarded, eight because of contact with their natural mother or maternal relatives, one because of multiple gastrointestinal anomalies, and one because no control subject whose history matched the bizarre series of events that complicated the Experimental subject's early life could be found. The remaining 58 subjects comprise the final Experimental group.

A like number of control subjects, apparently normal at birth, were selected from the records of the same foundling homes that received some of the Experimental subjects. The control subjects were matched for sex, type of eventual placement (adoptive, foster family, or institutional), and for length of time in child care institutions to within ±10 percent up to five years. (Oregon State law prohibited keeping a child in an institution more than five years. Subjects in institutions up to this maximum were counted as "institutionalized" regardless of final placement.) Control subjects for the Experimental children who went to foundling homes were selected as follows: When the record of an Experimental subject was located, the admission next preceding in time was checked, then the next subsequent, then the second preceding and so on, until a child admitted to the home within a few days of birth and meeting the above criteria was found. Those Experimental subjects who were never in child care institutions were matched with children who had spent less than three months in a foundling home. The above method of selection was used with the record search beginning with an Experimental child's year of birth. The above restrictions regarding maternal contacts were applied to the control group. Oregon State psychiatric hospital records were searched for the names of the natural parents (where known) of the control subjects. In two cases a psychiatric hospital record was located and the children of these persons were replaced by others. All of the children went to families in which both parental figures were present.

Exact matching was complicated by the subsequent admission of several subjects to other child care institutions and by changes of foster or even adoptive homes. However, these disruptions occurred with equal frequency and intensity in the two groups and are considered random.

Table 1 gives the sex distribution of the subjects and the causes of further losses. Fifteen of the 74 Experimental subjects died before achieving school age. This rate is higher than that experienced by the general population for the ages and years involved, but not significantly so.

Table 1.

	Experimental		Control	
	Male	Female	Male	Female
Number	33	25	33	25
Died, infancy or childhood	3	6		5
Lost to follow-up		2		3
Final Groups	30	17	33	17

FOLLOW-UP METHOD

Starting in 1964, it proved possible to locate or account for all of the original subjects except five persons, all females. During this phase of the research, considerable background information of psychiatric import was developed. The records of all subjects known to police agencies and to the Veterans' Administration were examined. Retail credit reports were obtained for most subjects. School records, civil and criminal court actions, and newspaper files were reviewed. The records of all public psychiatric hospitals in the three West Coast States were screened for the names of the subjects and the records located were reviewed. Enquiries were directed to psychiatric facilities serving other areas where subjects were living, and to probation departments, private physicians, and various social service agencies with which the subjects were involved. Finally, relatives, friends and employers of most subjects were contacted.

In addition to information obtained from the above sources, for most subjects the psychiatric assessment included a personal interview, a Minnesota Multiphasic Personality Inventory (MMPI), an I.Q. test score, the social class of the subject's first home, and the subject's current social class. As the subjects were located, they were contacted by letter and asked to participate in a personal interview. The interview was standardized, although all promising leads were followed, and was structured as a general medical and environmental questionnaire which explored all important psychosocial dimensions in considerable depth. Nearly all of the interviews were conducted in the homes of the subjects, which added to the range of possible observations. The short form of the MMPI was given after the interview. The results of an I.Q. test were available from school or other records for nearly all subjects. If a test score was not available, the Information, Similarities, and Vocabulary subtests of the Wechsler Adult Intelligence Scale (WAIS) was administered and the I.Q. derived from the results. Two social class values were assigned according to the occupational classification system of Hollingshead (4). One value was based on the occupation of the father or surrogate father of the subject's first family at the time of placement, and a second on the subject's present occupational status or, for married females, the occupation of the husband. The social class values move from 1 to 7 with decreasing social status.

All of the investigations and interviews were conducted by the author in 14 states and in Canada.

EVALUATION OF SUBJECTS

The dossier compiled on each subject, excluding genetic and institutional information, was evaluated blindly and independently by two psychiatrists. A third evaluation was made by the author. Two evaluative measures were used. A numerical score moving from 100 to 0 with increasing psychosocial disability was assigned for each subject. The scoring was based on the landmarks of the Menninger Mental Health-Sickness Rating Scale (MHSRS) (5). Where indicated, the raters also assigned a psychiatric diagnosis from the American Psychiatric Association nomenclature.

Evaluations of 97 persons were done. Seventy-two subjects were interviewed. Of the remaining 25 persons, six refused the interview (7.6 percent of those asked to participate), eight were deceased, seven were inaccessible (active in Armed Forces, abroad, etc.), and four were not

approached because of risk of exposure of the subject's adoption. It did not seem reasonable to drop all of these 25 persons from the study, since considerable information was available for most of them. For instance, one man was killed in prison after intermittently spending most of his life there. His behavioral and social record was available in prison records plus the results of recent psychological evaluations. A man who refused the interview was a known, overt, practicing homosexual who had a recent felony conviction for selling narcotics. All persons in the Armed Forces were known through letters from their Commanding Officers or medical officers to have been serving honorably without psychiatric or serious behavioral problems. One 21-year-old man, the least known of any of the subjects, had been in Europe for the preceding 18 months in an uncertain capacity. He is known to have graduated from high school and to have no adverse behavioral record. In a conference the raters agreed that it would be misleading to discard any cases, and that all subjects should be rated by forced choice.

The MHSRS proved highly reliable as a measure of degree of incapacity. The Intraclass Correlation Coefficient between the scores assigned by the respective raters was 0.94, indicating a high degree of accuracy. As expected, several differences arose in the assignment of specific diagnoses. In disputed cases a fourth psychiatrist was asked for an opinion and differences were discussed in conference. The only differences not easily resolved involved distinctions such as obsessive-compulsive neurosis versus compulsive personality or mixed neurosis versus emotionally unstable personality. All differences were within three diagnostic categories: psychoneurotic disorders, personality trait or personality pattern disturbances. The raters decided to merge these categories into one: "neurotic personality disorder." This category included all persons with MHSRS scores less than 75—the point on the scale where psychiatric symptoms become troublesome—who received various combinations of the above three diagnoses. In this way, complete agreement on four diagnoses was achieved: schizophrenia, mental deficiency, sociopathic personality, and neurotic personality disorder. One mental defective was also diagnosed schizophrenic and another sociopathic. Only one diagnosis was made for all other subjects.

RESULTS

Psychiatric disability was heavily concentrated in the Experimental group. Table 2 summarizes the results.

The MHSRS scores assess the cumulative psychosocial disability in the two groups. The difference is highly significant with the Experimental group, the more disabled by this measure. However, the difference is attributable to the low scores achieved by about one-half (26/47) of the Experimental subjects rather than a general lowering of all scores.

The diagnosis of schizophrenia was based on generally accepted standards. In addition to the unanimous opinion of the three raters, all subjects were similarly diagnosed in psychiatric hospitals. One female and four males comprised the schizophrenic group. Three were chronic deteriorated patients who had been hospitalized for several years. The other two had been hospitalized and were taking antipsychotic drugs. One of the latter persons was also mentally deficient: a brief history of this person follows.

A farm laborer, now 36 years old, was in an institution for mentally retarded children from age 6-16. Several I.Q. tests averaged 62. He was discharged to a family farm, where he worked for the next 16 years. Before his hospitalization at age 32 he was described as a peculiar but harmless person who was interested only in his bank account: he saved $5500 out of a salary averaging $900 per year. Following a windstorm that did major damage to the farm where he worked he appeared increasingly agitated. Two days later he threatened his employer with a knife and accused him of trying to poison him. A court committed him to a psychiatric hospital. When admitted, he talked to imaginary persons and assumed a posture of prayer for long periods. His responses to questions were incoherent or irrelevant. The hospital diagnosis was schizophrenic reaction. He was treated with phenothiazine drugs, became increasingly rational, and was discharged within a month. After discharge he returned to the same farm, but was less efficient in his work and spent long periods sitting and staring blankly. He has been followed as an out-patient since discharge, has taken phenothiazine drugs continuously, and anti-depressants occasionally. This man exhibited almost no facial expression. His responses to questions, though relevant, were given after a long and variable latency.

The age-corrected rate for schizophrenia is 16.6 percent, a finding consistent with Kallmann's 16.4 percent. (Weinberg's short method,

Table 2.

	Control	Experimental	Exact probability
Number	50	47	
Male	33	30	
Age, mean	36.3	35.8	
Adopted	19	22	
MHSRS, mean (Total group mean = 72.8, S.D. = 18.4)	80.1	65.2	0.0006
Schizophrenia (Morbid Risk = 16.6%)	0	5	0.024
Mental deficiency (I.Q.<70)	0	4	0.052
Sociopathic personality	2	9	0.017
Neurotic personality disorder	7	13	0.052
Persons spending >1 year in penal or psychiatric institution	2	11	0.006
Total years Institutionalized	15	112	
Felons	2	7	0.054
Armed Forces, number serving	17	21	
Armed Forces, number discharges, psychiatric or behavioral	1	8	0.021
Social group, first home, mean	4.2	4.5	
Social group, present, mean	4.7	5.4	
I.Q., mean	103.7	94.0	
Years school, mean	12.4	11.6	
Children, total	84	71	
Divorces, total	7	6	
Never married, >30 years age	4	9	

One mental defective was also schizophrenic; another was sociopathic.
Considerable duplication occurs in the entries below Neurotic Personality Disorder.

age of risk 15-45 years). Hoffman (*6*) and Op-pler (*7*) reported rates of from 7 to 10.8 per-cent, of schizophrenia in children of schizo-phrenics. No relationship between the severity and sub-type of the disease in the mother-child pairs was evident.

Mental deficiency was diagnosed when a sub-ject's I.Q. was consistently less than 70. All of these persons were in homes for mental defec-tives at some time during their life and one was continuously institutionalized. His I.Q. was 35. The other mentally deficient subjects had I.Q.s between 50 and 65. No history of CNS disease or trauma of possible causal importance was obtained for any of these subjects. The mothers of the mentally defective subjects were not dif-ferent from the other mothers and none were mentally defective.

Three behavioral traits were found almost ex-clusively within the Experimental group. These were: (1) significant musical ability, seven per-sons; (2) expression of unusually strong re-ligious feelings, six persons; and (3) problem drinking, eight persons.

The results with respect to the effects of in-stitutional care, social group, and type of place-ment will be discussed in a later paper. None of these factors had measurable effects on the out-come.

DISCUSSION

The results of this study support a genetic etiology of schizophrenia. Schizophrenia was found only in the offspring of schizophrenic mothers. The probability of this segregation being effected by chance is less than 0-025. Fur-thermore, about one-half of the Experimental group exhibited major psychosocial disability. The bulk of these persons had disorders other than schizophrenia which were nearly as malig-nant in effect as schizophrenia itself. An il-lustration is provided by the 8 of 21 Experimen-tal males who received psychiatric or behavioral discharges from the armed services. If three subjects who were rejected for service for the same reasons are added, the ratio becomes 11 : 24, or essentially 1 : 2. Only three of these 11 subjects were schizophrenic and one schizo-phrenic served honorably. Kallmann's (*1*) rate for first degree relatives and Slater's (*2*) for di-zygotic twins of schizophrenic persons who de-veloped significant psychosocial disability not limited to schizophrenia are slightly lower, though in the same range, as those found in the present study.

The association of mental deficiency with schizophrenia has been reported by Hallgren and Sjögren (*8*) who noted an incidence of low-grade mental deficiency (I.Q. = 50-55) in schizophrenic subjects of about 10.5 percent. Kallmann (*1*) found from 5-10 percent mental defectives among his descendants of schizo-phrenic persons, but did not consider the find-ing significant. The association of mental defi-ciency with schizophrenia, if such an association exists, remains uncertain.

Two sub-groups of persons within the im-paired one-half of Experimental subjects exhib-ited roughly delineable symptom-behavior complexes other than schizophrenia or mental deficiency. The personalities of the persons composing these groups are described in aggre-gate below.

The first group is composed of subjects who fit the older diagnostic category, "schizoid psy-chopath." This term was used by Kallmann (*1*) to describe a significant sub-group of his rela-tives of schizophrenic persons. Eight males from the present study fall into this group, all of whom received a diagnosis of sociopathic per-sonality. These persons are distinguished by anti-social behavior of an impulsive, illogical nature. Multiple arrests for assault, battery, poorly planned impulsive thefts dot their police records. Two were homosexual, four alcoholic, and one person, also homosexual, was a narcot-ics addict. These subjects tended to live alone—only one was married—in deteriorated hotels and rooming houses in large cities, and locating them would have been impossible without the co-operation of the police. They worked at ir-regular casual jobs such as dishwasher, race-track tout, parking attendants. When inter-viewed they did not acknowledge or exhibit evi-dence of anxiety. Usually secretive about their own life and circumstances, they expressed very definite though general opinions regarding so-cial and political ills. In spite of their suggestive life histories, no evidence of schizophrenia was elicited in interviews. No similar personalities were found among the control subjects.

A second sub-group was characterized by emotional lability and may correspond to the neurotic sibs of schizophrenics described by Al-anen (*9*). Six females and two males from the

Experimental group as opposed to two control subjects were in this category. These persons complained of anxiety or panic attacks, hyper-irritability, and depression. The most frequent complaint was panic when in groups of people as in church or at parties, which was so profoundly uncomfortable that the subject had to remove himself abruptly. Most subjects described their problems as occurring episodically; a situation that they might tolerate with ease on one occasion was intolerable in another. The women reported life-long difficulty with menses, especially hyper-irritability or crying spells, and depressions coincident with pregnancy. These subjects described themselves as "moody," stating that they usually could not relate their mood swings to temporal events. Four such subjects referred to their strong religious beliefs much more frequently than other respondents. Psychophysiological gastrointestinal symptoms were prominent in five subjects. The most frequent diagnoses advanced by the raters were emotionally unstable personality and cyclothymic personality, with neurosis a strong third.

Of the nine persons in the control group who were seriously disabled, two were professional criminals, careful and methodical in their work, two were very similar to the emotionally labile group described above, one was a compulsive phobia-ridden neurotic, and four were inadequate or passive-aggressive personalities.

The 21 Experimental subjects who exhibited no significant psychosocial impairment were not only successful adults but in comparison to the control group were more spontaneous when interviewed and had more colorful life histories. They held the more creative jobs: musician, teacher, home-designer; and followed the more imaginative hobbies: oil painting, music, antique aircraft. Within the Experimental group there was much more variability of personality and behavior in all social dimensions.

SUMMARY

This report compares the psychosocial adjustment of 47 adults born to schizophrenic mothers with 50 control adults, where all subjects had been separated from their natural mothers from the first few days of life. The comparison is based on a review of school, po-lice, veterans, and hospital, among several other records, plus a personal interview and MMPI which were administered to 72 subjects. An I.Q. and social class determination were also available. Three psychiatrists independently rated the subjects.

The results were:

(1) Schizophrenic and sociopathic personality disorders were found in those persons born to schizophrenic persons in an excess exceeding chance expectation at the 0.05 level of probability. Five of 47 persons born to schizophrenic mothers were schizophrenic. No cases of schizophrenia were found in 50 control subjects.

(2) Several other comparisons, such as persons given other psychiatric diagnoses, felons, and persons discharged from the Armed Forces for psychiatric or behavioral reasons, demonstrated a significant excess of psychosocial disability in about one-half of the persons born to schizophrenic mothers.

(3) The remaining one-half of the persons born to schizophrenic mothers were notably successful adults. They possessed artistic talents and demonstrated imaginative adaptations to life which were uncommon in the control group.

ACKNOWLEDGMENTS

The author is greatly indebted to Drs. Duane D. Denney, Ira B. Pauly, and Arlen Quan who evaluated the case histories and provided invaluable advice and encouragement. Drs. Paul Blachly, John Kangas, Harold Osterud, George Saslow, and Richard Thompson provided advice and/or facilities which greatly contributed to the success of the project. All of the above are faculty or staff members of the University of Oregon Medical School.

This research could not have been completed without the splendid cooperation of numerous officials of various agencies who provided indispensable information. I am especially indebted to the following: Dean R. Mathews, Waverly Baby Home; Elda Russell, Albertina Kerr Nurseries; Stuart R. Stimmel and Esther Rankin, Boys' and Girls' Aid Society of Oregon; Reverend Morton E. Park, Catholic Charities; George K. Robbins, Jewish Family and Child Services; Miss Marian Martin, State of Oregon, Department of Vital Statistics, all of Portland, Oregon.

Drs. Dean K. Brooks. E.I. Silk, Russel M. Guiss, J.M. Pomerov, Superintendents of Oregon State Hospital, Eastern Oregon State Hospital, Danmasch State Hospital, and Oregon Fairview Home, respectively. David G. Berger, Research Coordinator, Oregon State Board of Control; Stewart Adams, Research Director, Los Angeles County Probation Department; Robert Tyler, Research Information Director, California Bureau of Corrections; Evan Iverson, State of Washington, Department of Institutions; Anthony Hordern, Chief of Research, California Department of Mental Hygiene; Captain George Kanz, Oregon State Police; J.S. Gleason, Administrator, Veterans' Administration; and Lt. General Leonard D. Heaton, Rear Admiral E.C. Kenney, and Major General R.L. Bohannon, Chief Medical Officers of the Army, Navy and Air Force, respectively.

Renate Whitaker, University of Oregon Medical School, and Eliot Slater and James Shields of the Psychiatric Genetics Research Unit, Maudsley Hospital, London, reviewed the manuscript and made many helpful suggestions.

Finally, I wish gratefully to acknowledge the contribution made by the subjects of this research project, most of whom freely gave of themselves in the interest of furthering medical science.

References

(1) Kallmann, F.J. *The Genetics of Schizophrenia.* New York: J.J. Augustin, 1938.

(2) Slater, E. with J. Shields. Psychotic and neurotic illnesses in twins. Medical Research Council Special Report Series No. 278. London: H.M. Stationery Office, 1953.

(3) Alanen, Y.O. The mothers of schizophrenic patients. *Acta Psychiat Neurol Scand* Suppl. 1227, 1958.

(4) Hollingshead, A.B. and F.C. Redlich. (1958). *Social Class and Mental Illness: A Community Study.* New York: J. Wiley, 1958.

(5) Luborsky, L. Clinicians' judgments of mental health: a proposed scale. *Arch Gen Psychiat (Chic.)* 7:407, 1962.

(6) Hoffman, H. *Studien über Vererbung und Entstehung geistiger Störungen. II. Die Nachkominenschaft bei endogenen Psychosen.* Berlin, Springer, 1921.

(7) Oppler, W. Zum Problem der Erbprognosebestimmung. *Z Neurol,* 141:549-616, 1932.

(8) Hallgren, B. and T. Sjögren. A clinical and genetico-statistical study of schizophrenia and low grade mental deficiency in a large Swedish rural population. *Acta Psychiat Neurol Scand* Suppl. 140. Vol. 35, 1959.

(9) Alanen, V.O., J. Rekola, A. Staven, M. Tuovinen, K. Takala, and E. Rutanen. Mental disorders in the siblings of schizophrenic patients. *Acta Psychiat Scand* Suppl. 169 39:167, 1963.

PELLAGRA PREVENTION BY DIET AMONG INSTITUTIONAL INMATES

Joseph Goldberger,[1] C. H. Waring,[1] and W. F. Tanner[1,2]

In 1914, when the study herein reported was begun, American opinion as to the etiology and prophylaxis of pellagra may be said to have been very unsettled, if not chaotic. The spoiled-maize theory of the cause and as the basis for prevention, though stoutly held in some important quarters, was declining in favor; and the belief that the disease was an infection of some kind, supported as it was by such important studies as those of the Illinois and of the Thompson-MacFadden pellagra commissions (1, 2), was gaining a ready and rapidly widening acceptance. The state of mind, both lay and professional, is well indicated by the following from Lavinder (3), even though written five years earlier:

"There are several very good reasons just now why this question of communicability should have arisen to much importance in this country. . . . In the first place, the disease has arisen and grown to large proportions, apparently like the proverbial mushroom, almost in a single night. It is something new, a malady with which we are not familiar, and in some of its manifestations is repulsive, if not actually loathsome; indeed, some of the older writers, evidently struck with this fact, applied to it the name 'leprosy,' a term which, since the days of Moses, has been a synonym to mankind of all that is repulsive and loathsome in human disease. Then, too, it has been associated in our minds very frequently with mental alienation, a state naturally abhorrent to all; and its reported death rate has been very large indeed. Furthermore, the indefinite and pervasive character of its etiology, with the lack, not only of any specific treatment, but the apparent inefficacy of all treatment, has added further color to an already vivid picture.

"All these features have given to the disease an air of strangeness, not to say of actual mystery, which has made a strong appeal to the public mind and which has probably, to a certain extent, reacted upon the professional mind. The result in certain communities has been to produce a very uneasy state of feeling, almost an hysterical condition, at times actually bordering on panic."

The fear that the disease was communicable led here and there to the adoption of such drastic measures of control as isolation and quarantine.

The situation called urgently for renewed investigation with a view of testing these conflicting views and, if possible, establishing a sound basis for the prevention of the disease. Considering this problem, one of the present writers was struck by the possible significance of the long recognized exemption from the disease enjoyed by well-to-do people. In reflecting on this striking phenomenon and in considering the elements differentiating affluence from poverty, diet, in view of the conspicuous place it had always had in discussions of the disease, naturally arrested attention. It seemed possible that the well-to-do owed their exemption to their superior diet. Coupled with certain other epidemiological observations, this led him (4) to suggest that it might be well to attempt to prevent the disease by providing those persons subject to pellagra with a diet such as that enjoyed by the class practically free from it. Accordingly, in the fall of 1914, the Public Health Service undertook to put this hypothesis to the test. A report covering the work and results of the first year was published in 1915 (5). It was originally intended to make a detailed presentation of the study on its completion; but the confirmation of the published results of the first year by White (6), among Armenian refugees at Port Said, and by Stannus (7) among the inmates of Central Prison, Nyassaland, before this could be done, has rendered a detailed account superfluous.

Source: *Public Health Reports* 38(41): 2361-2368, 1923.
[1] Surgeons, United States Public Health Service
[2] During the first two years of the study at the Georgia State Sanitarium, Dr. David G. Willets, late assistant epidemiologist, United States Public Health Service, was associated with us. His premature separation was unhappily made necessary by the development in December, 1916, of what proved to be a fatal illness.

And this all the more as the later results, as will presently be seen, were in close harmony with and in complete confirmation of those of the first year. We therefore present now but a general summary of this study with brief mention of only the more important and significant details.

Since the study was carried on throughout along the lines adopted at its beginning, and since, as stated, later results were in close harmony with those of the first year, it will be helpful to review at the outset the methods and results of the first year.

First year. The test of the preventive value of diet was begun at two orphanages at Jackson, Miss., in September, 1914, and in two wards of the Georgia State Sanitarium later that same year. These institutions had been endemic foci of the disease for some years. During the spring and summer of 1914, 79 cases of pellagra had been observed among the children of one orphanage and 130 among those of the other. Besides a variable number of cases of pellagra annually admitted as such (see beyond), cases of intramural origin were of frequent occurrence at the sanitarium.

At the orphanages the diet of all the residents, and at the sanitarium that of a group of selected inmates of two wards set aside for the purpose, was modified in several respects, among others in that oatmeal almost entirely replaced grits as the breakfast cereal and the allowance of fresh animal protein foods (milk, meat, and, at the orphanages, eggs) and legumes was greatly increased. The allowance of maize was thus reduced but not abolished. Aside from these modifications in diet and increased watchfulness over the individual eating, all administrative routine and hygienic and sanitary conditions remained unchanged. Furthermore, in order, at the same time, to test the hypothesis of infection, no restrictions were imposed on new admissions by reason of any manifestations of pellagra or of a history of an attack of the disease, and thus association and contact with newly admitted active cases was permitted without hindrance and, from time to time, actually took place, particularly at the sanitarium, the opportunities there being better.

At about the end of the first year following the inauguration of the modified diet, it was found that, at the orphanages, of an aggregate

of 172 pellagrins who had completed at least the anniversary date of the 1914 attack under observation, only one had showed any evidence of a recurrence, and not a single case developed among an aggregate of 168 nonpellagrins who had been continuously under observation at least one year; and at the sanitarium of an aggregate of 72 pellagrins who had either remained continuously under observation up to October 1, 1915, or, at least, until after the anniversary date of the 1914 attack, not one presented recognizable evidence of a recurrence, although at the same time 47 percent of a comparable group of 32 pellagrins not receiving the modified diet had recurrent attacks of the disease.

Second year. The results of the first year afforded no support for the idea that pellagra was communicable, but very clearly indicated that the disease could be prevented by an appropriate diet. Nevertheless, by reason of the importance of the question involved, and in order to make the test and demonstration of preventability as convincing as possible, it seemed desirable to continue the investigation, as originally planned, for at least another year and, if possible, on a larger scale.

The study at the orphanages and at the asylum was accordingly continued and, in addition, was extended to include an orphanage at Columbia, S. C., and a third ward of insane pellagrins, with recent attacks, at the State Sanitarium.

It was extended to the Columbia institution on September 1, 1915. At this orphanage the disease, after its recognition there in 1907 or 1908, had prevailed from year to year in spite of various efforts to control it. With this purpose in view, a water carriage sewerage system had been installed in 1914 in place of the surface privies theretofore used, but without appreciable effect, for in 1915 the number attacked and the rate of recurrence were higher than ever, upward of 100 cases being recognized among the children by the orphanage physician (8). At the time of taking charge there were present 235 residents at this orphanage, of whom 106 had been reported to us as having had pellagra that year; and of these 15 still presented recognizable evidence of the attack.

At the sanitarium the additional ward of pellagrins was taken under observation and provided with the modified and supplemented diet about November 1, 1915.

The result of this more extensive test of the preventability of pellagra by dietary means was in the closest harmony with that of the first year. In not a single one of the individuals receiving the modified diet at the three orphanages and at the hospital for insane did pellagra develop either as an initial or a recurrent attack. So impressive was this outcome that it seemed unnecessary longer to continue the demonstration on so large a scale. Accordingly, the study at the orphanages was discontinued on September 1, 1916; but because of the much greater significance likely to attach to results of tests in the insane, that at the State Sanitarium was continued through a third year; that is, until December 31, 1917.

Third year. The third year's study at the sanitarium was continued with three wards under observation, one in the white and two in the colored service, as during the second year. The modifications of and supplements to the institution diet, the hygienic conditions, the administrative routine, the mingling with other inmates (including those with active pellagra) in the wards and in the recreation yards were continued as during the first and second year.

The result of the third year's study was exactly like that of the second year: no recurrence and no new case among those inmates taking the modified diet.

Result as a whole. The result of the investigation considered as a whole may be summed up as follows: The individuals under observation, disregarding those who were present for periods too brief to be significant, numbered 702,

of whom 414 were pellagrins and 288 nonpellagrins.

Two hundred and fifty of the pellagrins and 268 of the nonpellagrins were included in the study at the orphanages and were under continuous observation for at least one year. Of this group, 107 of the pellagrins and 85 of the nonpellagrins were under observation for a period of at least two years (Table 1).

Of the 414 pellagrins included in the study, 164 were observed at the sanitarium and were under observation until at least the first anniversary date of the attack, during which or shortly after which they entered the study. Of these 164, 109 were under observation until at least the second anniversary date, and, of the latter group, 57 until at least the third anniversary date. Resident on the same wards and receiving the same diet as these pellagrins, were nonpellagrins, 20 of whom (not including nurses and attendants) were under observation for at least one year, 16 of these for not less than two years, and, of the latter, 10 for not less than three years.

As has already been stated, but a single case of pellagra occurred among all these pellagrins and nonpellagrins. This one case, a recurrence in a boy at one of the Jackson orphanages, developed during the first year of the study. The boy continued under observation during the second year without again developing any evidence of the disease.

At this point mention may be made of the history of pellagra at one of the institutions subsequent to the discontinuance of the foregoing study. Immediately following our withdrawal, there was a return to the unmodified and unsupplemented institution diet. During the period of from three and one-half to nine

Table 1. Number of specified classes of individuals observed for pellagra during specified periods, according to orphanage of residence.

	Period of observation										
	At least one year				One year but less than two years				At least two years		
Class	Total	MJ[a]	BJ[a]	EC[b]	Total	MJ[a]	BJ[a]	EC[b]	Total	MJ[a]	BJ[a]
Pellagrins	250	59	99	92	143	22	29	92	107	37	70
Nonpellagrins	268	100	69	99	183	58	26	99	85	42	43

[a] Two orphanages at Jackson, Miss., indicated by "MJ" and "BJ."
[b] Orphanage at Columbia, S. C., indicated by "EC."

and one-half months following this, approximately 40 percent of those who were affected by the change in diet developed pellagra. Thereupon there were added to the institution diet, again under our direction, 4 ounces of fresh beef, about 7 ounces of sweet milk, and about 14 ounces of buttermilk per adult per day; and during an observation period of 14 months immediately succeeding the adoption of these supplements no evidence of pellagra developed in any of the group.

DISCUSSION

It appears, then, that at each institution at which the test was made, barring cases admitted as such during the progress of the test, pellagra promptly disappeared. And it is perhaps important to note that this was not merely a marked reduction in prevalence, but in each instance a complete disappearance of the disease. It may be noted also that the disease disappeared from the institutions at a time when it was highly prevalent at large in the corresponding States. Thus, judging by mortality reports, we find that in Mississippi there were 1192 deaths from pellagra in 1914, 1535 in 1915, 840 in 1916, and 1086 in 1917; that in South Carolina there were 1649 in 1915, 729 in 1916, and 714 in 1917. For Georgia no reports are available for this period, but admissions to the Georgia State Sanitarium will serve as a good index of the yearly prevalence in that State. In 1914, of 1427 patients admitted, 194, or 13.59 percent, were active cases of pellagra; in 1915, of 1683 admissions, 272, or 16.16 percent, were cases of pellagra; in 1916, of 1331 admissions, 111, or 8.34 percent, were pellagra; and in 1917, of 1219 admissions, 121, or 9.93 percent, were active cases.

Clearly, therefore, the disappearance of pellagra from the institutions under consideration must have been due to something not operative at large or operative only to an inappreciable degree. Recalling the conditions of the test— namely, that hygienic and sanitary conditions (excepting diet) continued unaltered, that admission of active cases and association of these with persons in the test continued without hindrance (and was particularly frequent and free at the sanitarium), that considerable groups of persons in four separate endemic foci in three widely separated localities were involved—the something that operated to bring this disappearance about must have been the one factor, diet, close upon the modification of which disappearance of the disease followed. Since both pellagrins and exposed nonpellagrins were carried for as long as two and three years without manifesting recognizable evidence of a return or of the development of an initial attack of the disease, and since in one group of these the disease reappeared on departing from and again disappeared on returning to what, for this purpose, is considered to have been an appropriate diet, the inference seems clearly warranted that not only may pellagra be completely prevented by diet, but that it may be prevented indefinitely as long as a proper diet is maintained and without the intervention of any other factor, hygienic or sanitary.

What food or foods, food factor or factors, in the diet are to be credited with the result under discussion, this experiment in itself does not definitely reveal. In planning the test diet we were guided by general observation of the character of the dietary of well-to-do people and the results of certain epidemiologic observations (5) which suggested that the disease was dependent upon a diet that was faulty and that this fault was, in some way, either prevented or corrected by including in the diet larger proportions of the fresh animal protein foods. The experiment may be therefore considered as, at most, suggesting that the fresh meat and milk of the diet were concerned in bringing about the protective effect, or, in other words, that fresh meat and milk supplied some factor or factors which operated to prevent the development of pellagra.

Since the results here reported are but a confirmation, on a more extended and more convincing scale, of those previously reported for the first year of this study, which alone and in connection with the results of certain other phases of the general investigation of which they are parts, have already been sufficiently considered (5, 9-13), both in their implications and in their relation to the results of the studies of other investigators, further discussion at this time seems uncalled for.

SUMMARY AND CONCLUSIONS

A report of a three years' study of the preventability of pellagra by means of diet, the result of the first year of which was reported eight years ago, is briefly presented.

The study was carried on for a year at one and for two years at two of three orphanages, and for three years in a section of the Georgia State Sanitarium, each of the institutions being recognized as an endemic focus of the disease.

The institution diet was in each instance modified by reducing the maize element and increasing the fresh animal protein foods—meat, milk (and at the orphanages, eggs), and legumes.

All other conditions, hygienic and sanitary, including association with active cases which from time to time were admitted, remained unchanged.

The individuals under observation, not counting those who were present for periods too brief to be significant, numbered 702 in all, of whom 414 were pellagrins and 288 non-pellagrins.

Among the pellagrins a single recurrent case was noted during the first year following the inauguration of the modified diet; none in the second nor in the third year. Among the non-pellagrins there was not a single case.

A return to the institution diet immediately after the discontinuance of the formal study at one of the institutions was shortly followed by an incidence of pellagra of approximately 40 percent among the affected group. Resumption of the modified diet was again followed during a period of observation of 14 months by complete disappearance of the disease.

During the study the disease disappeared from the institutions, although a considerable prevalence at large in the corresponding States continued.

The idea that pellagra is a communicable disease receives no support from this study.

Pellagra may be completely prevented by diet.

References

(1) Report of the Pellagra Commission of the State of Illinois. Springfield, Ill., 1912.

(2) Siler, J.F., P.E. Garrison, and W.J. MacNeal. *JAMA* 62:8-12, 1914.

(3) Lavinder, D.H. *Public Health Rep* 24:1617-1624, 1909.

(4) Goldberger, J. *Public Health Rep* 29:1683-1686, 1914.

(5) Goldberger, J., C.H. Waring, and D.G. Willets. *Public Health Rep* 30:3117-3131, 1915.

(6) White, R.G. *Report on an Outbreak of Pellagra Amongst Armenian Refugees at Port Said, 1916-17* Cairo, Egypt, 1919.

(7) Stannus, H.S. *Trans Roy Soc Trop Med Hyg* (London). 14:16, 1920.

(8) Rice, H.W. *Southern Med J* 9:778-785, 1916.

(9) Goldberger, J. *JAMA* 66:471-476, 1916.

(10) Goldberger, J. and G.A. Wheeler. *Hyg Lab Bull* (Washington, D.C.), 120, 1920.

(11) Goldberger, J. and G.A. Wheeler. *Arch Int Med* 25:451-471, 1920.

(12) Goldberger, J., G.A. Wheeler, and E. Sydenstricker. *Public Health Rep* 35:648-713, 1920.

(13) Goldberger, J. *JAMA* 78:1678-1680, 1922.

THE BIOLOGY OF EPIDEMICS[1]

W.W.C. Topley

Some, at least, among those who have shared with me the honor of being invited to deliver the Croonian Lecture must have shared also an uneasy feeling that they were under an obligation to refer, directly or indirectly, to some aspect of muscular motion, in accordance both with precedent and with the supposed intentions of the Founder. Uncertain of the facts, I consulted the Society's records, and found I need have no qualms. The Lecture was founded, not by Dr. Croone, but by his widow, who, after his decease, married Sir Edwin Sadleir. It was founded by her for the Advancement of Natural Knowledge on Local Motion, or (conditionally) on such other subject as, in the opinion of the President for the time being, should be most useful for promoting the objects for which the Royal Society was instituted.

A Report on the Croonian Lecture, issued by the Society in 1834, states the position clearly and concisely. The relevant passage reads:

"The epithet *Croonian* which has hitherto (with few exceptions) been applied to this Lecture, instead of that of *Sadleirian,* to which in justice to its Founder it seems to be entitled, appears to have arisen in the misconception of the Council....Having mistaken Dr. Croone as the Founder of the Lecture, they also mistook its nature and conditions; and instead of regarding it, as founded by Lady Sadleir, for promoting the general objects of the Society, they conceived it to be confined to the subject of Muscular Motion only; and the error, thus established, appears to have continued through subsequent years."

In the light of this evidence, I am a little uncertain as to whether I am delivering a Croonian or Sadleirian Lecture; but I have no doubt at all that, without any dispensation from the President, I am entitled to discuss any phenomena depending, not on muscular, but on local motion. I can think of no better or more ambitious aim for any student of epidemics than to attempt to reduce his problems to precisely these terms. There is ample evidence that local movements of populations, of parasites and hosts, of insect vectors, and especially the relation of these movements to one another, determine outbreaks of infective disease. We are far as yet from identifying all relevant movements, or the factors on which they depend; and of those we know, many are hard to measure. But there is no other hopeful method of approach.

The epidemiology of today is the child of parasitology. Medicine is its grandmother, once or twice removed. The universe of study which now faces the epidemiologist is not, in its essence, composed of a number of cases of a clinically recognizable disease, with a distribution that varies in an intriguing way in space and time. It is composed of a variety of biological species, some acting as parasites and some as hosts. The parasites may be viruses, or bacteria, or fungi, or protozoa, or worms. The hosts may be men, or animals, or insects, or plants. Some parasites, particularly certain helminths, pass through different life cycles in different hosts, so that they are dependent on at least two host species for their continued propagation. Many parasites can propagate themselves in the tissues of two or more animal species which act as alternative hosts. Certain biting insects act as vectors. Sometimes the parasite passes through an essential phase of a complex life cycle within the insect's tissues. Sometimes it is simply transferred from the blood of one host to that of another, perhaps with multiplication by binary fission during transit. Sometimes non-biting insects act as mechanical vectors of parasites, commonly from excreta to food; but in these instances they provide only one among many possible routes of infection. Even if we take the simplest case in which there is no insect vector, and in which, so far as we yet know, only one host, say man, and one parasite are concerned, we find that our universe is not composed of sick persons and the parasite that

Source: *Proceedings of the Royal Society of London* 130:337-359, 1942.
[1] The Croonian Lecture, delivered 17 July 1941; received 27 October 1941.

causes the disease, but that there are, among the infected hosts, all gradations from clinically typical cases, through mild and atypical infections, to what are known as healthy carriers, persons who display no signs or symptoms of illness but from whose tissues or excreta the causative parasite may be isolated.

It is clear that no amassing of clinical observations, however careful and acute, and no correlation of such observations with environmental factors, however complete the records and statistical analyses, could have solved such problems as these, or have shown us in any detail how and when we might intervene effectively. Such observations have supplied us with data that form an essential part of our field of study; but when, today, we are faced with correlations between certain diseases and certain conditions of climate, or housing, or occupation, we do not leave it at that, we transpose our picture into terms of the effect of these environmental conditions on the hosts, or vectors, or parasites concerned. We think, for instance, not in terms of marshes and malaria, but in terms of breeding places for mosquito larvae, and of how these are affected by light, shade, salinity, and a host of other factors. We try to discover which misquitoes bite which hosts and under what conditions, how far they fly, and where they hibernate, and when. We view the problem of plague in terms of rats and fleas, of typhus in terms of lice, of diphtheria in terms of carriers as well as cases, and so on. The medical or veterinary epidemiologist becomes a biologist whether he will or no. The biologist can study many of the problems of epidemiology with no more than a nodding acquaintance with human or veterinary medicine.

The very complexity of the natural systems with which the epidemiologist is faced often makeş it difficult to tell which of the correlations that he observes are biologically significant. This difficulty is not lessened by the fact that it is quite easy to invent hypotheses that would, if they were true, fit attractively into our puzzle. It is much less easy to determine whether they are true or not; and this step has been omitted with a rather surprising frequency.

One way of attempting to solve some of our problems is to turn our backs on the natural world, and to simplify our conditions until the number of variable factors reaches manageable proportions, and then to see what happens when we hold some factors constant and vary others. This is the method that Professor Greenwood and I, together with our colleagues Dr. Joyce Wilson and Dr. Bradford Hill, have been exploring for many years past (*1*). We have worked with mice, and with three diseases to which mice are naturally prone: pasteurellosis, a bacterial disease of the respiratory tract; mouse typhoid, an intestinal bacterial disease; and a virus disease, ectromelia. All these diseases spread from mouse to mouse by direct contact. The various precautions that we have taken to control our experimental conditions have been described elsewhere.

THE EFFECT OF VARYING THE RATE OF ADDITION OF SUSCEPTIBLE MICE

In most experiments we have started an epidemic among a group of mice, and then added a constant number of mice each day for many months, or for several years. The effect of varying the rate of addition of susceptible mice to infected herds, contact being continuous, may be briefly summarized as follows.

With low rates of addition, up to one or two mice each day, the death rate has shown wide and irregular fluctuations, with occasional intermissions. As the rate of addition rises, the curve of daily mortality assumes an undulating form, with no intermissions, and no clearly defined waves or peaks after the few initial fluctuations that always mark the earliest phase of epidemic spread under these conditions. The total population of the herd rises, at first steeply, then more slowly. In experiments carried on for many months or years it tends towards a relatively constant level. Figure 1 shows the first five months' experience in an epidemic of pasteurellosis, in which six mice were added daily to the herd. Figure 2 shows similar periods for two epidemics of ectromelia, in each of which three mice were added daily to the herd.

It may be noted that, in our limited experience, there is little correlation between the average daily death rate and the rate of addition of susceptible mice, provided that immigration is maintained at a steady rate. It follows that the effect of adding more mice each day is simply to increase the level of population at which equilibrium is attained.

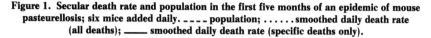

Figure 1. Secular death rate and population in the first five months of an epidemic of mouse pasteurellosis; six mice added daily. _ _ _ _ population; . . . . . . smoothed daily death rate (all deaths); _____ smoothed daily death rate (specific deaths only).

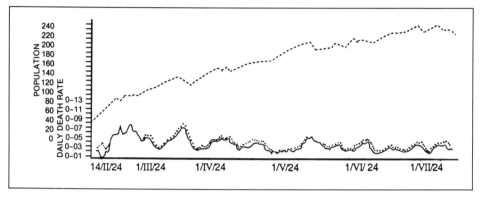

Figure 2. Two epidemics of ectromelia. Three mice added daily.

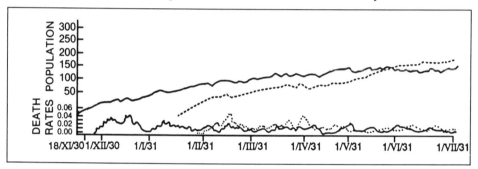

All our evidence suggests that, with rates of addition higher than have been practicable in our experiments, we should attain a steady rate of mortality and a stable population, the daily deaths equalling the daily additions. This means only that such a system has no inherent tendency to fluctuate, as epidemics fluctuate under natural conditions. There is no evidence that the parasite waxes or wanes in its relevant biological properties as it passes from host to host, or that the hosts pass through any periodic variation in resistance. Nor does the infection ever die out. We must search in other directions for the factors that determine the rise and fall of epidemic waves.

THE EFFECT OF CHANGING FROM CONTINUOUS TO DISCONTINUOUS CONTACT

In an experiment which has not yet been recorded in detail we varied the procedure described above by keeping the mice constituting an infected herd in separate cages, one mouse to a cage. We started the experiment with 25 mice infected with mouse typhoid and 100 normal companions. Each Monday, Wednesday, and Friday the mice were assembled in a single large cage for four hours, and on each of these days two normal mice were added to the herd. The course of events is shown in Figure 3. The herd was assembled on 19 April 1937. An epidemic started, but soon died down; and after about the 70th day deaths from mouse typhoid ceased to occur. The population was rising, and by the 149th day had reached 180. Since no death from mouse typhoid had occurred for approximately 80 days, it seemed that these conditions, though involving close contact between the mice for four hours on each of three days a week, were not such as to ensure an effective spread of infection. The conditions were therefore altered, and on the 149th day the mice were aggregated in a single large cage.

Figure 3. A, contact becomes continuous; B, contact becomes intermittent; C, contact becomes continuous.

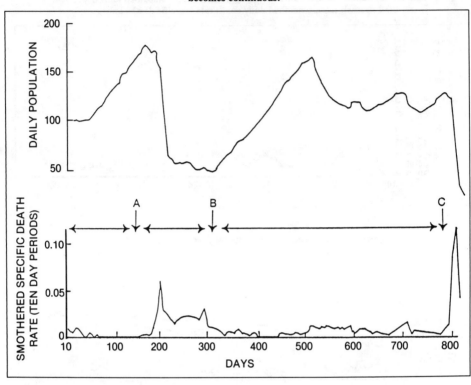

The response was almost immediate. Within a few days deaths from mouse typhoid recurred, and, within 35 days of aggregation, a major epidemic wave was well under way, reaching a peak 15 days later. After this wave had subsided, the mortality remained at a relatively high level, and by the 289th day of the experiment the total population had fallen from 180 mice to 44, in spite of the addition of 6 new entrants a week. On day 290 the herd was again separated into single cages, and allowed to mingle for four hours on each of three days a week. The response was as prompt as before, but in the reverse direction. The death rate sank, and the population mounted. These conditions were maintained from the 290th to the 767th day, a period of over one year and three months. During this period the death rate followed an irregular course. It seemed clear that intermittent contact of this degree, while it had been insufficient to maintain the initial epidemic spread when only a few of the mice were infected, was adequate to maintain a smouldering endemic prevalence after the massive infection of the herd that followed the first aggregation. On the 767th day the herd was aggregated in a single cage for a second time. Again there was a brisk response. A major epidemic wave started within 15 days, reaching a peak about 20 days later, and then fell sharply. Within 30 days the population fell from 150 to 20 mice. The experiment was shortly after brought to an end. Its interest lies in the striking response to simple changes in the continuity of contact without the introduction of any new source of infection.

THE EFFECT OF DISPERSAL ON AN INFECTED HERD

We have carried out a few experiments to test the effect of dispersing an infected herd into groups of varying size, no subsequent additions being made (2, 3). The results indicate that dispersal into relatively large groups, for instance the dispersal of 100 mice into four groups each of 25, has little effect once an epidemic has begun to spread. If the groups are smaller, if, for instance, a herd of 100 mice is dispersed into 10 groups of 10 mice apiece, the subsequent specific mortality is much lower than in a control herd of 100 mice maintained as a single unit, provided that dispersal is carried out in the initial phase of an epidemic. If, on the other hand, dispersal is delayed until an epidemic wave is well under way it has little effect, even though the dispersed groups are numerous and small. The withdrawal of mice from a herd, in which infection is continuously spreading, to isolation in single cages, always lowers the subsequent average mortality of these mice as compared with that of their contemporaries left in the herd, however long they have previously been exposed to risk (*4*).

GROUP-TO-GROUP INFECTION

In the same category of experiments depending on the controlled movements of infected and susceptible mice in relation to one another, we may include a small series of tests designed to answer a rather different question (*5*). In the many experiments in which we have added normal mice to an infected herd for periods of months or years, the infection has never shown any signs of dying out. It was clearly of interest to see how long an infection could be propagated if a small group of infected mice was placed in contact with a small group of normal mice for a relatively short period, the normal contacts removed after this exposure and placed in contact with another group of normal mice, and this process repeated as long as infection continued to pass from group to group. The results of these tests were in sharp contrast to those obtained when normal mice were added to a herd in which infection was spreading continuously. By the group-to-group method of contact, the period of contact between groups varying from 4 to 21 days, it was never possible to secure the passage of mouse typhoid or of pasteurellosis beyond the third successive group. We have not yet made similar experiments with ectromelia. Had the groups been larger, or the period of contact between them longer, continuous spread would probably have been secured. These experiments are merely another illustration of the dominance in the spread of infection of those factors that determine the probability of effective contact.

There is no difficulty in finding analogies to the events in our cages in the natural world outside them. As examples we may take some of the data collected by my colleague, Dr. Joyce Wilson, on behalf of the School Epidemics Committee of the Medical Research Council (*6*). They were obtained from 21 public schools for boys, and 10 public schools for girls. Complete card records were made, for the five years 1930-1934 inclusive, of all forms of sickness involving an absence from school on one or more days.

Taking the group of minor nasopharyngeal infections, colds, sore throats and so on, Figures 4, 5 and 6 show the attack rates for these disorders for each week of the Lent, Summer and Christmas terms in each year for the ten girls' schools. It will be seen that in every term, in every year, there was a primary peak incidence between the second and fourth week of term, usually between the third and fourth. Similar curves for any of the common infectious diseases, such as measles, tell an analogous story.

There can be no doubt that this termly distribution of infective disease is the direct result of the reaggregation of boys and girls after the dispersal of the holidays. It cannot be due to seasonal influences, since the same thing happens in each of the three terms, save that the peaks are higher in the Lent terms for those diseases that are prevalent in the late winter and early spring. Epidemics of this kind are, at the moment, part of the price that we must pay for education.

It is of some interest to trace the effect on these contact infections of the evacuation of children from our larger and more vulnerable cities which occurred on the outbreak of war. Figure 7 shows the weekly incidence of scarlet fever and diphtheria in England and Wales for the ten years 1931-1941. For measles and whooping cough, which have only recently been made notifiable, the weekly deaths in the 150 great towns have been taken over the same period. The vertical lines are drawn at 31 December each year.

It is obvious at a glance that the last three months of 1939 and the greater part of 1940 were periods of unusually low incidence so far as these diseases were concerned; and the change in the form of the yearly curves, with the exception of that for diphtheria, is as striking as the total fall in the cases or deaths. Scarlet fever, in 1940, fell to its lowest level in the early spring, instead of in the late summer. The ex-

Figure 4. Weekly attack rates (percent) for all nasopharyngeal infections (excluding influenza) for the five Lent terms 1930-1934 (girls' boarding schools).

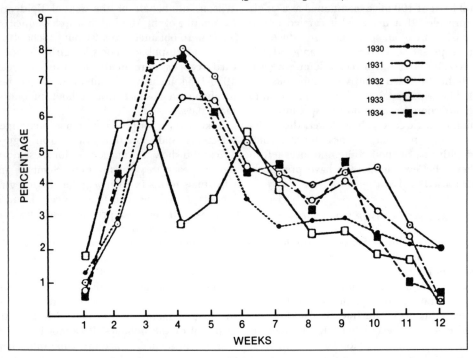

pected rise in the measles death rate in the winter of 1939-1940, and in the early spring of the latter year, is conspicuous by its absence; and the same is true of whooping cough during the early months of 1940. It might be argued that the abnormal curves for measles and whooping cough are due to the figures for these diseases being taken from the great towns. When the curve was drawn, monthly mortality figures for the country as a whole were not available; but Dr. Stocks, of the General Register Office, has kindly supplied me with the relevant quarterly figures for the period in question, and these show that the number of deaths

Figure 5. Weekly attack rates (percent) for all nasopharyngeal infections (excluding influenza) for the five summer terms 1930-1934 (girls' boarding schools).

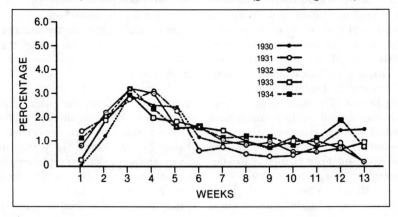

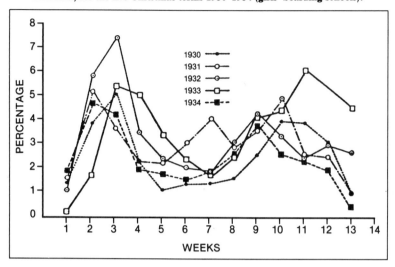

Figure 6. Weekly attack rates (percent) for all nasopharyngeal infections (excluding influenza) for the five Christmas terms 1930-1934 (girls' boarding schools).

in England and Wales was so low that no epidemic can have occurred. There are, however, many considerations that have to be taken into account in interpreting secular curves of this kind; and it is possible that the decrease in any of these diseases would have occurred apart from the war. The cumulative evidence does, however, suggest that the association with evacuation was not in each case fortuitous. Assuming this, it seems at least possible that school closure in towns, and the lack of school accommodation in the evacuation areas, contributed more to the result than the move from town to country per se.

At the same time that we were evacuating children from our larger towns, and decreasing their contacts in school, we were collecting a large part of our young adult males into huts and billets. Young adults are, for the most part, resistant to scarlet fever, diphtheria, measles and whooping cough; but they are susceptible to another disease, cerebrospinal meningitis, which is also spread by contact infection by way of the upper respiratory tract. Whenever we mobilize an army we may expect an outbreak of this disease during the first winter or spring, when the men spend a large part of their time in huts or billets. In spite of the low rates of other sickness in the army, this particular expectation was fulfilled. Figure 8 shows that a major epidemic of cerebrospinal meningitis oc-

curred in the early months of 1940. During the rest of the year the incidence remained higher than in any year of peace, and there was another epidemic wave, though on a smaller scale, in the early months of 1941. Fortunately, the new sulphonamide drugs had provided us, for the first time, with an effective remedy; and though the morbidity was high the case mortality was low.

The lesson to be drawn from this is, I think, the following. It is quite certain that movements of susceptible and infected hosts in relation to one another, and aggregations or dispersals of human or animal herds, apart from any introduction of new infection, are sufficient to induce major changes in the incidence of many infective diseases. In considering the relation of any environmental factors to the rise and fall of epidemic waves, it will always be wise to determine in what way they affect the movement and distribution of the hosts at risk.

Equally, when we attempt to lessen the incidence of an infective disease, it will be wise to consider carefully whether any practicable change in the habitual movements and distribution of infected and susceptible hosts will lessen the frequency of contact between them.

The same applies to the mechanical transference of parasites, through the air, by dust, by contaminated objects, by persons or animals who may transfer the parasites from host to host without themselves becoming infected, and so on. The system becomes more complex, the risks more numerous, and the necessary meas- ures of control more various, but the principle does not change. Any step that lessens the probability of effective contact, direct or indirect, is a

Figure 7. Weekly notified cases of scarlet fever and diphtheria in England and Wales (1931–1941) and weekly notified deaths for measles and whooping cough in great towns of England and Wales (1931–1941).

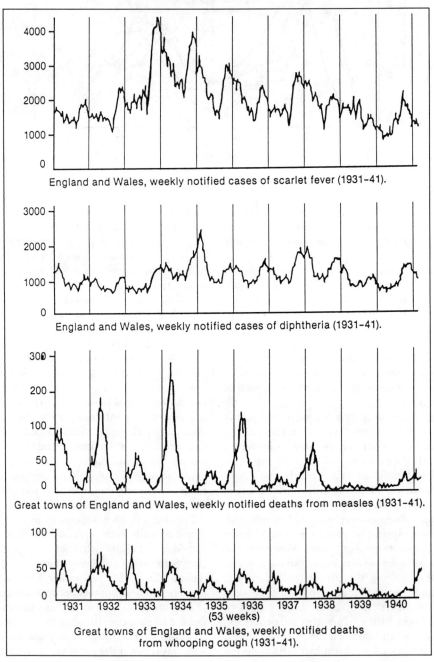

England and Wales, weekly notified cases of scarlet fever (1931–41).

England and Wales, weekly notified cases of diphtheria (1931–41).

Great towns of England and Wales, weekly notified deaths from measles (1931–41).

Great towns of England and Wales, weekly notified deaths from whooping cough (1931–41).

Figure 8. England and Wales, weekly notified cases of cerebro-spinal fever (1931–1941).

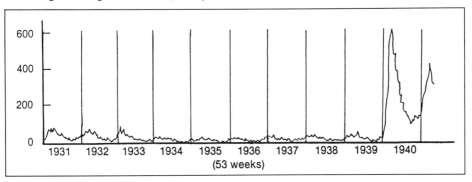

step in the right direction. This seems a platitude; and so it should be. But there are many instances in which the possibilities of action along these lines have not yet been fully exploited.

THE EFFECT OF NATURAL AND ARTIFICIAL IMMUNIZATION

In summarizing the results obtained in long-continued experimental epidemics, it was noted that there was no evidence of any periodic change in the resistance of the hosts at risk of a kind that would lead to fluctuations in the rate of mortality. This does not mean, of course, that the resistance of the mice is uniform on entry to the herd, or remains unchanged thereafter. The individuals of any host species vary in their innate resistance, and the average resistance of mice that have lived for long in an infected herd will be greater than the average resistance of mice on entry, if only because the more susceptible will have been sifted out by death.

Those who survive do not remain unchanged. The great majority of them react to a non-fatal infection by developing an immunity of the type that depends on the production, in the host's tissues, of antibodies that react specifically with certain constituents of the infecting microorganisms.

It would be easy to give any number of illustrations of this type of immunization from the world of natural events, but the data available for infected herds of mice are more complete, and therefore more easily represented in graphic form. Figure 9 is constructed from the

results obtained in a particular epidemic of mouse typhoid in which daily examinations were made of the excreta of all mice at risk, so that infection could be detected apart from death (7). The abscissae are days of cage age, not days in secular time. Mice dead of the disease are included among the infected, so that the difference between the broken and continuous curves represents mice infected but still alive. It will be seen that, by the 25th day of residence in an infected herd, 42 percent of entrants are dead, and 41 percent infected but alive. The data from many other epidemics indicate that infection rates of this order hold for most of our experiments, though there is naturally some variation. We can, at least, regard it as highly probable that most survivors of a few weeks' standing have acquired the specific infection, and with it the stimulus that we should expect to result in some degree of specific immunity. In considering how far our expectations are realized it will be convenient to select experiments in which the fate of normal entrants has been compared with that of mice artificially immunized with an appropriate vaccine, so that we may at the same time assess the extent to which we can gain the advantage of immunity without the risk of death.

Figure 10 shows the relevant findings in the case of mouse typhoid (8). The ordinates give the average expectation of life arbitrarily limited to 60 days. Here again, the abscissae are days of cage age, not days in secular time. The upper curve shows the limited expectation of life at all days of cage age from 0 to 50 of normal mice living in an uninfected herd to which three normal mice were added each day. As one would expect, the expectation of life

Figure 9. Percentage of infections and deaths among ninety mice exposed to mouse typhoid, for different cage ages.

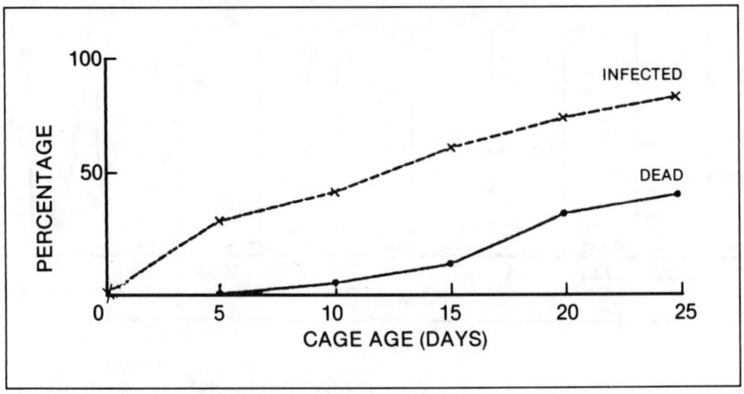

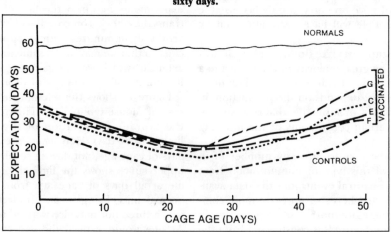

approximates closely to its maximum value throughout, though it is somewhat below it during the earlier days of cage life before the mutual antagonisms of new entrants and old inhabitants have been replaced by a reasonable degree of tolerance. The lower curves show the change in expectation of life with cage age of mice that were living, and dying, in a herd infected with mouse typhoid, to which groups of vaccinated and control non-vaccinated mice were added together at regular intervals. It will be seen that the controls fared badly. On entry they had less than half the normal expectation of life, and their expectation sank till about the 25th day, when it was only 9.3 days out of a possible 60. This fall is due to the fact that the expectation of life will be minimal on the day of cage age at which, on the average, the mice have become infected and are in the final stages of a fatal illness. The expectation of life then rises, in part because the more susceptible mice have been eliminated by death, in greater part, perhaps, because the survivors have been specifically immunized by a non-fatal infection.

The curves labelled *C*, *E*, *F* and *G* refer to mice artificially immunized by the injection of two doses of four different killed bacterial vaccines, all containing the essential antigenic constituents of *Bacterium typhi-murium*. It will be seen that, at all cage ages, they fare better than

Figure 10. Effect of vaccination in mouse typhoid; expectation of life limited to sixty days.

the non-immunized controls; but they never attain an expectation of life approaching the normal. It should, however, be noted that the mice in these experiments are exposed to a continuous risk of contact infection greater than would be encountered by any human population, except under very unusual conditions. The effectiveness of antityphoid inoculation in man has been amply proved by the experience in our armies.

Figure 11 shows similar curves for an epidemic of the virus disease ectromelia (*1*). The immunized mice in this instance were injected with two doses of a living but attenuated virus. The results here differ sharply from those obtained with mouse typhoid. On entry to the cage the control mice have an expectation of life even lower than that of the non-immunized entrants to the herd infected with mouse typhoid. But, after a slight fall, reaching its lowest point on the 8th day of cage age, the curve rises sharply, and by the 30th day has attained a value not far below the normal. Clearly, the natural immunization that follows a non-fatal attack of ectromelia is more effective than the natural immunization that follows an attack of mouse typhoid. Similarly, our vaccination has been far more effective. The immunized mice on entry to the cage have an expectation of life

of almost 50 days out of a possible 60. The expectation never falls significantly below that figure, and later rises above it. We have placed our immunized immigrants, from the start, in the same position as that reached by the surviving non-immunized controls after some 26 days of cage life, when they have passed through an experience to which more than half the normal entrants have succumbed. It should be noted that, in this experiment, the limited expectation of life declined between the 30th and 50th days of cage life; but this decline applied equally to the control and vaccinated mice.

It is clear that the process of natural immunization will result in changes in the proportions of resistant and susceptible hosts among any community exposed to the risk of infection by a particular parasite. After the subsidence of a major epidemic wave the proportion of susceptibles will be decreased to a level depending on the average risk of infection to which the community as a whole has been subjected. If no new susceptibles gain access, an equilibrium may persist in which a high infection rate is balanced by a high level of herd immunity. If, after such an equilibrium has been maintained for a considerable period, a relatively large number of susceptibles gain entrance within a short interval of time, another major outbreak

Figure 11. Effect of vaccination in extromelia: expectation of life limited to sixty days.

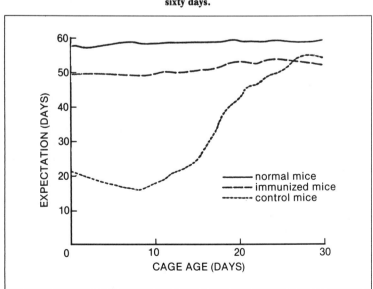

may occur, in which the newcomers suffer first and most severely, but in which some of the old survivors are also involved (9). This sequence of events has been observed both in experimental epidemics and in natural outbreaks of disease. If, on the other hand, susceptibles gain access in small numbers, continuously or intermittently, the course of events will depend in the main on the average risk of infection to which the newcomers are subjected. If it is very high, there will tend to be a persistent endemic prevalence, with occasional cases of disease, but no major outbreak. If it is low, the proportion of newcomers at risk may attain a relatively high level before a chance succession of infections sets a spark to the susceptible material and precipitates a new epidemic wave.

It is probable that changes in the spatial distribution of the hosts at risk, and changes in the proportion of susceptible and resistant hosts resulting from natural immunization, together account for many, perhaps most, of the periodic or repetitive fluctuations in prevalence observed under natural conditions in those epidemic systems in which infection is spread by direct contact, and in which no insect vectors or alternative hosts are involved.

It should be noted that the effectiveness of natural immunization varies, both in degree and duration, from one infective disease to another, and that, apart from variations of this kind, the immunity involved is in each case specific, not to the clinical disease as such, but to the chemical constitution of the parasite that causes it, or of the toxin that the parasite produces. The chemical components concerned are known as antigens, and it happens that microorganisms with different antigenic structures may produce indistinguishable symptoms and lesions in infected hosts, so that an acquired immunity towards a particular species or type of parasite may not be synonymous with immunity to the clinical disease of which it is one among several causes. There are, for instance, more than 30 different antigenic types of pneumococci that cause pneumonia in man, several types of the virus that causes foot-and-mouth disease in cattle, and, very unfortunately, more than one type of virus that causes human influenza.

We may now turn to factors of a different kind, which come into play at certain times, and in certain places, rather than as constant contributors to the course of events in any prolonged prevalence of infective disease.

THE EPIDEMIC POTENCY OF DIFFERENT STRAINS OF A SINGLE SPECIES OF PARASITE

Many field epidemiologists, and particularly the late Dr. Fred Griffith, have been convinced that the observed behavior of certain human infections, such as those due to hemolytic streptococci, demand the hypothesis of the existence of special epidemic strains of the parasites concerned, with heightened powers of producing disease by contact infection.

In an attempt to test this hypothesis experimentally, we have carried out a large number of trials by a method which differs from that employed in our long-term epidemics. We have assembled 100 mice in a single cage, and added to them 25 mice infected by the injection of a constant dose of the strain of bacterial parasite under test. We have watched events for 60 days, and then killed all surviving mice. We should not expect that experiments of this kind, even though carried out with a single strain of a particular bacterial parasite, would give us consistently replicable results, nor do they do so; but the variations are not so wide as might be feared.

Figure 12 shows the course of events in 13 such epidemics, the number of survivors among the 100 mice at risk being plotted against time (10). The ten upper curves were obtained in ten experiments carried out with a particular strain of *Bacterium typhi-murium*. It will be seen that this strain caused only a moderate mortality in the mice exposed to risk, though a large series of other tests had shown it to possess a relatively high virulence when injected directly into the tissues. The three lower curves were obtained in experiments carried out with a different strain of the same organism. It will be seen that this strain caused an appreciably higher epidemic mortality. The variations with each strain are considerable, but there can be no doubt as to the difference between them. The strain that failed to kill many of the mice did not fail to spread beyond those that it killed. In six of the ten experiments with this strain, the proportion of infected mice among the survivors killed on the 60th day varied from 23 to 40 percent. From the survivors of the remaining epidemics initiated with this

Figure 12. Course of events in thirteen epidemics, showing the number of survivors among 100 mice at risk being plotted against time.

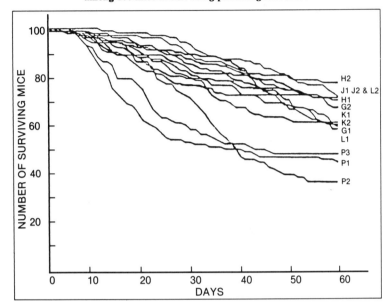

strain 100 mice were taken at random. The same number were taken from the survivors of the three more severe epidemics initiated with the other strain. These two herds were tested separately for resistance, by adding to each 25 mice infected with a third strain of *Bacterium typhi-murium*, known to produce a high epidemic mortality. As a control, three herds, each of 100 normal mice, were tested at the same time in the same way. On the 60th day 69 percent of the survivors from the mild epidemics remained alive, 66 percent of the survivors from the severe epidemics, and 36.7 percent of the normal mice that had not previously been exposed to risk.

The main interest of this experiment lies in the demonstration that one strain of a bacterial parasite may, as it spreads by contact, kill more hosts than it immunizes, while another may immunize more than it kills. We have, of course, long been aware that an effective specific immunity may be conferred by mild, or latent, infections; and Dudley's prolonged and detailed studies at the Royal Naval School at Greenwich (*11, 12*) provide a convincing demonstration of the epidemic immunization that accompanies any outbreak of diphtheria. It seems possible that infective strains, defined as those that have

a relatively high power of contact spread, may be subdivided into those with high and low ratios of killing to immunizing potency.

Experiments with various strains of *Pasteurella* (*1*) have given a still clearer illustration of the independence of virulence, as tested by the power to kill when bacteria are injected directly into the tissues, and epidemicity as tested by the numbers of mice that succumb to contact infection. Table 1 shows the results obtained with five different strains of *Pasteurella*, which are listed in the first column in descending order of epidemicity. It will be seen that strain P.64 caused the death of 73 of 100 mice by contact infection within 60 days, and infected 6 others without killing them. It was also highly virulent, 10 *Pasteurella* killing 4 of 5 mice on injection, and larger doses killing all mice receiving them. Strain P.62, within the margin of error of such experiments as these, is of the same order of epidemicity and virulence as strain P.64; but strain P.A. 39 and P.29 have the same high virulence as strain P.62, but are at low epidemicity, showing very little of contact spread. Strain P.58 has the same low epidemicity as strain P.A.39, but is also of low virulence. It is clear that the biological properties, whatever they may be, that enable a bacterium

Table 1.

Strain	Infectivity		Virulence: deaths among 5 mice per dose				
	Contact deaths	Survivors infected	10^5	10^4	10^3	10^2	10
P.64	73/100	6/27	5	5	5	5	4
P.62	62/100	7/38	5	5	4	4	2
P.29	26/100	0/74	—	5	4	4	2
P.58	18/100	1/82	3	1	0	1	0
P.A. 39	13/100	0/87	5	4	5	4	2

to multiply within the tissues, causing the death of the host, are different, and dissociable, from those that enable it to obtain a foothold in a new host, to which it is transmitted by natural contact infection. The nature of the factors involved is at present quite obscure, and offers a fertile field of study to the bacteriologist and to the biochemist.

It may be noted that all the evidence at present available is against the view that variations in the epidemicity or virulence of the infecting parasite play a part in the fluctuations in mortality that may occur during a long-continued epidemic, or that follow changes in the closeness or continuity of contact between infected and non-infected hosts. In this respect our own experience is in accord with the views expressed by Webster and his colleagues (13-23) whose independent studies at the Rockefeller Institute began soon after our own in this country. In observations lasting for more than 20 years we have only twice obtained evidence of a change of this kind occurring during experimental epidemics (1, 24). So far as our present evidence goes, it seems likely that the evolution within any parasitic species of a strain of high epidemicity is an occasional event, rather than part of a normal or periodic process.

THE EFFECT OF GENETIC DIFFERENCES IN RESISTANCE WITHIN A SINGLE HOST SPECIES

Just as different strains within a single parasitic species differ in their power of infecting, and killing, a particular species of host, so different strains, or races, within a single host species differ in their resistance to attack; and the dissociation of different infective powers that can be demonstrated in selected strains of a given parasite has an analogy in the dissociation of resistance toward different parasites, or to-

ward different activities of the same parasite, that can be demonstrated in selected strains of host.

Several observers have been able, by selective breeding, to produce strains of laboratory animals unusually resistant, or unusually susceptible, to particular bacterial parasites (25). In some instances, late generations of these selected strains, or mice belonging to inbred strains that have been found to be abnormally resistant, or abnormally susceptible, to a particular bacterial parasite, have been tested against other bacteria, viruses, or toxins. Thus, Gowen and Schott (26) tested two inbred strains of mice, Silver and S., against *Bacterium typhi-murium* and against the virus of pseudorabies. S. was approximately four times as resistant as Silver to *Bacterium typhi-murium*, but Silver was approximately twice as resistant as S. to pseudorabies. Webster (27) produced strains of mice abnormally resistant, or abnormally susceptible, to *Bacterium enteritidis* by selective breeding through several successive generations from mice that had survived infection with this organism. He then tested these selected strains against three other pathogenic bacteria, *Pasteurella*, Friedländer's bacillus, and the pneumococcus, and also against the virus of louping ill. The strain that was abnormally resistant to *Bacterium enteritidis* was also relatively resistant to the three other bacteria, but it was less resistant to the virus of louping ill than the strain that was abnormally susceptible to *Bacterium enteritidis*. Hill, Hatswell and Topley (28) produced a strain of mice abnormally resistant to the injection of a partially purified toxin isolated from *Bacterium typhi-murium*, by selective breeding in successive generations from mice that had survived large doses of this substance. Late generations of these toxin-resistant mice were tested against living bacilli of the same bacterial species, but proved no more resistant than unselected controls. It is clear, therefore, that genetic resistance, while not specific in the same sense as the resistance depending on antigen-antibody reactions, is limited in its range, and is an expression of the effect of different factors that may be inherited independently.

The racial differences in resistance depending on these factors, in man or in animals, will affect the natural spread of epidemics by increasing their severity in some quarters of the world, and lessening it in others. They may also, in areas inhabited by a mixture of races, lead to a differential incidence or death rate. It should, however, be emphasized that it is usually a matter of the greatest difficulty, when faced with recorded observations of this kind, to disentangle the effects of genetic factors, immunization by previous infection, and environmental influences.

The plant pathologist and the plant geneticist have gone further in this particular field, and have obtained results of the greatest interest. They have, for instance, demonstrated, in their studies on the stem rust of wheat, that the genetic resistance of selected host strains may be narrowly related to strain differences in the parasite (see *29*). A selected strain of wheat that is highly resistant to one strain of rust may be highly susceptible to another; so that the possibility that has here been opened to us of eliminating susceptible hosts by selective breeding depends on our ability to produce, by appropriate crossing, strains of wheat that are resistant to all the strains of rust by which they are likely to be attacked.

Apart from innate differences in resistance, and acquired differences in specific immunity, host resistance may be affected by a variety of other factors, by certain dietetic deficiencies, by exposure to severe climatic changes, and so on. It would take us too far afield to discuss these factors in any detail. We need only note that it is desirable to assess their relative importance by experiment, or by carefully controlled observations, before attempting to assign to them their respective roles in the natural course of events.

MORE COMPLEX SYSTEMS

We have so far limited our attention to the simplest form of epidemiological system, in which a single species of parasite reacts with a single species of host; though each species may

be divisible into biological races or types that differ significantly in their behavior.

In turning to more complex systems, we can do no more than note analogies. The most important natural modification in our simple system is, perhaps, the intervention of an insect vector; and of all human diseases conveyed by insect vectors malaria has pride of place.

So far as prevention is concerned, our main problem is still to reduce the probability of effective contact between a person infected with the malarial parasite and a person susceptible to it. But effective contact no longer means mere propinquity. The infected person must be bitten by a mosquito of the appropriate species at the appropriate time, when parasites at the right stage of development are present in the circulating blood, and this same mosquito must then bite a susceptible, non-infected host, again at the appropriate time, when the parasite has passed through its sexual cycle in the mosquito's tissues. In the absence of mosquitoes of an appropriate kind, and in adequate concentration, the malarial parasite cannot pass with effective frequency from host to host, however closely the hosts are aggregated; indeed, the aggregation or dispersal of infected and susceptible hosts now loses its significance, except insofar as it is related to the distribution of the insect vectors, to their powers of flight, and to their feeding habits.

I have neither the knowledge nor the time to discuss the fascinating story of the prevention of malaria by mosquito control. There are, however, two points in the epidemiology of malaria that may be noted, since they bear directly on the general principles that we have considered in relation to simpler systems.

The first concerns the malarial parasite itself, and the host's reactions to it. There was a tendency until quite recent years to assume that the problem of resistance to protozoal infections in general, and to malaria in particular, differed in some fundamental way from that of resistance to bacteria and viruses. In particular, little attention was paid to the possible effect of mechanisms depending on antigen-antibody reactions. This neglect, though a natural result of difficulties in technique, was always biologically unjustified, if only because the production of specific antibodies is a general phenomenon that follows the introduction into the animal tissues of any foreign protein, or any foreign chemical complex of which a protein is a part. It is possible that this property may be shared by other large and complex molecules that have no protein component. Recent studies in malaria, particularly on monkey malaria, and on the artificial infection of human subjects as a method of cure in certain mental diseases, have shown quite clearly that there is a specific acquired immunity depending not only on the species of malarial parasite, but on strain differences within a species that are clearly analogous to the different antigenic types of bacteria and viruses. The role of antigen-antibody reactions may well be less important in protozoal than in bacterial or virus infections, but it is, perhaps, equally probable that mechanisms other than those dependent on such reactions are more important in acquired resistance to bacteria and viruses than has been commonly supposed.

The second point concerns the insect vector. Just as we have seen that different biological races within a single parasitic species, quite apart from differences in antigenic type, differ significantly in their epidemiological behavior, and that different strains within a host species may show wide differences in genetic resistance, so we find that different strains, or races, of a single species of insect vector may differ profoundly in their efficacy as infecting agents, usually because of differing predilections for the blood of man and other animals (*30*).

Time forbids consideration of the further complexities that may be introduced into our epidemiological systems by the intervention of alternative or reservoir hosts, or of many other factors that we have left untouched; but there is one last point that should be underlined. Whenever we seek to lessen the frequency of an infective disease, we seek, in one way or another, and usually by synchronous attack along many different lines, to reduce the probability of a pathogenic parasite gaining access to a susceptible host. We need never, by our own action, reduce the probability to zero. The biological system on which any endemic or epidemic prevalence depends is in unstable equilibrium, shifting now to the advantage of the parasite, now to that of the host. As we reduce the frequency of effective contact, we reduce the mass of infective material on which the probability of further diffusion in part depends. If we can tip the balance far enough the system itself will do the rest, and the disease will be reduced to negligible proportions, or even disappear.

In conclusion I should wish to express my indebtedness to Mr. W.T. Russell, Mr. W.J. Martin and Mr. E. Lewis Faning for the help they have given me in obtaining certain statistical data, and in the preparation of some of the graphs.

References

(*1*) Greenwood, M., A.B. Hill, W.W.C. Topley, and J. Wilson. *Spec Rep Ser Med Res Coun, Lond*, No. 75, 1936.

(*2*) Topley, W.W.C. *J Hyg Camb* 21:20, 1922.

(*3*) Topley, W.W.C. and J. Wilson. *J Hyg Camb* 24:295, 1925.

(*4*) Greenwood, M., A.B. Hill, W.W.C. Topley, and J. Wilson. *J Hyg Camb* 39:109, 1939.

(*5*) Topley, W.W.C. and G.S. Wilson. *J Hyg Camb* 21:237, 1923.

(*6*) School Epidemics Committee, Med. Res. Coun. *Spec Rep Ser Med Res Coun Lond*, No. 227, 1938.

(*7*) Topley, W.W.C., J. Ayrton, and E.R. Lewis. *J Hyg Camb* 23:223, 1924.

(*8*) Greenwood, M., W.W.C. Topley, and J. Wilson. *J Hyg Camb* 31:257, 403.

(*9*) Topley, W.W.C. *J Hyg Camb* 20:103, 1921.

(*10*) Topley, W.W.C., M. Greenwood, and J. Wilson. *J Path Bact* 34:523, 1931.

(*11*) Dudley, S.F. *Spec Rep Ser Med Res Coun Lond*, No. 75, 1923.

(*12*) Dudley, S.F. *Spec Rep Ser Med Res Coun Lond*, No. 111, 1926.

(*13*) Webster, L.T. *J Exp Med* 37:231, 1923.

(*14*) Webster, L.T. *J Exp Med* 38:33, 45, 1923.

(*15*) Webster, L.T. *J Exp Med* 39:129, 837, 879, 1924.

(*16*) Webster, L.T. *J Exp Med* 40:109, 1924.

(*17*) Webster, L.T. *J Exp Med* 42:1, 1925.

(*18*) Webster, L.T. *J Exp Med* 43: 573, 1926.

(*19*) Webster, L.T. *J Exp Med* 51:219, 1930.

(*20*) Webster, L.T. *J Exp Med* 52:901, 909, 931, 1930.

(*21*) Webster, L.T. and C.G. Burn. *J Exp Med* 44:343, 359, 1926.

(*22*) Webster, L.T. and C.G. Burn. *J Exp Med* 45:911, 1927.

(*23*) Webster, L.T. and C.G. Burn. *J Exp Med* 46:855, 871, 1927.

(*24*) Topley, W.W.C., M. Greenwood, and J. Wilson. *J Path Bacteriol* 34:523, 1931.

(*25*) Hill, A.B. *Spec Rep Ser Med Res Coun Lond*, No. 196, 1934.

(*26*) Gowen, J.W. and R.G. Schott. *Am J Hyg* 18:674, 1933.

(*27*) Webster, L.T. *J Exp Med* 57:819, 1933.

(*28*) Hill, A.B., J.M. Hatswell, and W.W.C. Topley. *J Hyg Camb* 40:538, 1940.

(*29*) Craigie, J.H. Publication No. 666, Department of Agriculture, Dominion of Canada, 1940.

(*30*) Hackett, L.W. *Malaria in Europe*. Oxford University Press, 1937.

THE CONCLUSION OF A TEN-YEAR STUDY OF WATER FLUORIDATION[1]

David B. Ast[2] and Edward R. Schlesinger[3]

In areas where the potable water supplies contain the fluoride ion at optimum concentration at the source, the dental caries experience of children who ingest these water fluorides during the years of tooth development is about 60 percent less than among children in areas with fluoride-deficient water supplies (1). Adults who have used such water supplies continuously enjoy the dental benefits obtained during childhood (2).

Controlled water fluoridation for the prevention of dental caries, i.e., the addition of fluoride compounds in optimum concentration to fluoride-deficient supplies, has been studied since 1945 in three different areas. These studies have demonstrated that dental caries can be effectively reduced through controlled water fluoridation to the same extent as observed in areas where water contains the fluoride at the source. A recent review (3) presented the DMF (decayed, missing, or filled teeth) rates for six- to 10-year-old children after nine years of fluoride experience in Grand Rapids, Mich., Newburgh, N. Y., and Brantford, Ontario, and compared these data with those in Aurora, Ill., which uses a water supply with naturally occurring fluoride at 1.2 ppm F. At ages six to nine the rates in all four communities were found to be quite comparable and at age 10 the rates for the three communities fluoridating their water supplies approached the expectancy level noted in Aurora.

One of the most comprehensive of the studies, the Newburgh-Kingston Caries-Fluoride Study, has recently issued its final report based on 10 years of fluoridation experience. The report, consisting of three definitive papers

dealing with the history of the study and its pediatric and dental aspects, and a fourth paper dealing with fluoride metabolism, was presented before the New York Institute of Clinical Oral Pathology on December 12, 1955. These papers appear in the March 1956 issue of the Journal of the American Dental Association (4-7).

Prior to the initiation of controlled water fluridation programs in 1945, extensive epidemiological investigations (8, 9) had demonstrated (1) the occurrence of a defect of tooth enamel which discolored and, in extreme cases, caused pitting of the enamel; (2) the discovery that the stain or mottled enamel was caused by the ingestion of water-borne fluorides during the years of enamel calcification; (3) the direct relationship of the degree of mottling to the fluoride content of the water; (4) an inverse relationship of dental caries to fluorosed or mottled teeth; and (5) that where the water supply contained approximately 1 ppm F, the residents enjoyed considerable protection against dental caries without the hazard of disfiguring mottled enamel.

Cox and his co-workers (10) in 1939 suggested that the addition of fluorides to food and water to bring the fluoride content up to the optimum level could prevent dental caries if ingested during the years of tooth development. Ast (11) in 1942 outlined a plan to test the caries-fluorine hypothesis. He suggested a study of two comparable communities with fluoride-deficient water supplies, one of which should have its water supply supplemented with sodium fluoride to bring its fluoride content up to 1 ppm and the second to serve as a control.

This plan was considered by the New York State Department of Health. In 1944 a Technical Advisory Committee on the Fluoridation of Water Supplies was appointed to study the proposal. The committee was also asked to recommend the types of medical and dental examinations which should be made to determine the efficacy and safety of water fluoridation.

Source: *American Journal of Public Health* 46(3):265-271.
[1] Here, in capsule form, is a resumé of the Newburgh-Kingston Caries-Fluorine Study after a decade, with some additional information on the safety of water fluoridation.
[2] Director, Bureau of Dental Health, New York State Department of Health, Albany, New York.
[3] Associate Director, Division of Medical Services, New York State Department of Health, Albany, New York.

After a careful review of the literature and the objectives of the study, the committee recommended that a long-range study be undertaken. The cities of Newburgh and Kingston, each with a population of approximately 30 000, situated about 35 miles apart on the west bank of the Hudson River and using fluoride-deficient water supplies, were asked to participate in a 10-year study. Newburgh agreed to serve as the study area and to have its water supply supplemented with sodium fluoride to bring its fluoride content up to 1–1.2 ppm. Kingston agreed to serve as the control and continue to use its water supply with approximately 0.1 ppm F.

In June 1944, base-line pediatric and dental examinations were begun and on May 2, 1945, Newburgh's water supply was fluoridated. This process has been in continuous operation since that date. The base-line data showed that the children aged six to 12 in both cities had a similar dental caries experience. The Kingston rate was 20.2 DMF teeth per 100 permanent teeth and the Newburgh rate was 20.6. Periodic progress reports have demonstrated a downward trend in the dental caries experience among the children in Newburgh. In Kingston the caries rates have remained relatively unchanged.

In June 1955, clinical and intraoral dental roentgenographic examinations were completed after 10 years of fluoride experience. In Newburgh 1519 children aged 6 to 14, and 109 aged 16, who had had continuous residence there throughout the period of fluoridation were examined. The Kingston children examined included 2021 aged 6 to 14, and 119 aged

16. The clinical examinations were made in both cities by the staff senior dentist and the roentgenograms were taken by the staff senior dentist and dental hygienist. The films were developed and sent to the Dental Bureau office in Albany. There statisticians randomized the film series so that the interpreters did not know whether they were reading Newburgh or Kingston films.

The children aged 6 through 9 years in Newburgh had used fluoridated water throughout their lives. The 10- to 12-year-old children, who were under two years of age in 1945, had used fluoridated water during the partial calcification of the crowns of the first permanent molars and throughout the calcification of the second permanent molar crowns. The 13- to 14-year-old children were three to four years old in 1945. These children started drinking fluoridated water after the calcification of the crowns of the first molar teeth but prior to the eruption of these teeth, and throughout the period of calcification of the crowns of the second molars. The 16-year-old children were six years of age when fluoridation was started. At that time their first permanent molars were beginning to erupt into the mouth and the crowns of their second molars were almost fully calcified.

The DMF rate for the six- to nine-year-old children in Newburgh was 58 percent lower than that for the Kingston children. The 10- to 12-year-old children in Newburgh had a DMF rate 53 percent lower. At ages 13 to 14 the DMF rate was 48 percent lower, and at age 16 it was 41 percent lower, than the rates in Kingston (Table 1).

Table 1. DMF[a] teeth per 100 children ages 6-16, based on clinical and roentgenographic examinations, Newburgh[b] and Kingston, N.Y., 1954-1955.

Age[d]	Number of children with permanent teeth		Number of DMF teeth		DMF teeth per 100 children with permanent teeth[c]		
	Newburgh	Kingston	Newburgh	Kingston	Newburgh	Kingston	Per cent Difference K-N
6-9[e]	708	913	672	2136	98.4	233.7	− 57.9
10-12	521	640	1711	4471	328.1	698.6	− 53.0
13-14	263	441	1579	5151	610.1	1170.3	− 47.9
16	109	119	1063	1962	975.2	1648.7	− 40.9

[a] DMF includes permanent teeth decayed, missing (lost subsequent to eruption), or filled.
[b] Sodium fluoride added to Newburgh's water supply beginning May 2, 1945.
[c] Adjusted to age distribution of children examined in Kingston who had permanent teeth in the 1954-1955 examination.
[d] Age at last birthday at time of examination.
[e] Newburgh children of this age group exposed to fluoridated water from time of birth.

The first permanent molar is frequently referred to as the keystone of the dental arch and warrants special consideration because of its strategic position in the mouth. This tooth, because of its morphology and the early age at which it erupts into the mouth, frequently succumbs to dental caries early in life. It is therefore significant to note that among the six- to nine-year-old children in Newburgh the DMF rate for first permanent molars was 53 percent lower than that for the Kingston children in the same age group. The DMF rate in Newburgh at ages 10 to 12 was 30 percent lower, at ages 13 to 14 it was 14 percent lower, and at age 16 it was 4 percent lower, than in Kingston (Figure 1).

Of even greater significance is the observation that the children in Newburgh at age six to

nine had 68 percent fewer untreated carious first molars and 88 percent fewer first molars lost than did the Kingston children of the same ages. The 10- to 12-year-old children in Newburgh had a rate 45 percent lower for untreated caries and 78 percent lower for missing first molars. At ages 13 to 14 the differences were 26 percent for untreated caries and 42 percent for missing first molars, and at age 16 the differences were 41 percent for untreated caries and 32 percent for missing first molars (Table 2).

Another significant observation was that ingested water fluorides afford selective protection to the proximal (adjacent) surfaces of the teeth in comparison with the occlusal (biting) surfaces. This is highly important because the proximal surfaces present difficulties in both caries detection and correction. Frequently caries on the proximal surface of a tooth requires the cutting of much sound tooth structure in order to place an adequate filling in the tooth. At each of the age levels studied the percent of differentiable carious proximal surfaces among the Kingston children was about three times greater than that noted in the Newburgh children.

At ages six through nine all of the deciduous cuspids and deciduous molars are normally present in the mouth. If any of these teeth are missing it may reasonably be presumed that they were lost because of caries. Among the six to nine-year-old children in Newburgh, 25.5 percent had all these teeth present and caries free, as compared with 4.7 percent of the Kingston children (Table 3).

Dean's (12) epidemiological studies of endemic dental fluorosis demonstrated that there

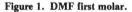

Figure 1. DMF first molar.

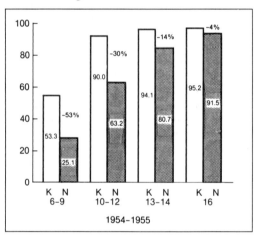

Table 2. Status of erupted first permanent molars in children ages 6-16, based on clinical and roentgenographic examinations, Newburgh[a] and Kingston, N.Y., 1954-1955.

	Percent of erupted first permanent molars[b]									
	Caries-free		DMF[d]		Filled		Untreated caries		Missing	
Age[c]	Newburgh	Kingston	Newburgh	Kingston	Newburgh	Kingston	Newburgh	Kingston	Newburgh	Kingston
6-9[c]	74.9	46.7	25.1	53.3	14.2	17.8	10.6	33.2	0.3	2.4
10-12	36.8	10.0	63.2	90.0	40.2	41.3	20.5	37.1	2.5	11.6
13-14	19.3	5.9	90.7	94.1	43.9	40.5	27.0	36.7	9.8	16.9
16	8.5	4.8	91.5	95.2	55.0	36.6	20.9	35.5	15.6	23.1

[a] Sodium fluoride added to Newburgh's water supply beginning May 2, 1945.
[b] Adjusted to the first permanent molar population in the Kingston 1954-1955 examination.
[c] Age at last birthday at time of examination.
[d] DMF includes permanent teeth decayed, missing (lost subsequent to eruption), or filled.
[e] Newburgh children of this age group exposed to fluoridated water from time of birth.

Table 3. Number and percent of children age 6-9 with caries-free deciduous cuspids, first and second deciduous molars, based on clinical and roentgenographic examinations, Kingston and Newburgh,[a] N.Y., 1954-1955.

Age[b]	Number of children examined		Number of children with all 12 teeth present and caries-free		Percent children with all 12 teeth present and caries-free	
	Kingston	Newburgh	Kingston	Newburgh	Kingston	Newburgh
6	216	184	24	68	11.1	37.0
7	255	208	12	58	4.7	27.9
8	277	213	5	53	1.8	24.9
9	192	129	3	13	1.6	10.1
Total	940	734	44	192	4.7	26.2
Adjusted rate[c]					4.7	25.5

[a] Sodium fluoride added to Newburgh's water supply beginning May 2, 1945.
[b] Age at last birthday at time of examination. Newburgh children of these ages exposed to fluoridated water from time of birth.
[c] Adjusted to the age distribution of Kingston children in the 1954-1955 examination.

was no disfiguring dental fluorosis at the level of about 1 ppm F. Unfortunately, the term mottled enamel or dental fluorosis is applied to all degrees of this condition. In its more severe forms it does produce discoloring stains and possibly pitting of the enamel. However, in the milder forms of fluorosis the enamel of the tooth has a high luster which enhances the beauty of the tooth rather than disfigures it. The detection of the early signs of dental fluorosis requires an examiner who has had extensive experience in areas of endemic fluorosis. The average dental practitioner would in all probability not detect the earliest signs of mottling.

In order to determine whether the children in Newburgh showed any signs of dental fluorosis a specially trained officer of the Public Health Service with long experience in the detection of the mildest of such lesions was requested to make the examinations. He examined 621 children aged 7 to 14 in Newburgh, of whom 438 had resided there continuously since the start of fluoridation. In Kingston 612 children of the same ages were examined. In addition to dental fluorosis, examinations were made for enamel opacities due to causes other than ingested fluorides. These other enamel opacities are generally developmental hypoplasias. They usually appear as circular white or colored patches and most of them are obvious even to the untrained eye.

Among the 438 children with continuous residence in Newburgh, 46 had questionable flu-

orosis, 26 had very mild, and six had mild fluorosis. There were no cases of moderate or severe mottling and in no instance was there any disfiguring discoloration. Thirty-six of the Newburgh children examined had non-fluoride opacities. Of the 612 children examined in Kingston, 115 had nonfluoride opacities. The relatively infrequent occurrence of nonfluoride enamel opacities in Newburgh compared with Kingston tends to confirm a previous report (13) that ingested water fluorides at the recommended concentration appear to reduce the occurrence of hypoplastic spots on the teeth.

The same groups of children examined for enamel opacities were also examined for evidence of gingivitis. A positive score was recorded only for flagrant gingivitis, thus making it possible to place greater emphasis on advanced disease and minimize examiner bias. There was slightly, but significantly, more gingivitis observed among the Kingston children than among those in Newburgh.

The final report on the pediatric findings of the Newburgh-Kingston study pointed out that all the scientific evidence available at the time the study was first proposed indicated the safety of drinking water containing about 1 ppm F at the source. There was no reason at that time to believe that fluorides, when added to the drinking water as part of the water treatment process, would act in any way differently from fluorides already present. Nevertheless, it was considered desirable to test this remote possibility under the carefully controlled conditions established for the long-term Newburgh-Kingston study.

Closely similar groups of children were studied in Newburgh and Kingston. In the final year of the study 500 of the children enrolled in Newburgh and 405 in Kingston were examined in the study clinic. The points of concentration in the examination were those related to possible systemic effects of fluoride ingestion as manifested by changes in growth and development or in abnormalities on the physical, laboratory, and roentgenographic examinations. Each child was given a general medical examination by a qualified pediatrician. Height and weight were measured. Roentgenograms were taken of the right hand, both knees, and the lumbar spine. Bone density and bone age (maturation of the skeleton) were estimated by independent observers who were not aware of the city of origin of the individual roentgenograms. Laboratory examinations, including hemoglobin level, total leucocyte count, and routine urinalysis were also made. No differences of medical significance could be found between the groups of children in the two cities. This indicated the absence of any findings suggestive of systemic effects from the drinking of fluoridated water during the period of most rapid growth. In addition, special detailed studies of the eyes and ears were performed on a smaller group of children; these included determination of visual acuity, visual fields, and hearing levels. The results of these special examinations were well within the range of expected prevalence of the conditions studied.

Reference was made to another recently published paper (*14*) which presented further evidence for the absence of systemic effects from fluoridated water. The purpose of this study was to determine whether any irritative effects on the kidneys follow prolonged use of fluoridated water. The quantitative excretion of albumin, red blood cells, and casts in 12-hour urine specimens in 12-year-old boys, using a modified Addis technic, was determined in the two cities. The differences in the results between the groups in the two cities tended to favor the Newburgh children, but no medical significance could be attributed to any of the differences.

The review of current knowledge of the metabolism of fluorides, particularly in the human body, applied this information in estimating the factors of safety in water fluoridation. Knowledge of blood fluoride levels, of the rate and mechanism of urinary excretion of fluoride, and of the magnitude and mechanism of bone deposition increases our understanding of some important biological effects of toxic doses of fluorides, such as acute fluoride poisoning, crippling fluorosis, osteosclerosis, and mottled enamel.

The blood fluoride level in experimental animals given lethal doses of fluoride rises to a peak in a half hour to an hour, falls rapidly within two to three hours, and returns to its normal level within 24 hours. The blood does not tend to accumulate fluoride, although the blood fluoride level in persons drinking fluoridated water is somewhat higher than in persons drinking fluoride-deficient water.

When human beings ingest small amounts of fluoride a significant fraction is promptly excreted in the urine. It is probable that when human beings ingest small amounts of fluoride equivalent to that of fluoridated water over a period of years, the daily urinary excretion is greater than half of the amount absorbed each day. The extraordinarily rapid and efficient urinary excretion of fluoride is attributable to a somewhat lower resorption of fluoride in the kidney tubules than is characteristic of chloride.

The other mechanism for removal of fluoride from the blood is by deposition in the bones, the amount of fluoride present in the hard tissues probably being directly dependent on the amount of fluoride taken into the body day after day. The mechanism of fluoride deposition is simple, the fluoride ion replacing the hydroxyl groups of the surface of the bone crystals. There is no indication that any notable biological disadvantage results from this. Fluoride deposition in bone is a reversible process.

With regard to acute fluoride poisoning there is at least a 2500-fold factor of safety in water fluoridation. The mechanics of water fluoridation are such that it is impossible to produce acute fluoride poisoning either by accident or intent.

Crippling fluorosis, characterized by a stiffening in the back due to calcification of the broad ligaments of the back, occurs with a daily intake of 20 to 80 milligrams of fluoride or more for 10 to 20 years. Since five gallons of fluoridated water at 1 ppm F contain 20 milligrams, it is obvious that crippling fluorosis can never be produced by drinking fluoridated water. The earliest evidence of osteosclerosis, a hypercalcification detectable by roentgen examination, does not occur with an intake of fluoride below eight to 10 times the level of fluoridated water.

The evidence with respect to heart disease, kidney disease, cancer, and possible influence of fluoride on the thyroid is also reviewed. Ample statistics are available to indicate no influence of fluoride intake on any of these at the levels found in any water supplies in the United States. Studies on experimental animals with the use of radioactive fluoride show that the thyroid gland does not concentrate fluoride as it does iodide. The presence of renal impairment in experimental animals and in human beings with long-standing kidney disease appears not to affect excretion of fluoride by the kidneys.

The comprehensive analysis of the Newburgh-Kingston Caries-Fluorine Study after 10 years of experience, added to the wealth of evidence previously reported, demonstrates conclusively two important facts—fluoridation is effective in reducing dental caries and it is a safe public health practice.

References

(*1*) Dean, H.T., F.A. Arnold, and E. Elvove. Domestic water and dental caries. *Public Health Rep* 57:1155, 1942.

(*2*) Russell, A.L. and E. Elvove. Domestic water and dental caries: VII. A study of the fluoride-dental caries relationship in an adult population. *Public Health Rep* 66:1389, 1951.

(*3*) Dean, H.T. Fluorine in the control of dental caries. *J Am Dent A* 52:1, 1956.

(*4*) Hilleboe, H.E. history of the Newburgh-Kingston Caries Fluorine Study. *J Am Dent A* Vol. 57, 1956.

(*5*) Schlesinger, E.R. et al. The Newburgh-Kingston Caries Fluorine Study: XIII. Pediatric findings after ten years. *J Am Dent A* Vol. 57, 1956.

(*6*) Ast, D.B., et al. The Newburgh-Kingston Caries Fluorine Study: XIV. Combined clinical and roentgenographic dental findings after ten years of fluoride experience. *J Am Dent A* Vol. 57, 1956.

(*7*) Hodge, H.C. Fluoride metabolism: Its significance in water fluoridation. *J Am Dent A* Vol. 57, 1956.

(*8*) Moulton, F.R., ed. *Fluorine and Dental Health.* Washington, D.C., American Association for the Advancement of Science, 1942.

(*9*) Moulton, F.R., ed. *Dental Caries and Fluorine.* Washington, D.C., American Association for the Advancement of Science, 1946.

(*10*) Cox, G.J., M.C. Matuschak, et al. Experimental dental caries IV. Fluorine and its relation to dental caries. *J Dent Res* 18:481, 1939.

(*11*) Ast, D.B. The caries-fluorine hypothesis and a suggested study to test its application. *Public Health Rep* 58:857, 1943.

(*12*) Dean, H.T. Endemic fluorosis and its relation to dental caries. *Public Health Rep* 53:1413, 1938.

(*13*) Zimmerman, E.R. Fluoride and nonfluoride enamel opacities *Public Health Rep* 69:1115, 1954.

(*14*) Schlesinger, E.R., D.E. Overton, and H.C. Chase. Study of children drinking fluoridated and nonfluoridated water: Quantitative urinary excretion of albumin and formed elements. *JAMA* 160:21, 1956.

THE INFLUENCE OF VITAMIN SUPPLEMENTATION OF THE DIETS OF PREGNANT AND LACTATING WOMEN ON THE INTELLIGENCE OF THEIR OFFSPRING[1]

Ruth F. Harrell,[2] Ella R. Woodyard,[2] and Arthur I. Gates[2]

This study is an attempt to determine whether the intelligence of children can be measurably affected by vitamin supplements to expectant and nursing mothers. While testing numbers of retarded children and taking their histories, one of the authors (Harrell) noted the high incidence of faulty nutrition in the prenatal lives of these mental defectives. The idea developed that a maternal diet qualitatively inadequate during pregnancy might be a factor militating against optimum development of the fetal nervous system.

The detrimental effect of early vitamin B complex deficiency on the learning ability of seventy day old rats was pointed out by Maurer and Tsai (1). Maurer et al. subsequently studied this problem in rats (2–4) and Balken and Maurer (5) made an attempt to extend their observations to humans. Bernhardt et al. (6–8) presented results suggesting that rats fed a stock diet learned in a superior manner when compared with animals subjected to depletion, the poorest learning occurring in those animals depleted most early. O'Neill (9–11) studied the effects of thiamine deficiency and excess, concluding that rearing white rats on these contrasting regimens produced significant differences in learning ability. Less than 3 µg. thiamine daily diminished maze learning below normal, whereas feeding over 100 µg. daily improved maze performance above normal. In the presence of excess thiamine no further improvement was observed following the addition of riboflavin, pyridoxine and calcium pantothenate. Before much of the work cited, the study by Poole et al. (12) led them to conclude, with regard to the feeding of human infants, that "all available data on vitamin B seem to indicate some close interaction in the infant between the metabolism and the development of external behavior." It, therefore, seems reasonable that vitamin supplementation of the diets of women with poor diets might cause improvement in the intelligence of their children.

PLAN

Daily dietary supplement tablets were provided to 2400 women, equally divided between a maternity clinic in Norfolk, Va. and one in Leslie County, Ky. The study was conducted simultaneously in both groups from October 1945 to June 1948. A "double-blind" technique avoided knowledge by the subjects or investigators of the nature of the supplements. Four tablets[3] were used in a carefully organized pattern of randomization.

Tablet A (group A) = 200 mg. ascorbic acid; Tablet B (group B) = 2 mg. thiamine, 4 mg. riboflavin, 20 mg. niacinamide, 15 mg. iron; Tablet C (group C) = inert placebo; Tablet D (group D) = 2 mg. thiamine.

In Norfolk the expectant mothers were interviewed on their first registration in the free maternity clinic. They were offered a "tonic" tablet, for daily use, with the explanation that it was expensive, but would be provided free if they would continue in the project, and would engage to bring their babies back for measurement at ages 3 and 4 years. The choice of the four types of supplementation was by rotation in order of new patient registration. No one who handled the materials knew which type was given to a patient. These women were seen in the clinic twice monthly, and were visited in

Source: *Metabolism* 5: 555-562, 1956.

[1] To be published in monograph form by Teachers College, Columbia University. This résumé edited by Elmer L. Severinghaus, Vice President for Clinical Research, Hoffmann-La Roche, Inc.

Acknowledgment is gratefully made to the Williams-Waterman Fund, Research Corporation, New York, for financial support of the experimental and statistical studies, and to Hoffman-La Roche, Inc., Nutley, N. J., for the generous supplies of vitamin tablets and placebos.

[2] From the Department of Psychology and Education, College of William and Mary, Williamsburg, Va.; Teachers College, Columbia University, New York, N.Y.

[3] Provided by Hoffman-La Roche, Inc.

their homes in addition twice monthly, by nurses of the King's Daughters Maternity Service. Compliance with the program for daily use of the supplements appears to have been satisfactory, since only 3 of the 1200 women were eliminated for apparent noncompliance and two more for professed inability to swallow the tablets. Supplies were issued for two weeks at a time. Nurses took vitamin tablets to those women who failed to keep clinic appointments.

In Leslie County the travel problems caused by poor roads or lack of roads, weather hazards and conventions of the area made it necessary to depend upon monthly visits to the clinic, with distribution of the supplements in quantities adequate for one month. When women failed to keep monthly clinic appointments the supplements were sent by nurse or often by mail. The total amount of supplementation achieved in the Kentucky group is therefore undoubtedly less than in the Norfolk group.

These two populations were thought to be reasonably homogeneous as to customs and economic situations within themselves, but were known to differ from each other in at least the following features:

Norfolk: 80 percent Negro; most mothers employed outside the home; urban, congested; diet poor, economically limited. The population sample was limited to the families at the lowest economic level in Norfolk, by the clinic arrangements.

Kentucky: all white, ancestry from Great Britain; employed mothers rare; rural; diet plain, but generally not conspicuously inadequate. The population sample was a representative one from the area, since almost all women in the Leslie County families are cared for by this nursing and midwife service.

TESTING OF CHILDREN

Intelligence testing was done by using selected portions of the Terman-Merrill Revised Stanford-Binet Scale, employing form L for 3-year-olds and for 4-year-olds. Although these tests did not appear perfectly suited to the children in either group, the difficulties were more evident in the rural Kentucky group where some of the pictures were of objects totally unfamiliar to these children. In Kentucky, practical difficulties limited the testing to the 3-year-old-children.

At the time of the original clinic registration each woman had agreed to bring back the expected child during the week of the third and the fourth birthday, for measurement of height and weight and for intelligence testing. In the week before each birthday a card was mailed to each mother, reminding her to bring the child in for his "birthday money" (one dollar) and a candy sucker. When the mother and child failed to appear, the visiting nurses made up to three attempts to find them. Failures to secure children for examination were limited in almost all cases to removals from the community. The high degree of transiency, known to be characteristic of Norfolk, accounts for the smaller number of children examined there than in Kentucky.

Physical handicaps hampered the obtaining of anthropometric data in Kentucky, since it was out of the question for the nurses to transport scales on their trips to the more remote homes. Also the attitude of these mountain people rendered it impossible to obtain as good medical histories as was desired. This attitude also made necessary the development of special approaches by the examiner in getting family, as well as child, cooperation in the intelligence testing. In both areas the principal causes which reduced the numbers of children examined from the initial groups of 1200 expectant mothers were removal from the community, deaths or failure to achieve a viable child at term. The desire to obtain some sort of diet history from each woman was frustrated by the demonstrated tendency to gross fabrication in the Norfolk group, and by the extraordinary individual reticence in the Kentucky mountain folk. Dietary histories were therefore abandoned early in the study.

RESULTS

In Norfolk, 612 women completed the program of taking supplements and 518 children were available for tests at age 3; 370 children were tested at age 4. The mean birth weights of these children did not differ significantly for the four groups which received the four different tablets. For the entire group the mean was 7.42 lb., the lowest recorded birth weight being 3.5 lb. The distribution of intelligence quotients in the 3-year-old and 4-year-old children is shown in Tables 1 and 2.

Table 1. Frequency distributions of intelligence quotients of 3-year-olds at Norfolk.

IQ	A	B	C	D	Total
			Group		
57				1	1
60					
3		1			1
6		1	1	1	3
9		1			1
72	1		3	4	8
5		2	4		6
8	5	5	1	1	12
81	12	3	8	4	27
4	5	1	4	4	14
7	4	6	11	8	29
90	12	5	13	7	37
3	11	5	9	9	34
6	11	7	9	11	38
9	13	11	23	16	63
102	16	8	6	6	36
5	11	12	10	7	40
8	16	12	8	14	50
111	5	6	9	5	25
4	12	7	4	10	33
7	8	3	2	7	20
120	1	2	4	4	11
3	5	4	2	2	13
6		1		1	2
9	1	1	1		3
132		6		1	7
5		1	1		2
8					
141				1	1
4					
7					
150					
3					
6					
9					
162				1	1
Total	149	111	133	125	518
Mean[a]	100.9	103.4	98.4	101.9	101.0

[a] Means were computed from scores listed above using the midscore of each step as the value of all scores at that step.

Table 2. Frequency distribution of intelligence quotients of 4-year-olds at Norfolk.

IQ	A	B	C	D	Total
			Group		
63				1	1
66			1		1
69	1		1	1	3
72	3		1	1	5
5	1	1	3		5
8	2	1	4	2	9
81	2	4	4	6	16
4	5	2	10	2	19
7	12	8	11	4	35
90	7	4	6	5	22
3	8	8	15	9	40
6	7	7	6	4	24
9	17	15	18	13	63
102	8	8	4	9	29
5	14	10	8	6	38
8	7	2	1	2	12
111	3	10	3	6	22
4	1	2	1	1	5
7	4	1	1	1	7
120		1		3	4
3	1	3		1	5
6	1	1			2
9		2			2
132					
5					
8					
141					
4					
7					
150		1			1
3					
Total	104	91	98	77	370
Mean[a]	97.9	101.7	93.6	97.9	97.7

[a] Means were computed from scores listed above using the midscore of each step as the value of all scores at that step.

Statistical studies of these data[4] by the analysis of variance technique show really significant differences in the IQs of the four groups. These differences are most obvious when comparing the three groups that received vitamins with the group that received the placebo. The intergroup differences of the supplemented groups, A, B and D, do not indicate significance. The mean IQs of the three groups receiving vitamins tend uniformly to favor the B group (mixed vitamins) as compared with the D group (thiamine alone) or A group (ascorbic acid alone).

The values shown in Table 3 under $F_{.99}$ are abstract numbers which indicate the greatest variance that would occur in 99 percent of a theoretic normal distribution (with the factors delimited as in our sample). Since the values of the variance ratio calculated from our observations, compared to $F_{.99}$ (the 1 percent level of confidence), are definitely greater than would be expected in a normal distribution, we are assured that the intergroup relationships have real significance, and are definitely not due to sampling errors or to chance. Where $F_{.95}$ is used

---

[4] Performed by R.E. Wheeler, Howard College, Birmingham, Alabama.

Table 3. Variance ratios of IQ scores for vitamin supplemented groups.

Source of variation	Variance ratio		
	Calculated F	$F_{.99}$	$F_{.95}$
Norfolk 4 year olds, IQ Test			
Groups A, B, C, D to total	7.78	3.84	
Groups A, B, D to C	16.6	6.71	
Groups A to B to D	3.02		3.03
Norfolk 3 year olds, IQ Test			
Groups A, B, C, D to total	4.24	3.82	
Groups A, B, D to C	9.66	6.69	
Groups A to B to D	1.00		3.02
Kentucky (groups A, B, C, D to total)			
IQ scores	1.36		2.61
Pictorial Vocabulary	.5		2.61
Bead Stringing	.8		2.61

for comparison with the calculated F, the differences are seen to be within the limits of chance and thus have no independent significance. ($F_{.95}$ indicates the 5 percent level of certainty.)

The difference between the mixed vitamin B group (group B) and the placebo group (group C), referring to the 4-year-old Norfolk children, is 8.1 points IQ (101.7—93.6); and in the 3-year-old children, 5.0 points IQ (103.4—98.4). Most psychologists and educators would regard a difference of 8 points IQ as clinically or educationally significant; a difference of 5 points IQ might be regarded as difficult to discern, but, nevertheless, significant in effect over periods of time, for example, in the elementary school period.

Attempts to detect significant intergroup clinical differences among the mothers were unsuccessful. These included analyzing data on age, parity, headaches, vomiting, hypertension, constipation, hemorrhages, urinary specific gravity and albumen, and incidence of venereal diseases. The failures to establish significant differences in these respects add to the probability of significance in the intelligence test comparisons with and without vitamin supplementation.

In Leslie County starting with 1200 women during pregnancy, 811 children were available for testing at age 3 years. Table 4 gives the distribution of intelligence quotients. The differences between the 4 groups are clearly insignificant. A higher mean intelligence is evident in this group than in the Norfolk group in spite of the fact that difficulties with the test operated to the disadvantage of the Kentucky group. The

birth weight data did not differ materially from those in the Norfolk group, nor was there any apparent intergroup difference correlated with the four supplements when taken by the mothers. No significant correlations could be established by analysis of variance or by scattergrams for the several features of maternal status during pregnancy or at delivery.

DISCUSSION

Supplementation of the diets of the mothers in this study began at times varying from the first to the ninth month of pregnancy. The mean duration of antepartum supplementation was 134 days in the Norfolk group, 114 days in Kentucky. It is therefore apparent that any benefits from supplementation were made available at highly variable times and usually for less than half the pregnancy. Attempts to apply statistical methods to the significance of differences in intelligence as correlated with the various durations of vitamin supplementation appear unjustified in view of the small numbers of cases available for any one supplement and any special fraction of time concerned. In view of the known effects of nutritional deficiencies in experimental animals during the first third of pregnancy, it is possible that more definitive results might be secured were it possible to institute supplementation from the earliest days of pregnancy. Furthermore, since the development of the central nervous system continues during the first two years of infancy, optimum results from nutritional improvement would involve a supplementation of the diets used

Table 4. Frequency distribution of intelligence quotients of 3 year olds in Kentucky.

IQ	Group A	B	C	D	Total
72.4	1				1
5.7			1		1
8	3		3	1	7
81	2	4	1	1	8
4	3	3	5	2	13
7	6	3	4	5	18
90	9	5	8	12	34
3	13	6	8	16	43
6	18	10	12	8	48
9	11	24	14	13	62
102	12	23	16	21	72
5	22	23	21	15	81
8	19	26	12	20	77
111	26	17	16	17	76
4	16	15	21	8	60
7	15	23	19	18	75
120	10	8	20	8	46
3	7	8	8	10	33
6	6	5	4	10	25
9	3	5	6	6	20
132	1	3	3		7
5		2	1		3
S140					
141			1		1
Total	203	213	204	191	811
Mean[a]	105.74	107.62	107.94	106.76	107.03

[a] Means were computed from scores listed above using the midscore of each step as the value of all scores at that step.

through infancy. The results obtained in this study must, therefore, be thought of as indicative, rather than as showing how much can be accomplished by dietary improvement.

The significantly higher mean IQs in the Kentucky studies, compared with those in Norfolk, have led to many speculations concerning the reasons for the differences. Attention should be called to the distinct handicaps imposed by these tests on the Kentucky group, which would have operated in the opposite direction, therefore making the difference between groups more convincing. Disregarding any other factors of importance, we must emphasize the obviously more adequate diet used conventionally in the Kentucky families. Although careful and detailed dietary surveys could not be included in this study, we are certain that in Kentucky the daily use of pork or fowl, succulent vegetables and fruits, both fresh and home preserved, furnished a significantly higher intake of water-soluble vitamins of the B complex and ascorbic acid, as well as vitamin A,

than the low economic level of the Norfolk group usually allowed. In other words, the baseline from which supplementation began was lower in Norfolk, and the finding of significant results is, therefore, more probable in this group. It would be expected that the effect of dietary improvement in any individual mother would be dependent upon the dietary pattern characteristic of that mother. Inadequacy of diet may be determined by economic handicaps, dietary customs, atypical tastes and numerous other factors which need not be listed here.

SUMMARY

The mean intelligence, determined by conventional testing methods at ages 3 and 4 years, in children born of 612 women in Norfolk, Va., was significantly higher in those whose mothers had received vitamin supplements during the latter part of pregnancy than in those whose mothers received an inert control tablet. Benefits were most apparent in the group receiving a supplement of thiamine, riboflavin, niacinamide and iron, less so for those receiving only thiamine or only ascorbic acid. The differences between these three groups, which received some vitamin supplement, were not significant at the 5 percent level of certainty, whereas the differences between the supplemental groups and the controls were significant at the 1 percent level of certainty. No significant differences were demonstrated in a similar study among Kentucky mountain women, where the usual and unsupplemented diet was found to be more nearly adequate than that used in the Norfolk homes.

References

(1) Maurer, S. and L.S. Tsai. Vitamin B deficiency in nursing young rats and learning ability. *Science* 70: 456-458, 1929.

(2) _____ and _____. Vitamin B deficiency and learning ability. *J Comp Psychol* 11: 51, 1930.

(3) _____. The effect of early partial depletion of vitamin B_1 upon learning in rats. *J Comp Psychol* 20: 309-318, 1935.

(4) _____. The effect of early depletion of vitamin B_2 upon performance in rats. IV. *J Comp Psychol* 20: 385-387, 1935.

(5) Balken, Eva R. and S. Maurer. Variations of psychological measurements associated with increased vitamin B complex feeding in young children. *J Exper Psychol* 17: 85-92, 1934.

(6) Beilly, J.S. and I.J. Kurland. Relationship of maternal weight gain and weight of the newborn infant. *Am J Obst Gynecol* 50: 202-206, 1945.

(7) Bernhardt, K.S. Protein deficiency and learning in rats. *J Comp Psychol* 22: 269-272, 1936.

(8) _____ and R.J. Herbert. A further study of vitamin B deficiency and learning with rats. *J Comp Psychol* 24: 263-267, 1937.

(9) O'Neill, P.H. 1946. The effects on subsequent maze learning ability of graded amounts of vitamin B_1 in the diet of very young rats. Unpublished doctoral thesis. Fordham University Library, New York.

(10) _____. The effect on subsequent maze learning ability of graded amounts of vitamin B_1 in the diet of very young rats. *J Genet Psychol* 74: 85-95, 1949.

(11) _____. If mother is short on B_1 child may not learn fast. *Science News Letter* Aug. 13, 1949.

(12) Poole, M. H., B. M. Hamil, T. B. Cooley and I. G. Macy. Stabilizing effect of increased vitamin B_1 intake on growth and nutrition of infants. Basic study. Research Laboratory. Children's Fund of Michigan for the Study of Growth. *Am J Dis Child* 54: 726-749, 1937.

A CONTROLLED STUDY OF THREE METHODS OF PROPHYLAXIS AGAINST STREPTOCOCCAL INFECTION IN A POPULATION OF RHEUMATIC CHILDREN[1]
II. RESULTS OF THE FIRST THREE YEARS OF THE STUDY, INCLUDING METHODS FOR EVALUATING THE MAINTENANCE OF ORAL PROPHYLAXIS

Alvan R. Feinstein,[2] Harrison F. Wood,[3] Jeanne A. Epstein,[4] Angelo Taranta,[5] Rita Simpson,[6]
and Esther Tursky,[7]
with the collaboration of Thomas Argyros, Julian Frieden, Raymond C. Haas,
Ilse Hirschfeld, Arthur J. Lewis, Carlos Manso, and Konrad Ulich

Oral and injectable agents are now being widely used to prevent streptococcal infections in patients who have had rheumatic fever (*1, 2*). The choice of treatment has generally been made arbitrarily because the comparative effectiveness of the available agents has not been adequately determined in clinical trials. For statistically valid results, any trial studies would need to ensure that the prophylactic agents were given to groups of patients whose numbers were large enough to be adequately comparable in certain crucial aspects of their rheumatic background.

A previous report presented the results of the first two years of observation on 405 patients in a prophylaxis clinic that was organized for this purpose (*3*). It described the operation of the study, and the details are here only briefly reviewed. The clinic contains 391 children and adolescents, all of whom were admitted after unequivocal attacks of rheumatic fever. The patients have been followed at monthly intervals with regular clinical, bacteriologic, and serologic examinations to detect streptococcal infections or rheumatic activity. At the beginning of the study they were divided into three groups by a statistical method of randomization ensuring that the patients in each group would be comparable in the most critical parameters of such a study: age, cardiac status, and duration of freedom from rheumatic activity. Each group was then assigned to one of three prophylactic regimens, as follows: sulfadiazine,[8] 1 gm a day by mouth in a single dose; buffered potassium penicillin G,[9] 200 000 units a day by mouth in a single dose, half an hour before breakfast; and benzathine penicillin G,[10] 1 200 000 units in 2 ml by intramuscular injection every four weeks.

In the first two years of the study, streptococcal infections occurred in each of the three groups with the following attack rates per patient year: parenterally injected penicillin, 7 percent; orally administered penicillin, 20 percent; and sulfadiazine, 24 percent. For this period, rheumatic fever recurred in each of the three groups with the following attack rates per patient year: parenterally injected penicillin, none; orally administered penicillin, 4.8 percent; and sulfadiazine, 2.7 percent.

Source: *The New England Journal of Medicine* 260(14): 697-702, 1959.

[1] From Irvington House and the departments of Medicine and Pediatrics, New York University College of Medicine. The Irvington House Prophylaxis Study is supported in part by the American Heart Association, the New York Heart Association, the Westchester Heart Association, the Sullivan County Heart Chapter, the United States Public Health Service, and Wyeth Laboratories.

[2] Instructor in medicine, New York University College of Medicine; clinical director, Irvington House.

[3] Assistant professor of pediatrics, New York University College of Medicine; medical director, Irvington House.

[4] Research associate, Irvington House Prophylaxis Clinic.

[5] Adjunct assistant professor of microbiology, New York University College of Medicine; senior research associate, Irvington House. (Work done during the tenure of a research fellowship of the American Heart Association and under a research grant from the John Polachek Foundation for Medical Research.)

[6] Statistician, Irvington House Prophylaxis Study.

[7] Head nurse, Irvington House Prophylaxis Study.

[8] Kindly supplied by Lederle Laboratories Division, American Cyanamid Company, Pearl River, New York.

[9] Kindly supplied as Pentids by E. R. Squibb and Sons, New York City.

[10] Kindly supplied as Bicillin by Wyeth Laboratories, Philadelphia.

The previous report indicated that a major problem in the evaluation of the data was the difficulty in deciding how faithfully the patients had maintained the oral prophylactic regimens (3). Since pills or tablets are often not taken, the previous superiority of the benzathine penicillin was conceivably due to the fact that it was injected, thus giving assurance that the prophylaxis was received. During the third year of the study, a specific technic was used to determine the answer to this question. These data are now presented, together with further data on streptococcal infections and rheumatic recurrences obtained during this interval.

METHODS

The third year of operation of the study continued in the manner described in the previous report. (3). The patients received monthly examinations. Streptococcal infections were detected by monthly throat cultures, by routine bimonthly determinations of antistreptolysin-O titers, and by serial measurement of antistreptolysin O, antihyaluronidase, and antistreptokinase titers in serums of several consecutive months when clinical or bacteriologic suspicion of an infection with Group A streptococci existed (4-6). The diagnosis of rheumatic fever recurrences was made according to the modified Jones criteria (7).

Two procedures were used to determine how faithfully patients maintained their oral prophylaxis. The first method consisted of a special interview, 10 to 15 minutes in duration, with each child. The interview included the child's parents whenever possible and was conducted throughout by the same physician (J.A.E.). The questions considered the nature of supervision, the place where the drug was kept at home, and the daily ritual that the child followed in taking it. Additional questions asked how many times each month the patient failed to take the assigned medication, and whether, with the passage of time, he had become any more or less faithful in his observance of the program. At each previous routine monthly Clinic visit, the examining physician had regularly questioned the patient about the number of pills missed that month, and these results could be compared with the answers given at the special interview. The second procedure of this special study sought to obtain more objective data. The

patient was supplied each month with a bottle containing a known number of pills (35 penicillin or 70 sulfadiazine tablets). When the bottle was returned at the end of the month, the remaining tablets were counted. The difference then represented the presumptive number of pills that had been consumed as rheumatic-fever prophylaxis.

It was recognized that both the interview and the pill-count technic had definite disadvantages. However, no more complex method gave promise of being more accurate or practical for large-scale screening of this type.

From the physician's interviews, prophylaxis was graded in a number of ways. It was considered "good" if less than five daily (nonconsecutive) doses were missed per month and if the history was believed to be reliable. It was considered "poor" if the patient missed five or more days per month. It was "questionable" if the patient missed four or less days per month but the reliability of the history was doubtful. With the use of the pill-count method, prophylaxis was considered "good" if a three-month average of the pills returned differed from the expected number by −3 to +4 for the penicillin tablets and by −3 to +9 for the sulfadiazine tablets. It was considered "poor" if this number differed by 5 or more for the penicillin tablets and by 10 or more for the sulfadiazine tablets. Some patients regularly failed to return their pill bottles, so that pill counts could not be obtained. The designation "too few pills" was used when the three-month average of those returned differed from the expected number by −4 or more. This was presumably due to destruction or loss of the medication or to its use by other members of the family.

The occurrence of streptococcal infections in each patient was then related to the fidelity with which oral prophylaxis was maintained. For this purpose, the patients whose prophylaxis maintenance had been questionable or poor were tabulated in a single category as not good and were compared with those whose maintenance had been good.

RESULTS

Streptococcal infections were classified in three ways: clinical infection, subclinical infection, and questionable infection or carrier state.

Table 1. Number of streptococcal infections in patients receiving three different prophylactic agents in the first three years.

Year	Prophylactic agent	Clinical infections	Subclinical infections	Carriers	Totals
Totals for 1st 2	Benzathine penicilline G[a]	6	6	—	12
	Potassium penicillin G[b]	11	26	1	38
	Sulfadiazine	17	22	7	46
3d	Benzathine penicillin G	6	3	2	11
	Potassium penicillin G	5	15	4	24
	Sulfadiazine	5	9	8	22
Totals for 1st 3	Benzathine penicillin G	12	9	2	23
	Potassium penicillin G	16	41	5	62
	Sulfadiazine	22	31	15	68
Totals		50	81	22	153

[a] For intramuscular injection.
[b] For oral administration.

The criteria used for these classifications were described in the previous report (3). Table 1 lists the total number of each type of infection due to Group A streptococci for the patients in the three prophylaxis groups. The data continue to show the same trends that were demonstrated previously: about two-thirds of the total number of streptococcal infections were not clinically evident; there were approximately equal numbers of infections in the penicillin and sulfadiazine groups; the number of infections in the group receiving injections was lower than that in either of the two groups receiving prophylaxis by mouth.

Table 2 gives the attack rates of streptococcal infections during the first three years of the study. The attack rates per patient year for the total period in each of the three groups were as follows: penicillin by injection, 7.3 percent; penicillin by mouth, 20.7 percent; and sulfadiazine, 21.1 percent.

Table 3 indicates how well oral prophylaxis was maintained, as evaluated by the interview technic. "Good" prophylaxis was achieved by 73

Table 2. Attack rates of infections with the group A streptococcus in the first three years.

Year[a]	Prophylactic agent	No. of patient yr.	No. of streptococcal infections	Rate per patient yr., %
Totals for 1st 2[b]	Benzathine penicillin G	190	12	6.3
	Potassium penicillin G	183	38	20.8
	Sulfadiazine	191	46	24.1
3d	Benzathine penicillin G	124	11	8.9
	Potassium penicillin G	117	24	20.5
	Sulfadiazine	131	22	16.8
Totals for 1st 3	Benzathine penicillin G	314	23	7.3
	Potassium penicillin G	300	62	20.7
	Sulfadiazine	322	68	21.1
Totals		936	153	

[a] During 1st 3 yr. 2 patients on injections of penicillin had 2 streptococcal infections; of those on penicillin tablets 9 had 2 infections, and 1 had 3; of those on sulfadiazine, 13 had 2 infections, 5 had 3, and 1 had 4.
[b] Additional data obtained since previous report (3) caused minor modifications in figures originally published.

Table 3. Evaluation of fidelity of maintenance of oral prophylaxis, with the use of the interview technic.

Fidelity of prophylaxis	Penicillin group		Sulfadiazine group		Totals	
	No. of patients	Percentage	No. of patients	Percentage	No. of patients	Percentage
Good	82	73	84	67	166	69
Questionable	22	19	33	26	55	23
Poor	9	8	9	7	18	8
Totals	113	100	126	100	239	100

percent of the patients on penicillin and by 67 percent of those on sulfadiazine. Table 4 indicates the same measurements with the use of the pill-count technic of evaluation. By these standards, good prophylaxis was maintained by 55 percent of the patients on penicillin and by 44 percent of those on sulfadiazine. The percentage of the former was less by the pill-count technic than by the interview method because of the difficulty in evaluating patients who failed to return their bottles or who returned bottles containing too few pills.

In Table 5 the patients have been classified according to the fidelity of oral-prophylaxis maintenance, and the prevalence of streptococcal infections in these patients over the three-year period has been simultaneously correlated. Additional data have been included to compare these results in patients receiving penicillin by injection, in whom the maintenance of good prophylaxis is assured. For patients who maintained good prophylaxis, as evaluated by the interview technic, streptococcal infections occurred in 29 percent of those on penicillin and in 20 percent of those on sulfadiazine. For the patients who maintained good prophylaxis as evaluated by the pill-count method, streptococcal infections occurred in 27 percent of those on

penicillin and in 21 percent of those on sulfadiazine. It should be noted that these results refer to the percentage of patients who had streptococcal infections, and are not given in terms of attack rates per patient years. The striking similarity of these data suggests that the two methods of evaluation used in this study may be considered reliable. By comparison, streptococcal infections occurred in 12 percent of the patients receiving injections of penicillin. This indicates that even when good oral prophylaxis was maintained, the patients receiving the agents by mouth had a larger number of streptococcal infections than those given injections. Of patients in the groups receiving the agents by mouth those who maintained good prophylaxis with sulfadiazine had fewer streptococcal infections than those who maintained good prophylaxis with penicillin.

Table 6 shows the number of recurrences of rheumatic fever that have taken place in the first three years of this study. There has been only one recurrence in the bicillin group, an attack rate of 0.3 percent per patient year. There have been 15 recurrences during the three hundred patient years on penicillin tablets, an attack rate of 5.0 percent. There have been six recurrences in the three hundred and

Table 4. Evaluation of fidelity of maintenance of oral prophylaxis, with the use of the pill-count technic.

Fidelity	Penicillin group		Sulfadiazine group		Totals	
	No. of patients	Percentage	No. of patients	Percentage	No. of patients	Percentage
Good	60	55	53	44.0	113	49.0
Questionable						
a. No bottle	11	10	15	12.5	26	11.5
b. Too few pills returned	27	25	37	31.0	64	28.0
Poor	11	10	15	12.5	26	11.5
Totals	109	100	120	100.0	229	100.0

Table 5. Streptococcal infections in the three-year period according to fidelity of oral prophylaxis as evaluated by two technics.

Technic of evaluation	Fidelity of prophylaxis	Prophylactic agent	No. of patients	No. of patients who had one or more strepto-coccal infections	Percentage of patients who had one or more streptococcal infections
Physician's interview	Good	Potassium penicillin G[a]	82	24	29
		Sulfadiazine	84	17	20
	Not good	Potassium penicillin G[a]	31	16	52
		Sulfadiazine	42	21	50
—	Good	Benzathine penicillin G[b]	116	14	12
Pill count	Good	Potassium penicillin G[a]	60	16	27
		Sulfadiazine	53	11	21
	Not good	Potassium penicillin G[a]	49	22	45
		Sulfadiazine	67	25	37

[a] By mouth.
[b] By intramuscular injection.

Table 6. Recurrences of rheumatic fever in the first three years of the study.

Prophylactic agent	Patient yr.	Recurrences	Rate per patient yr., %
Benzathine penicillin G	315	1	0.3
Potassium penicillin G	300	15	5.0
Sulfadiazine	322	6	1.9
Totals	937	22	
Average			2.3

twenty-two patient years on sulfadiazine, an attack rate of 1.9 percent. The overall total attack rate for the nine hundred and thirty-seven patient years of observation has been 2.3 percent per patient year.

DISCUSSION

The data obtained in the first three years of this study indicate that 1 200 000 units of benzathine penicillin G given intramuscularly every four weeks is more effective in preventing both streptococcal infections and rheumatic recurrences than either of the two methods of oral prophylaxis. Additional data obtained during the third year have enabled a classification of patients into those who maintain good oral prophylaxis and those who do not. The data indicate that the injections have prevented strepto-

coccal infections more effectively than the agents given by mouth, even when the latter are faithfully taken. This indicates that the superiority of benzathine penicillin G does not come about merely because its monthly injections give assurance that it is well maintained by the patient. It should be noted, however, that each monthly injection provided a dose that is usually capable of eradicating for Group A streptococci, a property that was not present in the dosage schedule used for the other two agents.

A more surprising finding emerges from the comparison of the two agents given by mouth. The data of the first three years indicate that sulfadiazine and potassium penicillin G have been approximately equal in the prevention of streptococcal infections, and that sulfadiazine has been superior to penicillin in the prevention of recurrences of rheumatic fever and in preventing streptococcal infections in patients who maintained good prophylaxis. The numerical data are not yet great enough in each category to give statistical significance to these results, which suggest that sulfadiazine is superior to penicillin as an agent for the oral prophylaxis of rheumatic patients. However, the data are adequate to indicate that, in the dosage schedules used, sulfadiazine has been at least as good as penicillin G for this purpose. No sulfonamide-resistant strains of streptococci have developed or been introduced during the course of this study.

These results are surprising because sulfadiazine is only bacteriostatic whereas penicillin is bactericidal. No immediate explanation for the clinical observations is available. It is possible that the orally administered penicillin is poorly absorbed or that the dosage used is too low to achieve adequate blood levels for bactericidal action. It should be noted that the attack rates in the present study for patients taking 200 000 units of penicillin G *once* daily are very similar to those observed by Massell et al. (*8*) in a somewhat similar study in which two different penicillin preparations were used, both given by mouth at a dosage of 200 000 units *twice* daily.

In its current recommendations for penicillin as an oral prophylactic agent in rheumatic patients, the Committee on Prevention of Rheumatic Fever and Bacterial Endocarditis of the American Heart Association lists the alternative schedules of 200 000 or 250 000 units once *or* twice daily (*9*). Because sulfadiazine has been demonstrated to be equal to 200 000 units daily of penicillin for this purpose, and because of the potentially important public-health ramifications of the present data, the protocol of the study has been augmented so that sulfadiazine can be tested against a double daily dose of penicillin. Accordingly, the present study will be extended beyond the original five years that were planned for it, and will add new groups of patients in whom this comparison can be made. Subsequent conclusions await the accumulation of further data.

SUMMARY

Three hundred and ninety-one children and adolescents, with unequivocal previous attacks of rheumatic fever, were followed in a special study clinic designed to compare the effectiveness of three prophylaxis regimens in the prevention of streptococcal infections and rheumatic recurrences. At the start of the study, a statistical method of random selection divided the patients into three groups comparable in age, cardiac status, and duration of freedom from rheumatic activity. Each group was assigned to one of the three agents under study: sulfadiazine, 1.0 gm per day by mouth; potassium penicillin G, 200 000 units per day by mouth; and injections of benzathine penicillin G, 1 200 000 units per month. The patients have been examined monthly since the beginning of the study. Streptococcal infections have been detected by careful bacteriologic and immunologic technics (using antistreptokinase and antihyaluronidase as well as antistreptolysin-O titers when necessary). Recurrences of rheumatic fever were diagnosed by means of the modified Jones criteria.

The data of the first three years of this study are now completed and show the following incidence of streptococcal infections per patient year in each group: sulfadiazine, 21.1 percent; penicillin given by mouth, 20.7 percent; and penicillin by injection, 7.3 percent. When the group of patients taking the agents by mouth was divided into those who maintained good prophylaxis and those who did not, it was found that the injections were still more effective than either preparation given orally for the prevention of streptococcal infections and that sulfadiazine had been more effective than the penicillin by mouth in patients who maintained good prophylaxis. The recurrence rate of rheumatic fever per patient year was as follows: sulfadiazine, 1.9 percent; penicillin tablets, 5.0 percent; and penicillin injections, 0.3 percent.

The data show unequivocally that injections are more effective than either sulfadiazine or penicillin by mouth, in the dosage schedule used, for the prevention of streptococcal infections and rheumatic fever. Of the two agents given orally, sulfadiazine has been as good as, and possibly superior to, penicillin. This observation has many ramifications for the mass-scale rheumatic-fever prophylaxis programs now in operation. The apparent superiority of sulfadiazine is now being tested against a double dose of penicillin in a new group of patients who have been added to the original study.

The statistical analyses were made by Mrs. Rita Simpson, B.S., aided by the consultant advice of Miss Marjorie Bellows, chief statistician of the American Heart Association. We are indebted to the Irvington House Prophylaxis Study Nursing Staff for its invaluable services, which were performed by Martha Yoza, R.N., Nancy Campbell, R.N., and Maureen Johnson, R.N., under the direction of Esther Tursky, R.N. Laboratory technical assistance was provided by Mrs. Florence Girsch, Mrs. Catherine Pszcola, Mrs. Ina Smith, Miss Edna Lindsey, Mrs. Hanna Schramm, and Mr. Kenji Nogaki.

References

(1) Stollerman, G.H. Prevention of rheumatic fever by use of antibiotics. *Bull NY Acad Med* 31:165-180, 1955.

(2) Wood, H.F. Prevention of rheumatic fever. *Am J Cardiol* 1:456-463, 1958.

(3) Wood, H.F. et al. Controlled study of three methods of prophylaxis against streptococcal infection in population of rheumatic children. I. Streptococcal infections and recurrences of acute rheumatic fever in first two years of study. *New Eng J Med* 257:394-396, 1957.

(4) Rantz, L.A. and E. Randall. Modification of technic for determination of antistreptolysin titer. *Proc Soc Exper Biol Med* 59:22-45, 1945.

(5) Harris, S. and T.N. Harris. Measurement of neutralizing antibodies to streptococcal hyaluronidase by turbidimetric method. *J Immunol* 63:233-247, 1949.

(6) Christensen, L.R. Methods for measuring activity of components of streptococcal fibrinolytic system and streptococcal desoxyribonuclease. *J Clin Investigation* 28:163-172, 1949.

(7) American Heart Association. Report of Committee on Standards and Criteria for Programs of Care of the Council on Rheumatic Fever: JONES criteria (modified) for guidance in diagnosis of rheumatic fever. *Mod Concepts Cardiovas Dis* 24:291-293, 1955.

(8) Massell, B.F. Prevention of rheumatic fever and rheumatic heart disease: Brief historical review and preliminary report of three controlled studies. *St. Francis Sanatorium Hosp Bull* 14:1-26, 1957.

(9) American Heart Association, Committee on Prevention of Rheumatic Fever and Bacterial Endocarditis. Prevention of rheumatic fever and bacterial endocarditis through control of streptococcal infections. *Mod Concepts Cardiovas Dis* (Supp. 12) 25:365-369, 1956.

THE DYNAMICS OF MALARIA

George Macdonald,[1] Caton B. Cuellar,[2] and Cecil V. Foll[3]

Previous studies on dynamic systems of transmission of malaria, and of eradication of infection following the interruption of transmission, have now been adapted for advanced techniques using the facilities offered by computers.

The computer programs have been designed for a deterministic model suitable for a large community and also for a stochastic model relevant to small populations in which infections reach very low finite numbers. In this model, new infections and recoveries are assessed by the daily inoculation rate and are subject to laws of chance. Such a representation is closer than previous models to natural happenings in the process of malaria eradication. Further refinements of the new approach include the seasonal transmission and simulation of mass chemotherapy aimed at a cure of *P. falciparum* infections.

These programs present models on which the actual or expected results of changes due to various factors can be studied by the analysis of specific malaria situations recorded in the field. The value of control methods can also be tested by the study of such hypothetical epidemiological models and by trying out various procedures.

Two specific malaria situations (in a pilot project in Northern Nigeria and in an outbreak in Syria) were studied by this method and provided some interesting results of operational value. The attack measures in the pilot project in Northern Nigeria were carried out according to the theoretical model derived from the basic data obtained in the field.

The present study originated in a desire to explore the belief that a powerful tool for the design of eradication and control programs, and for the analysis of difficulties in them, could be produced by the extension of dynamic studies using computer techniques. One of us has previously developed a system of dynamics of malaria (*1-6*). This system has been satisfying insofar as it has led to the enunciation of certain principles governing the epidemiology of malaria. However, development of quantitative dynamics has been meagre; the original author (*5*) showed that the system could be used quantitatively to reconstitute a model of an actual epidemic and thereby to define the factors which determined it, while Macdonald and Göckel (*7*) have explored some of the dynamics of diminishing parasite rates during the process of eradication. However, this development by desk techniques has been clumsy and has involved so much calculation as to be usable only for special purposes.

The practicability of quantitative dynamic studies has, however, been greatly changed by the facility of the computer whereby previously intractable aspects can now be handled with ease. It has seemed rational to pursue the previous studies with this technique, and it seems irrational not to use it to support technical knowledge and experience in the field by design techniques which can present the probable result of any suggested course of action or any number of variants on it. By doing this, the epidemiologist can refine his ideas and can have a guided method of choice between alternative lines of action, and with it a yardstick of expected results to guide evaluation month by month so that the earliest signs of deviation can be identified. For these reasons, a series of related computer programs have been developed.

THE FORM OF COMPUTER PROGRAMS

The previous model of the dynamic system of malaria was deterministic in that it represented

Source: *Bulletin of the World Health Organization* 38(5):743-755, 1968.

[1] Lately Director of the Ross Institute of Tropical Hygiene and Professor of Tropical Hygiene in the University of London. Professor Macdonald died on 10 December 1967.
[2] Research Assistant, Ross Institute of Tropical Hygiene, London.
[3] World Health Organization Field Research Project, Kankiya, Nigeria.

happenings in a large community within which neither population numbers nor case numbers ever reached very low finite numbers. Some of the main elements of this early model are set out in the Annex because it has been used as the basis of development of the computer programs which have been run on the ATLAS computer of the London University Institute of Computer Science. The simplest of these programs is a straight transfer of the basic deterministic model. It can fulfill those functions which were previously fulfilled but is infinitely easier to apply. For instance, instead of the very laborious simulation of an epidemic previously demonstrated by the author (5), it would be quite simple to run off a score of simulations with different parameters and then to see which most closely fitted the observed curve. Equally, the laborious calculations of the rates of fall of parasite rates with different low reproduction rates during the progress of attempted eradication (7) can now be reproduced or elaborated with minimal trouble.

However, the opportunity has been taken to introduce a number of sophistications in order to adapt the model better to the detailed study of various preventive measures and to the process of eradication which cannot be handled by a deterministic model that deals only in numbers which never reach very low finite levels. An incubation interval has been incorporated in all programs, to a small extent to introduce the timing influence which it exerts in nature, but principally to separate infections into two groups, overt and covert, the latter incubating in either the mosquito or man. It is only with this modification that a realistic representation can be made of drug treatment which affects overt infections and may leave others untouched.

A second sophistication has been the development of stochastic models representing happenings in finite populations and when cases grow small in number. In these stochastic models an inoculation rate, calculated daily, has been applied as a probability of infection to each separate parasite-free member of the community using a Monte Carlo technique and resulting in the conversion of an integral number of negatives into positives. A similar technique has been used in applying the recovery rate to positive cases. Both new infections and recoveries therefore occur in integral numbers deter-

mined by inoculation rates and recovery rates subject to the laws of chance. This has been the extent of the stochastic modification, no adjustment having been made elsewhere in the model or thought to be necessary. Some of the significant differences between the two types of programs are illustrated in Figure 1, which demonstrates the application of both techniques to predicting the possible course of events in disappearing malaria with reproduction rates ranging from 0 to 1.0. The deterministic lines represent proportions positive; accordingly they never reach zero, and are quite smooth. The stochastic graphs represent numbers of positives which in the end decline to zero; they are irregular, approximately following the deterministic line so long as cases are numerous, but deviating markedly from it when they become rare, under the influence of chance. The graphs therefore represent a single possible set of happenings and need to be under the influence of chance, and several replicates have to be made before a general picture can be assumed with certainty. They all have one characteristic, however, which is that the numbers of cases round-off rather abruptly and before this would have been expected from the deterministic curve. This is the representation of the statistical actuality of "fade-out" and may be assumed to be a natural happening in the process of eradication.

A further sophistication has been to provide for the introduction of curative or suppressive treatment of variable efficiency, and at variable intervals. Though programs have been developed in relation to both curative and suppressive treatment, the main usage has been in the simulation of mass chemotherapy aimed at the cure of falciparum infections. Further refinements developed for the precise simulation of field conditions include the development of seasonal programs in which two or three seasons governed by different epidemiological parameters can be simulated.

These programs have been developed in the EXCHLF language of the ATLAS computer and are not, therefore, widely interchangeable, though the authors would be happy to provide any worker who has access to this language and system with a copy. However, there is set out in the Annex a flow diagram from which it should be possible to construct a program in any language. It represents a model of seasonal ma-

Figure 1. Comparison of the stochastic and deterministic expectation of changes in the parasite rate following a reduction of a previously high reproduction rate (z).[a]

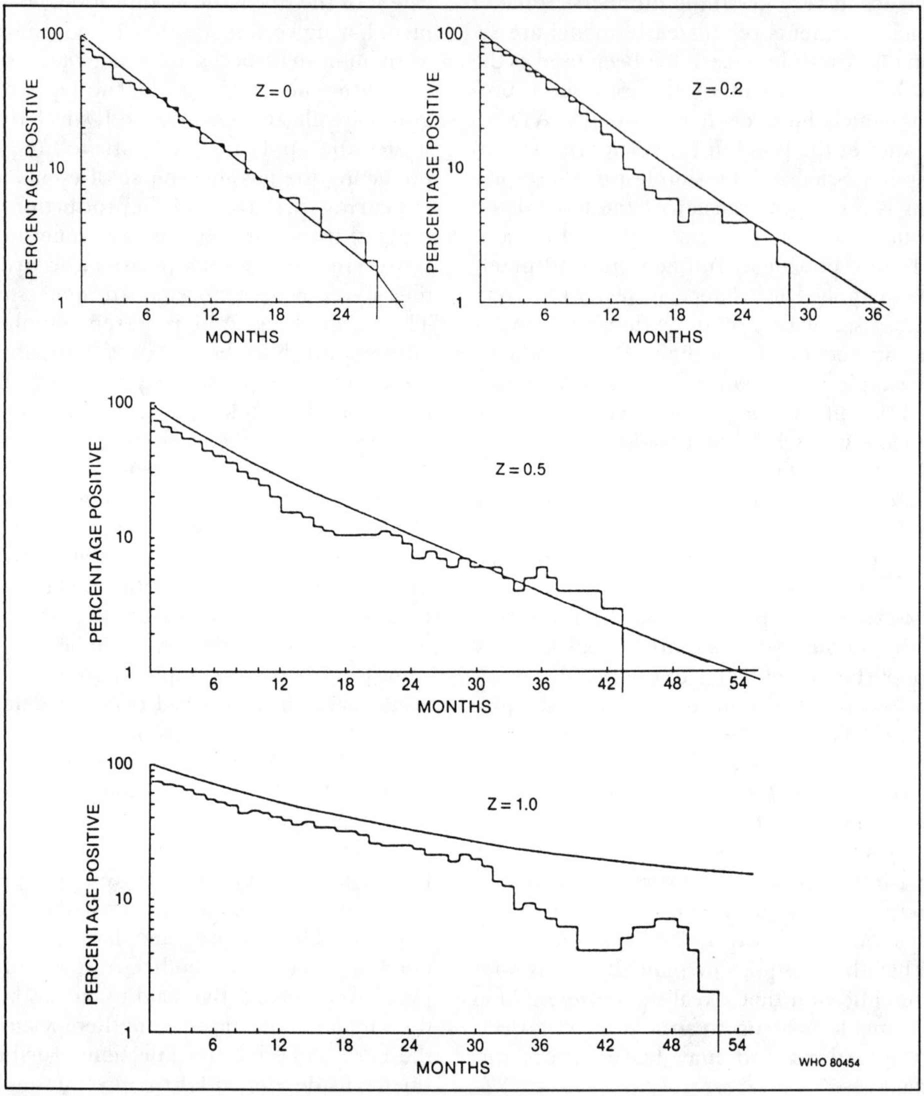

[a] Reduction to 0, 0.2, 0.5 or 1.0. The size of the stochastic community is 100.

laria, complete with incubation interval, stochastic handling and periodic curative mass treatment. The development of a simpler deterministic model or more sophisticated model should be simple on this basis.

The model requires four epidemiological parameters for its working: the man-biting habit of the mosquito, the probability of mosquito survival through a day, the recovery rate from malaria in man, and the reproduction rate prev-

alent under the given conditions. If actual or postulated values of these four parameters are fed in with the data stream a complete picture of malaria can be constituted. If three of them are known from field observations—normally the man-biting habit, the mosquito longevity, and the recovery rate—it is possible to do a large number of runs including a wide range of values of the fourth, the reproduction rate, producing corresponding curves in the prevalence of parasitemia. Known changes in the prevalence of parasitemia can then be matched against these specimens or "templets" and when a reasonable fit is obtained an appropriate value of the reproduction rate can be assigned to the natural happenings. This method has been extensively used on the basis of field data, including the three named parameters, and measurements of two successive parasite rates at several months' interval during the same season in the same group of people. It has been found to be readily workable and through it a complete reconstitution can be made of natural conditions for later use in testing the probable effect of preventive measures.

These four parameters are required because each of them enters into the expression which represents the dynamic curve of parasitemia. The reproduction rate is itself a composite expression including all the directly controlling factors, and also the mosquito numbers and the period of extrinsic development of the parasite. These need not be estimated separately; they can be included in the general representation of a reproduction rate which is much more accurately estimated by the indirect means described above than by any attempt at direct measurement of mosquito numbers and all the other factors involved.

A precise model requires a precise input of data which may be very difficult to achieve. In consequence, a large number of programs have been run to determine the degree of error in the final product produced by various misrepresentations of the input data. The man-biting habit and the probability of mosquito survival always occur in the expressions jointly as the stability index.[4] Variations in this index below the value of 1.0 have a quite negligible effect on the total picture and there is little effect when it is 2.0 or less. From this it can be taken as a working rule that if the man-biting habit is known to be under 0.1 or if the probability of mosquito survival is known to be under 0.75 the index can be given an assumed value of 1.0 and analysis continued without great consequent error, provided this assumed value is maintained throughout the operation. If these requirements are not fulfilled, further measurement of both is needed.

The recovery rate from falciparum malaria has previously been estimated at 0.005 and there is sound evidence (7) that it does not vary much from place to place and this may reasonably be put as a value for this parameter. Deviations from this value have been postulated but they cannot be great: values of 0.01 or 0.0025 would produce, on the one hand, a mercurial mobility of parasite rates in non-malarious seasons and, on the other, a stiff resistance to change, such as are outside our observation. This significance of possible differences has been studied and it has been shown that in the process of analysis, insertion of a deviant recovery rate results in the deduction of a markedly deviant reproduction rate, but if these two deviant values are then inserted in a model which is to be used for checking the effect of preventive measures, their deviations are almost complementary and little difference is seen in the final product. It is therefore fully justifiable to use a standard value of 0.005 for the recovery rate.

PRACTICAL APPLICATIONS

These programs have been designed to make models on which the actual or expected results of some change in the surrounding circumstances can be simulated and studied. They may be used in a number of ways and actual experience has been gained in the following forms of application.

(1) The testing of the potential value of the control mechanism by creating one or more hypothetical, though realistic, epidemiological models and trying out the suggested preventive measure with a number of variations in efficiency, timing, etc.

(2) The analysis of a specific malaria situation from the collection of observed field data.

(3) The design of specific control or eradication programs, carried out by a combination of the methods listed as (2) and (1) above; and the creation of a full model from the collection of field data and the superimposition thereon of different mechanisms of control. A great variety of potentially available mechanisms can thereby be tested and when the most appropriate has been selected a yardstick of expected progress

---

[4]Stability index = $a/(-\log_e p)$, representing the mean number of bites on man taken by an average mosquito during its entire lifetime, and determining the stability of epidemiological conditions (5). For definitions of a and p, see Annex.

can be prepared for later comparison month by month with actual progress.

(4) The study of outbreaks of malaria. Outbreaks occur nowadays mainly on the basis of nearly successful eradication programs starting from very low parasite rates. They differ from normal situations in that the type of data available for study is usually different and refers to incidence only.

Study of the Efficacy of Preventive Measures: Mass Treatment

A study has been made of the potential value of mass treatment as an adjuvant to or substitute for insecticidal attack. It has been envisaged as being given to a high proportion of the population of an area at approximately the same time and over a very brief period, probably one or two days. A search has been made of the literature to see whether the effects of such brief courses as either curatives or suppressives can be properly evaluated. It has been concluded that a single dose of a 4-aminoquinoline may be curative to a very high proportion of cases of falciparum malaria in people previously exposed to this infection (*8-15*). No similarly convincing or even generally coherent picture emerges of the effects of regimes of treatment which might be applied as mass therapy against vivax or other types of malaria. Programs have been prepared applicable to the cure or suppression of vivax malaria, but until some concept can be formed of the ratio in which these two occur there is little point in operating them. The studies have therefore been continued in relation to falciparum, in which context they are believed to be realistic. The efficiency of mass treatment has been deemed to be the product of the proportion of falciparum cases cured by the regime studied (typically 0.6 g of chloroquine base as an adult dose) and the proportion of the population to whom it is administered. A large number of programs have been operated on widely differing epidemiological backgrounds, with treatment at intervals of one month upwards and with efficiencies ranging from 50 percent to 90 percent. The general form of results is illustrated in Figure 2, which refers to the expected effect of an 80 percent effective mass treatment every two months against falciparum malaria of low stability (stability index = 1.0) and where the reproduction rate of malaria independently

of this mass treatment is as shown in the graphs. The first four of these are identical epidemiological conditions to those illustrated in Figure 1 and may be compared with them. The other three graphs extend this series to some higher reproduction rates. It will be noted that in the last of these where the reproduction rate is 4.0 the prevalence of parasitemia declines slowly and this is about the limit of reproduction rate within which mass treatment of this periodicity could ultimately eliminate infection. It is for the operator to decide how frequently mass treatment could be applied, but it is not likely that it could be applied at this efficiency at much shorter intervals. Reproduction rates of this low value are rare in nature and it follows that mass treatment could rarely be a substitute for insecticidal attack though it could be a valuable adjuvant. Figure 2 shows that it could be expected to accelerate the decline of parasitemia very greatly and so reduce greatly the time from the start of attack until surveillance levels were reached, while the last four graphs dealing with reproduction rates of 1.0 and upwards show that it could convert attack by insecticides which would otherwise be a total failure into complete and moderately early success. The conclusions which have been reached from this series of studies are as follows:

(1) Mass treatment could play a very effective part in the eradication of falciparum malaria but in most conditions only as an adjuvant to insecticidal attack.

(2) The value is not limited to conditions where insecticides have failed or might fail; the speed which it introduces constitutes a valuable factor in any program.

(3) The most effective time for the institution of mass treatment is during the period of minimal transmission. Where malaria is seasonal the greatest advantage is gained by the initiation of treatment early in the non-malarious or relatively non-malarious season, and this despite the absence of transmission or many clinical cases at that time.

(4) Mass chemotherapy applied at a time when the incidence of malaria is increasing, as in the early stages of an outbreak, is relatively ineffective and would have less value than is indicated by these examples.

(5) Preliminary analysis of the malaria situation along the lines which have been described is essential for the forecasting of the results of mass treatment. The data required from the field for this purpose are the man-biting habit

Figure 2. Expected effect of an 80% effective mass treatment every 2 months on malaria subject to reproduction rates (*z*) shown and a stability index of 1.0.[a]

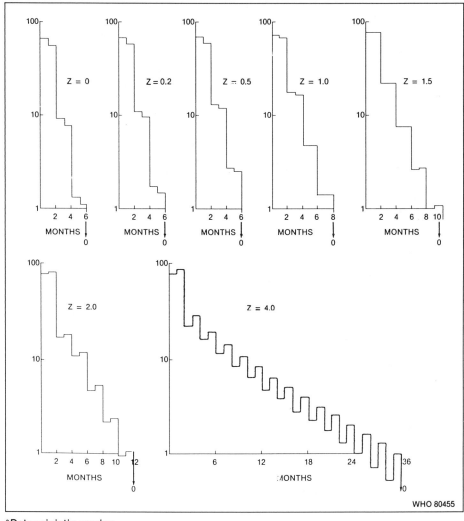

[a] Deterministic version.

of the vector (unless it is known to be under 0.1), the expectation of the survival of the mosquito (unless this is known to be under 0.75), and information on changes during each season in the prevalence of parasitemia—this could take the form of successive parasite rates in selected communities.

Analysis of a Particular Malaria Situation

The prevalence of malaria and its epidemiological characteristics in Kankiya, Northern Nigeria, have been studied for several years and described by Foll, Pant and Lietaert (*16*) and Foll and Pant (*17*). Malaria is normally holoendemic; it is seasonal, the more malarious season lasts four or five months, the less malarious one lasts seven or eight; transmission is by *Anopheles gambiae* and much of this takes place outdoors; the man-biting habit of this mosquito approaches 0.5. Falciparum malaria predominates. Several experimental control programs have been carried out but have failed to eliminate transmission entirely and this is thought to be due to the common outdoor resting habit of the mosquito and consequent escape from insecticides, with associated transmission. Under the influence of insecticides the probability of survival of the mosquito through one day is about 0.8 and this probability does not vary greatly between the seasons when insecticides are applied. Two consecutive parasite rates taken in children aged four to nine years at intervals of three months during the wet season were 82 percent and 94 percent, and successive examinations of one group during the dry season at intervals of six months gave rates of 68 percent and 42 percent. These rates are maximal for the area concerned within which there are localities in which they are much lower, but it seemed best to devise programs in relation to the most intense transmission that they are intended to meet.

Analysis of this situation has been carried out on the basis of the recorded man-biting habit and mosquito longevity with which a lengthy series of templets has been prepared, illustrating the expected changes in parasitemia over a wide range of reproduction rates. A very much abbreviated series of these is shown in Figure 3. Comparison with the observed changes showed that those in the wet season corresponded to a reproduction rate of 6.0 and those in the dry season to 1.0. These values have been reentered on a complete model with different lengths of wet and dry season from which it has been shown that with a dry season of seven months these parameters almost exactly reproduce the known epidemiological position with a parasite rate ranging from 48 percent to 89 percent, and this has been accepted as representing conditions at Kankiya.

Design of Specific Programs

It was suggested that periodic mass treatment as an adjuvant to insecticidal attack might make successful interruption of transmission possible. The output of a small selection of preliminary runs is illustrated in Figure 4, showing the expected effect of mass treatment of 60 percent, 70 percent and 80 percent efficiency applied at intervals of one month and two months, starting at the beginning of the dry season. It seemed from these preliminary runs that either

Figure 3. Abbreviated series of the "templets" run off as a guide in the analysis of the Kankiya malaria situation.

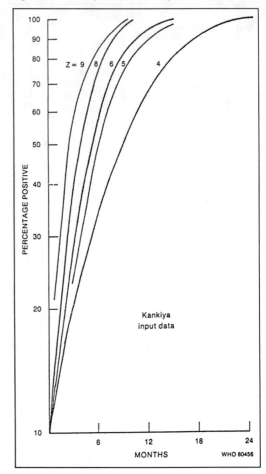

a 70 percent or 80 percent efficient treatment every two months might be adequate, but reliance could not be placed on less efficient or more widely spaced treatments. Operational considerations made it desirable to concentrate on the regime carried out every two months for which one of us (C.V.F.) estimated that he could secure an 80 percent or greater efficiency. This treatment was further explored in a number of stochastic and deterministic runs; the output for one of the former, covering a population of 1000, is shown in Figure 5. It seemed from these subsequent runs that there was a distinct probability that treatment started at the beginning of the dry season and repeated every two months might reduce the general parasite rate

Figure 4. Expected effect of 60%, 70% and 80% effective mass treatment given once a month[a] and once every 2 months[b] as an adjuvant to imagicidal attack to communities living under Kankiya holoendemic conditions.

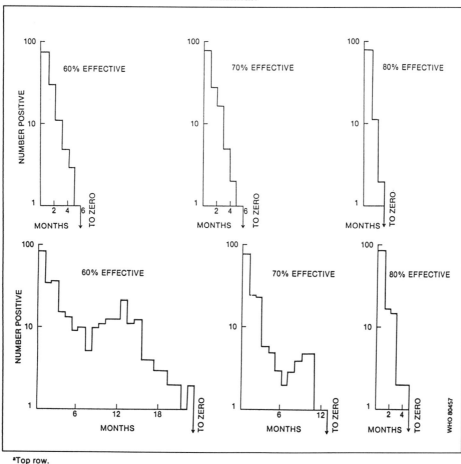

[a]Top row.
[b]Bottom row.

to under 1 percent in six months, at which time infection might have disappeared from several localities. If vigorous insecticidal attack was then applied, this position, it was concluded, could then be maintained or improved during the rains and further very greatly improved during the early part of the ensuing dry season.

This proposed regime of combined therapeutic and imagicidal attack has been put into operation by WHO with the consent and very active support of the Ministry of Health, Northern Nigeria. A particularly pleasing aspect of the work in Nigeria has been the assistance and encouragement that the team received from the Emir of Katsina, his Wambai, District Head,

and village headmen. It was started as an experimental scheme in an area of some 300 square miles (777 km^2) containing 52 000 people in which a comprehensive geographical reconnaissance was completed together with a house-to-house census of all occupants. The intention was to administer a curative dose of a combination of chloroquine and pyrimethamine to the entire population every two months for a total of seven treatments and to spray DDT three times a year at a dosage of the technical product of 2 g/m^2. This program was started in November 1966 and a coverage of 87.2 percent, 84.4 percent, 77.7 percent and 82.8 percent achieved in the first four rounds of

Figure 5. Expected effect of an 80% effective mass treatment applied as an adjuvant to imagicidal attack on a population of 1000 living under Kankiya holoendemic conditions.

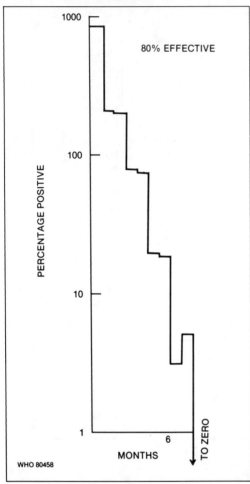

WHO 80458

Study of Outbreaks of Malaria

Study of Outbreaks of Malaria

of the parasite rate and of its subsequent increase with the predicted patterns justify the system of design.

Some outbreaks of malaria have occurred in the course of consolidation and it has been desirable to study them in order to determine by what means they might have been detected at an earlier stage or remedied more quickly. In the examples studied, there has been available a statement of the incidence of new cases over a period of some months without a full statement of the population at risk, so that calculation of the proportion infected has not been possible. However, if cases are known to be few in relation to the total population and the proportion infected to be small, this is not a significant barrier to analysis. A program has been adapted to produce, for any set of epidemiological parameters fed into it, a daily print-out of the resultant number of cases. This is necessarily run on a stochastic basis subject to the laws of chance, as is the natural epidemic, so that general resemblance rather than precise conformity between the simulated and the observed happenings is to be expected.

An outbreak of this type in the neighborhood of Damascus, Syria, has been reported to us by Dr. K. El Shami. Within the area studied, Zakieh, the outbreak arose from a known relapse case, which became overt on 23 May 1965, and continued without serious check until the end of August, during which time there had been 52 known secondaries. The vector was *Anopheles sacharovi*, a highly anthropophilic and long-lived species. The epidemic was analyzed in the way already described except that the daily incidence of cases in a long series of simulated models was compared with that in the observed, instead of the changes in parasite prevalence. From several runs it was concluded that a reproduction rate of 22 on the simulated model presented a very close approximation to the actual observed number of new cases, and the output from this run is shown, together with observed happenings, in Figure 6. Statistical analysis on the basis of the number of cases during each successive incubation interval, excluding the first during which none could occur, gives a probability exceeding 0.5 that the difference is due to chance alone; a comparable

mass drug administration. After the third round the parasite rate in the central indicator zone had been reduced from 24.2 percent to 1.0 percent, which can be compared with a predicted decrease to 0.5 percent. It was at this stage that wet weather conditions ensued and DDT should have been applied; unfortunately, owing to operational failures outside the experimental area, this was not possible. Active transmission under wet weather conditions was resumed for two months, with the increase in the parasite rate which had been predicted in this event. The experiment is therefore incomplete but both the close coincidence of the rate of fall

Figure 6. Daily incidence of new cases of malaria arising from a relapsed case occurring on 23 May in an observed epidemic near Damascus and in a simulated epidemic with parameters as shown in the text.

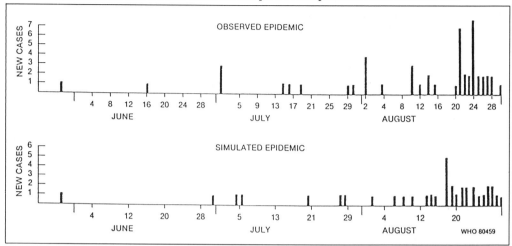

analysis on the basis of cases per week gives a probability exceeding 0.35.

A number of simulations of periodic case-finding activities, representing the cure of 60 percent, 70 percent or 80 percent of overt cases at discrete time intervals from 14 days upward gave extremely disappointing results, and it was concluded that none of these regimes could have effectively brought the outbreak to an end without the addition of special measures. The only case-finding with treatment mechanism which could have had this result would have been continuous, operating daily over a period of at least one incubation interval following the discovery of an overt case. This unexpected inadequacy of periodic detection and treatment was finally identified as being due to the relative proportions of overt and covert cases. The position on 21 August at the height of the epidemic was that there were then 21 overt infections and 34 incubating in the mosquito or man but not yet manifest. The conclusion was that in such cases the function of periodic active case-detection should be to detect cases, but that once a case had been detected the significance of passive case-detection, which could be continuous, was greatly enhanced.

Other similar problems relating to outbreaks of malaria on Assam tea estates during the consolidation phase have been approached in a similar manner.

ACKNOWLEDGMENT

The authors very gratefully acknowledge the facility of the use of the ATLAS computer at the University of London Institute of Computer Science.

References

(*1*) Macdonald, G. *Trop Dis Bull* 47:907, 1950.
(*2*) Macdonald, G. *Trop Dis Bull* 47:915, 1950.
(*3*) Macdonald, G. *Trop Dis Bull* 49:569, 1952.
(*4*) Macdonald, G. *Trop Dis Bull* 49:813, 1952.
(*5*) Macdonald, G. *Trop Dis Bull* 50:871, 1953.
(*6*) Macdonald, G. *The Epidemiology and Control of Malaria.* London, Oxford University Press, 1957.
(*7*) Macdonald, G. and C. Göckel. *Bull WHO* 31:365, 1964.
(*8*) Butts, D.C.A. *J Nat Malar Soc* 9:44, 1950.
(*9*) Villarejos, V.M. *Am J Trop Med* 31:703, 1951.
(*10*) Hoekenga, M.T. *JAMA* 149:1369, 1952.
(*11*) Covell, G., G.R. Coatney, J.W. Field, and Jaswant Singh. Chemotherapy of malaria. Geneva, World Health Organization: Monograph Series, No. 27, 1955.
(*12*) Clyde, D.F. *Br Med J* 2:1238, 1958.
(*13*) Clyde, D.F. *Am J Trop Med Hyg* 10:1, 1961.
(*14*) Clyde, D.F. *Malaria in Tanzania.* London, Oxford University Press, 1967.
(*15*) Pringle, G. and S. Avery-Jones. *Bull WHO* 34:269, 1966.
(*16*) Foll, C.V., C.P. Pant, and P.E. Lietaert. *Bull WHO* 32:531, 1965.
(*17*) Foll, C.V. and C.P. Pant. *Bull WHO* 34:395, 1966.

ANNEX: THE MATHEMATICAL MODEL

The deterministic form has been previously described and summarized by Macdonald (6), and part is here repeated for convenience. The symbols used are:

m = the anopheline density in relation to man;

a = the average number of men bitten by one mosquito in one day;

b = the proportion of those anophelines with sporozoites in their glands which are actually infective;

p = the probability of a mosquito surviving through one whole day;

n = the time taken for completion of the extrinsic cycle;

h = the proportion of the population receiving infective inocula in one day;

x = the proportion of people affected (that is showing parasitemia);

L = the limiting value of the proportion of men infected when equilibrium is reached;

r = the proportion of affected people, who have received one infective inoculum only, who revert to the unaffected state in one day;

t = time in days;

z_0 = the basic reproduction rate, or the number of infections distributed in a community as a direct result of the presence of a single, primary, non-immune case.

The system is based on the definition of an overall reproduction rate, z_0 above, and its daily element $z_0 r$ representing the number of infections distributed by a single case in one day. However, in a wholly independent system the reproduction rate itself becomes a function of x, the proportion of the population affected owing to the intervention of the mosquito vector in which infections may overlap when common, and thus limits the net number distributed.

The basic rate, usable only for static conditions and defined in relation to near-vanishing infections, is given by the following equation:

$$z_0 = \frac{ma^2bp^n}{r(-\log_e p)}, \qquad (1)$$

and the net rate, applicable in all conditions, is given by:

$$z = \frac{z_0\,(-\log_e p)}{ax - (\log_e p)}. \qquad (2)$$

The inoculation rate, which is largely a development of it, is:

$$h = \frac{z_0 rx(-\log_e p)}{ax - \log_e p}. \qquad (3)$$

It is, however, essential to realize that, when the occurrence of new cases is to be studied, they are the product of an inoculation rate dependent on values of x of some time previously. New overt infections are the product of a reservoir of cases separated in time by both the incubation period in the mosquito and that in man, by, indeed, the entire incubation interval (i). If allowance is to be made for the incubation interval this must be taken into account, and for this purpose the effective value of the inoculation rate is:

$$h = \frac{z_0 rx_{t-i}(-\log_e p)}{ax_{t-i} - \log_e p}, \qquad (4)$$

and it is this value of h which is here used in all programs. In working examples the value of i for falciparum infections has been put at 30, to allow also for delay in infectivity. For *vivax* infections a typical value of 20 has been estimated (5). In an example recently worked, a value of 16 was postulated, but fuller working suggested that 17 or 18 would have been more appropriate.

The basic differential has two forms applicable when $h < r$, and when $h > r$, the two merge when $h = r$. For program purposes they are best represented in incompletely simplified forms which facilitate a switch from one to another at the appropriate point, and it is well to emphasize the different time scale of the parasite rate;

when $h < r$,

$$\frac{dx}{dt} = h(1 - x_t) - (r-h)x_t, \qquad (5)$$

and when $h > r$,

$$\frac{dx}{dt} = h(1-x_t), \qquad (6)$$

the expression for h used being always that given in equation (4).

The limiting value of (5) is:

$$L_x = (-\log_e p)/a\cdot(z_0 - 1), \qquad (7)$$

and that of equation (6) is 1.0. In practice, any observed equilibrium is represented by equation (7).

The stability index (4) is:

$$a/(-\log_e p), \tag{8}$$

which represents the mean number of bites on man taken by a typical vector during its entire lifetime, a characteristic which determines stability because it represents the working of a density-dependent mechanism. The two elements, a and $-\log_e p$, always occur in expressions in such a way that they can be expressed as this ratio, or its reciprocal, and it is often convenient to refer to them jointly.

Computer Program: General Principles

The flow diagram (Figure 7) is an attempt to describe the layout of a program in such a way that it could be translated reasonably easily into any computer language. It has been divided into a number of subsections in order to avoid the confusion inevitably associated with a long diagram which has many loops. The diagram describes the dynamics of a stochastic malaria model which can be modified to include provision for periodical mass treatment or for seasonal changes in epidemiology, or for both.

The stochastic element, using a "Monte Carlo" technique, is described separately and before the main program (Figure 8). This description is then assumed, and in the main program the whole operation is described in the words "Monte Carlo the negatives" or elsewhere as "Monte Carlo the positives."

The program includes a stop after cases reach zero, and this is slightly complicated owing to the need to run it for a further complete in-cubation interval in order to check the absence of covert infections. The need for two time scales, t and $(t-1)$, has been met on ATLAS by the reservation of main variable space sufficient to cover every day for which the program might operate, typically 1899 cells representing five years. This has been simple on ATLAS, which is a very large machine, but some modification would probably be needed for smaller machines.

The Monte Carlo System

This is used in order to apply probability rather than certainty of a proportion to the conversion of negatives into positives, or *vice versa*. This probability is first decided, the inoculation rate in one case and $(r-h)$ in the other. The machine is then instructed to select a random number between 0 and 1.0; if this random number is equal to or less than the probability already determined, the conversion is judged to have taken place. If it exceeds the probability the case remains unchanged.

It may be noted that the machine's random numbers are in truth pseudo-random and repetition of this process in a subsequent program might result in the selection of the same "random" number. This difficulty has been overcome when multiple programs are to be operated by the insertion of a genuine random number into the data input with an instruction to the machine to run through its pseudo-random series for this number of times before starting on its selection.

Notes A, B, and C of Figure 7.

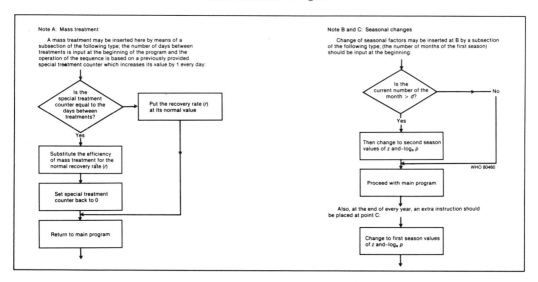

Figure 7. Flow diagram for the main computer program.[a]

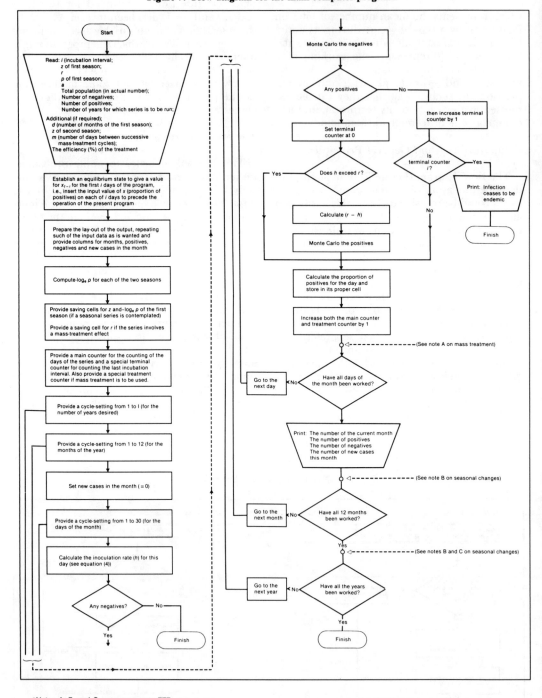

Figure 8. Flow diagram for the Monte Carlo system.

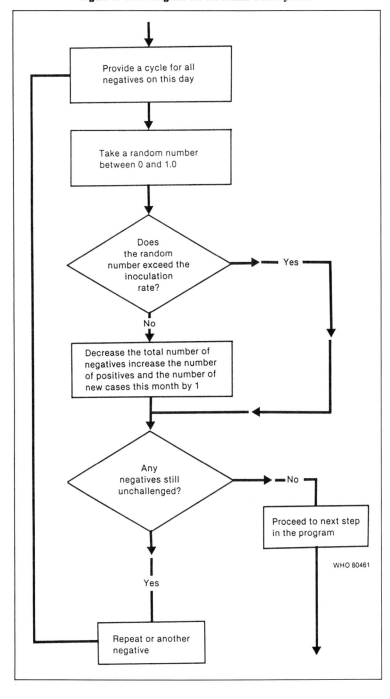

INCIDENCE OF CANCER IN MEN ON A DIET HIGH IN POLYUNSATURATED FAT

Morton Lee Pearce and Seymour Dayton[1]

In an eight-year controlled clinical trial of a diet high in polyunsaturated vegetable oils and low in saturated fat and cholesterol in preventing complications of atherosclerosis, 846 men were assigned randomly to a conventional diet or to one similar in all respects except for a substitution of vegetable oils for saturated fat. Fatal atherosclerotic events were more common in the control group (70 $v.$ 48; P < 0.05). However, total mortality was similar in the two groups: 178 controls $vs.$ 174 experimentals, demonstrating an excess of non-atherosclerotic deaths in the experimental group. This was accounted for by a greater incidence of fatal carcinomas in the experimental group. Thirty one of 174 deaths in the experimental group were due to cancer, as opposed to 17 of 178 deaths in the control group (P = 0.06).

INTRODUCTION

In 1969 we presented the results of an eight-year clinical trial designed to determine whether a diet which lowers serum-cholesterol levels can also reduce clinical manifestations of atherosclerosis (1). Fatal acute atherosclerotic events were significantly more common in the controls than in the experimental group. Despite this difference, total mortality was scarcely affected, indicating an excess of non-atheromatous deaths in the experimental group. We anticipated that these deaths would be due to a variety of competing causes in these elderly men. At first, we attempted to clarify this problem by examining non-atheromatous deaths in the last two years of the study. Our results were inconclusive, and when we published them, we left open the question of toxicity associated with feeding polyunsaturated fats in amounts larger than most populations consume. Subsequently we reviewed all our data with regard to deaths from causes other than atherosclerotic complications, especially when we read of experiments which associate unsaturated-fat feeding with an increased incidence of spontaneous and induced neoplasms in animals (2). When we found a higher than expected incidence of car-

cinoma deaths in the experimental group, we did a detailed retrospective record search in an effort to identify all malignancies in the study population, fatal and non-fatal. We also added the experience of the two years which followed returning experimental and control groups to the standard institutional diet.

METHODS

The experimental design and methods are given in detail in our 1969 report (1). In 1959 we started a controlled trial of a diet high in polyunsaturated fat and low in saturated fat and cholesterol. The participants, men living in a veterans' home, were assigned randomly to the control group (422 men) or to the experimental group (424 men). The efficacy of randomization was demonstrated by the compatibility of the two groups in respect of nearly all baseline observations (1). The efficacy of the randomization in respect of cigarette smoking has been analyzed in more detail elsewhere (3). The study was done "double blind" in that both groups were fed diets differing from the regular institutional diet but simulating conventional food, and the doctors evaluating clinical events or deaths did not know what the diet assignment was. Meals were served cafeteria style, and adherence to the diet was monitored by means of individual attendance records.

Sample diets were analysed periodically throughout the study. Average values are presented in Table 1. The experimental diet simu-

Source: *Lancet* March 6, 1971, pages 464-467.

[1] Research Service, Wadsworth Hospital Medical Service, and Domiciliary Medical Service of Veterans Administration Center, Los Angeles, and Department of Medicine, University of California—Los Angeles School of Medicine, Los Angeles, California 90024, U.S.A.

Table 1. Composition of diets.

Component	Control	Experimental
Total calories/day	2496	2496
Protein (g/day)	96.3	97.4
Fat calories (% of total)	40.1	38.9
Iodine value of fat	53.5	102.4
Cholesterol (mg/day)	653	365
Polyunsaturates		
(% total fatty acid)	10	39.5

lated a conventional United States diet, and nearly quadrupled the intake of polyunsaturated fat at the expense of saturated fat. Cholesterol intake was cut approximately in half. Beta-sitosterol content of the experimental diet was high, averaging 215 mg per day in several analyses.

Definitions of atheromatous deaths and events are presented in detail in our original report (1). Neoplasms were diagnosed on the basis of tissue reports, biopsy, and/or necropsy. Information about neoplasms was retrieved by reviewing clinical records and cytology, surgical-pathology, and necropsy reports. Retrieval of records from within this institution was almost complete. Although cancer-morbidity data were undoubtedly incomplete, chances of failing to identify a non-fatal malignancy were equal in the two groups. Mortality data are about 99 percent complete (1). Diagnoses were reviewed and recorded "blindfold" by M.L.P. and later reviewed by S. D. Death-certificate diagnoses were not accepted. (There was only one instance where a non-verified death-certificate diagnosis of cancer was found—a man in the experimental group with a death-certificate diagnosis of carcinoma of the larynx.) The various categories of neoplasms are shown in Table 2.

The experiment was divided into two phases—the 8½ years in which the control and experimental diets were fed (diet phase) and the period after the men had returned to the standard institutional diet (post-diet phase).

RESULTS

The unrestricted consumption of the two diets had no significant effect on average body-weight. Serum-cholesterol levels fell promptly in the experimental group and the mean stayed 12.7 percent below that of the control group. Fatal acute atherosclerotic events during the diet phase were more numerous in the control group (70) than in the experimental group (48), and the same was true of the combined definite

Table 2. Numbers and sites of fatal and non-fatal carcinomas and other neoplasms diagnosed during the diet phase and the two-year period after termination of the diet.

Site	Diet phase			Post-diet phase		
	Control		Experimental	Control		Experimental
Buccal and pharynx	6		10	1		0
Digestive and peritoneum:	6		12	6		3
Stomach		1	6	2		0
Other		5	6	4		3
Respiratory:	13		18	3		1
Lung and bronchus		12	16	2		1
Other		1	2	1		0
Genitourinary:	10		16	2		3
Prostate		8	11	2		1
Other		2	5	0		2
Other carcinoma	0		1	0		0
Total carcinomas, excluding skin	35		57	12		7
Skin carcinomas	21		10	4		2
Other malignancies[a]	3		3	1		1
Fatal benign tumor	0		0	0		1
Total	59		70	17		11

[a] These include lymphosarcoma, reticulum-cell sarcoma, rhabdomyosarcoma, angiosarcoma, lymphocytic leukemia, and astrocytoma.

clinical events (*1*). However, total mortality during the diet phase was not significantly different—178/422 controls compared with 174/424 in the experimental group.

During the diet phase (see Figure 1) there were 31 carcinoma deaths in the experimental group and 17 in the control group ($\chi^2 = 3.668$, $P < 0.06$). The carcinoma deaths are plotted from the time of randomization to the time of death. In the post-diet phase the excess continued for a year (3 experimentals, 0 controls), but in the second year the controls exceeded the experimentals (4 experimentals, 10 controls). Cancers, both fatal and non-fatal, counted from the time of randomization to the time of diagnosis are summarized in Table 2. There was a higher incidence of the more commonly occurring visceral carcinomas in the experimental

group. The contrary observation in regard to basal and squamous-cell skin cancers (none fatal) is largely due to two controls who had multiple lesions of this sort.

We examined the relationship of carcinoma deaths with a number of other variables (Table 3). The percentage of pre-existing definite cerebral infarcts was higher, and the baseline serum-cholesterol values were lower, than in men not dying of carcinoma, but neither difference was statistically significant. Cigarette smoking is analyzed in detail in Table 4. There is no apparent non-dietary explanation for the higher frequency of carcinoma deaths in the experimental group.

Figure 1. Cumulative carcinoma deaths in experimental and control groups from time of randomization to time of death.

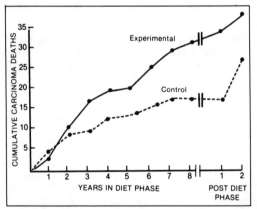

Table 3. Incidence of selected baseline variables in patients who died of carcinoma during the diet phase.

	Control group (17 carcinoma deaths)	Experimental group (31 carcinoma deaths)
Myocardial infarction, definite	2	5
Cardiac decompensation	2	5
History of angina pectoris	5	6
Cerebral infarction, definite	3	6
Age (yr.)	68.4	65.5
Serum-cholesterol (mg/100 ml)	224.5	221.2

There were more low adherers to diet in the experimental group with fatal carcinomas than in the controls (Table 5). This distribution is not significant by chi square, but the number in

Table 4. Deaths from carcinoma in diet phase adjusted for cigarette smoking.

	Control			Experimental		
Cigarette smoking	No. of men	Carcinoma observed	Carcinoma adjusted	No. of men	Carcinoma observed	Carcinoma adjusted
Unknown	57	2	1.74	42	1	1.15
>2 packs/day	13	0	0	7	0	0
1–2 packs/day	57	2	1.66	38	4	5.00
½—1 pack/day	129	6	7.02	173	19	16.53
<½ pack/day	62	3	2.61	46	4	4.68
Occasional	18	1	1.03	19	0	0
None	86	3	3.24	99	3	2.79
	422	17	17.30	424	31	30.15

Deaths are adjusted by multiplying the number of men affected in a given cigarette-smoking stratum of the control group by (C + E)/2C, in which C = number of controls in the stratum and E = number of experimental subjects. A corresponding calculation is made for the experimental group (*3*).

Table 5. Adherence to diet in patients with fatal carcinoma during the diet phase.[a]

Adherence (%)	Control group	Experimental group
0–10	2	10
10–20	1	2
20–30	1	3
30–40	0	0
40–50	3	3
50–60	3	3
60–70	0	4
70–80	2	2
80–90	4	1
90–100	1	3
	17	31

[a] Adherence, calculated from attendance records, is expressed as a percentage of the maximum number of meals which could have been taken in the study dining-hall.
$\chi^2 = 10.26$; $P > 0.3$.

each cell is small. The number of low adherers in the experimental group with fatal carcinoma is (at least in part) a reflection of the adherence pattern of the total experimental group, which is significantly lower than in the controls (Table 6). We also analyzed the data in this table by chi square for regression to take into account the ordered character of the percent adherence. The difference in adherence remains significant at the 1 percent level.

Table 6. Adherence to diet in the total study population.

Adherence (%)	Control group	Experimental group
0–10	82	120
10–20	47	46
20–30	31	42
30–40	21	30
40–50	42	23
50–60	40	33
60–70	32	32
70–80	42	37
80–90	50	31
90–100	35	30
	422	424

$\chi^2 = 21.78$; $P < 0.01$.

DISCUSSION

The experience of other investigators using similar diets has not been the same. In an eleven-year report on the Oslo diet-heart study, Leren noted seven cancer deaths in his experimental group and five in the control group (4). His criteria for a diagnosis of cancer are not given, and diets were not supervised after the fifth year. The six-year London trial of a diet high in soya-bean oil noted six cancer deaths in the control group and one in the experimental group. Again, cancer criteria are not given (5). The Helsinki group has not yet published cancer data (6). These differences in cancer experience may have been due to differences in patient population and in trial design. Our trial involved the longest period of dietary control of the studies cited. The high incidence of neoplasms which we report in both experimental and control subjects is due to factors not operative in the other studies—our subjects were much older than those in the other series, and we obtained a high necropsy-rate (80 percent of the men dying in the center and 65 percent of all deaths in the study during the diet phase).

Many of the cancer deaths in the experimental group were among those who did not adhere closely to the diet. This reduces the possibility that the feeding of polyunsaturated oils was responsible for the excess carcinoma mortality observed in the experimental group. However, there were significantly more low adherers in the entire experimental group than in the controls (Table 6). In both groups, the numbers of cancer deaths among the various adherence strata are compatible with random distribution (Table 5). A high incidence among high adherers would be expected if some constituent of the experimental diet were contributing to cancer fatality.

These observations present a dilemma. On the one hand, it is tempting to ignore the low-adherence segment of the study population. On the other hand, conclusions based on the better-adhering strata may be misleading because of bias. We cannot resolve this dilemma, and feel that the results must be examined in both ways.

Other trials of the effect of polyunsaturated-fat diets on the incidence of atherosclerotic complications have been negative in regard to an increased incidence of fatal cancer, and our own results are of borderline significance. However, our results must be viewed in the light of animal experiments which suggest that fat intake (especially unsaturated-fat intake) affects the incidence of certain types of neoplasm.

Overweight has been associated with a higher incidence of cancer than the incidence observed in normal or underweight people (*7, 8*) and fat consumption is strongly correlated with death from neoplasms of the breast, ovaries, and rectum, and from leukemia (*9*). Earlier work suggested that animals on fat-rich diets had an increased incidence of spontaneous and carcinogen-induced carcinomas (*10, 11*). Carroll et al. have investigated carcinogen-induced mammary carcinomas in rats (*2, 12*) and found that increasing the level of dietary fat enhances the yield of these neoplasms. Twenty percent corn oil diets had a greater effect than 0.5 percent corn oil, and a greater effect than 20 percent coconut oil, which is largely saturated. In another experiment they fed 20 percent corn oil after the administration of the carcinogen to half the animals and up to the time of carcinogen administration in the other half. There was a higher incidence in the animals which were given the corn oil diet after the carcinogen administration than in the group which was switched from the corn oil diet to a low-fat diet at the time of carcinogen administration. These observations suggest a promoting rather than an initiating process. Their metabolic significance remains speculative.

Aflatoxins contaminating cottonseed meal have been implicated in hepatic carcinoma in trout (*13*). It is most unlikely that they were present in our experimental diet since the commercial production of edible oils in the United States removes these substances (*14*).

Other explanations of our data should be considered. If elderly men are protected from atherosclerotic complications, they will die of something else, and cancer is the next most common cause of death in this population. Also, it is theoretically conceivable that a diet high in saturated fat protects against cancer, but both epidemiological data and animal experiments suggest otherwise. At any rate, if the experimental diet is cocarcinogenic, the responsible component still needs to be identified.

Our results and those from the literature are uncertain and confusing in respect of the role of polyunsaturated fats in an increased incidence of malignancies. The high incidence of fatal carcinomas in our experimental group is of borderline significance. A retrospective review of any large collection of data will suggest causal relationships which are chance occurrences. Tests of significance such as chi square have been formulated to evaluate pre-stated hy-

potheses, and their application to hypotheses which were made after scrutiny of data will tend to overstate the significance of observed differences. Furthermore, it is important to remember that no population under study has been consuming a diet high in polyunsaturated fats over long periods of time.

What is the practical application of our data? Certainly they should be considered in the design and performance of any new diet trial. A diet similar to our experimental one, but slightly lower in total fat and with polyunsaturates largely replaced by mono-unsaturates, would have a similar serum-cholesterol lowering effect. We think it premature to make a blanket prescription of a diet high in polyunsaturated fat for the entire population. However, the risks involved seem small compared with the high incidence of atherosclerotic complications in patients with certain hyperlipidemias (*15*), and the use of diets high in polyunsaturated fat is certainly justifiable in selected patients. A trial of a diet low in fat, and very low in unsaturated fat, would be of interest in selected human carcinomas, especially breast cancer.

Miss Nancy Chin helped in document and data management. Mrs. Dolores Adams and Prof. Wilfred J. Dixon provided assistance in data processing. This work was supported by the Veterans Administration, and by grants from the Arthur Dodd Fuller Foundation. Computing was done at the Health Sciences Computing Facility, U.C.L.A., supported by National Institutes of Health grant FR-3.

References

(*1*) Dayton, S., M.L. Pearce, S. Hashimoto, W.J. Dixon, and U. Tomiyasu. *Circulation* Vol. 40, suppl. No. II, 1969.
(*2*) Gammal, E.B., K.K. Carroll, and E.R. Plunkett. *Cancer Res* 27:1737, 1967.
(*3*) Dayton, S. and L.M. Pearce. *Lancet* 1:473, 1970.
(*4*) Leren, P. *Circulation* 42:935, 1970.
(*5*) Research Committee to the Medical Research Council. *Lancet* ii:693, 1968.
(*6*) Turpeinen, O., N. Miettinen, M.J. Karvonen, P. Roine, M. Pekarinen, E.J. Lehtosuo, and P. Alivirta. *Am J Clin Nutr* 21:255, 1968.
(*7*) Tannenbaum, A. *Arch Path* 30:509, 1940.
(*8*) Tannenbaum, A. and H. Silverstone. In *Cancer* (R.W. Raven, ed.) Vol. 1, p. 306. London, 1957.
(*9*) Lea, A.J. *Lancet* ii:332, 1966.

(10) Tannenbaum, A. *Cancer Res* 2:468, 1942.

(11) Watson, A.F. and E. Mellanby. *Br J Exp Path* 11:311, 1930.

(12) Carroll, K.K. and H.T. Khor. *Cancer Res* 30:2260, 1970.

(13) Sinnhuber, R.O., D.V. Lee, J.H. Wales, and J.L. Ayres. *J Natl Cancer Inst* 41:1293, 1968.

(14) Parker, W.A. and D. Melnick. *J Am Oil Chem Soc* 43:635, 1966.

(15) Slack, J. *Lancet* ii:1380, 1969.

THE LIPID RESEARCH CLINICS CORONARY PRIMARY PREVENTION TRIAL RESULTS I. REDUCTION IN INCIDENCE OF CORONARY HEART DISEASE[1]

Lipid Research Clinics Program

The Lipid Research Clinics Coronary Primary Prevention Trial (LRC-CPPT), a multicenter, randomized, double-blind study, tested the efficacy of cholesterol lowering in reducing risk of coronary heart disease (CHD) in 3806 asymptomatic middle-aged men with primary hypercholesterolemia (type II hyperlipoproteinemia). The treatment group received the bile acid sequestrant cholestyramine resin and the control group received a placebo for an average of 7.4 years. Both groups followed a moderate cholesterol-lowering diet. The cholestyramine group experienced average plasma total and low-density lipoprotein cholesterol (LDL-C) reductions of 13.4 percent and 20.3 percent, respectively, which were 8.5 percent and 12.6 percent greater reductions than those obtained in the placebo group. The cholestyramine group experienced a 19 percent reduction in risk (P<.05) of the primary end point—definite CHD death and/or definite nonfatal myocardial infarction—reflecting a 24 percent reduction in definite CHD death and a 19 percent reduction in nonfatal myocardial infarction. The cumulative seven-year incidence of the primary end point was 7 percent in the cholestyramine group v 8.6 percent in the placebo group. In addition, the incidence rates for new positive exercise tests, angina, and coronary bypass surgery were reduced by 25 percent, 20 percent, and 21 percent, respectively, in the cholestyramine group. The risk of death from all causes was only slightly and not significantly reduced in the cholestyramine group. The magnitude of this decrease (7 percent) was less than for CHD end points because of a greater number of violent and accidental deaths in the cholestyramine group. The LRC-CPPT findings show that reducing total cholesterol by lowering LDL-C levels can diminish the incidence of CHD morbidity and mortality in men at high risk for CHD because of raised LDL-C levels. This clinical trial provides strong evidence for a causal role for these lipids in the pathogenesis of CHD.

Coronary heart disease (CHD) remains the major cause of death and disability in the United States and in other industrialized countries despite recent declines in CHD mortality rates. It accounts for more deaths annually than any other disease, including all forms of cancer combined (1). Nationally, more than 1 million heart attacks occur each year and more than a half million people still die as a result. Coronary heart disease ranks first in terms of social security disability, second only to all forms of arthritis for limitation of activity and all forms of cancer combined for total hospital bed days. In direct health care costs, lost wages, and productivity, CHD costs the United States more than $60 billion a year.

This enormous toll has focused attention on the possible prevention of CHD by various means, especially through lowering of the

Source: *Journal of the American Medical Association* 251(3):351-364, 1984.
[1] From the Lipid Metabolism–Atherogenesis Branch, National Heart, Lung, and Blood Institute, Bethesda, Maryland. Funding for the study came from the following National Heart, Lung, and Blood Institute contracts and interagency agreements: N01-HV1-2156-L, N01-HV1-2160-L, N01-HV2-2914-L, N01-HV3-2931-L, Y01-HV3-0010-L, N01-HV2-2913-L, N01-HV1-2158-L, N01-HV1-2161-L, N01-HV2-2915-L, N01-HV2-2932-L, N01-HV2-2917-L, N01-HV2-2916-L, N01-HV1-2157-L, N01-HV1-2243-L, N01-HV1-2159-L, N01-HV3-2961-L, and N01-HV6-2941-L. The Lipid Research Clinics Program acknowledges the long-term commitment of the volunteer participants in this clinical trial. Lipid Research Clinics Coronary Primary Prevention Trial sites and key personnel are listed at the end of the article.

plasma cholesterol level. Observational epidemiologic studies have established that the higher the plasma total or low-density lipoprotein cholesterol (LDL-C) level, the greater the risk that CHD will develop (2). The view that LDL-C is intimately involved in atherogenesis, the basic pathophysiologic process responsible for most CHD, is sustained by reports from other epidemiologic studies as well as many animal experiments, pathological observations, clinical investigations, and metabolic ward studies (3).

Plasma total and LDL-C levels may be reduced by diets and drugs. However, before such treatment can be advocated with confidence and before it can be concluded that cholesterol plays a causal role in the pathogenesis of CHD, it is desirable to show that reducing cholesterol levels safely reduces the risk of CHD in man. Many clinical trials of cholesterol lowering have been conducted, but their results, although often encouraging, have been inconclusive.

The most appropriate clinical trial of the efficacy of cholesterol lowering would be a dietary study, because of the links between diets high in saturated fat and cholesterol typical of most industrialized populations, high plasma total and LDL-C levels, and a high incidence of CHD. However, the 1971 National Heart and Lung Institute Task Force on Arteriosclerosis recommended against conducting a large-scale, national diet-heart trial in the general population because of concern regarding the blinding of such a study, the large sample size, and the prohibitive cost, then estimated to range from $500 million to more than $1 billion (4). Accordingly, the Lipid Research Clinics Coronary Primary Prevention Trial (LRC-CPPT) was initiated in 1973 as an alternative test of the efficacy of reducing cholesterol levels. The choice of hypercholesterolemic men at high risk of CHD events developing reduced the necessary sample size to a feasible level; in this regard, women were not recruited because of their lower risk of CHD.

The use of the drug cholestyramine resin permitted a double-blind design. This drug, previously approved for general use by the Food and Drug Administration, was selected on account of its known effectiveness in reducing total cholesterol and LDL-C levels (5), the availability of a suitable placebo, its nonabsorbability from the gastrointestinal (GI) tract, its few sys-temic effects, and its low level of significant toxicity.

Reported herein is the outcome of the study with respect to its major response variables, definite CHD death and/or definite nonfatal myocardial infarction, and related data.

PARTICIPANTS AND METHODS

The design of the LRC-CPPT has been described in detail (6). Briefly, the LRC-CPPT was a double-blind, placebo-controlled clinical trial that tested the efficacy of lowering cholesterol levels for primary prevention of CHD. Twelve participating Lipid Research Clinics (LRCs) recruited 3806 middle-aged men with primary hypercholesterolemia (type II hyperlipoproteinemia) free of, but at high risk for, CHD because of elevated LDL-C levels. The men were randomized into two groups that were similar in baseline characteristics. The treatment group received the bile acid sequestrant cholestyramine resin, and the control group received a placebo; both groups followed a moderate cholesterol-lowering diet. To ensure comparability of all data across the 12 clinics over a ten-year period, a common protocol documenting all procedures in detail was strictly adhered to by clinical personnel, who were trained and certified in standardized procedures (7). All aspects of the conduct of the study were carefully monitored by the Central Patient Registry and Coordinating Center and by the Program Office. The progress of the trial and the possibility of serious side effects were reviewed twice a year by a Safety and Data Monitoring Board. Any protocol violations that were identified were brought to the attention of this board; none were regarded by them to put the trial into jeopardy.

Selection of Participants

The LRCs recruited men aged 35 to 59 years with a plasma cholesterol level of 265 mg/dL or greater (the 95th percentile for 1364 men aged 40 to 49 years who participated in a previous LRC pilot study) and with an LDL-C level of 190 mg/dL or greater. Men with triglyceride levels averaging greater than 300 mg/dL or with type III hyperlipoproteinemia were excluded.

The numerous sources of the volunteer participants and the techniques of their recruitment have been described (8, 9). Of the approx-imately 480 000 age-eligible men screened between July 1973 and July 1976, 3810 were eventually entered into the trial (10). Four, two in each treatment group, were subsequently removed when they were found to have type III hyperlipoproteinemia, and the results reported are for the 3806 type II participants. The participants were preponderantly college- or high school-educated whites. Their mean age was 47.8 years. Informed consent was obtained from each participant randomized into the study.

Participants were also excluded if they had any of the following clinical manifestations of CHD: (1) history of definite or suspect myocardial infarction; (2) angina pectoris, as determined by Rose Questionnaire; (3) angina pectoris during exercise electrocardiography; (4) various ECG abnormalities, according to the Minnesota code—left bundle-branch block, tertiary or secondary heart block, two or more consecutive ventricular premature beats, left ventricular hypertrophy, R-on-T-type ventricular premature beats, or atrial flutter or fibrillation; or (5) congestive heart failure. Men with a positive exercise test result in the absence of other manifestations of CHD were not excluded. Only men in good health and free of conditions associated with secondary hyperlipoproteinemia, such as diabetes mellitus, hypothyroidism, nephrotic syndrome, hepatic disease, hyperuricemia, and notable obesity, were selected. Men were excluded if they had hypertension or were receiving antihypertensive medication or had life-limiting or comorbid conditions such as cancer or nonatherosclerotic cardiovascular disease. Men who required long-term use of certain other medications were also excluded.

Screening (Prerandomization) Visits

The accrual phase consisted of four screening visits at monthly intervals. Physical examinations, lipid and lipoprotein level determinations, clinical chemistry measurements, medical history ascertainment, and resting and graded exercise ECGs were performed. At the second screening visit, a moderate cholesterol-lowering diet, which aimed to provide 400 mg of cholesterol per day and a polyunsaturated-to-saturated fat ratio of approximately 0.8 and which was designed to lower cholesterol levels 3 per-

cent to 5 percent, was prescribed for all potential participants (6).

A cholesterol-lowering diet was offered to potential participants because, when the LRC-CPPT began, it was the practice of many physicians to recommend such a diet to hypercholesterolemic patients. Although the cholesterol lowering expected from the diet given to both study groups had the potential to diminish the statistical power of the trial by reducing the subsequent incidence of CHD, it was hoped that such a diet, along with a nutritional counseling program, would facilitate recruitment of participants. Moreover, since the diet was introduced before randomization, it was possible to exclude men whose plasma cholesterol levels were highly sensitive to diet. Thus, men whose LDL-C levels fell below 175 mg/dL at the third or fourth screening visit were excluded. The maintenance of both treatment groups on the diet after randomization minimized the opportunity for confounding of the study because of differential dietary intakes. Dietary intake was assessed semiannually by means of a 24-hour dietary recall (11).

Randomization

At the fifth visit to the clinic, eligible participants were randomly divided by the permuted block method into two treatment groups within eight prognostic strata at each of the 12 clinics. The strata were based on high and low risk of CHD with respect to LDL-C level ($\geq$ or <215 mg/dL), ST-segment depression during exercise testing, and a logistic risk function of age, cigarette smoking, and diastolic blood pressure.

Only five of 83 variables compared at baseline showed statistically significant differences (height, weight, and two-hour postchallenge glucose, SGOT, and albumin levels) (10). Because the observed differences were small and the number of statistically significant differences is that expected by chance in comparisons involving a large number of variables, the randomization and stratification process was found to produce two almost identical groups.

Study Medication

Participants were prescribed either the bile acid sequestrant cholestyramine resin at 24 g/day (six packets per day, divided into two to four equal doses) or an equivalent amount of placebo, dispensed in identical sealed packets. Those unable to tolerate six packets per day were prescribed a reduced dosage. Rigorous steps such as unique marking of individual packets and boxes and continuous external auditing of medications were followed to ensure proper drug-allocation assignment. Medication adherence was monitored by means of a packet count (packets issued minus packets returned, divided by the number of days elapsed since the packets were issued).

Postrandomization Visits

Participants attended clinics every two months, at which time the study medication was dispensed, dietary and drug counseling was given, and end points and possible drug side effects, as well as possible confounding variables such as blood pressure and weight, were evaluated. Intervention by LRC-CPPT staff was restricted to prescription of the study medication and the diet. At annual and/or semiannual visits, resting and graded exercise ECGs, 24-hour dietary recalls, and complete physical examinations and medical histories were obtained. All participants initially entered were followed up to the completion of the trial irrespective of their levels of adherence and the frequency of their visits.

Lipid Measurements

Lipid levels were determined with high precision and accuracy. Comparability of the measurements of the 12 LRC laboratories was ensured by a rigorous quality control program especially designed for the LRC Program and maintained by the Lipid Standardization Laboratory. The lipid levels at the second screening (prediet) visit were used as the baseline to calculate the changes in levels of total cholesterol and LDL-C and triglyceride observed at subsequent visits. Since the measurement of HDL-cholesterol (HDL-C) levels at the second screening visit was not performed according to protocol at several clinics, the levels at the first screening visit were used as the baseline to calculate change in HDL-C levels.

End Points

The primary end point for evaluating the treatment was the combination of definite CHD death and/or definite nonfatal myocardial in-

farction. Appendix A gives the detailed definitions of these events as well as the definition of suspect CHD death and suspect nonfatal myocardial infarction. Other end points included all-cause mortality, the development of an ischemic ECG response to exercise (positive exercise test result), angina pectoris as determined by Rose Questionnaire, atherothrombotic brain infarction, arterial peripheral vascular disease (intermittent claudication as determined by Rose Questionnaire), and transient cerebral ischemic attack. Detailed definitions of these nonprimary end points have been published elsewhere (6).

The classification of cause of death was based on the examination of death certificates, hospital records, and interviews with physicians, witnesses of the death, and next of kin. The diagnosis of nonfatal myocardial infarction was based on ECGs, blood enzyme levels, and history of chest pain at the time of the clinical event. A physician at the clinic at which the potential end point occurred classified the end point. In addition, each potential end point was classified independently by two members of a blinded verification panel. If the three reviewers agreed, the diagnosis was accepted. If there was disagreement, the case was submitted for definitive classification to the LRC-CPPT Cardiovascular Endpoints Committee (6). Classification of deaths not caused by CHD was also performed by a blinded panel.

An intraoperative event was classified on the basis of ECG changes occurring during coronary bypass surgery or other cardiac surgery or during the recovery period extending from the time of surgery until discharge from the hospital.

Statistical Methods

The hypothesis of the LRC-CPPT was that lowering cholesterol (or LDL-C) levels would reduce the incidence of end points, and, hence, a one-sided test was used for the main hypothesis. The statistic reported is a stratified (using the eight baseline risk strata) log rank (Mantel-Haenszel) statistic (12). This statistic compares the life-table survival (or failure) curves in the two groups rather than the proportion of failures. In view of the necessity for periodic review, the data were analyzed many times, and conventional methods of computing statistical significance no longer applied. Several statistical methods were used to monitor the trial. These methods included a modification of the method of O'Brien and Fleming (*13*), the two-dimensional rank statistic of Majundar and Sen (*14*), and a modification of the method of Breslow and Haug (*15*). All of these methods essentially gave the same result, and, in view of its ease of presentation, the modified O'Brien and Fleming method was used for this article. As formulated by O'Brien and Fleming, the data are analyzed *k* times after an equal number of end points. In practice, the data for this trial were analyzed at 15 equal time intervals, and strictly speaking, the method of determining the critical value proposed by O'Brien and Fleming does not hold. The distribution of the statistic taking into account the actual times when the analyses were conducted was determined by simulation and the critical z value for a one-sided test with $\alpha = 0.05$ was found to be 1.87, as compared with the O'Brien-Fleming value of 1.83. The simulated critical value 1.87 is used in this report.

This method for determining significance was used for the primary end point of the study. Other statistical tests reported use the nominal level of significance. The reader is cautioned that interpretation of these nominal *P* values should include the possibility that some may be significant by chance because of the many comparisons made.

The Kaplan-Meier method was used for construction of the life-table plots (*12*). The percentage reduction of end points is reported as $(1 - RR) \times 100$, where RR is the estimated relative risk of an event in the cholestyramine group, compared with the placebo group. For end points where time of occurrence could be obtained precisely, the relative risk was estimated from the life tables. Where the actual time of occurrence (e.g., the onset of angina) could not be precisely determined, the relative risk was estimated from the 2×2 table defined by treatment and the occurrence of an end point. All relative risks were estimated, taking into account the baseline risk strata, unless otherwise noted.

To conform with the one-sided test of the main hypothesis, 90 percent confidence intervals for the estimated reduction in risk are reported. The Cox proportional hazards model (*12*) was used to adjust the treatment comparisons for other variables, such as blood pres-

sure. Tests of interaction in the proportional hazards model were accomplished by including cross-product terms in the model.

Homogeneity of treatment effect over risk strata was assessed by an efficient scores test based on the proportional hazards model, and included parameters for treatment and strata (*16*). Homogeneity of effect over clinic was similarly assessed.

RESULTS

Follow-up

All men were followed up for a minimum of seven and up to ten years. The average period of follow-up was 7.4 years. Between May 15 and Aug 27, 1983, contact was made with all of the men who were still living, including any who discontinued visits during the course of the trial. Thus, the vital status is known for all men originally entered into the study. In addition, every man or a close relative was questioned before and at the end of the study regarding previous hospitalizations for CHD or other reasons.

Adherence to Treatment

During the first year, the mean daily packet count for participants attending clinic was 4.2 in the cholestyramine and 4.9 in the placebo group, falling to 3.8 and 4.6, respectively, by the seventh year. Adherence to the diet as determined by a 24-hour dietary recall conducted at six-month intervals showed no important differences between the two treatment groups (Table 1). A rise of 2 kg in body weight occurred in each group during the seven years of the study.

Maintenance of Blind

No cases of medical emergency required the unblinding of participants or staff and no one asked to be told his treatment assignment.

Lipids and Lipoproteins

When the LRC-CPPT diet was introduced, total cholesterol levels fell 11.1 ± 0.65 (mean $\pm$ SE) mg/dL in the cholestyramine group and 12.6 ± 0.67 mg/dL in the placebo group (Table 2). Corresponding falls of 10.3 ± 0.61 and 11.7 ± 0.63 mg/dL occurred in LDL-C levels. During the first year of follow-up,

Table 1. Median daily dietary intake.

| | Placebo | | | | Cholestyramine resin | | | |
| | Pre-entry | | Postentry | | Pre-entry | | Postentry | |
Dietary Variable	Prediet	On-diet	1st year	7th year	Prediet	On-diet	1st year	7th year
Total calories	2264	2023	2056	2060	2278	2027	2058	2086
Cholesterol, mg	309	248	255	264	308	243	251	288
Total fat, g	95	79	83	87	97	80	82	89
Saturated fat, g	33	24	26	28	34	24	26	29
P/S[a] ratio	0.48	0.73	0.69	0.67	0.47	0.72	0.67	0.66

[a] Ratio of polyunsaturated fats to saturated fats.

Table 2. Mean plasma lipid and lipoprotein cholesterol concentrations.

| | Placebo | | | | Cholestyramine Resin | | | |
| | Pre-entry | | Postentry | | Pre-entry | | Postentry | |
Lipid	Prediet	On-diet	1st year	7th year	Prediet	On-diet	1st year	7th year
Total cholesterol, mg/dL	291.8	279.2	275.4	277.3	291.5	280.4	238.6	257.1
LDL[a] cholesterol, mg/dL	216.2	204.5	198.8	197.6	215.6	205.3	159.4	174.9
HDL[a] cholesterol, mg/dL	45.1	44.4	44.5	45.5	45.0	44.4	45.6	46.6
HDL cholesterol/total cholesterol	0.16	0.16	0.16	0.17	0.16	0.16	0.20	0.19
Triglycerides, mg/dL	158.4	153.2	162.0	173.5	159.8	156.3	172.2	182.9

[a] LDL indicates low-density lipoprotein; HDL, high-density lipoprotein.

there were additional falls of 41.8 ± 0.81 mg/dL and 45.9 ± 0.82 mg/dL in total and LDL-C levels in the cholestyramine group and 3.8 ± 0.51 mg/dL and 5.7 ± 0.48 mg/dL in the placebo group. By seven years, the total and LDL-C levels had fallen, from the pre-entry postdiet levels, 23.3 ± 0.99 mg/dL and 30.4 ± 0.99 mg/dL in the cholestyramine group and 1.9 ± 0.75 mg/dL and 6.9 ± 0.70 mg/dL in the placebo group. Almost all of the change in total cholesterol was in the LDL-C fraction. During treatment, the cholestyramine group experienced average plasma total cholesterol and LDL-C reductions of 13.4 percent and 20.3 percent, respectively, which were 8.5 percent and 12.6 percent greater (P<.001) than those obtained in the placebo group. (It should be noted that these percentage changes were computed for each individual and then averaged.) There was a 1.6 ± 0.19 mg/dL increase in HDL-C levels and a larger increase in triglyceride levels attributable to cholestyramine therapy. There also was a rise in triglyceride levels in the placebo group, although not as great as in the cholestyramine

group. Additional details are provided in the companion article (17).

Primary End Point

The cholestyramine group experienced 155 definite CHD deaths and/or definite nonfatal myocardial infarctions, whereas the placebo group had 187 such events (Table 3). When the stratified log rank test was used to take into account the stratification of participants at entry and their differing lengths of follow-up, the incidence rate of CHD was estimated to be 19 percent lower in the cholestyramine than in the placebo group. The z score for this difference was 1.92 with P<.05, after adjustment for multiple looks at the data. Both the fatal and nonfatal categories of the primary end points showed corresponding reductions. Thirty CHD deaths occurred in the cholestyramine group as compared with 38 CHD deaths in the placebo group, representing a reduction in risk of 24 percent. The cholestyramine group experienced 130 definite nonfatal myocardial infarc-

Table 3. Definite or suspect primary end points and all-cause mortality.

End point	Placebo (N = 1900)		Cholestyramine resin (N = 1906)		% Reduction in risk[a]	90% Confidence interval for % reduction in risk		z Score
	No.	%	No.	%				
Definite coronary heart disease (CHD) death and/or defimite nonfatal myocardial infarction	187[b]	9.8	155[b]	8.1	19	+3	+32	1.92[c]
Definite CHD death	38	2.0	30	1.6	24	...	...	...
Definite nonfatal myocardial infarction	158	8.3	130	6.8	19	...	...	...
Definite or suspect CHD death or nonfatal myocardial infarction	256[b]	13.5	222[b]	11.6	15	+1	+27	1.80
Definite or suspect CHD death	44	2.3	32	1.7	30	...	...	...
Definite or suspect nonfatal myocardial infarction	225	11.8	195	10.2	15	...	...	...
All-cause mortality	71	3.7	68	3.6	7	−23	+30	0.42

[a] Percent reduction in risk is defined as $(1\text{-}RR) \times 100\%$, where RR is the incidence rate ratio of an event in the cholestyramine group compared with the placebo. Percent reduction in risk and z score are adjusted for follow-up time and stratification.

[b] A subject experiencing a myocardial infarction and CHD death is counted once in this category. Hence, this line is not the sum of the following two lines.

[c] The .05-level, one-sided critical value of the z score adjusted for multiple looks at the data is 1.87.

tions, compared with 158 in the placebo group, with a 19 percent reduction in risk. The inclusion of the categories of suspect CHD death and suspect nonfatal myocardial infarction resulted in an overall reduction in risk of 15 percent, with a 30 percent reduction for fatal events and a 15 percent reduction for nonfatal events. The z score for this comparison ex-

ceeded the nominal 5 percent threshold (1.65) for statistical significance and was close to the modified O'Brien-Fleming threshold of 1.87 (see "Participants and Methods" section). Thus, the conclusion that treatment was beneficial is not essentially altered by the inclusion of suspect events. The separate category of intraoperative myocardial infarction (Table 4) also

Table 4. Other cardiovascular events.[a]

End point	Placebo (N = 1900)		Cholestyramine resin (N = 1906)		% Reduction in risk
	No.	%	No.	%	
Coronary disease					
Positive exercise test	345	19.8[b]	260	14.9[b]	25[c]
Angina (Rose Questionnaire)	287	15.1[b]	235	12.4[b]	20[c]
Coronary bypass surgery	112	5.9	93	4.9	21[c]
Congestive heart failure	11	0.8	8	0.4	28
Intraoperative myocardial infarction	7	0.4	5	0.3	29
Resuscitated coronary collapse	5	0.3	3	0.2	40
Cerebrovascular disease					
Definite or suspect transient cerebral ischemic attack	22	1.2	18	0.9	18
Definite or suspect atherothrombotic brain infarction	14	0.7	17	0.9	−21
Peripheral vascular disease					
Intermittent claudication (Rose Questionnaire)	84	4.4[b]	72	3.8[b]	15[c]

[a] Counts all events for each individual, including events occurring after a nonfatal myocardial infarction.

[b] Percent of those without condition at baseline.

[c] Percent reduction in risk is adjusted for stratification.

showed more cases in the placebo group (7 *v* 5), although the difference is not statistically significant. (One of the four type III participants excluded after the randomization experienced a nonfatal myocardial infarction; he was in the placebo group.)

The life-table failure rates in the two groups are plotted in . . . Figure 1. Very early in the follow-up period, the number of CHD events was higher in the cholestyramine group, but by two years the two curves were identical. Thereafter, there was a steady divergence of the two sets of event rates, and at seven years of follow-up the event rate was 8.6 percent in the placebo group and 7.0 percent in the cholestyramine group, a reduction of 19 percent.

The primary end points were examined within the risk strata defined at randomization. The hypothesis of homogeneity of effect across these strata was not rejected. Thus, although

differences were observed in the estimated relative risk among the strata, there was insufficient statistical evidence to claim that the treatment was more beneficial in one stratum than in another. The cholestyramine-treated group at seven clinics had at least 18 percent fewer primary end points than placebo-treated men. At four clinics there was essentially no treatment difference; only one clinic showed an excess of events in the drug group. The statistical hypothesis of homogeneity of effect among clinics also was not rejected; thus, the benefit of cholestyramine resin treatment cannot be attributed to effects in only a small number of clinics.

This stratified analysis provided an estimate of treatment benefit adjusted for baseline strata of what were considered to be the most important CHD risk factors when the study began. Adjustment for a more extensive list of baseline

Figure 1. Life-table cumulative incidence of primary end point (definite coronary heart disease death and/or definite nonfatal myocardial infarction) in treatment groups, computed by Kaplan-Meier method. N equals total number of Lipid Research Clinics Coronary Primary Prevention Trial participants at risk for their first primary end point, followed at each time point. N = 3806, 3753, 3701, 3659, 3615, 3564, 3520, 3466, 1816, 302.

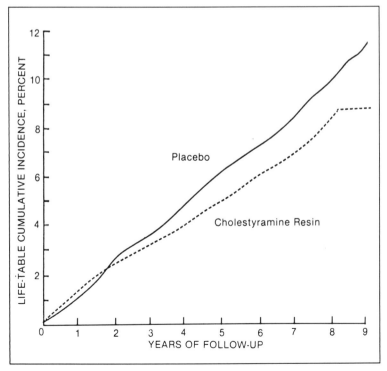

characteristics, including LDL-C, HDL-C, tri-glyceride, age, cigarette smoking, and systolic blood pressure, each considered as a continuous variable, as well as exercise test outcome, was performed by Cox proportional hazards analysis. The adjusted estimates of treatment effect (20.0 percent risk reduction) and z score (2.05) were slightly greater than those obtained in the stratified analysis. There was no significant interaction of the treatment effect with any of the seven baseline characteristics. Thus, the proportional hazards and stratified analyses both indicate that it is highly unlikely that the treatment benefit could have arisen from inequality of the two treatment groups with respect to CHD risk at baseline or from a particular subgroup of LRC-CPPT participants.

Other Cardiovascular End Points

The frequency of other cardiovascular end points in the two treatment groups is reported in Table 4. Each of the CHD categories having a large number of events showed a reduction in incidence similar to the 19 percent reduction in the primary end point. Thus, the cholestyramine group showed reductions of 20 percent (P<.01) in the incidence of the development of angina ascertained by the Rose Questionnaire, 25 percent (P<.001) in the development of a new positive exercise test result, and 21 percent (P = .06) in incidence of coronary bypass surgery. The two cerebrovascular disease categories did not provide a consistent or significant pattern of benefit, but the numbers were small. For peripheral vascular disease there was a 15 percent (P>.1) reduction in new intermittent claudication in the cholestyramine group. None of the other differences in Table 4 were statistically significant, possibly because of the small numbers.

All-Cause Mortality

Although the incidence of definite and of definite and suspect CHD death was reduced by 24 percent and 30 percent, respectively, in the cholestyramine group, that of all-cause mortality was reduced by only 7 percent (Table 3), reflecting an increase in deaths not caused by CHD. Table 5, patterned after a similar table reported in the World Health Organization Clofibrate Trial (18), breaks down the all-cause mortality into major categories. None of the differences are statistically significant. More details are provided in Appendix B. The only noteworthy difference (P = .08) was 11 deaths from accidents and violence in the cholestyramine group, compared with four in the placebo group. Of these, five in the cholestyramine and two in the placebo group were homicides or suicides, and six in the cholestyramine and two in the placebo group were accidents, mainly automobile. Each of the other major categories, including malignant neoplasms, differed only by one or two cases.

The possibility that a CHD event could have been the underlying cause of a violent or accidental death was examined. All of these deaths had been evaluated by the Cardiovascular Endpoints Committee without knowledge of treatment group, and none had met the study criteria of a CHD death. Furthermore, none had any clinical evidence suggestive of myocardial ischemia. Subsequent to the conclusion of the study, all of these deaths were carefully scrutinized for the possibility of a CHD event. Seven were due to homicide or suicide, and in none of these was there any reason to doubt the diagnosis. Autopsy information was available for seven of the eight accidental deaths; seven of these deaths were due to automobile or motorcycle accidents. None showed evidence of new

Table 5. Deaths in the Lipid Research Clinics Coronary Primary Prevention Trial.

Cause of death	Placebo	Cholestyramine resin
Coronary heart disease (CHD)	44	32
Other vascular	3	5
Malignant neoplasm	15	16
Other medical causes	5	4
Accidents and violence	4	11
Total, all causes other than CHD	27	36
All causes other than CHD, other vascular, and accidents and violence	20	20
Total, all causes	71	68

coronary thrombosis or acute myocardial infarction. Half had high blood alcohol levels. In four, this information and the circumstances of death made it virtually certain that CHD was not an underlying cause of death. In the other four, although the circumstances of death did not completely rule it out, a CHD episode was regarded as highly unlikely.

Possible Confounders

The results described previously show that the cholestyramine-treated group had a reduced rate of CHD. If during the course of the LRC-CPPT there were changes in CHD risk factors other than total cholesterol or LDL-C levels that were not the same in the two groups, this could pose an alternative explanation of the observed treatment benefit. Table 6 gives the pre-entry, first-year, and seventh-year mean values for selected variables that include the major known risk factors for CHD. For all of these major risk factors, the change from baseline was similar in the two groups, and, thus, they do not explain the treatment benefit. In addition, very

similar percentages of participants in both groups (e.g., placebo, 37 percent, *vs* cholestyramine, 38 percent, at year 7) reported taking at least one aspirin in the previous week. Slightly more placebo- than cholestyramine-treated participants reported the use of β-blockers at the end of the trial.

Side Effects and Toxicity

Many possible side effects to treatment were monitored throughout the trial. There were no noteworthy differences in non-GI side effects between the groups. Gastrointestinal side effects occurred frequently in the placebo- and cholestyramine-treated participants, especially the latter (Table 7). In the first year, 68 percent of the cholestyramine group experienced at least one GI side effect, compared with 43 percent of the placebo group. These diminished in frequency so that, by the seventh year, approximately equal percentages of cholestyramine and placebo participants (29 percent *vs* 26 percent) were so affected. Constipation and heartburn, especially, were more frequent in the cho-

Table 6. Selected variables before and during treatment.

Variable	Placebo			Cholestyramine resin		
	Pre-entry	1st year	7th year	Pre-entry	1st year	7th year
Mean systolic blood pressure, mm Hg	121	120	122	121	120	122
Mean diastolic blood pressure, mm Hg	80	79	78	80	78	78
Mean Quetelet index g/sq cm	2.6	2.6	2.7	2.6	2.6	2.7
Mean weight, kg	81	81	83	80	80	82
% current smokers	37	35	26	38	36	27
Mean cigarettes per day for current smokers	25	24	25	26	25	26
% regular exercisers	30	. . .[a]	27	31	. . .[a]	28
Median alcohol consumption, g/wk	61	58	51	64	57	53

[a] No assessment of exercise was done in the first year.

Table 7. Percent of participants reporting moderate or severe side effects.

Side effect	Placebo			Cholestyramine resin		
	Pre-entry	1st year	7th year	Pre-entry	1st year	7th year
Abdominal pain	5	11	7	5	15	7
Belching or bloating	10	16	6	10	27	9
Constipation	3	10	4	4	39	8
Diarrhea	6	11	8	5	10	4
Gas	22	26	12	22	32	12
Heartburn	10	10	7	10	27	12
Nausea	4	8	4	3	16	3
Vomiting	2	5	3	2	6	2
At least 1 gastrointestinal side effect	34	43	26	34	68	29

lestyramine group, which also reported more abdominal pain, belching or bloating, gas, and nausea. The side effects were usually not severe and could be dealt with by standard clinical means.

Little or no differences were seen between the two treatment groups for most of the clinical chemical tests monitored during the study (Appendix C). During the first year, serum alkaline phosphatase levels, iron binding capacity, SGOT levels, and the WBC count were higher in the cholestyramine group, while carotene and uric acid levels were lower (Table 8). These differences were generally less apparent by the seventh year; none was associated with clinically apparent disease.

The number of participants hospitalized for conditions other than CHD was monitored. The hospitalizations were classified, using the H-ICDA code, eighth revision (*19*), according to the primary diagnosis on the hospital discharge form. In particular, hospitalizations for GI tract disease were monitored (Appendix D). Of the many categories, the only difference with nominal statistical significance, using a test of comparison of proportions, was the primary diagnosis of deviated nasal septum, with more (16 *v* 6) cases in the cholestyramine group. Similar monitoring of all noncardiac operations or procedures was conducted. The only significant difference was a greater number in the cholestyramine group (40 *v* 23) of operations or procedures involving the nervous system. This excess mainly reflected more operations or procedures in the cholestyramine group for spinal disease (23 *v* 10), especially lumbar (19 *v* 9), and for decompression of the carpal tunnel (7 *v* 1).

Diagnoses and procedures involving the gallbladder were scrutinized in view of the ability of certain lipid-lowering drugs to produce gall-

stones and gallbladder disease. A few more hospitalized participants in the cholestyramine group had, as their main diagnosis, gallstones (16 *v* 11) and more cholestyramine-treated participants had an operation involving the gallbladder (36 *v* 25), but the differences were not significant. Gallstones, not necessarily as the main diagnosis, were reported in the cholestyramine group slightly more frequently than in the placebo group (31 *v* 30), as were other gallbladder and biliary tract diseases (28 *v* 23). No death attributable to gallbladder disease was recorded.

Appendix E indicates that the numbers of incident and fatal cases of malignant neoplasms were similar in the two groups: 57 incident cases in the placebo group, of which 15 were fatal; and 57 incident cases in the cholestyramine group, of which 16 were fatal. The cholestyramine group had a few more malignant neoplasms in some categories (e.g., buccal cavity and pharynx) and less in others (e.g., respiratory system) than the placebo group, but the numbers were small. When the various categories of GI tract cancers (buccal cavity-pharynx, esophagus, stomach, colon, rectum, and pancreas) were considered together, there were 11 incident cases and one fatal case in the placebo group and 21 incident and eight fatal cases in the cholestyramine group. The total number of incident colon cancers was identical.

COMMENT

Previous Trials of Cholesterol Lowering

The LRC-CPPT demonstrated that treatment with cholestyramine resin reduced the incidence of CHD. This result is in agreement

Table 8. Mean laboratory values influenced by cholestyramine resin.

Laboratory value	Placebo			Cholestyramine resin		
	Pre-entry	1st year	7th year	Pre-entry	1st year	7th year
Alkaline phosphatase, IU/L of serum	71	70	71	71	82	74
Carotene, µg/dL of serum	150	146	149	149	111	132
Iron-binding capacity, µg/dL of serum	355	355	324	357	371	334
SGOT, units/L of serum	30	31	35	30	34	36
Uric acid, mg/dL of serum	6.3	6.1	6.3	6.2	5.8	6.1
WBC count, per cu mm	6205	6178	6043	6327	6443	6299

with those of previous clinical trials of cholesterol lowering, which have shown a general trend of efficacy for selected CHD end points. However, the earlier trials have not been regarded as conclusive because of such factors as inadequate sample size, absence of a double-blind, failure to achieve identical treatment groups, inadequate cholesterol lowering, or questionable statistical procedures (*20, 21*).

Several major primary prevention trials of diet have reported encouraging, although not always significant, reductions in CHD incidence. They include the New York Anti-Coronary Club Study (*22*), the Los Angeles Veterans Administration Study (*23*), and the Finnish Mental Hospital Study (*24*). The interpretation of the results of these studies, as well as secondary prevention studies using diet, is clouded by the ascertainment bias that may result from a nonblinded design. Because of this and other shortcomings, these trials have also been regarded as inconclusive (*21*). Primary prevention of CHD by diet has been evaluated during concurrent reduction of other CHD risk factors. A 47 percent lower CHD incidence was observed in the hypercholesterolemic participants in the Oslo Study who were treated with a cholesterol-lowering diet and counseled to reduce their cigarette smoking (*25*). The investigators attributed most of the lower CHD incidence to the cholesterol reduction. The Multiple Risk Factor Intervention Trial (MRFIT) achieved too small an overall difference (2 percent) between the cholesterol levels of its two treatment groups to assess the effect of cholesterol lowering (*26*).

One major primary prevention trial of a lipid-lowering drug has been reported: the WHO Clofibrate Study obtained a 9 percent fall in serum cholesterol levels and a significant 20 percent reduction in the overall incidence of major ischemic heart disease events, similar in magnitude to the LRC-CPPT findings (*18*). However, unlike the LRC-CPPT, this decline was confined to nonfatal myocardial infarction, whereas the incidence of fatal heart attack was similar in both treatment and control groups. Of concern in this study was the increased incidence in all-cause mortality in the clofibrate group, which became more significant during a four-year posttrial follow-up (*18, 27*).

The Coronary Drug Project (CDP) was a major secondary prevention trial of several lipid-lowering drugs. Three of its groups (high-dose estrogen, low-dose estrogen, and d-thyroxine) had to be discontinued prematurely because of evidence of toxicity (*28, 30*). The nicotinic acid group, in which a 9.9 percent fall in cholesterol levels occurred, showed a 27 percent lower incidence of nonfatal myocardial infarction but little difference in fatal CHD (*31*). The clofibrate group, in which a 6.5 percent reduction in cholesterol levels occurred, had a 9 percent lower incidence of fatal and nonfatal CHD, but statistical significance was not attained (*31*). Two trials of clofibrate, the Newcastle Study (*32*) and the Scottish Society of Physicians Study (*33*), had previously reported a suggestion of benefit, especially in subjects with pre-existing angina, but the post hoc use of subgroups and discordance in placebo group events has led to questioning of the conclusions from these two studies (*34*).

The results of these various studies of lipid-lowering drugs for the prevention of CHD indicate that even though some evidence of reduction of CHD has attended their use, noteworthy and sometimes serious toxicity has occurred for each drug.

Side Effects and Clinical Chemistry Analyses

The use of cholestyramine resin resulted in several GI side effects, although these were also common in the placebo group. They were most evident in the initial stages of the study and could usually be handled by symptom-specific treatment, but sometimes they were the basis for cessation of, or reduction in, the drug dose. These side effects, which have been previously noted for cholestyramine resin, reflect the properties of a drug that is not metabolized in, or absorbed from, the GI tract. The monitoring of hospitalizations showed that the two treatment groups were similar for almost all of the large number of primary diagnoses and procedures. Of special interest is the absence of a significant increase in gallstones or cholecystectomy. This contrasts with clofibrate, which, unlike cholestyramine resin, is known to alter the lithogenicity of bile and has been associated in the WHO and CDP trials with an increased incidence of gallbladder disease (*18, 31*). The results of a systematic radiological study for gallstones in participants at two LRCs before and after the LRC-CPPT will be published.

A greater incidence of respiratory system hospitalizations and of operations and procedures on the nervous system was observed in the cholestyramine group. However, examination of the individual diagnoses or procedures within these categories failed to reveal any disorder for which there was a plausible explanation of an effect that could be attributed to cholestyramine resin. In view of the more than 60 diagnoses and procedures assessed, the two categories in which significant differences were found may represent chance occurrences.

Cholestyramine treatment altered results of several clinical chemistry studies, especially alkaline phosphatase, SGOT, and carotene. Such changes have been previously reported for cholestyramine use and, as in the present study, have not been associated with clinical disease (5).

Malignant Neoplasms

The total incidence of fatal and nonfatal malignant neoplasms was similar in both treatment groups. When the many different categories are examined, various GI tract cancers were somewhat more prevalent in the cholestyramine group. Other cancers (e.g., lung and prostate) were more frequent in the placebo group. The small numbers and the multiple categories prevent conclusions being drawn. However, in view of the fact that cholestyramine resin is confined to the GI tract and not absorbed, and [in view] of animal experiments in which cholestyramine resin has been found to be a promoter of colon cancer when a cancer-inducing agent was also fed orally (35), further follow-up of the LRC-CPPT participants is planned for cause-specific mortality and cancer morbidity.

CHD End Points

The LRC-CPPT shows that treatment with cholestyramine resin results in a significantly lower incidence of CHD as measured by the primary end point of the study. The benefit of treatment was not concentrated in any one subgroup or in a few clinics, but was widespread. Inspection of the life-table curves shows that benefit became apparent two years after initial treatment. This benefit was reflected in both categories of primary end points. The findings were not essentially altered when the men classified as having a "suspect" primary event were added to the definite CHD category, nor were they altered by the inclusion of the small number of intraoperative events in the primary endpoint category. The possibility was considered that some deaths attributed to violence or accidents were precipitated by a CHD event, especially since more of them occurred in the cholestyramine group. As described, an extensive review of autopsy and clinical evidence was convincing that it was extremely unlikely that an underlying CHD event had occurred in any of the accidental or violent deaths.

The evidence of reduction of CHD incidence is further strongly supported by the analysis of other CHD end points for which a sufficient number occurred. Other studies have reported that angina and a positive exercise test result identify subjects at increased risk for CHD. In the LRC-CPPT, angina at entry was an exclusion. A positive exercise test result at entry, in the absence of chest pain, was a significant independent predictor of a subsequent primary end point, using proportional hazards analysis (to be published). Thus, the development of angina or new positive exercise test results, although not primary study end points, seem to be valid indicators of CHD risk status. Incident cases of the development of angina or of a new positive exercise test result were substantially lower by 20 percent and 25 percent, respectively, in the cholestyramine group. A corresponding 21 percent reduction was observed in the number of participants progressing to coronary bypass surgery. Also of interest is the 15 percent reduction in intermittent claudication.

All-Cause Mortality

There was only a 7 percent reduction of all-cause mortality in the cholestyramine group, reflecting a larger number of violent and accidental deaths. Several other primary prevention trials have reported higher noncardiovascular mortality in their active treatment groups, resulting from a variety of medical causes (36). Excess mortality in the LRC-CPPT cholestyramine group was confined to violent and accidental deaths. Since no plausible connection could be established between cholestyramine treatment and violent or accidental death, it is difficult to conclude that this could be anything but a chance occurrence.

Confounding

The lower incidence in CHD events seen in the cholestyramine group does not seem to be attributable to changes in CHD risk factors other than cholesterol. The use of randomization and stratification procedures produced two treatment groups that, at entry, were similar with respect to all the major CHD risk factors, other minor or possible risk factors, and a variety of other measurements. The levels of CHD risk factors such as cigarette smoking, systolic and diastolic blood pressure, body weight, and reported levels of physical activity continued to be similar throughout the study. Both groups reported similar nutrient intakes and alcohol consumption.

Maintenance of Double-Blind

Many steps were taken to ensure that neither participants nor clinic staff knew to which treatment group participants had been assigned (7). No need arose during the study to identify a participant's treatment group to him or to clinical staff. The higher incidence of GI effects in the cholestyramine group, mainly in the first year, made it possible that some loss of the double-blind might have occurred, although the high prevalence of such side effects in the placebo group makes this less likely. A survey at the end of the study showed that approximately equal numbers of participants (cholestyramine group, 56.0 percent *v* placebo group, 54.6 percent) or clinic staff (cholestyramine group, 55.2 percent *v* placebo group, 52.9 percent) could correctly identify treatment assignments.

Implementation of Study Design

The extent to which the LRC-CPPT was able to implement its original design objectives (6) is noteworthy (Table 9). The study exceeded its original sample size goal of 3550 and successfully randomized 3806 participants into two similar treatment groups. Participants were followed up for an average of 7.4 years. Consistent with the initial study parameters, a 4.8 percent reduction in plasma total cholesterol levels attributed to diet was obtained in the placebo group. In the seventh year, men taking cholestyramine resin maintained a mean plasma total cholesterol level reduction of 13.9 percent, attributable to the combination of drug and diet. Thus, the additional reduction in cholesterol levels attributable to cholestyramine resin was only 9.1 percent, well below the desired 24 percent. Although the 27 percent of participants who were taking no drug by seven years was lower than the predicted 35 percent, a number of participants were not taking the full dose of six packets. Difficulties in adherence related to the bulk, texture, and side effects of the drug seem to explain much of the shortfall in cholesterol lowering. It can be effectively argued that additional deterrents to taking the drug were the participants' lack of knowledge, for seven to ten years, as to which treatment group they were in as well as of their cholesterol levels during treatment. Better cholesterol lowering with cho-

Table 9. Comparison of LRC-CPPT[a] design goals and actual experience.

Design feature	Goal	Experience
Sample size	3550	3806[b]
Duration of follow-up, yr.	7	7-10
Lost to follow-up	0	0
Reduction of plasma total cholesterol levels in placebo group	4%	4.8%
Nonadherers at yr. 7	35%	27%
Reduction of plasma total cholesterol levels in men adhering[c] to cholestyramine resin treatment	28%	13.9%[d]
7-yr. incidence of primary end point in placebo group	8.7%	8.6%
Reduction in primary end point	36%	19%

[a] LRC-CPPT indicates Lipid Research Clinics Coronary Primary Prevention Trial.
[b] After removal of four type III participants.
[c] A nonadherer is someone averaging less than half a packet of cholestyramine resin per day.
[d] Computed for seventh year.

lestyramine resin could be expected when it is used in a routine clinical context. In addition, knowledge that treatment with cholestyramine resin prevents CHD can be expected to motivate adherence.

The seven-year incidence of the combined primary end points in the LRC-CPPT placebo group, 8.6 percent, was almost identical to the 8.7 percent predicted in the original study design based on data derived from the Framingham Study (*37*). However, the actual incidence of definite CHD death was well below the predicted rate, whereas the rate of definite non-. fatal myocardial infarction was increased above the predicted rate. A lower-than-predicted CHD death rate has been a feature of several clinical trials, including the recent MRFIT study (*26*). Possible explanations include the stringent selection processes employed, resulting in an atypically healthier study population, better health monitoring and management during the course of the study, and the concurrent national decline in CHD mortality.

Implications of the LRC-CPPT

Caution should be exercised before extrapolating the CPPT findings to cholesterol-lowering drugs other than bile acid sequestrants. It has been shown that bile acid sequestration leads to a substantial reduction in plasma total and LDL-C levels by increasing the removal of LDL from the blood through increased activity of specific cell-surface LDL receptors (*38*). This mode of action is conceptually attractive inasmuch as it represents the enhancement of a physiological mechanism for the control of LDL levels. The mode of action, cholesterol-lowering potency, and possible toxicity of other cholesterol-lowering drugs must be taken into account before their use is advocated for the prevention of CHD.

The LRC-CPPT was not designed to assess directly whether cholesterol lowering by diet prevents CHD. Nevertheless, its findings, taken in conjunction with the large volume of evidence relating diet, plasma cholesterol levels, and CHD, support the view that cholesterol lowering by diet also would be beneficial. The findings of the LRC-CPPT take on additional significance if it is acknowledged that it is unlikely that a conclusive study of dietary-induced cholesterol lowering for the prevention of CHD can be designed or implemented.

The consistency of the reductions in CHD manifestations observed with cholestyramine resin in this controlled trial, which extend from the softer end points of angina, a positive exercise test result, and coronary bypass surgery to the hard end points of nonfatal myocardial infarction and CHD death, leaves little doubt of the benefit of cholestyramine therapy. These results could be narrowly interpreted to apply only to the use of bile acid sequestrants in middle-aged men with cholesterol levels above 265 mg/dL (perhaps 1 to 2 million Americans). The trial's implications, however, could and should be extended to other age groups and women and, since cholesterol levels and CHD risk are continuous variables, to others with more modest elevations of cholesterol levels. The benefits that could be expected from cholestyramine treatment are considerable. In the LRC-CPPT, treatment was associated with an average cholesterol fall of 8.5 percent beyond diet, and an average 19 percent reduction in CHD risk. Moreover, a companion article (*17*) that looks at cholesterol reduction and CHD more closely indicates that a 49 percent reduction in CHD incidence would be predicted for subjects who obtained a 25 percent fall in plasma cholesterol levels or a 35 percent fall in LDL-C levels, which are typical responses to 24 g of cholestyramine resin daily.

LIPID RESEARCH CLINICS

Baylor College of Medicine, Houston.
   Principal investigator: William Insull, MD; associate director (former principal investigator): Antonio M. Gotto, MD, PhD; CPPT director: Jeffrey Probstfield, MD; former CPPT directors: O. David Taunton, MD, Ellison Wittels, MD; key personnel: Susan Andrews, MA, Mohammed Attar, MD, Katherine Canizares, Janice Henske, MPH, RD, Tsai-Lien Lin, MS, Wolfgang Patsch, MD, Georgia White, RN.
University of Cincinnati Medical Center.
   Principal investigator: Charles J. Glueck, MD; CPPT director: Jane Third, MD; former CPPT directors: Ronald Fallat, MD, Moti Kashyap, MD, Evan Stein, MD; key personnel: Robert Adolph, MD, W. Fraser Bremner, MD, Jack Friedel, PhD, Rhea Larsen, RD, Susan McNeeley, MS, Paula Steiner, MS.
George Washington University Medical Center, Washington, DC.
   Principal investigator: John C. LaRosa, MD;

CPPT director: Valery Miller, MD; former clinical trials director: Marilyn Bassford-McKeown, RN; key personnel: Donna Embersit, Agnes Gordon Fry, RD, Richard Muesing, PhD, Diane Stoy, RN.

University of Iowa Hospitals, Iowa City.
Co-principal investigators: Francois Abboud, MD, Helmut Schrott, MD; former principal investigator: William E. Connor, MD; CPPT director: Helmut Schrott, MD; key personnel: Erling Anderson, PhD, Paul King, Nancy Merideth, RN, Karen Smith, MS, RD, Linda Snetselaar, PhD, RD, Marlys Svare, RN, Lori Ziegenhorn, PAC.

Johns Hopkins Hospital, Baltimore.
Principal investigator: Peter O. Kwiterovich, MD; CPPT director: Angeliki Georgopoulos, MD; former CPPT directors: William Benedict, MD, Michael Ezekowitz, MD, Lindsay Wyndham, MD; key personnel: Stephen Achuff, MD, Paul Bachorik, PhD, Frank A. Franklin, MD, PhD, Katherine Salz, RD, MS, Thomas Weber, MS.

University of Minnesota, Minneapolis.
Co-principal investigators: Ivan D. Frantz, Jr, MD, Donald B. Hunninghake, MD; CPPT director: Donald B. Hunninghake, MD; key personnel: Elizabeth Brewer, RD, Florine Campbell, RN, Kanta Kuba, MS, Monica LaDouceur, Lynn Lau, Arthur Leon, MD.

Oklahoma Medical Research Foundation, Oklahoma City.
Principal investigator: Reagan H. Bradford, MD, PhD; former CPPT director: Thomas F. Whayne, MD, PhD; key personnel: Betty Edge, RD, Gerald First, MD, Hans Kloer, MD, Arlene Meier, RN, Katherine Moore, RD, Carl Rubenstein, MD.

Washington University School of Medicine, St Louis.
Principal investigator: Gustave Schonfeld, MD; CPPT director: Anne Goldberg, MD; former CPPT directors: Boas Gonen, MD, Joseph Witztum, MD; key personnel: Thomas Cole, PhD, Wolfgang Patsch, MD, Joseph Ruwitch, MD, Stuart Weidman, PhD.

University of California at San Diego, La Jolla.
Principal investigator: Fred H. Mattson, PhD; former principal investigators: W. Virgil Brown, MD, Daniel Steinberg, MD, PhD; CPPT codirectors: Joseph Witztum, MD, Richard C. Gross, MD; key personnel: Joe Juliano, Jackie Sooter-Bochenek, MS, RD, Helen Stalmer, Eileen Taylor, RD, Edward Wade, MS, Magdalen Wong.

University of Washington, Seattle.
Principal investigator: Robert H. Knopp, MD; former principal investigators: William R. Hazzard, MD, Edwin L. Bierman, MD; CPPT director: James T. Ogilvie, MD; former CPPT director: Robert H. Knopp, MD; key personnel: John J. Albers, PhD, Elizabeth R. Burrows, RD, MS, Margaret R. Poole, RN, Gene B. Trobaugh, MD, G. Russell Warnick, MS.

Stanford University, Stanford, Calif.
Principal investigator: John W. Farquhar, MD; CPPT director: Daniel E. Feldman, MD, PhD; former CPPT directors: Thomas Maneatis, MD, Michael Stern, MD; key personnel: Denise Desmond, Judy Halloran, William L. Haskell, PhD, Lillian O'Toole, Anne Schlagenhaft, Stephen Sidney, MD, H. Robert Superko, MD, Phyllis Ullman, RD, Sharon Vanden Bossche, Peter D. Wood, DSc.

Universities of Toronto and McMaster, Toronto and Hamilton, Ontario, Canada.
Principal investigator: J. Alick Little, MD; CPPT coordinator: Josephine Bird, MD; CPPT directors: Randolph Lee, MD, David Stinson, MD, Maurice Mishkel, MD; former CPPT director: George Steiner, MD; key personnel: Carl Breckenridge, PhD, Gary Kakis, PhD, Norma Mishkel, Valerie McGuire, RPD, Joan McLaughlin, RPD, J. K. Wilson, MD.

Central Patient Registry and Coordinating Center, University of North Carolina, Chapel Hill.
Principal investigator: O. Dale Williams, PhD; former principal investigator: James E. Grizzle, PhD; director, CPPT division: C. E. Davis, PhD; assistant director, CPPT division: Melvin Jackson, MSPH; key personnel: Bruce Allen, MS, Carol Bittinger, MSPH, Lars-Goran Ekelund, MD, Karen Graves, PhD, Carol Hazard, MS, James Hosking, PhD, Sandra Irving, MS, John Karon, PhD, James Knoke, PhD, Kenneth Kral, MS, Joanne Kucharski, Robert McMahan, J. J. Nelson, MSPH, Patricia Scott, Ratna Thomas, MS, Mary Williams.

Central Electrocardiographic Laboratory, University of Alabama, Birmingham.
Principal investigator: L. Thomas Sheffield, MD; codirector: David Roitman, MD; key personnel: Carol Troxell.

Lipid Standardization Laboratory, Centers for Disease Control, Atlanta.
Director: Gerald R. Cooper, MD, PhD; codirector: Adrian Hainline, PhD; key personnel: Barbara L. Botero, Myron Kuchmak, PhD, Linnard Taylor, Carole Winn.

Central Clinical Chemistry Laboratory, Bio-Science Laboratory, Van Nuys, Calif.
Principal investigator: James Demetriou, PhD; former principal investigator: Frank Ibbott, PhD.

Nutrition Coding Center, University of Minnesota, Minneapolis.

Principal investigator: Marilyn Buzzard, PhD, RD; associate director: Joyce Wenz, MS, RD; former principal investigator: Victor Grambsch.

Drug Supply and Distribution Center, Mead-Johnson, Evansville, Ind.

Key personnel: John Boegnik, PhD.

Recruitment and Adherence Consultants, Stanford University, Calif.

Director: Stewart Agras, MD; former directors: Albert Stunkard, MD, Steven M. Zifferblatt, PhD; deputy director: Jacqueline Dunbar, PhD; key personnel: Melbourne Hovell, PhD, Gary Marshall, PhD, Barbara Newman, MA, Mary Southam, PhD.

Program Office: Lipid Metabolism-Atherogenesis Branch, Division of Heart and Vascular Diseases, National Heart, Lung, and Blood Institute, Bethesda, Md.

Chief: Basil M. Rifkind, MD; former chief: Robert I. Levy, MD; CPPT coordinator: Ronald S. Goor, MPH, PhD; former CPPT coordinator: Richard Havlik, MD; medical officer: David Gordon, MD, PhD; key personnel: Conrad Blum, MD, Virginia Keating, RD, MS, Kenneth Lippel, PhD, Gail Morrison, MD, Marjorie Myrianthopoulos, RD, Beverly Neal, Gary J. Nelson, PhD, Beth Schucker, MA, Alan Seplowitz, MD.

Safety and Data Monitoring Board.

Chairman: Basil M. Rifkind, MD; former chairman: Robert I. Levy, MD; members: James Dalen, MD, Harold Fallon, MD, William Friedewald, MD, PhD, James Grizzle, PhD, Proctor Harvey, MD, Robert I. Levy, MD, Caroline S. Lurie, Henry McGill, Jr, MD, William F. Taylor, PhD, Herman A. Tyroler, MD; former member: Steven M. Zifferblatt, PhD.

Cardiovascular Endpoints Committee.

Stephen Achuff, MD, Robert Adolph, MD, Edward Atwood, MD, Fraser Bremner, MD, Dennis Costello, MD, Robert DeBusk, MD, Brian Gaffney, MD, David Gordon, MD, PhD, Patrick Gorman, MD, Richard Miller, MD, Jeffrey Probstfield, MD, Barbara Roberts, MD, Donald Romhilt, MD, Douglas Rosing, MD, Carl Rubenstein, MD (chairman), Joseph Ruwitch, MD, Leonard Schwartz, MD, Brian Sealey, MD, Abid Sha, MD, L. Thomas Sheffield, MD, Gene Trobaugh, MD, John Wilson, MD.

The computations for this manuscript were done by David Christiansen, Ronald Parker, Cynthia Nash, Hope Bryan, Dawn Stewart, Gail Olson, Douglas Baber, Judi Connor, Doyle Hawkins, and Joanne Kucharski. Janet Bungay provided editorial assistance. Typing assistance was provided by Edna Wilkerson and Ernestine Bland.

References

(1) Levy, R.I. Review: Declining mortality in coronary heart disease. *Arteriosclerosis* 1:312-325, 1981.

(2) Gordon, T., W.P. Castelli, M.C. Hjortland, et al. The prediction of coronary heart disease by high-density and other lipoproteins: An historical perspective. In Rifkind, B.M., and R.I. Levy (eds.), *Hyperlipidemia—Diagnosis and Therapy*. New York, Grune & Stratton Inc., 1977, pp. 71-78.

(3) Stamler, J. Population studies. In Levy, R.I., B.M. Rifkind, B.H. Dennis, et al. (eds.), *Nutrition, Lipids, and Coronary Heart Disease*. New York, Raven Press, 1979, pp. 25-88.

(4) *Arteriosclerosis: A Report by the National Heart and Lung Institute Task Force on Arteriosclerosis*, Dept. of Health, Education, and Welfare publication (NIH) 72-137. Washington, D.C., National Institutes of Health, 1971, vol. 1.

(5) Levy, R.I., D.S. Fredrickson, N.J. Stone, et al. Cholestyramine in type II hyperlipoproteinemia: A double-blind trial. *Ann Intern Med* 79:51-58, 1973.

(6) The Lipid Research Clinics Program. The Coronary Primary Prevention Trial: Design and implementation. *J Chronic Dis* 32:609-631, 1979.

(7) *Protocol for the Lipid Research Clinics Type II Coronary Primary Prevention Trial*. Chapel Hill, N.C., University of North Carolina Department of Biostatistics, 1980.

(8) The Lipid Research Clinics Program. Participant recruitment to the Coronary Primary Prevention Trial. *J Chronic Dis* 36:451-465, 1983.

(9) The Lipid Research Clinics Program. Recruitment for clinical trials: The Lipid Research Clinics Coronary Primary Prevention Trial experience. *Circulation* 66(suppl. 4):1-78, 1982.

(10) The Lipid Research Clinics Program. Pre-entry characteristics of participants in the Lipid Research Clinics Coronary Primary Prevention Trial. *J Chronic Dis* 36:467-479, 1983.

(11) Dennis, B., N. Ernst, M. Hjortland, et al. The NHLBI nutrition data system. *J Am Diet Assoc* 77:641-647, 1980.

(12) Kalbfleisch, J.D., and R.L. Prentice. *The Statistical Analysis of Failure Time Data*. New York, John Wiley & Sons, 1980.

(13) O'Brien, P.C., and T.R. Fleming. A multiple testing procedure for clinical trials. *Biometrics* 35:549-556, 1979.

(14) Majundar, H., and P.K. Sen. Nonparametric testing for simple linear regression under progressive censoring with staggering entry and random withdrawal. *Communication in Statistics—Theory and Methods* A7:349-371, 1978.

(15) Breslow, N., and C. Haug. Sequential comparison of exponential survival curves. *J Am Stat Assoc* 67:691-697, 1972.

(16) Tsiatis, A.A. The asymptomatic joint distribu-

tions of efficient scores test for the proportional hazards model over time. *Biometrika* 68:311-315, 1981.

(17) The Lipid Research Clinics Program. The Lipid Research Clinics Coronary Primary Prevention Trial Results: II. The relationship of reduction in incidence of coronary heart disease to cholesterol lowering. *JAMA* 251:365-374, 1984.

(18) Committee of Principal Investigators, W.H.O. Clofibrate Trial. A cooperative trial in the primary prevention of ischaemic heart disease using clofibrate, report. *Br Heart J* 40:1069-1118, 1978.

(19) H-ICDA: *Hospital Adaptation of ICDA,* 2nd ed., 8th rev. Ann Arbor, Mich., Commission on Professional and Hospital Activities, 1973, vol. 1.

(20) Cornfield, J., and S. Mitchell. Selected risk factors in coronary disease: Possible intervention effects. *Arch Environ Health* 19:382-391, 1969.

(21) Davis, C.E., and R. Havlik. Clinical trials of lipid lowering and coronary artery disease prevention. In Rifkind, B.M., and R.I. Levy (eds.), *Hyperlipidemia—Diagnosis and Therapy.* New York, Grune & Stratton Inc., 1977, pp. 79-92.

(22) Rinzler, S.H. Primary prevention of coronary heart disease by diet. *Bull NY Acad Med* 44:936-949, 1968.

(23) Dayton, S., M.L. Pearce, S. Hashimoto, et al. A controlled clinical trial of a diet high in unsaturated fat in preventing complications of atherosclerosis. *Circulation* 39-40(suppl. 2):1-63, 1969.

(24) Turpeinen, O., M.J. Karvonen, M. Pekkarinen, et al. Dietary prevention of coronary heart disease. The Finnish Mental Hospital Study. *Int J Epidemiol* 8:99-118, 1979.

(25) Hjermann, I., K. Velve Byre, I. Holme, et al. Effect of diet and smoking intervention on the incidence of coronary heart disease: Report from the Oslo Study Group of a randomized trial in healthy men. *Lancet* 2:1303-1310, 1981.

(26) Multiple Risk Factor Intervention Trial Research Group. Multiple Risk Factor Intervention Trial: Risk factor changes and mortality results. *JAMA* 248:1465-1477, 1982.

(27) Committee of Principal Investigators, W.H.O. Clofibrate Trial. W.H.O. Cooperative Trial on primary prevention of ischaemic heart disease using clofibrate to lower serum cholesterol: Mortality follow-up report. *Lancet* 2:379-385, 1980.

(28) Coronary Drug Project Research Group. The Coronary Drug Project: Initial findings leading to modification of its research protocol. *JAMA* 214:1303-1313, 1970.

(29) Coronary Drug Project Research Group. The Coronary Drug Project: Findings leading to discontinuation of the 2.5 mg/day estrogen group. *JAMA* 226:652-657, 1973.

(30) Coronary Drug Project Research Group. The Coronary Drug Project: Findings leading to further modifications of its protocol with respect to dextrothyroxine. *JAMA* 220:996-1008, 1972.

(31) Coronary Drug Project Research Group. The Coronary Drug Project: Clofibrate and niacin in coronary heart disease. *JAMA* 231:360-381, 1975.

(32) Group of Physicians of the Newcastle Upon Tyne Region: Trial of clofibrate in the treatment of ischaemic heart disease: Five-year study. *Br Med J* 4:767-775, 1971.

(33) Research Committee of the Scottish Society of Physicians. Ischaemic heart disease: A secondary prevention trial using clofibrate. *Br Med J* 4:775-784, 1971.

(34) Friedewald, W.T., and M. Halperin. Clofibrate in ischemic heart disease. *Ann Intern Med* 76:821-823, 1972.

(35) Asano, T., M. Pollard, and D.C. Madsen. Effects of cholestyramine on 1,2-dimethylhydrazine-induced enteric carcinoma in germfree rats. *Proc Soc Exp Biol Med* 150:780-785, 1975.

(36) Oliver, M.F. Serum cholesterol: The knave of hearts and the joker. *Lancet* 2:1090-1095, 1981.

(37) Kannel, W.B., W.P. Castelli, T. Gordon, et al. Serum cholesterol, lipoproteins and the risk of coronary heart disease: The Framingham Study. *Ann Intern Med* 74:1-12, 1971.

(38) Goldstein, J.L., T. Kita, and M.S. Brown. Defective lipoprotein receptors and atherosclerosis: Lessons from an animal counterpart of familial hypercholesterolemia. *N Engl J Med* 309:288-296, 1983.

(39) Blackburn, H., A. Keys, E. Simonson, et al. The electrocardiogram in population study. *Circulation* 21:1160-1175, 1960.

Appendix A. Definition of primary end points.

Primary end points

I. Definite atherosclerotic coronary heart disease death—either or both of the following categories:
  A. Death certificate with consistent underlying or immediate cause plus either of the following:
   1. Preterminal hospitalization with definite or suspect myocardial infarction (see below).
   2. Previous definite angina or suspect or definite myocardial infarction when no cause other than atherosclerotic coronary heart disease could be ascribed as the cause of death.
  B. Sudden and unexpected death (requires all three characteristics):
   1. Deaths occurring within one hour after the onset of severe symptoms or having last been seen without them.
   2. No known nonatherosclerotic acute or chronic process or event that could have been potentially lethal.
   3. An "unexpected" death occurs only in a person who is not confined to his home, hospital, or other institution because of illness within 24 hours before death.
II. Criteria for definite nonfatal myocardial infarction—any one or more of the following categories using the stated definitions:
  A. Diagnostic ECG at the time of the event.
  B. Ischemic cardiac pain and diagnostic enzymes.
  C. Ischemic cardiac pain and equivocal enzymes and equivocal ECG.
  D. A routine Lipid Research Clinics ECG is diagnostic for myocardial infarction while the previous one was not.
III. Suspect atherosclerotic coronary heart disease death—one or both of the following categories:
  A. Death certificate with consistent underlying or immediate cause but neither adequate preterminal documentation of the event nor previous atherosclerotic coronary heart disease diagnosis.
  B. Rapid and unexpected death (requires all three characteristics):
   1. Death occurring between one and 24 hours after the onset of severe symptoms or having last been seen without them.
   2. No known nonatherosclerotic acute or chronic process or event that could have been potentially lethal.
   3. An "unexpected death" occurs only in a person who is not confined to his home, hospital, or other institution because of illness with 24 hours before death.
IV. Suspect myocardial infarction—any one or more of the following categories using the stated definitions:
  A. Ischemic cardiac pain.
  B. Diagnostic enzymes.
  C. Equivocal ECG and equivocal enzymes.
  D. Equivocal ECG alone, provided that it is not based on ST or T-wave changes only.

Glossary

I. Ischemic cardiac pain—severe substernal pain having a deep or visceral quality and lasting for half an hour or more.
II. ECG (classified by Minnesota Code) (*39*)
  A. Diagnostic—either of the following must be present:
   1. Unequivocal Q or QS pattern (code 1-1).
   2. Q or QS pattern (codes 1-2-1 to 1-2-7), plus any T-wave item (codes 5-1 to 5-3).
   Only the first criterion applies in the presence of ventricular conduction defects.
  B. Equivocal—any of the following must be present:
   1. Q or QS pattern (codes 1-2-1 to 1-2-7).
   2. ST junction and segment depression (codes 4-1 to 4-3).
   3. T-wave item (codes 5-1 to 5-2).
   4. Left bundle-branch block (code 7-1).
III. Enzymes
  A. Diagnostic enzymes—all of the following conditions:
   1. Creatine kinase, SGOT, or lactic dehydrogenase values determined coexistent with the event.
   2. The upper limit of normal for the local laboratory is recorded.
   3. The determined value for one or more enzymes is at least twice the upper limit of the local laboratory but does not exceed 15 times that value.
  B. Equivocal enzymes—all of the following conditions:
   1. Creatine kinase, SGOT, or lactic dehydrogenase values determined coexistent with the event.
   2. The upper limit of normal for the local laboratory is recorded.
   3. The determined value for one or more enzymes is elevated but does not fulfill criteria for diagnostic enzymes.

Appendix B. Deaths not attributed to coronary heart disease.

Cause of Death	Placebo	Cholestyramine resin
Cardiovascular (non-coronary heart disease)	3	5
Cerebrovascular	2	2
Peripheral vascular with gangrene	0	1
Surgical complications[a]	1	2
Malignant neoplasm[b]	15	16
Other illnesses	5	4
Infectious diseases[c]	3	2
Chronic obstructive pulmonary disease	1	1
Alcoholism	1	1
Trauma	4	11
Accidents	2	6
Homicide	0	1
Suicide	2	4
Total	27	36

[a] One placebo participant died while undergoing cardiac catheterization. Two cholestyramine resin participants died of complications ensuing from mitral valve replacement and from carotid endarterectomy.

[b] Listed by site in Appendix E.

[c] Three deaths (two in the placebo group) caused by pneumonia, one placebo death caused by staphylococcal septicemia, and one cholestyramine resin death resulting from an undetermined infectious cause.

Appendix C. Mean laboratory values not influenced by cholestyramine resin.

Laboratory value	Placebo			Cholestyramine resin		
	Pre-entry	1st year	7th year	Pre-entry	1st year	7th year
Albumin, g/dL of serum	4.3	4.2	4.2	4.3	4.2	4.2
Bilirubin, direct, mg/dL of serum	0.04	0.04	0.04	0.04	0.05	0.04
Bilirubin, total, mg/dL of serum	0.52	0.52	0.61	0.52	0.54	0.62
Calcium, mEq/L of serum	4.8	4.8	4.7	4.9	4.8	4.6
Chloride, mEq/L of serum	103	104	103	103	105	103
Creatinine, mg/dL of serum	1.03	1.02	0.98	1.03	1.01	0.98
Globulin, g/dL of serum	2.9	3.0	3.0	2.9	3.0	3.0
Glucose, mg/dL of serum	98	96	101	98	94	100
Hematocrit, %	46	45	45	46	45	45
Iron, μg/dL of serum	114	113	103	113	114	103
Phosphorus, mg/dL of serum	3.1	3.0	3.0	3.1	3.0	3.0
Potassium, mEq/L of serum	4.5	4.5	4.4	4.5	4.5	4.4
Sodium, mEq/L of serum	140	141	141	140	140	141
Thyroxine, μg of T_4/dL of serum	4.1	4.0	4.3	4.1	4.1	4.3
Total protein, g/dL of serum	7.2	7.2	7.3	7.2	7.2	7.3
Vitamin A, IU/dL of serum	228	234	267	229	236	270

Appendix D. Hospitalizations with a primary diagnosis[a] of gastrointestinal tract disease.

Primary Diagnosis[b]	Placebo	Cholestyramine resin
Intestinal infectious diseases	13	9
Neoplasm		
Benign	11	12
Malignant	11	15
Unspecified	0	1
Diseases of esophagus	5	6
Ulcer	20	30
Gastritis	5	12
Functional and other disorders of stomach	3	0
Appendicitis	4	11
Hernia	100	97
Intestinal obstruction	5	4
Enteritis and colitis	2	1
Diverticular disease of intestine	9	10
Anal fissure and fistula	9	5
Abscess of anal and rectal region	5	5
Peritonitis	0	1
Functional and other diseases of intestine	3	6
Liver disease	2	3
Gallstones	11	16
Other gallbladder and biliary tract disease	19	22
Pancreas	0	3
Hemorrhoids	27	29
Signs, symptoms, and ill-defined conditions	23	16

[a] Participants are counted only once within each category.
[b] By H-ICDA code, eighth revision, 1973.

Appendix E. Incident malignant neoplasms.

Primary site	Placebo (N = 1900) All cases	Deaths[a]	Cholestyramine resin (N = 1906) All cases	Deaths[a]
Buccal cavity-pharynx	0	0	6	0
Esophagus	1	0	2	2
Stomach	2	1	0	0
Colon	6	0	6	2
Rectum	2	0	4	1
Pancreas	0	0	3	3
Larynx	3	0	1	0
Lung	10	8	6	3
Leiomyosarcoma	1	1	0	0
Melanoma	5	1	0	0
Other skin	5	0	3	0
Prostate	11	1	7	1
Urinary bladder	3	0	7	0
Kidney	1	0	2	0
Brain	1	1	3	3
Thyroid	1	1	0	0
Thymus	0	0	1	0
Lymphatic tissue	1	0	4	1
Hematopoietic tissue	3	1	2	0
Unknown	1	0	1	0
Total	57	15	57[b]	16

[a] Four men with malignant neoplasms (two in each treatment group) died of nonneoplastic causes. They are counted among the incident cases but not among the deaths in this table.
[b] One cholestyramine group participant, who survived to the end of the study, had both a prostate carcinoma and a lymphoma; he is counted only once in the total.

PART IV

HEALTH SERVICES AND HEALTH POLICY

DISCUSSIONS

BUCK: We sometimes forget that the term etiological refers not only to causes of disease, but to causation in general; that a well-done investigation of factors affecting the outcome of illness or the prevention of disease uses the same rules of inference as an etiological study of disease causation. I realize it is awkward because etiology in most people's minds means only disease causation, pure and simple. But in terms of science I think we should be right in the way we classify things.

TERRIS: I agree, but I also think it is terribly important to differentiate between the evaluation of health services and etiological studies. The whole history of epidemiology has been the history of etiological studies. That has been the main emphasis. Now we are moving into an era when people want to take a really good look at what they are doing. We have come to the point where we now use observational studies and experiments to conduct etiological studies and to evaluate health services. In Latin America, for example, they want to use epidemiology to evaluate available health services, including medical care services.

LLOPIS: The problem is that the word evaluation might be too broad. We should distinguish between an evaluation of the outcome of health services and an evaluation of how health services provide medical care. Epidemiologic evaluation should be limited to an evaluation of the outcome.

TERRIS: Right, we are not interested in whether people are satisfied with health services. That is a different kind of evaluation; it's not an evaluation of outcome.

NAJERA: But even the process of or the satisfaction with health services could be evaluated epidemiologically, and the methodology would be basically the same. Increasingly, the term "health service research" is being used to describe this. As scientists we should emphasize that epidemiology is the main science in health service research.

TERRIS: In my opinion, epidemiology should stick to the evaluation of outcomes, the *effect* of health services on health. The rest is traditional health service research: it's sociological, political, or economic. The field of health service research has been taken over by the medical care people, and, as a result, we have all sorts of studies of resources, physicians, number of beds, financial issues. That's all that anyone studies now—costs. But the whole emphasis is wrong. What we want to have as the keystone of health service research are epidemiologic studies of outcomes. We should be very bold here and say just that.

NAJERA: In my opinion, there are three main uses of epidemiology: planning of health services, organization and management of health services, and research on causation and new study methods. Since the fifties or sixties everyone has agreed that epidemiology is the basic science for planning, organizing, and evaluating health services, but, save for evaluating vertical programs or a certain type of medical care, it has never really been used for this. Consequently, health services have evolved, for the most part, in a very anarchic way: changes have resulted from the needs, demands, and desires of doctors and other personnel, with a very limited evaluation of health problems or health outcomes. Not even in socialist countries has epidemiological knowledge of health status been used to plan services. This probably results from the difficulty in changing services that are already in place. This means that one of the objectives for epidemiologists is to find out how epidemiology can be used to improve existing services. In other words, can we suddenly curtail one type of service to create another type of service when the resources—the hospitals, the people— are already there? I think that this is a major limitation that has never been addressed, and until we do so we will lose a big part of the limited financial resources available. We have to be aware of costs. Epidemiology that doesn't look at costs scientifically is not epidemiology. Epidemiology should, therefore, not only take causation but health services into consideration. The whole thing is really on a continuum: the investigation of causes at one end and the investigation of outcomes at the other. If we don't consider health outcomes, we cannot really modify the services.

TERRIS: The process of taking health outcomes into consideration has already begun. For example, take the Lalonde Report in Canada and the United States Public Health Service's *Objectives for the Nation.* They are both revolutionary documents. A revolution is occurring, a revolution that is symbolized by a paper which Pineault, Contandriopoulos, and Lessard published in the *Journal of Public Health Policy,* called "The Quebec Health System: Medical Care Objectives or Health Objectives?" The Quebec paper is a brilliant discussion on objectives, on what the issues really are. Let me read to you their list of examples of medical-care objectives and of health objectives. For medical-care objectives they have: insure adequate availability of resources, make health services available to the population, insure the quality of care components (professional norms), achieve universality, maintain continuity, increase the degree of productivity. For the health objectives: reduce mortality from cardiovascular disease, reduce mortality and morbidity from accidents, reduce the incidence of childhood infectious diseases, increase the proportion of elderly maintaining an adequate degree of autonomy, reduce the incidence of sexually transmitted diseases. That's the issue. In the same journal, Tulchinsky wrote an article on Israel and made the same point: "Medical Care Objectives or Health Objectives?"

Let me give you an example of what this approach can mean. When we were in Havana for PAHO, we looked at the data collected by Cuban epidemiologists from the Institute of Cardiology. The data indicated that in Havana only about 25 percent of the population age 40 and over had serum cholesterol levels under 200, meaning that 75 percent had abnormal serum cholesterol levels. We expected that, because they have a high rate of coronary heart disease in Cuba. But the interesting thing was that the women had higher serum cholesterol levels than the men. This is very unusual, as you know. Then we looked at the mortality data and, sure enough, while in the United States the ratio of male to female mortality for ischemic heart disease is 2 to 1, in Cuba it is 1.3 to 1. Now we know why the mortality in Cuba is not so different between men and women. This kind of study by epidemiologists is terribly important. For Cuba, it means that when they try to do something about heart disease they have to pay a lot of attention to women; they also know that their problem is that three quarters of the population age 40 and over have abnormal serum cholesterol levels. If you go to India, however, you won't find this. Another good example are the studies in the Soviet Union that show that if you check serum cholesterol levels in the Central Asian Republics, there are not many people with high serum cholesterol. But if you do this in European Russia, in the RSFSR, it's like Europe; serum cholesterol levels are high. This is the kind of study where epidemiology can play a major role. It's applied epidemiology.

The real problem is that, in trying to carry through such a revolution, we run up against the medical profession, and the medical profession is committed to therapy. They cannot see prevention. It doesn't matter whether a country is underdeveloped, socialist, capitalist; this happens in every country in the world.

Epidemiologists should participate in studies to determine the best ways to deal with the problem of health service research. We have to lead that revolution in the public health profession. But it won't be easy.

NAJERA: Health service research has become more and more important in the organization of health services. But without epidemiology, health service research is just administration. It concentrates on better administration, better management techniques.

TERRIS: We should claim an aspect of health service research for epidemiology and make this aspect its primary emphasis. The economists have taken over the field and we've got to take it back from them.

BUCK: One thing I would like to see is the use of health statistics to suggest epidemiological research. Wouldn't it be nice if by using health statistics we could demonstrate that the major health problems of a country are not always those on which most of the money is spent, such as in the glamorous tertiary-care centers?

TERRIS: I have another recent experience related to this use of research to set up priorities. Not long ago, I spent a week in a Latin American country visiting with the Deputy Ministers of Health. They were all young clinicians with no public health training; they had youthful enthusiasm but not much background. I kept asking for the leading causes of death and they claimed they didn't know; they could only tell me what they saw in the hospitals. In desperation, I asked for the mortality statistics and they brought out the computer sheets. I looked at the data for the country's capital, since there, unlike the rural areas where they have very few doctors, the diagnosis would be reasonably accurate. They had excellent data for both men and women; everything was laid out on the computer sheets. Since we knew the size of the population, I spent the afternoon figuring out the mortality rates with a borrowed hand calculator. They had not done it because they were not trained to do this kind of thing. I then presented the data in a talk to the staff of the Ministry of Health. I was surprised to find that, young as the country's population was, the leading cause of death was heart disease. My audience couldn't believe it. The third leading cause of death, higher than infectious and parasitic diseases, was injuries. They couldn't believe that either. It was hard for them to accept the concept that injuries are important. They are doctors, and for doctors injuries are not diseases; they are another kind of medical problem. I couldn't convince them. The health officer responsible for the capital region said that the major emphasis still had to be on infectious disease. Well, it certainly should be a major emphasis, but not if they pay no attention to the injuries that kill more people than the infectious diseases. And let's not forget that heart disease is the leading cause of death in most of the countries of Latin America.

BUCK: We should stress the importance of evaluating health services in terms of specific health outcomes. When a final outcome is too difficult to observe, we can at least examine an intermediate outcome.

TERRIS: One of the ways to evaluate health services is to see who gets what, how needs are being met—even in cases where there is total access to care, where everyone has access. If you look at the way, for example, teachers use the health services versus the way manual workers use them, there is a tremendous difference. There is an educational and cultural difference.

BUCK: Well, I guess the most vivid illustration of that comes from the studies of social class that show differences in psychiatric treatment: the upper classes get psychotherapy; the lower classes get drugs because there isn't the rapport between the doctor and patient to make psychotherapy pleasant or feasible.

TERRIS: That is why we need nurses to work with the patients. That is why patients prefer nurse practitioners to doctors. Nurses are more down to earth and most doctors are so arrogant.

NAJERA: There was also a very nice study done in the United States which showed how medical school students lose their social conscience. According to the study, in the first year of medical school up to 80 percent of the students had very strong social interests. This is why many of them had chosen to study medicine in the first place. But by the time they graduated, the percentage had dropped to 20.

TERRIS: I would like to raise an issue that I think clinicians ought to understand: health should be approached in terms of continua, not in terms of hard-and-fast categories. This is a very important concept. Yet clinicians do not understand this because medical training is always rather rigid; it uses a yes/no logic with no room for gradation.

The issue of hypertension is a good way to illustrate this. My cardiologist, for example, is very happy to get my blood pressure just below 140/90. But all the studies show that the lower the blood pressure, the longer you live. There is no sharp dividing line between normal and abnormal. The same is true of serum cholesterol. In the early days of the Framingham study they seemed to be saying that 260 milligrams percent or above is bad, everything else is all right. But now they emphasize that it is a continuum: the lower you get the better. Below 200 does not seem to matter very much, but the minute you start going above 200 you are at risk.

Another way to illustrate the rigidity of medical training is with the difference between statistical normality and physiologic normality. For serum cholesterol levels, for example, statistical normality for American males age 40 is around 230, with two sigmas on each side; physiological normality is under 200. The two are very different, but this is not understood. In one of our epidemiology exercises we reproduce the lab report card from my hospital, which, like a lot of other places, gives the normal figures for serum cholesterol as 220 to 260, when actually it is under 200. Hospitals do this because they are going by statistical normality instead of physiologic normality. In dealing with cardiovascular diseases it is very clear that we are dealing with continua instead of rigid definitions, and the question of statistical versus physiological normality is also important. Yet no one has ever discussed these as philosophical issues, which they really are, they are basic concepts.

BUCK: I think these issues have been addressed in the course of the last decade, but they haven't made it into medical journals until much more recently.

TERRIS: They certainly are not addressed in medical schools, particularly not by clinicians. Ask clinicians what is hypertension: "It's above 140/90," they say. There is no concept that, compared to 100/70, anything above 120/80 is really hypertension.

BUCK: Careful, though. We know that the clinicians are partly right. To get blood pressure much below 140/90 or to get a North American's cholesterol below 200 may require measures so drastic that you will be doing more harm than good.

TERRIS: I do not agree. My doctor, who was always satisfied when my blood pressure was at 140/90, put me on a new drug and it came down to 130/80. It was not so hard, he just used a different drug. I had been trying to tell him to please do something like that. And as far as serum cholesterol is concerned, it does not take heroic measures. I used to have 245 milligrams percent and then I went on the prudent diet and it came down to 200, and it has stayed there ever since. Diet is critically important when it comes to serum cholesterol levels. Take the case of Vietnam: they live on a rice diet, and since they don't eat meat or fats, they don't have much heart disease. Another good example is Eastern Europe. Once they did not have meat, milk, and eggs. They worked hard to get them and their coronary disease rate rose sharply. There are, of course, individual genetic differences, but it is very hard to have high serum cholesterol when you are on a rice diet.

I think these are concepts which doctors and clinicians ought to understand, but it is difficult since the teaching is all black-and-white. Do you know what the medical students say when I give them my two hour exercise on cigarette smoking and lung cancer? They say that we are wasting their time. They do not want to learn all this junk that I am teaching them, it's too methodological. They just want to know whether cigarette smoking causes lung cancer, yes or no. That way they can answer the exam question. I can speak like an expert on this, because I have spent most of my life teaching medical students, and I can tell you I deserve a medal for that.

I have yet to meet a teacher of preventive medicine in a medical school who is happy. Once a teacher told me how happy she was teaching epidemiology at her university and how wonderful it was because the students were eating it up. A few months later there was a strike of the students against her teaching program. When I went to the medical school in Costa Rica and told them about this and about my own troubles they were so glad to find that they were not alone. I visited the famous medical school in New Delhi, India, and found posters all over the medical school building attacking community medicine in the most insulting terms. The federal government had decided that medical students should spend six months instead of three doing community medicine in the rural health service. You should have seen those posters. The students went on strike and won. The term was reduced from six months to four.

NAJERA: You cannot change the mentality of medical students. By then it is too late. The change must happen earlier.

TERRIS: That's true. I taught first- and second year medical students and it is already too late. By then they are learning microbiology, anatomy—big subjects. Why should they bother with this junk, they think. That is their attitude. And isn't it part of the problem of the future of epidemiology and public health also a prestige problem? If you go to a school of public health you don't have the prestige that you have in a medical school?

NAJERA: Well, at least in Spain, the problem is mainly financial. In the first place, the medical schools are the ones with the money; also, most people go into clinical work because they stand to make more money as clinicians in private practice. The people who go to the school of public health become government employees who make less money.

BUCK: That's the problem, isn't it? Low prestige means less money. We are so materialistic.

TERRIS: I saw something else in one European country where I talked with the young people in the department of social medicine. These people spend half their time doing clinical work. I asked them how they could do public health when they spent their time doing clinical work, and they answered that you have to combine theory and practice. I told them that that was the wrong practice for their theory. How can you do epidemiology or medical care research when half your time is spent taking care of patients? They don't realize that they are destroying public health when they do that. I bet you this happens in Latin America, too.

LLOPIS: Yes. This is one of the problems created by the expansion of the social security systems. The social security systems increased the medical care coverage. It is a medical approach. All activities have to do with patient care because people go there to be treated. As a result, physicians end up being sort of public health administrators. They become heads or directors of health centers and hospitals without the necessary training. And what results is similar to what the British used to say about the French social security system: nine doctors to supervise one.

BUCK: Do they still have fee for service?

LLOPIS: The main problem with social security in Latin America is exactly the problem of fee for service. Some of the professionals are salaried employees, but many enter into a fee-for-service contract with the social security agencies. Fee for service has created an overutilization of medical services as well as a number of unnecessary tests and other procedures.

NAJERA: Since most social security systems either have evolved from or are still essentially insurance systems, most of these problems are rooted in the insurance system. From an administrative point of view, social security systems look at health problems as nothing more than risks that must be covered. If the users are healthy, they still pay but don't get any service. If they are sick, the system delivers a service for an insurance-covered risk. Health problems are not an issue. There are only diseases.

BUCK: After this goes on for a while, the costs involved make prevention seem very attractive. So far, however, prevention has been directed almost entirely at individuals' bad habits rather than at changing the environment that fosters such habits. It is all pretty shortsighted.

TERRIS: My guess is that in Latin America today there is socio-political unrest among many epidemiologists without enough of an epidemiological structure to back it up. That is why you read papers full of sociological rethoric that I have tended to deride as being talk. But it isn't just talk. I think we are seeing the beginning of a movement. The whole emphasis now, interestingly enough, is on doing actual research. I think that in all these countries where people talk so much about social epidemiology, what is really happening is that they are not really clear on which way to go. Someone has to assume the job of providing them with an adequate epidemiological knowledge base.

NAJERA: I don't agree with your statement that people are doing social epidemiology just because they don't know what else to do, or because they are in the initial stages of a process. Even if we don't call this discipline socio-epidemiology, we must recognize that social factors are so enormously important to the development of disease that they should be analyzed and studied. I have no doubt that social factors have always been the most important factors in the development of most diseases. The difference with which a disease manifests itself in different social groups is evident, yet it is much easier to quantify other factors.

The problem may be that we don't have the right tools or the methodology to study social factors scientifically. Regardless, these limitations should not stop us from attempting it. We should intensify our efforts and ability to analyze the role of social factors like nutrition, occupation, salary, housing, and so on.

BUCK: What we do know is that the successful application of some results of epidemiological research to health care organization requires a change in medical education, basically a change in the selection of people for the health professions.

TERRIS: That is akin to saying that it requires changing the medical profession, and I've given up on changing the medical profession. Physicians are going to be therapeutically oriented no matter what you do. You'll waste a lot of time and effort trying to change that. I think we should take a clue from the tremendous change that took place in Canada and in the United States with respect to heart disease and stroke—without changing medical education.

BUCK: But we don't know all the reasons for this.

TERRIS: I know why. It had nothing to do with medical education. It had to do with primary prevention. We're not talking about secondary prevention, although it is true that the medical profession is very much involved in hypertension control as primary prevention for stroke. They've done very well in Canada and the United States, even though they're therapeutically oriented. You have to give them credit. But, in general, what happened in the United States and Canada had very little to do with the medical profession. It had to do with the fact that the epidemiologists found out about serum cholesterol and hypertension and smoking, and the newspapers and magazines spread this information throughout the country. The well-to-do and well-educated people who read and who are very health conscious said, "By God, we're going over to unsaturated fats." Now they go to the supermarket and buy sunflower oil and corn oil margarine; they stay away from fatty foods; they exercise; they stop smoking; and they get their blood pressure taken care of. It was almost all done by the people themselves, without too much help either from public health or from the medical profession. It was all primary prevention. Before this everyone said that health education could never do anything. Yet we now know that even without an organized program of health education, a revolution occurred. In only ten years there was a 25 percent decline in coronary heart disease and a 38 percent decline in stroke in the United States. So I don't think that we need to worry so much about changing medical education. What we need is a strong commitment, from both the government and from non-government agencies like the Cancer Society and the Heart Association, to educate the public and get money for primary prevention programs. Forget about trying to educate the doctors; they'll come along. That's my opinion.

NAJERA: And yet these are all examples of changes that do not reach the whole population; they benefit only the upper class. It will be very difficult for this type of health education and this type of prevention to reach everyone if the structure of the population doesn't change. Yours is not the only solution. Sure, we need prevention, we need primary prevention, it's the most important thing—but we also need something else.

TERRIS: What else do you need?

NAJERA: Oh, several things. Among them is changing the physicians.

TERRIS: Don't waste your time.

NAJERA: We have to try to make a physician who, being concerned with treatment, also thinks in terms of the community rather than just in terms of individuals. We also need to change the organization of health services. In Spain we are trying very hard to do this because we feel that this could be the start of something new.

TERRIS: You mean if you have a National Health Service, you'll get this? Do you know what happens in National Health Services? I have met directors of health who were the medical directors of hospitals. They didn't know anything about public health, yet they held key positions in the ministries of health. And I have been in countries where the leading people in public health were all physicians. They were very proud of the fact that every one of them, including the Minister himself, did clinical work one afternoon or one day a week. They really believe this is good "theory and practice." I know of one Minister of Health who was a cardiac surgeon, and guess what got emphasized in his National Health Service? Cardiac surgery and intensive care units; tertiary care. This is what we are up against, everywhere in the world.

NAJERA: I'm not only strongly advocating a National Health Service, I am also talking about a change in the organization of the health services towards a community oriented approach.

TERRIS: What do you mean by community oriented?

NAJERA: Benefitting most of the people, having a positive approach to health, being prevention oriented—and ensuring that health services are in the interest of the community. For me, there is a great difference between what is community oriented and what is only prevention oriented.

TERRIS: What's the difference?

NAJERA: What is just prevention oriented isn't necessarily directed towards everyone. For example, the target might be diseases that primarily affect the rich. These may be prevented very quickly, but these changes don't touch the whole community. In the same way, the evaluation of a tuberculosis or polio program is only a partial evaluation: it is not aimed at the health services as a whole. But the community will always have an interest in prevention, and this is why I prefer to say community oriented. In my opinion, the big change in the future will be to have epidemiologists use their expertise to perform more comprehensive evaluations of the importance of disease and its causes in the different social classes, occupational groups, age groups, and so forth. Otherwise, what you have described can happen: a mortality reduction for diabetes, or coronary heart disease, or whatever, will not really have reduced mortality or morbidity in all population groups.

TERRIS: A talk I gave recently on Canadian health directly answers your comment on the community and prevention. I said that to prevent the major causes of illness, disability, and death, you need a well funded campaign led by Canada's local, provincial, and national health departments. Well funded, in this case, requires only a small fraction of the many billions of dollars which Canada now spends for the treatment of these preventable diseases. Implementing this program—and this is the key point—would mean not only achieving better health for the Canadians, but also achieving equity in health. Just as the Canadian National Health Insurance Program was established to assure equity in medical care (that's what you want to do with a National Health Service in Spain), so must we pursue this aim in the more fundamental goal of improving health status. The available evidence indicates that, both in the United States and Canada, lifestyle modification has been more effective in the more highly educated groups, those who have been to college. That's why it's important to make every effort—that's where you need the money and the programs—to reach the less educated groups in order to get equity in health. And I'm not just talking about the poor, but about the majority of the less educated people; in other words, 80 percent of the Canadian population. But that's not just community oriented, it is total population oriented.

NAJERA: Yes, it is. When I use the term community I mean it to include everyone. Regarding equity in health, I must say that your success with the lifestyle modification among the more highly educated groups certainly has not been because of the equity of the health education system.

TERRIS: There has been no health education system. That's the problem.

NAJERA: Here you have something that has been successful with one group and has failed with others. You say we need to spend more money; that it is essential to make every effort to reach the less educated. But the question is how? These people have other problems that depend on other factors. Even if they stopped smoking, what then of the factories, the whole economy which depends on tobacco? Up to now, the impact on smoking cessation has been minimal, so much so that the tobacco industry doesn't mind.

TERRIS: Not in the United States. That's not true. Tobacco companies are in trouble.

NAJERA: Well, they still sell cigarettes outside the United States, in the Third World. And the same is true of other products, dairy products, for example.

TERRIS: You know what my proposal is? That it would be worthwhile to put a lot of money—and the United States is wealthy enough to do it—into subsidizing farmers to get out of growing tobacco so that they could grow other crops.

NAJERA: Now we are coming to the changes that I meant. We need to stop growing tobacco, maybe we need to reduce the production of dairy products, or change agriculture, but we also need to change housing and occupational risks. We need so many changes of this nature, and I don't believe that they can all be achieved through health education.

TERRIS: I agree with you.

NAJERA: In order to achieve this level of change I think we need to have the community—the people—participate in running the health services at the decision making level. Therefore, the big change is in implementing a community oriented approach. We want the people themselves to think of what health services they need. It's only at this level that we will be able to venture into changing the economy, into doing intersectoral development.

LLOPIS: But, don't you need to use health education to have the community's cooperation?

NAJERA: I don't like the term health education because it has the connotation of something that is being imposed on someone—the teacher who knows and the child that doesn't. I think it fails because this may be good for children, but not for adults. Adults do not want to be educated in this sense. They like to discuss things. This is why I don't use the term health education; I prefer community involvement, because it stresses that you have to get people involved in the discussion.

TERRIS: The error you make is to consider health education in a very simplistic way by saying that the role of health education is to get people to change behavior. That's not the role of health education; that's only half its role. The main role of health education is to get political support from the people. In the United States, if we had said in the early days that smoking in restaurants would be restricted, people would have laughed at us. It took twenty-five years of informing people about the dangers of smoking, and then it wasn't the health people that demanded the restriction, people did. They were the ones that said that they did not want to be next to someone who smokes. So, health education is an organizing resource. It's not what you think it is, because you cannot get community involvement unless the community understands the issues.

NAJERA: The community will understand them.

TERRIS: They will understand only through health education.

NAJERA: They will understand immediately, if they are involved in the process, if their interests are the priority.

BUCK: I think you have to go further. I agree with the mechanisms for diffusion of change, because I think it's the only way. But you also made reference to factors such as housing, and remember that in our historical section we talked a great deal about the studies of health and social class. It's not just historical. It seems to be true that at the present time, almost any study you do of any kind of morbidity or mortality shows that the inverse social class gradient continues. There are important environmental causes for this gradient, and they're not all a matter of lifestyle. I'm all for changing lifestyles in a healthy direction. But in doing that you cannot neglect the other causes: housing, education, and occupation; the conditions under which people live, learn, and work today. We may no longer have the satanic mills of the Industrial Revolution, but we still have lots of jobs where there's no creativity, where work is boring, and where there is a fear of unemployment if you object to anything. It's been shown that some of the lifestyle problems are generated by environmental problems, particularly occupational ones. That may be one of the reasons why less educated people are not as likely to stop smoking or to do other things that we would like them to do. Studies by the Social Research Institute in Michigan have found that people on piece work, people on shift work—especially the kind that goes against the body's natural rhythms—are much more often smokers. So I think we have to go beyond lifestyle. We have to consider how people live and this comes down to what you were saying about involving the people themselves. People have to be encouraged to associate some of their environmental problems with their health. The trade-union movement has been rather slow to do this. Their interests are only recently beginning to veer in this direction.

NAJERA: What you said about occupation is very interesting. In my opinion, it is the most important thing right now. This is what I mean when I talk of involving the people rather than just giving them health education. Health education implies teaching them about alternative lifestyles as if the educators were imposing responsibilities on the individuals. By doing that, what is most important for people, their working conditions, is being neglected. This is the most important issue for them, and so it should be for us. In my opinion, the lifestyle approach (smoking, cholesterol, etc) shifts attention to less important things. All the efforts made since the 1950s in the area of chronic diseases have, in general, done nothing but shift attention from the big occupational problems that have been there since before the Second World War. Working conditions were improved more between the wars than they have been after the Second World War. It seems as if we have slowed down on this. We talk about cigarette smoking and all that, which would be fine if someone was also paying attention to the problems of occupation, low salaries, etc.

TERRIS: I want to dissent very seriously from your line of reasoning. I think it leads to an absolute blind alley. It's a dereliction of duty on the part of the intellectuals, if you'll forgive me for saying this. I've been in a number of socialist countries that emphasize community involvement, and in those countries the workers play an important part in dealing with problems. I'm sorry to say that are also backward in noninfectious disease control. I speak advisedly; I've been there and I know this is true. The reason they are backward is because they still emphasize medical care; they have not yet developed public health. They have not really worked on these issues. They've got all the involvement you want, but they still don't have public health leadership and health education of the public on what the issues really are.

NAJERA: But it is not real community involvement. Community involvement means that the community makes decisions and sets priorities for an overall development in which health is one important area. It is easy to talk about this but very difficult to achieve it.

BUCK: Just a word before I forget where you're leading us, Terris. You are just making a big leap to the conclusion that in those countries occupational and environmental conditions are O.K. All you have really said is that socialism does not insure an environment conducive to health. I agree. But that does not argue against the importance of the environment.

TERRIS: You both imply that the major causes of death and disease are related to occupation. I don't buy that at all.

BUCK: Occupation and other environmental factors.

TERRIS: The main cause of disease and death in the industrial countries, and increasingly in the developing countries, is heart disease, where we know what the risk factors are, and occupation is not involved.

BUCK: You cannot prove that, Terris. You cannot prove that.

TERRIS: Yes, I can. It's cigarette smoking, saturated fats, hypertension, lack of exercise.

BUCK: Look, we can only predict about half the coronary cases. There is a 50 percent variation in the incidence of coronary disease that we have yet to account for. We can't prove it's occupation. Nor can you deny that it might be.

TERRIS: It could be genetic.

NAJERA: Also, we don't know which factors in occupation, nor can we quantify their influence. As we were saying, what about work that is not pleasant?

LLOPIS: I guess this is the role of epidemiology: to explain how every factor participates in the causation of disease. This is, in part, what papers like the Lalonde Report were saying. These papers attempt to find the best way to apply epidemiology—to define the main areas involved in disease causation and to evaluate the impact of promotion, prevention, and rehabilitation measures on health.

BUCK: I think this point takes us back to some of the classic papers that we have selected. The role of epidemiologists, acting as epidemiologists rather than as citizens trying to change policy (because there is an argument about the borderline between the professional's and the citizen's role), will be more important if they study what I will call the "right things." Epidemiologists should not constantly keep their studies within the framework of personal attributes and lifestyles, they should go back to the kind of things that made Cassel's work so influential. Cassel and his group pointed the way towards epidemiological studies of environmental phenomena, cultural phenomena, not just physical things in the environment. This area is greatly neglected in epidemiology, partly because the flow of funds is now very much toward the study of specific risk factors. But I say that epidemiologists, if they want to turn things around while still acting within their profession, should be much more diversified in what they study. In particular, they should be willing to extend themselves into far more powerful and subtle studies of environmental causes of ill health.

NAJERA: The role of epidemiology is to understand, in a comprehensive way, what is happening with health. This is my main general criticism of the lifestyles approach. It is a partial approach because it only looks at, say, coronary heart disease, without looking at the web of causation.

TERRIS: What do you mean when you say comprehensive? Give me the facts. We have a lot of facts which we can use to dramatically reduce morbidity and mortality and we should move on that. That's the main task of public health at the present time, not just the task of epidemiology.

NAJERA: But that approach will only take you so far. Look at us, supposedly highly educated people; we cannot move further because special interests will not allow the shutting down of tobacco factories, tobacco growing fields, dairy farms and industries, and so on. Besides, the majority of the population cannot choose lifestyles. The word style implies the possibility of choice, and choice is not an option for more than 80 percent of the population of the world.

TERRIS: If we get enough public support we not only can, we will succeed against special interests.

BUCK: I'll just interject one example of where these things belong and they're not as intangible as you allege. Take blood pressure. None of us would disagree about its importance as a risk factor. But there are some occupational observations which suggest that not only the task of the worker but also the milieu of the occupational environment can exert a profound influence on blood pressure and other physiological factors. They're tiny studies and we need more of them. They're not encouraged nearly as much as they should be, I think, partly because of this unbalanced view of causation that you're addressing.

TERRIS: We don't have good hypotheses on the causes of hypertension. We really don't. All of the social class studies have been very unproductive. There are very minor differences by social class. The big difference is between whites and blacks, and there are no good hypotheses for why that is so. You say that it's occupational, but you don't have any basis for saying that at all. You have nothing that shows that.

BUCK: The reason we don't have any very solid basis is that the research is not sufficiently refined in terms of occupational classification.

NAJERA: You were asking why I used the term comprehensive. Comprehensive epidemiological studies take into account every imaginable factor. For instance, consider the health services. We take for granted that our health services are good and we don't look at them as possibly iatrogenic, as factors that may cause disease. Then we start studying, let's say, coronary heart disease, without taking into consideration what the health services are doing with coronary heart disease. We also have to review many of our diagnoses. What is hypertension? Is it a risk factor? Is it a disease? What does hypertension really mean? We have to review and revise these diagnoses. We cannot have a partial approach; we cannot study hypertension without studying coronary heart disease, or studying stroke, or even diabetes. We must consider the interrelation of those factors so we can understand the web; again the web.

TERRIS: What I am proposing is a very specific program since we now have been given powerful tools by the epidemiologists to attack some of the most important plagues of mankind—heart disease, cancer, stroke, injuries, chronic obstructive lung disease, cirrhosis of the liver. These are among the major causes of death and we now have weapons to greatly reduce many of them. To stand by and refuse to put the main emphasis on that, it seems to me, is a dereliction of duty. That doesn't mean that we should not study and act upon the other problems like occupational disease, toxic wastes, the environment. We should. That's another role we should fulfill. But not to attack, at this point, the major causes of illness and death for the benefit of humanity is a dereliction of duty.

BUCK: Actually though, the right time to move is when the epidemiological knowledge is solid enough that it deserves to have an effect on public opinion. In the meantime we should be moving on the research front to areas of less certainty but greater potential.

TERRIS: We should do that all the time. I'm not objecting to that. What I'm saying is that the main task of public health at the present time is to fight noninfectious disease with the very powerful tools we've been given. I consider health education a part of politics. We now have all sorts of laws in the United States that you would never have believed possible. It really is remarkable that mandatory seat-belt laws and motorcycle helmet laws, laws that infringe on personal liberties, have been passed. We're going to have compulsory labeling of saturated fats, and sooner or later we will have subsidies of unsaturated fats and taxes on saturated fats. There will be all sorts of techniques we will work out to deal with these problems.

NAJERA: I think that can be important, but you are talking of the role of public health. We agree that this is part of its role, but we should be talking of the role of epidemiology. Epidemiology is always research, epidemiology is what is next, epidemiology is fundamental.

TERRIS: You're not a public health man?

NAJERA: Yes, I am, but we are talking of the role of epidemiology—
where we should go, how we should study the problems
again and again. The application is public health. And it
will be real public health if it results from epidemiology, if it
is arrived at through the epidemiologic method.

TERRIS: The role of epidemiology in health services is to study the
best methods for getting the outcomes. In other words,
epidemiology must move to become the central feature of
health services research. From now on, we should not think
of health service research in terms of medical care research, but in terms of public health research.

SICK INDIVIDUALS AND SICK POPULATIONS

Geoffrey Rose[1]

THE DETERMINANTS OF INDIVIDUAL CASES

In teaching epidemiology to medical students, I have often encouraged them to consider a question which I first heard enunciated by Roy Acheson: "Why did *this* patient get *this* disease at *this* time?" It is an excellent starting point, because students and doctors feel a natural concern for the problems of the individual. Indeed, the central ethos of medicine is seen as an acceptance of responsibility for sick individuals.

It is an integral part of good doctoring to ask not only, "What is the diagnosis, and what is the treatment?" but also, "Why did this happen, and could it have been prevented?" Such thinking shapes the approach to nearly all clinical and laboratory research into the causes and mechanisms of illness. Hypertension research, for example, is almost wholly preoccupied with the characteristics which distinguish individuals at the hypertensive and normotensive ends of the blood pressure distribution. Research into diabetes looks for genetic, nutritional, and metabolic reasons to explain why some people get diabetes and others do not. The constant aim in such work is to answer Acheson's question, "Why did *this* patient get *this* disease at *this* time?"

The same concern has continued to shape the thinking of all of us who came to epidemiology from a background in clinical practice. The whole basis of the case control method is to discover how sick and healthy individuals differ. Equally, the basis of many cohort studies is the search for "risk factors," which identify certain individuals as being more susceptible to disease; and from this we proceed to test whether these risk factors are also causes, capable of explaining why some individuals get sick while others remain healthy, and applicable as a guide to prevention.

To confine attention in this way to within-population comparisons has caused much confusion (particularly in the clinical world) in the definition of normality. Laboratory "ranges of normal" are based on what is common within the local population. Individuals with "normal blood pressure" are those who do not stand out from their local contemporaries, and so on. What is common is all right, we presume.

Applied to etiology, the individual-centered approach leads to the use of relative risk as the basic representation of etiologic force, that is, "the risk in exposed individuals relative to risk in nonexposed individuals." Indeed, the concept of relative risk has almost excluded any other approach to quantifying causal importance. It may generally be the best measure of etiologic force, but it is no measure at all of etiologic outcome or of public health importance.

Unfortunately, this approach to the search for causes, and the measuring of their potency, has to assume a heterogeneity of exposure within the study population. If everyone smoked 20 cigarettes a day, then clinical, case control, and cohort studies alike would lead us to conclude that lung cancer was a genetic disease, and in one sense that would be true, since if everyone is exposed to the necessary agent, then the distribution of cases is wholly determined by individual susceptibility.

Within Scotland and other mountainous parts of Britain (Figure 1, left section) (1), there is no discernible relation between local cardiovascular death rates and the softness of the public water supply. The reason is apparent if one extends the inquiry to the whole of the U.K. In Scotland, everyone's water is soft, and the possibly adverse effect becomes recognizable only when study is extended to other regions that have a much wider range of exposure (r = −0.67). Even more clearly, a case control study of this question within Scotland would have

Source: *PAHO Epidemiological Bulletin* 6(3):1-8, 1985. This article was reprinted with permission from the author. It was first published in the *International Journal of Epidemiology* 14:32-38, 1985.

[1] Department of Epidemiology, London School of Hygiene and Tropical Medicine, London, U.K.

Figure 1. Relation between water quality and cardiovascular mortality in towns of the U.K. *(1)*.

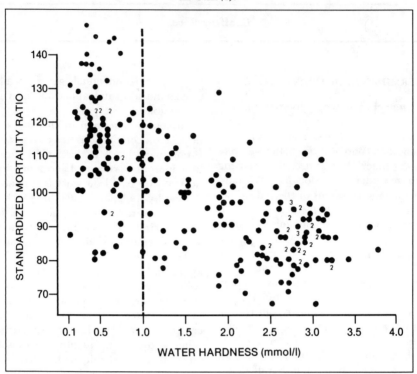

been futile. Everyone is exposed, and other factors operate to determine the varying risk.

Epidemiology is often defined in terms of study of the determinants of the distribution of the disease, but we should not forget that the more widespread is a particular cause, the less it explains the distribution of cases. The hardest cause to identify is the one that is universally present, for then it has no influence on the distribution of disease.

THE DETERMINANTS OF POPULATION INCIDENCE RATE

I find it increasingly helpful to distinguish two kinds of etiologic question. The first seeks the causes of cases and the second seeks the causes of incidence. "Why do some individuals have hypertension?" is a quite different question from "Why do some populations have much hypertension, whilst in others it is rare?" The questions require different kinds of study and they have different answers.

Figure 2 shows the systolic blood pressure distributions of middle-aged men in two populations—Kenyan nomads *(2)* and London civil servants *(3)*. The familiar question, "Why do some individuals have higher blood pressure than others?" could be equally well asked in either of these settings, since in each the individual blood pressures vary (proportionately) to about the same extent, and the answers might well be much the same in each instance (that is, mainly genetic variation, with a lesser component from environmental and behavioral differences). We might achieve a complete understanding of why individuals vary, and yet quite miss the most important public health question, namely, "Why is hypertension absent in the Kenyans and common in London?" The answer to that question has to do with the determinants of the population mean, for what distinguishes the two groups has nothing to do with the characteristics of individuals; it is rather a shift of the whole distribution—a mass influence acting on the population as a whole. To find the deter-

Figure 2. Distributions of systolic blood pressure in middle-aged men in two populations *(2, 3)*.

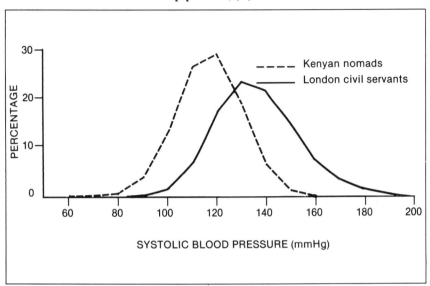

minants of prevalence and incidence rates, we need to study characteristics of populations, not characteristics of individuals.

A more extreme example is provided by the population distributions of serum cholesterol levels *(4)* in East Finland, where coronary heart disease is very common, and Japan, where the incidence rate is low; the two distributions barely overlap. Each country has men with relative hypercholesterolemia (although their definitions of the range of "normal" would no doubt disagree), and one could research into the genetic and other causes of these unusual individuals, but if we want to discover why Finland has such a high incidence of coronary heart disease, we need to look for those characteristics of the national diet which have so elevated the whole cholesterol distribution. Within populations it has proved almost impossible to demonstrate any relation between an individual's diet and his serum cholesterol level, and the same applies to the relation of individual diet to blood pressure and to overweight. But at the level of populations it is a different story; it has proved easy to show strong associations between population mean values for saturated fat intake *versus* serum cholesterol level and coronary heart disease incidence, sodium intake *versus* blood pressure, or energy intake *versus* over-

weight. The determinants of incidence are not necessarily the same as the causes of cases.

HOW DO THE CAUSES OF CASES RELATE TO THE CAUSES OF INCIDENCE?

This is largely a matter of whether exposure varies similarly within a population and between populations (or over a period of time within the same population). Softness of water supply may be a determinant of cardiovascular mortality, but it is unlikely to be identifiable as a risk factor for individuals, because exposure tends to be locally uniform. Dietary fat is, I believe, the main determinant of a population's incidence rate for coronary heart disease, but it quite fails to identify high-risk individuals.

In the case of cigarettes and lung cancer, it so happened that the study populations contained about equal numbers of smokers and non-smokers, and in such a situation case control and cohort studies were able to identify what was also the main determinant of population differences and time trends.

There is a broad tendency for genetic factors to dominate individual susceptibility, but to explain rather little of population differences in incidence. Genetic heterogeneity, it seems, is mostly much greater within than between populations. This is the contrary situation to that seen for environmental factors. Thus migrants, whatever the color of their skin, tend to acquire the disease rates of their country of adoption.

Most noninfectious diseases are still of largely unknown cause. If you take a textbook of medicine and look at the list of contents you will still find, despite all our etiologic research, that most are still of basically unknown etiology. We know quite a lot about the personal characteristics of individuals who are susceptible to them, but for a remarkably large number of our major noninfectious diseases, we still do not know the determinants of the incidence rate.

Over a period of time we find that most diseases are in a state of flux. For example, duodenal ulcer in Britain at the turn of the century was an uncommon condition affecting mainly young women. During the first half of the century, the incidence rate rose steadily and it became very common, but now the disease seems to be disappearing, and yet we have no clues to the determinants of these striking changes in incidence rates. One could repeat that story for many conditions.

There is hardly a disease whose incidence rate does not vary widely, either over time or between populations at the same time. This means that these causes of incidence rate, unknown though they are, are not inevitable. It is possible to live without them, and if we knew what they were, it might be possible to control them. But to identify the causal agent by the traditional case control and cohort methods will be unsuccessful if there are not sufficient differences in exposure within the study population at the time of the study. In those circumstances all that these traditional methods do is to find markers of individual susceptibility. The clues must be sought from differences between populations or from changes within populations over time.

PREVENTION

These two approaches to etiology—the individual and the population-based—have their counterparts in prevention. In the first, preventive strategy seeks to identify high-risk susceptible individuals and to offer them some individual protection. In contrast, the "population strategy" seeks to control the determinants of incidence in the population as a whole.

The "High-Risk" Strategy

This is the traditional and natural medical approach to prevention. If a doctor accepts that he is responsible for an individual who is sick today, then it is a short step to accept responsibility also for the individual who may well be sick tomorrow. Thus, screening is used to detect certain individuals who hitherto thought they were well but who must now understand that they are in effect patients. This is the process, for example, in the detection and treatment of symptomless hypertension, the transition from healthy subject to patient being ratified by the giving and receiving of tablets. (Anyone who takes medicines is by definition a patient.)

What the "high-risk" strategy seeks to achieve is something like a truncation of the risk distribution. This general concept applies to all special preventive action in high-risk individuals—in at-risk pregnancies, in small babies, or in any other particularly susceptible group. It is a strategy with some clear and important advantages (Table 1).

Table 1. Prevention by the "high-risk strategy": advantages.

1. Intervention appropriate to individual
2. Subject motivation
3. Physician motivation
4. Cost-effective use of resources
5. Benefit-risk ratio favorable

Its first advantage is that it leads to intervention that is appropriate to the individual. A smoker who has a cough or who is found to have impaired ventilatory function has a special reason for stopping smoking. The doctor will see it as making sense to advise salt restriction in a hypertensive. In such instances the intervention makes sense because that individual already has a problem which that particular measure may possibly ameliorate. If we consider screening a population to discover those with high serum cholesterol levels and advising them on dietary change, then that intervention is appropriate to those people in particular; they have a diet-related metabolic problem.

The "high-risk" strategy produces interventions that are appropriate to the particular individuals advised to take them. Consequently, it has the advantage of enhanced subject motivation. In our randomized controlled trial of smoking cessation in London civil servants, we first screened some 20 000 men and from them selected about 1500 who were smokers with, in addition, markers of specially high risk for cardiorespiratory disease. They were recalled and a random half received antismoking counseling. The results, in terms of smoking cessation, were excellent because those men knew they had a special reason to stop. They had been picked out from others in their offices because, although everyone knows that smoking is a bad thing, they had a special reason why it was particularly unwise for them.

There is, of course, another and less reputable reason why screening enhances subject motivation, and that is the mystique of a scientific investigation. A ventilatory function test is a powerful enhancer of motivation to stop smoking; an instrument which the subject does not quite understand, that looks rather impressive, has produced evidence that he is a special person with a special problem. The electrocardiogram is an even more powerful motivator, if you are unscrupulous enough to use it in prevention. A man may feel entirely well, but if those little squiggles on paper tell the doctor that he has got trouble, then he must accept that he has now become a patient. That is a powerful persuader. (I suspect it is also a powerful cause of lying awake in the night and thinking about it.)

For rather similar reasons, the "high-risk" approach also motivates physicians. Doctors, quite rightly, are uncomfortable about intervening in a situation where their help was not asked for. Before imposing advice on somebody who was getting on all right without them, they like to feel that there is a proper and special justification in that particular case.

The "high-risk" approach offers a more cost-effective use of limited resources. One of the things we have learned in health education at the individual level is that once-only advice is a waste of time. To get results we may need a considerable investment of counseling time and follow-up. It is costly in use of time, and effort, and resources, and therefore it is more effective to concentrate limited medical services and time where the need—and therefore also the benefit—is likely to be greatest.

A final advantage of the "high-risk" approach is that it offers a more favorable ratio of benefits to risks. If intervention must carry some adverse effects or costs, and if the risk and cost are much the same for everybody, then the ratio of the costs to the benefits will be more favorable where the benefits are larger.

Unfortunately, the "high-risk" strategy of prevention also has some serious disadvantages and limitations (Table 2).

Table 2. Prevention by the "high-risk strategy": disadvantages.

1. Difficulties and costs of screening
2. Palliative and temporary—not radical
3. Limited potential for (a) individual
                        (b) population
4. Behaviorally inappropriate

The first centers around the difficulties and costs of screening. Supposing that we were to embark, as some had advocated, on a policy of screening for high cholesterol levels and giving dietary advice to those individuals at special risk. The disease process we are trying to prevent (atherosclerosis and its complications) begins early in life, so we should have to initiate screening perhaps at the age of ten. However, the abnormality we seek to detect is not a stable lifetime characteristic, so we must advocate repeated screening at suitable intervals.

In all screening one meets problems with uptake, and the tendency for the response to be greater among those sections of the population who are often least at risk of the disease. Often there is an even greater problem; screening detects certain individuals who will receive special advice, but at the same time it cannot help also discovering much larger numbers of "borderliners," that is, people whose results mark them as at increased risk but for whom we do not have an appropriate treatment to reduce their risk.

The second disadvantage of the "high-risk" strategy is that it is palliative and temporary, not radical. It does not seek to alter the underlying causes of the disease but to identify individuals who are particularly susceptible to those causes. Presumably in every generation there will be such susceptibles, and if prevention and control efforts were confined to these high-risk individuals, then that approach would need to be sustained year after year and generation after generation. It does not deal with the root of the problem, but seeks to protect those who are vulnerable to it, and they will always be around.

The potential for this approach is limited— sometimes more than we could have expected— both for the individual and for the population. There are two reasons for this. The first is that our power to predict future disease is usually very weak. Most individuals with risk factors will remain well, at least for some years; contrariwise, unexpected illness may happen to someone who has just received an "all clear" report from a screening examination. One of the limitations of the relative risk statistic is that it gives no idea of the absolute level of danger. Thus, the Framingham Study has impressed us all with its powerful discrimination between high- and low-risk groups, but when we see (Figure 3) *(5)* the degree of overlap in serum cholesterol level between future cases and those who remained healthy, it is not surprising that an individual's future is so often misassessed.

Often the best predictor of future major disease is the presence of existing minor disease. A low ventilatory function today is the best predictor of its future rate of decline. A high blood pressure today is the best predictor of its future rate of rise. Early coronary heart disease is better than all the conventional risk factors as a predictor of future fatal disease. However, even if screening includes such tests for early disease, our experience in the Heart Disease Prevention Project (Table 3) *(6)* still points to a very weak ability to predict the future of any particular individual.

This point came home to me only recently. I have long congratulated myself on my low levels of coronary risk factors, and I joked to my friends that if I were to die suddenly, I should be very surprised. I even speculated on what other disease—perhaps colon cancer—would be the commonest cause of death for a man in the lowest group of cardiovascular risk. The painful truth is that for such an individual in a Western population the commonest cause of death—by far—is coronary heart disease! Everyone, in fact, is a high-risk individual for this uniquely mass disease.

There is another, related reason why the predictive basis of the "high-risk" strategy of prevention is weak. It is well illustrated by some data from Alberman *(7)*, which relate the occurrence of Down's syndrome births to maternal age (Table 4). Mothers under 30 years are individually at minimal risk, but because they are so

Figure 3. Percentage distribution of serum cholesterol levels (mg/dl) in men aged 50 to 62 who did or did not subsequently develop coronary heart disease (Framingham Study) *(5)*.

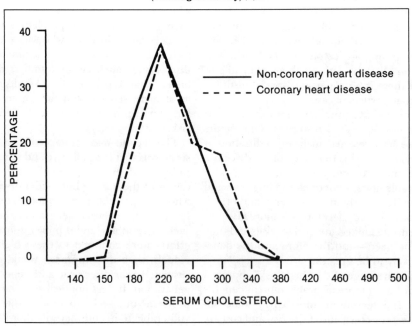

Table 3. Five-year incidence of myocardial infarction [MI] in the U.K. Heart Disease Prevention Project.

Entry characteristic	% of men	% of MI cases	MI incidence rate %
Risk factors alone	15	32	7
"Ischemia"	16	41	11
"Ischemia" + risk factors	2	12	22
All men	100	100	4

Table 4. Incidence of Down's syndrome according to maternal age (7).

Maternal age (years)	Risk of Down's syndrome per 1000 births	Total births in age group (as % of all ages)	% of total Down's syndrome occurring in age group
< 30	0.7	78	51
30–34	1.3	16	20
35–39	3.7	5	16
40–44	13.1	0.95	11
≥45	34.6	0.05	2
All ages	1.5	100	100

numerous, they generate half the cases. High-risk individuals aged 40 and above generate only 13 percent of the cases.

The lesson from this example is that *a large number of people at a small risk may give rise to more cases of disease than the small number who are at a high risk.* This situation seems to be common, and it limits the utility of the "high-risk" approach to prevention.

A further disadvantage of the "high-risk" strategy is that it is behaviorally inappropriate. Eating, smoking, exercise, and all our other lifestyle characteristics are constrained by social norms. If we try to eat differently from our friends, it will not only be inconvenient, but we risk being regarded as cranks or hypochondriacs. If a man's work environment encourages heavy drinking, then advice that he is damaging his liver is unlikely to have any effect. No one who has attempted any sort of health education effort in individuals needs to be told that it is difficult for such people to step out of line with their peers. This is what the "high-risk" preventive strategy requires them to do.

The Population Strategy

This is the attempt to control the determinants of incidence, to lower the mean level of risk factors, to shift the whole distribution of exposure in a favorable direction. In its traditional "public health" form, it has involved mass en-

vironmental control methods; in its modern form it is attempting (less successfully) to alter some of society's norms of behavior.

The advantages are powerful (Table 5). The first is that it is radical. It attempts to remove the underlying causes that make the disease common. It has a large potential—often larger than one would have expected—for the population as a whole. From Framingham data one can compute that a 10 mm Hg lowering of the blood pressure distribution as a whole would correspond to about a 30 percent reduction in the total attributable mortality.

Table 5. Prevention by the "population strategy": advantages.

1. Radical
2. Large potential for population
3. Behaviorally appropriate

The approach is behaviorally appropriate. If nonsmoking eventually becomes "normal," then it will be much less necessary to keep on persuading individuals. Once a social norm of behavior has become accepted and (as in the case of diet) once the supply industries have adapted themselves to the new pattern, then the maintenance of that situation no longer requires effort from individuals. The health education phase aimed at changing individuals is, we hope, a temporary necessity, pending changes in the norms of what is socially acceptable.

Unfortunately, the population strategy of prevention has also some weighty drawbacks (Table 6). It offers only a small benefit to each individual, since most of them were going to be all right anyway, at least for many years. This leads to the *Prevention Paradox (8)*, "A preventive measure which brings much benefit to the population offers little to each participating individual." This has been the history of public health—of immunization, the wearing of seat belts, and now the attempt to change various lifestyle characteristics. Of enormous potential importance to the population as a whole, these measures offer very little—particularly in the short term—to each individual, and thus there is poor motivation of the subject. We should not be surprised that health education tends to be relatively ineffective for individuals and in the short term. Mostly people act for substantial and immediate rewards, and the medical motivation for health education is inherently weak. Their health next year is not likely to be much better if they accept our advice or if they reject it. Much more powerful as motivators for health education are the social rewards of enhanced self-esteem and social approval.

There is also in the population approach only poor motivation of physicians. Many medical practitioners who embarked with enthusiasm on antismoking education have become disheartened because their success rate was no more than 5 or 10 percent; in clinical practice one's expectation of results is higher. Grateful patients are few in preventive medicine, where success is marked by a nonevent. The skills of behavioral advice are different and unfamiliar, and professional esteem is lowered by a lack of skill. Harder to overcome than any of these, however, is the enormous difficulty for medical personnel to see health as a population issue and not merely as a problem for individuals.

In mass prevention each individual has usually only a small expectation of benefit, and this small benefit can easily be outweighed by a small risk *(8)*. This happened in the World Health Organization clofibrate trial *(9)*, where a cholesterol-lowering drug seems to have killed more than it saved, even though the fatal complication rate was only about 1/1000/year. Such low-order risks, which can be vitally important to the balance sheet of mass preventive plans, may be hard or impossible to detect. This makes it important to distinguish two approaches. The first is the restoration of biological normality by the removal of an abnormal exposure (e.g., stopping smoking, controlling air pollution, moderating some of our recently acquired dietary deviations); here, there can be some presumption of safety. This is not true for the other kind of preventive approach, which leaves intact the underlying causes of incidence and seeks instead to interpose some new, supposedly protective intervention (e.g., immunization, drugs, jogging). Here, the onus is on the activists to produce adequate evidence of safety.

CONCLUSIONS

Case-centered epidemiology identifies individual susceptibility, but it may fail to identify the underlying causes of incidence. The "high-risk" strategy of prevention is an interim expedient, needed in order to protect susceptible individuals, but only for so long as the underlying causes of incidence remain unknown or uncontrollable; if causes can be removed, susceptibility ceases to matter.

Realistically, many diseases will long continue to call for both approaches, and fortunately competition between them is usually unnecessary. Nevertheless, the priority of concern should always be the discovery and control of the causes of incidence.

Table 6. Prevention by the "population strategy": disadvantages.

1. Small benefit to individual ("Prevention Paradox")
2. Poor motivation of subject
3. Poor motivation of physician
4. Benefit-risk ratio worrisome

References

(1) Pocock, S. J., A. G. Shaper, D. G. Cook, *et al.* British regional heart study: Geographic variations in cardiovascular mortality and the role of water quality. *Brit Med J* 283:1243-1249, 1980.

(2) Shaper, A. G. Blood pressure studies in East Africa. In: Stamler, J., R. Stamler, and T. N. Pullman (eds.). *The Epidemiology of Hypertension.* New York, Grune and Stratton, 1967, pp. 139-145.

(3) Reid, D. D., G. Z. Brett, P. J. S. Hamilton, *et al.* Cardiorespiratory disease and diabetes among middle-aged male civil servants. *Lancet* 1:469-473, 1974.

(4) Keys, A. *Coronary Heart Disease in Seven Countries.* American Heart Association Monograph Number 29. American Heart Association, New York, 1970.

(5) Kannel, W. B., M. J. Garcia, P. M. McNamara, *et al.* Serum lipid precursors of coronary heart disease. *Human Pathol* 2:129-151, 1971.

(6) Heller, R. F., S. Chinn, H. D. Tunstall Pedoe, *et al.* How well can we predict coronary heart disease? Findings in the United Kingdom Heart Disease Prevention Project. *Brit Med J* 288:1409-1411, 1984.

(7) Alberman, E. and C. Berry. Prenatal diagnosis and the specialist in community medicine. *Community Med* 1:89-96, 1979.

(8) Rose, G. Strategy of prevention: lessons from cardiovascular disease. *Brit Med J* 282:1847-1851, 1981.

(9) Committee of Principal Investigators. A co-operative trial in the primary prevention of ischemic heart disease. *Br Heart J* 40:1069-1118, 1978.

EVALUATION OF 1954 FIELD TRIALS OF POLIOMYELITIS VACCINE

T. Francis, Jr., J.A. Napier, R. B. Voight, F. M. Hemphill, H. A. Wenner, R. F. Korns, M. Boisen, E. Tolchinsky, and E. L. Diamond

PLAN OF STUDY

Establishment of Study Population and Participants

Selection of Field Trial Areas

The selection of areas in which to carry out the field trials sought to meet the geographic peculiarities of poliomyelitis and to anticipate the areas in which the disease would be most prevalent. The National Foundation for Infantile Paralysis [NFIP] with extensive study had developed a basis for concluding that, in the aggregate, counties demonstrating consistently high reported poliomyelitis attack rates during the previous five-year period were more likely to have attack rates in excess of the national average during the study period. The 100 counties with populations from 50 000 to 200 000, and with consistently the highest reported incidence of poliomyelitis 1946 through 1950, were observed to have an attack rate of 31 per 100 000 population in 1951 compared with a rate of 20 per 100 000 in other counties of similar population. In 1952 these same counties had a reported poliomyelitis attack rate of 58 per 100 000 compared with 38 for the other counties. Moreover, in 1952 the counties had an average of 42 paralytic cases per 100 000 population in the 6-9 year age group, which was well above that of the remainder of the country. This factor, plus consideration of the age distribution of the population and the seasonal pattern of poliomyelitis in the area, led to a listing of counties of this size in order of priority for consideration by the state and local health officers concerned, as a basis for selecting the actual trial areas. Many practical administrative matters influenced these officials in making their final selections, including the availability

of an adequately organized county health department to carry out the program.

Selection of Study Plans

1. Observed Control Study. The plan of procedure announced by the National Foundation for Infantile Paralysis and its Advisory Committee was to administer vaccine to children in the second grade of school; the corresponding first and third graders would not be inoculated but would be kept under observation for the occurrence of poliomyelitis in comparison with the inoculated second graders. This has been designated the "Observed Control" study. The plan poses difficulties to objectivity in that knowledge of the vaccination status of a patient is readily determinable and the introduction of even unintentional bias can result; its adequacy would depend upon a high incidence and severity of disease, a high degree of effectiveness of vaccine, and the care with which the data were collected. A number of states, however, had already made their decision to participate on this basis. When finally arranged, the procedure was followed in 127 areas of 33 states with total population in the first, second, and third grades of 1 080 680. The areas represent complete counties with exception of Kansas City and the town units of Connecticut.

2. Placebo Control Study. Since the problem was to measure the degree of effectiveness, if any, of an untried product, it was important to have data which could provide an accurate gauge of the effect, free of possible bias in diagnosis and reporting. There was introduced, therefore, a second plan corresponding in pattern to that usually employed in scientific investigations. Children of the first, second, and third grades would be combined. One half would receive vaccine; the other matching half, serving as strict controls, would receive a solution of similar appearance which should have no influence on immunity to poliomyelitis. Each

Source: *American Journal of Public Health* 45(5), 1955.

child would receive the same lot of material, labeled only by code, for all three inoculations. Only the Evaluation Center would have the key. A single lot of each material was, so far as possible, to be used in a given area. The children in the study would be observed thereafter and all reports relating to a case of poliomyelitis would be made on a concealed or blindfold basis without knowledge of the nature of the inoculum. Although the operative procedures of the placebo plan would require much more work and care, a number of well-populated states indicated their preference for it and the "Placebo Control" study was incorporated into the field trial. It comprised 84 areas of 11 states with population in the first, second, and third school grades of 749 236. Here again, areas represented counties except for the combined areas of New York City and the town units of Massachusetts.

In a short time, plans for collecting and recording information on the involved population were devised by the staffs of the Vaccine Evaluation Center and of the NFIP. A Manual of Procedures provided detailed instructions for the registration, vaccination, and follow-up of the children. Great efforts were made to acquaint the responsible administrative groups in the study areas with the need for accuracy, uniformity, completeness in performance, and recording. It was clearly emphasized that all areas were part of a coordinated study with the Vaccine Evaluation Center serving as the central agency to which all records would come for assimilation and analysis.

It was readily agreed, as a condition for participation, that local preliminary estimates or reports would not be made until the Center had made a report of the total experience. This was necessary in order to avoid the possibility of early and unreliable estimates of the effectiveness of the vaccine, based on small numbers and subject to great irregularity.

Identification of the Study Population

It is obviously essential in a study of a phenomenon arising in a limited, selected population that the members of that population be clearly recorded, and their status with respect to the study be established. They constitute the denominator against which all effects are to be measured; hence, any child in the group who

Table 1. Distribution of study population by participation status and vaccination status, placebo areas.

Study Population	Number	Percent
Total in grades 1, 2, and 3	749 236	100.0
Total requests to participate	455 474	60.8
Complete series of injections:		
Vaccine	200 745	26.8
Placebo	201 229	26.9
Incomplete injections:		
Vaccine	8484	1.1
Placebo	8577	1.1
Absent at first clinic or withdrew	36 439	4.9
Number not requesting participation	280 868	37.5
Participation status not recorded	12 894	1.7

subsequently would be reported to have poliomyelitis could be specifically identified. A series of records with cross-references was then prepared.

1. Registration. The basic record is a Registration Schedule (Form FT-3) on which was entered the name of each child in a first, second, or third grade class of a participating school. Since each sheet and line was numbered uniquely, a person could be permanently identified on that basis. Address, date of birth, sex, color, previous history of poliomyelitis or disability were to be recorded. Furthermore, data with respect to participation and inoculation were subsequently to be used as a cross check of data on other forms. The same procedure applied to the placebo and observed areas alike. It was necessary in some of the observed areas to emphasize repeatedly that these records were required for the first and third graders who were not inoculated but who constituted the control population. The registration thus obtained constituted the total study population.

2. Participation Request. Each child was to receive a form briefly telling of the pattern of study—observed (FT-1) or placebo (FT-2)—on which a parent could make written request for the child to participate in the study, whether to be inoculated or not. It also gave permission for the collection of specimens of blood, if needed. When a specifically signed request was returned, this fact was to be entered in the proper space on the Registration Schedule. Specific refusals were entered, and when the form was not returned or returned not signed, that was to be appropriately recorded as "no". Certain irregularities were encountered in the observed areas since only one grade was subject to vaccination; for example, request forms were sometimes used only for those control children who were to give samples of blood, so that yeses and noes in those groups could not be fully defined.

3. Vaccination Record. This form (FT-4) was filled out for each person who received an inoculation or from whom blood was taken. It duplicated the identification contained in the Registration Schedule and the name of the signer of the request form. Three injections of 1 cc each were to be given intramuscularly at 0, 1, and 5 weeks, respectively. The date of each inoculation, the lot or code number of the material given, the name of the physician and date blood drawn was recorded. Space was provided for recording any evidence of reactions. When the vaccination series was not completed, the reason was to be stated. The dates of inoculation and of blood specimens were also entered on the Registration Schedule, permitting a check for accuracy or inconsistencies.

After a careful check of the registration records with enrollment figures for the first three grades in each participating school, submitted to the Center at the time of the vaccination clinics, and persistent effort on the part of the Center staff through correspondence and personal visits to more than 30 trial areas during the course of the summmer and fall, complete registration was obtained from all schools in the placebo areas except for six schools where the children whose parents refused participation were not included. In the observed areas complete records were obtained from all except twenty-six schools with a total estimated enrollment in the first three grades of 916 or .08 percent of the total observed area study population.

These essential records were prepared in triplicate. When vaccinations were completed

and the blood specimens collected, they were to be edited locally and the first two copies sent to the State Health Department which, after review, would send the original copy of the Registration Schedule and the Vaccination Record to the Evaluation Center. . . .

4. Procurement of Blood Specimens. The only data with respect to the antibody response of humans to vaccine of the nature employed in the field trial were those reported by Dr. Salk. But there was only a small number of laboratories in position to undertake studies on the scale projected and few with experience in extensive serologic testing. In order to gain information of the responses to different lots of material subjected to transportation and variable field conditions, it was decided in consultation with experts in the laboratory investigation of poliomyelitis to obtain specimens of blood prior to inoculation from a two percent sample of children who were to receive vaccine, and from controls, and from these same persons again two weeks after vaccinations were completed.

Table 2. Number of blood specimens collected at pre- and post-vaccination bleedings and third bleedings in November.

	First bleedings		Second bleedings		Third bleedings
	No.	%	No.	%	No.
Placebo areas	14 475	100.0	12 382	100.0	11 870
Vaccinated	7220	49.9	6210	50.1	a
Placebo	7255	50.1	6172	49.9	a
Observed areas	26 406	100.0	20 046	100.0	20 931
Vaccinated	9789	37.1	7870	39.2	a
Controls	16 617	62.9	12 176	60.8	a

[a] Data by vaccinated and control population not yet available.

By titration of the sera for antibody levels by means of tissue cultures of monkey kidney or HeLa cells, evidence would be provided regarding the occurrence of antibodies to the different types of poliomyelitis virus in the various parts of the country and the changes in titer induced by vaccine. It would give a view of the variation in the potency of lots of vaccine or of the same lot in different areas. Moreover, the results could be measured in persons without demonstrated antibody to any type in comparison with a reinforcing effect in persons who already possessed some antibody. The specimens from control subjects would also provide a base line for measuring any concurrent changes which might take place in the population through natural exposures, and permit accurate conclusions as to the antigenic activity of the vaccine. It was also urged that blood specimens be obtained from the same persons again at the end of the poliomyelitis season of 1954; this was carried out in November. The laboratories would be uninformed as to whether the specimens were from a vaccinated or control child and the tests would largely be done on an unselected basis. . . .

5. *Reactions.* Because of the natural concern with reactions which might occur with a new product in large-scale use, the Manual of Procedures emphasized the need to record any untoward reactions which appeared to be related or coincidental to the administration of vaccine. A further notice from the Evaluation Center asked for notification by phone of any circumstance of significant severity which might be related to the inoculations.

During the course of the vaccination of children in Pittsburgh by Dr. Salk, a concurrent study was carried out in March and April of 1954 by the Evaluation Center concerning cause of absenteeism in vaccinated children as compared with their classmates who had not received vaccine. The bulk of these data had been collected by Dr. Salk before the Center entered the study. They were analyzed and, in addition, a system was developed for recording absences from school and verifying the cause of absenteeism through the school health service.

Significant illnesses were investigated further through personal consultation with the attending physician and the family. Initially the experience in 20 public schools during each of five weeks following vaccination was recorded for 3246 vaccinated children and 1773 non-vaccinated children. Total absences during this period were 2270 for the vaccinated and 1611 for the non-vaccinated. When absenteeism is analyzed by interval after the vaccination, the only apparent difference between the two groups exists in the first week. Absenteeism is somewhat higher in the non-vaccinated group, 31.5 percent compared to 22.9 percent. It seems likely that this is due to the fact that children who were absent were by that fact alone not included in the vaccinated population at the time of clinic.

Information on reason for absence was tabulated in similar fashion for each of the five weeks following vaccination for those receiving vaccine and those not receiving vaccine. Here again, according to the 29 itemized causes, no significant difference was observed between the two groups. Only one case of nephritis occurred and that in a non-vaccinated child during the first week after first clinic.

It seemed advisable to extend these studies further to an additional group of schools for more thorough follow-up as to extent and cause of absence. The procedure was identical with that described above, although greater effort was put into obtaining accurate medical information on the causes of absenteeism. In the five schools studied, there were 969 vaccinated children and 486 non-vaccinated; of the latter, 380 had not requested vaccination and 106 had requested but were absent on the day of the first

Table 3. Distribution of study population by participation status and vaccination status, observed areas.

Study population	Number	Percent of second grade	Percent of total population
All grades — Total	1 080 680		100.0
Requests	567 210		52.5
Second grade — Requests	245 895	69.2	22.8
Complete vaccinations	221 998	62.4	20.5
Incomplete vaccinations	9904	2.8	0.9
Absent or withdrew	13 993	3.9	1.3
First and third grades — Requests	321 315		29.7
All grades — Participation not requested	332 870		30.8
Participation not recorded	180 600		16.7

clinic. Study of the total absenteeism by week and by days within weeks during the three-week period after the clinic merely served to confirm the earlier observation that absenteeism was identical in the two groups. The only difference, again, was observed in the first week when absences occurred among 16.1 percent of the vaccinated compared with 41.6 percent among the non-vaccinated. This was accounted for largely by children who had requested participation but were absent on the clinic day. Again, detailed examination of the reasons for absence failed to reveal any significant differences between these two groups during any of the weeks of study. The one case of kidney disease which came to attention occurred in a non-vaccinated child. The great bulk of remaining causes of absence might be defined as respiratory in nature and did not differ in the two groups. The findings from these two studies were made available to those concerned with final decision as to whether the field trials were to be conducted as planned, and served as additional assurance at that time of the safety of the product. . . .

Vaccinating Procedure and Assignment of Controls

Placebo Areas

The materials to be used in placebo areas were supplied in boxes containing six vials of 10 cc content; three of them contained vaccine and three contained placebo, each set of three labeled with a code number unique to that set. A vial was entered with a new, sterilized needle attached to a freshly sterilized 5.0 cc syringe. That volume of fluid was withdrawn and the needle left in place. Then with a new needle for each injection, 1.0 cc of the material was given to each of five children in the left triceps muscle. A new syringe was then used to remove the remaining 5.0 cc from the vial which was given as before to five additional children. (In a few areas, separate syringes and needles were used for each child.) The exact code number of the material given was recorded. Following the same procedure, the next ten children received the material from a vial bearing the second code number, indicating that it was different from the first. The remaining four vials were then returned to storage until the next clinic when the same children would again receive their inoculations from the specific vials with the same code numbers as before. This required careful attention to procedure and to identification of each child. Provision had to be made for consultation with the Evaluation Center for replacements or additions when shortage developed, without revealing the code or the nature of material in question.

The classroom groups of the first, second, and third grades constituted the basic clinic unit and remained so through the three inoculations. Consequently those receiving vaccine or the corresponding placebo were segments of the same group and the controls were clearly designated. In general, only one lot of vaccine or placebo was used in a placebo study area or in a school. Because of supply problems this was not completely uniform, and in 14 placebo areas more than one lot was employed. Even then, the uniformity in the 206 schools of those areas was maintained and the controls for each lot of vaccine were clearly designated on the 22 997 records according to corresponding codes.

In 346 schools, with small classes, the numbers were insufficient to complete the use of a 10 cc vial—the required procedure; thus, 1529 children received only placebo. This was balanced by 1761 children in 387 other small schools who received only vaccine. But it is important to emphasize that the equal distribution of vaccine and placebo held at every level. Moreover, according to our records, out of a total of 1 237 446 injections in 419 035 persons inoculated in placebo areas, only 748 persons received a mixed series of vaccine and placebo.

Observed Areas

In observed study areas where only those second grade children whose parents requested participation were vaccinated, the problem of establishing the control population was more complex. After careful consideration of various alternatives, it was decided that the total first and third grade study population compared to the vaccinated second grade population would be the most critical measure that could be applied to measure the efficacy of the vaccine. This was also the original premise on which various state health offices agreed to participate in the study. In observed areas there was a greater number of instances in which more than one lot of vaccine was used in an area, which came about partly as a supply problem and partly from a decision to use, for the third inoculation, lots which appeared upon test to be stronger antigenically in combination with those which appeared to be only moderately so. This resulted in as many as seven or eight different lot combinations being used in some areas. Naturally, it resulted in further irregular lot combinations being used in a single school. There were 268 schools out of 7925 in observed areas where this occurred, involving a study population of 51 157 of whom 11 533 were vaccinated, or five percent of the total complete vaccinations in observed areas. Since it was impossible to determine the proper controls for each lot combination in these schools, they have been given a separate designation in the report as "mixed lots within schools" for both the vaccinated and control populations.

In 765 other observed area schools there were a few children who received a lot combination different from the major series used in the school. In these schools involving a vaccinated group of 39 914 children where only one, two, or three second graders received a series of lots different from the rest of the vaccinated group, the total first and third grade populations were taken as the control populations for the major lot combinations and specific controls for the 1144 children receiving odd combinations were not established.

Staff Supervision

During the vaccination period, April 26 to June 15, members of the Evaluation Center staff visited 32 of the 44 participating states to inspect or correct procedure and to ensure proper recording and understanding. It was necessary to prepare additional memoranda specifically restating the requisite information and the need for uniformity and completeness of the data to be supplied in the records. The problems of vaccine replacement and the completing of inoculations in migrant children were also handled. In the field more than 150 000 persons assisted in the total program, including clinicians, epidemiologists, health officers, physical therapists, public health nurses, virologists, school teachers and administrators, and local volunteer recorders and clerks.

Instructions for the reporting and investigation of cases of poliomyelitis occurring in the study population were reinforced with specific memoranda, and forms for use in this phase of the field trial were drawn up and distributed to the trial areas.

Identification and Verification of Reported Cases in the Study Population

The second phase of the study was that of determining the occurrence of poliomyelitis among members of the study population, of identifying the patient, and of establishing diagnosis by integration of clinical, epidemiologic, and laboratory data which could contribute reliable, objective information. It was apparent that with the large number of different professional personnel involved in the widespread study, variability could be expected. By seeking uniformity of understanding and performance it was hoped that the variations could be reduced, and that 211 different patterns could be avoided even though the Evaluation Center was completely dependent upon the ability, willingness, and collaboration displayed at the local level where the cases of poliomyelitis would occur.

To reduce the need for discrimination locally, to encourage completeness of reporting and uniformity of procedure, a single plan was instituted for the investigation of all cases in the entire study population; that is, cases arising in any member of the first, second, and third grades during the spring of 1954, whether inoculated or not, whether participation had been requested or not. Every case, paralytic, nonparalytic, suspect or doubtful was to be reported to the Center and subjected to the same degree of study, recognizing at the same time diagnostic problems of the early acute phase and variation in medical interpretation. All cases in families containing a member of the study population were also to be reported but subjected to limited investigation except as special studies.

Reporting of Cases

Because there may reasonably be delay between the onset of a case of poliomyelitis and its diagnosis as poliomyelitis, it was urged that the local agencies try to reduce any further delay in reporting of cases to the health department or program director.

As a means of following the occurrence of poliomyelitis in each of the trial areas as closely as possible, both in the study population and in the family associates of study members, a weekly reporting system was established as of May 1, 1954, whereby all reported cases of poliomyelitis in each trial area were submitted to the Vaccine Evaluation Center weekly on Form VEC-11 which called for the name, age, date of onset as given, city of residence, grade if enrolled in school, and type of case. Each area was also asked to report all deaths from all causes in the study population on these weekly reports. This plan proved to be too slow and local health officers were subsequently requested to notify the Evaluation Center by collect telegram immediately upon notification of a case. It was then possible promptly to send back to the Health Department schedules listing the further information to be obtained and the date on which each item was due.

In addition to this reporting system, arrangements were made with the National Foundation for Infantile Paralysis to obtain photostat copies of all NFIP medical care, hospital admission, and discharge records for children in the age group five through nine in each of the trial areas. These records were cross-checked with the VEC-11 reports submitted by the local health officers as a means of spotting any eligible cases which had not been reported. In each instance, if notification to the Center of the usual reportable clinical case was not forwarded by the local health office, correspondence was initiated by the Center to determine if the case was in the study population.

The total of cases reported from each trial area each week was compared with the standard reports issued by the United States Public Health Service as a means of determining if adequate coverage was being obtained from the trial areas. The need to find cases in study members who migrated to other trial areas or communities outside the trial areas was strongly emphasized, and many cases which would otherwise have been lost to the study were thus recovered.

Through these methods assurance was gained that the Center was informed of a high percentage of all cases in the study population considered to have poliomyelitis even though delays in notification and investigation inevitably occurred. Not more than a half dozen cases were disclosed to have escaped the established procedures for identification and these were essentially migrant children.

Investigation of Case

Upon report of a case of poliomyelitis, the health department needed to arrange promptly for the successive steps in investigation. Since a high percentage of patients was admitted to the hospitals (88.9 percent in placebo, 85.9 percent in observed areas) not always in the same county, various means of carrying out the requirements were devised. The responsibility, however, remained with the local director of the study. In a number of instances the state or district authorities assumed all responsibility. Great assistance was provided in a number of areas by the Epidemiologic Intelligence officers of the USPHS assigned through Dr. Alexander Langmuir to state health departments and laboratories participating in the study.

1. Clinical-Epidemiological Report. As soon after onset—or report—as possible, a summary of the clinical history and examination, including spinal fluid, of the case was to be made on the proper form (FT-6) together with the diagnosis at that time. On the same form the family history with respect to concurrent illness or previous poliomyelitis was to be recorded. Administration of gamma globulin to family members was also to be recorded. This information constituted the first official record received at the Evaluation Center and contained the tentative diagnosis. It provided also a basis on which to proceed with subsequent studies or to eliminate the patient from consideration if obviously his illness was due to another cause. Much of this was done by staff physicians but public health nurses also contributed a large part. No case was accepted as part of the study unless this record was received; thus, for every case disclosed by any means an FT-6 record was obtained.

2. Laboratory Specimens. As early as possible a specimen of stool (or two) and a specimen of blood were to be collected from the patient and sent promptly to the laboratory functioning for that area. They were accompanied by forms (FT-9) identifying the patient and the dates of collection. Copies of the forms were to be sent to the Center—if not received, it was assumed the specimens had not been collected and the health officer was notified of the deficiency.

After three to four weeks a second specimen of blood was to be obtained and, together with the first sample, antibody titrations for diagnosis of poliomyelitis were made. The stool was to be studied for the presence of poliomyelitis or other virus. In some areas studies of familial associates were also carried out by the laboratory and the local health authorities.

The complete laboratory report was made directly to the Center on Form FT-10, although preliminary reports were sometimes made by letter.

At first, the same serological procedure was employed for the testing of sera of patients in the study areas as was used for study of pre- and post-vaccination sera. Later it was agreed that it should be more sensitive and titrations were made with twofold dilutions and four tubes per dilution to reach the endpoint. In some instances this was preceded by a preliminary screening. In addition, Dr. Wenner and Dr. Frisch provided to all laboratories supplies of standard human sera with titers in the range ordinarily encountered in man. Additional spot checks for variability in laboratory results were made at different times by a single pair of sera sent to all laboratories.

Virus isolations, from stool specimens primarily, were attempted in monkey kidney cells or HeLa cells and generally a negative specimen was retested at least once. The information gradually accumulated to indicate that HeLa cells might be less sensitive and again exchange of specimens among a series of laboratories was made to test this probability— which proved to be correct. Subsequently, when HeLa cells were used, passages were to be made three times before considering the test negative. In some instances specimens were also tested by the inoculation of monkeys. In a number of instances serologic tests were carried out against mumps, choriomeningitis, and encephalitis viruses as well.

In addition, the laboratories frequently played a large part in collection of specimens, of maintaining the attention of health and hospital personnel in the continued need for proper specimens and prompt delivery. There is little doubt that the present experience will have done much toward prompt laboratory diagnosis of poliomyelitis.

3. Examination by Physical Therapist. On the recommendation of clinical consultants it was decided that an expert examination of the patient's muscular status should be made 10 to 20 days after onset of illness. At that time the febrile stage of the disease is commonly past and further progression of paralysis is unlikely. Furthermore, spasm and tenderness are generally diminished and a reasonable measure of disability can be obtained. Again, in an effort to gain uniformity, the physical therapists who agreed to participate had received or did receive a two weeks' course of orientation in an abridged system of muscle examination and in grading of muscles or muscle groups according to a uniform system of recording disability which gave a score of involvement based on muscle mass and severity of dysfunction. . . .

Accordingly, at the time the other procedures for study of a patient were instituted, the local health officer was to notify the designated therapist of the identity and location of the patient with a request that the examination be made at the proper time. The examiner was not informed of the patient's vaccination status and was to conduct the examination on all cases reported to be poliomyelitis whether considered to be paralytic or not. At that time it was requested that provision be made for a review and interpretation of the case by a physician especially skilled in the clinical aspects of poliomyelitis. This was to be recorded on the same form and became the established clinical diagnosis. Provision for securing this specialist's report was again left to local authorities and done under a variety of arrangements, often through the local medical society. In many of the hospitals to which the patients were admitted the specialist was readily obtained. When completed, the examination record (FT-7) was to be returned to the local health department and forwarded to the Evaluation Center.

It was further agreed that the examination should be repeated 50 to 70 days after onset. By this time the patient may have experienced the major proportion of muscular recovery but, on the other hand, defects not clearly localized earlier may have become more apparent as activity or use of the muscles increased. The other interferences of the acute stage will be sent so that residual injury can be more accurately measured. The specialist's interpretation of the entire character and course of the case would be expected at this time as well. This form (FT-8) transmitted to the Center by way of the State Health Department, was the last of the field investigations which provided the basis for clinical classification of the patient.

The cross-responsibilities and communication difficulties often resulted in delays in receipt of the reports, even when completed expeditiously by the physical therapist. The consultant's diagnosis and comments were often difficult to obtain and the records of muscle evaluation not infrequently were simply not forwarded promptly.

4. Fatal Cases. It was requested that any fatality in the study population be reported by telephone to the Evaluation Center and that every effort be made to obtain a complete autopsy, central nervous system tissue, and other specimens for laboratory study. Early in May, a special message was sent to all study areas asking that any fatal cases in inoculated children up to four weeks after last injection be given special attention. The Evaluation Center and the regional laboratory were to be notified immediately, and a complete post-mortem examination should be sought and made by a well-qualified pathologist with specimens provided to the laboratory. Clinical and epidemiological reviews were to be made. The Center offered to assist in obtaining the desired personnel if necessary and to meet expenses incurred in fulfilling the requirements.

5. Steps to Maintain Completeness of Investigation. The substantial amount of correspondence required very early in the trials concerning proper field follow-up and collection of specimens pointed up the fact that clarification of the needs was necessary beyond the printed instructions. Meetings were held in May and June in study areas with state and local health officials, state and local NFIP representatives, and interested hospital personnel in 32 of the 44 states in the trials. At these meetings staff members of the Evaluation Center reviewed the requirements for follow-up and the local plans for this phase of the operation.

By July the pattern of the deficiencies in case studies had become quite apparent, and steps were taken to correct them. Physician's interpretation and signature as required on the FT-7 and FT-8 forms were frequently missing. Therefore, a form letter was developed which provided a convenient means for promptly requesting the missing information. Each participating laboratory was sent a list of all cases on record in their area and all reported specimen collections. Thereafter, a postcard reporting this information to the laboratory on all newly reported cases became standard operating procedure so that the laboratories would have a complete record of cases from whom specimens should be anticipated.

A system of logging each case by area was also put into effect at the Center. The log served several purposes. It provided a complete and compact record wherein receipt of the various forms required by the follow-up could be posted. At intervals during the latter part of the year a summary of the incomplete records in the log was mailed to each state health officer for any cases in his areas.

In an effort to point up the importance of getting qualified review and interpretation of reported cases on the FT-7 and FT-8 forms a general letter was mailed to all state health officers on August 27, re-emphasizing the need for a specialist's comments and interpretation on the back of the physical therapists' forms and asking that the professional status of the physician be indicated below his signature. In this letter the states were again reminded to furnish the Center the names and qualifications of the specialists they had selected for this purpose if they had not already done so.

Late in September it became evident that on receipt of case records attention to all phases of the investigation should be re-emphasized to the field and that the waiting period for each of the forms should be reduced. A form (VEC-31) was developed for this purpose as a Special Attention note sent on each case, showing the dates on which each report was due in the office of the Evaluation Center. The request for specialist's comments, signature, and status was stressed by a quote from the VEC letter on this subject clipped to the VEC-31 forms.

After the middle of November lists again were prepared showing missing data and sent to state health officers requesting immediate action. Telephone calls were made to a number of the areas.

As of December 31, a tally of the incomplete study cases showed that there were approximately 290 incomplete study cases out of a total of 1103 reported. An intensive follow-up by telegram, telephone, letter, and field visit was made during January, and the open cases were reduced to 78 as of January 31. The last of the delinquent reports was not received until March 9, 1955.

Formulation of Criteria for Diagnostic Interpretation

It became apparent early in the examination of case records that a substantial body of data would need to be reviewed before generalizations and limits of variation could be established. Moreover, this must be done by repeated examination of the accumulating data without respect to the vaccination status of the patient. The policy was adopted that effort should be made to establish criteria on the basis of objective analysis, to formulate them clearly, and to apply them to each case before any attempt was made to divide cases into vaccinated or control groups. Consequently, attention and effort was concentrated on obtaining complete and reliable data. The data from each report were reduced to punched cards from which in turn mass listings and tabulations could be made for study. Since there was a minimal interval of three months between the onset of a case and receipt of the final report, the complete data accumulated slowly. Nevertheless, as significant amounts became available the compiled data were subjected to careful study. Once again, it is important to emphasize that this was not an evaluation of data from a single investigative unit, but from many sources; and while the procedures employed were basically standardized, qualitative and quantitative variation was quite evident. Interpretation must, of necessity, accept that fact.

Definition of Paralytic Status and Severity

The physical therapist's examination was recorded on two forms (FT-7 and FT-8) which listed muscles or muscle groups on the basis of their anatomical mass, rather than by functional importance. The examiner was to enter a standardized estimate of the degree of impairment for each unit, grading from normal through five increasing degrees of severity: good, fair, poor, trace, or no power. Involvement of muscles supplied by cranial nerves and of the muscles of respiration was recorded with limited score without grade of severity. It became evident that special problems existed: the neck and abdominal muscles are obviously affected by muscular spasm and pain; asthenia of illness made the significance of minor muscular weakness difficult to determine. It was necessary, then, to adopt criteria uninfluenced by other data, defining what extent of involvement would be required in order to consider a patient to be "paralytic" and, conversely, what would categorize the patient as "nonparalytic". In reaching the conclusions, Doctors Bennett, Green, Hodes, Top, and Wright gave continuously of their time and expert judgment. They intensively reviewed tabulated data of muscle examinations, both early and late, unexposed and hence uninfluenced by other clinical details, the laboratory findings or the vaccination status of the cases.

A. Minimal criteria for classification of a reported case as paralytic were then adopted.
1) The following would be excluded: a) Abdominal and neck muscles graded, bilaterally, good or fair. b) Other muscles graded bilaterally good. c) Record of hoarse voice without supporting evidence or comment. A check mark indicating deviation of the palate without supporting evidence or comment. d) All ratings of good would be eliminated from scoring.
2) The following would be accepted as significant: a) Spotty asymmetrical involvement with a grading of good recorded on either first or second muscle examination, in muscles characteristically affected by poliomyelitis: deltoid, triceps, finger extensors, opponens pollicis, gluteus medius, quadriceps, gastrocnemius, anterior tibialis. They would comprise Grade I of paralytic (spinal) without score. b) A grade of fair of a single muscle or single miracle group. It would receive the appropriate score. c) Definite indication of facial, laryngeal, pharyngeal involvement alone, or of palate with supporting evidence. It was decided to consider bulbar involvement independent of score.

Any of these involvements may have completely disappeared by time of the second examination or may be first recognized at time of the second examination. The physician's diagnosis and comments were of major value in these reviews.

The elimination of all good muscles from scoring, as well as muscles innervated by cranial nerves, and respiratory muscles would provide for a maximal score of 440. However, all tabulations have been arranged so that any scoring system can be employed for further analysis.

B. Further examination of the data resulted in the following classification of spinal paralytic involvement on what appeared to be group characteristics. Grade I might be termed "minimal paralytic without a score", and frequently such cases were questionable clinically. Grade II might be termed "minimal with a score".

Grade	Score
I	0
II	1-19
III	20-89
IV	90-199
V	200 +

C. An effort was also made to assign grades of severity to bulbar involvement apart from those specifically excluded.

Grade 1—listing of involvement by physical therapist without comment, minimal or doubtful.

Grade 2—one area of involvement with supporting comment or two areas commonly related—definite.

Grade 3—distinct difficulty swallowing including previous grades in combination. Other moderate involvement.

Grade 4—required tracheotomy in addition—or at times respirator.

Involvement of diaphragm and intercostals with or without use of respirator was considered independently.

Cases with spinal and bulbar involvement could be classified into grades of spinal involvement with the accompanying bulbar severity designated.

This, then, was adopted as the basis of classification according to paralytic status with which the data from other clinical reports and laboratory data would be integrated to furnish a final diagnosis. In 37 instances (9 percent) in the placebo areas the 10 to 20 day examination of the musculature was not done, and in 11 (3 percent) the second was not obtained; in the observed areas 81 (14 percent) first examinations and 19 (3 percent) of the second were not done.

Interpretation of Laboratory Investigations

Since the laboratories engaged in the diagnostic studies were also busily engaged in the testing of pre- and post-vaccination sera, and since a number of them had to develop facilities for the work, certain delays in obtaining the results of their studies were anticipated. By the end of October a limited number of complete reports had been received. The examination of stool specimens for virus had proceeded ahead of the serologic studies which of necessity awaited the receipt of a sample of convalescent blood. At the time the books had finally to be closed to new entries, the number of reports had mounted progressively so that the following record existed for cases occurring after mid-June 1954.

It must be recognized that omissions represent specimens which were unsatisfactory, others not received, as well as those which were not collected so that the uncompleted laboratory examinations represented a small number.

The results of tests for virus isolations were classified as positive, negative, no specimen or unsatisfactory, virus other than poliomyelitis, poliomyelitis virus of type unidentified, or test not done. From 72 patients viruses were recovered which have not been identified as poliomyelitis. Whether they are primary or coincidental infections is not completely determinable at this time.

Table 4. Status of laboratory data on all cases in study population.

Areas	Cases	Stool not done or not collected		Serology not done or not collected		No lab reports	
		No.	%	No.	%	No.	%
Placebo	428	56	13.1	80	18.7	14	3.3
Observed	585	101	17.3	92	15.7	44	7.5

Interpretation of serological studies was more complex. The reported results of neutralization tests done in tissue culture were subjected to analysis. The levels of titers obtained varied moderately among the laboratories.

From 426 patients, a typed poliomyelitis virus was recovered and in 376 of the instances serological tests were also done.

Reported isolations	Total		I		Virus type II		III	
	No.	%	No.	%	No.	%	No.	%
No. with virus recovered	426	100.0	238	55.9	53	12.4	135	31.7
No. with serologic test	376	88.3						

299 tests (79.5%) with paired sera—first obtained 14 days or less after onset.

67 tests (17.8%) with single or paired sera—first obtained 15 days or later after onset.

10 tests (2.7%) with single serum—obtained 14 days or less after onset.

Of the 299 tests in which the first serum was collected less than 15 days after onset, only 44 percent revealed a fourfold or greater rise in antibody to the homologous virus, but in 67 percent of these tests antibody to only the homologous virus was present in the patient's serum. In the other 67 tests the first serum or the only serum was obtained 15 days or more after the onset; they are considered to represent only the convalescent phase serologically. But when they were added to the previous group

the percentage of total with antibody to only specific type of virus isolated from the patient was still 67 percent. It is reasonable to conclude that the solitary antibody had resulted from the current virus infection, particularly since it specifically agreed with the type of virus recovered. It indicates, furthermore, prior to this illness those persons had no antibody to any of the three types of poliomyelitis virus. On the basis of these observations, while a rise in titer was considered a definite positive, a substantial level of antibody to the homologous virus only in first and second specimens, or in a late serum alone, without rise in titer was considered probably positive.

It is of interest, moreover, that in these data there is no indication that infection with one type of virus induces antibody to heterologous types in persons without previous experience, at least under the conditions of measurement employed.

When the first serum was obtained before the tenth day, a fourfold or greater rise was demonstrated in 47 percent of the second sera; thereafter, the frequency diminished progressively.

It is also clear that if the initial titer were 32 or less, in 78 percent of the second sera a fourfold or greater increase was noted while in only one-third of those with initial titers of 128 or more was this rise observed. Hence, the presence of titer of 32 or more to the homologous, even with low titers to other types, was considered suggestive. In the absence of virus isolation the probable and suggestive interpretation may be less secure because an illness resembling polio-

Table 5. Serologic rises in cases with virus isolation.[a]

Collection of first blood—days after onset	Total	4x rise; homologous type only	No rise or irregular changes	4x rise to more than one type	% 4x rise; homologous type only
Total	358	145	191	20	40.7
0–4	76	33	38	5	43.4
5–9	147	71	65	11	48.3
10–14	76	28	45	3	36.8
15–29	44	11	33	0	25.0
30 or more	13	2	10	1	15.4

[a] Includes only cases with two specimens of serum.

myelitis might occur in a patient who had earlier acquired antibody against a single type of virus, but it can be accepted that if the acute illness now observed was poliomyelitis the type of virus is, by these criteria, serologically indicated.

The following criteria for interpretation of serologic results were drawn up:

Table 6. Serologic rises in cases with virus isolation according to level of first serum specimen.[a]

Level of first serum	Total	4x rise; homologous type only	No rise	% 4x rise
16 or less	46	40	6	87
32 or less	80	62	18	77.5
64 or less	108	79	29	73.1
128 or more	150	51	99	34

[a] Excludes 18 cases with unsatisfactory serological tests, 6 cases with no antibody in acute or convalescent serum, 20 cases with fourfold rise to more than one type, and 54 cases with first blood collected after 14 days.

A. With Poliomyelitis Virus Isolated:

1) Positive. Fourfold or greater rise to homologous type only.

2) Probably positive. Antibody present at level of 16 or more in first and second sera to homologous type only without rise; in convalescent serum 15 days or later when earlier specimen was not obtained.

3) Suggestive: a) Level of 32 or more to homologous type; present at low levels to heterologous type. b) Twofold rise to homologous type only.

4) Indeterminate: a) Only acute stage serum available; less than 10 days. b) Multiple antibodies; no distinctive change, or irregular changes up or down. c) Fourfold rise to more than one type.

5) Negative: a) No antibody to any type in first and second sera or in second serum alone. b) Low levels, 4 to 8, to one or more types; no rise.

6) Inconsistent. Did not agree with type of virus reported.

7) Reports of serologic evidence of other etiology.

B. No Isolation of Poliomyelitis Virus or No Test for Virus:

1) Positive. Fourfold or greater rise to one type of virus only.

2) Possibly positive or suggestive—the criteria called probably positive under A above, when limited to one type only with or without twofold rise. Also—high level to one type with or without two-fold rise and low levels to other types.

3) Suggestive: a) Level of 32 or more to homologous type; present at low levels to heterologous type. b) Twofold rise to homologous type only.

4) Indeterminate: a) Only acute stage serum available; less than 10 days. b) Multiple antibodies; no distinctive change, or irregular changes up or down. c) Fourfold rise to more than one type.

5) Negative: a) No antibody to any type in first and second sera or in second serum alone. b) Low levels, 4 to 8, to one or more types; no rise.

6) Inconsistent. Did not agree with type of virus reported.

7) Reports of serologic evidence of other etiology.

C. When other virus alone is reported, criteria B were followed. It is not certain at present to what extent those reports represent other viruses alone, or mixtures. The latter have been demonstrated in some instances. In addition, typings have sometimes been obtained only after monkey passage.

D. In some laboratories studies of the family associates have been conducted. When virus was isolated from the family and not from the patient, criteria A were employed.

Integration of Data for Final Diagnosis

Although the frequency with which virus was isolated tended to increase with increasing clinical severity of illness, the failure to recover virus from a significant number of characteristic paralytic cases indicates that lack of virus isolation is not sufficient at this time to eliminate the patient from classification as poliomyelitis. Consequently, a combination of clinical findings, muscle evaluation, and laboratory data have been utilized in arriving at the final classification—but it should be re-emphasized that this was done without information of the vaccination status of the patient. The criteria for classifying illness other than paralytic polio (see pages 847, 848) were then formulated

A. Not Poliomyelitis: Those cases where the clinical record and comments or later communication indicated other disease.

Cases with lack of common symptoms or signs of poliomyelitis and examination of spinal fluid negative or not done.

Cases in which orphan viruses, or Coxsackie virus only were isolated, or serological evidence of active infection with mumps virus.

Cases with no antibody to poliomyelitis virus detected.

B. Non-paralytic Poliomyelitis: It is recognized that this is a difficult group to define, shading gradually into cases in the minimal paralytic class. They were cases called poliomyelitis by the physician, exhibiting characteristic clinical features, with positive spinal fluid, with or without virus isolation or positive serology but without presenting significant evidence of muscular impairment.

C. Doubtful Poliomyelitis: There remains a group which on careful review of all data leaves a decision in doubt as to whether they are poliomyelitis.

D. Fatal Cases: In these instances great effort was made to obtain an adequate record of the patient's history and course, to urge post-mortem examination, and to obtain a complete report. When possible histological sections were obtained for review by consultants. In some instances the examination was conducted after embalming and specimens for laboratory study were only then obtained. In others, the post-mortem was done without obtaining laboratory specimens; in others, no autopsy was done.

Diagnosis of poliomyelitis was based upon history of characteristic severe disease, histologic evidence described by a well-qualified pathologist, with or without isolation of virus.

Cases were considered not to be poliomyelitis on the basis of history indicating specifically other disease, major pathologic evidence at post-mortem of other disease, and lack of characteristic changes in the bulb or spinal cord. No poliomyelitis virus was recovered from these cases.

Controls in Observed Control Areas

The data from many investigations have indicated that infection with poliomyelitis virus occurs at an earlier age in lower socioeconomic groups than in the higher. Certain factors related to these characteristics might be involved in the decision as to whether parents requested participation of their children in the vaccination program and thus affect the composition of the groups. Therefore, differences in susceptibility related to these variations among the participants and non-participants might be encountered in the study population. Accordingly, at the request of the Evaluation Center, the Survey Research Center, University of Michigan, in December 1954, conducted a survey of the educational level, health consciousness, living conditions, and community activities of a portion of the study population in 10 of the 11 placebo control states. A sample of 1300 families of study members was carefully selected so as truly to represent the total study population of these areas. Eleven hundred two families were interviewed; 665 being participants, 56 who requested participation initially but failed to attend clinic, and 381 who did not request participation.

Interviews were conducted by trained interviewers who had no specific knowledge as to the underlying purpose of the study and hence were not biased in their questioning, nor were the respondents aware that the questioning was related to poliomyelitis or the field trial in any way.

Among other things the schedule of questions dealt with the following items of information: size of family, frequency of illness, use of medical services, parental appraisal of child's health, attitude toward prophylactic inoculations and extent of their use in the study child, knowledge about poliomyelitis, physical facilities of the home, parents' extra-household or community activities, parental occupation and educational level, age of mother, annual income, and an assessment of living conditions and of the type of neighborhood. There is much of interest in the details of this survey report; however, for the purpose here, it is sufficient to summarize by itemizing those factors which seemed to be positively correlated with participation in the field trial. The following differences in the participating groups compared with non-participants were significant at the 99 percent level of confidence.

1. The frequency of vaccination against smallpox, diphtheria, and whooping cough strongly correlated with participation.
2. Participants more frequently stated that "shots always work" than non-participants.

3. Mothers of participants were more likely to spend two or more evenings a week in outside activities than were mothers of non-participants.

4. Mothers of participants were more likely to have completed high school than mothers of non-participants.

5. A much smaller percentage of participants had family incomes under $4500. Participation rate increased steadily with increasing income.

6. Finally, the interviewer's rating of the quality of the respondent's neighborhood and condition of his house was highly correlated with participation status. Participants lived in better neighborhoods, and their homes were better kept.

Another refinement in the analysis dealt with the extent of participation according to the same characteristics but subclassified as to whether the child was a member of a high, medium or low participation school. These findings have interest in connection with the question of motivation but add little clarification of the basic question. The results together with an appreciation of the possible existence of other unknown factors bearing on poliomyelitis incidence, which might influence to a different extent the participants and non-participants, led certain consultants of the Evaluation Center to suggest that in observed control areas the unvaccinated members of the second grade be combined with the vaccinated population to form the test group for comparison with the combined first and third grade populations as controls. However, it was deemed preferable by the staff of the Evaluation Center, before analyses were begun, to employ as the control population in observed areas that which was originally announced to the states at the time they enrolled in the study, namely, a comparison of the poliomyelitis experience in vaccinated second grade children with the combined experience in the total first and third grades. It is difficult to combine incidence in vaccinated and unvaccinated populations and have a clear view of the effect in the vaccinated alone.

Other alternative procedures were considered and discarded, such as the use as control that portion of the first and third grades which signified willingness to participate, through submission of a parental consent form. This would seem to be the ideal group for comparison with the vaccinates. Unfortunately, the accuracy of data on participation status of first and third grade children varied greatly from area to area.

SUMMARY OF ESTIMATES OF EFFECTIVENESS OF VACCINE

In an effort to give summary expression to the differences observed between the incidence of poliomyelitis in vaccinated and control subjects through the different stages of analysis which have been presented the accompanying table was compiled. It is arranged in four stages of analysis which sought progressively to eliminate certain cases which might be considered less conclusively established as poliomyelitis. . . .

As a first step, the data comprising the total cases reported, total cases of poliomyelitis, total non-paralytic, and total paralytic in both placebo and observed control areas were subjected to this examination. Through these stages of purification there is a progressive increase in the percentage of effectiveness displayed. There was no significant difference in the non-paralytic cases and any estimate of possible effect on their rate of occurrence was unreliable. When they and the cases considered not to be poliomyelitis are removed so that paralytic cases only remain, an estimate of 72 percent effectiveness was obtained in the placebo areas and 62 percent in the observed areas.

Because the data indicate that the cases classified as bulbo-spinal paralytic are somewhat more definite clinically and yield a higher percentage of virus recoveries, the second stage was to separate the spinal paralytic cases from the bulbo-spinal. The number of pure bulbar cases was too small to work with properly. In placebo areas effectiveness calculated against spinal paralytic cases was 60 percent with a lower limit of 39 percent; against the bulbo-spinal patients it was 94 percent with a lower limit of 81 percent—an extremely successful effect. In observed areas the calculated effectiveness was about the same against the spinal cases but only 50 percent and a lower limit of 19, in the bulbo-spinal group. These variations emphasize the influence of small numbers in addition to any differences in severity of risk among placebo and observed study populations.

Because the group classified as paralytic poliomyelitis, especially in the mild grades, may

Table 7. Estimates of effectiveness of vaccine at successive stages of analysis.

Diagnostic classification	Placebo study areas					Observed study areas				
	No. of cases		Signif-icance level	Percentage effectiveness		No. of cases		Signif-icance level	Percentage effectiveness	
	Vacc'd	Controls		Est.	Lower limit	Vacc'd	Controls		Est.	Lower limit
I. Total cases reported	82	162	<0.001	49	36	76	439	<0.001	44	32
Total poliomyelitis	57	142	<0.001	60	49	56	391	<0.001	54	32
All paralytic	33	115	<0.001	72	61	38	330	<0.001	62	51
All non-paralytic	24	27	NS	—	—	18	61	NS	—	—
II. Paralytic-Spinal	28	70	<0.001	60	39	20	199	<0.001	66	53
Bulbo-Spinal	2	36	<0.001	94	31	15	100	<0.001	50	19
III. Laboratory confirmed										
Spinal	3	45	<0.001	82	65	7	127	<0.001	83	64
Bulbo-Spinal	2	23	<0.001	91	68	9	71	<0.01	60	23
IV. All virus positive										
Total	15	70	<0.001	80	65	20	210	<0.001	69	56
Type I	13	39	<0.001	68	41	14	114	<0.001	62	33
Type II	0	6	<0.05	100	33	2	34	<0.01	80	33
Type III	2	25	<0.001	92	72	4	62	<0.001	78	47

The difference in distribution of non-paralytic cases is not significant at any stage of analysis.
Because of small numbers the bulbar and fatal cases are omitted.
All fatal cases occurred in controls.

contain cases which are not related to poliomyelitis virus, the next tests were conducted with cases which had been demonstrated by laboratory studies to have undergone infection with poliomyelitis virus. They represented a higher degree of confidence in diagnosis. The cases were again divided into spinal and bulbo-spinal groups. The effectiveness of vaccine measured against the incidence of spinal-paralytic cases was the same in placebo and observed areas, 82 and 83 percent respectively, and the corresponding lower limits of estimated effect were 65 and 64, respectively. Enforcement of laboratory criteria apparently eliminated a substantial number of cases which were less influenced by vaccination and in reality, may contain cases which are not poliomyelitis. As in the preceding analysis, the effectiveness measured by bulbo-spinal cases in placebo areas was 91 percent but that in observed areas was but 60 percent and the significance of difference between vaccinated and control groups was sharply reduced.

The next step was to seek a measurement of the effectiveness of vaccine in all cases of poliomyelitis from whom a specifically identified type of virus was recovered. Serologic data alone were not accepted. In this manner the effectiveness of vaccine against infection with the different types might be evaluated. In the placebo areas effectiveness of 68 percent against Type I, 100 percent with .05 significance against Type II, and 92 percent against Type III were demonstrated. This clearly agrees with the previous demonstrations that the lots of vaccine were generally less effective against disease caused by Type I virus. In cases related to identified virus of all three types an effectiveness of 80 percent was noted. A measure of the effectiveness of different lots of vaccine is not included here although definite differences exist. These data represent the composite results obtained with the various lots of vaccine used in the placebo areas.

In the observed areas the same trend was noted with respect to individual types or to the total but, as in most of the foregoing data, the calculated effectiveness was less than in the placebo areas.

From these data it is not possible to select a single value giving numerical expression in a

**Figure 1. Trend of paralytic cases among vaccinated children and their control groups
June 19, 1954 to December 31, 1954.**

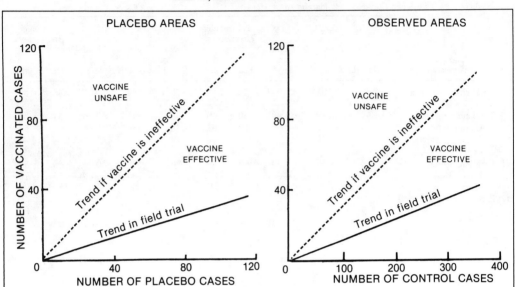

complete sense to the effectiveness of vaccine as a total experience. If the results from the observed study areas are employed the vaccine could be considered to have been 60-80 percent effective against paralytic poliomyelitis, 60 percent against Type 1 poliomyelitis, and 70 to 80 percent against disease caused by Types II and III.

There is, however, greater confidence in the results obtained from the strictly controlled and almost identical test populations of the placebo study areas. On this basis it may be suggested that vaccination was 80-90 percent effective against paralytic poliomyelitis; that it was 60 to 70 percent effective against disease caused by Type I virus and 90 percent or more effective against that of Type II and Type III virus. The estimate would be more secure had a larger number of cases been available.

THE SURVEILLANCE OF COMMUNICABLE DISEASES OF NATIONAL IMPORTANCE[1]

Alexander D. Langmuir[2]

In the introduction to his comprehensive report on the cholera epidemic of 1848-1849, William Farr *(1)*, that greatest of statistical epidemiologists, wrote, "If a foreign army had landed on the coast of England, seized all the seaports, . . . ravaged the population through the summer and . . . in the year it held possession of the country slain fifty-three thousand two hundred and ninety-three men, women and children, . . . the task of registering the dead would be inexpressibly painful; and the pain is not greatly diminished by the circumstance that in the calamity to be described the minister of destruction was a pestilence." He continued as follows:

In following cholera through its fatal way, the inquirer meets with some grounds for consolation. He sees places on every side which the epidemic passed over, leaving the inhabitants in the serene enjoyment of health and complete immunity. And the hope is perhaps not fallacious that an examination of the results of the . . . (invasion) may be the means of mitigating, if not preventing . . . (another); for whatever may be the immediate cause of cholera it will appear evident that in England it is only seriously fatal under certain known conditions which admit to a great extent to remedy.

He then goes on to admonish the reader not to accept the opinions expressed in the report as "ultimate results," but to place full reliance on the tabular data "because they have been derived directly from the returns."

These rather lengthy quotations, in Farr's flowery style, only inadequately reveal his true character. Throughout his forty years of public service as superintendent of the Statistical Department of the Registrar General's Office, his extraordinary productivity demonstrated his abiding faith that natural laws govern the occurrence of disease, that these laws can be discovered by orderly epidemiologic inquiry and that, when discovered, the causes of epidemics "admit to a great extent to remedy."

His was no ivory-tower existence. He accepted the responsibility of seeing that action was taken on the basis of his analyses. Through his weekly, quarterly, annual, and special reports he became an active protagonist in the great controversies of his time. He believed in the democratic tradition that making the facts known to those who need to know them is the basis of achieving effective action.

Farr's example set a standard for the development of vital statistics services throughout the world. Since his time only rarely, if ever, has his standard been met in terms of immediate, imaginative, practical use of statistics for the definition of current problems and their effective control.

During the past decade an effort has been made in this country to recapture some of the old and vital spirit of William Farr through the Program for the Surveillance of Communicable Diseases of National Importance. It is a distinct honor, which I deeply appreciate, to be granted the opportunity, as Cutter Lecturer for 1962, to recount the development of the present concepts of surveillance, to describe some of the main problems that have been encountered and to deign to look at some that can be anticipated in the near future. A glance at the scope of subjects embraced in the distinguished group of previous Cutter Lectures indicates that even in this age of worship of those symbols of modern medicine, the intravenous catheter and the milliequivalent, a paper dealing with the general practice of epidemiology is nonetheless within the spirit of this lectureship.

The term surveillance has been chosen advisedly to describe this program. The term is not new to public health, but its usual connotation has had application to individuals rather

Source: *New England Journal of Medicine* 268:182–192, 1963.
[1] The Cutter Lecture on Preventive Medicine, presented at Harvard School of Public Health, Boston, May 16, 1962.
[2] Chief, Epidemiology Branch, Communicable Disease Center, Public Health Service, United States Department of Health, Education, and Welfare.

than to diseases. Surveillance, when applied to a person, means close observation to detect the early signs of infection without restricting his freedom of movement. It implies maintaining a responsible alertness, making systematic observations and taking appropriate action when indicated. It does not involve the restrictions of either isolation or quarantine.

Surveillance, when applied to a disease, means the continued watchfulness over the distribution and trends of incidence through the systematic collection, consolidation and evaluation of morbidity and mortality reports and other relevant data. Intrinsic in the concept is the regular dissemination of the basic data and interpretations to all who have contributed and to all others who need to know. The concept, however, does not encompass direct responsibility for control activities. These traditionally have been and still remain with the state and local health authorities.

Elements of the present concept of surveillance are apparent in the early history of the United States Public Health Service and its Hygienic Laboratory. The brilliant field studies on plague, tularemia, Rocky Mountain spotted fever, poliomyelitis, pellagra, brucellosis, typhus and influenza developed in response to local problems of national importance. The halting efforts to establish an effective morbidity reporting system and the progressive but slow achievement of the Death Registration Area, which did not include the whole country until 1933, were basic steps toward a national surveillance program. However brilliant, these field studies were not systematic, and the morbidity and mortality reporting systems were largely conceived to have long-term documentary importance rather than to be epidemiologically significant indicators of current problems.

A fundamental change in the relation of the Public Health Service with the states was initiated in 1946 with the formation of the Communicable Disease Center. Starting with the war emergency organization known as Malaria Control in War Areas, the Center was conceived as becoming a large, well equipped and broadly staffed agency with the primary function of aiding the states in the control of communicable diseases *(2)*.

To discharge this responsibility, the Communicable Disease Center needed a systematic source of information regarding the communicable disease problems of the nation. The surveillance program has developed out of this need and has been shaped by the various problems and emergencies that have been encountered.

Summaries of experience with four diseases—malaria, poliomyelitis, influenza and hepatitis—will be illustrative.

THE MALARIA STORY

The first major national program that the Communicable Disease Center undertook was the Malaria Eradication Program, which was based on use of DDT indoor residual spraying in each of the 13 traditionally malarious states. Long experience and extensive surveys during the mid-1930s had established malaria as a deeply rooted endemic problem in rural sections of the Atlantic and Gulf Coastal Plains and of the Mississippi Delta area. Furthermore, many thousands of veterans of World War II returning from Africa, the Mediterranean, and the Pacific theaters were introducing peculiarly persistent, relapsing strains of *Plasmodium vivax*. Many of these veterans while on furlough, or after separation from the service, were returning to areas of long known endemicity. The fear of a resurgence or cyclical return of malaria was real to many experienced malariologists. The availability of DDT presented a challenging opportunity. A major control program was undertaken in collaboration with the states.

Actually, this extensive DDT spraying program was in operation well before effective epidemiologic services had been organized. A full, current evaluation of the extent of the problem had not been made. When epidemiologic studies were initiated in 1947 quite surprising findings were revealed. Simple appraisals of the morbidity and mortality reports indicated that these traditional measures were grossly erroneous. The highest reported incidence occurred in Mississippi, South Carolina, and Texas, but these three states followed the practice of requesting weekly reports of malaria by numbers of cases seen rather than by name of individual patient. Such a system encourages exaggeration. Efforts to substantiate the diagnoses by laboratory study consistently failed. Beginning in 1947, Mississippi changed its reporting requirements. The incidence dropped from 17 764 cases to only 914 in the first year, and appraisals among even these cases revealed that only a very few could be verified.

It became imperative to adopt new criteria to evaluate the presence of malaria. Laboratory findings were sufficient to confirm the existence of a bona fide case, but the occurrence of two or more cases in an epidemiologic relation to each other was the ultimate basis for determining endemic presence. These new criteria soon revealed that malaria had disappeared as an endemic disease from the South, probably before the DDT program had gotten underway *(3)*.

The major events of this extraordinary malaria story are revealed in Figure 1. The high, sustained level of 100 000 cases a year during the 1930s is generally believed to represent gross underreporting. Extensive WPA surveys at that time confirmed parasitemic rates or spleen indexes of 50 percent or higher, indicating extensive, largely unreported endemic infection.

As just mentioned, however, at some time between 1935 and 1945 malaria mysteriously disappeared, much more rapidly than either the reported morbidity or the mortality indicated. The slight rise in the morbidity curve in 1945 reflects the influx of infected veterans, but the steep decline in 1947 and subsequently is artificial and reflects the elimination of erroneous reports. The major decline clearly occurred earlier.

The sharp peak in the curve in 1951 and 1952 reflects the Korean War and the occurrence of several thousand cases among veterans who returned before the primaquine treatment for all returning servicemen was instituted.

In the past five years the incidence of reported malaria in the whole country has remained below 100 cases a year. Now, the states carry out a detailed epidemiologic investigation on each case and report to the Communicable Disease Center as part of an established and continuing Malaria Surveillance Program. Almost all the cases can clearly be accounted for as

Figure 1. Reported malaria morbidity and mortality in the United States, 1932-1961. (Source: Cases and Deaths, National Office of Vital Statistics.)

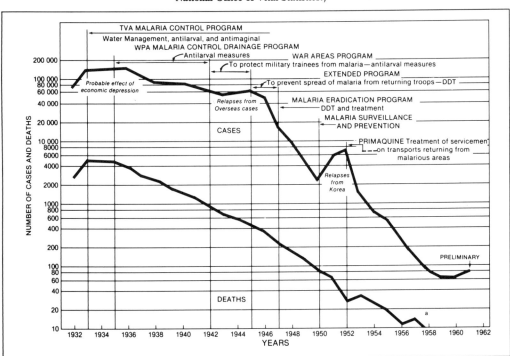

[a]In succeeding years starting with 1958 the total reported deaths were as follows: 1958 - 0, 1959 - 1, 1960 - 0, 1961 - 1.

importations. They occur throughout the country without relation to previously endemic areas. Only an occasional confirmed case arises that is explainable in no other way than being of indigenous origin.

The malaria story in this country should be a sobering one to epidemiologists and health administrators. Here, a disease deeply entrenched in large areas of the South disappeared within a single decade, largely, if not wholly, through natural processes rather than through planned public health measures. Even the fact of its disappearance was not appreciated until after a major control program had been in operation for several years. This experience was a major factor emphasizing the necessity of a more current and comprehensive system of surveillance.

POLIOMYELITIS

Early in its history the Communicable Disease Center became actively involved with poliomyelitis. A major first effort centered on fly control, both as an epidemic measure and a long-term control procedure. In 1953, a nationwide evaluation of gamma globulin was sponsored; the results showed the extremely limited usefulness of this measure for practical control *(4)*. In 1955, however, major plans for national surveillance of poliomyelitis developed.

With the heightening enthusiasm that the Francis Field Trial of the formaldehyde-inactivated vaccine would be successful an effort was made to anticipate the new problems that would be encountered. Two main ones were visualized: the possible failures of potency; and the confusion caused by other diseases simulating poliomyelitis. The thought that a problem of safety existed was considered but discarded. After all, this had been of serious concern the previous year, and the Francis Field Trial had been a massive human demonstration of safety.

Within two weeks of the announcement of the results of the Field Trial, a national crisis involving vaccine safety was at hand. On the evening of April 25, one case from Chicago and, during the day of April 26, five additional cases of paralytic poliomyelitis from various parts of California were reported among children who had received poliovaccine produced by a certain manufacturer. The interval between inoculation and onset of symptoms ranged from four to nine days. In each case first

paralysis had developed in the inoculated limb.

The explanation of these cases was not evident. Several different production lots were implicated. The detailed production protocols were in order. The intervals between inoculation and paralysis seemed short even for inoculation poliomyelitis in laboratory animals. The possibility that nonspecific provocation of paralysis had been induced among naturally infected children or that the six cases were merely coincidental infections unrelated to the vaccine was considered. Some epidemiologists, however, recognized the ominous signs of a common-source epidemic and feared the occurrence of many more cases in a predictable wave determined by the period of use of the implicated vaccine and the incubation period of inoculation poliomyelitis.

The Surgeon General, on the morning of April 27, requested the manufacturer to recall all outstanding lots of vaccine pending full inquiry. In this crisis the necessity for prompt and detailed epidemiologic case data on all vaccine-associated cases was crucial. On April 28 the Surgeon General directed the establishment of the Poliomyelitis Surveillance Program in the Communicable Disease Center.

All state health officers were requested to arrange for the prompt investigation of all cases of poliomyelitis occurring within their jurisdiction and to report details, particularly those related to prior poliomyelitis vaccination, by telephone or telegraph to the Poliomyelitis Surveillance Unit established in Atlanta. Virologists, clinicians and epidemiologists in official and academic positions also contributed to this national clearinghouse of information.

On May 1 the first Poliomyelitis Surveillance Report was mailed to a list of over 200 persons, including all those who had contributed data and all others who had responsibility or concern in poliomyelitis control. The report consisted primarily of a listing of the significant data on each vaccine-associated case. Thus, each reader could make his own analyses and reach his own conclusion upon which reliance could be placed, because, to quote Farr, the tabular data "had been derived directly from the returns."

For the next month a daily listing of information on new cases and corrections and supplements to previously reported data on old cases was issued to all persons on the mailing list. In addition, a weekly summary and analysis of the findings was prepared and distributed. These reports and analyses provided regular materials for news releases issued in the Office of the Surgeon General.

On April 27 the decision to request withdrawal of the vaccine was made on the basis of reports of six vaccine-associated cases. On the evening of May 1, four days later, when the first surveillance report was issued, 22 cases, associated with one brand of vaccine, had been recorded, and, in addition, three cases had been associated with a different brand.

On May 7 the count had risen to 42 cases associated with one brand and seven cases associated with other vaccines. These cases were sharply concentrated in California and Idaho, where most of the particular vaccine had been used in clinics for schoolchildren in the first and second grades. However, a small amount of the vaccine had been distributed commercially throughout a large part of the country, and cases associated with the vaccine had been reported from 11 additional states.

The common-source character of the problem was becoming abundantly clear. More than 80 percent of the cases could now be related to one brand of vaccine, which comprised less than 10 percent of the total vaccine distributed. The small number of cases reported in association with other brands of vaccines occurred at a frequency well within normal expectancy for the time of the year. These did not reveal localization of first paralysis to the site of inoculation, and the intervals from inoculation to onset were scattered and did not peak in a normal incubation-period curve. A relation of these vaccines to the cases, therefore, was not indicated.

Thus, each day as more information accumulated, the problem came into sharper focus. It became increasingly clear that a particular brand of vaccine was involved rather than the vaccines of all manufacturers. Although a thorough review of all production and safety procedures was clearly demanded and, in fact, was already in progress at the time, the other vaccine manufacturers were encouraged to stay in production. If the surveillance program had not been in existence and the epidemiologic pattern had not been so distinct, many and perhaps all vaccine manufacturers would probably have ceased production altogether.

By the end of the first week in May it seemed that the problem had been reasonably confined, and the occurrence of less than 100 total vaccine-related cases could be predicted with reasonable confidence. There were, however, disturbing reports, the significance of which was not clear. In California and Idaho health officials were making inquiries about the frequency of ill-defined minor febrile illnesses that seemed to be occurring among vaccinated children a few days to a week after inoculation. Although these illnesses were clinically quite nondescript, the time of their occurrence was unusual for a nonspecific type of vaccine reaction. The possibility that they represented abortive infections with the Mahoney strain of poliovirus and were thus infectious to others was a disquieting thought.

On May 8 a twenty-eight-year-old housewife from Tennessee, while visiting in Atlanta, was diagnosed as having poliomyelitis. She had not received vaccine, but her two children had been inoculated with the suspect brand of vaccine two weeks earlier and had had attacks of "tonsillitis," for which they had been given penicillin. On May 10 a similar case occurred in Atlanta.

It was a most remarkable and fortuitous coincidence that both these cases occurred in Atlanta, where only a little of the involved brand of vaccine had been used. Actually, the information was reported informally to the Communicable Disease Center before it reached local health officials. Immediate checks were made with the epidemiologists in California and Idaho, where the largest number of such contact cases would be expected to occur if they were going to occur at all. By noon on May 10, Atlanta time, no such cases were known, but, by evening, both states knew that they had a problem. The timely alert from Atlanta illustrates the importance of the two-way flow of information that is intrinsic to national surveillance.

The major events of April and May, 1955, are summarized in Figure 2, which shows the epidemic curves of the vaccinated and family-contact cases along with an explanation of the early predictions of the extent of the problem.

The middle curve shows the dates of onset of paralysis of the 61 vaccine-associated cases. The first occurred on April 23, and the peak was on April 27. However, new cases continued into May, with a few, perhaps of doubtful vaccine relation, appearing at the end of May. The 80 paralytic family-contact cases are somewhat more disperse. The first two cases had onsets on April 30 and May 1 and were followed by cases throughout May and into June. The later appearance and greater dispersal of the family-contact cases can presumably be related to the double incubation period involved. There is the time necessary for the inoculated child to incubate the infection to the point of becoming a spreader, and then there is the time of the normal incubation in the infected contact.

The predicted curves were determined by application of the experimental data of Bodian on the incubation period of inoculation poliomyelitis in cynomolgus macaques, shown in the top curve in Figure 2, to the hypothetical distribution of the use of the vaccine. This distribution

Figure 2. Poliomyelitis associated with vaccine of one manufacturer, April–June 1955.

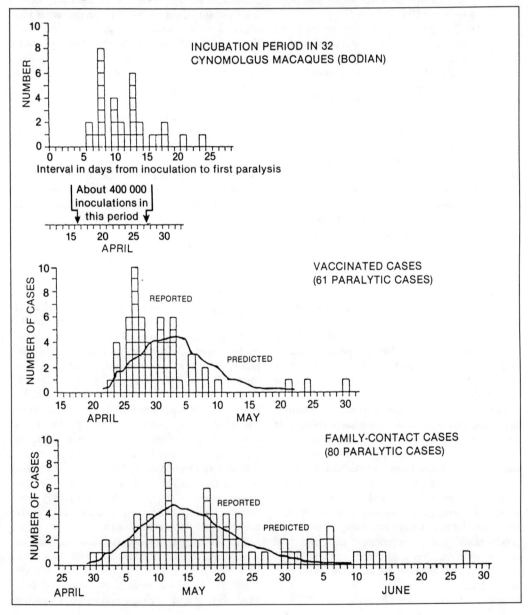

was not known precisely, but the vaccine first became available on April 14 and was withdrawn on April 27. About 400 000 doses were distributed during this interval. For simplicity, a horizontal distribution of use of this vaccine was assumed.

By the end of the first week of May the shape of the epidemic curve of the 42 cases so far reported justified the conclusion that a total of less than 100 vaccine-associated cases would occur. By the end of the second week of May, when nine family-contact cases had been recorded, a rough prediction that the total would reach or somewhat exceed 100 was made. Actually, the final totals were, for vaccine-associated cases, 79, with 61 paralytic, and for family-contact cases, 105, with 80 paralytic (5).

Much attention has been devoted to the poliomyelitis events of the spring of 1955 for two reasons: they have been reported from the epidemiologic point of view only to a limited extent; and the experience during the emergency and the relations that developed of necessity between the Communicable Disease Center and the states and many other collaborating laboratories and agencies throughout the country were decisive in the formation of the Communicable Disease Center Surveillance Program.

The surveillance of poliomyelitis has continued. Regular reports are issued weekly during the poliomyelitis season and at intervals of three to four weeks in the winter. The mailing list has expanded to include more than 700 persons. All the states cooperate to the fullest extent by submitting an individual case record giving, in addition to general identifying data, the critically important vaccine history. Approximately sixty days later the state submits a supplementary report giving verification of diagnosis, presence and extent of residual paralysis and laboratory data when known. The reporting is believed to be essentially complete. In the past several years sixty-day residual reports have been submitted on more than 90 percent of the total number of cases originally reported. The regular tabulations and analyses of these data have been of inestimable value in guiding both day-by-day decisions and broad future plans for progress toward the control and eventual elimination of poliomyelitis.

The progress in the past seven years since release of the vaccine is depicted in Figure 3. All the problems originally anticipated in planning for poliomyelitis surveillance, notably the questions of potency and of diseases simulating poliomyelitis, have been encountered in full measure. These problems have been faced and resolved.

Before the subject of poliomyelitis is set aside, however, one broad question deserves mention because it involves the niceties of epidemiologic analysis that are always interesting and often

Figure 3. Annual incidence rates of poliomyelitis in the United States, 1935–1961 (Source: National Office of Vital Statistics).

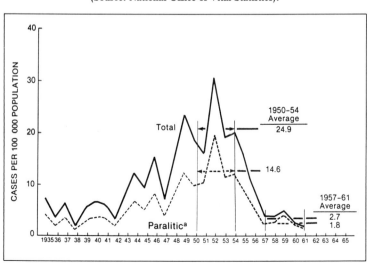

aParalytic cases prior to 1951 assumed to be 50% of total.

argumentative. Figure 2 shows the rising trend of poliomyelitis that began in the early 1940s and continued upward to the early 1950s. In the past seven years the trend has been sharply downward, with a slight interruption in 1958 and 1959.

The interpretation of this curve is in question. Can the decline of the past seven years be confidently attributed to the widespread use of poliovaccine, or is there some other explanation such as a spontaneous decline due to a long-term natural periodicity of unknown character? Such an idea could suggest that the vaccine program had little or no effect. It would also indicate that poliomyelitis might recur in severe epidemic form during the next cycle. The question is valid, and the implications serious.

It is my opinion that there is no sound basis for the hypothesis of long-term cycles in poliomyelitis in large populations. To be sure, in limited populations, such as single states or small countries, epidemics of great severity have occurred in certain years preceded and followed by periods of relatively low incidence. In large populations such as the whole United States or other continental land masses, however, no cyclical pattern has been manifest. On the contrary, the increasing trends of poliomyelitis in the 1940s and 1950s were part of a worldwide phenomenon related to the advancing standard of living and the increasing birth rate that followed the Great Depression. The commonly accepted explanation is that with better housing, suburban living, greater access to soap and water and greatly improved care of infants, the time of first exposure to the once ubiquitous polioviruses has been progressively postponed to an age where the risk that paralysis will develop is greater. Nothing has happened in this country during the past seven years to change these basic ecologic relations. On the contrary, there has been progressive improvement in the standard of living.

Hence, all the evidence would have supported the prediction of a continuing upward trend in incidence during the late 1950s and early 1960s if no other factor such as the poliovaccine program had been introduced to affect the picture. No evidence supports a decline. Therefore, to select the five-year average incidence from 1950 to 1954 as a level for comparison with current figures is conservative. This average for paralytic cases was 22 706,

giving a rate of 14.6 per 100 000. The average for the five-year period 1957 to 1961 was 3249 cases, giving a rate of 1.8. This constitutes a reduction in rates of 87.4 percent. This reduction very substantially, if not entirely, can be attributed to the poliovaccine program.

INFLUENZA

Beginning with the work of Frost *(6)* during and after the 1918 pandemic of influenza, the Public Health Service has had a long interest in the descriptive epidemiology of influenza. The extended studies of Collins *(7)* involving both morbidity surveys and analyses of excess mortality are notable. Incidentally, Farr *(8)* used this technique in 1847. It was only in 1957, however, that the Public Health Service undertook a position of active leadership in an attempt to control influenza.

With the reports of epidemic influenza originating within China and spreading out from Hong Kong, and with the identification of the A_2 (Asian) strain as being immunologically distinct, the long anticipated world pandemic was clearly at hand. The Surgeon General directed that a comprehensive national program be undertaken *(9)*. This included urging the pharmaceutical manufacturers to embark on a crash program of production of monovalent vaccine using the new Asian strain. The American Medical Association, the American Hospital Association and the Association of State and Territorial Health Officers joined in conducting an educational program for physicians, hospital staffs and health workers to prepare for the anticipated emergency. A program of influenza surveillance assigned to the Communicable Disease Center was an intrinsic part of this national plan.

In mid-June all epidemiologists on the staff of the Center were alerted to emergency field duty. All state health department laboratories and many laboratories collaborating in the WHO International Influenza Center for the Americas conducted by the Virus and Rickettsia Laboratory of the Communicable Disease Center were also alerted. The central services of the Laboratory and the availability of standard strains and diagnostic antisera were made generally known.

On July 9 the first formal influenza surveillance report was issued as a joint undertaking of the Epidemiology and Laboratory branches of the Communicable Disease Center. Thereafter, the report came out twice weekly throughout the summer months, and then weekly when the epidemic was under way. The report presented extensive summaries of descriptive epidemiologic data as the information came in. Laboratory findings were added as they became available. Summaries of the international spread of the infection were a major feature.

Maintaining surveillance over a disease such as epidemic influenza involving up to tens of millions of cases on a national basis presented special statistical problems. The reporting and counting of individual cases, a practice still followed in some areas, is obviously cumbersome, slow, and of limited value. Several more effective indexes were used. These included the following:

Simple narrative reports of epidemics and outbreaks.

Newspaper reports of the recognized prevalence of influenza in a city or a county as measured by closing of schools or increased absenteeism in industry.

Systematic reports of absenteeism among the employees of a large, nationwide public-service industry.

Current analyses of excess mortality from influenza and pneumonia reported weekly by 108 cities.

Current analyses of acute-respiratory-illness rates in the National Health Survey.

The full account of the 1957 pandemic of Asian influenza has been published (9–11). The first outbreaks were recognized early in June among the crews of naval ships at Newport, Rhode Island, and independently at several bases in California. Spread was most apparent in California when sharp outbreaks occurred in shore-based naval personnel and among groups of students attending youth-guidance camps and special conferences where large numbers of persons were congregated in crowded places.

On June 26 a group of 1688 delegates from 43 states and a foreign country convened at a church conference in Grinnell, Iowa. The college facilities used normally housed about 800 students. A group of 100 delegates from California had chartered a railroad coach for the trip. Cases of influenza developed en route. On arrival, these 100 delegates were carefully and systematically intermingled among the remaining 1600 in a true spirit of togetherness.

The ensuing epidemic was explosive. By July 1 about 200 clinical cases of influenza had occurred. The conference was wholly disrupted, and the separate delegations, each now well seeded with the infection, began returning to their homes, thus further disseminating the new strain of virus throughout the country.

The Grinnell conference undoubtedly was only a single, if vivid, example of the manner of spread and of the extensive seeding of the new virus that must have occurred. Throughout the summer, however, with few exceptions influenza outbreaks remained confined to crowded population groups. They did not tend to spread on a community-wide basis.

One of these exceptions occurred in Tangipahoa Parish, Louisiana, where schools open early in August so that the children can be released for strawberry-picking time in the spring. Sudden outbreaks developed in these schools within two weeks of opening. This experience was a harbinger of events to follow when the normal pattern of school attendance began in early September (12).

The advance seeding had been sufficient. By mid-September epidemics, largely among schoolchildren, appeared simultaneously in all parts of the country. No longer was it possible to trace spread as it had been, so vividly, in June and July. Reports received by the Influenza Surveillance Unit revealed that the epidemic had involved the whole country by the middle of December.

The experiences in 1957 with the Asian-influenza pandemic, and with the subsequent epidemics, have refocused attention on the necessity of taking organized action for more effective control. Influenza-pneumonia mortality in 108 cities of the United States is shown in Figure 4 for the period from mid-1956 to April, 1962. The two waves of mortality of the Asian pandemic in 1957–58 stand out. Only a small excess mortality occurred the next year. This was related to activity, both of the A_2 and B strains. From January to March, 1960, a sharp influenza A_2 epidemic occurred. It was particularly severe in Southern California, which had been largely spared in 1957. The winter of 1960–61 was essentially free of epidemic influ-

Figure 4. Pneumonia-influenza deaths in 108 United States cities (prepared by Dr. Robert E. Serfling, Chief, Statistics Section, Epidemiology Branch, Communicable Disease Center).

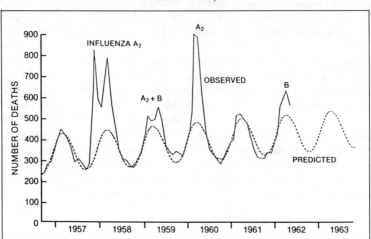

enza, but, during the winter of 1961–62, influenza B was widely epidemic; in fact, the severity of this epidemic as measured by excess mortality was the highest of any influenza B epidemic since 1936.

Although influenza-pneumonia mortality is the most sensitive index for describing influenza epidemics, these figures do not truly reflect the full toll of the disease. Influenza is often fatal to the aged and the chronically ill, although a wide variety of diagnoses may appear on the death certificates. Excess total mortality is, without doubt, a more accurate measure of the costs in terms of death attributable to influenza. Taking the six-month period from October to March, 1957–58, and the three-month period from January to March, 1960, together, excess total mortality amounts to 86 000 deaths. Approximately two thirds of these patients were sixty-five years of age or older, and 25 percent were from forty-five to sixty-four years of age. Only a third of the cases were classified in the death records as influenza pneumonia; half were charged to cardiovascular-renal disease, and 15 percent to all other causes.

This impressive fact of 86 000 excess deaths is the basis for the recommendation of the Surgeon General's Advisory Committee on Influenza Control to urge the annual immunization of the aged and the chronically ill. Since it is recognized that many recent studies have dem-

onstrated the protective value of present influenza vaccines, it is most reasonable to assume that the immunization of those at greatest risk of dying would provide a firm measure of protection. It is not visualized that mass immunization campaigns are warranted, but rather annual immunization of the aged and chronically ill should become an accepted routine of good medical and geriatric practice.

HEPATITIS

The story of hepatitis from the public health point of view illustrates the degree to which the rigidities of tradition, the fickleness of fashion and the lack of systematic epidemiologic data can fetter progress. This disease, or rather this mixture of specific diseases, has long been recognized as a major military health problem, sometimes decisive in campaigns, yet only in the past 10 to 15 years have health authorities accepted the problem as coming within their sphere of activity. Not until 1950 did the disease become commonly reportable, and only in 1954 was it universally reportable in all states.

Beginning in 1950, the Communicable Disease Center took an active part in epidemiologic field investigations of hepatitis. Many outbreaks spread by contact, and a few waterborne epidemics were described. Efforts were made to evaluate gamma globulin in the prophylaxis of the disease, with limited success. Some retrospective analysis of morbidity and mortality statistics helped to characterize the problem *(13)*, but no systematic surveillance was undertaken until 1960. At first, quarterly reports summarizing current trends and reporting significant news were issued; more recently a monthly schedule of reporting has been attempted.

Events of considerable consequence have occurred in profusion during the past two years. The year 1961 was a record year, with 72 000 cases being reported. The seriousness of serum hepatitis resulting from faulty sterilization techniques was vividly shown in an outbreak involving over 40 cases and 15 deaths in one physician's practice. The importance of raw shellfish, both oysters and clams, as an occasional factor in the spread of infectious hepatitis was established for the first time in this country. These and other events have come to recognition at least in part as a result—and in several cases as a direct result—of the surveillance program, at both the state and national levels.

Figure 5 shows the incidence of reported cases of hepatitis from 1954 to the present. Note the seasonal swing, with highest frequency occurring during winter months and lowest frequency during the summer. A seven-year periodicity is also evident; peaks occurred in 1954 and 1961. Such a rhythmic pattern would have been fascinating to William Farr and all subsequent epidemic theorists, because relatively simple natural laws must govern such a regular phenomenon if only they could be divined.

A comparison of morbidity and mortality trends reveals one epidemiologic conclusion

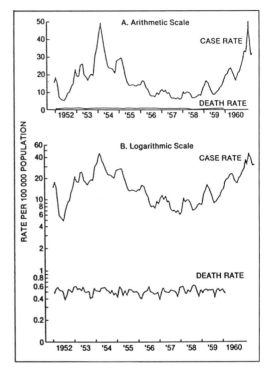

Figure 6. Case and death rates of viral hepatitis in the United States, 1952-1960 (monthly rate adjusted to an annual base).

that is surprising to many. Figure 6 shows the reported monthly incidence rates, on both arithmetic and logarithmic scales, for cases and deaths ascribed to viral hepatitis from 1952 to 1962. Although the seasonal swing may vary as much as 3:1, and the range from peak to trough in the long-term periodicity varies as much as 7:1, the mortality rate throughout this period is essentially constant. No seasonal or periodic variation is apparent.

It is well recognized that the swings in the incidence curve reflect swings in the prevalence of infectious hepatitis. Included in the data also, of course, are an unknown number of cases of serum hepatitis probably occurring at a fairly constant rate. The constancy of the mortality curve reveals that most, if not all, deaths attributable to hepatitis must result from serum hepatitis and that infectious hepatitis is rarely, if ever, fatal.

In the late winter of 1961 Dr. William Dougherty, state epidemiologist in New Jersey, reported that the age incidence of hepatitis in his state was predominantly adult. He at first as-

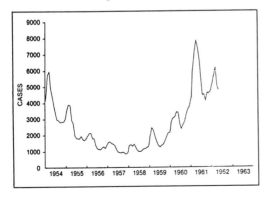

Figure 5. Reported cases of infectious hepatitis in the United States since 1954, according to four-week periods.

cribed this observation to his recent emphasis on reporting of communicable diseases by hospitals. Further investigation was recommended by the Communicable Disease Center, and it soon became apparent that the observation was real. Pediatricians were not seeing the disease; internists were. More intensive field investigations in selected areas of high adult incidence revealed that a high proportion of the patients, 50 percent or more, gave a history of consuming raw clams twenty to forty days before onset. Control data regarding similar eating of raw clams among adults residing in the same neighborhoods revealed consumption rates in the range of 15 percent or less.

The investigation was then expanded progressively to other areas, with similar results. Thus, raw clams could be incriminated, but the tracing of the sources of these contaminated clams proved more difficult. A joint team from New Jersey and the Communicable Disease Center, directed by Dr. D. A. Henderson, began tracing sources of several hundred cases. Slowly, the evidence focused on Raritan Bay. On May 1 this area was officially closed to the further taking of raw shellfish *(14, 15)*.

THE FUTURE

It is clearly not the function of surveillance to predict the long-range future, but it is only prudent to anticipate the immediate problems that can be expected on the basis of presently known facts and presently accepted concepts, erroneous though some must be. The limitations of time force the restriction of comments to the four examples presented.

Malaria is no longer a problem in this country and will not be unless major changes in the standard of living occur. A level of approximately 100 confirmed cases a year will continue and might increase depending on the flow of travelers—military and civilian, American nationals and foreigners—to and from all parts of the world. The World Health Organization and the foreign aid program of the United States are now committed to a campaign of world eradication of malaria. The present Malaria Surveillance Program might serve as one rough index of the success of this effort.

Poliomyelitis now enters a new phase. The orally administered vaccines are being used ex-

tensively in a wide variety of campaigns. The immunity of the population will be materially enhanced. If vaccines are used widely enough, and wisely, the downward trend should be accelerated, although this may be difficult to measure. The fear of many epidemiologists, however, is that the immunization of the one most important segment of the population, the infants and preschool children, will be neither sufficiently complete nor maintained indefinitely. The present enthusiasm may wane. After only a few years isolated concentrations of poorly immunized children may start and grow in size. Epidemics, perhaps of unprecedented severity, may be expected to develop in such groups. The tools are at hand through mass administration of oral vaccine to stop such outbreaks, but promptness of recognition, accuracy of diagnosis and speed of administrative action will be necessary if dozens or even hundreds of cases are to be prevented. When a case of confirmed poliomyelitis occurs in the future, the reaction should be similar to that now associated with smallpox.

Influenza will continue its cyclical pattern of epidemics throughout the world and will continue to claim its periodic toll of excess deaths, many of which are preventable. More widespread acceptance of the practice of immunization of the aged and chronically ill should be encouraged. Extending the program to increasingly larger numbers of persons—for example, to those between forty-five and sixty-four years of age—is a logical further step. Methods for ensuring the proper antigenic components of the vaccine—that is, proper for the ensuing epidemics, not the past ones—present a real challenge to the influenzologists.

Hepatitis will continue to decline in incidence during the next three years and then will increase again in accord with its seven-year cycle. No practical measures are yet available to influence this characteristic phenomenon. Obviously, an effective vaccine, when developed, would be such a control measure. The steady level of deaths resulting from serum hepatitis presents a very real challenge to those who use the surveillance approach. Simple shoe-leather epidemiology should characterize and define this problem. Surveillance of adult hepatitis, including studies designed to distinguish serum hepatitis from infectious hepatitis, should sharpen the detection of future outbreaks resulting from faulty sterile technics and other now obscure causes.

CONCLUSIONS

In limiting comments on surveillance to four examples, I had no thought of derogating other important national problems from consideration. Mention should be made that surveillance, in some form, has been maintained and continues over smallpox, diphtheria, viral encephalitis, enterovirus infections, anthrax, rabies, psittacosis, and brucellosis. Exploratory studies are now well under way for surveillance of salmonella infections, at least with a selected group of volunteering states and other interested agencies. Pilot studies on the surveillance of staphylococcal and gram-negative hospital-acquired infections have been in progress for several years. Efforts to establish systematic surveillance programs for such basically important problems as measles, streptococcal infections and the acute respiratory viral infections, other than influenza, have not yet been started. That these are national problems is unquestioned. Their surveillance clearly falls within the scope of the responsibilities of the Communicable Disease Center. Much remains to be started.

In this lecture I have endeavored to indicate that many communicable diseases of national importance continue to exist. Although somewhat out of fashion, they are clearly unfinished business. In approaching these problems, the principles of William Farr are as fully applicable today as they were a century ago. The basis of effective surveillance is the current and accurate two-way flow of information among all those who need to know.

When major health problems arise, someone must make decisions. This is not the primary responsibility of the epidemiologist. Administrative and political as well as technical considerations must also be brought to bear. It is the epidemiologists' function to get the facts to the decision makers.

Good surveillance does not necessarily ensure the making of the right decisions, but it reduces the chances of wrong ones.

References

(*1*) Farr, W. Cholera epidemic, 1848–1849. In *Vital Statistics: A memorial volume of selections from the reports and writings of.* Edited by N.A. Humphrey. London, E. Sanford, 1885, pp. 333, 334.

(*2*) Andrews, J.M. United States Public Health Service, Communicable Disease Center. *Pub Health Rep* 61:1203, 1210. 1946.

(*3*) Andrews, J.M., G.E. Quinby, and A.D. Langmuir. Malaria eradication in United States. *Am J Pub Health* 40:1405–1411, 1950.

(*4*) United States Department of Health, Education, and Welfare, Public Health Service. *An Evaluation of the Efficacy of Gamma Globulin in the Prophylaxis of Paralytic Poliomyelitis as Used in the United States, 1953: Report of the National Advisory Committee for Evaluation of Gamma Globulin in Prophylaxis of Poliomyelitis.* Washington, D.C., Government Printing Office, 1954. (*Public Health Monograph* No. 20.)

(*5*) Langmuir, A.D., N. Nathanson, and W.J. Hall. Surveillance of poliomyelitis in United States in 1955. *Am J Pub Health* 46:75–88. 1956.

(*6*) Frost, W.H. Epidemiology of influenza. In *Papers of Wade Hampton Frost*, M.D.: A contribution to epidemiological method. Edited by K. F. Maxcy. New York: Commonwealth Fund, 1941, pp. 321–339.

(*7*) Collins, S.D. Review and study of illness and medical care with special reference to long-time trends. *Pub Health Monogr* No. 48, 1957, pp. 1–86.

(*8*) Farr, W. Cholera epidemic, 1848–1849. In *Vital Statistics: A memorial volume of selections from the reports and writings of.* Edited by N.A. Humphreys. London, E. Sanford, 1885, page 330.

(*9*) Burney, L.E., et al. Asian variant: influenza: type A. *Pub Health Rep* 73:99–178, 1958.

(*10*) Trotter, Y., Jr., et al. Asian influenza in United States, 1957-1958. *Am J Hyg* 70:34–50, 1959.

(*11*) International Conference on Asian Influenza. University of California School of Medicine and Institute of Allergy and Infectious Diseases, National Institutes of Health, U. S. Public Health Service. *Am Rev Resp Dis* 83:1–219, 1961.

(*12*) Dunn, F.L., D.E. Carey, A. Cohen, and J.D. Martin. Epidemiologic studies of Asian influenza in Louisiana parish. *Am J Hyg* 70:351–371, 1959.

(*13*) Sherman, I.L., and H.F. Eichenwald. Viral hepatitis: Descriptive epidemiology based on morbidity and mortality statistics. *Ann Int Med* 44:1049–1069, 1956.

(*14*) Dougherty, W.J. and R. Altman. Viral hepatitis in New Jersey, 1960–1961. *Am J Med* 32:704–736, 1962.

(*15*) Henderson, D.A. Relationship of infectious hepatitis to consumption of raw clams from Raritan Bay. Paper presented at Conference in the Matter of Pollution of the Interstate Waters of Raritan Bay (New Jersey-New York) and Its Tributaries, New York City, August 22 and 23, 1961.

SELECTIVE EPIDEMIOLOGIC CONTROL IN SMALLPOX ERADICATION[1]

William H. Foege,[2] J. Donald Millar,[3] and J. Michael Lane[4]

A change of strategy was instituted in the West and Central Africa Smallpox Eradication Program in the fall of 1968. High priority was given to eliminating smallpox foci rather than limiting activities to mass vaccination. The progress of the program since September 1968 shows that the change in emphasis resulted in active surveillance activities which discovered more smallpox cases than the official reporting system. All known smallpox outbreaks were investigated in 1969. Vaccination totals did not suffer from the change in emphasis. The attack on smallpox foci successfully prevented the expected seasonal increase in 1969 and resulted in an interruption of smallpox transmission throughout West and Central Africa.

INTRODUCTION

The belief that smallpox is one of the more contagious infectious disease (1, 2) has often resulted in systematic nationwide vaccination campaigns to increase immunity in all geographic areas, whether or not the area is infected with smallpox. Many eradication programs in the past were planned solely on the basis of population characteristics and neglected the distribution of smallpox within the population. Eradication programs were equated with mass vaccination programs. As recently as 1964, a World Health Organization Expert Committee stated "the target must be to cover 100 percent of the population" (3). An epidemiologic approach based specifically on interrupting transmission had received little attention in endemic countries.

Recent field observations have demonstrated that smallpox is not one of the more contagious diseases. Infected persons rarely transmit the disease to an average of more than two or three persons and most transmission occurs within the infected household. In addition, smallpox typically involves only a small percentage of villages at a given time. Examination of a smallpox endemic district in India revealed that at no time were more than 1 percent of the villages (20 of 2331) involved with smallpox, and at the lowest point only seven villages (0.3 percent) had cases of smallpox present (4). The slow development of outbreaks and the clustering of outbreaks indicate that an epidemiologic approach to interrupting transmission might have particular merit. Finally, the seasonal occurrence of smallpox is such that, at certain times of the year, during the period of low incidence, the interruption of transmission should be most readily accomplished.

In January 1967, 20 countries of West and Central Africa began a coordinated regional program of smallpox eradication with technical and material support from the Agency for International Development, the Centers for Disease Control, and the World Health Organization. By July 1968, 47 million persons had been vaccinated in the 20-country area, approximately 40 percent of the population. Based on the well established seasonal pattern, smallpox in West and Central Africa was expected to reach a seasonal low in September and October. During the period 1960–1967, the ratio of cases reported in September to cases reported during the following 11 months averaged 1:27. The ratio of cases reported in April (the seasonal high) to cases reported during the next 11

Source: *American Journal of Epidemiology* 94(1):311–315, 1971.

[1] From the Smallpox Eradication Program, Centers for Disease Control, Atlanta, Georgia.

[2] Director, Smallpox Eradication Program, Centers for Disease Control, Atlanta, Georgia.

[3] Director, State and Community Services Division, Centers for Disease Control, Atlanta, Georgia.

[4] Assistant to the Director, State and Community Services Division, Centers for Disease Control, Atlanta, Georgia.

months was 1:5. Thus, the most efficient use of epidemic control teams could be made during the fall, the period of lowest transmission.

A decision was made to undertake epidemiologic control activities as a priority measure even if mass vaccination efforts were reduced. In early September 1968, epidemiologic control activities were coordinated in eight nations (Nigeria, Togo, Dahomey [now Benin], Mali, Upper Volta, Niger, Guinea, and Sierra Leone), all of the countries in the 20-country region which were infected with smallpox. A neologic term, "eradication escalation," was used to identify these activities and is used in this report because to persons involved in the West and Central Africa Smallpox Eradication Program it became synonymous with a set of methods.

METHODS

Four principal methods were employed during the eradication escalation effort: active surveillance, outbreak investigation, outbreak control, and rapid communication of disease intelligence.

Surveillance

Participating countries employed a variety of techniques to locate smallpox cases. The usual disease-reporting system was utilized as a method for determining where control teams should work. Since this approach requires waiting for reports of smallpox, it constitutes a passive surveillance system. In addition, active surveillance techniques were used, here defined as attempts to find smallpox cases not reported through the usual system. Newspapers, radio, and letters were used to alert the public and solicit information about smallpox cases. Widely dispersed informal surveillance systems were developed through the cooperation of other health services (malaria, leprosy), other government personnel (teachers, rural mail carriers, agricultural project personnel), local authority figures (village and area chiefs), and volunteer agencies, such as missions. Several countries instituted special active surveillance projects in areas suspected to have smallpox. Visits by project personnel were made to each village leader in the suspicious area or exhaustive house-to-house searches were performed to locate patients and immunize unvaccinated persons.

Outbreak Investigation

Vigorous attempts were made to locate all sources of smallpox infection. Reported cases were promptly investigated, the full extent of each outbreak was delineated, and the target area for epidemic control efforts was defined. This area included villages, markets, and compounds which were contiguous with the infected village, or which received frequent visitors from the infected village. The events which produced the outbreak were established and, insofar as it was possible, the chain of infection was traced to determine the source of the original case. Laboratory specimens were collected to verify the diagnosis of smallpox.

Outbreak Control

Various outbreak control techniques were used. The objective was to vaccinate a geographically or sociologically contiguous "area" around each patient. The extent of this area was determined by the outbreak investigation. The approach is intermediate between selective vaccination of close personal contacts (practiced to control imported smallpox in many non-endemic countries) and the indiscriminant mass vaccination campaigns which must be performed in the absence of adequate outbreak investigation.

Communications

Unofficial weekly telegraphic reports were sent to the Smallpox Eradication Program headquarters at the Centers for Disease Control in Atlanta and to its Regional Office in Lagos, Nigeria, to facilitate rapid communication of smallpox information. The cables reported the weekly number of smallpox cases, their geographic location, and the status of control activities. These data were circulated in an informal weekly report and distributed to the involved countries, enabling health officials to take rapid preventive measures or to intensify active surveillance activities when outbreaks threatened their borders.

RESULTS

Smallpox Incidence

The 1968 monthly smallpox reports were consistently below the corresponding monthly mean for 1960–1967 (Figure 1). The decline of reported cases from May through August 1968 was reversed in September, reflecting the intensified surveillance activities which identified many cases not ordinarily detected by the official reporting network. Reports decreased in November and continued to decline in early 1969, despite improvement in disease reporting. The usual dry season epidemic did not appear. In contrast, cases declined, reaching zero in November 1969.

Figure 2 compares the decline of smallpox cases with the decline in smallpox susceptibles as the result of mass vaccination. Susceptibles are defined as individuals who had not been vaccinated since the inception of the program; smallpox cases are expressed as the ratio of cases reported by month in 1968–1969 to the monthly average of reported cases during 1960–1967. After October 1968, smallpox declined much more rapidly than did the number of smallpox susceptibles, undoubtedly due to the eradication escalation activities.

In Sierra Leone, with the highest smallpox rates in the world in 1968, only 66 percent of the population had been vaccinated by May 1969, when smallpox disappeared from the country. In Mali, 51 percent of the population had been vaccinated by February 1969 when smallpox disappeared.

Surveillance

The institution of active surveillance enabled countries to accurately assess the level of actual smallpox incidence, define endemic foci, and improve the effectiveness of control activities. Table 1 shows the influence of active surveillance activities on reported smallpox cases. During the first six months of 1968, less than 5 percent of known smallpox cases were detected by active surveillance techniques. By contrast, between 57 and 67 percent of all cases reported by these countries between October 1968 and January 1969 were detected by active surveillance procedures.

Outbreak Investigations

A major factor in the success of the eradication escalation strategy was the prompt and in-

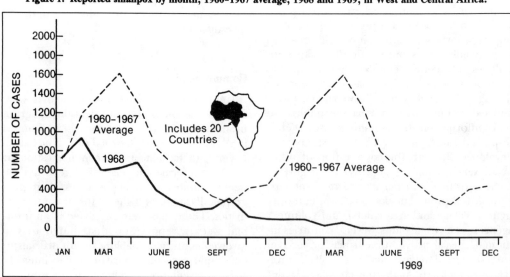

Figure 1. Reported smallpox by month, 1960–1967 average, 1968 and 1969, in West and Central Africa.

Source: WHO

Figure 2. Percentage of population not vaccinated in the Smallpox Eradication Program area compared with the ratio (%) of reported smallpox cases to the expected smallpox cases, where expected cases are based on the 1960-1967 monthly averages.

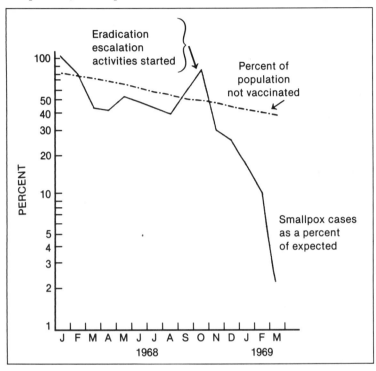

Table 1. Smallpox reports received through official reporting systems and by active surveillance in selected countries[a] of West and Central Africa, January 1968 to January 1969.

Time period	Cases reported through official reporting system	Cases discovered through active surveillance	Total cases	% detected through active surveillance
Jan-Jun 1968	3865	195	4060	4.8
(monthly average)	(644)	(33)	(677)	
Jul-Sept 1968	612	216	828	26.1
(monthly average)	(204)	(72)	(276)	
October 1968	88	177	265	66.8
November 1968	69	146	215	67.9
December 1968	60	80	140	57.2
January 1969	54	76	130	58.4

[a]Dahomey, Ghana, Guinea, Mali, Niger, Northern States Nigeria, Sierra Leone, Togo, and Upper Volta.

tensive response to each outbreak. A smallpox outbreak is defined as one or more cases occurring in an area previously free of smallpox, or cases occurring in smallpox-infected areas which are epidemiologically related. In 1968 and 1969 marked improvement occurred in the response to reported outbreaks. Table 2 indicates a steady improvement in the percentage of reported outbreaks which were investigated. In 1969 all outbreaks were investigated.

Table 2. Number of reported smallpox outbreaks and percentage investigated, January 1968 to January 1969.[a]

Time reported	No. of reported outbreaks	No. investigated	% investigated
January–June 1968[b]	109	86	78.7
(Monthly average)	(18)	(14)	
July–September 1968	91	77	84.6
(Monthly average)	(30)	(26)	
October–December 1968	71	69	97.2
(Monthly average)	(24)	(23)	
January 1969	28	28	100.0

[a]Dahomey, Ghana, Guinea, Mali, Niger, Northern States Nigeria, Sierra Leone, Togo, and Upper Volta.
[b]Incomplete for Northern States Nigeria

Effect of Eradication Escalation on the Mass Vaccination Campaign

Because of the emphasis placed on the eradication escalation activities and the diversion of vaccinators and supervisors from the mass vaccination campaign, it was feared initially that ongoing vaccination activities would be crippled. Table 3 demonstrates that the converse was true. Investigation and control activities diverted only a small proportion of project personnel to outbreak control activities. The participating countries frequently acquired short-term personnel to augment the program during the initial critical months.

DISCUSSION

Mass vaccination campaigns in themselves are often inadequate to eradicate smallpox (5). Smallpox eradication programs have resulted in vaccination numbers exceeding the estimated population, and yet smallpox remained endemic.

Dixon, while dismissing the notion that smallpox eradication can be achieved by vaccinating 80 percent of the population within four or five years, points out that "if more study were given to the foci of smallpox, it might be possible to eradicate the disease from an area by vaccinating a far smaller proportion of the total population" (6).

Epidemiologic control methods were advocated over a century ago in England, when it was clear that mass vaccination methods were not eliminating smallpox. In 1896, the Royal Commission pointed out the need for "a complete system of notification" to diminish the prevalence of smallpox (7). Despite repeated references in the literature, the practical concept of surveillance and epidemiologic control has developed slowly and has thus far had greatest application in non-endemic countries attempting to detect and eliminate importations.

The use of these techniques in smallpox endemic countries is a logical extension if endemic countries are viewed as non-endemic areas with

Table 3. Comparison of number of smallpox vaccinations, fourth quarter 1967 and fourth quarter 1968.

| | No vaccinations performed | | |
	Fourth quarter 1967	Fourth quarter 1968	% increase
Countries participating in eradication escalation activities[a]	4 546 424	6 092 684	34
Other West African countries	2 137 504	2 287 581	7
Total	6 683 928	8 380 265	25

[a]Minus Sierra Leone. Sierra Leone did not begin its vaccination campaign until 1968.

"islands" of endemicity, each equivalent to an importation. Removal of the islands is reasonable at any time, but particularly crucial at the seasonal trough period when the fewest islands exist.

"Selective epidemiological control" *(8)* has been successful in West and Central Africa. Intelligent use of vaccination based on knowledge of where the disease is and when, where, and to whom the disease is likely to spread is more economical in time, vaccine, and personnel than blind mass vaccination. Mass vaccination campaigns should continue in endemic areas, but we consider the use of surveillance, investigation, and selective epidemiologic control techniques to be of equal and, under certain circumstances, of even greater importance than systematic mass vaccination activities.

References

(1) Top, F.H., Sr. *Communicable and Infectious Diseases*. 6th edition. St. Louis, C.V. Mosby Co., 1968, pp. 165–173.

(2) Felsenfeld, O. *The Epidemiology of Tropical Diseases*. Springfield, Ill. Charles C. Thomas, 1966, pp. 336–343.

(3) WHO Expert Committee on Smallpox. *First Report*. WHO Technical Report Series 283:20, 1964.

(4) National Institute of Communicable Diseases of India. *Evaluation of the National Smallpox Eradication Program in Karnal District,* Haryana, New Delhi, 1968.

(5) Henderson, D.S. *Surveillance—The Key to Smallpox Eradication*. Presented at the WHO Inter-Regional Course on Methods of Epidemiological Surveillance. Prague, August 1968.

(6) Dixon, C.W. *Smallpox*. London, J. & A. Churchill Ltd., 1962, p. 359.

(7) *Royal Commission on Vaccination: A Report.* London, 1896.

(8) Dick, G. Smallpox. A reconsideration of public health policies. *Progr Med Virol* 8:1–29, 1966.

CHANGES IN FIVE-YEAR BREAST CANCER MORTALITY IN A BREAST CANCER SCREENING PROGRAM[1]

Sam Shapiro,[2] Philip Strax,[3] Louis Venet,[4] and Wanda Venet[5]

This paper provides additional data based on more extensive experience than previously reported regarding the impact of periodic breast cancer screening with mammography and clinical examination on mortality from breast cancer (1, 2). The new observations, covering a follow-up period of five years, reinforce the first preliminary reports that women in such a screening program have substantially lower mortality from breast cancer than a similarly constituted control group. During the five years of follow-up, there were 40 deaths due to breast cancer among the 31 000 women aged 40-64 years invited for screening, almost two-thirds of whom accepted, as compared with 63 among the 31 000 women in the control group. Reduction in mortality is concentrated entirely among women over 50 years of age; under age 50, mortality from breast cancer does not differ between the study and control groups. Clinical examination of the breast and mammography contribute independently to the early detection of breast cancer under screening conditions, but detection by mammography has been of special importance in reducing mortality from breast cancer, in the short-run, at least.

METHODOLOGY

In December 1963, the Health Insurance Plan of Greater New York (HIP), a prepaid, group-practice plan, started a long-term randomized trial directed at the question, "Does periodic breast cancer screening with mammography and clinical examination result in a reduction in mortality from breast cancer in the female population?" (3,4). Two systematic random samples, each consisting of 31 000 women aged 40 to 64 years with at least one year's membership in HIP were selected. Study group women were offered a screening examination and three additional examinations at annual intervals. All screening examinations have been completed.

Women in the control group followed their usual practices in receiving medical care. No special effort was made to encourage them to have general physical examinations. On the other hand, they were not discouraged from having such examinations, which are part of their benefits in HIP.

Each screening examination consisted of a clinical (usually conducted by a surgeon) and X-ray examination and an interview with the patient to obtain relevant demographic information and a health history. The clinician conducted his examination with no knowledge of the roentgenographic findings and recorded his observations and recommendations for follow-up medical care on study forms designed for this purpose.

Cephalocaudad and lateral X-ray views of each breast were taken by specially trained technicians using a modified Egan technique (5,6). Mammograms were separated from the clinical report for independent readings by two of the radiologists on the staff. Final responsibility for resolving differences rested with the chief radiologist on the study team. Later, clinical information derived from the screening examination was reviewed in conjunction with the radiologic findings by the chief clinician on the project staff, and a recommendation was made for routine examination one year later, early recall because of suspicious findings, biopsy, or aspiration.

Surgical and pathological findings in breast cancer cases are obtained from hospital charts. The project's coordinating pathologist reviews

Source: *Seventh National Cancer Conference Proceedings, September 27–29,* American Cancer Society, 1972.

[1] This study was supported in part by contracts PH43-63-69 and NIH 69-88 from the National Institutes of Health.

[2] Director, Department of Research and Statistics, Health Insurance Plan of Greater New York.

[3] Associate Clinical Professor of Preventive Medicine, New York Medical College; Director of Radiology, LaGuardia Hospital, New York.

[4] Associate Director of Surgery, Chief of Breast Service, Beth Israel Medical Center; Associate Clinical Professor of Surgery, Mt. Sinai School of Medicine, New York.

[5] Director of Operations, HIP Mammography Study, Health Insurance Plan of Greater New York.

slides and conducts special studies of tissue blocks when they are available. Each case of microscopically confirmed carcinoma of the breast is investigated to establish whether a mastectomy was performed prior to the woman's entry into the study (if so, she is excluded from the study), the type of surgery performed, the histologic type, nodal involvement, and size of lesion.

Deaths are identified through intensive follow-up of all confirmed breast cancer cases, and by matching death records on file in various health departments against the total file of records for study women (including those who refused screening examinations) and for control women in order to locate deaths attributed to breast cancer. As a final check in this process, several months after the fifth anniversary of the women's entry date, an attempt is made for each study and control group woman, even if she is no longer enrolled in HIP, to determine her survival status and any history of breast surgery. The techniques being used include a mail survey, medical and enrollment record review, and a check against the records of death from all causes for unresolved cases.

A critical requirement in the various follow-up procedures is to identify breast cancer cases and deaths with similar degrees of success in the study and control groups. The evidence is reassuring. Three-fourths of the women in both groups are still enrolled in HIP at the end of five years, and the enrollment and medical record systems should provide comparable information for study and control women. The mail survey designed to locate missing breast cancer cases appears to be almost equally effective in the study and control groups; the response rates are 84 percent and 82 percent for the two groups, respectively.

SCREENING PARTICIPATION

About 20 200 women, or 65 percent of the study group, appeared for their initial screening examinations. Information obtained through surveys of subsamples of the total study and control women demonstrates the comparability of these two groups (Table 1). However, study women who refused screening differ from those examined in several respects: e.g., they are slightly older; have lower educational attainment; are less likely to be multiparous or pre-

Table 1. Selected characteristics (%) of study and control groups of women entering study during 1964.

Characteristic[a]	Total	Study group[b] Examined	Study group[b] Not examined	Control group[c]
Total	100.0	100.0	100.0	100.0
Age, yr.				
40-44	24.2	25.3	22.3	24.5
45-49	23.7	24.1	22.9	23.6
50-54	22.5	22.4	22.7	21.9
55-59	18.4	17.8	19.3	18.7
60-69	11.2	10.4	12.8	11.3
Religion				
Protestant	29.1	28.0	31.1	29.2
Catholic	38.1	36.3	41.4	37.9
Jewish	32.8	35.7	27.5	32.9
Education				
Elementary school	22.6	19.5	28.3	22.1
High school	46.5	46.8	45.9	45.0
College	30.9	33.7	25.8	32.9
Marital status				
Never married	8.7	7.5	10.9	9.3
Ever married	91.3	92.5	89.1	90.7
Prior pregnancies				
Never pregnant	20.3	19.4	21.9	23.0
1-3	61.9	61.5	62.7	58.6
4 or more	17.8	19.1	15.4	18.4
Had or now having menopause				
No	29.1	33.4	21.2	25.9
Yes	70.9	66.6	78.8	74.1
Ever had lump in breast				
No	90.5	89.1	93.0	88.2
Yes	9.5	10.9	7.0	11.8

[a] "Not stated" categories, ranging from less than 1 percent to maximum of 4 percent of total, are distributed in same manner as "knowns."
[b] Data for age are based on total counts. For all other characteristics, data are based on 10 percent sample of examined group and 20 percent sample of non-examined group.
[c] Based on 20 percent sample of control group.

menopausal; and a lower proportion report ever having had a lump in the breast (7).

Successive rounds of annual reexaminations were restricted to participants in the initial screenings when it became clear from a pilot study that only a negligible proportion of the refusers (less than 5 percent) could be converted to participants. Of the 20 200 women who participated in the initial examinations, 80 percent appeared for their first annual reexamination, 74 percent for their second annual reexamination, and 69 percent for their third annual reexamination. Table 2 indicates that 60 percent of the participants in the screening program had all four examinations (initial plus three annual rescreenings), 28 percent had two or three examinations, and 12 percent only the first examination (*8*). The rate of participation was influenced to only a minor degree by demographic, health status, or attitudinal characteristics determined at the initial screening examination, several of which are shown in Table 2.

Table 2. Participation in repetitive breast cancer screening examinations by selected characteristics, women with initial screening examination.

Characteristic[a]	Sample size[b]	Percent by number of screening examinations[c]		
		1	2 or 3	4
Total	3232	12	28	60
Age				
40-49	1539	11	27	61
50-59	1294	13	27	60
60-64	399	12	32	56
Religion				
Protestant	735	12	31	57
Catholic	1194	14	30	56
Jewish	1156	10	24	66
Education				
Less than high school	1359	15	31	54
Completed high school	852	10	27	63
College	1003	10	25	66
Health self rating				
Excellent	711	14	25	61
Good	1684	11	27	62
Fair or poor	828	13	32	55
Ever had lump in breast				
Yes	376	12	25	63
No	2850	12	28	60
Exams just make you worry				
Agree	487	16	29	55
Disagree	2556	11	28	62
Not sure	166	16	32	52

[a] Characteristics as of initial screening examination.
[b] Subsample of women with initial screening examination who were included in a study of health behavior and other related health issues.
[c] Relates to participation in annual series of screening examinations; all women had at least one examination; maximum number is four.

BREAST CANCER DETECTION

Rates

Table 3 gives numbers and rates of breast cancers histologically confirmed during a five-year period of follow-up after entry into the study. This interval includes an average of one and one-half years follow-up after the last round of screening examinations was completed.

In the aggregate, 296 breast cancers have been diagnosed among the 31 000 study women and 284 breast cancers diagnosed in the control group. The prevalence rate of breast cancer among screened women, as determined from the results of the initial examinations, is 2.72 per 1000 women screened. The detection rate among women who appeared for annual re-screening examinations is 1.51 per 1000 person-years. Breast cancers diagnosed among screened women whose biopsies did not result from findings at the screening examinations occurred at a rate of 0.92 per 1000 person-years. These cases were detected anywhere from two to three months to almost five years after the woman's last screening examination. When these cases are added to those detected at various examinations, the average annual incidence rate of histologically confirmed breast cancers among women who had at least one screening examination is estimated at 2.25 per 1000 person-years.

Incidence rates among study group women who refused screening and among control

Table 3. Breast cancer detection rates, five years of observation from date of entry.

Population	Breast cancers	
	No.	Rate per 1000[a]
Study-screened	223	2.25
Detection due to initial exam.[b]	55	2.72
Detection due to annual reexam.	77	1.51
Detection not due to screening[c]	91	0.92
Study-refused screening	73	1.37
Control	284	1.86

[a] Rate of detection due to initial screening is per 1000 women examined; other rates are per 1000 person-years.
[b] 20 211 women had initial screening examination.
[c] Includes only cases diagnosed in course of regular medical care; case detection not due to follow-up of screening findings.

group women are 1.37 per 1000 and 1.86 per 1000, respectively. The relatively low rate in the group not accepting screening examinations suggests that study women with a higher risk for breast cancer tended to self-select themselves for screening.

Age at diagnosis differs slightly among the various categories of women. In the total screened group the average age is 54.5 years (54.9 for cases detected through screening, 54.0 for cases diagnosed through regular medical care). Average age at diagnosis is 53.3 years for study women who refused the screening examination and 54.5 years for the women of the control group.

Clinical and mammography examinations contributed independently to the detection of breast cancers on screening (Table 4). The relative contribution of mammography and clinical examinations to case detection was very different among women under 50 years of age at diagnosis as compared with those over 50. In the younger age group, omission of clinical examinations would have resulted in failure to detect 61 percent of the breast cancers during screening, whereas only 19 percent would have been missed by omission of mammography. At ages over 50, the two modalities made similar contributions to the detection of breast cancers.

Table 4. Breast cancers detected on screening by age group and modality.

Modality[a]	Total	Age at diagnosis 40-49	50-59	60 or older
	Number			
Total	132	31	65	36
Mammography only	44	6	27	11
Clinical only	59	19	26	14
Clinical and mammography	29	6	12	11
	Percent[b]			
Total	100.0	100.0	100.0	100.0
Mammography only	33.3	19.4	41.5	30.6
Clinical only	44.7	61.3	40.0	38.9
Clinical and mammography	22.0	19.4	18.5	30.6

[a] Initial evidence for biopsy recommendation made independently by the two modalities.
[b] Percentages in this and subsequent tables may not add to 100.0 due to rounding.

AXILLARY NODAL INVOLVEMENT

Figure 1 and Table 5 show that among breast cancers detected through screening, the proportion with no histological evidence of axillary nodal involvement is high (70 percent). Mammography and clinical examinations contributed equally to this situation. In the group of

Figure 1. Percent of breast cancers with no histological evidence of axillary node involvement.

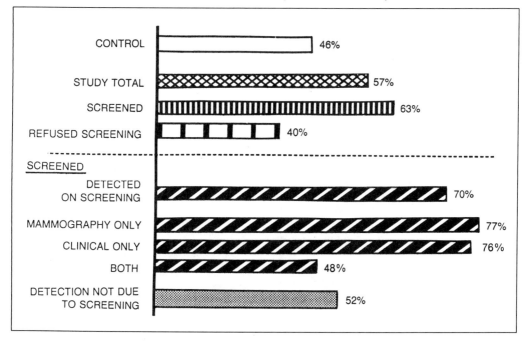

Table 5. Percent distribution of breast cancers by histologic evidence of axillary node involvement or other evidence of metastases.

		Axillary node metastasis (histology)		Unknown[a]	
Population	Number	Negative	Positive	Other evidence of metastasis[b]	Extent of disease unknown
Study (screened or refused screening)	296	57.1	34.5	4.4	4.1
Study, screened	223	62.8	32.3	1.3	3.6
Detection due to screening	132	70.5	22.7	1.5	5.3
Mammography only	44	77.3	15.9	—	6.8
Clinical only	59	76.3	18.6	—	5.1
Clinical & mammography	29	48.3	41.4	3.4	6.9
Detection not due to screening	91	51.6	46.2	1.1	1.1
Study, refused screening	73	39.7	41.1	13.7	5.5
Control	284	45.8	42.3	7.0	4.9

[a] Breast biopsy or simple mastectomy only or nodal histology unknown.
[b] Local advanced disease (skin, chest wall fixation, etc.), supraclavicular metastasis, radiographic or histologic confirmation of distant metastases.

cancers diagnosed among screened women in whom screening was not responsible for case detection, the proportion with no nodal involvement was 52 percent. The figure is 40 percent for study women who refused screening, as compared with 46 percent for control group women, a difference that could readily be due to chance factors. For the total group of study women, the proportion with no evidence of nodal involvement was 57 percent. Definitive information about axillary node involvement in the remaining cases was not always available. However, as seen in Table 5, the control group contains a substantially higher proportion of cases with positive axillary nodes or other evidence of advanced disease than the total study group.

Histologic Type and Therapeutic Modalities

A large majority of the breast cancers (80 percent) in both the study and control groups were of the duct cell histologic type. Intraductal-type cases were twice as frequent in the study group (28 cases or 9 percent) as in the control group (15 cases or 5 percent). Seventeen of the 28 intraductal type of cancers in the study group were detected during screening as a result of abnormal mammograms only. Three cases of lobular carcinoma *in situ* were found in the study group and three in the control group.

Information on type of surgery performed and use of local radiation therapy, pre- or postoperatively, suggests that there were no major differences in primary medical management of

breast cancer cases between the study and control groups (Table 6). By far the most frequent surgical procedure in each of the subgroups was radical mastectomy. As would be expected from the data on stage of disease at diagnosis in Table 5, the proportion with radical mastectomy is somewhat higher among the breast cancer cases

Table 6. Percent distribution of breast cancers by type of surgery and use of local radiation therapy.

		Study		
Treatment modality	Control	Total	Screened	Not screened
Number	284	296	223	73
Type of surgery				
Radical[a]	73.9	83.4	87.0	72.6
Modified radical[b]	14.1	9.8	9.4	11.0
Other[c]	12.0	6.8	3.6	16.4
Local radiation therapy				
Yes[d]	49.7[e]	36.1[e]	33.2	45.2
No	49.7	63.2	66.8	52.1

Note: Percentages for "unknown" type of surgery or local radiation therapy not shown separately.
[a] Includes extended radical mastectomy; eight study cases, two control cases.
[b] Includes simple mastectomy with axillary dissection.
[c] Consists of biopsy only, excision of simple mastectomy cases.
[d] Includes a small number of preoperative local radiation therapy cases; two study cases, five control cases.
[e] Adjustment to take into account differences between study and control cases in their distributions by evidence of axillary node involvement and other evidence of metastasis results in the following with local radiation therapy—total study, 39.4 percent; control, 45.8 percent.

in the screened study group (87 percent) than among cases diagnosed in the not screened study group (73 percent) or the control group (74 percent). An appreciably lower proportion of the study group women with breast cancer had local radiation therapy than was observed in the control group. However, most of the difference is due to the relatively large proportion of cases with no evidence of axillary node involvement in the study group (see adjusted figures in footnote e, Table 6).

MORTALITY FROM BREAST CANCER

Death Rates

One of the primary methods used to measure the effect of screening on mortality is to compare deaths from breast cancer in the study group with deaths from breast cancer in the control group. This corresponds to a com-

parison between two populations in their breast cancer mortality based on vital statistics. Since the study and control groups are random selections of equal size from the HIP membership, comparisons involving numbers of deaths during defined time periods provide the same information as rates.

Only deaths that occurred during the five-year period after date of entry (beginning of observation for a woman) are included. In view of the follow-up procedures previously described, this is the interval during which the highest degree of comparability in ascertainment of deaths could be expected for the study and control groups. Further, the effect of attenuation that results from the increasing number of breast cancers detected among screened women after completion of the screening program should be relatively small in the five-year period.

Figure 2 shows that there were 63 deaths in

Figure 2. Deaths due to breast cancer: 5-year follow-up after entry into study.

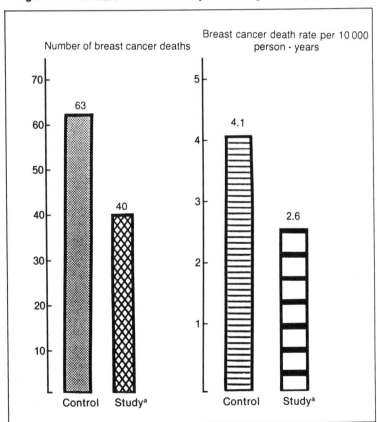

aIncludes deaths among women screened and those who refused screening

Table 7. Breast cancer deaths by interval from start of observation to end of five years of follow-up.

Interval since start of observation[a]	No. of person-years		No. of breast cancer deaths	
	Control	Study	Control	Study[b]
Total	152 742	151 660	63	40
First two years	61 781	61 337	8	11
Third year	30 567	30 350	12	6
Fourth year	30 327	30 114	18	8
Fifth year	30 067	29 859	25	15

[a] Starting point is date of entry to study or control group.
[b] Includes women screened and women who refused screening.

which breast cancer was the underlying cause among the women in the control group; the corresponding number of deaths among the study group of women, screened and not screened combined, was much smaller, 40 (difference statistically significant at the $0.01 < P < 0.05$ level). Table 7 and Figure 3 indicate that in the first two years of follow-up, breast cancer mortality was similar for the study and control groups. But in each of the following years, study group women were far less likely to die from breast cancer than the control women. The rela-

tively few cancer deaths in the first two years of follow-up is explained by the fact that only breast cancers diagnosed for the first time after the start of the study are included.

Breast cancer death rates are almost identical in the study and control groups at ages under 50 years (Table 8). Major differentials are found in the two age groups 50-54 and 55-59 years. A lower breast cancer death rate is also observed among study women 60 years and over, but in view of the small number of cases involved, the difference is not statistically significant.

Figure 3. Five-year cumulative number of breast cancer deaths by interval from start of observation.

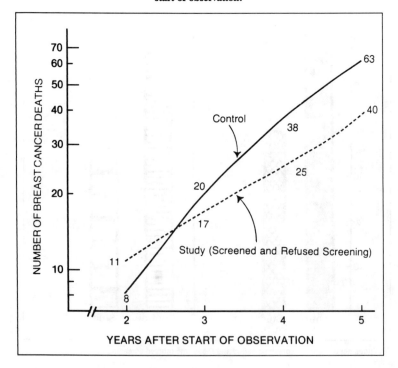

Table 8. Breast cancer deaths by age at death, five years of follow-up.

	Breast cancer deaths			
	Number		Rate per 10 000 person-years	
Age at death	Control	Study[a]	Control	Study[a]
Total	63	40	4.1	2.6
40-49 years	12	13	2.4	2.5
(40-44)	(2)	(1)	—	—
(45-49)	(10)	(12)	—	—
50-59 years	34	16	5.0	2.3
(50-54)	(16)	(9)	—	—
(55-59)	(18)	(7)	—	—
60-69 years	17	11	5.0	3.4

[a] Includes women screened and women who refused screening.

Case Fatality Rates

Another approach being taken to determine whether screening has an impact on breast cancer mortality is to examine probabilities of death among women with breast cancer during specified periods following histologic confirmation of breast cancer. These case fatality rates include all deaths among women with breast cancer regardless of the cause of death. Case fatality rates are obtained from life-table values calculated separately for breast cancer cases in the control group and for the following three subcategories of cases in the study group— those identified through screening, those diagnosed among screened women in the course of receiving regular medical care, and those detected among women who refused to participate in the screening program. Allowance is made for the lead time in diagnosing breast cancer gained through the particular program of screening that was conducted (9). Average lead time is estimated at about one year and case fatality over $x + 1$ years of follow-up breast cancers detected through screening is equated to the experience over x years among the other breast cancer cases. Combinations of subcategories of study women reflect this allowance of lead time. Case fatality rates have been derived for periods up to five years following breast cancer diagnosis.

The short-run picture seems clear. As seen in Figure 4 and Table 9, there is a substantially lower five-year case fatality rate among the 296 breast cancer patients in the study group than among the 284 cases in the control group: 28 percent vs. 42 percent. Figure 5 indicates that the margin between case fatality rates was relatively small in the first year after diagnosis, but the differential soon increased and remained fairly constant throughout the interval of two to five years.

In these comparisons the study group includes not only the screened women but also the study women who refused screening. The case fatality rate among the refusers is 35 percent. If this category is excluded from the study group and attention is limited to women screened one or more times, the rate becomes 26 percent (Figure 4). This low figure is entirely related to the favorable prognosis among women with breast cancer detected through screening.

If case fatality is restricted to the 132 breast cancer cases detected through screening, the rate is 17 percent. Only one death occurred during the period of follow-up in this report among the 44 patients with breast cancers detected on screening through mammography alone. Of the remaining 88 cases of breast cancer detected through screening, 16 deaths have occurred. Ten of these cancers were detected by the clinician only, and six by both the radiologist and the clinician. The corresponding case fatality rates in Table 10 indicate quite clearly that while both the clinical examination and mammography contributed to the relatively favorable picture for the total group of cases detected through screening, the addition of mammography to the screening program was of particular importance in accounting for the very low rate among the screened women.

An issue that will draw increasing attention as experience accumulates concerns the nature of the breast cancers detected among screened women in the normal course of receiving medical care. All but 3 of the 91 women involved were negative in the screening examination and 48 of the breast cancers were detected within one year after screening. It might be speculated that these 91 breast cancers are heavily weighted with more rapidly developing cases and in time would show a relatively high case fatality rate. However, at this point, the five-year case fatality rate in the category (39 percent) does not differ significantly from the rate for the control group (42 percent).

Figure 4. Five-year case fatality rates among women with breast cancer.

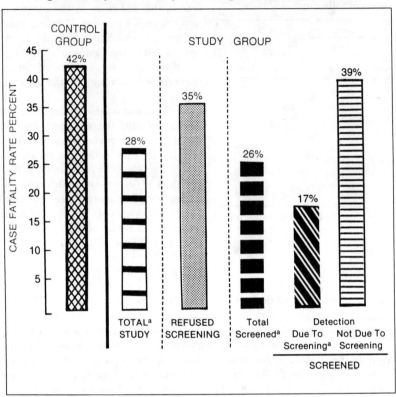

ᵃAllowance made for 1 year lead time in cancer detection due to screening.

Table 9. Five-year case fatality rates among confirmed breast cancer cases, rates per 100.

Population	Five-year case fatality rate	Control compared with study groups		
		Difference	Standard error of difference	p^a
Control	42.1	—	—	—
Study (screened and refused screening)	27.9	14.1	6.6	.03
Screened, total	25.8	16.3	6.3	.01
Detection due to screening	16.9	25.2	5.2	<.01
Detect. not due to screening	38.7	3.4	8.0	.67
Refused screening	34.5	7.6	7.5	.31

Note: Rates for study group cases allow for one year average lead time in cancer detection due to screening.
ᵃ Probability that difference as large or larger is due to chance factors.

Another question is whether the reduction in case fatality rates in the study population reflects only the higher proportion of breast cancers with no axillary node involvement. Data in Table 11 suggest that this may not be the case, although at this stage of data collection the differences are not statistically significant. Fatality rates are lower in the study group (screened and refused screening combined) than in the control group, both among women with no histologic evidence of axillary node involvement and among the other cases.

Consistent with the observations based on mortality due to breast cancer discussed in the earlier section, case fatality rates do not suggest any improvement related to the screening pro-

Figure 5. Cumulative case fatality rates among women with breast cancer by interval of follow-up after diagnosis.

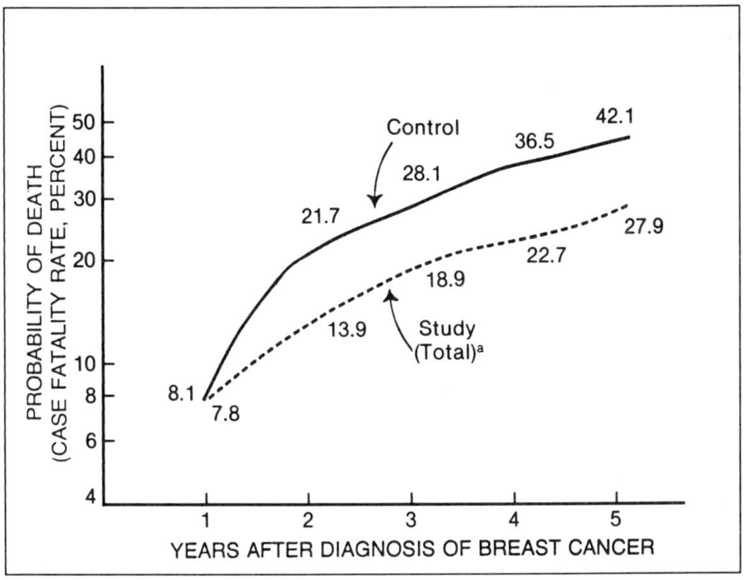

[a]Includes women screened and those who refused screening. Allowance made for 1 year lead time in cancer detection due to screening.

Table 10. Case fatality rates among breast cancer cases detected on screening by modality, rates per 100.

Modality[a]	Case fatality rate[b]
All cases detected on screening	16.9 (± 3.9)
Mammography only	2.3 (± 2.2)
Clinical only	22.0 (± 6.4)
Clinical and mammography	29.1 (± 10.7)
Cases positive on both modalities Plus	
Mammography only cases	12.4 (± 4.6)
Clinical only cases	24.1 (± 5.5)

[a] Initial evidence for biopsy recommendation made independently by the two modalities.

[b] Rates for all modalities obtained from life-table values covering a six-year follow-up period, which is equated with five-year period for cases not detected through screening. Numbers in parentheses refer to standard error due to sampling variability.

Table 11. Five-year case fatality rates among confirmed breast cancer cases by stage of disease at diagnosis.

Population	No evidence of node involvement[a]	Evidence of metastasis[b]
Rates per 100		
Control	26.1	60.8
Study[b]	17.4	45.2
Difference	8.7	15.6
Standard error of difference	7.9	10.6
Probability that difference as large or larger is due to chance factors	0.27	0.14

[a] Rates for study group cases allow for one year average lead time in cancer detection due to screening.

[b] Evidence of node involvement (histology) or other evidence of advanced diseases.

gram among women with breast cancer diagnosed at ages 40-49 years (Table 12). Considerably lower case fatality rates are observed at both ages 50-59 and 60 and over.

General Mortality

Mortality due to causes other than breast cancer is being determined through the follow-up

procedures described previously. At the time this report was prepared, all available means for identifying deaths, including the mail survey five years after entry into the study and files of death records, had been applied for women with entry dates ending December 1965, representing 82 percent of the 31 000 women in the study group and the same percent of the 31 000 women in the control group. As seen in Figure 6, the death rate (excluding deaths due to breast cancer) is identical for the study and control groups. From Tables 13 and 14, it is clear that in each age group, the study group (screened and refused screening) and the control group had very similar mortality experience during the five years of follow-up. Further, there is close correspondence between the two groups in the numbers of deaths in each major category of cause of death (other than breast cancer).

Another observation that may be made from the data in Figure 6 and the tables concerns the selectivity among the study women in accepting the invitation to participate in the breast cancer screening program. It is now apparent that this

process resulted in the study group separating itself into two distinctly different mortality risk groups; those who were screened have a substantially lower death rate than those who refused screening. This holds for each age group and for each of the cause of death categories given in Table 14. It will also be noted that the differences in the cause categories "circulatory system" and "other" are relatively far greater than in the category "malignant neoplasms (other than breast)."

DISCUSSION

The randomized clinical trial described above has now reached a stage where the evidence that repetitive screening with clinical examination and mammography leads to a reduction in five-year breast cancer mortality is quite convincing. A critical element of the investigation is that comparisons can be made between the experience of the total group of 31 000 women offered screening (referred to as the study group) whether or not they accepted, with that of a comparable control group not offered screening, thereby avoiding the usual problem of selectivity in who appears for screening (*10, 11*).

Over the short-run period of five years of follow-up, the study group of women have about a one-third lower mortality from breast cancer than those in the control group. This holds whether the comparison is based on deaths due to breast cancer during the five

Table 12. Five-year case fatality rates among confirmed breast cancer cases by age at diagnosis.

Population	Under 50	50-59	60-69
Rates per 100			
Control	31.8	48.8	41.5
Study[a]	39.4	24.2	21.0
Difference	−7.6	24.6	20.5
Standard error of difference	13.9	8.5	13.0
Probability that difference as large or larger is due to chance factors	0.59	<0.01	0.11

[a] Rates for study group cases allow for one year average lead time in cancer detection due to screening.

Table 13. Number and rate of deaths from all causes, excluding breast cancer, by age at death; five-year follow-up after entry.

Age at death	Control	Study		
		Total	Screened	Refused screening
Number				
All ages	680	670	338	332
40-49	98	106	53	53
50-59	294	296	147	149
60-69	288	268	138	130
Rates per 10 000 person-years				
All ages	54.3	53.9	41.5	77.4
40-49	23.6	25.3	18.9	38.4
50-59	52.5	53.0	40.2	77.2
60-69	103.8	100.4	81.7	132.6

Note: Data refer to mortality over a five-year period among women whose entry dates ended Dec. 31, 1965, representing 82 percent of total population in the study and control groups.

Figure 6. Death rate from all causes, excluding breast cancer, 5 years follow-up after entry into study.

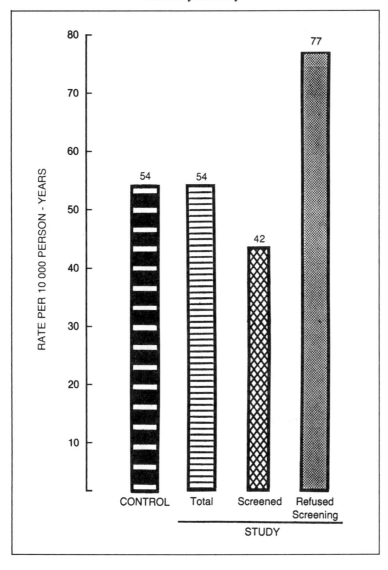

years following entry to the investigation—63, control vs. 40, study; or on case fatality rates for the five years of follow-up after diagnosis—42 percent, control vs. 28 percent, study one year's lead time in diagnosis of breast cancer due to screening taken into account). The screening program appears to have resulted in a reduction in breast cancer mortality at ages 50 and over but not at ages 40-49 years.

The differential between control and study cases in their fatality rates is almost entirely due to the exceptionally low rate (17 percent) among the cases detected through screening. Both the clinical examination and mammography contributed to this favorable situation but mammography, with a fatality rate of only 2 percent among cases it detected in the absence of a positive clinical finding during screening, was especially important. Whether the picture that seems to be emerging about mammography's role in reducing mortality among women with breast cancer is only a short-term phenom-

Table 14. Number and rate of deaths by cause of death, excluding breast cancer; five-year follow-up after entry.

Cause of death	Control	Study		
		Total	Screened	Refused screening
Number				
All causes (excl. breast cancer)	680	670	338	332
Malignant neoplasms	217	201	119	82
Digestive system	79	75	41	34
Genitourinary system	62	48	29	19
Other	76	78	49	29
Circulatory system	312	299	136	163
Other	151	170	83	87
Rate per 10 000 person-years				
All causes (excl. breast cancer)	54.3	53.9	41.5	77.4
Malignant neoplasms	17.3	16.2	14.6	19.1
Digestive system	6.3	6.0	5.0	7.9
Genitourinary system	4.9	3.9	3.6	4.4
Other	6.1	6.3	6.0	6.8
Circulatory system	24.9	24.0	16.7	38.0
Other	12.1	13.7	10.2	20.3

Note: Data refer to mortality over a five-year period among women whose entry dates ended Dec. 31, 1965, representing 82 percent of total population in the study and control groups.

enon remains to be determined. A point to be borne in mind is that the gain of one year's lead time that enters into the calculation of case fatality rates for breast cancers detected on screening is an average, and the possibility that this average is longer for mammography-detected cases than for those detected clinically is in fact part of the underlying assumption in introducing mammography into the screening program. However, it is of interest that in the age group, 40-49, where the case fatality rate did not change as a result of screening, mammography was relatively ineffective in breast cancer detection. This is in contrast to the observation that at ages 50 and over, omission of either the clinical examination or mammography would have resulted in a signficantly lower breast cancer rate at screening.

Another finding that will be of considerable importance, if longer periods of follow-up support it, is that the lowered mortality in the study population is not entirely due to the increased proportion of cases in this group detected with no evidence of axillary node involvement. Lower case fatality rates are observed among the study group of women compared with the control group's rates, regardless of the stage of the disease at time of diagnosis. The differen-

tials are not statistically significant and the two categories, "no evidence of axillary node involvement" and "evidence of metastases" used in this study are very broad. However, persistence of the differentials over a long period of time would raise the question of whether a reduction in mortality might result from earlier detection even in cases where metastasis has already occurred.

In any event, the five-year results of this investigation project the development of practical programs to screen for breast cancer as a high priority issue. In view of the costs, manpower, and technical requirements, it would be unrealistic to expect a rapid spread of screening programs to cover major segments of the female population. But one might hope for two types of activities to be carried out simultaneously over the next few years: 1) expansion of the availability of breast cancer screening, either in conjunction with multiphasic examinations or in the form of single purpose examinations, and 2) further research that would lead to more efficient screening modalities, increased use of paramedical personnel, and identification of women at high risk for breast cancer who would become special targets for screening programs.

ACKNOWLEDGMENTS

The authors appreciate the help and cooperation of the clinicians and radiologists of the 23 medical groups associated with the project and the pathologists in the hospitals involved. Important contributions were made by Raymond Fink, Ph.D., in the design and conduct of the study and Ruth Roeser, M.S., and Mary Tang, M.S., in the analytical phase. Acknowledgment is also made for the fine contributions of Dr. Stanley Gross who was the coordinating pathologist for the study and Drs. Maurice M. Pomeranz, Mortimer J. Lacher, and Filomen Lopez who aided in the review and analysis of the medical and radiologic reports of screening observations.

References

(*1*) Shapiro, S., P. Strax, and L. Venet. Periodic breast cancer screening in reducing mortality from breast cancer. *JAMA* 215:1777-1785, 1971.

(*2*) Venet, L., P. Strax, W. Venet, and S. Shapiro. Adequacies and inadequacies of breast examinations by physicians in mass screening. *Cancer* 28:1546-1551, 1971.

(*3*) Shapiro, S., P. Strax, and L. Venet. *Periodic Breast Cancer Screening in Pre-symptomatic Detection and Early Diagnosis*. London, Sir Isaac Pitman & Sons, Ltd., 1968, pp. 203-236.

(*4*) Strax, P., L. Venet, S. Shapiro, and S. Gross. Mammography and clinical examination in mass screening for cancer of the breast. *Cancer* 20:2184-2188, 1967.

(*5*) Clark, R.L., M. M. Copeland, R. L. Egan, H. S. Gallagher, H. Geller, J. P. Lindsay, L. C. Robbins, and E. C. White. Reproducibility of the technic of mammography (Egan) for cancer of the breast. *Am J Surg* 109:127-133, 1965.

(*6*) Egan, R. L. Mammography, an aid to diagnosis of breast carcinoma. *JAMA* 182:839:843, 1962.

(*7*) Fink, R., S. Shapiro, and J. Lewison. The reluctant participant in a breast cancer screening program. *Public Health Rep* 83:479-490, 1968.

(*8*) Fink, R., S. Shapiro, and R. Roeser. Impact of efforts to increase participation in repetitive screenings for early breast cancer detection. *Am J Pub Health* 62:328-336, 1972.

(*9*) Hutchison, G.B. and S. Shapiro. Lead time gained by diagnostic screening for breast cancer. *J Nat Cancer Inst* 41:665-681, 1968.

(*10*) Day, E. and L. Venet. Periodic Cancer Detection Examinations as a Cancer Control Measure. In *Fourth National Cancer Conference Proceedings*. Philadelphia, J. B. Lippincott Co., 1961, pp. 705-707.

(*11*) Gilbertsen, V. A. Survival of asymptomatic breast cancer patients. *Surg Gynecol Obstet* 122:81-83, 1966.

DOES SCREENING BY "PAP" SMEARS HELP PREVENT CERVICAL CANCER?
A CASE-CONTROL STUDY[1]

E. Aileen Clarke[2] and Terence W. Anderson[3]

The Papanicolaou (Pap)-smear history of 212 cases of invasive cervical cancer was compared with that of 1060 age-matched controls drawn from neighbors. In the five years before the year of diagnosis 32 percent of the cases had been screened by Pap smear, compared with 56 percent of the controls. This difference was statistically highly significant ($p<0.0001$) and indicated a relative risk of invasive cancer of 2.7 in women who had not been screened by Pap smear, compared with those who had. Differences in Pap-smear history between cases and controls persisted when the data were stratified by age, income, education, marital history, smoking habit, employment status, and access to medical care. These results support the belief that the Pap smear is an effective screening procedure for invasive cervical cancer.

INTRODUCTION

There is still some uncertainty about the efficacy of screening programs which use the Papanicolaou (Pap) smear in reducing the incidence of invasive cervical cancer. This uncertainty will probably persist until a properly randomized trial has been carried out, but unfortunately such a trial is impractical (1). Several non-randomized studies have given encouraging results (2-5), but such studies are liable to self-selection bias, with the screened women tending to be of higher socioeconomic status than the unscreened and thus less likely to get cervical cancer (1, 6).

In 1973 a task force of the Ontario Ministry of Health on cytological services (7) observed that an assessment of the effectiveness of Pap-smear screening could be made by a retrospective (case-control) study in which failure to participate in a screening program was examined as a potential risk factor for invasive cervical cancer. Since no such case-control study of Pap-smear screening had ever been done, the task force recommended that the Ontario Cancer Treatment and Research Foundation consider funding such a study in the Toronto area, the findings of which are reported here.

METHOD

Toronto area residents, aged 20 to 69 and admitted to the Princess Margaret Hospital with newly diagnosed invasive carcinoma of cervix between Oct. 1, 1973, and Sept. 30, 1976, were eligible for the study. Of the 323 eligible, only 212 could be interviewed. Of the 111 patients who were not interviewed, 26 had died, 29 were considered by the attending physician to be too ill to be interviewed, 32 could not speak English, 2 had moved away, and 22 refused to be interviewed.

Five age-matched (± 10 years) controls were obtained for each case. They were also matched by neighborhood and by type of dwelling (house or apartment) in the expectation that this would lead to reasonably close socioeconomic matching. Controls were obtained by door-to-door calls, which started at the fourth door to the right of the case and proceeded systematically round the residential block or through the apartment building.

Cases were interviewed at home after their initial hospital treatment. Most interviews were completed within three months of discharge

Source: *The Lancet* Saturday 7 July, 1979, pages 1-4.
[1] This study was supported by Grant 302 from the Ontario Cancer Treatment and Research Foundation.
[2] Division of Epidemiology and Statistics, Ontario Cancer Treatment and Research Foundation.
[3] Department of Preventive Medicine and Biostatistics, University of Toronto, Ontario, Canada.

from hospital and within six months of initial diagnosis. An explanatory letter to the patient described the investigation as a study of the use by women of medical tests available in the community; mention of cancer was deliberately omitted. Controls were interviewed at home as soon as possible after the interview of the case and almost always within a month.

A personal and medical questionnaire sought information on social and economic factors and on details of past visits to physicians, especially visits involving gynecological examinations and Pap smears and whether such visits were prompted by symptoms. Cases and controls usually answered the entire questionnaire; however, some refused to answer questions on certain topics, notably income and sexual history.

Two hundred and three (96 percent) of the cases and 880 (83 percent) of the controls gave permission for their past or present physicians to be approached for information concerning their Pap smears. Eighty-six percent of the physicians contacted gave information on dates and results of Pap smears, and on whether the tests were done as a routine or were prompted by symptoms.

A screening Pap smear was defined as a smear taken at either a routine "preventive" examination, or during a visit for an unrelated medical problem, but in either instance there were no gynecological symptoms such as bleeding, discharge, or pelvic pain.

Two types of statistical analysis were performed. In the first the matching of cases and controls was preserved, and relative risk (odds ratio) was calculated by matched-pair analysis (8). (According to Ontario Cancer Registry data, the age-standardized incidence-rate for invasive cervical cancer in Ontario in 1971 was 19.9/100 000. With a disease which has such a low frequency, odds ratio and relative risk should be virtually identical). In the second the matching was broken, and standard contingency tables were used (9). Breaking of the matching led to more conservative (lower) estimates of relative risk, but it had the advantage of simplicity and fuller use of the data, especially where an item of information was not available for the case and all five controls. The bulk of the analysis is therefore presented in this matter. Standardized overall (summary) relative risks for stratified variables were calculated after testing for heterogeneity (10, 11).

RESULTS

Information obtained at the interview showed that during the five years preceding the year of diagnosis 67 (32 percent) of the 212 cases had had one or more screening Pap smears, compared with 591 (56 percent) of the 1060 controls. This difference gave women who had not been screened a relative risk of invasive cervical cancer of 2.7 (p<0.0001) compared with those who had (95 percent confidence limits, 2.0–3.7). When the matching on individual cases and controls was maintained, the relative risk was increased to 3.3. (Both estimates of relative risk were statistically very highly significant, with p values of <0.000 000 0001, but for brevity p values in this paper will be limited to <0.0001).

When all Pap smears were considered (i.e., smears done because of symptoms as well as screening smears) 89 (42 percent) of the cases and 682 (64 percent) of the controls had had smears done in the five years before the year of diagnosis. These findings gave a slightly lower estimate of relative risk of 2.5 (p<0.0001).

The results so far appear to provide strong evidence that the Pap smear is an effective screening procedure for invasive cervical cancer, but the observed difference in Pap-smear histories between cases and controls may be due to bias that was not adequately controlled by matching for age and neighborhood. Several possible sources of bias were therefore examined.

Age and Socioeconomic Status

Despite the loose age-matching of the controls (±10 years), the mean age of the cases was close to that of the controls (52.4 vs 51.5). Cases and controls were neighbors, but both educational attainment and total family income were significantly lower in the cases; the highest mean grade achieved in school was 9.9 in the cases, compared with 11.1 in the controls (p<0.05), and 54 percent of the cases had a combined family income below $10 000, compared with only 41 percent of the controls (p<0.001).

All three variables (age, income, and education) were strongly associated with a history of having a screening Pap smear (see Table 1), a positive history being commonest in the younger age-groups, and in those with the

Table 1. Frequency of screening by Pap smear among cases and controls during the five years before the year of diagnosis of the index case in relation to age, income, and education.

	Frequency of Pap-smear screening in:		Relative risk
	Cases	Controls	
All subjects	67/212 *(32%)*	591/1060 *(56%)*	2.7[b]
Age			
20–34	7/16 *(44%)*	66/107 *(62%)*	2.1
35–44	18/36 *(50%)*	124/185 *(67%)*	2.0
45–59	31/102 *(30%)*	266/460 *(58%)*	3.1[b]
60+	11/58 *(19%)*	134/304 *(44%)*	3.4[c]
Total[a]	67/212 *(32%)*	590/1056 *(56%)*	2.8[b]
Income ($ p.a.)			
<6000	9/45 *(20%)*	81/184 *(44%)*	3.1[d]
6–9999	9/41 *(22%)*	65/124 *(52%)*	3.9[d]
10–14 999	12/37 *(32%)*	128/217 *(59%)*	3.0[d]
15 000+	16/35 *(46%)*	160/226 *(71%)*	2.9[d]
Total[a]	46/158 *(29%)*	434/751 *(58%)*	3.2[b]
Highest grade achieved			
<9	22/78 *(28%)*	109/251 *(43%)*	2.0[e]
9–11	19/64 *(30%)*	200/339 *(59%)*	3.4[b]
12+	19/43 *(44%)*	214/328 *(65%)*	2.4[e]
Total[a]	60/185 *(32%)*	523/918 *(57%)*	2.5[b]

[a] Total figures vary because of missing values. Total relative risk is standardized to the distribution of the characteristic in the combined population of cases and controls.
[b] p<0.0001   [c] p<0.001   [d] p<0.01   [e] p<0.05

highest levels of income and education. However, within each level the relative risk of cervical cancer in those who failed to have a Pap smear remained consistently high (2.0–3.9), and most risks were statistically significant. Standardized overall estimates were all highly significant.

Other Known Risk Factors

As might be expected, there were also significant differences between cases and controls regarding some of the other known risk factors for carcinoma of the cervix. Thus, the proportion of divorced and separated women among the cases was 16 percent, significantly higher than the 6 percent among controls (p<0.0001). The mean age at marriage was 22.1 years in cases, compared with 23.1 in controls (p<0.05), and in those women for whom the information was available (167 cases, 801 controls) the mean age at first intercourse was 20.0 years in cases vs 21.5 in controls (p<0.001). However, the overall (standardized) relative risk of cervical cancer associated with failing to have a Pap smear remained virtually unchanged when standardized

for marital status (2.7), age at marriage (2.7), or age at first intercourse (2.6); in each case it remained highly significant (p<0.0001).

Multiple regression equations were calculated for various combinations of screening Pap smear, age, income, education, age at marriage, and age at first intercourse. History of Pap smear accounted for more of the variance than any other variable, while adjustment for the other variables led to either no change or to a slight increase in the relative risk of cervical cancer.

Selection of Cases

The cases interviewed may not have been a representative sample of all new cases of cervical cancer in the Toronto area since they came from only one cancer hospital and since some of the more seriously ill ones were not interviewed. However, selection bias is not likely to have been a serious problem in this study—firstly, because Ontario Cancer Registry shows that nearly 80 percent of invasive cervical cancers in the Toronto area are first treated at the Princess Margaret Hospital; secondly, the Data Dissemination Committee of the Ontario Health Insurance Plan, without revealing the identity of patients, kindly supplied us with information on the first 100 eligible cases, which showed that the proportion of cases who had had a Pap smear before their first symptom was almost exactly the same in those not interviewed (33 percent) as in those interviewed (31 percent).

Selection of Controls

To obtain the 1060 neighborhood controls, 12 991 households were approached, a success-rate of approximately 1 in 12. On average, 8 of the 11 failures were due to there being no one at home at the time the interviewer called, 2 to there being no woman of the right age, and 1 to either the woman's inability to speak English or refusal to participate.

We have attempted to get some idea of the possible bias introduced by this non-random selection process by separating out those controls who were enrolled immediately after the case (or another control) had been interviewed—i.e., controls obtained without an intervening failure. There were 232 such controls, of whom 122 (53 percent) had had a screening Pap smear. This was lower than the overall figure of 56 percent, but the difference was not statistically significant. Substitution by this figure in the calculations reduced the relative risk to 2.4 (p<0.0001).

Employment

More cases than controls were regularly employed at the time of the interview (38 percent vs 29 percent), and this could account for some of the difference in Pap-smear frequency since working women might have less opportunity to visit a doctor. In fact, however, regular employment was associated with a higher proportion of screening Pap smears, both in the cases (36 percent vs 28 percent) and the controls (62 percent vs 52 percent). Furthermore, the relative risk associated with failure to have a Pap smear was identical (2.9, p<0.001) whether the analysis was restricted to cases and controls who were regularly employed or to those who were not.

Access to Medical Care

The low frequency of Pap-smear screening among the cases, particularly among the elderly and those with lower levels of income and edu-

cation (see Table 1), might simply reflect less contact of any sort with the medical-care system. The data were therefore reanalyzed, only those cases (154; 73 percent) and controls (936; 88 percent) who had visited a physician at least once during the five years before the year of diagnosis being included. Among these subjects 44 percent of the cases had been screened compared with 63 percent of the controls, and the relative risk was 2.2 (p<0.001). When those who had visited a physician were stratified by age, income, and education as in the table, the relative risk for every group remained greater than one and most were still statistically significant. The overall relative risks remained high after standardization for age (2.3), income (2.0), and education (2.0), and all remained highly significant (p<0.001). Interestingly, some of the highest relative risks were still seen in the elderly (2.8, p<0.01) and the poor (3.5, p<0.01), largely because of the very low frequency with which Pap smears had been done in the cases.

Smoking

A woman's smoking history may give some indication of her concern with her own health (and thus her liability to volunteer for a screening program) but allowance for smoking habit had little effect on the relative risk. Among ex-smokers the relative risk associated with failure to have a Pap smear was 3.6 (p<0.001); for current smokers it was 2.6 (p<0.0001), and for those who had never smoked it was 2.8 (p<0.001).

Adenocarcinoma

Since the Pap smear may be less effective as a screening procedure for adenocarcinoma of the cervix than for squamous-cell carcinoma (12), cases were subdivided according to histological diagnosis. Of the 13 cases of adenocarcinoma, 69 percent had been screened, compared with 62 percent of their matched controls; the relative risk was only 0.7 (p>0.1). For patients with squamous-cell carcinoma alone the relative risk was 3.1 (p<0.0001). The inclusion of the adenocarcinomas in this study will therefore have tended to produce an underestimation of the efficacy of the Pap smear.

Hysterectomy

Two hundred and twenty-one controls had had a total hysterectomy before the diagnosis was made in the index case. If these 221 controls are not considered, 489 (58 percent) of the remaining 839 controls had been screened, and the relative risk of cancer rose to 3.0 (p<0.0001). The inclusion of hysterectomized controls in the main analysis has therefore also tended to produce an underestimation of the relative risk.

Recall

A potential source of error in any case-control study is faulty memory, cases being more likely than controls to recall the details of their past health. Information provided by personal physicians for 170 cases and 730 controls (80 percent and 69 percent of the totals) showed that 48 cases (28 percent) and 418 controls (57 percent) had been screened in the previous five years and that the relative risk of cervical cancer was 3.4. Of these same individuals 35 percent of the cases and 60 percent of the controls had reported being screened; these figures made the relative risk 2.8. If the information from the physicians' records was the more accurate, cases and controls had overestimated their past frequency of Pap smears by seven percent and three percent respectively; since this overestimation reduces the true difference between the groups, the use of interview-based information has tended to minimize the true risk.

Interviewer Bias

Since the interviewers knew who were cases and who were controls, some of the differences found between the two groups may be due to interviewer bias. However, on the point that was likely to have been the most sensitive to interviewer bias—the past history of Pap smears—the information from physicians' records led to an even higher estimate of relative risk.

DISCUSSION

Ideally, a case-control assessment of this kind should be a mirror-image of a randomized controlled trial, with perfect matching of all characteristics except the one of interest—the exposure to the screening procedure. In practice, with matching carried out after the event, one can never be sure that all relevant characteristics have been recognized or properly measured, so that this type of study can therefore never be as convincing as a randomized trial. However, the

persistence of such highly significant relative risks within the several subdivisions of the present data makes it unlikely that any important confounding variables could have been overlooked. Furthermore, when the possible "volunteer" bias was reduced by restricting the comparison to those women who had had at least one visit to a physician during the previous five years there were still substantial and highly significant differences between cases and controls.

As with any other screening procedure, the Pap smear itself has no preventive value, and there must be appropriate follow-up and treatment of abnormal smears. A substantial proportion of those cases who had invasive cancer despite one or more Pap smears during the previous five years had had at least one abnormal smear, which implies that follow-up may not have been adequate. These cases will be examined in more detail in another report.

In conclusion, although it may well now be too late to do a formal randomized trial of the efficacy of Pap-smear screening in the control of invasive cervical cancer, we believe that this study has provided more convincing evidence in its favor than has previously been available.

We thank the physicians who cooperated in the project and in particular Dr. R. S. Bush, Dr. H. A. Bean, Dr. W. E. C. Allt, Dr. F. A. Beale, and Dr. J. F. Pringle of the Princess Margaret Hospital; the interviewers (Mrs. M. Beagrie [coordinator], Mrs. A. Rosenberg, Mrs. R. Chepa, Mrs. V. Cundari, Mrs. T. Galbraith, Mrs. K. Gillespie, and Mrs. S. Tinker); Prof. P. N. Corey for advice on statistical methods; Ms. A. McTiernan, Ms. A. Weir, and Ms. J. Kidd for statistical and clerical help; and Dr. D. Cannell, Dr. D. W. Thompson, and the late Dr. K.J.R. Wightman for their encouragement and support.

References

(1) Apostolides, A. and M. Henderson. Evaluation of cancer screening programs. *CA* 39:1779-1787, 1977.

(2) Christopherson, W.M., J.E. Parker, W.M. Mendez, and F.E. Lundin, Jr. Cervical cancer death rates and mass cytology screening. *CA* 26:808-811, 1970.

(3) Boyes, D.A., G. Knowelden, and A.J. Philips. L'appreciation des mesures de contrôle du cancer. *Bull Cancer* 1:83-88, 1973.

(4) Timonen, S., U. Nieminen, and T. Kauraniemi. Cervical cancer. *Lancet* i:401-402, 1974.

(5) Mac Gregor, E.J. and S. Teper. Mortality from

carcinoma of the cervix uteri in Britain. *Lancet* ii:774-779, 1978.

(6) Task Force on Cytological Screening. Cervical cancer screening programs. *Can Med Assoc J* 114:1003-1033, 1976.

(7) *Ontario Council of Health Task Force on Cytological Services. Cytological Services in Ontario.* Ontario, Ontario Council of Health, 1973.

(8) Pike, M.C. and R.H. Morrow. Statistical analysis of patient-control studies in epidemiology. *Br J Prev Soc Med* 24:42-44, 1970.

(9) Fleiss, J.L. *Statistical methods for rates and proportions.* New York, John Wiley and Sons, 1973, pages 109-129.

(10) Mantel, N. and W. Haenzel. Statistical aspects of the analysis of data from retrospective studies of disease. *J Natl Cancer Inst* 22:719-748, 1959.

(11) Mantel, N. Chi-square tests with one degree of freedom: extension of the Mantel-Haenzel procedure. *Am Stat Assoc J* 58:690-700, 1963.

(12) Spriggs, A. and M.M. Buddington. Protection by cervical smears. *Lancet* i:143, 1976.

MEASURING THE QUALITY OF MEDICAL CARE THROUGH VITAL STATISTICS BASED ON HOSPITAL SERVICE AREAS: 1. COMPARATIVE STUDY OF APPENDECTOMY RATES[1]

Paul A. Lembcke[2]

The changing character of medical and public health problems in recent years has intensified the need for new methods of measuring the quality of medical care. The term "quality of medical care" may mean different things to different people. It is usual to express the quality of medical care in terms of qualifications of personnel, adequacy of equipment, and the technical excellence of medical services performed, and it is assumed that such factors are correlated positively with results favorable to the patient. Granted that a well trained professional staff working in a well equipped and organized institution will deliver a better quality of medical care generally than a poorly trained staff working with inadequate resources, it is true nevertheless that such measurements are at best only relative and indirect, and are not adequate scientific methods.

The old chestnut, "The operation was a success but the patient died," is a homely illustration of the fact that attention is sometimes directed to the wrong criteria of success of medical treatment. The best measure of quality is not how well or how frequently a medical service is given, but how closely the result approaches the fundamental objectives of prolonging life, relieving distress, restoring function, and preventing disability. For example, unnecessary surgical operations, no matter how well done, do not contribute to such objectives, and any considerable number of unnecessary operations for a given disease or condition would indicate a poor quality of care for that condition.

Measurements of quality should be expressed in terms that are uniform and objective, and that permit meaningful comparisons between communities, institutions, groups and time periods, and with general standards. Unfortunately, there are as yet few simple and easy methods to meet the need for such type of measurement, and much thought and experimentation will be required to develop them.

The present comparative study of appendectomy rates in a number of hospital service areas is directed to only one small segment of the whole problem, and there is no thought that the quality of medical care generally can be characterized by the single index of appendectomy rate. This study is but one type of experimental approach to the general problem of methodology, and is the first of a series that have been undertaken in the hope of developing improved methods of measuring the quality of care of certain hospitalized illnesses through vital statistics based on hospital service areas.

THE HOSPITAL SERVICE AREA: DEFINITION AND USEFULNESS

The hospital vital statistics in this study of appendectomy incidence are based on the general population rather than on hospital discharges, beds, etc. The region covered consists of the 11 counties in western New York State that are served by the voluntary Council of Rochester Regional Hospitals. In the 7400 square miles of the region, there are 33 general and 14 special hospitals serving a population of 860 000.

Mortality rates for a large number of diseases, and morbidity rates for most of the communicable diseases and for neoplastic disease, are collected by the state department of health for cities, counties, villages, and townships. Medical statistics of the type usually derived from hospital records are not collected, and even if they were, presentation as city or county rates, etc., would not be particularly helpful unless, as in the study of Sinai and Paton, a single county were served principally by one hospital (1).

Source: *American Journal of Public Health* 42:276-286, 1952.
[1] Presented before the Medical Care Section of the American Public Health Association at the Seventy-ninth Annual Meeting in San Francisco, Calif., November 1, 1951.
[2] Associate Professor of Public Health Administration, School of Hygiene and Public Health, Johns Hopkins University, Baltimore, Md.

The situation was rather different in the region under study. For example, in one county, four different cities or villages had general hospitals. These hospitals varied considerably from one another in respect to size, type of medical staff, and occupation, etc., of the population served. In such circumstances, county-wide statistics based on hospital data would submerge and hide differences that otherwise might appear if the statistics were based on the population of geographic areas principally served by the hospital or hospitals in the locality.

Similar problems are encountered when a hospital's services extend over city, county, or state boundaries.

Studies of the place of residence of all patients, except newborn infants, who were hospitalized in 1946, served to outline 23 distinct and mutually exclusive hospital service areas in this region (2). Not only the hospitals in the region, but all surrounding hospitals as well, were studied to take into account residents of the region who might have been hospitalized outside. As shown in Table 1, the hospital service areas varied markedly, from one having a population of 3566 served by a 15 bed hospital, up to the Rochester metropolitan area, having a population of 457 965 and served by six general hospitals with about 1850 beds. The median is a hospital service area of 17 000 population served by a 50 bed hospital.

The hospital service areas defined by this method of residence studies do not correspond to cities or counties, but their outlines were

Table 1. Appendectomies and appendicitis deaths and population in 23 hospital service areas in and around Rochester, N. Y.

Hospital service area	Population (1)	Primary appendectomies, 1948						Deaths per 100 000	
		In area hospitals (2)	Other hospitals (3)	Total (4)	Rate per 1000		P^a (7)	1948 (8)	Average, 1944-1948 (9)
					Crude (5)	Age-sex adjusted (6)			
A	8862	3	19	22	2.5	2.9	.50	—	—
B	12 108	30	7	37	3.1	2.9	.43	8.3	6.6
C	13 277	33	4	37	2.8	2.9	.45	4.9	3.0
D	20 620	42	13	55	2.7	3.0	.60	—	2.9
E	8227	20	4	24	2.9	3.0	.75	—	—
R	457 965	1402	47	1449	3.2	3.2	—	1.8	2.8
F	18 906	60	4	64	3.4	3.5	.54	—	1.1
G	18 234	31	21	52	2.9	3.5	.49	5.5	5.5
H	15 249	50	2	52	3.4	3.5	.50	6.6	2.6
I	4352	12	2	14	3.2	3.6	.69	—	—
J	19 561	62	12	74	3.8	3.8	.17	—	4.1
K	18 081	66	7	73	4.0	4.0	.09	5.5	4.4
L	7663	23	8	31	4.0	4.1	.25	—	—
M	11 019	33	10	43	3.9	4.1	.16	9.1	3.6
N	7498	29	4	33	4.4	4.2	.18	—	5.3
O	11 133	21	26	47	4.2	4.5	.04	—	5.4
P	19 877	77	10	87	4.4	4.9	b	—	10.1
Q	24 766	103	16	119	4.8	5.3	c	4.0	3.2
S	3566	14	4	18	5.0	5.5	.07	—	—
T	73 718	400	8	408	5.5	5.7	c	2.7	4.9
U	30 916	189	5	194	6.3	6.2	c	6.5	4.5
V	17 120	99	10	109	6.4	6.9	c	—	4.7
W	34 619	229	9	238	6.9	7.1	c	2.9	5.2
Total	857 332	3028	252	3280	3.8	4.0	—	2.2	3.5

[a] Probability of difference between age-sex-adjusted rate and "standard" rate of 3.2 being due to chance variation.
[b] Less than 0.001.
[c] Less than 0.0001.

made to conform to township lines, these being the smallest units for which detailed population data are available through the U.S. Census. With the exception of the three hospital service areas designated as A, G, and O in Table 1, each hospital service area accounted for 75 to 95 percent of all hospitalizations of persons who resided therein. (The exceptions were due to a very small staff in the one hospital in Area A; to concurrent hospital reorganization in Area G; and to the situation in Area O of a somewhat specialized hospital drawing patients from many states.) The Rochester hospital service area, R, was served by six hospitals; four areas— D, H, T, and W—had two hospitals; and the other 18 had one hospital each. Except in the Rochester hospital service area, almost without exception all physicians active in medical practice are active members of the medical staff of the one hospital, or if two, both hospitals, serving their area.

The significance of hospital service areas for medical care statistics is that in most instances a hospital medical staff can be held pretty directly responsible for a very high percentage of the medical care given to residents of that area, whether in hospital, home, or physician's office. Once responsibility is fixed, changes that may be necessary can be brought about with relative ease because the hospital medical staff is a well defined group of physicians, subject through their own action and that of the hospital to educational and regulatory influences.

The situation is quite similar in the two-hospital areas described above, but in large communities with many hospitals, hospital service area statistics are not of such direct value. Question may be raised as to the responsibility of local physicians and hospitals for the 5 to 25 percent of medical care that residents obtain outside of their local hospital service area. In many instances the local physician and hospital must share such responsibility because they will make or should have made the preliminary working diagnosis and referral to the outside physician or hospital.

It has been noted in selected instances that hospitals and their medical staffs have been moved by hospital service area statistics of this type to make a searching investigation and institute educational or disciplinary measures which have resulted in marked reductions in certain types of surgery. This method would seem worthwhile if it accomplished nothing more than a reduction of unnecessary surgery, but it is hoped that positive results also may be forthcoming; for example, the finding of a delay in hospitalization for early cancer stimulating an improvement in diagnostic ability and facilities.

CALCULATION OF APPENDECTOMY INCIDENCE

The incidence of appendectomies in various hospital service areas was selected as the subject of the first of a series of studies because surgical removal of the appendix is a common operation done almost exclusively in hospitals.[3] Data were obtained from all hospitals in and adjoining the region. No matter where the operations were done, they were allocated to the place of usual residence of the patient, thus making it possible to compare resident rates. Operations done solely for the removal of the appendix were designated as primary appendectomies and these form the main subject of this study. When the appendix was removed at the time of any other operation, it was classified as a secondary appendectomy.

In making this study, early in 1949, great care was taken to insure that figures for primary appendectomies were complete and that all data were comparable. The project was discussed on several occasions with groups of medical staff members, administrators, and medical record librarians representing the hospitals of the region. With few exceptions, the data were collected in the hospital jointly by hospital personnel, a field worker, and the author. Data from hospitals outside of the region were collected in some instances by the field worker, and in others they were supplied by the medical record departments of such hospitals. In many cases,

---

[3] Appendectomy is an important operation, too. An estimated 600 000 primary appendectomies are done each year in the United States, costing perhaps $100 to $150 million for medical and hospital care, and resulting in as much as $50 million loss of income to wage earners. Six hundred thousand appendectomies would require 3 million or more hospital days, tying up more than 10 000 hospital beds having a capital replacement value of $150 to $200 million. This amount of care would require the equivalent of full-time service by about 2500 doctors, 6000 nurses, and 10 000 other hospital employees.

the operating room journal was consulted origi-nally, and in all cases it was referred to as a check on the index of operations, where such existed. Data recorded on separate cards for each patient included: name of hospital; pa-tient's residence, age or year of birth, and sex; whether primary or secondary appendectomy; whether recovered or died. A very interested and helpful attitude was shown by all hospitals both in and outside of the region.

Primary appendectomies in 1948 numbered 3280 among the 857 332 residents of the 23 hospital service areas, a crude rate of 3.83 per 1000 population per year. In addition, 1372 secondary appendectomies were recorded in the hospitals of the region, a crude rate of 1.60. The crude primary and secondary rates to-gether were 5.43 per 1000 population. This figure is roughly one-third of the average birth rate of the past 20 years, suggesting that if the same rates were to hold, the average expectancy of having the appendix removed at some time during life is about one in three.

Table 1 shows for each hospital service area its population and the respective numbers of primary appendectomies done in and outside of the hospital service area. Because the hospi-tal service areas differed somewhat in age and sex composition, rates were adjusted, as shown in column 6, to those that would be expected if the age and sex distribution of each hospital service area were the same as that of New York State at the Census of 1940.

The age-sex-adjusted primary appendec-tomy rates range from 2.9 to 7.1 per 1000 pop-ulation. As a "standard" for comparison, there has been chosen the rate of 3.2 per 1000 among the 457 965 persons in the Rochester hospital service area. This area was chosen because it has a large population, lending stability to rates, and because it contains a medical school and teaching hospital, and several other hospitals generally believed to be well staffed and equipped. Because of the small population groups in many hospital service areas, minor differences from the "standard" may be due to chance variation. The probability that the ob-served difference was due to chance variation is shown in column 7 of the table. Assuming that probability of 0.05 or less is needed for statis-tical significance, seven hospital service areas show rates above the "standard" by amounts that are statistically significant.

SECONDARY APPENDECTOMIES

The secondary appendectomy rates in the different hospital service areas were not associ-ated directly or inversely with the primary ap-pendectomy rates for the corresponding areas. The only correlation noted was that the ratio of secondary to primary appendectomy rates in-creased as the size of the hospital increased. This relationship probably is due chiefly to the fact that relatively fewer abdominal operations other than appendectomy are done in the smaller hospitals, thus limiting the opportunity to do secondary appendectomies. It is inferred also that in the larger hospitals, where the sur-gical teams are on the average larger, faster, and more skillful, there is a greater tendency to re-move the appendix secondary to some other abdominal operation.

The 20 years intervening between the peak incidence of primary appendectomies at age 20 years and that of secondary appendectomies at age 40 makes it seem unlikely that secondary appendectomies can qualify as preventive in any large degree. Ninety-one and six-tenths percent of secondary appendectomies were in females. The crude rate per 1000 population was 0.2 for males and 2.6 for females.

RELATIONSHIP BETWEEN PRIMARY APPENDECTOMY RATES AND APPENDICITIS DEATH RATES

The chief purpose of surgical removal of the appendix is to prevent death from appendicitis. In the past, when annual appendicitis death rates were 14 to 16 per 100 000 population, the importance of this disease as a cause of death prompted a rather widely held belief that ap-pendectomy should be done on the slightest suspicion in order to save life, an attitude often expressed among physicians by the familiar, "When in doubt, take it out."

In the absence of contrary evidence, it is as-sumed that the incidence and severity of appen-dicitis over the period of one year are approx-imately the same throughout the rather homogeneous, circumscribed area covered in this study. If the surgical treatment of appen-dicitis is a lifesaving measure, one would expect to find under these conditions an association of high appendectomy rates and low appendicitis mortality rates.

Such an association is not apparent, however, in columns 6 and 8 of Table 1. In fact, the 19 resident appendicitis deaths reported to the state department of health in 1948 are so few in number that the difference between the combined rate of 2.78 appendicitis deaths per 100 000 population for the eight hospital service areas with the highest appendectomy rates and the rate of 1.75 for the "standard" is not statistically significant. However, if one considers the average appendicitis mortality over the five year period 1944-1948, a statistically significant difference is found between the "standard" of 2.75 for that period and the appendicitis death rate of 5.10 for the eight highest areas.

Of course, it is not known whether the hospital service areas with the highest appendectomy rates in 1948 occupied the same relative position in the four preceding years. It does seem reasonable to infer, however, that within the upper and lower limits of the appendectomy rates observed in this study, a low incidence of surgical operations for appendicitis was not associated with high appendicitis death rates.

COMPARISON OF APPENDECTOMY RATES

In a later section of this paper the possibility is suggested that in the future the surgical treatment of appendicitis may be largely supplanted by antibiotic therapy alone, and that appendectomy may become as obsolete as mastoidectomy. In the meantime, it is necessary to answer the question, "In the present state of our knowledge, what is a reasonable annual rate for primary appendectomy?" The difficulties in answering this question may be eased somewhat by the results of further investigation in some of the hospital service areas studied. For example, the figures shown in Table 1 prompted a study by the medical staff of the hospital serving the area designated as U in the table. They found that among 16 physicians with surgical privileges, one-half of the primary appendectomies were done by only two, neither of whom received referred cases; and that clearcut indications for surgical operation were lacking in a large proportion of patients operated on by the two physicians. There can be no reasonable doubt that many unnecessary operations have been done on residents of this hospital service

area. Similar findings were obtained in several other areas and hospitals.

A curious difference between hospital service areas with high and those with low appendectomy rates is found when urban and rural rates are computed for the six hospital service areas containing cities. In the Rochester hospital service area, the urban and rural appendectomy rates were 2.71 and 2.86 per 1000, respectively, and average annual appendicitis mortality rates for the period 1944-1948 were 2.73 per 100 000 for the urban population and 2.80 for the rural. The results in Hospital Service Area J were similar, although somewhat higher. In the four hospital service areas having high total rates, the urban appendectomy rate was 8.11 per 1000 and the rural rate was 3.44. The corresponding mortality rates were 5.26 for the urban and 3.94 for the rural area. This difference in urban-rural rates is not due to the different age distribution of the various population groups. A reasonable inference is that in areas served by hospitals where operations are not controlled strictly, the simple fact of greater accessibility to hospital and medical care is a deciding factor.

Few references to appendectomy incidence in the general population were found in the literature. Those that were found tended to correspond with the overall rates in this study.

In a questionnaire survey of 2968 college students averaging 19.5 years of age, Stiles and Mulsow (3) elicited a history of previous appendectomy in 9.6 percent of males and 10.9 percent of females. Comparable cumulative percentages were developed from the data in this study, using 1948 age-specific rates and New York State life table data (4). At the 1948 rates, 12.2 percent of males and 17.2 percent of females in all 23 hospital service areas would have had primary appendectomy by age 20. In the "standard" area, however, comparable figures were much lower—7.7 percent for males and 8.4 for females.

The Navy reported for 1949 a total of 3831 appendectomies in a mean strength of 535 410 persons of median age 23.2, a rate of 7.2 per year (5). In a 10 year period at the University of Minnesota, Fowler and Boehner (6) found an annual incidence of 4 per 1000 among 15 000 students averaging about age 20. Such a rate was no more than one-half the actual incidence, they thought, because many students had appendectomies done outside the student health service. In the Greater Cleveland area, general population rates based on cases confirmed as acute appendicitis by pathological examination were about 1.5 per 1000 annually in the period 1932-1941, according to Green and Watkins (7).

There can be little doubt that the "standard" annual appendectomy rate of 3.2 chosen for this study would be considerably lower if only laboratory-confirmed cases were counted, or if the operation were performed only on the strict indications that are observed in teaching hospitals. For example, if the teaching hospital in Rochester is considered to serve a general population group proportionate in size to the number of its general beds, the rate would be only 0.8 per 1000.

Against the acceptance of such a hypothesis, it may be argued that patients with relatively simple diseases such as appendicitis tend to go to non-teaching hospitals, and that beds in teaching hospitals are tied up by patients with unusual diseases. However, if as many as one-half the beds in the teaching hospital were considered unavailable for simple conditions, the appendectomy rate for the hypothetical population group served still would be very low.

The data available do not provide an entirely satisfactory answer to the question of a "standard" rate, chiefly because the care given by the teaching hospital cannot be related to a population group distinct from that served by other hospitals. A more explicit answer should be sought by studying an area that is served by one hospital which is, or closely resembles, a teaching hospital; or an insured group served by such a hospital. The first type of study seems preferable because it would cover more fully the various age, educational, economic, national, and occupational segments of the general population, and such a study is now being conducted by the author.[4]

---

[4] Data now available permit calculation of the crude primary appendectomy rate among the 18 000 persons residing in the Cooperstown, N. Y., hospital service area served primarily by the Mary Imogene Bassett Hospital. The annual average resident rate over the five year period 1946-1950 was 1.9 per 1000 general population. Of the 171 primary appendectomies on which this rate is based, 81 percent were done in the Mary Imogene Bassett Hospital, and 19 percent in hospitals outside of the Cooperstown hospital service area.

DISCUSSION OF THE METHOD

Vital statistics based on hospital service areas have limited but definite usefulness. At the present time they seem to be best suited to the development and comparison of rates for diseases and operations that are handled almost entirely in hospitals. In the field of surgery particularly, the use of such statistics may point up the need for, and initiate a chain of events culminating in, the reduction of unnecessary surgery. A shortcoming of the method is found in large cities and other hospital service areas served by several hospitals, in which case it seems impossible to relate the service of one hospital to a population group not served to any great extent by other hospitals in the area.

In this study, epidemiological factors of age and sex were explored to bring out the differences, if any, between hospital service areas with high and with low primary appendectomy rates. It was hoped that if characteristic differences appeared, they could be applied directly to the data for an individual hospital to indicate whether the number of appendectomies probably was too high or low. Unfortunately for this purpose, age distribution was not characteristic for any one type of area, and the preponderance of females in the high appendectomy rate areas as opposed to the other areas (57 percent females in the "high" areas, 52 in the "standard" area, and 48 in the teaching hospital) was not sufficiently large and consistent to be helpful.

Outlining hospital service areas and obtaining data for comparative rates on diseases and operations involves considerable field work and requires the cooperation of a number of surrounding hospitals. The time and effort involved are not beyond the resources of the average hospital service area, but the work is of course greatly reduced for all if a number of adjoining areas and their hospitals participate. There may be reluctance on the part of some hospitals to open their records to study by the representative of another hospital, and for this reason it would seem desirable to have studies made under the aegis of a hospital association, educational institution, or state agency. To obtain uniform data it is desirable that the initial studies throughout the area or areas be made by one individual who would visit the various hospitals, but it seems probable that subsequent studies of the same type could be made simply and cheaply, with little or no field work, through reports by hospitals to a central agency.

THE ROLE OF SURGICAL OPERATION IN THE TREATMENT OF ACUTE APPENDICITIS

Some of the data cited earlier suggest that the influence of appendectomies on appendicitis death rates generally is not clear beyond question. Seeking further information on this subject, the reports of the New York State Department of Health and the Metropolitan Life Insurance Company (8), were consulted, with the results shown in Figure 1. Data from several other cities and states also showed the same striking, downward trend in mortality in recent years. This trend, associated with the antibiotic era, also raised the question of the efficacy of surgical operation in the treatment of acute appendicitis.

Appendicitis as an important disease entity first began to attract attention about 1886, following the report of Fitz (9). The dramatic nature of the disease soon gained wide professional and public attention, and it would seem that recognition of deaths from this cause should have been reasonably complete in the early 1900s in view of the fact that surgical operation offered a ready means of verification of diagnosis. Nevertheless, a steady increase in mortality was noted, from an average of 10.7 per 100 000 population for New York State in the period 1900-1904, to a 15.4 average in 1930-1934. The increase may well have been only apparent, in view of improved diagnosis in recent years; the true cause probably will never be known. A slight decline occurred around 1933 or 1934, following an all-time high in the years immediately preceding. This first decline may have been due to improved surgical treatment, especially in the relief of intestinal disten-

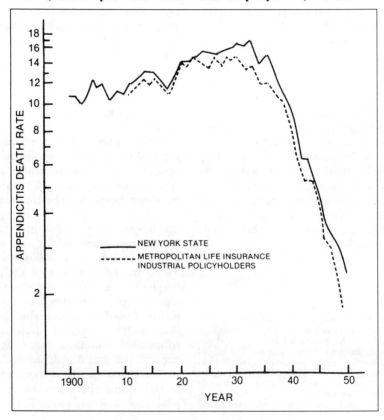

Figure 1. Appendicitis death rate per 100 000 population, New York State, 1900-1950, and Metropolitan Life Insurance industrial policyholders, 1911-1950.

tion, and correction of water and electrolyte imbalance, or it may have been due to unknown causes that produced decreases in the 1907-1910 and 1916-1919 periods. However this may be, the death rate has fallen precipitately since the sulfonamides and other antibiotics became available.

What was the value of surgical operation up to the advent of the antibiotic era? The great majority of physicians seem to have felt that appendectomy was a lifesaving procedure, and believed much as Homans did in 1932 when he wrote, "There is now no question of the value of early operation, nor is the physician backward in promptly recommending it (*10*). But some doubt existed. After quoting Willis (*11*) to the effect that apparently the mortality of the disease was not diminishing, Homans went on to speculate over this paradox of increasing mortality with increasing surgical treatment: "The reason lies perhaps in the inherent difficulty, in many instances, of making a diagnosis, and in a false feeling of security, on the part of many persons, lay and medical, that the problem of appendicitis has been solved."

At the same time, there were a few clinicians who felt that surgical operation tended to spread infection that had reached the peritoneum, and that severely ill patients did not tolerate well the shock of operation. Reynolds reports that the Ochsners, father and son, were outspoken in favor of conservative treatment in the presence of active infection of the peritoneum (*12*). Adams and Bancroft (*13*) felt that conservative treatment of appendiceal peritonitis in children at the University of Minnesota was responsible for reducing the case fatality rate from 10.1 percent in 1920-1929 to 4.5 percent in 1930-1934. (They did, however, remove the appendix after active infection had subsided.)

Looking backward from today's vantage point, it seems unlikely that surgery alone contributed much to the reduction of appendicitis mortality. It seems more likely that, in the earlier years, general supportive treatment such as prevention of dehydration, relief of abdominal distention, and good nursing care may have been of benefit, as it was in many other types of infection. Substantial reduction in appendicitis mortality appears to be attributable almost entirely to treatment with the sulfonamides and other antibiotics. In the Navy in World War II,

when surgical facilities were lacking, appendicitis was often treated successfully with penicillin or other antibiotics only (*14, 15*). Recent studies such as those of Yaeger, Ingram, and Holbrook (*16*) on aureomycin in experimental peritonitis in dogs; Yaeger, Lynn, and Barnes (*17*), Crile (*18*), and Joslin and Drake (*19*) on the use of aureomycin and penicillin in peritonitis of appendiceal origin in children and adults, strongly support the importance of the antibiotics, even though most of the human cases were subjected to surgery routinely, without regard to presence or absence of abscess, after antibiotic therapy was completed.

The question of whether surgery is needed in addition to antibiotic therapy is still open. As was true of the early advocates of conservative management, Crile and Fulton (*15*) seem to feel that surgery may be dangerous where the peritoneum is involved. They point out that in the majority of cases, acute appendicitis is self-limited and subsides spontaneously and completely in 48 hours. They consider that the majority of so-called "ruptured" appendices are periappendiceal abscesses that are ruptured by the surgeon during the operation. Also, they believe that if the patient is first seen when the infection has extended into the free peritoneal cavity, immediate operation is unlikely to improve chances of recovery. These observations and inferences suggest that surgical treatment of appendicitis should be required only rarely because, according to Crile (*18*) only 5 percent of cases go on to the stage of appendiceal peritonitis, and if treated with antibiotics only one-half of the peritonitis cases will require surgical treatment—usually for drainage of residual abscess. It seems possible also that considerably less than 5 percent of cases of acute appendicitis would progress to peritonitis if they were treated promptly with antibiotics. Surgical treatment for the relief of symptoms due to fecaliths, stenosis, or external constricting agents should be required very rarely, according to Jennings, Burger, and Jacobi (*20*), who found only 14 such cases in a total of 1680.

The findings of this study, and the publications cited, are interpreted as strongly suggesting that the antibiotics are the essential factor in successful treatment of appendicitis with peritonitis, and uncomplicated appendiceal infections as well. In view of the possibility of a great reduction in the amount of surgical treatment of appendicitis, with all of its attendant benefits, controlled clinical study is proposed to compare the efficacy of antibiotic therapy alone with the efficacy of surgical treatment with or without concurrent antibiotic therapy.

SUMMARY AND CONCLUSIONS

1. Resident vital statistics derived from hospital records and based on the total population of a hospital service area represent one useful type of measurement of the quality of medical care. Clearly demarcated, mutually exclusive areas served principally by one or more hospitals can be defined by residence studies of hospital patients, and detailed population data for such hospital service areas can be assembled from that supplied by the U. S. Census for small subdivisions.

2. The outstanding values of resident vital statistics based on hospital service areas are: (1) rates are comparable between areas and with a standard; (2) responsibility for results is associated closely with the hospital medical staff and governing board; (3) the likelihood of corrective action is enhanced by the objectivity of the rates.

3. This method is best applied to diseases and operations associated almost exclusively with hospitals. Limitations on the effectiveness of the results are encountered when a hospital service area is served in large part by several hospitals.

4. Application of this method to a study of primary appendectomies in 23 hospital service areas would seem to indicate that considerably more operations of this type are done than are necessary in the light of our present knowledge—excesses of from 25 to 100 percent in various areas.

5. The findings of this study, together with observations by others reported in the recent medical literature, are interpreted as showing that the antibiotics are the essential factor in the currently successful treatment of acute appendicitis, with or without peritonitis, and that the value of surgery is questionable in most cases. In view of these findings, a controlled clinical study of the relative efficacy of surgery with or without antibiotic therapy, and of antibiotic therapy alone, is recommended.

References

(1) Sinai, N. and D.E. Paton. *Hospitalization of the People of Two Counties.* Bureau of Public Health Economics Research Series No. 6, Ann Arbor, Mich., University of Michigan, School of Public Health, 1949.

(2) *The Regional Hospital Plan—The First Year's Experience.* Council of Rochester Regional Hospitals, 1946.

(3) Stiles, K.A. and F.W. Muslow. Incidence of appendicitis from a survey of college students. *Am J Digest Dis* 13:39-40, 1946.

(4) *State Regional Life Tables, 1939-41.* National Office of Vital Statistics, Public Health Service, Washington, D.C., Federal Security Agency, 1948.

(5) Statistics of Diseases and Injuries in the U.S. Navy. Bureau of Medicine and Surgery, Dept. of the Navy, 1949.

(6) Fowler, L.H. and J.J. Boehner. Appendicitis in college students. *Staff Meeting Bull Hosps University of Minnesota* 11:344-361, 1940.

(7) Green, H.W. and R.M. Watkins. Appendicitis in Cleveland. *Surg Gynecol Obstet* 83:613-624, 1946.

(8) *Stat Bull Metropol Life Insur Co* Vol. 32, 1951.

(9) Fitz, R.H. Perforating inflammation of the vermiform appendix. *Trans Assoc Am Physicians* 1:107-144, 1886.

(10) Homans, J. *A Textbook of Surgery* Baltimore, Md., Thomas, 1932.

(11) Willis, A.M. Mortality in appendicitis. *Surg Gynecol Obstet* 42:318-322, 1926.

(12) Reynolds, J.J. Conservative management of appendiceal peritonitis. *New Orleans M & S J* 87:32-39, 1934.

(13) Adams, J. and P.M. Bancroft. The conservative management of appendiceal peritonitis in children. *J Pediat* 12:298-312, 1938.

(14) Berkely, W.L. and H.C. Watkins. Chemotherapy in the management of acute appendicitis. *U.S. Nav M Bull* 42:1-6, 1945.

(15) Crile, G., Jr. and J.R. Fulton. Appendicitis with emphasis on use of penicillin. *U.S. Navy M Bull* 45:466-473, 1945.

(16) Yeager, G.H., C.H. Ingram, and N.A. Holbrook, Jr., Comparison of effectiveness of newer antibiotics in experimental peritonitis. *Ann Surg* 129:797, 1949.

(17) Yeager, G.H., W.D. Lynn, and T.G. Barnes. Treatment of peritonitis of appendiceal origin with aureomycin. *South Surgeon* 16:1192, 1950.

(18) Crile, G., Jr. Peritonitis of appendiceal origin treated with massive doses of penicillin. *Surg Gynecol Obstet* 83:150-162, 1946.

(19) Joslin, B.S. and M.E. Drake. Aureomycin in the treatment of ruptured appendices in children. *Pediatrics* 7:684-690, 1951.

(20) Jennings, J.E., H.H. Burger, and M. Jacobi. Acute appendicitis: A clinical and pathological study of 1680 cases. *Arch Surg* 44:896, 1942.

CASE-FATALITY IN TEACHING AND NON-TEACHING HOSPITALS, 1956-1959.

L. Lipworth,[1] J. A. H. Lee,[1] and J. N. Morris[1]

In 1957 the Social Medicine Research Unit of the Medical Research Council first showed that there were differences in case-fatality of certain conditions between teaching and non-teaching hospitals. That report was the beginning of a series and went back to 1957. Now the latest available figures have been studied and the story has been brought up to 1959. It is clear that the differences persist.

It has previously been shown that there was a higher case-fatality in appendicitis, hyperplasia of prostate, and other conditions in non-teaching hospitals of the National Health Service than in teaching hospitals (1, 2). These studies were based on data collected in 1951-1955 by the General Register Office in the national Hospital Inpatient Enquiry which they made jointly with the Ministry of Health. Collection of data has continued, and analysis of the years 1956-1959 is now presented.

The hospitals participating in the Enquiry report an effectively random 10 percent sample of their "discharges." The proportion of beds included in the Enquiry has increased from 79 percent of the total teaching hospital beds in England and Wales and 67 percent of the non-teaching in 1956, to 95 percent and 97 percent, respectively, in 1959.

RESULTS

Table 1 shows the conditions where the authors feel that comparison is most valid. Numbers are substantial and the diagnostic label is unequivocal. The Appendix Table includes all the data available to us, except for diabetes which is dealt with separately. "Immediate admissions" and "other admissions" are, in general, distinguished in the data, the latter referring largely to cases from the 'waiting list' and transfers from other hospitals. The proportion of older patients is greater in the non-teaching hospitals, and direct standardization for *age* was used to adjust for this. Standardization for *sex* was also done where applicable.

The condition of the patient on admission must be a factor in determining the case-fatality, but analysis of the deaths by length of stay in hyperplasia of the prostate in 1956-1957 does not show a high early mortality in non-teaching hospitals which might be expected with admission of excess numbers of moribund patients (Table 2). On the other hand, in ischemic heart disease, the higher case-fatality among "other admissions" in non-teaching hospitals may largely be due to the tendency to refer cases in terminal cardiac failure to this type of hospital. Again, the concentration of specialized units in the teaching hospitals must affect the "other admissions" to them, in the form of transfers of seriously ill patients for special treatment. Figures supplied to us for 1957 show that 101 cases of head injury admitted "immediately" were transferred elsewhere within three days, 95 of these from non-teaching hospitals, and six from teaching hospitals. The same analysis revealed that the latter had 68 "other admissions" for this condition, of whom 13 died. It is unreasonable to assume that a large proportion of these were badly injured patients transferred to neurosurgical units.

The cases included in the Enquiry do not always have their full diagnosis reported, being returned simply as "peritonitis," for example, or "retention of urine." These "Symptom" diagnoses therefore are also given in the Appendix Table where relevant; they do not affect the teaching/non-teaching hospital difference.

In diabetes, Table 3, even a marked acidosis may not be mentioned in the return, and in any event it is difficult to find a workable definition for incipient diabetic coma. The statistics in this emergency are thus of doubtful value. "Diabetes with other complications" is likewise a

Source: *Medical Care* 1:71–76, 1963.
[1]From the Social Medicine Research Unit, Medical Research Council, London Hospital, E.1.

Table 1. Case-fatality in teaching and non-teaching hospitals for certain conditions.

Condition	Teaching hospitals		Non-teaching hospitals	
	Deaths	Case fatality %	Deaths	Standardized Case fatality[a] %
(A) Immediate admissions 1956-1959				
Ischemic heart disease	378	23	4060	29 (P<.001)
Peptic ulcer[b]				
(a) With perforation	33	8.1	316	10
(b) Without perforation	61	5.0	594	5.3
All immediate admissions	94	5.8	910	6.4
Appendicitis				
(a) With peritonitis	10	2.8	121	4.3
All immediate admissions	14	0.44	186	0.60
Hernia of abdom. cavity with obstruction	23	6.1	312	9.7 (P<.01)
Gall bladder (Cholelithiasis, Cholecystitis and Cholangitis)	16	2.6	207	3.6
Hyperplasia of prostate				
(a) With acute retention 1957-1959	16	10	270	14
(b) Without mention of acute retention 1957-1959	20	9.5	262	12
All immediate admissions, 1956-1959	46	9.4	636	13 (P<.05)
Skull fractures and head injuries	68	2.7	602	3.4 (P<.05)
(B) "Other" Admissions				
Peptic ulcer with operation	16	1.3	106	2.3 (P<.05)
Gall bladder (Cholelithiasis, Cholecystitis and Cholangitis)	10	1.1	81	1.5
Hyperplasia of prostate	21	3.5	190	6.0 (P<.01)

[a] The standardized case fatality was derived by "direct" standardization on the age and sex distribution of the teaching Hospital admissions.
Where differences are statistically significant the probability level is shown.
[b] Admissions with hematemesis or melena are not separated in the data supplied.

very broad category and the rest of diabetes cases were not available in a form distinguishing "immediate" and "other admissions." A separate table has therefore been presented.

Hyperplasia of Prostate

Analysis of case-fatality in this condition is for many reasons particularly worthwhile. Table 2 has given details by "length of stay." In Table 4 the case-fatality for different age groups in both types of hospital during 1956-1957 is shown. In Table 5 non-teaching hospitals of different size are compared for 1957. Case-fatality does not appear to be greater in the smaller hospitals.

DISCUSSION

Two main lines of explanation may be proposed. Firstly, it is possible that the difference in case-fatality represents superior treatment in the teaching hospitals. Secondly, the non-teach-

Table 2. Case-fatality of hyperplasia of prostate in teaching and non-teaching hospitals by duration of stay[a] 1956-1957.

Duration of stay in days	Teaching hospitals, case-fatality, %	Non-teaching hospitals, case-fatality,[b] %
0-3	0.2	1.0
4-7	1.3	1.4
8-21	1.3	4.2
22-28	1.3	1.2
29 +	2.1	2.5
All durations	6.2	10.2

[a] The deaths in each period have been related to the number of original admissions.
[b] Standardized by age and mode of admission.

ing hospital patients may be socially or otherwise at an initial disadvantage. It has already been shown that, proportionate to their number of beds, teaching hospitals had more consultants and other staff. Hospital staffing is at present under review as a result of the Platt Reports and some improvement may result from this.

We know of no recent published evidence of social differences between the patients of the two types of hospital. If these were substantial they could well be a factor; thus it is well known that chronic bronchitis is more prevalent in the lower social classes. This aspect needs more study. In the meantime there is little evidence

Table 3. Case-fatality of diabetes mellitus in teaching and non-teaching hospitals, 1956-1959.

Condition	I.C.D. No.[a]	Teaching hospitals			Non-teaching hospitals			
		Cases	Deaths	Case-fatality, %	Cases	Deaths	Case-fatality, %	Standardized case-fatality, %
(a) Diabetic acidosis or coma admitted immediately	260.1	132	6	4.5	734	130	18	14 (P<.001)
(b) Diabetes with other complications specified as diabetic	260.2-260.5	274	19	6.9	1215	155	13	13 (P<.01)
All complicated diabetes admitted immediately	260.1-260.5	406	25	6.2	1949	285	15	14 (P<.001)
Remainder of diabetes		1000	42	4.2	6777	298	4.4	3.7
All diabetes	260	1406	67	4.8	8726	583	6.7	5.9
All diabetes < 45 years of age		435	3	.69	2244	37	1.6	1.6

[a] International Statistical Classification of Diseases, Injuries and Causes of Death, World Health Organization (1957) as modified by the General Register Office.

Table 4. Case-fatality of hyperplasia of prostate in teaching and non-teaching hospitals showing different age groups, 1956-1959.

Age	Teaching hospitals			Non-teaching hospitals			Non-teaching hospital standardized[a]
	Cases	Deaths	Rate %	Cases	Deaths	Rate %	
Immediate Admissions							
45 years	1	—	—	26	2	7.7	
45-54	16	—	—	122	1	0.8	
55-64	103	2	1.9	906	41	4.5	
65-74	224	21	9.4	1834	200	11	
75 +	143	23	16	1721	392	23	
Total	487	46	9.4	4609	636	14	13%
Other Admissions							
45 years	6	—	—	35	—	—	
45-54	45	—	—	121	1	0.8	
55-64	206	3	1.5	761	13	1.7	
65-74	233	6	2.6	1111	68	6.1	
75 +	112	12	11	682	108	16	
Total	602	21	3.5	2710	190	7.0	6.0%

[a] As in Table 1.

Figure 1. Case-fatality in teaching and non-teaching hospitals of hyperplasia of prostate, 1953–1959. Standardized for age and mode of admission.

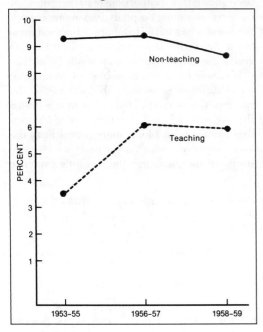

Figure 2. Case-fatality in teaching and non-teaching hospitals of appendicitis with peritonitis, 1953–1959. Standardized for age and sex.

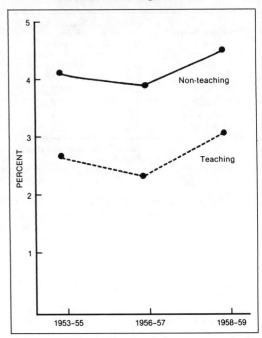

Table 5. Case-fatality of hyperplasia of prostate in non-teaching hospitals by size of hospital, 1957.

	200 beds and less	201–500 beds	Over 500 beds
Deaths	52	70	15
Case-fatality[a]	9.9%	13%	9.7%

[a] All ages and types of admission: not standardized: "Acute Hospitals." The equivalent teaching hospital case-fatality for 1957 was 6.4%

that the differences observed previously have diminished, still less disappeared (Figures 1 and 2).

We are grateful to the General Register Office for the many special tabulations of the data they made for us, and to Mrs. P. M. Parker of the Social Medicine Research Unit for much of the computing.

References

(1) Lee, J. A. H., S. L. Morrison, and J. N. Morris. Fatality from three common surgical conditions in teaching and non-teaching hospitals. *Lancet* ii:785-790, 1957.

(2) Lee, J. A. H., S. L. Morrison, and J. N. Morris. Case-fatality in teaching and non-teaching hospitals. *Lancet* i:170-171, 1960.

(3) Platt, R. *Medical Staffing Structure in the Hospital Service.* London, H.M.S.O., 1961.

Appendix. Case-fatality in teaching and non-teaching hospitals for all data examined.

Condition	I.C.D. No.	Teaching hospitals			Non-teaching hospitals			
		Cases	Death	Case-fatality, %	Cases	Deaths	Case-fatality, %	Standardized Case-fatality, %
(A) Immediate Admissions 1956-59								
Ischemic heart disease								
(a) Coronary embolism or thrombosis, coronary arteriosclerosis, other heart disease specified as involving coronary arteries	420.1	1568	369	24	11 716	3927	34	30
(b) Arteriosclerotic heart disease, angina pectoris without mention of coronary disease	420.2	100	9	9	925	133	14	12
All ischemic heart disease	420	1668	378	23	12 641	4060	32	29 (P<.001)
Non-specific mesenteric lymphadenitis	468.1	161	0	0	1217	1	.082	0 (—)
Peptic ulcer								
(a) Without perforation								
—gastric	540.0	547	35	6.4	4626	340	7.3	6.6
—duodenal	541.0	628	22	3.5	5405	242	4.5	4.1
—gastrojejunal	542.0	36	4	11	184	12	6.5	5.4
All ulcers { 540.0 541.0 542.0		1211	61	5.0	10 215	594	5.8	5.3 (N.S.)
(b) With perforation								
—gastric	540.1	86	16	19	738	120	16	17
—duodenal	541.1	315	17	5.4	1606	192	12	8.5
—gastrojejunal	542.1	6	0	0	30	4	13	8.6
All ulcers { 540.1 541.1 542.1		407	33	8.1	2374	316	13	10 (N.S.)
(c) All immediate								
—gastric	540	633	51	8.1	5364	460	8.6	8.0
—duodenal	541	943	39	4.1	7011	434	6.2	5.3
—gastrojejunal	542	42	4	9.5	214	16	7.5	6.4
All ulcers	540-542	1618	94	5.8	12 589	910	7.2	6.4 (N.S.)
Appendicitis and peritonitis								
Acute appendicitis with peritonitis	550.1	362	10	2.8	2435	121	5.0	4.3
Peritonitis (cause not stated)	576	48	16	33	486	198	41	35
Appendicitis without mention of peritonitis { 550.0 551 552		2821	4	0.14	26 791	65	0.24	0.22
All immediate appendicitis admissions	550-552	3183	14	0.44	29 226	186	0.64	0.60 (N.S.)
Hernia of abdominal cavity								
With obstruction	561	375	23	6.1	2899	312	11	9.7
Without obstruction	560	515	9	1.8	4211	81	1.9	1.6
All immediate admissions	560-561	890	32	3.6	7110	393	5.5	4.7 (N.S.)
Gall bladder cholelithiasis, cholecystitis, and cholangitis	584 585	613	16	2.6	5389	207	3.8	3.6 (N.S.)
Hyperplasia of prostate and retention of urine in males								
Hyperplasia of prostate with acute retention of urine 1957-59[b]	610	158	16	10	1754	270	15	14
Retention in males cause not stated 1957-59	786.1	40	1	2.5	480	45	9.4	7.8

Appendix. (Continued.)

Condition	I.C.D. No.	Teaching hospitals			Non-teaching hospitals			
		Cases	Death	Case-fatality, %	Cases	Deaths	Case-fatality, %	Standardized Case-fatality, %
Hyperplasia of prostate without acute retention of urine 1957-59	610	210	20	9.5	2107	262	12	12
All immediate admissions of hyperplasia of prostate 1957-59	610	368	36	9.8	3861	532	14	13
All immediate admissions 1956-59	610	487	46	9.4	4609	636	14	13 (P<.05)
Retention of urine	786.1	78	3	3.8	804	73	9.1	7.3 (N.S.)
Skull fractures and head injuries (Except fracture of face bones)	800 801 803 804 850-856	2508	68	2.7	18 288	602	3.3	3.4 (P<.05)
(B) Other Admissions 1956-59								
Ischemic heart disease	420	380	36	9.5	1556	550	35	25 (P<.001)
Non-specific mesenteric lymphadenitis	468.1	22	0	0	108	0	0	0 (—)
Peptic ulcer —gastric	540	369	9	2.4	1531	50	3.3	3.1
With —duodenal	541	773	6	0.78	2747	55	2.0	1.9
operation—gastrojejunal	542	46	1	2.2	97	1	1.0	1.2
—All ulcers	540-542	1188	16	1.3	4375	106	2.4	2.3 (P<.05)
Without —gastric	540	273	2	0.73	1283	34	2.7	2.1
operation—duodenal	541	424	2	0.47	1760	20	1.1	0.83
—gastrojejunal	542	14	0	0	50	0	0	0
All ulcers	540-542	711	4	0.56	3093	54	1.7	1.3 (P<.05)
All non- —gastric	540	642	11	1.7	2814	84	3.0	2.6
immediate—duodenal	541	1197	8	0.67	4507	75	1.7	1.5
—gastrojejunal	542	60	1	1.7	147	1	0.68	0.72
All ulcers	540-542	1899	20	1.1	7468	160	2.1	1.9 (P<.01)
Appendicitis	550-552	810	2	0.25	9625	16	0.17	0.19 (N.S.)
All hernia of abdominal cavity	560 561	3872	10	0.26	22 621	74	0.33	0.29 (N.S.)
Peritonitis	576	12	2	17	83	25	30	22 (N.S.)
Gall bladder cholelithiasis, cholecystitis, and cholangitis	584 585	924	10	1.1	4953	81	1.6	1.5 (N.S.)
Hyperplasia of Prostate	610	602	21	3.5	2710	190	7.0	6.0 (P<.01)
Retention of urine	786.1	17	0	0	127	6	4.7	3.2 (P<.05)
Skull fractures and head injuries (Except fractures of face bones)	800 801 803 804 850-856	260	36	14	813	46	5.7	4.4 (P<.001)

[a] Admissions with hematemesis or melena are not separated in the data supplied.
[b] "Breakdown" in sub-categories shown is only available for 1957-59.

   I.C.D. No. refers to the international statistical classification of diseases (seventh revision, 1955) adopted by the World Health Organization.

   Tests of statistical significance were applied to all totals and the results are as shown.

   The Standardized case fatality was derived by direct standardization on the age and sex distribution of the teaching hospital admissions.

   Terminology used in the "breakdown" of ischemic heart disease (immediate admissions) and under other sub-headings is that used in the General Register Office.

REHABILITATION OF NURSING HOME RESIDENTS[1]

Howard R. Kelman[2] and Jonas N. Muller[3]

Comparisons of the self-care status of treated and untreated patients before and after a one-year period of treatment suggest that the rehabilitation potential of a disabled public assistance population tested by the provision of maximum medical rehabilitation programs is very low.

BACKGROUND AND PURPOSE OF STUDY

Public concern for the medical and social well-being of more than 4500 public assistance recipients in proprietary nursing homes in New York City led to consideration of the efficacy of the application of complete medical rehabilitation services to this group. It had been hoped that, with such services, some patients might demonstrate sufficient potential to improve self-care levels or even to return to community living. Other studies concerned with the education of nursing home personnel in rehabilitation concepts and a few medical rehabilitation programs dealing with selected, small numbers of nursing home residents have claimed encouraging results in some communities (1-3). Surveys of such populations in New York State by rehabilitation physicians, however, estimated that only 5 percent of this population had significant rehabilitation potential (4).

Therefore, before attempting the development of a large-scale effort in New York City, it was felt that the rehabilitation potential of this population should be assessed and the possibilities and problems of bringing optimum rehabilitation services to patients in nursing homes determined. There seemed to be little doubt that a few patients who would benefit from rehabilitation treatment could be selected from among this population. However, concern was with the larger group of patients—specifically, the entire group with self-care deficits resulting from physical disabilities. The specific questions which this study sought to investigate, then, were:

1. Would a large-scale medical rehabilitation program offered to physically impaired patients residing in nursing homes or provided to patients by transferring them from the nursing home to rehabilitation hospitals significantly alter the level of self-care activities of this population?

2. Could population subgroups who would differ significantly in their response to rehabilitation treatment be identified retrospectively? In this study, rehabilitation services were to be used as a research instrument to determine whether the self-care skills of a physically impaired population unselected from the point of view of anticipated rehabilitation benefit could be sufficiently improved or maintained as a result of rehabilitation services to justify the wider application of such services to such nursing home populations.

RESEARCH METHODS AND PROCEDURES

In order to investigate these questions, an experimental design employing matched samples of randomly assigned treated and untreated patient groups was compared before and after a year's treatment. The change criteria were levels of function in ambulation, dressing, feeding, toileting, and transfer skills.

Patients residing in proprietary nursing homes were systematically reviewed by qualified physiatrists. All patients with self-care deficiencies were to be included in the study population except those *in extremis* or totally incapacitated. In addition, those patients with no manifest

Source: *Geriatrics* June 1962, pages 402–411.

[1] This report is based on a recently concluded three-year study of the rehabilitation potential of a physically disabled public assistance nursing home population in New York City. The results of a scientifically controlled experimental attempt to provide medical rehabilitation services to a sample of this population will be discussed.

[2] Assistant Professor, Departments of Physical Medicine and Rehabilitation and Preventive Medicine, New York Medical College, New York City.

[3] Professor and Chairman, Department of Preventive Medicine, New York Medical College, New York City.

self-care deficiencies were not considered eligible.

All eligible patients were randomly assigned to treatment or control groups. Initial self-care levels were then determined at an independent hospital by a special testing team otherwise unconnected with the treatment program. Therapeutic teams were organized to develop programs for patients assigned to the treatment groups and were not given information concerning the results of the initial pretreatment evaluations. The self-care evaluations were repeated at the hospital testing site by the evaluation group at the end of a year of treatment and/or observation. The testing group was not given information as to whether the patient had been treated or not.

Pretreatment psychologic and physiatric studies of all patients were performed, and relevant social and demographic background data were obtained from the records (5,6). These data and the correlation noted with the self-care change variables will be reported later.

REHABILITATION TREATMENT PROGRAMS

Two rehabilitation treatment programs were established.

Program 1. Patients assigned to this group (group B) received rehabilitation services in the nursing home by mobile medical rehabilitation teams. All patients assigned to this group were fully evaluated by the teams, which included physiatrists, occupational and physical therapists, rehabilitation nurses, social case workers, and social group workers. On the basis of this team evaluation, individualized therapeutic programs for approximately 100 patients were devised and carried out in the nursing homes by members of two teams. When patients had derived maximum benefit from their services, the teams instituted maintenance programs for the duration of the study treatment period. Additional consultation services for diagnosis and treatment, as well as prostheses and appliances, were obtained from the cooperating official agencies, who also retained medical responsibility for the patient. The primary nursing responsibility remained with the nursing home personnel. In this sense, the attempt was made to graft the additional rehabilitation services onto the existing medical, nursing, and social services normally made available to patients.

Program 2. Patients assigned to this second group (group C) were to be referred to one of five cooperating rehabilitation hospitals. The referral process was initiated by the project social work staff, which was responsible for obtaining the cooperation of the patient and family members and for making the necessary arrangements for the transfer of the patient to the hospital site and his return to the nursing home upon completion of rehabilitation efforts at the hospital. Maintenance services, after return to the nursing home, were supplied to these patients by the two mobile therapeutic teams for the duration of the study treatment period.

NURSING HOME AND POPULATION CHARACTERISTICS

Nursing Homes. All nursing homes from which patients were selected for the study were licensed and had no restrictions as to severity of patient disability. For practical reasons relating to the organization of staff effort, it was decided to sample populations in nursing homes in Manhattan. It was found necessary to sample populations in 15 such homes in order to secure the necessary study population. The nursing homes ranged in size, that is, bed capacity, from 50 to 353 beds (Table 1). In each of these

Table 1. Bed capacity and number of welfare clients of proprietary nursing homes included in project.

Nursing home (no.)	Bed capacity[a]	Welfare clients[a] (no.)
1	58	41
2	135	103
3	134	120
4	60	30
5	83	78
6	353	327
7	272	226
8	67	19
9	50	31
10	328	255
11	180	109
12	248	157
13	180	156
14	240	142
15	59	50
Total	2447	1844

[a] Census, August 1958. Source—New York City Interdepartmental Health Council.

homes, the majority of residents were recipients of public assistance.

Structurally, the homes were not originally designed as facilities for sick people. The majority were converted multi-story brownstone dwellings or apartment buildings. One had formerly been a Y.M.C.A. residence, and another had served some other institutional purpose. These nursing homes presented a fairly typical picture of the wide range of both physical characteristics and standards which have been reported and described by others (7). Living quarters and patient areas were frequently quite crowded and often poorly ventilated and lighted. Passageways between the beds and from the rooms to toilet facilities and to elevators were very narrow and winding in some homes, while in other homes the corridors were quite adequate. The presence of handrails and other assistive devices in bathrooms and other areas was variable.

The proprietary aspects of the nursing homes required maximum utilization of beds and bed space in order to insure a reliable return on the investment dollar. The organization and quality of staff, as well as the main emphasis of effort, reflected an overall philosophy of care devoted to custody rather than to treatment. Considerations of cheerfulness, privacy, and attention to decor appeared to be of lesser importance.

The general rules governing patient care and management were to create conditions which made management possible and easy. Thus, restrictions were imposed on the patients' ambulation activities. Little organizational effort of a consistent character was given to encourage patient self-help. There were no regular programs of toilet training, for the most part. Incontinent patients were frequently left in bedclothes. Staff turnover at the attendant and aide levels was quite high. Interest, as well as skill, in dealing with patients and patient-care problems was also extremely variable, ranging from considerable interest to expressions of annoyance and hostility.

Population. The population selected for the study had largely neuromuscular and musculoskeletal disabilities (Table 2). The modal age for the group was in the 70s, with somewhat more women than men (Table 3). The group contained a somewhat larger number of Negroes and New York City-born white persons than might be expected of this generation of New Yorkers.

Most patients appeared to be chronically ill, with chronic diseases. They had been generally dependent for financial, medical, and social services upon the public assistance agency long before changes in their physical condition or in their community-living situations required removal from the community to the institution. For many patients, their current nursing home stay was one in a series of hospitalizations and placements since their separation from their usual community-living arrangements.

Socially, the population seems to have been drawn from persons who had been in the lower socioeconomic levels during their adult lives and who had limited educational attainments. Approximately a third of the group had never married. Among those who had been married and were now widowed, there were few available

Table 2. Number of patients by assigned group according to diagnostic category.

Diagnostic category	Assigned group[a]				Total	
	A	B	C	D	Number	Percent[b]
Hemiplegia and paraplegia	35	35	35	35	140	34
Lower extremity fracture	18	17	18	12	65	16
Arthritis	15	15	14	14	58	14
Amputation	15	14	14	12	55	13
Other neurologic conditions	8	8	8	8	32	8
Cardiac conditions	4	4	4	2	14	3
Other	11	11	10	11	43	11
Total	106	104	103	94	407	100

[a] A = Control group; B = Nursing home treatment group; C = Rehabilitation center treatment group; D = Control group.
[b] All percentages are approximate.

Table 3. Age and sex distribution of study population.

Age (years)	Female		Male		Total	
	No.	Percent	No.	Percent	No.	Percent
Under 69	62	26	76	46	138	34
70-79	81	34	65	39	146	36
80+	93	40	26	15	119	30
Total	236	100	167	100	403[a]	100
	(59%)		(41%)			

[a] Discrepancy between total number in this table and in succeeding tables is due to lack of information on small numbers of patients.

responsible children. Relatively few patients had intact, interested, immediate family or other close kinship ties. Our data also suggest that many patients had had some previous exposure to rehabilitation care in the course of their earlier hospitalizations (*8*).

RESULTS

The findings of this study will be discussed here only in relation to the population's rehabilitation potential. The results of the early attempt to select an appropriate population are of significance in reviewing this question.

Eligibility and Prognoses. Shown in Table 4 is the distribution of the population screened and the numbers of patients found eligible for inclusion in the study. Analysis of those not considered eligible for inclusion indicated that nearly 60 percent of the total population screened were rejected for lack of manifest physical impairments limiting self-care or ambulation independence. An additional 20 percent were not considered eligible, despite the presence of self-care deficiencies, because of medical contraindication, poor survival prognosis beyond one year, or total incapacitation. The remaining population, approximately 20 percent, constituted the group included in the study. Thus it would appear that no more than 20 percent of the physically impaired nursing home public assistance population could be considered available for medical rehabilitation programs designed to improve or maintain physical self-care and ambulation skills. Even within this "available" pool of patients, it is of interest to note that 42 percent of the selected population had neuromuscular and 44 percent had musculoskeletal disabilities (Table 2).

Table 4. Number and group assignment of study population according to nursing home.

Nursing home	Number of patients screened	Number of eligible patients	Assigned group			
			A	B	C	D
1	36	10	3	3	4	
2	105	39	12	15	12	
3	123	26	11	7	8	
4	29	6	0	3	3	
5	80	16	6	3	7	
6	356	80	29	25	26	
7	255	50	15	18	17	
8	19	4	0	3	1	
9	38	14	5	6	3	
10	279	52	18	16	18	
11	130	16	7	5	4	
12	171	32				32
13	167	31				31
14	162	25				25
15	57	6				6
Total	2007	407	106	104	103	94

Shown in Table 5 are the medical and rehabilitation prognoses offered by the screening physiatrists. In only 25 percent of the cases were good rehabilitation prognoses given and only 21 percent of the population had medical prognoses which implied a possible return to full activity. Only 43 patients, approximately 10 percent of the sample, were regarded as having reasonable medical and rehabilitation prognoses for return to full activity.

The limited numbers of disabled persons available for rehabilitation treatment in this population and the still smaller proportion with good medical and rehabilitation prognoses support earlier survey and study reports by physiatrists of a low rehabilitation potential for physically impaired nursing home populations (4,9).

Pretreatment Independence. Despite these early physiatric findings in the nursing home, the results of the independent pretreatment self-care tests, as shown in the figure, indicated that rather high proportions of this population were independent or nearly independent in four out of five self-care criteria areas. Except for dressing—an activity which was discouraged by both the social conditions of living and the imperatives of patient management in the nursing home—this population's measured levels allowed for little possibility of showing improvement over time. For most of the population, only maintenance or worsening in self-care levels was possible.

An interesting by-product of this test finding was the marked contrast between the high levels of self-care skills obtained at the test site away from the nursing home and the low levels of self-care skills reported by our clinical teams in their day-to-day observations of this patient group in the nursing home. One interpretation of this discrepancy would suggest that the major rehabilitation problem was the lack of employment of physical self-care skills already present in this population in the nursing home rather than a need to restore physical function to perform self-care tasks. Questions may also be raised concerning differences in function under different conditions as well as differences between test results and the ability to sustain activity in daily life.

Comparisons. Comparisons of the differences between initial and post-treatment self-care statuses indicate that neither of the two rehabilita-

Figure 1. Distributions of initial self-care status.

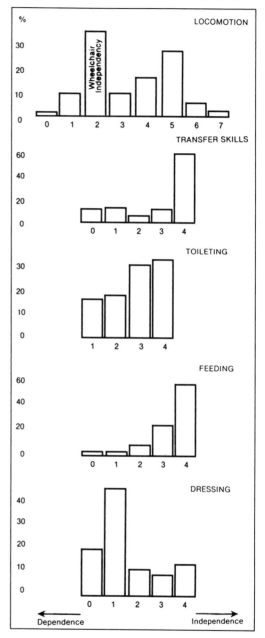

tion treatment programs significantly altered levels of self-care status favorably (Table 6). Comparison of all treated patients, regardless of the type of program, with all untreated patients does not change the interpretation of the results. Thus, by this test, our population

Table 5. Pretreatment estimated rehabilitation potential of study population according to medical prognosis.

| | Rehabilitation potential | | | | | | | | | |
| | Good | | Fair | | Poor | | Totals | |
Medical prognosis	No.	Percent	No.	Percent	No.	Percent	No.	Percent
Return to full activity	43	42	31	14	12	13	86	21
Return to limited activity	58	57	188	85	61	67	307	74
No change	1	1	3	1	18	20	22	5
Total	102	100	222	100	91	100	415[a]	100
		(25%)		(53%)		(22%)		

[a] In a few cases, more than one rank was given.

Table 6. Percent distribution of differences between initial and final self-care scores according to assigned group (excluding losses).

| | | Self-care areas | | | | | | | | | | | | | | |
| | | Locomotion | | | Transfer skills | | | Dressing | | | Feeding | | | Toileting | | |
Group	Difference[a]	−	0	+	−	0	+	−	0	+	−	0	+	−	0	+
A (control)		20	50	30	12	69	19	14	60	25	11	77	12	18	49	33
B (nursing home)		23	48	29	13	72	15	18	59	23	12	65	23	26	51	23
C₁ (hospital transfer)[b]		13	55	32	10	73	17	17	50	34	7	72	21	10	67	23
C₂ (hospital refusal)[c]		18	63	19	11	56	33	18	67	15	11	78	11	12	44	44
D (control)		20	39	41	13	74	13	33	55	11	8	79	13	32	51	17
All groups		20	49	31	10	70	20	21	58	21	10	74	16	22	52	26

[a] + = first score<second score
   0 = first score = second score
   − = first score>second score.
[b] Group C patients transferred to hospitals for rehabilitation treatment.
[b] Group C patients who refused transfer to hospitals and were not treated.

showed no greater potential for gain or mainte- nance in status when medical rehabilitation care was supplied than when it was not.

Attempts were also made to look for group differences by comparing patients rather than attributes or traits. This was done by arith- metically combining, for each patient, the scores of the pretreatment evaluations and then com- paring this sum with the sum of the posttreat- ment scores. The results are shown in Table 7. Here, too, no consistent pattern favorable to the therapeutic programs was obtained. Part of this result may be due to the previously noted high levels of initial self-care status and the outstand- ing population characteristic of failure to show significant change (more than + or − 1 score unit) in measured self-care levels. In Table 8, the distribution of obtained score differences for the entire population is shown. The percent- age of persons who receive identical scores ini-

Table 7. Change in patient self-care status by assigned group (excluding losses).

| Change in status[a] | Assigned group | | | | Total all groups |
	A	B	C	D	
Improved +	20	16	16	25	77
Same 0	13	15	11	20	59
Worsened −	31	29	22	16	98
Total	64	60	49	61	234

[a] Change is defined as difference between arithmetic sum of initial scores and final scores.

tially and at the end of one year's treatment varies from 50 percent in locomotion to 74 per- cent in feeding. The percentage showing change of more than one score unit, + or −, varied from 6 to 26.

The data also were looked at to see whether the rehabilitation programs favorably influ-

Table 8. Distribution of differences between initial and final test scores for all groups (excluding losses) according to self-care area.

Difference in scores	Locomotion		Transfer skills		Toileting		Feeding		Dressing	
	No.	Percent	No.	Percent	No.	Percent	No.	Percent	No.	Percent
−4	3	1.2	4	1.7	0	0	3	1.2	0	0
−3	12	4.9	8	3.4	2	.9	2	0.8	6	2.5
−2	27	11.0	14	5.7	12	4.9	4	1.6	9	3.7
−1	35	14.3	17	7.0	49	20.2	30	12.3	37	15.0
0	120	48.9	169	69.8	125	51.7	180	74.1	143	58.1
+1	28	11.4	21	8.7	45	18.5	18	7.4	32	13.0
+2	12	4.9	4	1.7	8	3.3	5	2.1	12	4.5
+3	7	2.9	4	1.7	1	0.4	1	0.4	7	2.9
+4	1	0.4	1	0.4	0	0	0	0	0	0

enced patient hospitalizations and mortality. The evidence does not allow for an interpretation that either numbers of hospitalizations or patient deaths were favorably influenced by the therapeutic programs. These findings would appear to confirm the early pretreatment estimates made by the screening physiatrists of the restricted rehabilitation and medical prognoses of this group.

Reactions to Treatment. The clinical response of this population to the two therapeutic programs developed in this study provides additional evidence bearing on the question of its rehabilitation potential. The most general conclusion which can be drawn is that the goals of more independent self-care and ambulation were not considered by this population as being relevant to their immediate concerns and problems. This was illustrated most dramatically by the resistance shown by those patients (group C) designated to be transferred from the nursing home to hospital rehabilitation centers. Less than half of this group agreed to participate in the program, and they did so only after intensive efforts on the part of the project casework staff. The reasons given for such "lack of cooperation" related to patients' concerns for their future well-being, negative and hostile attitudes toward hospitals, fear of losing their present nursing home situation, and "disillusionment" with rehabilitative care received in the past.

Pretreatment orientation and planning sessions were held with the administrative staffs at these rehabilitation centers. Nevertheless, most patients were not regarded by the therapeutic personnel as good candidates for rehabilitation.

Attempts were made to insure that each patient so referred received an adequate therapeutic trial before being referred back to the nursing home. Still, there were frequent questions from the operational staffs at these hospital centers as to the validity of referral of these patients to their facilities.

The impressions of our therapeutic teams who treated patients in the nursing home also pointed up the apathy, lack of motivation, and reluctance of patients to participate in the formal physical exercise and conditioning programs. Many patients questioned the relevancy of these exercises to their immediate needs, though they enjoyed the social interaction the therapeutic sessions entailed. There was evidence that few patients carried out the exercise programs when our staff was not present unless the nursing home staff itself provided the stimulation and the initiative. The population's immediate concerns were with their everyday complaints and worries. The quality of food, interpersonal difficulties with other patients, and bodily aches and pains were the problems they were anxious to have our staff deal with.

SUMMARY

A medical rehabilitation program was offered to a physically impaired population (1) with a background of chronic disease and disability and a long history of economic and social dependency; (2) drawn from the lower socioeconomic strata in our society, with few meaningful family ties and attachments; and (3) with many previous hospitalizations and placements in other institutional facilities. Many of the patients had been exposed to rehabilitation in the past.

The population was medically "fragile," with a poor prognosis for survival or improvement in medical condition. The patients' everyday concerns with the problems of living in a nursing home and with their medical conditions preempt serious consideration of what they tend to regard as possibly irrelevant goals, namely, increased independence or self-reliance in the activities of daily living. A test of the potential for improved self-care through the application of a maximum rehabilitation team effort suggests that such potential is extremely limited in this segment of the public assistance population of New York City's proprietary nursing homes.

This project was supported by the National Institutes of Health (RG 5547-"Rehabilitation of Nursing Home Patients"), the New York State Department of Health, and the Benjamin Rosenthal Foundation. Jerome S. Tobis, M.D., formerly professor and chairman of the Department of Physical Medicine and Rehabilitation, New York Medical College, and now chief of the Division of Physical Medicine and Rehabilitation, Montefiore Hospital, New York City, and Jonas N. Muller, M.D., were the senior investigators.

Major assistance in planning and execution of program 1 was rendered by the New York City Departments of Welfare, Hospitals, and Health and the New York State Health Department.

The rehabilitation centers used in program 2 were located at Bellevue, Bird S. Coler, Goldwater Memorial, and Elmhurst hospitals in New York City and the New York State Rehabilitation Hospital at West Haverstraw, New York.

References

(1) Hackley, J.A. Instructing nursing home personnel in rehabilitation techniques. *Public Health Rep* 74:989, 1959.

(2) Park, W.E. and M.I. Moe. Rehabilitation care in nursing homes. *Public Health Rep* 75:605, 1960.

(3) Soller, G.R. Training nursing home aides. *Public Health Rep* 75:283, 1960.

(4) Reynolds, F.W., M. Abramson, and A. Young. Rehabilitation potential of patients in chronic disease institutions. *J Chron Dis* 10:152, 1959.

(5) New York Medical College, Departments of Physical Medicine and Rehabilitation and Preventive Medicine. Study of rehabilitation potential of nursing home population—Report of progress of first year. Mimeographed copy. October 1959.

(6) Muller, J.N. Rehabilitation evaluation—some social and clinical problems. *Am J Public Health* 51:403, 1961.

(7) Solon, J., and others. Nursing homes, their patients and their care. A study of nursing homes and similar long-term care facilities in 13 states. Washington, D.C., U.S. Government Printing Office, 1957. (Public Health Monograph No. 46, Public Health Service Publication No. 503.)

(8) Kelman, H.R. Experiment in rehabilitation of nursing home patients. Submitted for publication.

(9) Moskowitz, E. and others. Controlled study of rehabilitation potential of nursing home residents. *NY J Med* 60:1439, 1960.

THE ICEBERG: "COMPLETING THE CLINICAL PICTURE" IN GENERAL PRACTICE[1]

J. M. Last[2]

There is much interest in the role of the general practitioner in early detection of chronic disease and in its prevention. In this paper I have used epidemiological methods to show the nature and size of some of the problems in England and Wales, by adjusting the relevant data to a hypothetical "average general practice."

The practice has been given a list of 2250 (the nearest round number to the average list of general practices in England and Wales in 1960—1), and the age and sex distribution of England and Wales in 1960 (2) (Table 1). I have estimated the number of patients in this practice who would be "known" to have certain diseases according to morbidity statistics (2–16).

Table 1. Population distribution in the average general practice.

	Age group (yr.)				
	0–14	15–44	45–64	65+	Total
Male	264	441	276	104	1085
Female	251	446	304	164	1165
Total	515	887	580	268	2250

By the methods described by Morris (17), I have tried to "complete the clinical picture" by estimating the numbers of people with undetected or potential disease who might be found on search. These numbers are mostly based on surveys of whole communities for a particular condition, and I have assumed that the hypothetical average general practice will contain the same proportion of people with these conditions. Table 2 shows the experience of a year in the practice, with disease known to the general practitioner on the left, and the undetected cases on the right. The annual number of new cases and the age-groups of all patients, with data on precursors and associated signs for some diseases, are given.

Official sources have been used to compile the "vital statistics" given in Table 3 and for the estimate of certain other events in the practice.

COMMENT ON TABLES

Subclinical Disease

Community surveys have shown that epilepsy (14), psychoneurotic illness (8), chronic bronchitis (3), and rheumatoid arthritis (10), are more prevalent than is suggested by the morbidity statistics of 106 general practices in England in 1955-1956 (11). No doubt there are undiscovered cases of these diseases in most general practices. Some of these potential patients may be people living with a disability which has been recognized, and for which they have not sought treatment in the year of the inquiry. But this can hardly be true of diabetics and the tuberculous, where the figures support the dictum that for every known case there is another undiscovered.

Detection of *diabetes* has been made easier by the use of glucose-oxidase paper strips, a simple and reliable method of urine-testing. Community studies (4, 15) show that middle-aged and elderly patients are most likely to have unrecognized diabetes, and the general practitioner has many opportunities to test their urine. Those with symptoms can be helped, and some complications perhaps reduced.

The figures for *tuberculosis* (2, 6, 18) prove that this disease is still a clinical and public health problem. The highest rates of infection are among elderly men and delinquent and psychopathic members of the community (6), some of whom are likely to be found in the average general practice.

Source: *The Lancet* July 6, 1963, pages 28-31.

[1] Work done while holding a grant from the Postgraduate Medical Foundation, University of Sydney, at the Medical Research Council Social Medicine Research Unit, The London Hospital, London, E.1.

[2] School of Public Health and Tropical Medicine, University of Sydney, Australia.

It is hardly surprising that half the cases of *urinary infection* in women remain undetected. If the suggestion is correct, that bacteriuria may precede chronic pyelonephritis and hypertension (7), the general practitioner may help to prevent these serious conditions by detecting and treating patients with "symptomless" bacteriuria. Simple methods of detection have been described (19) though there is not yet agreement about their value (20).

Table 2. Experience of one year in the average general practice; both sexes, all ages, unless specified.

Disease recognized by the practitioner		Total present in the practice, including undetected and potential disease	
Pulmonary tuberculosis (2, 11, 18)		Previously unsuspected pulmonary tuberculosis, patients aged 15 and over, would be detected at mass radiography	
Cases	6–7		
New notifications per annum	1		
Deaths per annum (1 in 7 years)	0–12	phy	2–3
Cancer (23)		Suspect, probably inactive pulmonary tuberculosis	3–4
New cases per annum	7		
" " " " lung	1	Cancer (6,11)	
" " " " breast (3 in 4 years)	0–75	Cases	11–12
" " " " stomach (3 in 4 years)	0–74	Lung cancer, males aged 55+, would be first detected at mass radiography (1 in 2 years)	0.5
" " " " prostate and rectum (1 in 2 years)	0–52	Precancerous lesion (16)	
" " " " cervix (1 in 4–5 years)	0–22	Carcinoma-in-situ	2–3
		Hemoglobin concentration (9)	
Anemia (all forms) (11)		Males, below 12.5 g. per 100 ml. aged	
Males 15–44	1	15–44	10
45–64	1	45–64	23
65+	1	65+	23
		Females, below 12 g. per 100 ml. aged	
Females 15–44	12	15–44	114
45–64	7	45–64	37
65+	5	65+	35
		Glycosuria and "diabetic" blood-sugar	
Diabetes mellitus (4)	14	curve	29
Aged 45+	12	Undetected cases aged 45+	15
Urinary infections (11)		" "	14
Females, aged 15+	20	Significant bacteriuria (11)	
		Females aged 15+	40
Staphylococcal diseases (11)		Nasal carriers of Staph. aureus (13)	500–1500
Overt skin infection	110	" " " " " (penicillin-resistant)	100– 300
Glaucoma (11)		Early chronic glaucoma (5)	
Aged 45+	3	Aged 45+	17
Hypertension and hypertensive heart-disease (11)		Casual diastolic blood-pressure 100 mm. Hg. and over (12)	
Males aged 45+	8	Males aged 45+	30
Females aged 45+	24	Females aged 45+	131
Bronchitis (11)		Symptoms and signs of bronchitis (3)	
Males aged 45–64	24	Males aged 45–64	47
Females aged 45–64	19	Females aged 45–64	24
Rheumatoid arthritis (11)		"Definite" and "probable" rheumatoid arthritis (10)	
Aged 15+	11	Aged 15+	25
Epilepsy (11)	7–8	Epilepsy (14)	13–14
Psychiatric disorders (11)		"Conspicuous psychiatric morbidity" (7)	
Males 15+	27	Males 15+	58
Females 15+	62	Females 15+	102
Radiological evidence of pulmonary tuberculosis (6)	12–14		

Table 3. Some annual events in the average general practice.

Vital Statistics (2)		
Births		39
Illegitimate births	2	
Marriages		17
Divorces	1	
Deaths		26
Diseases of circulatory system	10	
Malignant neoplasms	5	
Vascular lesions of nervous system	4	
Bronchitis	1	
Violence	1	

Contact with other parts of N.H.S. (1, 11, 35, 36)		
Hospital		
All admissions		208
No. of patients		96
Peptic ulcer	3–4	
Acute appendicitis	3–4	
Abdominal hernia	5	
Uterovaginal prolapse	2	
Arthritis	1–2	
Tonsillectomy	9–10	
Injuries	14	
Head injuries	2–3	
Fractured femur	1	
New outpatients		641
Casualty		277
Other departments		364
Traumatic and orthopedic	51	
General surgery	46	
E.N.T.	32	
Ophthalmic	31	
General medical	31	
Mental Hospital:		
All admissions	5	

First admissions	2–3
New outpatients	8
Diagnostic Services:	
Referred to hospital pathological laboratory	59
Referred to hospital X-ray department	99
Referred to hospital mass radiography by practitioner	10
Annual number examined by mass radiography	177
Domiciliary visits by consultants	16
Domiciliary Services:	
Health visitor	600 visits
Home nurse	1134 visits to 45 patients
Home help	16 patients
Maternal and Child Welfare:	
Patients attending antenatal clinic	17
Patients attending postnatal clinic	2
Domiciliary confinements:	
Attended by midwife	14
Doctor booked	12
Attended by doctor	2
First attendance infant welfare clinic	31
Seen by school medical service	107

Miscellaneous (1, 29, 37)	
Receiving National Assistance	100
Supplied for first time with full dentures (all teeth just extracted)	17
Casualties on the roads	17
Receiving war pensions	25
Registered blind	5

The significance of the figure for glaucoma, based on several American surveys (5), may be debatable. Undetected cases of early chronic glaucoma will occur in the average general practice, if the incidence of the disease is comparable with American experience. These cases could be detected by a combination of techniques—measurement of visual acuity, perimetry, fundoscopy, and measurement of ocular tension—all within the competence of the well-trained and well-equipped general practitioner. The incentive is the prevention of blindness; the average general practice at present has five blind patients and at least one of these has glaucoma.

The problem of the *Staphylococcus* is demonstrated by this method of presentation; while there are about 110 cases annually of (presumably) staphylococcal skin infection in the average general practice (boils, carbuncles, impetigo, styes, and so on), there may be between 500 and 1500 nasal carriers of *Staph. aureus*—perhaps a fifth of them penicillin-resistant (13).

Anemia

If recent community surveys (9) record the true prevalence of anemia, the average general practitioner deals with only about one patient in seven of those who are anemic. In the course of a year many of the 200 with anemia in the practice will consult their doctor for incidental disease, if not because they have symptoms due to the anemia itself; and many are probably working below full efficiency. A small minority, especially of the elderly, have grave disease of which anemia is an early sign (21). Clinical examination alone will detect with certainty only those with severe anemia, below 60 percent Hb (9 g. per 100 ml.) (22); only laboratory tests will detect all who need treatment. The average general practitioner requests only 59 examinations annually, or just over one a week. (The figure includes all pathological investigations, blood, urine, and feces tests, and many must be for antenatal cases.) Without adding an insuperable burden to the hospital laboratory service, he could ask for more hemoglobin estimations for women of childbearing age, the group most likely to be anemic. Better still, could he not himself undertake such simple tests as estimation of hemoglobin? This can be done with reasonable accuracy using simple equipment, such as grey-wedge hemoglobinometer, though there is argument about the reliability of observations on capillary blood. Changes in the method of payment for medical services might encourage this work.

Cancer

There will be some seven new cases of cancer each year in the average general practice (23). The commoner forms are listed in Table 2.

The presence of two or three cases of carcinoma-in-situ of the uterine *cervix (16)* is a strong argument for better facilities for exfoliative cytology. The most vulnerable women (middle-aged multipara, particularly in the lower social classes) are more likely to attend their family doctor with complaints that justify pelvic examination and offer an opportunity to take a cervical smear, than they are to visit clinics set up for the purpose. The general practitioner is also in a good position to encourage people to attend special cancer-detection clinics, where these exist. The efficacy of the technique of cervical cytology in reducing the incidence of invasive cancer of the cervix is being convincingly demonstrated (24).

About three new cases of cancer of the *breast* will occur every four years in the average general practice. Many of the vulnerable women are likely to attend their general practitioner under circumstances that from time to time offer an opportunity to examine their breasts, thus reinforcing whatever measures some women may take for themselves; and if this opportunity were taken, some cancers might be detected earlier than otherwise. The incidence of the disease makes clear the need for educa-

tion of patients in the technique of self-examination.

Opportunities for rectal examinations are less common, but the knowledge that there will be one new case of cancer of either the *rectum* or the *prostate* every two years (as well as an unknown number of cases of benign hypertrophy of the prostate) may be an incentive to make this examination more often.

At present there is one new case of *lung* cancer every year in the average general practice in England and Wales—and one death. The probability that this case need not have occurred if all men in the practice were non-smokers, and the lower incidence of the disease among ex-smokers than among those still smoking (26), should encourage health counseling. It should also encourage the doctor to set his patients a good example. Of the cases that occur, perhaps one in alternate years might first be detected at mass miniature radiography if all men in the practice over the age of 55 were radiologically examined (6), though it may be hard to decide how often such an examination would be justifiable, and whether it should be confined to vulnerable groups, such as heavy smokers.

Too little is known about the causes of cancer for much of it to be considered preventable; but by always remembering the possibility, and by using ordinary clinical skills of history-taking and physical examination, with diagnostic aids such as cervical cytology and radiology when appropriate, the general practitioner can engage in "secondary prevention"—the earlier detection which will more surely lead to successful treatment.

THE ICEBERG PHENOMENON

Disease known to the general practitioner represents only the tip of the iceberg; Morris (17) has shown that differences below the surface may be qualitative as well as quantitative. A good example of this is coronary artery disease in middle-aged men (Table 4).

The numbers are mostly approximate, and there is considerable overlap in data about the submerged parts of the iceberg. The prognostic significance of several of the factors included in the table has been clearly demonstrated (25), and several lines of action are implied—namely, search for vulnerable individuals; health counseling, where appropriate; and epidemiological research.

Table 4. Coronary-artery disease in men aged 45–64.

Visible:
  1 Death (*2*).
  5 Cases (*11*).
Submerged:
  11 E.C.G. evidence of left ventricle hypertrophy (*38*).
  15 Casual diastolic blood-pressure 100 mm. Hg or over (*12*).
  24 Serum-cholesterol 300 mg. per 100 ml., or over (*39*).
  28 Healed infarcts (*40*).
  52 Smoking more than 20 cigarettes per day (*25*).
  55 Obese, more than 10% over ideal weight (*41*).
  140 Moderate to severe atheroma of coronary arteries (*42*).
  ??? Insufficient exercise.
      Worried by responsibility.
      Other emotional stress.
  276 At risk.

Although mass serum-cholesterol estimations are hardly justifiable until we have a cheap micromethod, ordinary clinical examination could detect more men with high blood-pressure, some of whom might need treatment. Cheap, and easily portable, transistorized electrocardiographs could be used by general practitioners to "screen" vulnerable groups in their practice—for example, men who are overweight, who lack opportunity or incentive to take exercise, or who smoke too much. These should benefit from the good counsels of their family doctor. The question marks in the table indicate suitable subjects for research in general practice; no one has any clear idea about the leisure activities of middle-aged men, nor about the relation, if any, between these and health. Is the vicarious stress of watching competitive sports related to the incidence of stress disease, such as hypertension?

Patients who commit suicide are at the tip of another iceberg. In the average general practice there will be one suicide (*2*) in four years, and, when it was still an indictable offense, one attempted suicide came before the courts (*27*) in the same period. But each year at least two more people will have made suicidal attempts (*28*). A still larger number have depressive illness severe enough to make them wish to end their lives. These people do not always get appropriate medical treatment, many with milder depression are even less likely to do so.

OTHER EVENTS

Social Pathology

The figures for illegitimate births and for divorce are given in Table 3. Others can be derived from various sources. Each year one adult criminal will be sent to prison, and five or six children under the age of 17 will be charged with offenses (*27*). About 100 people in the practice will receive National Assistance (*29*). Twenty-five to fifty people over retiring age will live alone (*30*) and about 40 children under the age of 15 come from broken homes (*31*). There will probably be between five and ten problem families (*32*); and there will be four chronic alcoholics with mental and physical complications, and about another dozen who are addicted to alcohol (*33*). Each year ten abortions will escape the notice of the medical profession, compared with the three or four who receive proper medical care (*34*). Many of these numbers are only crude estimates, and regional and social variations could cause wide deviations from the average.

Uncommon Events

In the same way figures can be adjusted to show how seldom some conditions will turn up in the average general practice. Diseases which were common a generation ago are now rare; the average general practitioner might wait eight years to see a case of rheumatic fever in a child under the age of 15; 60 years to see a case of typhoid or paratyphoid fever, and as long as 400 years to see a case of diphtheria (*18*). He will probably see a patient with schizophrenia once in two years (*35*), a patient with leukemia or other malignant disease of the lymphatic and hemopoietic system once in four years, and a patient with a cerebral tumor once in eight to ten years (*2*).

The diversity of activities in the average general practice, and the range of tasks expected of the average family doctor have been shown. Changing conditions of practice in recent years should not allow his clinical skills to atrophy.

COMMUNICATIONS

If the general practitioner is to draw together the various parts of the National Health Service, much will depend on the efficiency of his lines of communication. The number of contacts with the hospital services (Table 3) is probably inflated because some patients will attend more than one hospital and some will be admitted to the same hospital more than once in a year. The contrast between the figure of 208 derived from the report on the health and welfare services (*1*) and of 96 from the morbidity statistics from general practice (*11*) makes this clear. Even so nearly 1000 contacts between the practice and the hospital services each year must represent a formidable number of letters and/or telephone calls. Considering the quantity of communications, it is hardly surprising that their quality is sometimes defective.

The discrepancies in the figures for domiciliary obstetrics cannot only be due to the division of the obstetric services into three parts. Whatever else may be said about this, it is clear that if in the average general practice a doctor is present at only 2 out of the 14 home confinements that take place each year, opportunities are being lost to cement a firm doctor-patient relationship. Postnatal care may be no more satisfactory, but here the data are incomplete.

SUMMARY

A model has been used to show a year's experience in an average general practice, particularly of the chronic diseases.

A considerable amount of undetected disease, some of which is serious and some controllable, might be found fairly easily without adding greatly to the burden of the day's work.

Ordinary clinical skills and new diagnostic aids may be used to detect cases of actual and potential disease in general practice.

The detection and control of diabetes, some forms of hypertension and their sequelae, glaucoma, anemia, some kinds of cancer, and coronary-artery disease have been discussed.

This investigation was suggested by Prof. J. N. Morris. To him and other colleagues at the M.R.C. Social Medicine Research Unit, I am grateful for much helpful criticism.

References

(*1*) Ministry of Health. *On the State of the Public Health.* London, H.M. Stationery Office, 1961.

(*2*) Registrar General. Statistical Review of England and Wales, Part I, Tables, Medical. London, H.M. Stationery Office, 1961.

(*3*) College of General Practitioners. *Br Med J* ii:973, 1961.

(*4*) College of General Practitioners. *Br Med J* i:1497, 1962.

(*5*) David, W.D. Publication No. 666. Washington, D.C., U.S. Public Health Service, 1959.

(*6*) Heasman, M.A. *Stud Med Popul Subj* No. 17, 1961.

(*7*) Kass, E.H. *Ann Intern Med* 56:46, 1962.

(*8*) Kessel, W.I.N. *Br J Prev Soc Med* 14:16, 1960.

(*9*) Kilpatrick, G.S. *Br Med J* ii:1736, 1961.

(*10*) Lawrence, J.S., V.A. Laine, and R. de Graaff. *Proc Roy Soc Med* 54:454, 1961.

(*11*) Logan, W.P.D. and A.A. Cushion. *Morbidity Statistics from General Practice.* H.M. Stationery Office, 1958.

(*12*) Miall, W.E. and P.D. Oldham. *Clin Sci* 17:409, 1958.

(*13*) Munch-Petersen, E. *Bull WHO* 24:761, 1961.

(*14*) Pond, D.A., B.H. Bidwell, and L. Stein. *Psychiatr Neurol Neurochir* 63:217, 1960.

(*15*) Walker, J.B. and D. Kerrige. *Diabetes in an English Community.* Leicester, 1961.

(*16*) Wilson, J.M.G. *Monthly Bull Min Health P H L S* 20:214, 1961.

(*17*) Morris, J.N. *Uses of Epidemiology* Edinburgh, 1957.

(*18*) Ministry of Health. *On the State of the Public Health* H.M. Stationery Office, 1961.

(*19*) Simmons, N.A. and J.D. Williams. *Lancet* i:1377, 1962.

(*20*) Smith, L.G. and J. Schmidt. *JAMA* 181:431, 1962.

(*21*) Semmence, A. *Br Med J* ii:1153, 1959.

(*22*) McAlpine, S.G., A.S. Douglas, and R.A. Robb. *Br Med J* ii:983, 1957.

(*23*) Ministry of Health. *On the State of the Public Health.* H.M. Stationery Office, 1960.

(*24*) Boyes, D.A., H.K. Fidler, and D.R. Lock. *Br Med J* i:203, 1962.

(*25*) Royal College of Physicians. *Smoking and Health.* London, 1962.

(*26*) Dawber, T.R. *Proc R Soc Med* 55:265, 1962.

(*27*) Criminal Statistics 1960. H.M. Stationery Office, 1961.

(*28*) *Lancet* i:1171, 1962.

(*29*) Annual Abstract of Statistics No. 98. H.M. Stationery Office, 1961.

(*30*) Townsend, P. *Bull WHO* 21:583, 1959.

(*31*) Illsley, R. and B. Thompson. *Sociol Rev* 9:27, 1961.

(*32*) Philp, A.F. and N. Timms. *Problem of the Problem Family.* London, 1957.

(*33*) *Lancet* i:1169, 1962.

(*34*) Tietze, C. *Am J Obstet Gynecol* 56:1160, 1948.

(*35*) Registrar General. Supplement on Mental Health, 1960. H.M. Stationery Office, 1961.

(*36*) ———Report on the Hospital Inpatient Inquiry, 1956-1957. H.M. Stationery Office, 1961.

(*37*) Road Research, 1960. H.M. Stationery Office, 1961.

(*38*) Kagan, A., T.R. Dawber, W.B. Kannel, and N. Revotskie. *Fed Proc* 21(suppl. 11):52, 1962.

(*39*) Social Medicine Research Unit (M.R.C.). Unpubl. data.

(*40*) Morris, J.N. and M.D. Crawford. *Br Med J* ii:1485, 1958.

(*41*) Metropolitan Life Insurance Company. Statistical Bulletin, January 1960, p. 4.

(*42*) Hill, K.R., F.E. Camps, K. Rigg, and B.E.G. McKinney. *Br Med J* i:1190, 1961.

THE BURLINGTON RANDOMIZED TRIAL OF THE NURSE PRACTITIONER: HEALTH OUTCOMES OF PATIENTS

David L. Sackett, Walter O. Spitzer, Michael Gent, and Robin S. Roberts, in collaboration
with W. Ian Hay, Georgie M. Lefroy, G. Patrick Sweeny, Isabel Vandervlist, John C. Sibley,
Larry W. Chambers, Charles H. Goldsmith, Alexander S. MacPherson,
and Ronald G. McAuley[1]

In a randomized trial of nurse practitioners as providers of primary clinical services, attention was devoted to the "outcomes" of clinical effectiveness and safety. These outcomes—expressed in physical, emotional, and social function—were assessed with newly developed methods that could be applied easily and objectively by nonclinicians to the two groups of patients under study: patients receiving conventional care and patients receiving care from nurse practitioners. Besides showing the comparability of these groups at the start of this study, these measurements showed similar levels of physical, emotional, and social function in the two groups after one year of receiving either nurse-practitioner or conventional care. Since the numbers of patients were large enough for a statistical detection of even small differences, the results indicate that the nurse practitioners were effective and safe. This study provides a base from which to explore the "process" of delivering primary clinical services by nurse practitioners.

The availability and distribution of clinical manpower in Ontario, the increasing demand for primary clinical services, and the projected economic implications of this demand indicate the need for determining the feasibility of using the nurse practitioner as a source of primary clinical care (1). This feasibility could be determined by measurements of the "process" of providing clinical services (for example, patients seen, procedures performed, money spent, attitudes of patients and clinicians) or by measurements of "outcomes" among patients receiving these services (end-results measures such as mortality and physical, emotional, and social function), or by some combination of both. We believe that "process" measurements are meaningful only after proper "outcome" studies have shown that the clinical services under scrutiny are effective and safe. Accordingly, we have supplied the strategy of the controlled clinical trial to the health care delivery setting, and we have adapted or developed a series of health outcome measures and applied them to patients in the trial.

Using the World Health Organization definition of health as a starting point, we have sought indexes of positive physical, emotional, and social health for use as "outcome" measurements. For the purposes of this trial, these outcome measurements had to be objective, positive in orientation, and capable of application to several hundred patients by nonclinical interviewers. Satisfactory measures of physical function that had been developed elsewhere (2-4) were incorporated into a household survey. However, we were unable to find satisfactory positive measures of emotional and social function that were reasonably objective and could be employed and scored by nonclinicians. As a result, our research group had to develop and validate, in an independent investigation, the emotional and social function measurements used in this study.

METHODS

The basic design of the Burlington Randomized Trial is described in detail elsewhere (1). In summary, 1598 families receiving clinical services from two family physicians in a middle-class suburb were randomly allocated, in a ratio of 2:1, to a conventional group (designated RC),

Source: *Annals of Internal Medicine* 80:137-142, 1974.
All from the Faculty of Health Sciences, McMaster University, Hamilton, Ontario, Canada.

923

in which they continued to receive their primary clinical services from a family physician working with a conventional nurse, or to a nurse practitioner group (designated RNP). Patients in the RNP group received their first-contact, primary clinical services from one of two nurses who had successfully completed an educational program that stressed clinical judgment in the evaluation and management of conditions arising in primary care *(5)*. Accordingly, the nurse practitioner either totally managed each patient's office visit by providing reassurance or specific therapy, or requested consultation from the associated physician.

Outcome Measures

Four "outcome" measures were applied to members of the RC and RNP groups.

Mortality. A surveillance system identified deaths of RC and RNP patients during the one-year experimental period. Decedents were categorized by age, sex, cause of death, and group assignment, and crude mortality rates were generated. On two separate occasions, the clinical records for each decedent were assembled, purged of any notation that would indicate the experimental group to which they had been randomized, and submitted to the President of the Ontario College of Physicians and Surgeons. Members of this professional body, which serves a licensing and disciplinary function for physicians in the province, reviewed each case to determine whether, in their opinion, the death could have been prevented.

Physical Function. Specific "outcome" measurements were applied to the same patients (drawn by random sampling from each of the families in the study and designated the "interview cohort") both before and at the end of the experimental period, to permit "paired" comparisons in which patients could serve as their own controls. The measurement of physical function determined the patient's mobility, vision, hearing, and ability to execute activities of daily living. The three indexes of physical function were (1) the proportion of patients with unimpaired mobility, vision, and hearing on the day of the interview; (2) the proportion of patients able to execute their usual daily activities during the 14 days before the interview; and (3) the proportion of patients free from an illness

or injury requiring them to remain in bed for all or part of a day during the 14 days before the interview.

These indexes of physical function were determined both before and at the end of the one-year experimental period.

Emotional Function. It was necessary to develop measures of emotional and social function that were positive in their orientation, clinically valid, and capable of mass application and scoring by nonclinicians; they were developed in an independent Health Index Study *(6, 7)*. Briefly, in the Health Index Study an interview containing questions judged to relate to important dimensions of emotional and social function was conducted on a random sample of patients, who were simultaneously assessed by a physician for their functional status. In work to be published elsewhere, various analytic strategies, including discriminant function analysis, identified a subset of these questions, which correlated with the clinician's clinical assessment of function, and these questions were applied in the Burlington Trial to the interview cohort at the end of the experimental period.[2]

The emotional function questions were concerned with feelings of self-esteem, feelings toward relations with other individuals, and thoughts about the future. By using weighting factors derived from the Health Index Study, the responses to each question were combined into a composite emotional function index for each of the Burlington Trial patients in the interview cohort at the end of the experimental period. This index runs from 0.0 (poor emotional function) to 1.0 (good emotional function).

Social Function. A composite index of social function was derived from each member of the Burlington Trial who was in the interview cohort at the end of the experimental period. This composite index, also developed in the Health Index Study *(6, 7)*, considered the patient's interaction with others (as manifested by visits with, or telephone calls from, relatives, friends, social agencies, or other individuals); subjective feelings of happiness; and interactions with police, the courts, or welfare agen-

---

[2] See NAPS Document #02178 for 228 pages of questionnaire instruments used in this project.

cies. As in the case of emotional function, the answers to individual social-function questions were weighted and combined into a composite social-function index running from 0.0 (poor social function) to 1.0 (good social function).

Statistical Analyses

Similar to the pharmacologic randomized clinical trial, in which a new drug is compared with a "standard" drug in widespread current use, in our trial clinical outcomes among patients in the RNP group were compared with those of patients receiving "conventional" or "standard" care in the RC group. Since it was our thesis that the outcomes of RNP care would be equivalent to those resulting from RC care, the hypothesis that the RNP care was effective and safe would be supported if *no* statistically significant differences could be shown between the outcomes of the RNP and RC groups. In the analysis of these data, as in the testing of a phenotypic genetic model against a set of observations, the investigator wishes to minimize the chances of accepting the null hypothesis (no difference in outcomes) when it is false. Accordingly, the "alpha" level of the test of statistical significance, used when one wants to show "true" differences between comparison groups, is replaced in prominence by the "beta" level of the test of significance, a particularly important measure of the possibility that one is "missing" a true difference. In assessing observed differences between the RNP and RC groups, we have indicated the results of tests of statistical significance in terms of the probability with which we have "missed" a true difference between the groups, in either direction, of 5 percent or more at the start of the experimental period (a "two-tailed" test). At the end of the period we have applied a more precise "one-tailed" beta level of the test to determine the likelihood that we have missed a true deterioration among RNP patients, one in which they are less healthy by 5 percent or more than RC patients.

RESULTS

Of 1598 families, only seven refused their assignments (two families from the RC group and five from the RNP group). Furthermore, during the one-year experimental period, only 0.9 percent of RC families and 0.7 percent of

RNP families left the practice because of dissatisfaction. By the final two months of the experiment, the proportion of RNP patient visits managed entirely by the nurse practitioners had stabilized at 67 percent.

Comparability of the RC and RNP Interview Cohorts at the Start of the Trial

Table 1 summarizes the distributions of family size, sex, age, and annual household income for the RC and RNP cohorts just before the one-year experimental period. The groups are highly similar, and none of the observed differences approach statistical significance. The initial similarity of the RC and RNP groups is further supported in Table 2, which summarizes the physical function of members of the RC and RNP groups just before the one-year experimental period. Large and identical portions of patients in the RC and RNP groups had unimpaired mobility, vision, and hearing on the day of the interview. Similarly large and comparable proportions of patients in each group had been able to carry out their usual daily activities throughout the 14 days before this interview. A review of the "beta" levels for the

Table 1. Comparison of the RC and RNP interview cohorts at the start of the trial.[a]

	RC	RNP
Number of patients in the interview cohort	614	340
Mean number of persons per family	2.8	2.7
Males, %	42	43
Females, %	58	57
Age in years, %		
0 to 4	5	4
5 to 9	5	5
10 to 14	8	7
15 to 19	5	8
20 to 39	33	29
40 to 59	31	35
60 to 69	7	8
70 and over	6	4
Annual household income, %		
Less than $4000	4	4
$4000 to $7999	15	13
$8000 to $9999	13	12
$10 000 to $13 999	28	24
$14 000 to $17 999	15	14
$18 000 or more	16	23

[a] RC = patients receiving conventional care; RNP = patients receiving care from nurse practitioners.

Table 2. Physical function prior to the experimental period.

	RC[a]	RNP[a]	β[b]
	%		
Unimpaired mobility, vision, and hearing	86	86	0.03
Unimpaired in usual daily activities	87	89	0.09
Free from bed disability	86	83	0.22

[a] RC = patients receiving conventional care; RNP = patients receiving care from nurse practitioners.
[b] Indicates probability that we have failed to detect a *real* difference of ≥5% in physical function between RC and RNP patients.

differences between RC and RNP patients, given in the third column of Table 2, shows that RNP patients may have been less healthy than RC patients, in terms of bed disability, before the start of the experimental period.

Mortality

It was anticipated during the design of the trial that the number of deaths during the experimental period would be small. As shown in Table 3, there were only 18 deaths in the RC group and 4 deaths among RNP patients. The mean age at death was similar for decedents in the RC and RNP groups, and the difference in crude death rates for the two groups was not statistically significant. On the two occasions

Table 3. Mortality during the study.

	RC group[a]	RNP group[a]
	no.	
By cause at death		
Cancer	8	2
Myocardial infarction[b]	4	1
Other cardiovascular disease	4	—
Other	2	1
By age at death		
10 to 29 years	2	—
30 to 49 years	3	1
50 to 69 years	7	2
70 years and over	6	1
Mean age at death	59.3 years	57.0 years
Total deaths	18	4
Death rate per thousand	6.0	2.7

[a] RC = patients receiving conventional care; RNP = patients receiving care from nurse practitioners.
[b] Includes sudden death.

when the clinical records of decedents were reviewed by appointees of the Ontario College of Physicians and Surgeons, no deaths of RNP patients were judged to have been preventable.

Physical Function at the End of the Experimental Period

Table 4 summarizes the measurements of physical function for 521 patients in the RC group and 296 patients in the RNP group at the end of the experimental period. The proportions of individuals in the two experimental groups with unimpaired physical function, unimpaired usual daily activities, and freedom from bed disability were again virtually identical, and a similar pattern emerges when this analysis is limited to those members of the interview cohort who had these measurements both before and after the one-year experimental period. The last column in Table 4 indicates the probability that patients in the RNP group are less healthy by 5 percent or more, in terms of physical function, than those in the RC group, and it is seen that we are unlikely to have missed a deterioration among RNP patients, had it occurred during the trial.

Table 4. Physical function at the end of the experimental period.[a]

	RC group	RNP group	β[b]
Unimpaired mobility, vision, and hearing	88	86	0.10
Unimpaired in usual daily activities	90	90	0.02
Free from bed disability	87	86	0.05

[a] RC = patients receiving conventional care; RNP = patients receiving care from nurse practitioners.
[b] Indicates probability that we have failed to detect a *real* deterioration of physical function among RNP patients ≥ 5%.

Emotional Function at the End of the Experimental Period

Figure 1 is a histogram of the distribution of emotional function indexes for patients in the RC and RNP groups. The mean emotional function index for RC patients at the end of the experimental period was 0.583 (SD, 0.187) and for the RNP patients, 0.577 (SD, 0.187). These results indicate closely similar levels of emotional function in the two groups of patients; the likelihood that we have missed a deteriora-

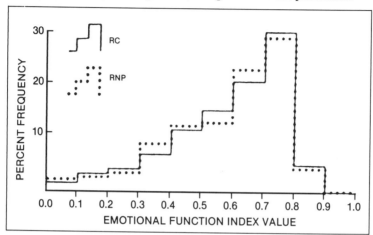

Figure 1. Emotional function at the end of the experiment. RC = patients receiving conventional care; RNP = patients receiving care from nurse practitioners.

tion of 5 percent or more among RNP patients is shown by the beta value of only 0.068.

Social Function at the End of the Experimental Period

Figure 2 is a histogram of social function index values for RC and RNP patients; the respective mean social function index values are 0.832 (SD, 0.249) and 0.839 (SD, 0.274). The likelihood that a drop of 5 percent or more in the social function of RNP patients has been "missed" is 0.008.

DISCUSSION

The close comparability of mortality rates and of measurements of physical, social, and emotional function between the RC and RNP patients supports the conclusion that patients randomly assigned to receive first-contact primary care from a nurse practitioner enjoy favorable health outcomes, which are comparable to those of patients receiving conventional care. Before concluding that the nurse practitioner is both effective and safe, however, it is important to consider three potential pitfalls in the design and execution of this randomized trial, which may have created these favorable findings in a spurious fashion.

The first potential pitfall results from the absence of a "no treatment" control group. It could be argued that neither the nurse practi-

tioner nor the family physician have any clinically significant impact on health outcomes and that this trial has merely compared equally ineffective, "neutral" alternatives for the delivery of primary care. We have deliberately excluded a "no treatment" control group for two reasons. First, we concluded with our collaborators that it would be unethical to withhold clinical services from a control group of patients in this investigation, just as it has been judged unethical to withhold treatment from control groups in randomized clinical trials of surgical and chemotherapeutic approaches to cancer *(8)*. Our trial is analogous to the trial in which therapy with a new pharmacologic agent is compared with current "standard" therapy. Second, primary care practices of this magnitude, studied over this duration of time, generate a volume of clinical conditions (both statistically and clinically significant in number) whose outcomes are profoundly affected by the skill of detection and the appropriateness of management. This is substantiated, for example, by the numbers of patients identified as requiring the diagnosis and treatment of occlusive cardiovascular and infectious disorders, both in this and in other investigations of primary care *(1, 9, 10)*.

The second potential pitfall, "volunteer bias," was avoided by incorporating random allocation into the experimental design, and the comparability of the RC and RNP groups at the start of the trial, as shown in Tables 1 and 2, attests to the success of this procedure. Further-

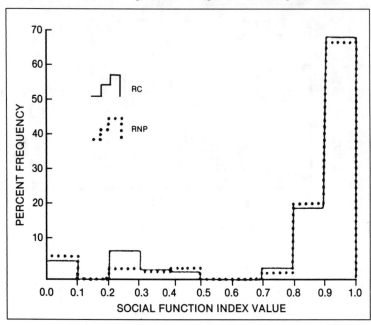

Figure 2. Social function at the end of the experiment. RC = patients receiving conventional care; RNP = patients receiving care from nurse practitioners.

more, as indicated by the extremely high rates of participation and follow-up, it is appropriate to compare the RC and RNP patients throughout the experimental period.

However, a third major potential pitfall remains: the measurements and indexes of function we used to assess health outcomes among patients. It is theoretically possible that our measures of physical, social, and emotional function may be insensitive to small but clinically significant changes in health status, which could have occurred during the experiment. If so, this insensitivity could mask a deterioration in the health status of patients assigned to the RNP group; for example, these indexes of function may remain fixed at relatively high levels until a substantial deterioration in health status has occurred and only then begin to show discernible declines.

The "paired" comparisons of physical function in the same patients, both before and at the end of the experimental period, suggest that this third potential pitfall has also been avoided. These paired comparisons (Table 5) indicate that the majority of patients with impaired physical function at the start of the trial no longer were impaired at the end of the experi-

Table 5. Paired comparisons of physical function among patients assessed both before and at the end of the experimental period.

	RC group[a]		RNP group[b]	
	no.	%	no.	%
Patients impaired at start who were unimpaired at end of the trial				
Mobility, vision, hearing	39/71	55	18/41	44
Usual daily activities	58/67	87	27/34	79
Bed disability	55/73	75	39/51	76
Patients impaired at end who were unimpaired at start of the trial				
Mobility, vision, hearing	32/64	50	19/42	45
Usual daily activities	42/51	82	23/30	77
Bed disability	51/69	74	28/40	70

[a] Patients who continued to receive primary clinical services from a family physician working with a conventional nurse.
[b] Patients receiving care from nurse practitioners.

mental period; similarly, from 45 percent to 82 percent of patients whose physical function was impaired at the end of the trial were free of impairment at its start. We have therefore concluded that these measures of physical function are quite sensitive to short-term variations in physical function. It is extremely unlikely that a clinically important deterioration in health status of the RNP group could go undetected.

This search for answers to questions of effectiveness and safety in using the nurse practitioner as a provider of primary clinical services required the measurement of health outcomes among patients, and the development and application of such measures may be difficult. This is not the case if the end-result is a "hard" one, such as the death of a study subject. Although disagreement and a resulting misclassification can occur in assigning a cause of death, the fact of death is indisputable. The measurement of health outcomes becomes more difficult as one moves toward "softer" end-results, such as discrete clinical events. Despite the slow evolution of strategies and tactics for clinical measurement, sufficient experience has been gained to indicate the feasibility of measuring clinical outcomes *(11)*.

Outcome measurement becomes quite formidable, however, when the innovative clinical maneuver results in the multidimensional, functional state the World Health Organization defines as health. Not only are well-developed and easily applied health-outcome indexes very few in number, "observer variation" and disagreement extend to the rationale, definitions, and justification for the indexes themselves, as well as to the subsequent measurement process.

Nonetheless, the high degree of patient cooperation and the successful measurement of physical, social, and emotional function by non-clinicians have reinforced our earlier conviction that it is possible to design and execute randomized clinical trials of innovations in the delivery of broad categories of clinical services. These favorable and comparable health outcomes, besides answering the questions of effectiveness and safety, are a solid base from which to analyze other data collected before, during, and after the experimental period. The quality of clinical care provided, the attitudes of clinicians and patients toward this innovation, and the economic issues affecting the introduction of nurse practitioners as providers of primary clinical care can now be explored.

ACKNOWLEDGMENTS

The authors acknowledge, with thanks, the enthusiasm, patience, and persistence of Mrs. Betty Bidgood and her team of household interviewers in the Health Sciences Field Survey Unit, who carried out the measurements of physical, social, and emotional function used in this trial.

Grant support: DM34 and PR146, Ministry of Health, Ontario, Canada.

Received 5 November 1973; accepted 19 November 1973.

References

(1) Spitzer, W.D., D.L. Sacket, J.C. Sibley, et al. The Burlington randomized trial of the nurse practitioner. Methods and principal results. *N Engl J Med* In press.

(2) Bruett, T.L. and R.P. Overs. A critical review of 12 ADL scales. *Phys Ther* 49:857-862, 1962.

(3) The staff of the Benjamin Rose Hospital. Multidisciplinary study of illness in aged persons. I. Methods and preliminary results. *J Chron Dis* 7:332-345, 1958.

(4) Holland, W.W. Health services in London. *Br Med J* 2:233, 1972.

(5) Spitzer, W.O. and D.J. Kergin. Nurse practitioners in primary care. I. The McMaster University Educational Program. *Can Med Assoc J* 108:991-995, 1973.

(6) Macpherson, A.S. The Measurement of Mental Health in a General Population (M.Sc. dissertation). Hamilton, Ontario, McMaster University, 1972.

(7) Chambers, L.W. An Index of Social Function (M.Sc. dissertation). Hamilton, Ontario, McMaster University, 1972.

(8) Glaser, E.M. Ethical aspects of clinical trials. In *The Principles and Practice of Clinical Trials*, edited by E.L. Harris and J.D. Fitzgerald. Edinburgh, E & S Livingstone, Ltd., 1970, pages 23-30.

(9) Fry, J. *Profiles of Disease*. Edinburgh, E & S Livingstone, Ltd., 1966.

(10) McFarlane, A.H., G.R. Norman, and W.O. Spitzer. Family medicine: The dilemma of defining the discipline. *Can Med Assoc J* 10:397-401, 1971.

(11) Sackett, D.L. Design, measurement and analysis in clinical trials. Presented at the Symposium on Platelets, Drugs, and Thrombosis, Hamilton, Ontario, Canada, October 16–18, 1972. In press.

HEALTH SERVICE "INPUT" AND MORTALITY "OUTPUT" IN DEVELOPED COUNTRIES

A.L. Cochrane,[1] A.S. St. Leger,[2] and F. Moore[2]

SUMMARY

The relationship between age-specific mortality rates and some indices of health facilities and some environmental and dietary factors has been studied in 18 developed countries. The indices of health care are not negatively associated with mortality, and there is a marked positive association between the prevalence of doctors and mortality in the younger age groups. No explanation of this doctor anomaly has so far been found. Gross national product per head is the principal variable which shows a consistently strong negative association with mortality.

Health services in developed countries, both state and private, are based upon many common assumptions about what constitutes adequate health care. Doctors and their paramedical colleagues in different developed countries receive similar educations to more or less the same standards, and their approaches to clinical and preventive medicine are unlikely to differ in fundamental principles. However, these countries show marked differences in their mortality rates and in health costs per head. In this paper, we seek to discover some factors to explain these differences in mortality.

MATERIALS AND METHODS

We employed the following criteria in selecting our countries:

1. Gross national product (GNP) exceeding $2000 per caput. We made an exception for the Republic of Ireland (GNP $1949 per caput).
2. Population of more than two million.
3. Data available for 1970, but, if not, data for 1969 or 1971 accepted if available.
4. We excluded countries where genetic factors may account for a substantial proportion of the difference in mortality between them and our other countries. This excluded Japan.

The data recorded on our countries are of two types: "Input" and "Output." The input variables were selected according to two criteria: firstly, availability; and, secondly, an expectation that the variables might be related to the health of the communities. There are three types: health care indices, dietary consumption, and other demographic or economic variables. The output is measured by age-specific mortality rates up to the age of 64; we excluded the older ages because these are less likely to be associated with environmental factors.

The set of input variables is far too large in relation to the number of countries, and it was necessary to reduce the numbers to produce a more manageable set of relevant variables. This was accomplished by studying scatter diagrams of the mortality rates against each of the input factors, and by examining the correlation matrix of all the variables. Regression analysis of the output variables also helped to determine which variables may explain differences in mortality. Our criteria for the inclusion of factors in the subsequent analysis were:

1. The intrinsic importance of the variable; that is, we included variables such as prevalence of doctors, and availability of hospital beds, which many people consider to be self-evidently related to mortality.
2. A factor had to show a large product-moment correlation with at least one mortality rate, or it had to show a consistent pattern of association with several mortality rates.

Source: *Journal of Epidemiology and Community Health* 32:200-205, 1978.
[1] Rhoose Farm House, Rhoose, South Glamorgan, Wales.
[2] MRC Epidemiology Unit, Cardiff, Wales.

930

3. A factor had to contribute a large proportion to the sums of squares of regression in a consistent manner in spite of changes in the composition of the other variables in the regression.

With only 18 countries, and many possible input variables, problems arise if we seek to apply standard methods of statistical inference, such as significance testing, to the data. If no allowance is made for multiple comparisons, then a correlation coefficient must exceed ±0.44 in order to be significantly different from zero at the 5 percent level of significance (assuming normality, etc.). It is arguable, however, that problems of statistical inference may not be relevant to our 18 countries because these cannot be regarded as being a random sample from some large set of developed countries. We think that there are so many possible sources of error in this sort of data, and so many pitfalls in interpretation, that a slavish adherence to significance testing, if relevant, would give our results a spurious and perhaps misleading aura of precision. We have used the criteria set out above in our analysis, and we have placed particular emphasis on the crite-

rion of consistency. We believe that the results outlined in the next section are both interesting and amusing, and we make no apology for the necessarily subjective nature of some stages in our analysis.

RESULTS

On the basis of the criteria listed earlier, we had a set of 18 countries which are shown in Table 1.

The input and output variables, their median values, and their ranges across the 18 countries, are shown in Tables 2 and 3.

Table 1. Countries used in the study.

Australia	Republic of Ireland
Austria	Italy
Belgium	Netherlands
Canada	New Zealand
Denmark	Norway
England and Wales	Scotland
Finland	Sweden
France	Switzerland
German Federal	United States of
Republic	America

Table 2. Input variables.

	Minimum	Median	Maximum
Health service indices			
Doctors[a]	10.2	13.7	18.5
Nurses[a]	6.7	35.4	56.0
Acute hospital beds[a]	39.5	52.3	97.7
Pediatricians[b]	3.9	23.6	68.8
Obstetricians[b]	12.6	27.3	50.8
Midwives[b]	10.2	106.0	399.7
% Gross national product spent on health	4.7	5.2	7.1
Dietary indices			
Cigarette consumption per caput per annum	630	2440	3810
Alcohol consumption in liters per caput per annum	3.7	7.2	17.5
Calories per caput per day	2805	3195	3410
Grams protein per caput per day	83.9	90.5	108.2
Grams total fat per caput per day	124.3	148.3	173.8
Grams sugar per caput per day	75.8	120.0	138.5
Economic and demographic factors			
Average population per km²	1.6	77.2	324.2
Gross national product per caput	1949	4236	6652
Education index	10.0	16.3	49.4
Intervention index (% of health expenditure covered by public expenditure)	40.5	80.7	94.8

[a] Per 10 000 population.
[b] Per 10 000 live births.

Table 3. Output variables.

Mortality rates	Minimum	Median	Maximum
Maternal per 100 000 live births	8.5	21.5	54.5
Perinatal per 1000 live births	16.5	22.9	31.7
Infant per 1000 live births	11.0	18.2	29.6
1– 4 years per 10 000 population	5.3	8.5	10.2
5–14 years per 10 000 population	3.2	4.1	4.7
15–24 years per 10 000 population	6.8	8.8	13.0
25–34 years per 10 000 population	8.0	10.9	15.9
35–44 years per 10 000 population	16.9	22.9	32.2
45–54 years per 10 000 population	43.6	56.2	72.8
55–64 years per 10 000 population	107.9	150.0	183.2

The principal findings on examination of the raw correlations (Table 4) were as follows:

1. The correlation between prevalence of doctors and pediatricians and mortality is large and positive in the younger age groups, it is positive in young adult life, and it only becomes negative in the two oldest age groups.
2. The correlation between alcohol consumption and mortality shows a similar pattern to that for doctors, but with a particularly strong correlation between alcohol consumption and maternal mortality.
3. The prevalence of nurses shows a negative association with maternal, perinatal, infant, and early childhood mortality. Their association with other mortality rates is positive or negligible.
4. The prevalence of acute hospital beds shows an erratic association with mortality rates; most of the associations are weak.
5. Cigarette consumption has a positive association with all the death rates, and this association is strongest in the two age groups 45 to 54 and 55 to 64.
6. The dietary factors, other than sugar consumption, have consistently positive associations with mortality. In particular, total calorie intake and protein consumption are strongly positively associated with all mortality rates.
7. Sugar consumption has a large negative association with maternal mortality and

Table 4. Correlation coefficients between the death rates and the input variables.[a]

| | | | | | | Mortality rates | | | | |
| | | | | | | Age groups (years) | | | | |
	Maternal	Perinatal	Infant	1–4	5–14	15–24	25–34	35–44	45–54	55–64
Doctors	0.45	0.60	0.67	0.37	0.42	0.32	0.23	0.04	−0.27	−0.20
Nurses	−0.39	−0.53	−0.50	−0.28	0.37	0.12	0.06	0.19	0.27	0.11
Beds	0.04	−0.32	−0.10	0.07	0.18	0.37	0.06	−0.02	−0.14	−0.14
Pediatricians	0.40	0.47	0.51	0.23	0.31	0.35	0.37	0.15	−0.11	−0.12
Obstetricians	0.04	0.18	0.18	−0.17	0.29	0.48	0.54	0.36	0.09	0.04
Midwives	−0.10	−0.15	−0.14	−0.29	−0.33	−0.57	−0.28	0.00	0.26	0.28
% GNP on health	−0.12	0.01	−0.10	−0.23	0.27	0.39	0.30	0.00	0.23	0.36
Cigarettes	0.17	0.22	0.22	0.11	0.31	0.36	0.35	0.32	0.46	0.49
Alcohol	0.68	0.52	0.61	0.33	0.32	0.26	0.27	0.09	−0.18	−0.14
Calories	0.41	0.59	0.58	0.58	0.41	0.31	0.30	0.31	0.38	0.52
Protein	0.43	0.37	0.33	0.44	0.20	0.47	0.50	0.50	0.49	0.43
Fat	0.10	0.29	0.23	0.32	0.46	0.43	0.37	0.21	0.10	0.16
Sugar	−0.61	−0.57	−0.56	−0.40	−0.31	−0.17	−0.20	−0.05	0.26	0.21
Population density	0.17	0.24	0.21	0.07	−0.03	−0.30	−0.35	−0.45	−0.30	−0.10
GNP per caput	−0.29	−0.48	−0.46	−0.41	0.18	0.25	0.17	−0.13	−0.36	−0.53
Education index	−0.13	−0.22	−0.20	0.28	−0.43	−0.79	−0.61	−0.47	−0.27	−0.21
Intervention index	−0.15	0.15	−0.02	−0.13	0.12	0.44	0.48	0.30	0.26	0.07

[a] The input variables are defined in Table 2.

with mortality in the younger age groups, and the association remains negative up to 44 years of age.

8. Gross national product per head is negatively associated with mortality except in the age groups 5 to 14 and 15 to 24 years.

9. The intervention index (percent of health care provided by public funds) has a consistently negative association with all mortality rates, and these associations are large in the age groups 15 to 24 and 25 to 34 years. There is reason to believe, however, that in the 25 to 34 age group this correlation may be spurious, because the United States of America, with a high mortality rate and a low index, stands far away from the other countries, which appear to form a random cluster. Exclusion of the USA halves the correlation coefficient.

The correlations for smoking and for GNP per head accord with expectation, and lead us to suppose that our method of study gives sensible results. Many of the other results are confusing, and interpretation is made more difficult by the cross-correlations among the input variables.

Regression analysis is a useful aid to sorting out the relationships between sets of moderately intercorrelated variables. There are too many input variables relative to the output variables to allow one large analysis, so we performed a series of regression analyses on various overlapping subsets of the input variables in order to seek a small subset, should it exist, of variables with the most explanatory power. The main findings from these analyses were:

1. None of the health service factors were consistently negatively related to mortality. Prevalence of doctors was positively associated with mortality in all age groups except 45 to 54 years, and the association was particularly marked for infant mortality, being even stronger than that suggested by the raw correlations.

2. The main factors consistently negatively associated with mortality were GNP per head, population density, sugar consumption, and the intervention index.

3. The principal factors, other than doctors, which were mainly positively associated with mortality were cigarette consumption and alcohol consumption.

4. Consumption of calories and protein showed very much weaker associations with mortality than their unadjusted cor-

relations suggested, particularly when the regression equations contained GNP per head. The correlations of GNP with protein and of GNP with calorie consumption are -0.29 and -0.30, respectively. Gross national product per head appeared to have an independent association with the mortality rates over and above the association which may be attributed to its cross-correlation with the dietary variables. We therefore retained GNP per head and rejected protein and calorie consumption as contributing little additional explanatory power. Incidentally, total calorie intake and sugar consumption have a correlation coefficient of 0.02, and the correlations between sugar consumption and fat and protein consumption are -0.12 and -0.04, respectively. It therefore follows that the contribution to the regression made by sugar consumption is unlikely merely to reflect a general dietary contribution.

On the basis of these analyses, we were able to select seven variables, each of which appeared to have some independent effect upon mortality in at least one age group. The set of variables as a whole had most of the explanatory power of our input data. The resulting regression equations seemed to be reasonably stable in the sense that adding other variables singly, in turn, to the set of seven did not bring about major alterations in the first seven regression coefficients. Table 5 displays the results of regressing mortality rates on the chosen seven variables. The figures in the first seven columns are the percentage change in a given death rate (denoted by the row) for a 1-standard-deviation increase in the input variable (denoted by the column) from its mean value, all other input variables being fixed at their mean values. This enables a comparison to be made, for example, between the effects of the prevalence of doctors, of maternal mortality, and of GNP, on the same mortality rate; or between the effect of prevalence of doctors on maternal mortality and that of GNP on infant mortality. The figures described above are not regression coefficients but they are derived from them. The legitimacy of the comparisons depends partly upon the stability of our regression equations over the input variables at our disposal and over others unknown to us, and partly on the fact that all the regression equations being com-

Table 5. Regression analysis of mortality rates on the seven variables with greatest explanatory power.

Mortality rate	Doctors	GNP	Cigarettes	Alcohol	Population density	Intervention index	Sugar consumption	% Total sums of squares explained by 7 variables
Maternal	1	−15	25	18	−3	2	−29	72
Perinatal	8[a]	−11[a]	8[a]	0	0	−2	−8[a]	90
Infant	17[a]	−16[a]	10[a]	5[a]	−2	0	−4	97
Age groups (years)								
1– 4	3	−8[a]	1	1	1	−6	−5	55
5–14	1	1	5	−1	−2	−2	−6	42
15–24	0	0	2	0	−7[a]	−16[a]	−8	79
25–34	−4	1	5	0	−7	−10[a]	−11	65
35–44	−3	−5	4	−1	−9[a]	−9	−8	57
45–54	−3	−7	7	−3	−4	−4	−3	55
55–64	−1	−9[a]	7	−3	−1	−3	−3	62

The figures in the first seven columns are the percentage changes in the death rates following a one-standard-deviation increase in the input variables, the other input variables remaining fixed.

[a] *t* value for inclusion of variable in regression exceeds 2. Note, however, that even when not formally "significant" the values given are best estimates.

pared have an identical set of independent (input) variables. The final column of Table 5 displays the percentage of the total (corrected) sums of squares of a given death rate explained by the set of seven variables.

The findings for infant mortality are particularly interesting. The seven variables explain 97 percent of the variance in infant mortality rates. In fact GNP per head alone explains 21 percent of the variance, while the prevalence of doctors alone explains 45 percent of the variance. Doctors and GNP per head together explain 82 percent of the variance. Doctors and GNP per head are not themselves highly correlated (r = 0.2) in these developed countries.

Other points of interest in Table 5 are the positive association between alcohol consumption and maternal and infant mortality; the positive association between cigarette consumption and mortality, which is strongest with infant, perinatal, and maternal mortality, and is also strong in the two oldest age groups; and the negative association between population density and mortality in young adults. Gross national product is negatively associated with mortality in all age groups except 5 to 34 years, where it becomes negligible. Sugar consumption is negatively associated with mortality in all age groups. The intervention index becomes prominent in the age groups 15 to 24 and 25 to 34 years, although, as noted earlier, caution is required in interpreting it in the latter age group. Caution is also advisable in interpreting the re-

sults for maternal mortality, because this is a very uncommon cause of death in our 18 developed countries.

We repeated a similar correlation and regression analysis on a smaller set of variables based upon data in 1960. Our main findings from the 1970 data concerning GNP per head, doctors, and some other health care variables, were replicated on the 1960 data. Our analysis of the 1960 data, although cursory, does suggest that our findings are fairly stable over time and cannot too easily be dismissed as a chance curiosity.

DISCUSSION

In the previous sections, we have remarked on the statistical difficulties associated with this study. We must now examine the broader issue of the general validity of studies which seek to draw inferences about the relationship between diet, environment, and mortality on the basis of a statistical comparison of countries.

The first objection to our study is that we have a highly selective collection of countries. This is indeed so, but this circumstance was forced upon us by the lack of developed countries for which extensive and reliable information was available. We may nevertheless claim the advantage that because our selected countries are all "Western" or "European" in their styles of life and outlook, they may be expected to be fairly homogeneous with respect to many variables which we have been unable to consider. A more serious methodological objection is that both the mortality rates and the input variables are averaged across each country, so that we cannot examine or allow for the undoubted heterogeneity of these factors within each country. We do not even have the comfort of knowing that their frequency distributions within each country are identical, and this throws greater doubt upon the representativeness of the simple averages. It may well be that these difficulties serve to dilute or underestimate any true associations, in which case any positive findings that we display are of enhanced interest. We cannot, however, dismiss the possibility that these problems cause entirely false associations. We do not claim that any of the associations are causal, although in one or two cases this hypothesis is attractive.

The striking relationship between the prevalence of doctors and mortality in the younger age groups deserves serious consideration. Stewart (1), Hinds (2), and Richardson (3) have each commented on this association but have not found a totally convincing explanation. We have examined the possibility that this association could be explained in terms of other variables in our data set, but as Table 5 shows, we were unable to make the doctor anomaly go away. In spite of the possibility that there is some variable unknown to us which is cross-correlated with doctor prevalence and is capable of explaining the anomaly, we shall attempt a few explanatory hypotheses.

One possibility is that each country, consciously or unconsciously, adjusted the supply of doctors to meet the demand of medical problems. We attempted to test this by seeing whether the increase in the number of doctors between 1960 and 1970 was related to infant mortality in 1960. No such relationship was found.

Another hypothesis is that increasing doctor prevalence increases "dependency," but even Ivan Illich (4) never suggested that the dependency was lethal. Similarly, "iatrogenesis" might be suggested as a linking factor, but the wrong age groups are affected and the effect on mortality is too large.

Two factors suggest that the doctor and mortality relationship is not causal. Firstly, there is no evidence of a relationship between doctor prevalence and infant mortality rates when the regions of England and Wales are studied (5).

Secondly, the correlation and regression coefficients are still positive, but much weaker, if doctors are replaced by obstetricians and pediatricians, both of whom are likely to influence infant mortality more strongly than other doctors.

In general, however, we must admit defeat and leave it to others to extricate doctors from their unhappy position.

It is also difficult to explain the roles of population density and the intervention index (proportion of health service spending coming from government funds), both of which are strongly negatively associated with mortality in young adults. An interpretation of the effect of the intervention index is that the more nationalized the health services, the more effective is delivery of health care for potentially lethal illness. This may well be so, but in referring to our analysis, great caution is necessary before drawing this inference. Why should the intervention index be most strongly associated with deaths in young adults? A tentative explanation might be that deaths in young adults are primarily due to accidents, particularly road accidents, and non-fatal outcome following an accident may be dependent upon an efficient accident service. Private medicine would not be interested in funding an accident service which by its nature must often provide treatment before questions of fees are broached, and therefore this may be highly dependent upon public financing. If state financing of health services in developed countries is truly effective, however, then the intervention index should be strongly associated with other causes of death, particularly perinatal and infant mortality; and this we have not found. We originally thought that the population density effect could be explained by a negative association with road accidents but this is not so, and, in the light of other findings, we can hardly argue that nearness to medical help is important.

The results for gross national product per caput accord with expectations. Its association with mortality is strongest in the youngest and oldest age groups, and its negative sign is consistent with the idea that increasing overall wealth reduces mortality. In the intermediate age groups, its negligible association with mortality is consistent with the view that older children and young adults, having survived thus far, are little affected, with respect to mortality, by those social and environmental factors which correlate with wealth. This view is, of course, tenable only for societies in which overall wealth exceeds subsistence level, as is true of all our 18 developed countries.

It is not surprising that cigarette consumption should be associated with mortality rates in the older age groups. The strong association with infant and perinatal mortality is not easy to explain, although it is perhaps now generally recognized that smoking in pregnancy has a deleterious effect on the fetus but we cannot claim to have shown this.

Our finding that sugar consumption is not positively associated with mortality is inconsistent with the belief that unrefined sugar is generally harmful, and associated with coronary heart disease in particular (6). We would not, however, wish to place too much weight upon our own findings. In any case, severe doubts about the harmful role of sugar have been raised by other workers in studies designed to test this issue (7, 8).

We believe that one overall conclusion may be drawn from this study. It is that health service factors are relatively unimportant in explaining the differences in mortality among our 18 developed countries. There is nothing new in this. The case has been argued particularly well by Fuchs (9). As a corollary to this, it could also be argued that there is probably a considerable element of inefficiency in the way some developed countries spend so much more than others on health services. As to the overall value of the results, we consider them to be interesting and provocative, and perhaps capable of generating worthwhile new hypotheses which may be tested in appropriate studies.

We thank Robert Maxwell and many international organizations for help with this study.

Reprints from A.L. Cochrane, Rhoose Farm House, Rhoose, South Glamorgan.

References

(1) Stewart, C.T. Allocation of resources to health. *J Hum Resour* 6(1):103-122, 1971.

(2) Hinds, M. W. Letter. *N Engl J Med* 291:741, 1974.

(3) Richardson, J. The Dependency Hypothesis—That More Doctors Will Result in Lower Quality Health. Research paper No. 113, School of Economics and Financial Studies. Sydney, Macquarie University, 1976.

(4) Illich, I. *Medical Nemesis—the Expropriation of Health.* London, Calder and Boyars, 1975.

(5) West, R.R. and C.R. Lowe. Regional variations in need for and provision and use of child health services in England and Wales. *Br Med J* 2:843-846, 1976.

(6) Yudkin, J. Diet and coronary thrombosis. *Lancet* 2:155-162, 1957.

(7) Bennett, A.E., R. Doll, and R. W. Howell. Sugar consumption and cigarette smoking. *Lancet* 1:1011-1014, 1970.

(8) Medical Research Council. Working Party on the relationship between dietary sugar intake and arterial disease. *Lancet* 2:1265-1271, 1970.

(9) Fuchs, V.R. *Who shall live?* New York, Basic Books, 1974.

APPENDIX

Sources of Data and Indices

Mortality data and population density data	World Health Organization. *World Health Statistics Annual. Vol. 1. Vital Statistics and Causes of Death for 1970.* Geneva, WHO, 1973.	Alcohol (liters per head per year)	Produkschap voor Gedistilleerde Dranken. *Hoeveel alcoholhoudende dranken worden er in de wereld gedronken?* Netherlands, Schiedam, 1975.
Doctors, nurses, and beds per 10 000 population	World Health Organization. *World Health Statistics Annual. Vol. 3. Statistics of Health Personnel,* etc. Geneva, WHO, 1973 (with help from Dr. Robert Maxwell).	Manufactured cigarettes per adult (aged over 15) per annum	Tobacco Research Council. *Tobacco consumption in various countries.* London, Tobacco Research Council, 1972.

GNP per head (we used data for 1960 and 1970 at constant 1973 prices as we hope to study changes later)	International Bank for Reconstruction and Development, Washington, 1977 (through the kindness of Dr. Schrieber).	Percentage of health expenditure covered by public expenditure (intervention index)	OECD Paris Working Party on Economic Policy (through the kindness of Dr. J. P. Poullier).
% GNP spent on health	United Nations *Year Book of National Accounts.* Statistics for 1970. London, Office of Health Economics. Dr. Robert Maxwell.	Education index. "Percentage of the cohort continuing education after age 18" (both sexes)	UNESCO, Paris (through the kindness of Dr. S. Fauchette).
		Dietary data	OECD. *Food consumption statistics 1955–1973.* Paris, OECD, 1975.

TEN-YEAR RESULTS OF A RANDOMIZED CLINICAL TRIAL COMPARING RADICAL MASTECTOMY AND TOTAL MASTECTOMY WITH OR WITHOUT RADIATION[1]

Bernard Fisher, Carol Redmond, Edwin R. Fisher, Madeline Bauer, Norman Wolmark, Lawrence Wickerham, Melvin Deutsch, Eleanor Montague, Richard Margolese, and Roger Foster[2]

ABSTRACT

In 1971 we began a randomized trial to compare alternative local and regional treatments of breast cancer, all of which employ breast removal. Life-table estimates were obtained for 1665 women enrolled in the study for a mean of 126 months. There were no significant differences among three groups of patients with clinically negative axillary nodes, with respect to disease-free survival, distant-disease-free survival, or overall survival (about 57 percent) at 10 years. The patients were treated by radical mastectomy, total ("simple") mastectomy without axillary dissection but with regional irradiation, or total mastectomy without irradiation plus axillary dissection only if nodes were subsequently positive. Similarly, no differences were observed between patients with clinically positive nodes treated by radical mastectomy or by total mastectomy without axillary dissection but with regional irradiation. Survival at 10 years was about 38 percent in both groups.

Our findings indicate that the location of a breast tumor does not influence the prognosis and that irradiation of internal mammary nodes in patients with inner-quadrant lesions does not improve survival. The data also demonstrate that the results obtained at five years accurately predict the outcome at 10 years. We conclude that the variations of local and regional treatment used in this study are not important in determining survival of patients with breast cancer.

Current controversy regarding the surgical treatment of primary breast cancer relates to the comparative merits of breast preservation and breast removal. A little more than a decade ago there was intense disagreement over whether the same outcome would occur if mammary cancers were managed by breast-removing operations that were less extensive than radical mastectomy. Anecdotal information reported by surgeons who performed less extensive operations because of dissatisfaction with the results of more radical procedures (1–3), as well as new information about the biology of

breast cancer and tumor metastases (4), suggested that possibility.

Recognizing the need for data to resolve the clinical controversy and to determine whether results relative to patient outcome were concordant with recently formulated biologic principles, the National Surgical Adjuvant Breast Project initiated a randomized trial in August 1971. The specific aims of that trial were to determine (1) whether in patients with clinically negative axillary nodes total mastectomy, followed by delayed axillary dissection in those who subsequently had positive axillary nodes, was as effective as radical mastectomy; (2) whether the outcome of total mastectomy followed by postoperative regional irradiation was equivalent to that of radical mastectomy; and (3) whether total mastectomy with delayed axillary dissection in patients with subsequently positive nodes was as efficacious as total mastectomy and radiation. For patients with clinically positive nodes the objective was to ascertain

Source: *The New England Journal of Medicine* 312 (11): 674–681, 1985.

[1] Supported by Public Health Service grants from the National Cancer Institute (NCI-U10-CA-12027 and NCI-U10-CA-34211) and by a grant from the American Cancer Society (ACS-RC-13).

[2] All from the National Surgical Adjuvant Breast Project Headquarters, Room 914 Scaife Hall, 3550 Terrace St., Pittsburgh, PA 15261, where reprint requests should be addressed to Dr. Bernard Fisher. (See Appendix I for a list of participating institutions and principal investigators.)

whether radical mastectomy and total mastectomy followed by radiation produced an equivalent outcome. Previous studies of results (life-table estimates) at three years *(5)* and at five years *(6)* have failed to demonstrate a significant difference in outcome among the three treatments in patients with clinically negative nodes and between the two treatments in patients with clinically positive nodes. This report presents the 10-year findings of our trial.

METHODS

Between July 22, 1971, and September 6, 1974, 1765 patients at 34 U.S. and Canadian institutions participating in the National Surgical Adjuvant Breast Project were enrolled in the trial and randomly assigned to treatment. A total of 100 patients (5.7 percent) were judged to be ineligible. The findings presented below are from the 1665 eligible patients, who were enrolled in the study for an average of 126 months (range, 108 to 145). Ineligible patients were excluded from these analyses since, at the time the study was begun, ineligible patients were not routinely followed. For 30 (3.6 percent) of the 834 patients still alive at the time of this evaluation, no follow-up data were available from the previous 12 months. The distribution of those 30 patients was similar throughout all groups. This report summarizes the results of 120 months of observation. Detailed descriptions of patient-entry information, eligibility and ineligibility criteria, the plan of investigation, operative and irradiation procedures, and other aspects of the study have been presented elsewhere *(5, 7)*. Comparability of the treatment groups with respect to patient and tumor characteristics has also been documented. The following briefly summarizes the salient features of the study design.

Women with primary, operable, potentially curable breast cancer were considered eligible for the trial if their tumors were confined to the breast or breast and axilla and were movable in relation to the underlying muscle and chest wall. If axillary nodes were palpable, they had to be movable in relation to the chest wall, neurovascular bundle, and overlying skin. All patients in the study consented to participate. If they met specific criteria described in the protocol, their clinical nodal status was documented. Patients judged to have clinically nega-

tive nodes were randomly assigned so that one third were treated by conventional radical mastectomy, one third by total mastectomy and regional irradiation, and one third by total mastectomy alone. Patients with clinically positive axillary nodes were randomly assigned so that one half underwent radical mastectomy, and one half total mastectomy and regional irradiation. A nodal biopsy was performed in patients with clinically negative axillary nodes who had undergone a total mastectomy without irradiation and subsequently had clinical evidence of axillary-node involvement in the absence of other manifestations of disease. If the nodes were reported as positive for tumor, a delayed axillary dissection was performed. Patients with positive axillary nodes after total mastectomy and radiation were considered to have had a treatment failure. The protocol did not stipulate specific criteria for their treatment.

Radiation was administered with supervoltage equipment at a dose of 4500 rad in 25 fractions to both the internal mammary and supraclavicular nodes at a depth of 3 cm. In patients with clinically negative axillary nodes, a dose of 5000 rad in 25 fractions was delivered to the midaxilla, with most of the dose delivered from the anterior supraclavicular portal, and the rest from a posterior axillary portal. Patients with clinically positive axillary nodes received an additional boost of 1000 to 2000 rad through a direct appositional portal. Tangential fields were employed to treat the chest wall with a tumor dose of 5000 rad in 25 treatments calculated at a depth of two thirds of the distance between the skin of the chest wall and the base of the tangential fields at midseparation. This usually produced a brisk erythema with limited patches of moist desquamation.

Statistical Analysis

The end points considered for the overall treatment comparisons were disease-free survival, distant-disease-free survival, and overall survival. Times to those end points were calculated from the date of mastectomy. Recurrences of tumor in the chest wall and operative scar were classified as local treatment failures. Recurrences in the internal mammary, supraclavicular, and subclavicular nodes in all patients and in the ipsilateral axillary nodes of patients treated by radical mastectomy or total mastectomy and regional irradiation were considered to be regional treatment failures. Patients with clinically negative nodes who were treated by total mastectomy and subsequently had positive nodes requiring an axillary dissection were not deemed to have had a treatment failure at that time unless the nodes could not be completely removed. The decision not to consider delayed nodal involvement a treatment failure was stipulated in the protocol before the start of the study. Such an event was not included in the determination of disease-free survival. Distant disease was evaluated in two ways: when it occurred as a first treatment failure and when it occurred as any distant treatment failure—i.e., the first or subsequent local or regional failure. Patients were considered to be free of disease at a point in time if they were alive and had no local, regional, or distant evidence of breast cancer and no other primary tumor.

The major goal of this study was to determine whether treatments used as alternatives to radical mastectomy increased the risk of tumor recurrence or death. Actuarial life-table estimates and associated standard errors *(8)* were calculated for each treatment group and each end point. Comparisons of the survival distributions were made within each nodal group by means of the summary chi-square (log-rank) test *(9, 10)*. A two-sided P value ≤0.05 was considered to be significant. Standard errors for specific points selected from the life tables are provided in the text.

RESULTS

Disease-Free Survival

There were no significant differences (P = 0.2, Figure 1A) in disease-free survival over the entire period of follow-up among the groups of patients with clinically negative nodes treated by radical mastectomy, total mastectomy plus radiation, or total mastectomy alone. At 10 years 47 ± 2.6, 48 ± 2.7, and 42 ± 2.6 percent of each group, respectively, were alive and free of disease. When disease-free survival was examined in terms of events occurring during the first and second five-year periods of follow-up, it was observed that any differences among groups occurred within the first five years after surgery (P = 0.08, Figure 1B). At the end of the fifth year the disease-free survival was 60 ± 2.5 percent for the radical-mastectomy group, 65 ± 2.5

percent for the patients undergoing total mastectomy plus radiation, and 56 ± 2.5 percent for those treated by total mastectomy alone. An additional 15 percent of patients in all three groups had a treatment failure between the 5th and 10th year. There were no differences in the probability of failure among the three groups during the second five years (P = 0.8, Figure 1C). In each group, approximately 75 percent of patients who were free of disease at the end of 5 years remained free of disease at the end of the 10th year. The differences noted during the initial five years were due to the higher incidence of local or regional disease occurring as the first evidence of disease in the total-mastectomy group, not because of an increase in distant disease occurring as a first treatment failure (Figure 2). The group treated by total mastectomy and radiation had a lower incidence of local and regional recurrence than did the other two groups.

There was no significant difference in disease-free survival between the two groups with clinically positive nodes, either overall (P = 0.2, Figure 1A) or during the first (P = 0.2, Figure 1B) or the second (P = 0.9, Figure 1C) five-year period. Only 45 ± 2.9 percent of patients treated by radical mastectomy and 40 ± 2.9 percent of those undergoing total mastectomy plus irradiation were free of disease at the end of the 5th year, and by the 10th year only 29 ± 2.7 and 25 ± 2.6 percent, respectively, remained free of disease. Nearly two thirds of the patients who were free of disease at the end of the fifth year remained so during the next five years. There was little difference between the two groups with respect to the occurrence of local, regional, or first distant disease (Figure 3).

The total incidence of events—i.e., first treatment failures, second cancers, and unrelated deaths—did not differ significantly among the three groups of patients with clinically negative nodes or between the two groups with clinically positive nodes (Table 1). The proportion of first distant treatment failures, as well as the distribution of distant disease according to site, was similar for the three negative-node groups and for the two positive-node groups. There was little difference in the sites of first distant disease between the negative-node and positive-node groups. Of 532 reported distant failures, one half (51.5 percent) were in two organ systems, 29.3 percent in the skeletal system, and

Figure 1. Survival free of disease through 10 years (A), during the first 5 years (B), and during the second 5 years for patients free of disease at the end of the 5th year (C). Patients were treated by radical mastectomy (solid circle), total mastectomy plus radiation (X), or total mastectomy alone (open circle). There were no significant differences among the three groups of patients with clinically negative nodes (solid line) or between the two groups with clinically positive nodes (broken line).

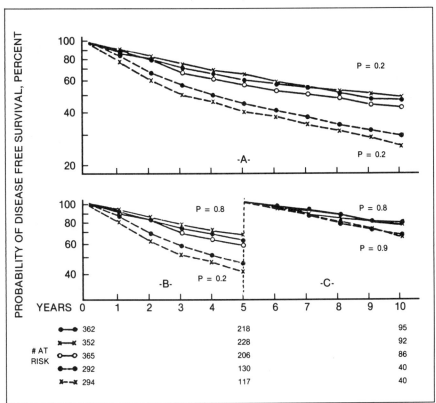

22.2 percent in the respiratory system. Tumors in the opposite breast (metastases or second primary tumors) accounted for 13.7 percent of distant treatment failures and were found in 4.4 percent of all patients. Second primary cancers (not in the breast) were found in 3.5 percent of all patients. They were fairly evenly distributed among the treatment groups. Of the 60 cancers, 5 were hematopoietic in origin. Four of the five occurred in patients treated by total mastectomy plus radiation (0.6 percent of the total number of such patients, as compared with 0.1 percent of patients not receiving radiation). The other 55 second cancers were visceral in origin and were distributed throughout all groups. Local recurrences were fewer in the total-mastectomy groups receiving radiation.

Whereas no major differences in the occurrence of regional disease were observed among the negative-node groups, there were differences between the two positive-node groups. Patients treated with radical mastectomy had a lower incidence of ipsilateral axillary-node recurrence (1.0 percent) than did patients undergoing total mastectomy and irradiation (11.9 percent). On the other hand, supraclavicular-node recurrences were higher in the radical-mastectomy group (5.8 vs. 0 percent).

Distant-Disease-Free Survival

There were no significant differences in the probability of survival free of any distant disease occurring as a first treatment failure or

Figure 2. Local or regional and distant treatment failures as the first evidence of disease in patients with clinically negative nodes who were treated by radical mastectomy (solid circle), total mastectomy and radiation (X), or total mastectomy alone (open circle). There were no significant differences in distant disease occurring as a first treatment failure among the three groups, whereas local and regional disease was best controlled in the group receiving radiation.

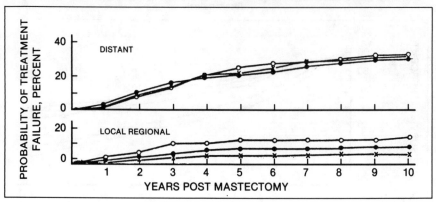

Figure 3. Local or regional and distant treatment failures as the first evidence of disease in patients with clinically positive nodes who were treated by radical mastectomy (solid circle) or total mastectomy and radiation (X). There was no significant difference in distant or local and regional disease between the two groups.

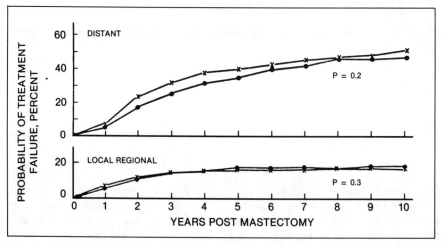

after local or regional disease among the three groups of patients with clinically negative nodes (P = 0.6, Figure 4A). At 10 years the probability was 58 ± 2.7 percent for the radical-mastectomy group, 57 ± 2.8 percent for patients treated by total mastectomy plus radiation, and 55 ± 2.7 percent for those undergoing total mastectomy alone. When the groups were examined according to the first and second five-year postoperative intervals, no significant differences were found among the three groups during the first

period (P = 0.3, Figure 4B). At five years 68 ± 2.5 percent of the radical-mastectomy group, 71 ± 2.4 percent of the group receiving total mastectomy plus radiation, and 65 ± 2.6 percent of the group treated by total mastectomy alone were free of any distant disease. Similarly, for patients who survived the first five years free of distant disease, there were no significant differences among the three groups in the recurrence of distant disease during the second five-year interval (P = 0.4, Figure 4C);

between 80 and 85 percent of patients who were disease-free at 5 years remained free of any distant disease at the end of the 10th year.

Among patients with clinically positive nodes, there was no significant difference in distant-disease-free survival between those undergoing radical mastectomy and those treated by total mastectomy plus radiation (P = 0.8, Figure 4A). At five years the distant-disease-free survival was 53 ± 3.0 percent for patients treated by radical mastectomy and 51 ± 3.0 percent for those

treated by total mastectomy plus radiation (P = 0.4, Figure 4B). At 10 years the corresponding figures were 39 ± 3.1 and 40 ± 3.1 percent. The probability of any distant disease occurring during the second five-year interval was similar for the two treatment groups (P = 0.4, Figure 4C).

The occurrence of a distant treatment failure as the first evidence of recurrent disease did not differ significantly among the negative-node (Figure 2) and positive-node (Figure 3) treatment groups.

Table 1. Distribution of first treatment failure, second cancers, and death from unrelated causes, according to treatment.[a]

Event	Patients with Clinically Negative Nodes			Patients with Clinically Positive Nodes	
	RM (N = 362)	TMR (N = 352)	TM (N = 365)	RM (N = 292)	TMR (N = 294)
Total	197 (54.4)	183 (52.0)	214 (58.6)	205 (70.2)	217 (73.8)
Local	16 (4.4)	4 (1.1)	28 (7.7)	21 (7.2)	5 (1.7)
Chest wall	11 (3.0)	3 (0.9)	19 (5.2)	17 (5.8)	2 (0.7)
Scar	3 (0.8)	1 (0.3)	6 (1.6)	1 (0.3)	1 (0.3)
Both	2 (0.6)	0 (0.0)	3 (0.8)	3 (1.0)	2 (0.7)
Regional	9 (2.5)	12 (3.4)	15 (4.1)	22 (7.5)	35 (11.9)
Axilla	5 (1.4)	11 (3.1)	4 (1.1)	3 (1.0)	35 (11.9)
Supraclavicular	4 (1.1)	1 (0.3)	11 (3.0)	17 (5.8)	0 (0.0)
Internal mammary	0 (0.0)	0 (0.0)	0 (0.0)	0 (0.0)	0 (0.0)
Subclavicular	0 (0.0)	0 (0.0)	0 (0.0)	0 (0.0)	0 (0.0)
>1	0 (0.0)	0 (0.0)	0 (0.0)	2 (0.7)	0 (0.0)
Distant	96 (26.5)	109 (31.0)	107 (29.3)	104 (35.6)	116 (39.4)
Opposite breast[b]	11 (3.0)	18 (5.1)	19 (5.2)	13 (4.4)	12 (4.1)
Integumentary	2 (0.6)	2 (0.6)	1 (0.3)	2 (0.7)	2 (0.7)
Skeletal	30 (8.3)	28 (8.0)	31 (8.5)	33 (11.3)	34 (11.6)
Respiratory	22 (6.1)	24 (6.8)	22 (6.0)	23 (7.9)	27 (9.2)
Hemic and lymphatic	8 (2.2)	8 (2.3)	7 (1.9)	5 (1.7)	6 (2.0)
Digestive	4 (1.1)	8 (2.3)	7 (1.9)	11 (3.8)	11 (3.7)
Genitourinary	3 (0.8)	1 (0.3)	1 (0.3)	1 (0.3)	1 (0.3)
Nervous	2 (0.6)	0 (0.0)	1 (0.3)	0 (0.0)	3 (1.0)
Endocrine	0 (0.0)	0 (0.0)	0 (0.0)	0 (0.0)	1 (0.3)
Cardiac and sense organs	0 (0.0)	0 (0.0)	0 (0.0)	0 (0.0)	0 (0.0)
>1	14 (3.9)	20 (5.7)	18 (4.9)	16 (5.5)	19 (6.5)
Combinations	12 (3.3)	9 (2.6)	13 (3.4)	22 (7.5)	17 (5.7)
Local and regional	3 (0.8)	0 (0.0)	3 (0.8)	1 (0.3)	1 (0.3)
Local and distant	5 (1.4)	2 (0.6)	3 (0.8)	9 (3.1)	6 (2.0)
Regional and distant	0 (0.0)	1 (0.3)	2 (0.5)	7 (2.4)	6 (2.0)
Widespread	3 (0.8)	2 (0.6)	3 (0.8)	2 (0.7)	2 (0.7)
Unknown	1 (0.3)	4 (1.1)	2 (0.5)	3 (1.0)	2 (0.7)
Second cancers (nonbreast)	16 (4.4)	15 (4.3)	11 (3.0)	7 (2.4)	11 (3.7)
Hematopoietic	0 (0.0)	2 (0.6)	1 (0.3)	0 (0.0)	2 (0.7)
Solid	16 (4.4)	13 (3.7)	10 (2.7)	7 (2.4)	9 (3.0)
Dead, no evidence of disease	48 (13.2)	34 (9.6)	40 (11.0)	29 (9.9)	33 (11.2)
Alive, event-free	165 (45.6)	169 (48.0)	151 (41.4)	87 (29.8)	77 (26.2)

[a] Values are numbers of treatment failures, with percentages of patients shown in parentheses. RM denotes radical mastectomy, TMR total mastectomy plus radiation, and TM total mastectomy.
[b] Includes second primary tumors.

Figure 4. Survival free of distant disease through 10 years (A), during the first 5 years (B), and during the second 5 years for patients free of distant disease at the end of the 5th year (C). Patients were treated by radical mastectomy (solid circle), total mastectomy and radiation (X), or total mastectomy alone (open circle). There were no significant differences among the three groups of patients with clinically negative nodes (solid line) or between the two groups with positive nodes (broken line).

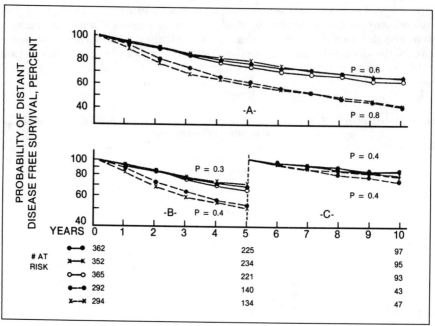

Overall Survival

Over the entire period of follow-up there was no significant difference in overall survival among the three negative-node groups (P = 0.5, Figure 5A). At 10 years overall survival was 58 ± 2.6 percent for the radical-mastectomy group, 59 ± 2.7 percent for patients treated by total mastectomy plus radiation, and 54 ± 2.7 percent for those undergoing total mastectomy alone. The probability of survival during the first five years after surgery did not differ significantly among treatments (P = 0.9, Figure 5B). Survival at five years was 75 ± 2.3 percent for patients treated by radical mastectomy, 75 ± 2.3 percent for those undergoing total mastectomy plus radiation, and 74 ± 2.3 percent for those treated by total mastectomy alone. Survival during the second five-year interval also did not differ significantly among treatment groups (P = 0.3, Figure 5C). About 75 percent of the patients with negative nodes who were alive at 5 years remained alive at 10 years.

There was no significant difference between the two positive-node groups with respect to survival for the whole 10-year period (P = 0.7, Figure 5A), during the first 5 years (P = 0.3, Figure 5B), or during the second 5 years (P = 0.4, Figure 5C). At the end of the fifth year 62 ± 2.8 percent of the radical-mastectomy group and 58 ± 2.9 percent of those treated by total mastectomy and radiation were alive. By the end of the 10th year only 38 ± 2.9 and 39 ± 2.9 percent, respectively, were alive. About 65 percent of patients with positive nodes who were alive at five years survived an additional five years.

Tumor Location and Survival

Survival was examined in terms of the location of the primary tumor in the breast, with adjustment for intralymphatic extension, cell reaction, clinical tumor size, and histologic grade. Among patients with clinically negative nodes, whether their tumors were lateral or medial-central in location, there was no significant

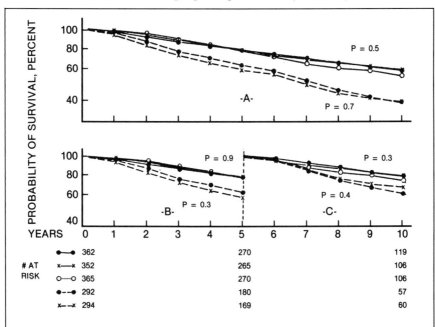

Figure 5. Survival through 10 years (A), during the first 5 years (B), and during the second 5 years for patients alive at the end of the 5th year (C). Patients were treated by radical mastectomy (solid circle), total mastectomy and radiation (X), or total mastectomy alone (open circle). There were no significant differences among the three groups of patients with clinically negative nodes (solid line) or between the two groups with positive nodes (broken line).

difference (P = 0.6 in both cases) in outcome among the three treatment groups (Figure 6) at any time. Among patients with clinically positive nodes, the treatment did not significantly affect survival in those with lateral (P = 0.8) or medial-central lesions (P = 0.3). No differences in outcome were observed when all patients with lateral tumors were compared with all those having medial-central tumors.

Occurrence of Positive Axillary Nodes after Total Mastectomy

Sixty-five (17.8 percent) of the 365 patients with clinically negative nodes who underwent total mastectomy without radiation subsequently had histologically confirmed, positive ipsilateral axillary nodes, which were removed by a delayed axillary dissection. These nodes had been shown to contain tumor before the occurrence of any other event. The median time from mastectomy to axillary dissection was 14.7 months, with a range of 3 to 112.6. More than three fourths (78.5 percent) of such dissec-

tions occurred within 24 months after total mastectomy; only three (4.6 percent) occurred during the second five years of follow-up. The hazard rate over time indicates that the highest risk of axillary-node involvement was concentrated in the first 24 months after operation. Over the rest of the 10-year period, a continuous but low risk remained evident.

DISCUSSION

We first reported results from this prospective randomized clinical trial comparing radical mastectomy with alternative treatments for primary breast cancer in 1977, when the average follow-up time was 36 months (26 to 62 months) (5). The findings at 10 years (average time in the study, 126 months) confirm and extend the earlier results. They continue to indicate no significant difference in disease-free, distant-disease-free, or overall survival among patients without clinical evidence of axillary-node involvement who were treated by three distinctly different treatment regimens: radical mastec-

Figure 6. Relation of treatment to survival according to tumor location. Patients were treated by radical mastectomy (solid circle), total mastectomy and radiation (X), or total mastectomy alone (open circle). The outcome for patients with clinically negative or positive nodes and lateral tumors or medial and central tumors was not affected by the treatment.

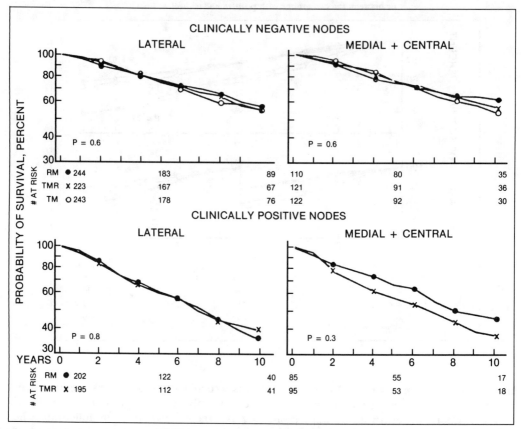

tomy, total ("simple") mastectomy with local and regional radiation, or total mastectomy with subsequent removal of axillary nodes if they became clinically positive. Among patients with clinical evidence of nodal involvement treated either by radical mastectomy or total mastectomy plus local and regional radiation, there continues to be no significant difference between the two treatment groups.

It has previously been reported that 40 percent of the patients in this trial who were judged to have clinically negative nodes and who underwent a radical mastectomy had histologic evidence of positive nodes *(11)*. Consequently, since this was a randomized trial, it can be justifiably assumed that approximately 40 percent of the patients with negative nodes in the other two treatment groups had tumor-positive lymph

nodes as well. In patients treated by total mastectomy alone, positive nodes might have been expected to serve as a source of further tumor dissemination, resulting in an increase in distant treatment failure and a higher mortality if temporal considerations are seminal in the metastatic process. Since such events did not occur, there is support for our concept that regional lymph nodes are indicators rather than instigators of distant disease. Moreover, just as unremoved nodes were not deleterious, our findings indicate that their removal did not adversely affect prognosis, refuting the view that it may be beneficial not to remove regional nodes in patients with clinically perceptible cancers *(12)*.

Particularly interesting was the observation that even though positive nodes were not removed in 40 percent of patients with clinically negative nodes who were treated by total mastectomy alone, only 18 percent subsequently required an axillary dissection for detectable nodes, and these patients had no evidence of recurrent disease. The need for a delayed dissection in these patients (the 18 percent) was the only discernible disadvantage of not routinely performing an axillary dissection.

The lack of necessity for carrying out an axillary dissection in a higher proportion of patients treated by total mastectomy may have been due to the occurrence of another event before the detection of axillary nodal involvement—i.e., tumor recurrence or death—or to microscopic tumor foci in nodes that had not yet progressed to the point of being clinically detectable. Although the risk of positive axillary nodes is highest during the first two postoperative years, a small risk persists for as long as 10 years. Thus, a few additional patients may well have nodal involvement in the future. Even though the present study cannot provide an explanation for the discrepancy between the proportion of patients with histologically positive nodes that were not removed and the proportion with nodes requiring subsequent dissection, there has been no difference in survival between patients with histologically positive nodes that were untreated and those with nodes that were removed or irradiated.

Many investigators insist on the need for an increasingly prolonged period of follow-up before one can accept or draw conclusions from the results of breast-cancer clinical trials. The conventional five years of follow-up is no longer considered adequate by many physicians. The current findings indicate that the 5-year results of our study accurately predicted the outcome at 10 years. At the end of the first five years there were no significant differences in distant-disease-free or overall survival among the three treatment groups with clinically negative nodes and between the two groups with clinically positive nodes. The slight difference in disease-free survival during the initial five-year period among the three negative-node treatment groups was related to a variation in the incidence of local and regional disease rather than to distant treatment failure. No such difference was evident between the two positive-node groups. Patients with negative nodes who completed the fifth postoperative year free of disease had the same estimated probability of remaining disease-free (free of disease overall or free of distant disease) and of surviving during the second five years regardless of the treatment. The findings were the same for the positive-node groups. The rate of treatment failure, overall or distant, was lower in the second five-year period than in the first regardless of nodal status or treatment. There was no difference, however, in the death rate between the first and second five-year periods. Patients with positive nodes who were free of distant disease at the end of five years had about the same probability of remaining free of distant disease during the next five years as did the negative-node group. Thus, the 5-year results were highly predictive of the outcome at 10 years, and conclusions based on the early results remain valid. We do not mean to imply that patients surviving for five years are not at risk for subsequent failure. The risk of failure in the next five years is not, however, related to the initial local and regional treatment. It will be important to discern whether the same conclusion remains valid during the third five-year period.

The current findings confirm the validity of our previous results and our conclusion that the location of tumor in the breast does not influence the prognosis and does not provide justification for varying local and regional therapy *(13)*. Our results fail to support the view that radiation of internal mammary nodes in patients with inner-quadrant lesions improves survival *(14,15)*. No survival benefit was noted in our patients with clinically negative or positive nodes who were treated by total mastectomy and regional radiation that included internal mammary nodes.

Almost all available information on patterns of metastases in patients with breast cancer has been derived from autopsy studies *(16–20)*. Relatively few data from breast-cancer clinical trials document the incidence and organ site of the first treatment failure in patients who received no systemic therapy after surgery *(21–23)*. Our current findings indicate that variations of primary treatment within a group of patients with the same clinical nodal status failed to alter the distribution of first treatment failures that were distant in location. Moreover, the distribution overall and in specific organ sites was remarkably uniform regardless of the therapy and the nodal status. As expected, radiation therapy altered the pattern of local treatment failure by decreasing both tumor recurrence in the chest wall and supraclavicular-node involvement. Radiation was not as effective as surgery for controlling tumor recurrence in axillary nodes in patients with clinically positive nodes. Despite the beneficial effect of radiation for local and regional disease control, survival was not improved.

In conclusion, this report provides firm evidence from a randomized controlled study of nearly 2000 women followed for over 10 years that variations in local and regional treatment—from radical to conservative—all involving removal of the breast, result in the same outcome. Our study also indicates that axillary dissection in conjunction with total mastectomy is useful for disease-staging purposes and is therapeutic only in that it reduces the possibility of subsequent regional recurrences. Axillary dissection does not alter the incidence of systemic recurrence or patient survival. As previously indicated *(24)*, our findings, by repudiating radical mastectomy, contradict the anatomic and mechanistic principles that have provided the scientific basis for the operation. They lend support to investigations that have culminated in a new conception of the biology of breast cancer, particularly in terms of tumor spread. Finally, negation of radical mastectomy and the principles on which it is based eliminates most of the biologic considerations against the performance of breast-conserving operations. The first results from our trial of breast conservation further support the concept that variations in local and regional treatment do not alter the survival of patients with breast cancer *(25)*.

References

(1) Fisher, B. The surgical dilemma in the primary therapy of invasive breast cancer: A critical appraisal. *Curr Probl Surg* 1:53, 1970.

(2) McWhirter, R. The value of simple mastectomy and radiotherapy in the treatment of cancer of the breast. *Br J Radiol* 21:599-610, 1948.

(3) Handley, R.S. The technic and results of conservative radical mastectomy (Patey's operation). *Prog Clin Cancer* 1:462-470, 1965.

(4) Fisher, B. Laboratory and clinical research in breast cancer—a personal adventure. *Cancer Res* 40:3863-3874.

(5) Fisher, B., E. Montague, C. Redmond, et al. Comparison of radical mastectomy with alternative treatments for primary breast cancer. A first report of

results from a prospective randomized clinical trial. *Cancer* 39:2827-2839, 1977.

(6) Fisher, B., C. Redmond, E.R. Fisher, et al. The contribution of recent NSABP clinical trials of primary breast cancer therapy to an understanding of tumor biology—an overview of findings. *Cancer* 46:1009-10025, 1980.

(7) Fisher, B., E. Montague, C. Redmond, et al. Findings from NSABP Protocol No. B-04—comparison of radical mastectomy with alternative treatments for primary breast cancer. I. Radiation compliance and its relation to treatment outcome. *Cancer* 46:1-13, 1980.

(8) Cutler, S.J. and F. Ederer. Maximum utilization of the life table method in analyzing survival. *J Chronic Dis* 8:699-712, 1958.

(9) Mantel, N. Evaluation of survival data and two rank order statistics arising in its consideration. *Cancer Chemother Rep* 50:163-170, 1966.

(10) Peto, R. and J. Peto. Asymptomatically efficient rank invariant test procedures. *J R Stat Soc* (A) 135:185-206, 1972.

(11) Fisher, B., N. Wolmark, M. Bauer, C. Redmond, and M. Gebhardt. The accuracy of clinical nodal staging and of limited axillary dissection as a determinant of histologic nodal status in carcinoma of the breast. *Surg Gynecol Obstet* 152:765-772, 1981.

(12) Crile, G., Jr., Simplified treatment of cancer of the breast: Early results of a clinical study. *Ann Surg* 153:745-761, 1961.

(13) Fisher, B., N. Wolmark, C. Redmond, et al. Findings from NSABP Protocol No. B-04: Comparison of radical mastectomy with alternative treatments. II The clinical and biologic significance of medial-center breast cancers. *Cancer* 48:1863-1872, 1981.

(14) Host, H. and I.O. Brenhovd. The effect of post-operative radiotherapy in breast cancer. *Int J Radiat Oncol Biol Phys* 2:1061-1967, 1977.

(15) Wallgren, A., O. Arner, J. Bergström, et al. The value of preoperative radiotherapy in operable mammary carcinoma. *Int J Radiat Oncol Biol Phys* 6:287-290, 1980.

(16) Lee, Y-T.N. Breast carcinoma: Pattern of metastasis at autopsy. *J Surg Oncol* 23:175-180, 1983.

(17) Hagemeister, F.B., Jr., A.U. Buzdar, M.A. Luna, and G.R. Blumenschein. Causes of death in breast cancer: A clinicopathologic study. *Cancer* 46:162-167, 1980.

(18) Cifuentes, N. and J.W. Pickren. Metastases from carcinoma of mammary gland: An autopsy study. *J Surg Oncol* 11:193-205, 1979.

(19) Amer, M.H. Chemotherapy and pattern of metastases in breast cancer patients. *J Surg Oncol* 19:101-105, 1982.

(20) Abrams, H.L., R. Spiro, and N. Goldstein. Metastases in carcinoma: Analysis of 1000 autopsied cases. *Cancer* 3:74-85, 1950.

(21) Fisher, B., R.G. Ravdin, R.K. Ausman, et al. Postoperative radiotherapy in the treatment of breast cancer: Results of the NSABP clinical trial. *Ann Surg* 172:711-732, 1970.

(22) Fisher, B., N.H. Slack, P.J. Cavanaugh, et al. Postoperative radiotherapy in the treatment of breast

cancer: Results of the NSAP clinical trial. *Ann Surg* 172:711-732, 1970.

(23) Valagussa, P., G. Bonadonna, and U. Veronesi. Patterns of relapse and survival following radical mastectomy: Analysis of 716 consecutive patients. *Cancer* 41:1170-1178, 1978.

(24) Fisher, B. Breast-cancer management: Alter-

natives to radical mastectomy. *N Engl J Med* 301: 326-328, 1979.

(25) Fisher, B., M. Bauer, R. Margolese, et al. Five-year results of a randomized clinical trial comparing total mastectomy and segmental mastectomy with or without radiation in the treatment of breast cancer. *N Engl J Med* 312:665-673, 1985.

APPENDIX. List of participants in protocol no. 4 of the national surgical adjuvant breast project.

Institution	Responsible surgeon	Responsible radiation oncologist	Responsible pathologist
Albert Einstein College of Medicine	Herbert Volk	N.A. Ghossein	John Molnar
Boston City Hospital (Tufts)	C. William Kaiser	Merrill Feldman	Leonard Berman
Creighton University	Claude H. Organ	J.R. Zastera	Wade Bardawil
Downstate Medical Center (SUNY)	Bernard Gardner	Joseph Bohorquez	Yale Rosen
Ellis Fischel State Cancer Hospital	William Donegan	James Thomson	Carlos M. Perez-Mesa
Fitzsimons General Hospital	Richard M. Hirata	Terry Powell	William Starke
French and Polyclinic Medical School	James McManus	George Schwarz	William Finkelstein
Geisinger Medical Center	C.W. Konvolinka	David Beiler	C. James Favino
Harbor General Hospital (UCLA)	John R. Benfield	Richard Small	Frank M. Hirose
Harrison S. Martland Hospital	Benjamin F. Rush, Jr.	John Mallams	Michael Lyons
Hennepin County General Hospital	Claude R. Hitchcock	Manoucher Azad	John I. Coe
Jewish General Hospital	Richard G. Margolese	J.J. Hazel	Claude LaChance
Louisiana State University	Isidore Cohn, Jr.	Joseph V. Schlosser	Ronald A. Welsh
Medical College of Pennsylvania	Donald Cooper	Janet Parker	Gerald Justh
Medical College of Virginia	Walter Lawrence, Jr.	E. Richard King	Saul Kay
Metropolitan Hospital	John F. Weiksnar	William Henkin	Eugene Schwartz
Michael Reese Hospital	Richard H. Evans	Lionel Cohen	Miriam L. Christ
Montefiore Hospital	Richard G. Rosen	Flora Mincer	Norwin Becker
Mount Sinai Medical Center (New York)	Gerson J. Lesnick	John Boland	Mamoru Kaneko
St. Vincent's Hospital (New York)	Thomas Nealon, Jr.	George Schwarz	William E. Delaney III
Temple University	Willis Maier	Marie LoPonte	Paul Putong
University of Arkansas	Kent Westbrook	Eleanor Deed	H.K. Leathers
University of California (San Diego)	Marshall J. Orloff	Carl Von Essen	Sidney Saltzstein
University of Illinois	Tapas K. Das Gupta	Edwin J. Liebner	Jose Manaligod
University of Iowa	Richard L. Lawton	Howard B. Latourette	Frederick W. Stamler
U.S. Naval Hospital (San Diego)	T. James Guzik	Quintus Crews	Frances Wachter
University of Pennsylvania	Francis E. Rosato	Lawrence Davis	Horatio T. Enterline
University of Pittsburgh	Bernard Fisher	John Parsons	Robert Totten
University of Rochester	W. Bradford Patterson	Eileen Paterson	Robert Cooper, Jr.
University of Texas (San Antonio)	Anatolio B. Cruz, Jr.	Peter Zanca	George Bannayan
University of Texas (Galveston)	Edward B. Rowe	Marvin H. Olson	Richard Marshall
University of Vermont	Roger S. Foster	G. Stephen Brown	David Duffell
Washington University	Harvey Butcher	Carlos A. Perez	Walter Bauer
Wayne State University	Alexander J. Walt	Alan Scheer	Barbara Rosenberg

FAILURE OF EXTRACRANIAL-INTRACRANIAL ARTERIAL BYPASS TO REDUCE THE RISK OF ISCHEMIC STROKE:[1] RESULTS OF AN INTERNATIONAL RANDOMIZED TRIAL

The EC/IC Bypass Study Group[2]

ABSTRACT

To determine whether bypass surgery would benefit patients with symptomatic atherosclerotic disease of the internal carotid artery, we studied 1377 patients with recent hemisphere strokes, retinal infarction, or transient ischemic attacks who had atherosclerotic narrowing or occlusion of the ipsilateral internal carotid or middle cerebral artery. Of these, 714 were randomly assigned to the best medical care, and 663 to the same regimen with the addition of bypass surgery joining the superficial temporal artery and the middle cerebral artery. The patients were followed for an average of 55.8 months.

Thirty-day surgical mortality and major stroke morbidity rates were 0.6 and 2.5 percent, respectively. The post-operative bypass patency rate was 96 percent. Non-fatal and fatal stroke occurred both more frequently and earlier in the patients operated on. Secondary survival analyses comparing the two groups for major strokes and all deaths, for all strokes and all deaths, and for ipsilateral ischemic strokes demonstrated a similar lack of benefit from surgery.

Separate analyses in patients with different angiographic lesions did not identify a subgroup with any benefit from surgery. Two important subgroups of patients fared substantially worse in the surgical group: those with severe middle-cerebral-artery stenosis (n = 109, Mantel-Haenszel chi-square = 4.74), and those with persistence of ischemic symptoms after an internal-carotid-artery occlusion had been demonstrated (n = 287, chi-square = 4.04).

This study thus failed to confirm the hypothesis that extracranial-intracranial anastomosis is effective in preventing cerebral ischemia in patients with atherosclerotic arterial disease in the carotid and middle cerebral arteries.

The first extracranial-to-intracranial (EC-IC) arterial anastomosis was performed in 1967 (1), and during the next decade the technique was widely applied. In order to test its ability to reduce the rate of subsequent stroke among patients with symptomatic atherosclerotic lesions of the internal carotid or middle cerebral arteries, an international multicenter randomized trial was initiated in 1977. The trial protocol and the entry characteristics of the study patients have been described elsewhere (2), and this report describes the primary results.

OBJECTIVE AND ORGANIZATION

This study was a randomized trial to determine whether anastomosis of the superficial temporal artery to the middle cerebral artery decreased the rate of stroke and stroke-related death among patients with symptomatic disease of the internal carotid and middle cerebral arteries.

METHODS

Patients were eligible for the trial if, within three months before entry, they had had either one or more transient ischemic attacks or one or more minor completed strokes in the carotid distribution. The arteries appropriate to the patient's symptoms had to have one or more of the following artherosclerotic lesions: (1) stenosis or

Source: *The New England Journal of Medicine* 313(19):1191–1200, 1985.

[1] Supported by a grant (R01 NS 14164) from the U.S. National Institutes of Health.

[2] A list of the participating centers, investigators, and study committee members appears in the Appendix.

occlusion of the trunk or major branches before the bifurcation or trifurcation of the middle cerebral artery; (2) stenosis of the internal carotid artery at or above the C-2 vertebral body (i.e., at a place inaccessible to carotid endarterectomy); or (3) occlusion of the internal carotid artery. A number of exclusion criteria were established, and the details have been published *(2)*. Adherence to these criteria was checked by a central review of all entry data. The decision to exclude ineligible patients was made by persons blinded to both the assigned treatment of the patients and their outcome status after randomization.

Randomization was performed by a telephone call to the Methods Center in Canada or Japan, where staff using a computer-generated randomization schedule first registered the patient and then informed the caller of the randomly assigned treatment. Patients randomly assigned to surgery underwent microsurgical end-to-side anastomosis of the superficial temporal or occipital artery to a cortical branch of the middle cerebral artery. Acetylsalicylic acid (325 mg four times a day) was prescribed for all the patients throughout the trial unless contraindicated or not tolerated. Its continued use and the control of hypertension were stressed and monitored in the follow-up visits every three months.

The entry films were reviewed by the principal neuroradiologist at the Central Office, who estimated and recorded the degree of stenosis of the lesion being studied. Surgical patients underwent postoperative angiography, and from these films the adequacy of the anastomosis was rated at the Central Office with a score from 0 to 12.

Patients who initially accepted their random assignment to medical therapy but later underwent EC-IC bypass on the randomized side and patients who accepted random assignment to surgical therapy and then declined the therapy were termed "crossovers." Strokes occurring in such patients whether before or after their crossing over were charged to the original treatment limb in the primary analysis.

The primary study events were the postrandomization occurrences of fatal or nonfatal stroke. The best current means for diagnosis (including CT scanning where available) were used to differentiate ischemic stroke from hemorrhage. The severity of the stroke, in terms of the impairment of functional status, was rated on a stroke-severity scale described elsewhere *(2)*. This scale summarized the signs, symptoms, and functional impairment of study patients as follows: 1) symptoms only; 2) signs only; 3) both symptoms and signs; 4) minor impairment (but patient still independent) in one or more of five domains (swallowing, self-care, ambulation, communication, and comprehension); 5 to 9) major impairment (loss of independence) in one of five domains, respectively; 10) reduced level of consciousness; and 11) death. Adjudication of the cause of death and of the occurrence and severity of strokes was performed independently by a nonparticipating neurologist and a neurosurgeon blinded to the patients' treatment category.

The targets for sample size and duration of follow-up were selected to permit the trial to demonstrate a 33 percent net surgical reduction in the five-year risk of fatal and nonfatal stroke with a single-sided alpha of 0.05 and a beta of 0.10 (a power of 90 percent). It was agreed that this degree of risk reduction constituted a clinically important surgical benefit, which, if achieved in the trial, would justify advocating the EC-IC bypass procedure.

The primary analysis, comparing surgical and medical groups for the occurrence of all fatal and nonfatal strokes, and secondary analyses employing other end-point combinations were performed by survival analysis with use of the Mantel-Haenszel chi-square statistic. The results of interim analyses, performed at half-year intervals as previously described *(2)*, were maintained in confidence by the principal epidemiologic investigator and chief biostatistician at the Methods Center and were not released to participating investigators.

RESULTS

Entry of Patients

A total of 1495 patients were entered between August 1977 and September 1982; of these, 118 (7.9 percent) were subsequently excluded because they did not meet entry criteria *(2)*. Participating centers were asked to provide lists of eligible patients not entered in the trial, as well as of patients who underwent bypass surgery outside the trial protocol. These lists included 115 eligible patients who refused to enter the trial and 52 patients whose clinicians insisted that they undergo bypass surgery; for 11 other patients, no reason was given. The mean age of the patients who were eligible but not entered was 58 years—similar to that of the trial patients. Of the 1377 eligible patients, 714 (52 percent) were randomly assigned to medical and 663 (48 percent) to surgical therapy. Randomization created balanced treatment groups with respect to important prognostic characteristics and underlying vascular lesions (Table 1). Although 74 percent had some abnormalities on neurologic examination at entry, 93 percent had either minimal or no functional impairment.

Table 1. Entry characteristics of 1377 study participants.

| Characteristics | Treatment group | |
	Medical	Surgical
No. of patients	714	663
Age (mean yr)	56	56
Sex (%)		
Male	82	81
Female	18	19
Randomization diagnosis (%)		
Transient ischemic attack	34	33
Minor stroke	66	67
Other medical problems (%)		
Hypertension	48	52
Diabetes	18	17
Angina pectoris	8	10
Prior myocardial infarction	9	11
Intermittent claudication	11	13
Medications at entry (%)		
Platelet antiaggregants	57	54
Antihypertensive agents	31	33
Blood pressure at entry (mean mm Hg)		
Systolic	144	145
Diastolic	85	85
Most distal angiographic lesion (%)[a]		
Middle cerebral artery		
Stenosis	13.0	14.4
Occlusion	11.1	12.1
Internal carotid artery		
Stenosis (above C-2)	16.7	15.4
Occlusion, no symptoms[b]	38.7	37.0
Occlusion, recurrent symptoms	20.6	21.1

[a] Refers to the most distal angiographic lesion for which the patient was randomized, ignoring the proximal part of tandem lesions.

[b] No symptoms were experienced between angiographic demonstration of the occlusion and randomization.

A final assessment was obtained for all patients between December 1984 and May 1985. The final adjudication of all end points was completed by June 6, 1985.

Follow-up Performance

No patient was lost to follow-up, none were withdrawn, and the average duration of follow-up among surviving patients was 55.8 months (range, 28 to 90). A total of 21 428 individual follow-up assessments were completed from a potential total of 24 160. The completeness of follow-up was similar in the smaller (<25 patients) and the larger centers: 86 and 92 percent, respectively. Less than 10 patients each were randomized from 19 centers. Their pooled contribution was only 101 patients (7 percent of the total).

Nine medical patients (1.3 percent) crossed over and underwent EC-IC bypass on the same side as the lesion for which they had been randomized. Another six medical patients (0.8 percent) underwent EC-IC bypass on the opposite side. Of the 663 patients randomly assigned to the surgical group, 652 (98 percent) underwent surgery, which was performed an average of nine days after randomization.

Repeat angiograms were obtained in 92 percent of the patients at a median time of 32 days after surgery, and on the final review 96 percent of these studies revealed patent anastomoses. The graft patency rates were 95 percent in the smaller and 96 percent in the larger centers, and they were high in all three regions: 94 percent in North America, 97 percent in Europe, and 98 percent in Asia. Fourteen percent of the original stenotic lesions of the middle cerebral artery had progressed to occlusion as seen on the postoperative angiograms. Three patients (0.5 percent of those in whom there were postoperative studies) had strokes within a day after postoperative angiography that were considered complications of the radiologic procedure. Two of the three recovered without a serious permanent deficit. Removing these three patients from the analysis did not change the results.

Medical regimens likely to affect the risk of stroke were equally applied to both groups: Aspirin was used for an average of 75 percent of the follow-up period among medical patients, as compared with 74 percent among surgical patients; hypertension received equally effective control in the two groups.

Perioperative Morbidity and Mortality

The perioperative period was defined as the period from randomization to 30 days after the actual surgery was completed. In this period a total of 81 patients (12.2 percent) had cerebral and retinal ischemic events ranging from trifling symptoms to fatal strokes. Major stroke (Grades 5 to 11 on the stroke-severity scale) occurred in 30 patients (4.5 percent). Seven of the 30 major strokes were fatal, accounting for the perioperative mortality of 1.1 percent. Ten of the 30 major strokes (3 of which were fatal) occurred after the patient was assigned to surgical treatment, but before surgery was performed. During surgery and in the subsequent 30 days, 20 major strokes occurred—16 nonfatal (2.5 percent) and 4 fatal (0.6 percent).

Because the average delay from randomization to surgery was nine days and all events in the additional 30-day postsurgery period were counted against surgery, a comparison was made in the medical group of ischemic events that occurred during the first 39 days after ran-

domization. In the medical cohort of 714 patients, a total of 24 patients (3.4 percent) had some kind of cerebral or retinal ischemic event, 9 (1.3 percent) had major strokes, and 1 died of myocardial infarction. Comparing the rate of major perioperative strokes in the surgical group (4.5 percent) with the spontaneous-stroke rate in the medical group (1.3 percent) showed an excess of 3.2 percent in fatal or non-fatal strokes in the surgical group.

Events

The primary study question was: "Does anastomosis of the superficial temporal artery to the middle cerebral artery, despite perioperative stroke and death, reduce the rate of subsequent events of stroke and stroke-related death in the patients studied?" The answer is no. Fatal and nonfatal strokes occurred both more frequently and earlier in patients randomly assigned to surgery (Figure 1). We were able to test and reject, with a statistical power greater than 99 percent, our original hypothesis of a surgical benefit consisting of a one-third reduction in fatal and nonfatal stroke. In fact, the Mantel-Haenszel chi-square analysis gen-

Figure 1. Results of the primary analysis (all strokes, both fatal and nonfatal), showing the failure of bypass between the superficial temporal artery and the middle cerebral artery to reduce stroke in the surgical (663 patients) as compared with the medical cohort (714 patients) after an average follow-up of 55.8 months. The analysis uses Kaplan–Meier cumulative-failure curves.

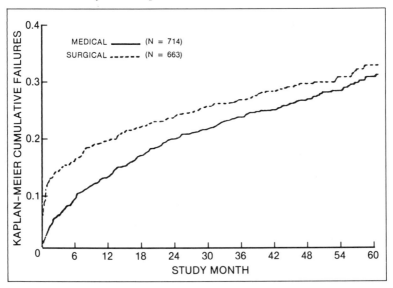

erated a point estimate of the average effect of surgery over the entire trial of a 14 percent increase in the relative risk of fatal and nonfatal stroke. Figure 1 shows that this risk was much more than 14 percent early in the trial and much less toward the end of the trial. The 90 percent confidence limits for this average effect of surgery run from a 34 percent relative increase in the risk of stroke to a 3 percent relative decrease; thus, we can reject (P = 0.05) a surgical benefit of 3 percent or more in the relative risk of fatal and nonfatal stroke.

Moreover, we have examined the influence of a number of potentially confounding base-line factors, identified before this analysis, with the Cox proportional-hazards model and have found that none of them explain away this negative result. These factors include the geographic region or size of the participating center; the site, type (stenosis or occlusion), or extent of the arteriographic lesion present at entry; whether the qualifying event occurred in the right or left hemisphere; the entry data or time from the first qualifying symptoms; the presence of prior stroke or functional impairment at entry; the smoking habit or presence of comorbid conditions at entry (diabetes, prior myocardial infarction, angina pectoris, intermittent claudication, or hypertension); and age, sex, and employment status at entry.

We have also examined the potential impact of the 118 ineligible patients excluded from the trial. All but six (three surgical, three medical) were followed until the end of the trial. The outcomes observed among these 67 surgical patients and 51 medical patients included 6 fatal strokes (3 surgical, 3 medical), 11 nonfatal strokes (5 surgical, 6 medical), and 16 other causes of death (7 surgical, 9 medical). These outcomes did not alter the trial's conclusion when they were added to the outcomes observed among eligible cases.

There was no evidence that surgery decreased the number of strokes. Eighteen percent of the medical patients and 20 percent of the surgical patients had a single stroke each. Two or more strokes occurred in 10 percent of the medical patients and 11 percent of the surgical patients.

A set of "secondary" analyses was also specified before data analysis, and the results of these [analyses] are shown in the four panels of Figure 2. In Figure 2A, the analysis was restricted to strokes of sufficient severity to kill or cause a major impairment (Grades 5 to 11 on the stroke-severity scale). Surgical patients had a 30-day postoperative rate of major nonfatal stroke of 2.5 percent; the death rate during this period was 0.6 percent. Again, no surgical benefit was observed, and these negative results could not be explained by the previously described base-line factors.

Figure 2B shows the results of a "management" or "intention to treat" analysis (3) that included all strokes and all deaths (from any cause) after random assignment. Again, no surgical benefit was observed, and stroke and death were found to occur earlier in the surgical group. These negative results could not be explained by the previously described base-line factors. In Figure 2C the analysis is restricted to the location and type of strokes most likely, on biologic grounds, to benefit from the bypass procedure: ipsilateral ischemic strokes of any severity judged to be due to cerebral or retinal infarction. Again, stroke and stroke death occurred earlier in the surgical group, no surgical benefit was observed, and these negative results could not be explained by the previously described base-line factors. In Figure 2D the analysis is restricted to major (Grades 5 to 11) ipsilateral strokes. The rate of stroke and stroke death according to survival analysis was the same in the medical and surgical groups, and once more the negative results could not be explained by the previously described base-line factors.

The functional status of all the study patients, both at their last evaluation and throughout the trial, is shown in Tables 2 and 3. Identical proportions of medical and surgical patients achieved each level of function at the end of the trial, and no difference was found in the percentage of follow-up time spent in each functional-status level for the two treatment groups.

The result was negative when the analysis was extended to determine whether surgery improved the prognosis and recovery in patients who had severe ipsilateral stroke subsequent to performance of the bypass. When the patients' functional status immediately after their first serious stroke was compared with their functional status one or more years later (mean, 3.5 and 3.8 years for the medical and surgical groups, respectively), equal proportions of medical and surgical patients were found to

Figure 2. Results of secondary analyses, showing the failure of bypass in the total surgical cohort, as compared with the total medical cohort, to reduce the occurrence of major stroke and stroke death (A), all strokes and all deaths (B), all ischemic strokes ipsilateral to the side of symptoms for which randomization was carried out (C), and major ischemic strokes ipsilateral to the side of such symptoms (D).

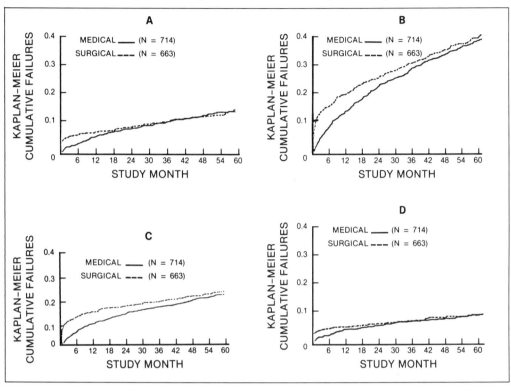

Table 2. Final functional status of all study patients.

	Treatment group	
Impairment[a]	Medical	Surgical
No. of patients	714	663
	percent	
None	56	57
Minor	19	19
Major	5	7
Death	20	17
Cerebrovascular	4.8	4.7
Myocardial infarction	4.5	3.8
Sudden death	2.7	1.5
Other cardiovascular	2.1	3.2
Other	5.6	3.8

[a] Impairments include difficulty in function (minor) or inability to function without assistance (major) in any domains, including communication, comprehension, swallowing, self-care, and ambulation.

have improved, remained at the same level of function, deteriorated, or died (Table 4).

Table 5 summarizes the analyses of fatal and nonfatal strokes among patient subgroups of special clinical interest, considering (1) the site and severity of arteriographic lesions; (2) internal-carotid-artery occlusion with and without continuing symptoms after its demonstration and before randomization; (3) patients with recent onset of frequent transient ischemic attacks; and (4) the size and location of the participating centers. In no case was a statistically significant surgical benefit found; in fact, most of these analyses revealed a higher number of strokes in the surgical groups than would be expected if surgery had no effect, indicating that these subgroups of surgical patients fared worse than their medical counterparts. This was particularly noticed in the subgroups of patients with severe middle-cerebral-artery ste-

Table 3. Percentage of total follow-up time spent at each functional status level.

Impairment[a]	Treatment group	
	Medical	Surgical
No. of patients	714	663
	percent	
None	61	61
Minor	23	23
Major	5	6
Death	11	10

[a] Impairments include difficulty in function (minor) or inability to function without assistance (major) in any domains, including communication, comprehension, swallowing, self-care, and ambulation.

Table 4. Final functional status in 78 patients after the first major ipsilateral ischemic stroke.[a]

Change from stroke to final assessment	Treatment Group	
	Medical	Surgical
No. of patients	42	37
Better	14	14
Same	6	6
Worse	5	5
Dead	17	12
Mean time from stroke to final assessment for surviving patients (yr)	3.5	3.8

[a] Among patients in whom status could be determined for at least one year after the first major stroke.

Table 5. Fatal and nonfatal stroke among clinically interesting subgroups.[a]

Patients[b]	Medical Group			Surgical Group			Mantel-Haenszel chi-square
	No.	Observed	Expected	No.	Observed	Expected	
	number of patients						
All patients	714	205	218.3	663	205	191.7	1.72
Excluding those with ICA occlusion, no symptoms[c]	438	133	148.0	418	148	133.0	3.23
Including only those with							
ICA occlusion, no symptoms[c]	276	72	69.9	245	57	59.1	0.13
ICA occlusion, symptoms[d]	147	51	61.7	140	64	53.3	4.04
Including only severe[e]							
ICA stenosis	72	26	27.1	77	29	27.9	0.10
MCA stenosis	59	14	20.5	50	22	15.5	4.74
Including only							
Bilateral carotid occlusion	43	17	17.4	31	14	13.6	0.02
MCA occlusion	79	18	16.9	80	16	17.1	0.15
1st TIA within 3 mo. of entry and total TIAs >3	87	27	31.5	109	41	36.5	1.32
Center size							
Smaller (<25 patients)	350	98	112.1	337	113	98.9	3.81
Larger (≥25 patients)	364	107	105.9	326	92	93.1	0.02
Geographical region							
North America	352	115	126.8	327	120	108.2	2.37
Europe	247	60	64.9	230	63	58.1	0.77
Asia	115	30	26.8	106	22	25.2	0.78

[a] Values listed under the heading "Observed" indicate the observed number of patients in each treatment group who had a stroke. Those listed under "Expected" indicate the number of patients in each treatment group who would be expected to have a stroke if surgery had no effect, taking into account differences in sample size and duration of follow-up.
[b] ICA denotes internal carotid artery, MCA middle cerebral artery, and TIA transient ischemic attack.
[c] No symptoms were experienced between angiographic demonstration of the occlusion and randomization.
[d] Symptoms were experienced between angiographic demonstration of the occlusion and randomization.
[e] Severe stenosis is stenosis of 70 percent or more of the luminal diameter.

nosis (chi-square = 4.74) and in the patients known to have internal-carotid-artery occlusion but with continuing symptoms after its demonstration (chi-square = 4.04). These subgroup analyses were repeated for the other end-point combinations shown in Figure 2, again with no evidence of a surgical benefit.

All the foregoing analyses were repeated, ignoring events that occurred between randomization and surgery and excluding the 11 patients who, although randomly assigned to surgery, did not undergo it. This "best-case scenario," which can be criticized on methodologic grounds for biasing the results in favor of surgery, failed to generate evidence of surgical benefit.

An analysis compared all stroke and stroke-death outcomes in the 200 surgical patients whose low scores (0 to 4 of a possible 12 points) on the angiographic bypass-rating scale reflected a poor angiographic appearance of the bypass graft and the 225 surgical patients whose high scores (9 to 12 points) reflected the best angiographic appearance of the graft. There was no evidence of a better outcome in those with an excellent bypass as assessed at postoperative angiography than in those with a small or nonpatent anastomosis.

A comparison was made of the occurrence of stroke after bypass surgery according to the

numbers of patients submitted by the centers (Figure 3). No trend was identified to indicate that patients fared better if the center contributed a larger rather than a smaller number of patients.

The effect of surgery on transient ischemic attacks was determined by comparing the frequency of attacks in the three months before entry with the number recorded in the three-month period that ended at the conclusion of the first year in the study. Among the 207 medical patients and 175 surgical patients who entered the trial with transient ischemic attacks and did not die or have a stroke in the first year of follow-up, nearly identical proportions (80 percent in the medical and 77 percent in the surgical group) had at least a halving of the frequency of transient ischemic attacks at one year. Stroke or death had occurred at the end of one year in 13.8 percent of the medical patients who were entered because of transient ischemia and 20.3 percent of the comparable surgical patients.

DISCUSSION

The possibility that microsurgical bypass of stenosed or occluded major arteries in the anterior (carotid) circulation to the brain might pre-

Figure 3. Analysis of the effect of surgery according to center size, for all fatal and nonfatal strokes, showing that the average difference between the observed and expected number of strokes was similar in small and large centers. Each participating center is represented by a dot on the scattergram.

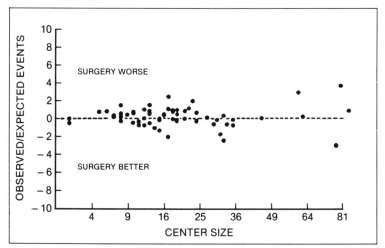

vent subsequent important ischemic events provided the rationale for this trial. It was recognized that the cerebral and retinal ischemic events experienced by the patients could be either of hemodynamic origin, resulting from poor circulatory perfusion, or caused by artery-to-artery emboli, and that in many of them it would not be possible to tell which mechanism was responsible *(4,5)*. However, advocates of the operation postulated that it might benefit patients with ischemia due to either of these causes by improving cerebral perfusion, providing additional collateral circulation, or in patients with ischemia of embolic origin, providing a sufficient increase in perfusion to promote early passage and disintegration of the embolus.

The results indicate with strong statistical power that fatal and nonfatal strokes were not prevented by anastomosis of the superficial temporal to the middle cerebral artery. A surgical benefit as small as 3 percent (clinically insignificant) can be rejected at the 0.05 confidence level. This negative result held for all patients and for individual subgroups, whether the patients had transient ischemic attacks or minor strokes, whether their lesions were occlusive or stenotic, and whether they involved the internal carotid artery, the middle cerebral artery, or both.

We believe that our conclusion that EC-IC surgery fails to prevent stroke or even reduce transient ischemic attacks is both statistically powerful and clinically credible because our study involved (1) a large number of patients with a long period of follow-up, (2) a uniformity of disease process in the population studied, (3) a randomization method that produced balanced treatment groups, (4) a complete and accurate record of all entry and event data, (5) external "blinded" adjudication of eligibility and event data, (6) a uniformity of ancillary treatment for the total patient population, and (7) the achievement of effective anastomoses with acceptably low morbidity and mortality.

As in the previous studies of internal mammary ligation *(6)* and the gastric freeze *(7)*, this negative result from a randomized trial is at variance with previously published reports on case series. Direct comparisons are impossible, because no other published series study has incorporated a concomitantly randomized control group. Studies have been reported that have used the patients as their own controls and have documented improvements in regional cerebral blood flow *(8–12)*, metabolic function in studies using positron-emission tomography *(13–16)*, "neuropsychological" indexes *(17–19)*, or electroencephalographic findings *(20)*. The randomized trial reported here focused on clinical end points and not on these "substitute" physiologic or psychological measurements. Without any established clinical correlation, such surrogate end points fail to provide hard data about the clinical benefit of anastomosis of the superficial temporal to the middle cerebral artery.

The effect of surgery was examined in certain subgroups that have been claimed to constitute particularly promising clinical entities likely to benefit from the procedure (Table 5). In the face of an overall result showing no benefit, we could not expect to identify statistically significant surgical benefits in these subgroups. However, if surgery was efficacious we should expect to find at least some strong trends that would justify more-focused trials. Nevertheless, no positive trends toward surgical benefit emerged in any of the subgroups analyzed. When data were analyzed for fatal and nonfatal strokes in patients with occluded internal carotid arteries, who had continued to have ischemic events between the proof of the occlusion and randomization (n = 287), they were found to have fared worse (chi-square = 4.04) after surgery than with medical therapy—a finding that failed to support the suggestion that such patients were promising candidates for bypass surgery *(21)*. The reason that this subgroup fared worse with surgery is unknown. Evidence has been adduced that a number of patients with internal-carotid-artery occlusion have a potential for thromboembolism through the external carotid artery, the embolus passing through either the natural or the iatrogenic communications between the external and the internal carotid arteries *(22–24)*. It is not certain, however, why this path for thromboembolism would have been more often followed in the surgical than in the medical cohorts. The increased flow through the external carotid artery created by an anastomosis may be a possible explanation. No trend to surgical benefit was found in the larger group of 521 "more stable" patients with occlusion of the internal carotid artery who had no events between the time their occlusions were demonstrated and randomization.

Patients with cerebral ischemia associated with severe stenoses of the intracranial internal carotid or middle cerebral artery had also been postulated as particularly likely to benefit from bypass surgery. Case series of 105 patients with internal-carotid-artery stenosis *(25)* and 47 patients with middle-cerebral-artery stenosis *(26)* were compared with historical controls, and surgical benefit was believed to be demonstrable. Our randomized trial contained larger numbers of both lesions (149 with severe internal-carotid-artery stenosis and 109 with severe middle-cerebral-artery stenosis). There was no difference in outcome between medical and surgical treatment of patients with severe inaccessible carotid stenosis. Moreover, the 50 patients with severe middle-cerebral-artery stenosis subjected to surgery fared considerably worse than did the 59 identical patients in the medical group, whether analysis was for the primary outcome of fatal and nonfatal stroke (chi-square = 4.74) or for any of the other combinations of end points. This is consistent with the progression of a stenosed middle cerebral artery to occlusion after a successful bypass procedure from the superficial temporal to the middle cerebral artery, described in an early report *(27)*. A few clinicoradiologic reports have cautioned that intracranial stenosis of the internal carotid artery or middle cerebral artery presents a potential hazard in terms of bypass surgery *(28–31)*. A morbidity and mortality rate of 9.8 percent was reported in a series of 47 patients with middle-cerebral-artery stenosis and 18 patients with middle-cerebral-artery occlusion *(26)*. In another series of 18 patients with stenotic lesions (7 in the middle cerebral artery, 11 in the internal carotid artery), postoperative ischemic complications developed in 7 (39 percent) *(28)*. A thrombus may form in the proximal stenosed portion of the artery when a bypass provides alternative means of distal perfusion; the obliteration of the stenosed middle cerebral artery results in infarction in the territory of its ganglionic branches. The results of this trial and the finding in the postoperative angiograms of a 14 percent conversion from stenosis to occlusion of the middle cerebral artery lend support to these earlier biologic observations.

The ability of surgery to reduce or eliminate transient ischemic attacks was not a primary issue in this study, but careful records of the occurrence and frequency of such attacks were kept on all patients. The frequency fell equally among medical and surgical patients, and there was no evidence to suggest a benefit from surgery in reducing or eliminating transient ischemic attacks. Previous claims of surgical benefit for transient ischemia have come from uncontrolled observations that have overlooked the fact that transient ischemic events occur in flurries and that there is a tendency toward spontaneous remission *(32, 33)*. Thus, one observer reporting on his uncontrolled series stated that "86 percent of the 400 patients had symptomatic relief" *(34)*. In the present randomized trial, reduction in the number of transient ischemic attacks was noted in 77 percent of the surgical patients but—what is more important—in an equal number (80 percent) of the medical patients. Patients with large numbers of transient ischemic attacks (so-called "crescendo TIA") did not have fewer strokes after surgery than with medical therapy alone.

In spite of the participation of many surgeons, the total 30-day morbidity from major strokes in the surgical group was 2.5 percent, and the 30-day surgical mortality rate was 0.6 percent. This performance compares favorably with that of the most experienced surgeons and that reported in the larger series. Zumstein and Yasargil (the latter is the innovative pioneer of the procedure joining the superficial temporal to the middle cerebral artery) reported on a recent series of 100 patients who underwent the procedure and had a surgical morbidity rate of 2.0 percent and a mortality rate of 3.0 percent *(35)*. One of the North American pioneers of this bypass procedure reported a five-year experience in 70 patients, with permanent neurologic worsening in 3 patients (4.2 percent), temporary neurologic disability in 3, and death within 1 to 17 days of the procedure in 3 *(36)*. An earlier review of most of the work published to 1978 reported a permanent neurologic morbidity of 2.4 percent, a transient morbidity of 4.3 percent, and an average operative mortality of 4.3 percent *(37)*. One surgeon reported on 400 patients and cited a 2 percent "permanent neurologic morbidity rate" and a "present operative mortality rate" of 2.5 percent *(34)*. A group of surgeons from a single institution reported a 4 percent morbidity and a 1 percent mortality rate in 415 such procedures carried out in 403 patients *(38)*. Another study in which one surgeon performed 150 procedures reported a morbidity rate that "slightly exceeded

20 percent" and a postoperative mortality of 6.3 percent *(39)*.

The patency of the bypass was confirmed by angiograms in 96 percent of the patients in the trial. This achievement is difficult to compare with other published rates, because most of them did not use angiography, opting instead for Doppler ultrasound examinations or measures of regional cerebral blood flow as evidence of patency *(40)*. Dural supply and not cortical perfusion can give false positive readings in Doppler examinations *(41)*. Regional studies of cerebral blood flow that are not supported by angiography are likewise open to error *(42)*. Zumstein and Yasargil reported a patency rate of 94.3 percent in 100 patients over a recent 10-year period *(35)*. In another series of 400 patients, 96 percent of the grafts were found to be "apparently open" by Doppler and ultrasound auscultation *(34)*. The effect of surgical experience in improving performance was reflected in the results from three periods in one center *(38, 43)*: 25 percent patency in 8 patients between 1971 and 1973; 95 percent patency in 58 patients between 1974 and 1976; and 99 percent patency in 403 patients between 1974 and 1982. Once again, patency was evaluated largely by Doppler velocity flow probe *(38, 44)*.

The impact of the adequacy of the bypass procedure was addressed by comparing the 200 patients who had the worst postoperative angiograms and the 225 with the best angiograms, each angiogram having been measured and assigned a multifactorial score. This analysis demonstrated that those with luxuriant perfusion fared no better than those with a small or nonfunctioning anastomosis. To be sure, a number of factors contribute to the adequacy of a bypass, including the degree of disease extending into the artery used for the bypass, the degree of pressure differential between the donor and recipient arterial beds, the amount of available collateral supply, and the technical adequacy of the anastomosis. Nonetheless, we judge it reasonable to conclude from this analysis that the achievement of a luxuriant flow through the anastomosis was not a critical factor in determining the benefit or lack thereof from bypass.

This trial was not designed to measure benefit in neurologic function. Many anecdotal reports have proposed a benefit from bypass from the superficial temporal to the middle cerebral artery in these circumstances on the basis of the theoretical consideration that a "penumbra" of ischemic tissue, or an area of "misery perfusion," surrounds recent or evolving areas of cerebral infarction—a concept supported by the measurement of hemodynamic and metabolic changes with positron-emission tomography *(39, 40, 45, 46)*. Anastomosis from the superficial temporal to the middle cerebral artery, performed in a few patients with mild neurologic impairment, has been reported to be followed by improved local cerebral-perfusion pressure in some and by improved local blood flow in others. No patients have been reported in whom these improved functions detected by positron-emission tomographic observations have been associated with dramatic clinical improvement *(47)*.

The 37 patients randomly assigned to surgery in this study who went on to have serious ipsilateral ischemic infarction despite the bypass surgery did not have a better functional recovery by the end of the trial than did the 42 comparable patients in the medical group. These results in patients in whom the bypass procedure was performed before the strokes occurred do not provide support for the suggestion that an early anastomosis from the superficial temporal to the middle cerebral artery after an incipient, evolving, or developed carotid-territory stroke would be likely to promote recovery of a sufficient number of neurons to reduce the ultimate disability. Futhermore, two thirds of all the patients were entered in the study after a nondisabling stroke. The lack of difference in functional outcome for the surgical and the medical groups with mild or moderate stroke does not encourage the proposition that bypass surgery will hasten or improve neurologic recovery after an ischemic lesion.

We are indebted to Linda Hill, Diane Woelfle, and Rebecca Taylor for assistance in the preparation of the manuscript.

APPENDIX

The EC/IC Bypass Study Group consisted of the following investigators, committees, and participating centers (members of the Executive Committee are indicated by an asterisk): *Central Office* (University of Western Ontario), London, Ont.: principal investigator, H.J.M. Barnett; principal neurosurgical investigator,

S.J. Peerless; principal neuroradiological investigator, A.J. Fox; senior staff, B. Valberg, J. Peacock. *Methods Center* (McMaster University), Hamilton, Ont.: principal epidemiologic investigator, D.L. Sackett; chief epidemiologist, R.B. Haynes; chief statistician, D.W. Taylor; senior staff, C.Collis, J. Mukherjee, P. Flanagan. *Steering Committee:* University of Western Ontario, H.J.M. Barnett (chairman), S.J. Peerless, A.J. Fox, B. Valberg, V.C. Hachinski; McMaster University, D.L. Sackett, D.W. Taylor, R.B. Haynes, J. Mukherjee. *Monitoring Committee:* M. Goldstein (chairman 1977–1982; National Institute of Neurological and Communicative Disorders and Stroke)*, M.D. Walker (chairman 1982–present, National Institute of Neurological and Communicative Disorders and Stroke)*, J.B. Benedict (National Institute of Neurological and Communicative Disorders and Stroke)*, W. Weiss (National Institute of Neurological and Communicative Disorders and Stroke), J.R. Marler (National Institute of Neurological and Communicative Disorders and Stroke), J.P. Whisnant (Mayo Clinic). H.G. Schwartz (Washington University), A. Heyman (Duke University-Medical Center). W.H. Feindel (Montreal Neurological Institute).

Participating Centers (in order of number of eligible patients entered): University of Western Ontario, London, Ont.: H.J.M. Barnett*, C.W. McCormick, V.C. Hachinski, S.J. Peerless*, G.G. Ferguson; neuroradiologists, J. Allcock, A.J. Fox*; additional contributors, K. Meguro, R. Cote, D. Moulin, P.C. Gates, S. Lauzier. University of Toronto, Toronto, Ont.: R. Wilson, G. Sawa, H. Schultz, M.C. Chiu. University of Tennessee, Memphis, Tenn.: A. Heck, J. Robertson*, B. Gerald; National Institute of Neurosurgery, Budapest, Hungary: L. Ronai, E. Pasztor* (sponsoring neurosurgeon), J. Vajda, M. Horvath, I. Nyary, G. Deak. University of Essen, Essen, Federal Republic of Germany; A. Buch, H.M. Mehdorn, C. Nahser. Universita di Firenze, Florence, Italy; L. Amaducci*, D. Inzitari, S. Briani (deceased), R. Gagliardi, A. Nori. Neurochirurgia und Neurologica University Klinik Giessen, Federal Republic of Germany: O. Busse, E. Grote, C. Hornig, R. Schonmayr. Kyoto University Medical School, Kyoto, Japan: M. Kameyama, I. Akiguchi, H. Shio, H. Handa (sponsoring neurosurgeon), Y. Yonekawa*. Hopital Pellegrin, Bordeaux, France: J.M. Orgogozo, J.J. Pere, J.P. Castel, J.M. Caille. New York University, New York: W.K. Hass*, E.S. Flamm*. University of Pecs, Pecs, Hungary: M. Bodosi, G. Gacs, F.T. Merei. Westeinde Ziekenhuis Den Haag, Holland: J.Th.T. Tans, C.A.F. Tulleken*, P. Hoogland. Univer-

sity of Mississippi, Jackson; A.F. Haerer, R.R. Smith. Institute of Brain and Blood Vessels, Gunma, Japan: G. Araki, K. Nagata, M. Mizukami, C. Yunoki. Tokyo Medical and Dental University, Tokyo, Japan: H. Tsukagoshi, U. Ito, Y. Inaba (sponsoring neurosurgeon), T. Fujimoto, K. Komatsu. Neurochirurgische University Klinik Universitatsspital, Zurich, Switzerland: H. Zumstein, H. Keller, B. Zumstein, H.G. Imhof. Upstate Medical Center, Syracuse, N.Y.: A. Culebras, C.J. Hodge. Case Western Reserve University, Cleveland, Ohio: D.L. Jackson, K. Chandar, R. Spetzler, R.B. Daroff, L.A. Hershey. University of Tokushima, Tokushima, Japan: S. Yasuoka; K. Matsumoto (sponsoring neurosurgeon). S. Ueda. Neurological Institute of Savannah, Savannah, Ga.: O.E. Ham, E.P. Downing, F.P. Wirth. Universita di Milano, Milan, Italy: P. Perrone, G. Cabrini. State University of New York at Buffalo, Buffalo, N.Y.: E.J. Manning, D. Ehrenreich, L.N. Hopkins, University of Minnesota, Minneapolis: M.C. Lee, D. Erickson. Royal Victoria Infirmary, Newcastle-upon-Tyne, England: D.A. Shaw, D. Bates, G. Venables, R. Sengupta. Veterans General Hospital, Taipei, Taiwan: Fu-Li Chu, Han-Hau Hu, W. Wen-Jang Wong, A.L. Shen*. Johns Hopkins University, Baltimore: T.J. Preziozi, M.H. Epstein. University of Oregon, Portland: B. Coull, F. Yatsu*, F. Waller, C. Tanabe. Sophia Hospital Zwolle, The Netherlands: W.G.M. Teunissen, P.W. Gelderman. Universita degli Studi, Naples, Italy: R. Cotrufo, P. Conforti, F. Tomasello, V. Albanese. Neurosurgical University Hospital, Belgrade, Yugoslavia: M. Panic, B. Milosavljevic, S. Domonji. Fujita-Gakuen University School of Medicine, Nagoya, Japan: M. Nomura, T. Kanno, H. Sano. Harvard Medical School, Boston, Mass.: P. Kistler, R. Crowell*. University of Pavia, Pavia, Italy: G. Brambilla, D. Locatelli, R. Rodriguez, P. Paoletti. University of North Carolina, Chapel Hill: J.N. Hayward, S.C. Boone, J.D. Mann. Emory University School of Medicine, Atlanta: H. Karp, R. Schnapper, A. Fleischer. University of Iowa, Iowa City: H. Adams, C. Gross. University of Texas, Dallas: E. Ross, D. Samson. Legnano General Hospital, Legnano, Italy: G. Tonarelli, I. Piazza. Tufts New England Medical Center, Boston: M. Pessin, R.M. Scott. University of Missouri, Columbia: J Byer, C. Watts, M. Dittmore. University of Mainz, Mainz, West Germany: G. Kramer, G. Meinig. University of South Alabama, Mobile: J.P. Mohr*, C.S. Kase, H.C. Mostellar. National Cardiovascular Center, Osaka Japan: T. Yamaguchi, T. Sawada, H. Kikuchi. Mayfield Neurological Institute, Cincinnati: R. Reed, J. Tew. Dalhousie University, Halifax, Nova Scotia: T.J. Murray, C.W. McCormick, W.J. Howes, M. Riding. Cleveland Clinic, Cleveland, Ohio: A. Furlan, J. Little, D. Dohn. Institute of Brain Diseases, Tohoku University, Sendai, Japan: H. Saito, J. Suzuki (sponsoring neurosurgeon), N. Kodama. T. Yoshimoto. University of California, San Francisco: M.S. Edwards. Hokkaido University Hospital, Sapporo, Japan: K. Tashiro, M. Tsuru (sponsoring neurosurgeon), Y. Nakagawa. North Manchester General Hospital, Manchester, England: D. Shepherd, G.M. Yuill, C. Bannister, I.W. Turnbull. Henry Ford Hospital, Detroit: R. Teasdall, J. Ausman. Research Institute of Brain and Blood Vessels, Akita, Japan: T. Kutsuzawa, N. Nakajima, T. Kobayashi, N. Yasui, Z. Ito (deceased). University of Cincinnati, Cincinnati, Ohio: C. Olinger, R. Singh, G. Khodadad. Duke University Medical Center, Durham, N.C.: W.C. Olanow, R.H. Wilkins. Ciudad Sanitaria v. del Rocio. Seville, Spain: R. Alberca-Serrano, F. Morales-Ramos. Barrow's Neurological Institute, Phoenix, Ariz.: A. Yudell, R. Thompson, P. Carter. Mississippi Baptist Medical Center, Jackson: W. Bowlus, L. Mahalak, D. Stringer. Neurological Institute, Tokyo Women's Medical College, Tokyo, Japan: S. Maruyama, K. Kitamura, M. Kagawa. University of Pittsburgh, Pittsburgh, Pa.: O. Reinmuth*, R. Heros. University of Nagasaki Medical School, Nagasaki, Japan: H. Matsumura, M. Takamori, K. Mori (sponsoring neurosurgeon), H. Ono, Osaka University Medical School, Osaka, Japan: M. Imaizumi, S. Yoneda, H. Mogami, T. Hayakawa. Nassau County Medical Center, East Meadow, N.Y.: R. Carruthers, R. Decker. Naval Regional Medical Center, Oakland, Calif.: A. Chalmers, T.H. Rockel, R. Hodosh. University of Arizona, Tucson: J. Laguna, P. Weinstein. Tokyo University Medical School, Tokyo, Japan: T. Takasu, T. Eguchi, H. Sugiyama, N. Basugi, T. Asano. Queens University, Kingston, Ont.: H.B. Dinsdale, P. Murray. Albert Einstein College of Medicine, Bronx, N.Y.: L.J. Thal. Hopital Neurologique, Lyon, France: D. Deruty. Daniel Freeman Memorial Hospital, Inglewood, Calif.: B. Dobkin. Scarborough General Hospital. Scarborough, Ont.: M.R. Goldman. Long Island-Jewish Hillside Medical Center, New Hyde Park, N.Y.: M. Nathanson.

Writing Committee for this paper: H.J.M. Barnett, D.L. Sackett, D.W. Taylor, S.J. Peerless, R.B. Haynes, P.C. Gates, A.J. Fox, J. Mukherjee, B. Valberg, V. Hachinski, S. Lauzier, J.M. Orgogozo.

References

(1) Yasargil, M.G., ed. *Microsurgery Applied to Neuro-Surgery.* Stuttgart, Georg Thieme, 1969, pages 105–115.

(2) EC/IC Bypass Study Group. The International Cooperative Study of Extracranial/Intracranial Arterial Anastomosis (EC/IC Bypass Study): methodology and entry characteristics. *Stroke* 16:397–406, 1985.

(3) Sackett, D.L. and M. Gent. Controversy in counting and attributing events in clinical trials. *N Engl J Med* 301:1410–1412, 1979.

(4) Barnett, H.J.M. Pathogenesis of transient ischemic attacks. In *Cerebrovascular Diseases* (P. Scheinberg, ed.) New York, Raven Press, 1976, pages 1–21.

(5) Barnett, H.J.M. Progress toward stroke prevention. *Neurology* (NY) 30:1212–1225, 1980.

(6) Barsamian, E.M. The rise and fall of internal mammary ligation in the treatment of angina pectoris and the lessons learned. In *Costs, Risks, and Benefits of Surgery* (J.P. Bunker, B.A. Barnes, and F. Moseler, eds.). New York, Oxford University Press, 1977, pages 212–220.

(7) Miao, L.L. Gastric freezing: an example of the evaluation of medical therapy by randomized clinical trials. In *Costs, Risks, and Benefits of Surgery* (J.P. Bunker, B.A. Barnes, and F. Moseler, eds.). New York, Oxford University Press, 1977, pages 198–211.

(8) Norrving, B., B. Nilsson, and J. Risberg. rCBF in patients with carotid occlusion: Resting and hypercapnic flow related to collateral pattern. *Stroke* 13:155–162, 1982.

(9) Tsuda, Y., K. Kimura, Y. Iwata, et al. Improvement of cerebral blood flow and or CO_2 reactivity after superficial temporal artery-middle cerebral artery bypass in patients with transient ischemic attacks and watershed-zone infarctions. *Surg Neurol* 22:595–604, 1984.

(10) Yonas, H., D. Gur, B.C. Good, et al. Stable xenon CT blood flow mapping for evaluation of patients with extracranial-intracranial bypass surgery. *J Neurosurg* 62:324–333, 1985.

(11) Yonekura, M., G. Austin, and W. Hayward. Long-term evaluation of cerebral blood flow, transient ischemic attacks, and stroke after STA-MCA anastomosis. *Surg Neurol* 18:123–130, 1982.

(12) Laurent, J.P., P.M. Lawner, and M. O'Connor. Reversal of intracerebral steal by STA-MCA anastomosis. *J Neurosurg* 57:629–632, 1982.

(13) Powers, W.J., W.R.W. Martin, P. Herscovitch, M.F. Raichle, and R.L. Grubb, Jr. Extracranial-intracranial bypass surgery: Hemodynamic and metabolic effects. *Neurology* (NY) 34:1168–1174, 1984.

(14) Baron, J.C., M.G. Bousser, A. Rey, A. Guillard, D. Comar, and P. Castaigne. Reversal of focal "misery perfusion" syndrome by extra-intracranial arterial bypass in hemodynamic cerebral ischemia: A case study with 150 positron emission tomography. *Stroke* 12:452–459, 1981.

(15) Grubb, R.L., Jr., R.A. Ratcheson, M.E. Raichle, A.B. Fliefoth, and M.H. Gado. Regional cerebral blood flow and oxygen utilization in superficial tem-

poral-middle cerebral artery anastomosis patients and exploratory definition of clinical problems. *J Neurosurg* 50:733–741, 1979.

(16) Gibbs, J.M., R.J.S. Wise, K.L. Leenders, and T. Jones. Evaluation of cerebral perfusion reserve in patients with carotid-artery occlusion. *Lancet* 1:182–186, 1984.

(17) Binder, L.M., C.T. Tanabe, F.T. Waller, and N.E. Wooster. Behavioral effects of superficial temporal artery to middle cerebral artery bypass surgery: Preliminary report. *Neurology* (NY) 31:422–424, 1982.

(18) Younklin, D., J.P. Hungerbuhler, M. O'Connor, et al. Superficial temporal-middle cerebral artery anastomosis: Effects on vascular neurologic and neuropsychological functions. *Neurology* (NY) 35:462–469, 1985.

(19) Drinkwater, J.E., S.K. Thompson, and J.S.P. Lumley. Cerebral function before and after extraintracranial carotid bypass. *J Neurol Neurosurg Psychiatry* 47:1041–1043, 1984.

(20) deWeerd, A.W., M.M. Veering, P.C.M. Mosmans, A.C. van Huffelen, C.A.F. Tulleken, and E.J. Jonkman. Effect of the extra-intracranial (STA-MCA) arterial anastomosis on EEG and cerebral blood flow: A controlled study of patients with unilteral cerebral ischemia. *Stroke* 13:674–679, 1982.

(21) Whisnant, J.P., T.M. Sundt, Jr., and F.C. Fode. Long-term mortality and stroke morbidity after superficial temporal artery-middle cerebral artery bypass operation. *Mayo Clin Proc* 60:241–246, 1985.

(22) Barnett, H.J.M. Delayed cerebral ischemic episodes distal to occlusion of major cerebral arteries. *Neurology* (Minneap) 28:769–774, 1978.

(23) Barnett, H.J.M. and S.J. Peerless. Collaborative EC/IC bypass study: The rationale and a progress report. In *Cerebrovascular Diseases* (J. Moossy and O.M. Reinmuth, eds.). New York, Raven Press, 1:271–288, 1981.

(24) Conley, F.K. Embolization of a superficial temporal artery to middle cerebral artery bypass: Case report. *Neurosurgery* 12:342–345, 1983.

(25) Weinstein, P.R., R. Rodriguez y Baena, and N.L. Chater. Results of extracranial-intracranial arterial bypass for intracranial internal carotid artery stenosis: Review of 105 cases. *Neurosurgery* 15:787–794, 1984.

(26) Andrews, B.T., N.L. Chater, and P.R. Weinstein. Extracranial-intracranial arterial bypass for middle cerebral artery stenosis and occlusion: Operative results in 65 cases. *J Neurosurg* 62:831–838, 1985.

(27) Chater, N.L. and P.R. Weinstein. Progression of middle cerebral artery stenosis to occlusion without symptoms following superficial temporal artery bypass: Case report. In *Microvascular Anastomoses for Cerebral Ischemia* (J.M. Fein and O.H. Reichman, eds.). New York, Springer-Verlag, 1974, pages 269–271.

(28) Gumerlock, M.K., H. Ono, and E.A. Neuwelt. Can a patent extracranial-intracranial bypass provoke the conversion of an intracranial arterial stenosis to a symptomatic occlusion? *Neurosurgery* 12:391–400, 1983.

(29) Nakagawa, Y., M. Tsuru, S. Mabuchi, K-h. Echizenya, M. Satoh, and T. Kashiwaba. EC-IC bypass surgery for the middle cerebral artery stenosis: Outcomes and postoperative angiography. In *Cerebral Revascularization for Stroke* (R.F. Spetzler, L.P. Carter, W.R. Selman, and N.A. Martin, eds.). New York, Thieme-Stratton, 1985, pages 449–457.

(30) Awad, I., A.J. Furlan, and J.R. Little. Changes in intracranial stenotic lesions after extracranial-intracranial bypass surgery. *J Neurosurg* 60:771–776, 1984.

(31) Furlan, A.J., J.R. Little, and D.F. Dohn. Arterial occlusion following anastomosis of the superficial temporal artery to middle cerebral artery. *Stroke* 11:91–95, 1980.

(32) Tanahashi, N., J. Stirling Meyer, et al. Long-term assessment of cerebral perfusion following STA-MCA bypass in patients. *Stroke* 16:85–91, 1985.

(33) Barnett, H.J.M. Stroke prevention and treatment: Milestones, perspectives and challenges. In *Cerebrovascular Diseases* (F. Plum and W. Pulsinelli, eds.). New York, Raven Press, 1985, pages 27–41.

(34) Chater, N. Neurosurgical extracranial-intracranial bypass for stroke: With 400 cases. *Neurol Res* 5(2):1–9, 1983.

(35) Zumstein, B., and M.G. Yasargil. Verbesserung der Hirndurchblutung durch mikrochirurgische Bypass-Anastomoses. *Schweiz Rundschau Med* (Praxis) 70:1866–1873, 1981.

(36) Reichman, O.H. Complications of cerebral revascularization. *Clin Neurosurg* 23:318–335, 1976.

(37) Samson, D.S., and S. Boone. Extracranial-intracranial (EC-IC) arterial bypass: Past performance and current concepts. *Neurosurgery* 3:79–86, 1978.

(38) Sundt, T.M., Jr., J.P. Whisnant, N.C. Fode, D.G. Piepgrass, and O.W. Houser. Results, complications, and follow-up of 415 bypass operations for occlusive disease of the carotid system. *Mayo Clin Proc* 60:230–240, 1985.

(39) Kletter, G. *The Extra-intracranial Bypass Operation for Prevention and Treatment of Stroke*. New York, Springer-Verlag, 1979, pages 117–128.

(40) Gratzl, O. and P. Schmiedek. STA-MCA bypass: Results 10 years postoperatively. *Neurol Res* 5(2):11–18, 1983.

(41) Ausman, J.I. and F.G. Diaz. Correlation of noninvasive Doppler and angiographic evaluation of extra-intracranial anastomoses. In *Microsurgery for Cerebral Ischemia* (S.J. Peerless and C.W. McCormick, eds.). New York, Springer-Verlag, 1980, pages 125–127.

(42) Halsey, J.H., Jr., R.B. Morawetz, and U.W. Blaustein. The hemodynamic effect of STA-MCA bypass. *Stroke* 13:163–167, 1982.

(43) Sundt, T.M., Jr., R.G. Siekert, D.G. Piepgrass, F.W. Sharbrough, and O.W. Houser. Bypass surgery for vascular disease of the carotid system. *Mayo Clin Proc* 51:677–692, 1976.

(44) Conforti, P., F. Tomasello, and V. Albanese. *Cerebral Revascularization by Microneurosurgical Bypass*. Padua, Italy, Piccin Nuova Libraria, 1984, pages 124–128.

(45) Lee, M.C., J.I. Ausman, J.D. Geiger, et al. Su-

perficial temporal to middle cerebral artery anastomosis: Clinical outcome in patients with ischemia of infarction in internal carotid artery distribution. *Arch Neurol* 36:1–4, 1979.

(46) Rhodes, R.S., R.F. Spetzler, and R.A. Roski. Improved neurologic function after cerebrovascular accident with extracranial-intracranial arterial bypass. *Surgery* 90:433–438, 1981.

(47) Powers, W.J. and M.E. Raichle. Positron emission tomography and its application to the study of cerebrovascular disease in man. *Stroke* 16:361–376, 1985.

PART V

PERSPECTIVE AND PROSPECTS

DISCUSSIONS

TERRIS: It might be useful to set down the tasks of epidemiology for the near future.

First, I think epidemiology should expand the scope and intensity of etiologic studies in diseases of unknown etiology, in occupational and environmental hazards (which are not diseases but hazards), and in the epidemiology of positive health (everything that goes into positive health: vigor, vitality, and performance; the effects of nutrition, physical exercise, rest and recreation, social relations, participation in decision making, etc.).

Second, it should provide epidemiological assistance in disease prevention to the public health movement by determining the population groups at greatest risk through, for example, surveys of serum-cholesterol levels, smoking prevalence, and blood pressure, as well as by obtaining data on the morbidity and mortality of these groups so that the greatest efforts may be directed to them. Epidemiologists should also carry out experimental studies to determine which measures are most effective in achieving results in prevention, monitor results of public health programs for prevention, and evaluate these programs in terms of outcomes.

Finally, epidemiology should study the medical care system, its procedures—such as clinical procedures—and technology in terms of both positive and negative effects on the population's health, as well as carry out experimental studies with different forms and methods of organization and various clinical procedures to determine which can improve the population's health most effectively.

BUCK: I think that's a coherent blending of all our points of view, but I have one question to ask. I'd like you to explain the at-risk business in your second point. It seems that you categorize people in terms of accepted etiological factors and then you end up looking at data on their morbidity and mortality. Are you trying to check whether these really are etiological factors?

TERRIS: Well, cancer of the cervix, for example, is a disease of poor people, not rich people. I have a friend in New York City who has a middle-class clientele. He takes a Pap smear on every woman, thousands upon thousands. He has never found anything; he is wasting his time. Obviously, the Pap smear program should not be concentrated on the rich people, but on the working class, on the poorest people. We know that their risk is much greater. The Pap smear should also be administered to promiscuous groups—prostitutes and people in jails, for instance. They've done studies that show much more cancer of the cervix in prisoners.

LLOPIS: Yes, that is a problem with any test. You also have a lot of venereal disease testing in groups that are not at risk.

BUCK: I agree with you entirely, Terris. It's just that your wording made me think that you were talking about more than just targeting disease screening toward people with the highest morbidity and mortality.

TERRIS: Let me give you another example. We know that smoking is more common in urban than in rural populations, so attention should focus on the urban areas rather than the rural. We also know that in very large countries, health problems may vary from region to region. In the Soviet Union, for example, you know that you don't have to worry about serum cholesterol levels in people in the East; it's in the West where they have the problem. Austria and Czechoslovakia have high serum cholesterol levels too, because for a hundred years they've been eating a diet rich in saturated fats. You want to find out which part of the population is at greater risk so you can direct your efforts there. This should be done not only in terms of morbidity and mortality, now we also have to do it in terms of risk factors. That's really what I meant. It's what we've always done in the infectious diseases. For example, I remember a big campaign in the United States in the 1940s to do mass chest X-ray surveys of factory workers because they had the highest incidence of tuberculosis.

NAJERA: I like the outline. When we talk about the role of epidemiology regarding high-risk groups, I think we should go beyond the known high-risk groups and try to find new ones. I think we should insist that high-risk groups be defined by their mortality and morbidity. And we should encourage general studies. The type of vital statistics or population data that we now have do not always allow us to study the population according to occupation or social class. We should insist on more precise demographic data. At present it is hard to determine groups, since categories are not well defined or heterogeneous. This affects the precision of epidemiological research.

Another point I want to make is that our health services have developed so much, especially in medical care, that whole populations have become "medicalized". We call it a health system, but it's really disease oriented, a medical-care system. There is too much "medical" in our health system. Perhaps it's time to add a fourth dimension to the basic epidemiologic triad of time, place, and person. We should include the particular health system that serves a population. In classifying populations, especially countries, PAHO has always grouped them by geography—Caribbean Area, South America, Central America, and so on. This lumps together countries as different as Nicaragua and Honduras. Sure, they're neighbors, but their health systems are different, so different, that they should not be in the same category. These differences even exist within the same country. Even where you have a national health system like in England, sometimes there are social-class differences in the utilization of the system. I think this is very important because care or prevention is determined by how people utilize the health services. I think it's time to consider the health system as an important fourth dimension in all epidemiological studies.

TERRIS: My own feeling is that what you're talking about now is health service research as a totality, but we are talking about the role of epidemiology. I think that if we don't limit ourselves to outcome studies, to studies of the effect of health services on disease and health status, then, all of a sudden, we're doing everything. We're no longer doing just epidemiology. Who is using the services? I think health service research should determine this. As you say, even in England with a National Health Service, the poor are not getting as much as the well-to-do for a lot of reasons. Among the reasons may be that the poor don't fully understand what the health services can do for them. But this is a general health service research problem. The study of utilization is part of the totality of health services research. I think we have to stick to the role of epidemiology because we don't really have a role now. Nobody pays attention to us.

BUCK: I agree with everything you're saying. I think it might help if we remember the historical roots of epidemiology: the study of causes and effects. Effects include the outcomes of health care. It's no distortion of the original epidemiological approach to insist that we have a role in etiological studies of outcome. There's no departure there.

NAJERA: What I want to say is that the utilization of health services is a very important dimension of the epidemiology of chronic diseases, that the role of epidemiology is not limited to etiology. Consider, for instance, the difference in the evolution of hypertension in people who have access to health services and people who don't. This is what I want to emphasize. People also differ depending on the type of health service they have, the amount of "medicalization" they receive, and whether they are followed-up or not. I think our health services have become so complicated and sophisticated that they are now a health factor. And many times they are a negative factor, which is why we could also include the importance of iatrogenic diseases.

LLOPIS: I think we also have to say something about evaluating new technologies in terms of outcome and survival, because technology is very expensive. This evaluation is extremely important for Latin American countries because they are big consumers of imported technology.

NAJERA: I think this point is very important. Who decides which technologies are important to those countries that do not produce them directly? Why are they used or imported or put into the system? Whose priorities do they represent? Epidemiology provides the only answer to this, but at present technology manufacturers and health ministries govern these decisions. Technology may be a solution to some problems, but at a very high cost. Besides, there may be other, more important, problems. So, I think this is the place for epidemiology.

Another point is the role of epidemiology in defining social classes. What is social class? We should be interested in the origin of social classes from a labor point of view—what people earn, where they work. We should be interested in how social classes influence the development of disease. Epidemiology should be used to define groups, which we can call social classes, that are subject to different conditions. We should utilize epidemiology to reclassify professions or occupations or ways of living in order to arrive at a better definition of social classes.

We have said before that the health system in England is not so good. True, it's not so good, but it's better than the one in the United States or Spain. We have nothing and something is so much better than nothing. But still it is not good enough. So why not utilize epidemiology to find out how it can be improved?

BUCK: You make a good point about social class and occupational categorization, and I agree that the British system of occupational statistics may have many imperfections, of which they are probably aware, but, as you say, most countries don't have one at all. My own country is a case in point. Canada could have occupational mortality data because the principal lifetime occupation is recorded on the death certificate. But for some reason this does not enter the statistical system; it probably doesn't enter the United States system for a similar reason.

TERRIS: The reason in the United States is that the dominant ideology insists that there are no social classes in the United States. Didn't you know that this is supposed to be the country without social classes?

BUCK: Well, you are giving a philosophical reason.

TERRIS: They don't want to study social classes.

NAJERA: What is the reason in Canada?

BUCK: We don't want to study them, either. It's the same reason.

NAJERA: The countries without social classes!

BUCK: The point is that before we can fully understand the social class factor we need to have this kind of data from a variety of countries.

I would like to emphasize again that there should be more studies like Cassel's. Cassel was one of the modern investigators who reestablished a mode of research which probably has classical origins. This mode starts with the rich hypothesis of a cause that can lead to many illnesses. I believe that we have some diseases which are interchangeable manifestations of a big cause. If all our research is disease specific, we may miss these big causes. There's a lot we don't know, because for every disease you look at, even when you appear to have quite a bit of its etiology figured out, there is always a substantial unexplained variation in frequency. It may be that the unexplained variation arises differently for each disease, but it may equally well be that much of it comes from a common source. That common source would be a big cause. One reason why we neglect this approach is that funds are raised within disease-specific boundaries.

NAJERA: I think that you have raised a very, very, important point—the definition of disease. Maybe it's not so necessary for acute diseases, but it is for chronic diseases. In order to help the study of disease, we need to think a lot about redefining diseases from a clinical and epidemiological point of view. I always use the example of fevers before the nineteenth century. Most acute diseases of the time were simply classified as fevers. Why couldn't we say that we are now in the same position with respect to tumors, or cancer, or what we call cardiovascular diseases? We need to use epidemiology to arrive at better definitions, in a practical sense. This is also one of the roles of epidemiology: to redefine health problems. This is one thing that the World Health Organization could incorporate into the Tenth Revision of the *International Classification of Diseases*. We are now at the end of the twentieth century and there has been very little change since the end of the nineteenth century when the first international classification was adopted. We have a little more sophisticated technology, but we haven't had any conceptual change.

TERRIS: I would like to touch on some of the issues discussed earlier. I think that despite all the criticism that the English system of defining social classes has received, it is pretty good. It has produced more epidemiology and more hints, more inferences, than any other system you can think of. It shouldn't be decried. For example, if you look at some of the long-term English and Scottish studies of child development, the interesting thing is that they took Class III, the skilled workers, and divided it into manual workers and white-collar workers. The results were fascinating because they turned out to be two different classes. The Class III manual workers were more like the semi-skilled workers (Class IV) and unskilled workers (Class V), while the Class III white-collar workers were more like the upper classes (I and II). What you really had was the difference between brain workers and manual workers within the class of skilled workers.

Another point that ought to be made is that the mental disease area needs a lot of attention. Not much work has been done in it. Earlier we talked about the problems of maladaptation and lack of well-being. In addition to the serious psychiatric problems, we also need to focus on those people who are neurotic, who are unhappy, people who are not really a part of their society, people whose whole life consists of working and then going home to watch television. In short, people who are not really living. This kind of problem has to do with well-being, with the problem of positive health and performance that we should address.

BUCK: You've really put your finger on it. Cassel, for example, did not confine himself to illness manifested in emotional disturbances. The studies he did of rapidly urbanized Appalachian Valley people, or the ones he did of Maoris who moved from remote islands to New Zealand, indicated that profound social changes were associated not only with what we would call psychological disturbances, but also with cardiovascular disease and many other allegedly physical diseases. I imagine that no one here is going to dispute the psychosomatic relationship. We shouldn't wall off physical from psychological disease.

TERRIS: I will. Although I think it exists, I believe it's been oversold.

BUCK: But we only have to look at the anatomy of the human body, its physiology, to realize that it's all of a piece, don't we?

TERRIS: It may be all of one piece, but I think there's been a lot of theorizing based on that without actual demonstration.

BUCK: I agree with you in that. But my point is that we need more demonstration. Quite apart from the possible effects of cultural phenomena upon all diseases, it is still important to look at psychological disturbances. Look at the amount of ill health and violence related to child abuse that gets transmitted from one generation to another. It's a very serious part of our ill health and we just don't know where to try to break the cycle. I think this issue is profoundly illustrative of the kind of psychological malaise that doesn't reflect its true nature in any mortality rate that we have.

TERRIS: Well, if you take drug addiction or alcoholism, you find that they're really social diseases. They occur mostly in blacks, Chicanos, Puerto Ricans—in the most oppressed groups of U.S. society. And child abuse is found mostly among blue collar workers, again in the most dispossessed parts of our society.

BUCK: Some believe you find it everywhere, but that it's not diagnosed the same in all classes.

NAJERA: Here is an interesting point to make. Take drug abuse, for instance. We find it in the poor, but thirty years ago it occurred among the rich. We should ask why drug abuse has moved from high-income to low-income groups in society. Someone has done something that has put drugs in the hands of another part of society. We should be interested in the reasons behind that.

  The role of the family is also a very important point to investigate. It may open a completely new door for epidemiology. Or the role of women in the prevention of diseases, or infant mortality, or problems generally related with reproduction. Even though it still has a long way to go, the role of women has changed drastically in the past 20 to 60 years, depending on the country. In many countries, we say women are already equal to men, but it's not true. Women still have very far to go. The objective should be not only to get more women into traditionally male-dominated jobs, women also must be allowed to participate in all decision making. These issues shouldn't apply to just a few women, all women should have the same opportunities as men. But it is all still very difficult: defining their psychological or occupational role, determining the place they occupy. We have been studying the effect that women's changing roles have had on the family from the thirties to now. It is very interesting to see these effects and their impact on some things like infant mortality. We often take for granted that only diseases like diabetes are clearly linked with sex differences and that everything else is the same because the differences do not appear in mortality statistics or are not statistically significant. We should analyze the behavior of different diseases in each sex. We should ask ourselves, for example, why women always constitute 60 percent or more of the patients in clinics or consultations. Is it because they are not working or because they get sick more? What are the effects of this on the children? We don't analyze these things deeply enough because we always look at mortality; we should also pay more attention to positive health. What is positive health in the working man or woman, especially if he or she is not a blue collar worker? What is a healthy life in a housewife? For women, what is the compounded effect of work at home and bad work outside the home? These are all interesting new areas of study.

BUCK: All this makes me want to say that epidemiologists may be ready to return to some of their older liaisons. Earlier we mentioned the period in which we worked closely with sociologists. I'm not sure, but I think that we have been departing a little bit from that relationship. What made me think of this was Yuri Brockson-Brynner's recent book, *The Handbook of Evaluation Research,* which has a chapter on the evaluation of the Head Start Operation, a pre-school enrichment program for disadvantaged children. This very long and detailed review makes the point that the most deprived families, those living under the most appalling circumstances, showed no effect of enrichment, not even a transitory one. The author then cites some references suggesting that if one made more fundamental environmental changes for those people—as opposed to just home tutoring, parent intervention, extra schooling—there might be a possibility of change. I am just trying to lead up to the thought that perhaps epidemiologists interested in broad aspects of disease etiology should ally themselves with psychologists and sociologists. Maybe we are getting a bit too entrenched in biology to make our full impact. Furthermore, some people in these other fields may even be assisted a little bit by our expertise. But even if they don't need us, we might find our ideas enriched by associating with them.

NAJERA: In 1983, in a PAHO seminar in Buenos Aires, we analyzed the uses of epidemiology, especially in research. Let's remember that epidemiology is a science. Let's not forget who is supposed to benefit from it, and try to keep it free from the interests of the most powerful part of society. If we don't do something to free ourselves of these interests, we cannot expect to really focus on these deprived parts of the society that are supposed to be the objects of our studies. Even though we may want to focus on them, something distracts us. Somehow we always find reasons or we don't find funds to conduct the appropriate studies.

TERRIS: In the United States and England we have a well-established tradition of epidemiological research, and PAHO has sent people from many Latin American countries to get some of the best training in the world at elite institutions in these two countries. When these people returned home, however, not very much happened in their countries in terms of research. For some reason they got involved in teaching, or whatever. Somehow we should also make it our task to indicate that the job of an epidemiologist is to stop talking and do some work, research work. If epidemiologists don't do some decent research studies, they're not fulfilling their jobs. And we have to emphasize this, because this seems to be a real problem in Latin America. I think it probably is so in most of the developing world that doesn't have a tradition of research. This is where it must be developed.

BUCK: I think you're right. Perhaps the problem with many of these people is that when they go back home, if they don't have a "critical mass" to return to, they become loners. This is very hard, it's very demoralizing. You have to have great intellectual curiosity to keep on doing research when you have nobody to talk to about it. It's doubly hard if you are surrounded by people who try to divert your energies from research. The solution to this problem is a difficult one. On the one hand, you don't want to put all these people in one spot and deprive the rest of the country of their training. On the other hand, you don't want to scatter them like seeds either. Nobody ever plants a single seed in a garden hoping to get a bed of flowers. You usually plant several in a spot, don't you?

NAJERA: What probably happens in Latin America, as in many other regions, is that epidemiology is seen with fear because it can show the real problems, the social roots of most of our health problems. That is why epidemiological work and epidemiological research are not encouraged at all. Epidemiologists are told that there is no money, they are told that they must be practical. Well this is an instance where being practical means not being practical! If you don't do any research, if you don't develop your own epidemiological services, you are not being practical. What you are doing is serving somebody else. This is what is happening. Epidemiologists are trained in the United States or in England and then they are absorbed by the health services or ministries—the bureaucratic machinery that wants to be practical. They arrive there as a little piece of the machinery and are completely absorbed by it. They end up doing what the bosses want them to do.

TERRIS: But couldn't this discussion put forth the concept of the critical mass and the centers of excellence in epidemiologic research? Let's emphasize that there really should be an attempt to create these research centers in epidemiology where you can try to get a critical mass.

BUCK: Even though I raised the question of a critical mass, I'm now a little fearful of it. The danger is that in an entrepreneurial scientific world there will be a few centers that will just collect every talent together and impoverish the rest of the country. Would it be possible to get a critical mass without undue centralization? Maybe a critical mass doesn't have to be all that big. Because when it gets really big, it leads to research by committee.

TERRIS: Four or five people in one place, that's enough of a critical mass.

BUCK: Yes, that could avoid the gargantuan "center of excellence" complex. One should try to avoid it, because, in small countries especially, there's always a center that would like to contain the whole country's resources.

NAJERA: The critical mass is a very difficult problem to discuss. If we use rates when we compare countries, we should also use rates when we talk of critical masses of epidemiologists. For instance, the United States is one country, but it has 250 million inhabitants. You would need all of South America to reach a population of 250 million. South America's population is divided into several countries, each one working separately. So, the problem of having a critical mass for investigation or research is complicated by the fact that all the countries, except for four or five, have populations of fewer than 20 million people. Most have quite small populations and each one wants to have everything.

TERRIS: The other thing that happens is that in a cardiology institute, for example, they will have one epidemiologist, very well trained in the London School of Hygiene. Then, in a neurology institution or in a peripheral vascular disease institute you will also find one lone epidemiologist. In each institute there will be an epidemiologist surrounded by 100 clinicians. But if you have one epidemiologist surrounded by hundreds of clinicians and laboratory people, he is dead, he won't do anything. What they should do is keep an epidemiologist in each institute, but also let them be part of a collective, of a center where there are two, three, or more individuals not affiliated with institutes, people who are the theoreticians in the group. That way, they can meet regularly with the epidemiologists from all of the institutes, and they can talk to each other. What people really need is to talk to each other, to discuss problems. There should be mechanisms developed for epidemiologists from different centers to get together and discuss what they're doing.

NAJERA: In Spain we founded an epidemiological society where we try to get together.

TERRIS: What is the experience in Latin America? Are there centers?

LLOPIS: Most countries have centers, but most of these centers are not part of the health services. Another problem is that although many people call themselves epidemiologists, many of them are not working in the discipline. Most of the time they administer disease control programs, and this follows the tradition of the practice of epidemiology in Latin America. Research is not a priority. This close association with disease control programs is not bad by itself. It is just that if it involves only administration, and epidemiology is not used at all, then instead of the person being in charge of control, control takes charge of the person.

BUCK: I think we should comment on trends in epidemiology training because these are important issues to talk about. I would discourage a trend towards rigid specialization within epidemiology. I'm saying this because we mentioned clinical epidemiology before. Although some specialization may occur in the course of an epidemiologist's work and contacts, it is a great error to institutionalize fragmentation in a field that is still relatively young. I get really scared by the use of "big E" and "little e", or "hard" and "soft" as though it might be pornography, or "clinical" and "classical" epidemiology. I think we ought to do everything we can to suppress excessive specialization. It has been the ruination of medicine and could equally be the ruination of our own discipline.

NAJERA: I think it goes against the essence of epidemiology to divide it into branches. Epidemiology has to be comprehensive. You cannot really be an epidemiologist if you are not thinking about all aspects of health. Although epidemiologists may be in contact with a specific type of work, or apply epidemiology to a specific group of diseases or a specific group in the population, they must never lose sight of the whole problem of health.

  The improvement of epidemiology training should start before graduation, it should start in the medical schools. To get people into epidemiology, you need maybe two things: a scientific interest and a community interest. What medical schools do now is to take students and make them only interested in individuals, they turn students into typical, biological, individual-oriented physicians, serving only very specific health problems. We should change something there. The social interest must be fostered and nurtured. If we do this, then we will have a more scientific physician who is more community oriented, a physician who can then be trained as a real epidemiologist.

LLOPIS: I have been involved in many training programs for epidemiologists, especially in surveillance, and on the whole they all have been highly disappointing. In my opinion, we have to change our whole approach. I think we shouldn't start with training programs, but rather with research programs. I don't believe that any effort we make toward training people will be successful if they have no place to work or to develop their skills and interests when they come back. People should be trained in cooperative research programs so that we could have both things at the same time: a place where they return to work that may provide the critical mass and this center of excellence that we were talking about. If we don't do this, we will have the same problems we have had for many decades and we will not achieve very good results.

TERRIS: I'd like to address a number of problems, and I'm going to speak from my own experience since that's what I know. They're beginning to develop a school of public health in one of the Asian countries. As part of that effort, the National Institute of Hygiene and Epidemiology asked me to give a course in fundamentals of epidemiology, the same one that I've been giving at the graduate summer session of the University of Minnesota for twenty years. I had 28 students, half of them men, half women. All of them were physicians, except one or two statisticians—this is also typical of the developing countries, hardly anyone except physicians. They were all people who were working in epidemiology in the medical school or the ministry or the various institutes, yet they didn't know any epidemiology. (I've been told this is also typical.) What they are taught as epidemiology is infectious disease prevention, so they know a lot about the clinical aspects of infectious diseases and the control methods for infectious diseases, but they don't know how to do an epidemiologic study. They don't have the faintest idea how to do it. This story, I think, illustrates one of the great problems in epidemiology training.

The main task, all over the world, is to teach epidemiology essentially in terms of methods of study and methods of research. What are the basic concepts? What are the basic research methods?

The second point, also based on my own experience, is not very original. I learned this from John Fox and Henry Gelfand at Tulane, where I taught. Although we gave lectures at Tulane, we did not teach primarily by lecture, we taught primarily by exercises. I know you are familiar with my disease-oriented exercises, *The Bank of Epidemiology Exercises.* Each exercise traces the development of the epidemiology of a specific disease such as polio, or coronary heart disease, or tuberculosis. I think it's a very important approach because the exercises use data from real research problems. It's not just lectures. My impression is that most epidemiology taught in the Third World is lecture-teaching. I believe lecture-teaching goes in one ear and out the other, unless you try to work with data and think the problem through.

The third point I want to make is that we're kidding ourselves if we think we're going to get anywhere if we don't encourage research. I agree absolutely with Llopis that what people have to do is to learn by doing. They must get into a research situation and learn, and the only way that will happen is if money is provided. It's the main reason for the tremendous development of epidemiology in the United States, greater than in any other country, much greater than in England since they never had our resources. We wasted millions of dollars on epidemiological research of all levels of quality, just as we did with medical research. We poured money in. Take MRFIT, it cost many millions of dollars. In Latin America, you don't have to pour that kind of money in, you don't have it. But I think PAHO's idea is to put aside a certain amount of money in grants for Latin American countries to do research. For epidemiological research in Latin America, PAHO would be like the United States' National Institutes of Health (NIH). This is very important. Finally, we, the epidemiologists, must try to convince the governments and the health departments, the Ministries of Health, to put money into epidemiology. We must woo them.

LLOPIS: The problem with increasing financial resources is that at this point most funds go to health care. In some instances, more than 80 percent of the money goes to pay salaries. There is very little chance of redistributing resources, and this is because we have been poor planners, we have squandered what little money was available.

NAJERA: I think this problem of training is very complicated. What Llopis said about having a place that people can come back to and do research is probably the most important thing. You not only need to have services, you also need to have research in order to attract people and keep them interested in the field. But still, I would like to come back to the issue of undergraduate training, because if we don't do something at that stage it will be very difficult to change people that have already been trained to think in terms of individuals and reshape them into epidemiologists. In 1962, I started comparing the curricula of medical faculties in many countries of the world, mostly in the so-called developed countries. I was trying to find the place for epidemiology, for prevention and community medicine. I found out that practically no curriculum had any emphasis on prevention or on community health during the undergraduate years. Since then, very little has changed in most countries.

TERRIS: It's gotten worse.

NAJERA: I remember that at that time I came up with a proposal to incorporate epidemiology into the medical curriculum. First I proposed introducing what I called "community anatomy", meaning demography, at the beginning of the curriculum, at the same time students were taught individual anatomy. The objective was to plant in the students' minds the idea that there were not only individuals, that these individuals live together in a community. This community has a shape and an age distribution and so on, and it can be studied through demography. Then, as they studied individual physiology, I proposed introducing sociology as "community physiology." Finally, epidemiology would be introduced at the same time that they studied general pathology. In other words, as they understand the disease process in the individual they should also understand the disease process in the community. But my proposal has never been applied anywhere. There have been many attempts to change the graduate medical curriculum, but I don't think any of them has been really radically planned.

TERRIS: My experience has convinced me that we are deluding ourselves if we think we are going to change most medical students. However, I firmly believe that we should have departments of community, preventive, and social medicine in medical schools. But, if it were up to me, if I were starting all over again, I would not ask for a compulsory course in epidemiology for all students. Instead I would want to have an attractive elective course in epidemiology for interested students. In the United States, only 5 to 10 percent of all students are socially conscious, really socially conscious, and they are the ones who are going to go into public health. Some will start out as clinicians, will suddenly get the bug, and come in. These are the ones that must be found among the medical students and then be taught and encouraged toward public health and graduate training in public health.

BUCK: I agree with you entirely about the elective course. But the problem is that you can't get people to come to a movie unless you show a preview. If there is no core course in epidemiology, how can you attract interested students to the elective course?

TERRIS: I think you're right. The emphasis should not be on trying to teach this to everyone, but on getting the introductory course to pick up the interested people and work with them. Otherwise you're kidding yourself. I really was a big failure, and every time I visited a school that said it had a successful epidemiology training program, I found, after I talked with them a while, that epidemiology was a failure there too.

BUCK: I've always thought I was a big failure, too. But the other day, for reasons I won't bore you with, I sat down and tried to figure out the number of people I knew that I had influenced for sure. It was a very small number, but if multiplied by itself it might be enough. It's like using the net reproduction rate which measures how many daughters will be born to a cohort of newborn girls. If the average is one, you achieve replacement. So we could figure out how many epidemiologists we have to produce to get enough. First, of course, we have to decide how many would be enough. We obviously don't have to turn 50 percent of every medical class into epidemiologists. It might be very dangerous if we did.

NAJERA: Well, there is another possible solution to this problem that my father proposed many years ago. He taught in Argentina after having good experience as an epidemiologist in the Spanish Health Services. His idea was that it was impossible to get medical students to go into epidemiology; that this was a futile effort. He proposed that what society needed was a completely new career, that public health and epidemiology should be independent disciplines. They should include sociology, economics, demography, and all the subjects that we know we need, but with much less medicine. At least not so much otolaryngology, or opthalmology, or surgery, or anatomy.

BUCK: I used to think that this was an attractive solution. But if we look at the Soviet Union we see that it may not work. Their medical curriculum is divided into separate streams, so that some students go into stomatology, some go into clinical medicine or pediatrics, and some into public health. Now, nothing much seems to have come out of that streamed arrangement, maybe because the public health stream does not contain enough instruction in epidemiology.

NAJERA: The example of the Soviet Union is not valid because the curriculum divisions are still all specialties of medicine, and that is not really the point. What my father proposed was a completely different, a distinct career. So much so that you could not go from public health into clinical practice. This would be like going from medicine to engineering. The curriculum might have some medical content, mainly the basic sciences and general pathology or knowledge of the process of disease, but there would not be much clinical content. Another approach, the premedical setup in England, has not been successful either, because it never was ambitious enough. In Spain, we have something like that in one of our schools, in Alicante, but again, it doesn't go far enough. They take first-year students and give them this pre-introduction to health aspects, but then they go on to the clinical and medical component more or less as usual.

TERRIS: I think that what is happening in the United States is very interesting from this point of view. In the old days, in my generation, to be an epidemiologist you had to be a physician and a male. Now we have Ph.D programs in epidemiology. My guess is that in the schools of public health most of the successful Ph.D candidates are not physicians and at least half are women. What is also happening is that the whole field of public health and medical care administration, both in the schools of public health and in practice, is now becoming an area not for physicians, but for people trained in public health and medical care administration. This is what is happening in the United States. There is nothing theoretical about it, it has just happened this way.

NAJERA: Perhaps this will be a way of evolving into the new profession I talked about. In Spain you still have to be a physician, but now we have more women than men in the field of prevention and epidemiology. There has been a shift in that.

BUCK: I think there is a potential problem here. Unless you provide the non-medical people with much more than methodological courses in epidemiology and statistics, especially if their background is very general, these courses will not really prepare them for creative epidemiological research, nor for administrative positions in public health or health care administration. Milton Roemer had the right idea when he said that students should be given a rich mixture of human biology, economics, political science, administrative theory, statistics, and epidemiology. This is not the same thing as the streamed medical curriculum, because it offers much more than you can offer today in a medical school.

NAJERA: Maybe with the help of these non-medical epidemiologists we are going to be able to change our definition of disease; without them we are stuck.

TERRIS: I would like to emphasize a point I made when we discussed why the London School of Hygiene was so important to the movement of transition from the old to the new epidemiology. That is that the key factor in the whole process was the close collaboration of epidemiologists with statisticians. You see, there is not going to be good research

if there isn't a team of medical or non-medical epidemiologists—and in Latin America it's going to be mostly
medical, let's not delude ourselves on this point—and statisticians working very closely together. Medical epidemiologists are not sufficiently sure of themselves on
methodology; they need the statisticians. There are dangers in working with the statisticians, they can cause difficulties, but we need them. I think this is crucial. The critical
mass must include both epidemiologists and statisticians.
Of that I'm convinced.

LLOPIS: At present, we are worried about the future of the schools
of public health in Latin America. The Rockefeller Foundation, which has a long history of supporting public health
in the region, now says that it is much more concerned with
medical schools than with public health schools. So much
so that they are funding clinical epidemiology programs
through medical schools in several Latin American countries.

BUCK: I think we all know the problem, but our reaction to it must
be active rather than passive. We have to present a cogent
and logically impeccable alternative.

TERRIS: The Rockefeller Foundation people are selling this program, with real money to back it up, all over Asia, Africa,
and Latin America. They are going to divert promising
people into doing drug trials. Both the Rockefeller Foundation program and the Robert Wood Johnson Foundation's "clinical scholars" program avoid public health
schools like the plague. I think it is an absurdity. Here we
have the Third World with all its terrible problems of
famine, malnutrition, infant diarrhea, malaria, and all the
other infectious and noninfectious diseases, and all this
money is being spent to teach clinicians how to do clinical
trials. These foundations operate under a false banner.
They are misusing the term epidemiology. Why? Because
of the great prestige of epidemiology in the world today,
because of the fact that the schools of public health are the
outstanding centers of teaching and research in epidemiology. This is threatening. They want the medical
schools to continue to be dominant; they want the clinicians
to keep their political power; they want to make sure that
health services don't infringe on the narrow professional
interests of the clinicians.

BUCK: The strangling of preventive medicine in medical schools is
fostered by the doctrine that prevention is everybody's business. It should be, but the danger is that what is everybody's

business becomes nobody's business. When the role models in the medical school faculty are not oriented toward prevention, then the abolition of a department of preventive medicine is dangerous.

TERRIS: Although clinical epidemiology should be epidemiology, it is not. It is clinical trials. This is useful: it is about time clinicians became a little more scientific about what they do. Also, I think that some of the people who are being trained to do drug trials will realize that epidemiology is more important than drug tests and then will become genuine epidemiologists and public health workers. But still, the real reason for the program is political. As I said before, clinicians in the United States and elsewhere are afraid that non-clinicians will run the health services. This is why the Robert Wood Johnson Foundation has a clinical scholars program and the Rockefeller Foundation has a clinical-epidemiology program. They want clinicians to know enough epidemiology, public health, and medical-care organization to step in as the leaders and run the show. And some of these people, with their medical arrogance, do not hesitate to denigrate schools of public health because they are multidisciplinary.

BUCK: It is all right to criticize deficient schools of public health. But the approach of these foundations is equivalent to prescribing euthanasia, and that is inappropriate. If a school of public health is depleted, stagnated, it should be strengthened, not killed.

TERRIS: This book will help. It gives a picture of the domain, the scope of epidemiology.

LLOPIS: On the other hand, we have made the point that the schools of public health need updating.

TERRIS: That should be a major role for epidemiologists to concentrate on in the future: get the schools of public health into the new era.

LLOPIS: Yes, and PAHO should take a leadership role in updating and reshaping Latin America's epidemiology programs.

TERRIS: If in ten years PAHO hasn't updated the schools of public health in Latin America, we will come back and haunt them.

LLOPIS: It cannot wait 10 years. We have to haunt them now.

APPENDIX: LIST OF CONTRIBUTORS[a]

Dr. Helen Abbey
Professor of Biostatistics
Johns Hopkins School of Hygiene and
Public Health
Baltimore, Maryland U.S.A.

Dr. Dionisio Aceves Saínos
Director de Normas para la Prevención de
Enfermedades Infecciosas y Parasitarias,
Subsecretaria de Servicios de Salud,
Secretaría de Salud
México, D.F., México

Dr. E. D. Acheson
Chief Medical Officer
Department of Health and Social Security
Alexander Fleming House
London, England

Prof. Anders Ahlbom
Department of Epidemiology
National Institute of
Environmental Medicine
Stockholm, Sweden

Dr. Rolando Armijo
Ex Professor of Epidemiology
School of Public Health
University of California
Walnut Creek, California, U.S.A.

Dr. Mary Jane Ashley
Professor and Chairman
Department of Preventive Medicine and
Biostatistics
Faculty of Medicine
University of Toronto
Toronto, Ontario, Canada

Dr. Frederico S. Barbosa
Diretor
Escola Nacional de Saúde Publica
Manguinhos, Rio de Janeíro, Brasil

Prof. D.J.P. Barker
Director of MRC Environmental
Epidemiology Unit
University of Southampton
Southampton General Hospital
Southampton, England

Dr. Hugo Behm
Apartado 293
San Pedro Montes de Oca
Costa Rica

Dr. Ettore Biocca
Direttore dell' Istituto di Parassitologia della
Universitá di Roma
Rome, Italy

Dr. Paul A. Blake
Chief, Enteric Diseases Branch
Division of Bacterial Diseases
Center for Infectious Diseases
Centers for Disease Control
Atlanta, Georgia U.S.A.

Dr. Carlos Bloch
Centro de Estudios Sanitarios y Sociales
Asociación Médica de Rosario
Rosario, Argentina

Dr. Francis Bolumar
Departamento de Medicina Preventiva
Facultad de Medicina
Universidad de Alicante
Alicante, Spain

Dr. Philip S. Brachman
Professor, Master of Public Health Program
Emory University School of Medicine
Atlanta, Georgia U.S.A.

Dr. Luis Cayolla da Motta
Profesor de Epidemiología
Escola Nacional de Saúde Publica
Lisbon, Portugal

Dr. Tom D.Y. Chin
Professor and Chairman
The University of Kansas Medical Center
School of Medicine
Department of Preventive Medicine
Kansas City, Kansas, U.S.A.

Dr. Joan Clos
Concejal Director, Area de Salud
Barcelona, Spain

Dr. John Frank
Department of Preventive Medicine and
Biostatistics
Faculty of Medicine
University of Toronto
Toronto, Ontario, Canada

[a] The posts listed are those the contributors held at the
time the articles were selected.

986

Dr. Julio Frenk Mora
Director General
Instituto Nacional de Salud Pública
México, D.F., México

Dr. George Friedman-Jiménez
Mt. Sinai Medical Center
Division of Environmental and
Occupational Medicine
New York, New York, U.S.A.

Dr. John Fry
Beckenham, Kent,
England

Dr. Truls W. Gedde-Dahl
Department of Infectious Diseases
National Institute of Public Health
Oslo, Norway

Profesor Miguel Gili-Miner
Cátedra de Medicina Preventiva y Social
Facultad de Medicina
Universidad de Sevilla
Seville, Spain

Dr. Carlos Luis González
Calle El Parque
Quinta María Elisa
La Lagunita, El Hatillo
Caracas, Venezuela

Dr. Germán González Echeverri
Profesor de Epidemiología
Facultad Nacional de Salud Pública
Universidad de Antioquia
Medellin, Colombia

Dr. Michael B. Gregg
Deputy Director
Epidemiology Program Office
Centers for Disease Control
Atlanta, Georgia, U.S.A.

Dr. Rodrigo Guerrero
Universidad del Valle
División de Salud
Cali, Colombia

Dr. B. Scott Halstead
Associate Director
Health Sciences Division
The Rockefeller Foundation
New York, New York, U.S.A.

Professor Walter W. Holland
Department of Community Medicine
United Medical and Dental Schools
St. Thomas' Campus
London, England

Dr. Donald R. Hopkins
Deputy Director
Centers for Disease Control
Atlanta, Georgia, U.S.A.

Dr. Michael A. Ibrahim
Dean and Professor of Epidemiology
University of North Carolina
School of Public Health
Chapel Hill, North Carolina, U.S.A.

Dr. Philip J. Landrigan
Director, Division of Environmental
and Occupational Medicine
Department of Community Medicine
Mount Sinai School of Medicine
New York, New York, U.S.A.

Dr. John M. Last
Professor of Epidemiology
School of Medicine
University of Ottawa
Ottawa, Ontario, Canada

Prof. W. Harding le Riche
University of Toronto
Faculty of Medicine
Toronto, Ontario, Canada

Dr. Martha S. Linet
Associate Professor
Department of Epidemiology
Johns Hopkins School of
Hygiene and Public Health
Baltimore, Maryland U.S.A.

Dr. Vicente E. Mazzáfero
Profesor Titular de la Cátedra de Salud
Pública
Facultad de Medicina
Universidad de Buenos Aires
Buenos Aires, Argentina

Dr. Ernesto Medina Lois
Director, Escuela de Salud Pública
Facultad de Medicina
Universidad de Chile
Santiago, Chile

Dr. J. Donald Millar
Director, National Institute for
   Occupational Safety and Health
Centers for Disease Control
Atlanta, Georgia, U.S.A.

Dr. Arnold S. Monto
Department of Epidemiology
University of Michigan
School of Public Health
Ann Arbor, Michigan, U.S.A.

Dr. Nubia Muñoz
Division of Epidemiology and Biostatistics
International Agency for Research on Cancer
Lyon, France

Dr. Rafael Nájera
Director
Centro Nacional de Microbiología,
   Virología e Immunología Sanitarias
Madrid, Spain

Dr. Aníbal Osuna
Prados del Este
Calle San Pablo
Quinta Elba
Caracas, Venezuela

Dr. Zoran M. Radovanovic
Professor of Epidemiology and Head,
   Institute of Epidemiology
Faculty of Medicine
Belgrade, Yugoslavia

Dr. Karel Raska
V. Ondrejove 2
Prague, Czechoslovakia

Dr. Conrado Ristori
Departmento de Programación
Ministerio de Salud
Santiago, Chile

Dr. Leon S. Robertson
Institute of Social and Policy Studies
Department of Epidemiology and
   Public Health (Injuries)
Yale University School of Medicine
New Haven, Connecticut, U.S.A.

Dr. Antonio Ruffino Netto
Profesor Titular de Medicina Social
Departamento de Medicina Social
Facultade de Medicina
Ribeirão Preto, São Paulo, Brazil

Dr. Susana Sans
Médica epidemióloga
Departamento de Medicina Preventiva y
   Salud Pública
Facultad de Medicina
Universidad Autónoma de Barcelona
Barcelona, Spain

Dr. Philip E. Sartwell
Emeritus Professor of Epidemiology
The Johns Hopkins University
Baltimore, Maryland, U.S.A.

Dr. Wolfgang Schmidt
Addiction Research Foundation
Toronto, Ontario, Canada

Dr. Andreu Segura
Societat Catalana de Salut Pública
Barcelona, Spain

Mr. Sam Shapiro
Past Director,
Health Services Research and
   Development Center
Professor Emeritus, Department of Health
   Policy and Management
The Johns Hopkins University
School of Hygiene and Public Health
Baltimore, Maryland U.S.A.

Dr. Jack Siemiatycki
Professor,
Université du Quebec
Institut Armand-Frappier
Laval-des-Rapides, Quebec, Canada

Profesor Antonio Sierra López
Cátedra de Medicina Preventiva y Social
Facultad de Medicina
La Laguna, Tenerife
Canary Islands, Spain

Prof. Sir Kenneth L. Standard
Department of Social and Preventive
   Medicine
University of the West Indies
Mona, Kingston, Jamaica

Dr. Mervyn Susser
Gertrude H. Sergievsky Professor of
   Epidemiology
Director, Gertrude H. Sergievsky Center
Columbia University
New York, New York, U.S.A.

Dr. Moyses Szklo
Professor and Director
Chronic Disease Epidemiology Program
Johns Hopkins School of Hygiene and
  Public Health
Baltimore, Maryland, U.S.A.

Prof. Benedetto Terracini
Profesor de Epidemiología de Cáncer
Departamento de Ciencias Biomédicas y
  Oncología Humana
Universidad de Turín
Turin, Italy

Dr. David B. Thomas
Professor and Member
Program in Epidemiology
Fred Hutchinson Cancer Research Center
Seattle, Washington, U.S.A.

Dr. Yolanda Torres de Gálvis
Profesora Titular de Epidemiología
Facultad Nacional de Salud Pública
Medellin, Colombia

Professor Dimitrios Trichopoulos
Director of Hygiene and Epidemiology
University of Athens Medical School
Athens, Greece

Dr. Carl W. Tyler, Jr.
Director,
Epidemiology Program Office
Centers for Disease Control
Atlanta, Georgia, U.S.A.

Dr. Yoshikazu Watanabe
Managing Director
International Medical Foundation
  of Japan
Tokyo, Japan

Dr. Karl A. Western
Assistant Director for International
  Research
National Institute of Allergy and
  Infectious Diseases
Bethesda, Maryland, U.S.A.

Dr. Christine L. Williams
Associate Professor of Pediatrics, and
  Community and Preventive Medicine
Director, Maternal and Child Health
New York Medical College
Valhalla, New York, U.S.A.

Dr. Warren Winkelstein
Professor and Chairman
School of Public Health
Department of Biomedical and
  Environmental Health Sciences
University of California
Berkeley, California, U.S.A.

Dr. Emilio Zapatero
Jefe del Servicio de Documentación y
  Publicaciones
Consejería de Bienestar Social
Junta de Castilla y León
Valladolid, Spain

NOTES

NOTES

NOTES